New Crops

NEW CROPS

Proceedings of the Second National Symposium

NEW CROPS
Exploration, Research, and Commercialization

Indianapolis, Indiana, October 6–9, 1991

In Cooperation With
Association for the Advancement of Industrial Crops

Society Sponsors
American Society for Agronomy
American Society for Horticultural Sciences
Crop Science Society of America
Society for Economic Botany
The International Society for Horticultural Science

Institutional Sponsors
The Indiana Business Modernization and Technology Corporation
United States Department of Agriculture
Indiana New Crops and Plant Products Center, Purdue University
Center for Alternative Plant and Animal Products, University of Minnesota

Industrial Sponors
Dow Elanco
The Proctor and Gamble Company
Petoseed Co., Inc.

NEW CROPS

Edited by

Jules Janick
and
James E. Simon
Purdue University

JOHN WILEY AND SONS, INC.
New York / Chichester / Brisbane / Toronto / Singapore

This text is printed on acid-free paper.

Copyright © 1993 by John Wiley & Sons, Inc.

All rights reserved. Published simultaneously in Canada.

Reproduction or translation of any part of this work beyond that permitted by Section 107 or 108 of the 1976 United States Copyright Act without the permission of the copyright owner is unlawful. Requests for permission or further information should be addressed to the Permissions Department, John Wiley & Sons, Inc., 605 Third Avenue, New York, NY 10158-0012.

This publication is designed to provide accurate and authoritative information in regard to the subject matter covered. It is sold with the understanding that the publisher is not engaged in rendering legal, accounting, or other professional services. If legal advice or other expert assistance is required, the services of a competent professional person should be sought.

Library of Congress Cataloging in Publication Data:

National Symposium NEW CROPS: Exploration, Research, and
  Commericalization (2nd : 1991 : Indianapolis, Ind.)
    New crops / edited by Jules Janick and James E. Simon.
        p.   cm.
    "Proceedings of the Second National Symposium NEW CROPS—
  Exploration, Research, and Commercialization, Indianapolis,
  Indiana, October 6–9, 1991, in Cooperation with the Association for
  the Advancement of Industrial Crops; society sponsors, American
  Society for Agronomy . . . [et al.]"—P. preceding t.p.
    Includes indexes.
    ISBN 0-471-59374-5
    1. New crops—Congresses.   I. Janick, Jules, 1931–
  II. Simon, James E.   III. Association for the Advancement of
  Industrial Crops.   IV. American Society for Agronomy.   V. Title.
  SB160.N38   1991
  630—dc20   93-17949
                                                                    CIP

Printed in the United States of America

10 9 8 7 6 5 4 3 2 1

CONTENTS

List of Contributors xi
PREFACE xx
FOREWORD xxi

PART I: POLICY & PROGRAMS

POLICY
National New Crops Policy—John W. Conrad 2
International New Crops Policy—J. Trevor Williams and N. Haq 5
New Crops and the International Agricultural Research Centers—Robert B. Bertram 11
International Conflicts in New Crops Policy—Cary Fowler 22

INTERNATIONAL DEVELOPMENTS
New Crop Development in Europe—Louis J.M. van Soest 30
Characterization and Processing Research on New Crops for Increased Industrial Applicability of New and Traditional Crops: A European Perspective—Willem M.J. van Gelder,
    F.P. Cuperus, J.T.P. Derksen, B.G. Muuse, and J.E.G. van Dam 38
Potential New Specialty Crops from Asia: Azuki Bean, Edamame Soybean, and Astragalus—
    Thomas A. Lumpkin, J.C. Konovsky, K.J. Larson, and D.C. McClary 45
New Crop Development in New Zealand—James A. Douglas 51
New Horticultural Crops in New Zealand—Errol W. Hewett 57
Genetic Resources in Africa—Jack R. Harlan 64

REGIONAL DEVELOPMENT
New Crops Research: Northeastern Regional and National Federal Efforts—George A. White 68
New Horticultural Crops for the Southeastern United States—Mary Lamberts 82
Development of New Agronomic Crops in the Midwest—Edward S. Oplinger 92
Development of New Crops in the Western United States—Dick L. Auld 95
The Western Regional Plant Introduction Station: A Source of Germplasm for New Crop
    Development—V.L. Bradley, R.C. Johnson, R.M. Hannan, D.M. Stout, and R.L. Clark 99
Determining Amaranth and Canola Suitability in Missouri Through Geographic Information
    Systems Analysis—Robert L. Myers 102
Preliminary Agronomic Evaluation of New Crops for North Dakota—Marisol T. Berti and
    A.A. Schneiter 106
Public Sponsored New Crops Research and Development Projects in Virginia—
    Gregory E. Welbaum 109

CENTERS
Center for Alternative Plant and Animal Products—Programs in Information Exchange and
    Research—Daniel H. Putnam, Ervin A. Oelke, and Laura McCann 114
Interdisciplinary Teamwork for New Crop Development in Missouri—Robert L. Myers 120
IMPACT and the East Asian Crop Development Program—Thomas A. Lumpkin,
    Bill B. Dean, and Desmond A. O'Rourke 122
Indiana Center for New Crops and Plant Products—Jules Janick 127

PART II: RESEARCH & DEVELOPMENT

EXPLORATION

Peppers: History and Exploitation of a Serendipitous New Crop Discovery—
W. Hardy Eshbaugh 132

Exploration and Introduction of Ornamental Landscape Plants from Eastern Asia—
Stephen A. Spongberg 140

Plant Exploration for New Forage Grasses—Kay H. Asay 147

Exploration and Exploitation of New Fruit and Nut Germplasm—Maxine M. Thompson 155

The Search for New Pharmaceutical Crops: Drug Discovery and Development at the National
Cancer Institute—Gordon M. Cragg, Michael R. Boyd, John H. Cardellina II,
Michael R. Grever, Saul Schepartz, Kenneth M. Snader, and Matthew Suffness 161

A Novel Method for Selection and Domestication of Indigenous Useful Plants in Amazonian
Ecuador—J. Friedman, D. Bolotin, M. Rios, P. Mendosa, Y. Cohen, and M.J. Balick 167

BIOTECHNOLOGY

Fatty Acid Synthesis Genes—H. Maelor Davies, L. Anderson, J. Bleibaum, D.J. Hawkins,
C. Fan, A.C. Worrell, and Toni A. Voelker 176

Bioassembly of Storage Lipids in Oilseed Crops—David C. Taylor, Ljerka Kunst, and
Samuel L. MacKenzie 181

Engineering New Sources of Domestic Natural Rubber—Katrina Cornish, Zhiqang Pan, and
Ralph A. Backhaus 192

CEREALS AND PSEUDOCEREALS

Pearl Millet: New Feed Grain Crop—David J. Andrews, John F. Rajewski, and
K. Anand Kumar 198

The Use of Protogyny to Make Hybrids in Pearl Millet—David J. Andrews, Barnabas Kiula,
and John F. Rajewski 208

Amaranth Rediscovered—Gilbert F. Stallknecht and J.R. Schulz-Schaeffer 211

Row Spacing and Population Effects on Yield of Grain Amaranth in North Dakota—
T.L. Henderson, A.A. Schneiter, and N. Riveland 219

Quinoa—Duane L. Johnson and Sarah M. Ward 222

Blue Corn—Duane L. Johnson and Mitra N. Jha 228

Teff: Food Crop for Humans and Animals—Gilbert F. Stallknecht, Kenneth M. Gilbertson,
and J.L. Eckhoff 231

Wild Rice: Domestication of a Native North American Genus—Ervin A. Oelke 235

Structure and Chemical Composition of Developing Buckwheat Seed—Ralph L. Obendorf,
Marcin Horbowicz, and Douglas P. Taylor 244

Storage, Processing, and Quality Aspects of Buckwheat Seed—G. Mazza 251

GRAIN LEGUMES

Food and Grain Legumes—Fredrick J. Muehlbauer 256

An Interdisciplinary Approach to the Development of Lupin as an Alternative Crop—
Daniel H. Putnam 266

White Lupin: An Alternate Crop for the Southern Coastal Plain—Paul L. Mask, D.W. Reeves,
E. van Santen, G.L. Mullins, and G.E. Aksland 277

The Potential of Zero Tannin Lentil—A. Matus, A.E. Slinkard, and A. Vandenberg 279

FORAGES

Native North American Grasses—Kenneth P. Vogel and K.J. Moore 284
African Grasses—Glenn W. Burton 294

OILSEEDS

Canola Seed Yield in Relation to Harvest Methods—Casimir A. Jaworski and
    Sharad C. Phatak 300
Rapeseed, a New Oilseed Crop for USA—Matti Sovero 302
Evaluation of Several Species of Oilseeds as Spring Planted Crops for the Pacific Northwest—
    Dick L. Auld, R.M. Gareau, and M.K. Heikkinen 308
Camelina: A Promising Low-Input Oilseed—Daniel H. Putnam, J.T. Budin, L.A. Field, and
    W.M. Breene 314
Perilla: Botany, Uses and Genetic Resources—David M. Brenner 322
Quinoa: A Potential New Oil Crop—Michael J. Koziol 328

INDUSTRIAL CROPS

Guayule: A Source of Natural Rubber—Dennis T. Ray 338
Evaluation of Rubber and Resin Content in Lines of Guayule Collected from Nuevo Leon
    Province in Mexico—Sathyanarayanaiah Kuruvadi, Alfonso López Benitez, and
    F. Borrego 343
Rubber and Resin Content in the Bark and Wood Portions of the Root Stem and Branches in
    Guayule—Sathyanarayanaiah Kuruvadi and Diana Jasso de Rodriguez 345
Interspecific Hybridization Between *Parthenium argentatum* Gray and *Parthenium
    lozanianum*—Alfonso López Benitez, F. Ramirez, S. Kuruvadi, and F. Borrego 347
Salt Tolerance in Relation to Ploidy Level in Guayule—Ali Estilai and Michael C. Shannon 349
Growth of Direct Seeded and Transplanted Guayule Seedlings—James L. Fowler and
    Robert Tinguely 352
Impact of Seeding Rate and Planting Date on Guayule Stand Establishment by Direct Seeding
    in West Texas—Michael Foster, Greg Kleine, and Jaroy Moore 354
Chrysothamnus: A Rubber-Producing Semi-Arid Shrub—D.J. Weber, W.M. Hess, R.B. Bhat,
    and J. Huang 355
Variation and Broad Sense Heritability of Branching Frequency of Jojoba—
    Damian A. Ravetta and David A. Palzkill 358
Irrigation Effects on Growth, Cold Tolerance of Flower Buds and Seed Yield of Jojoba—
    J.M. Nelson and D.A. Palzkill 360
Vernonia and *Lesquerella* Potential for Commercialization—David A. Dierig and
    Anson E. Thompson 362
Development of a Cosmetic Grade Oil from *Lesquerella fendleri* Seed—James G. Arquette
    and James H. Brown 367
Breakthroughs Towards the Domestication of *Cuphea*—Steven J. Knapp 372
Castor: Return of an Old Crop—Raymond D. Brigham 380
Potential of Fanweed and Other Weeds as Novel Industrial Oilseed Crops—Patrick M. Carr 384
Marigold Flowers as a Source of an Emulsifying Gum—Ana L. Medina and
    James N. BeMiller 389
Sweet Sorghum for a Piedmont Ethanol Industry—Glen C. Rains, John S. Cundiff, and
    Gregory E. Welbaum 394

FIBER CROPS

- Kenaf: An Emerging New Crop Industry—Charles S. Taylor 402
- Response of Kenaf to Multiple Cutting—Frank E. Robinson 407
- Kenaf in Irrigated Central Washington—David W. Evans and An N. Hang 409
- Utilization of Methanol Stress for Evaluating Kenaf Quality—Charles G. Cook and Andrew W. Scott, Jr. 411
- The Effects of Metolachlor and Trifluralin on Kenaf Yield Components— Charles L. Webber III 413
- Kenaf: Production, Harvesting, Processing, and Products—Charles L. Webber III and Robert E. Bledsoe 416
- The Milkweed Business—Herbert D. Knudsen and Richard D. Zeller 422
- Milkweed Cultivation for Floss Production—Merle D. Witt and Herbert D. Knudsen 428
- Black Locust: An Excellent Fiber Crop—James W. Hanover 432
- Development of *Hesperaloe* Species (Agavaceae) as New Fiber Crops— Steven P. McLaughlin 435
- Sweetgrass: History, Basketry, and Constraints to Commercialization—Robert J. Dufault, Mary Jackson, and Stephen K. Salvo 442

FRUITS AND NUTS

- Commercialization of Caramola, Atemoya, and Other Tropical Fruits in South Florida— Jonathan H. Crane 448
- Rambutan and Pili Nuts: Potential Crops for Hawaii—Francis T. Zee 461
- Introduction and Evaluation of Pejibaye (*Bactris gasipaes*) for Palm Heart Production in Hawaii—Charles R. Clement, Richard M. Manshardt, Joseph DeFrank, Francis Zee, and Philip Ito 465
- *Garcinia hombrioniana*: A Potential Fruit and an Industrial Crop— Hj. Serudin D.S. Hj. Tinggal 472
- New Products from *Theobroma cacao*: Seed Pulp and Pod Gum—Antonio Figueira, Jules Janick, and James N. BeMiller 475
- Golden Berry, Passionfruit, and White Sapote: Potential Fruits for Cool Subtropical Areas— Richard McCain 479
- Development of (*Cereus peruvianus*) Apple Cactus as a New Crop for the Negev Desert of Israel—Julia Weiss, Avinoam Nerd, and Yosef Mizrahi 486
- Pitayas (Genus *Hylocereus*): New Fruit Crop for the Negev Desert of Israel—Eran Raveh, Julia Weiss, Avinoam Nerd, and Yosef Mizrahi 491
- Domestication and Introduction of Marula (*Sclerocarya birrea* sbsp. *caffra*) as a New Crop for the Negev Desert of Israel—Avinoam Nerd and Yosef Mizrahi 496
- Chinkapin: Potential New Crop for the South—Jerry A. Payne, George P. Johnson, and Gregory Miller 500
- Pawpaw (*Asimina triloba*), A Fruit For Temperate Climates—M. Brett Callaway 505
- Saskatoon Berry: A Fruit Crop for the Prairies—G. Mazza and C.G. Davidson 516
- The Potential for Domestication and Utilization of Native Plums in Kansas—William Reid and Karen L.B. Gast 520
- Commercialization of the Cloudberry (*Rubus chamaemorus* L.) in Norway—Kåre Rapp, S. Kristine Næss, and Harry Jan Swartz 524

VEGETABLES

- New Directions in Salad Crops: New Forms, New Tools, and Old Philosphy— Edward J. Ryder and William Waycott 528

Root Vegetables: New Uses for Old Crops—Wanda W. Collins 533
New Opportunities in the Cucurbitaceae—Timothy J. Ng 538
Specialty Melons for the Fresh Market—James E. Simon, Mario R. Morales, and
    Denys Charles 547
Germination, Fruit Development, Yield and Post Harvest Characteristics of *Cucumis
    metuliferus*—A. Benzioni, S. Mendlinger, M. Ventura, and S. Huyskens 553
Evaluation of *Cucumis metuliferus* as a Specialty Crop for Missouri—Dyremple B. Marsh 558
Luffa Sponge Gourds: A Potential Crop for Small Farms—Jeanine M. Davis and
    Charles D. DeCourley 560
Population Density and Soil pH Effects on Vegetable Amaranth Production—Bharat P. Singh
    and Wayne F. Whitehead 562
Comparison of Somatic and Sexual Interspecific Hybridization for the Development of New
    Brassica Vegetable Crops—Richard H. Ozminkowski, Jr. and Pablo S. Jourdan 565
Evaluating Chinese Cabbage Cultivars for High Temperature Tolerance—I-Mo Fu,
    Carol Shennan, and Gregory E. Welbaum 570
Brussels Sprouts as an Alternative Crop for Southwest Virginia—Gregory E. Welbaum 573
Fennel: A New Specialty Vegetable for the Fresh Market—Mario R. Morales,
    Denys J. Charles, and James E. Simon 576
Essential Oil Content and Chemical Composition of Finnochio Fennel—Denys J. Charles,
    Mario R. Morales, and James E. Simon 579
Effect of Nitrogen Nutrition on Roselle—E.G. Rhoden, P. David, and T. Small 583
Dry Edible Beans: A New Crops Opportunity for the East North Central Region—
    Glenn H. Sullivan and Lonni R. Davenport 585
Plant Configuration and Population Effects on Yield of Azuki Bean in Washington State—
    An N. Hang, D.C. McClary, G.C. Gilliland, and T.A. Lumpkin 588
Herbicides for Azuki Production—Dean C. McClary, A.N. Hang, G.C. Gilliland,
    J.M. Babcock, T.A. Lumpkin, A.G. Ogg, and L.K. Tanigoshi 590
Range of Yield Components and Phenotypic Correlations in Tepari Beans (*Phaseolus
    acutifolius*) Under Dryland Conditions—Sathyanarayanaiah Kuruvadi and
    Isaac Sanchez Valdez 594
Pigeonpeas: Potential New Crop for the Southeastern United States—Sharad C. Phatak,
    Ram G. Nadimpalli, Suresh C. Tiwari, and Harbans L. Bhardwaj 597

FLORAL AND LANDSCAPE CROPS
New Hybrid Ornithogalums and Orchids—Robert J. Griesbach, F. Meyer, and H. Koopowitz 602
New Bedding Plants—Lowell C. Ewart 604
A Program for the Selection and Introduction of New Plants for the Urban Landscape—
    Bruce Macdonald 608
Cliff Brake Fern: A Native Texas Fern with Landscaping Potential—Ramsey L. Sealy and
    Steve Bostic 612

AROMATIC, SPICES, MEDICINAL, & OTHERS
Herbs, Spices, and Condiments—Nicolas Verlet 616
A Planning Scheme to Evaluate New Aromatic Plants for the Flavor and Fragrance
    Industries—Brian M. Lawrence 620
Monarda: A Source of Geraniol, Thymol, Linalool, and Carvacrol-rich Essential Oils—
    G. Mazza, F.A. Kiehn, and H.H. Marshall 628
New Aromatic Lemon Basil Germplasm—Mario R. Morales, Denys J. Charles, and
    James E. Simon 632

Nitrogen Application Affects Yield and Content of the Active Substances in Camomile Genotypes—Wudeneh Letchamo 636
Effect of Water Stress and Post-harvest Handling on Artemisinin Content in the Leaves of *Artemisia annua* L.—Denys J. Charles, James E. Simon, Clinton C. Shock, Erik B.G. Feibert, and Robin M. Smith 640
Evaluation of Various Parts of the Paw Paw Tree, *Asimina triloba* (Annonaceae), as Commercial Sources of the Pesticidal Annonaceous Acetogenins—Sunil Ratnayake, J. Kent Rupprecht, William M. Potter, and Jerry L. McLaughlin 644
Tagetes minuta: A Potential New Herb from South America—Jacqueline A. Soule 649
Soft-shell Crayfish: A New Crop for the Midwest—Paul B. Brown 654

PART III: PATHS TOWARD COMMERCIALIZATION

INDUSTRY OUTLOOK

New Crops from a Seed Company Perspective—Carrol D. Bolen 658
Tomato Processing: Old Crops in New Areas—William Reinert 660
Pesticide Chemicals: An Industry Perspective on Minor Crop Uses—Robert F. Bischoff 662
Medicinal Plants and the Pharmaceutical Industry—James A. Duke 664
Phytomedicines as a New Crop Opportunity—Loren D. Israelsen 669

COMMERCIALIZATION

AAIC Panel Discussion—Commercializing Industrial Crops: The Industrial Component
Introduction—Anson E. Thompson 674
Cooperative Research and Development Agreements Under the Technology Transfer Act of 1986—James T. Hall 674
Role of the New Uses Council—Raymond L. Burns 677
Commercializing New Crops: Measuring the Opportunity—Keith A. Walker 678
Perspective from a Small Industrial Company—James H. Brown 680
Perspective from a Large Industrial Company—Joseph S. Boggs 681
Perspective from an Independent Industrial Consulting Company—R. Martin O'Shea 683
Perspective from Europe—Louis J.M. van Soest 684
Open Discussion—Moderator: Duane L. Johnson 686
Summary and Conclusions—Joseph C. Roetheli 693

Index to Species, Crops, and Crop Products 695
Index to Authors 709

List of Contributors

G.E. Aksland
Department of Agronomy and Soils
Auburn University
Auburn, Alabama 36849-5633

W.R. Andersen
Brigham Young University
275 WIDB
Provo, Utah 84602

L. Anderson
CALGENE
1920 Fifth St
Davis, California 95616

David J. Andrews
Agronomy Department
University of Nebraska
Lincoln, Nebraska 68583-0915

James Arquette
Jojoba Growers & Processors, Inc.
2267 S. Coconino Dr.
Apache Juntion, Arizona 85220

Kay Asay
USDA/ARS/FRRL
Utah State University UMC 6300
Logan, Utah 84322-6300

Dick L. Auld
Department of Agronomy
 Horticulture and Entomology
Texas Tech University
Lubbock, Texas 79409-2122

J.M. Babcock
Department of Crop and Soil
 Sciences
Washington State University
Pullman, Washington 99164-6420

Ralph A. Backhaus
USDA/ARS/WRRC/PBT
800 Buchanan St
Albany, California 94710

M.J. Balick
Institute of Economic Botany
The New York Botanical Garden
Bronx, New York 10458

James N. BeMiller
Whistler Center for Carbohydrate
 Research
Purdue University
West Lafayette, Indiana 47907

A. Benzioni
The Institutes for Applied Research
Ben-Gurion University of the Negev
P.O.B 1025
Beer-Sheva 84110, Israel

Marisol T. Berti
Crop and Weed Sciences
 Department
North Dakota State University
Fargo, North Dakota 58105

Robert Bertram
Bureau for Science & Technology
USAID
Room 513 SA 18
Washington, DC 20523

Harbans L. Bhardwaj
Agricultural Research Station
Fort Valley State College
Fort Valley, Georgia 31030-3298

B.H. Bhat
Department of Botany and Range
 Science
Brigham Young University
Provo, Utah 84602

Robert F. Bischoff
Dow Elanco Quad IV
9002 Purdue Rd
Indianapolis, Indiana 46268-1189

Robert E. Bledsoe
Ladonia Maarket Center
#4 South Side Square
Ladonia, Texas 75449

J. Bleibaum
CALGENE
1920 Fifth St
Davis, California 95616

Joseph S. Boggs
Procter and Gamble Company
11530 Reed Hartman Highway
Cincinnati, Ohio 45241

Carrol D. Bolen
Pioneer Hi-Bred International, Inc.
11252 Aurora Avenue
Des Moines, Iowa 50322

D. Bolotin
Department of Botany
The George S. Wise Faculty of Life
 Sciences
Tel-Aviv University
Tel-Aviv, Israel

F. Borrego
University Autónoma Agraria
 Antonio Narro
Saltillo, Coahuila, Mexico

Steve Bostic
Austin Community College
712 Keasbey
Austin, TX 78751

Michael R. Boyd
Natural Products Branch
National Cancer Institute
Fredrick Cancer R&D Center
Fredrick, Maryland 21702

V.L. Bradley
USDA/ARS
59 Johnson Hall
Washington State University
Pullman, Washington 99164-6402

W.M. Breene
Center for Alternative Plant and
 Animal Products
University of Minnesota
Borlaug Hall
St. Paul, Minnesota 55108

David Brenner
Plant Introduction Station
Iowa State University
Ames, Iowa 50011

Raymond Brigham
Texas Agriculture Experiment
 Station
Texas A&M University
Route 3, Box 219
Lubbock, Texas 79401

James H. Brown
Jojoba Growers & Processors, Inc.
2267 S. Coconino Dr.
Apache Juntion, Arizona 85220

Paul B. Brown
Purdue University
1159 Forestry Building
West Lafayette, Indiana 47907-1159

J.T. Budin
Center for Alternative Plant and
  Animal Products
University of Minnesota
Borlaug Hall
St. Paul, Minnesota 55108

Raymond L. Burns
New Uses Council
112 West Sixth Suite 408
Topeka, Kansas 66603

Glenn W. Burton
USDA/ARS
Department of Agronomy
Costal Plain Experiment Station
Tifton, Georgia 31793

M. Brett Callaway
Department of Plant and Soil
  Science
Kentucky State University
Atwood Research Facility
Frankfort, Kentucky 40601

John H. Cardellina II
Natural Products Branch
National Cancer Institute
Fredrick Cancer R&D Center
Fredrick, Maryland 21702

Kenneth D. Carlson
USDA/ARS
1815 North University Street
Peoria, Illinois 61604

Patrick M. Carr
Carrington Research Center
Box 219
Carrington, North Dakota 58421

Denys J. Charles
Purdue University
1165 Horticulture Building
West Lafayette, Indiana 47907-1165

Charles R. Clement
Department Horticulture–CTAHR
University Hawaii
3190 Maile Way
Honolulu, Hawaii 96822

R.L. Clark
USDA/ARS
59 Johnson Hall
Washington State University
Pullman, Washington 99164-6402

Y. Cohen
Department of Botany
George S. Wise Faculty of Life
  Sciences
Tel Aviv University
Tel Aviv, Israel

Wanda W. Collins
North Carolina State University
Horticulture Science Box 7609
Raleigh, North Carolina 27695-7609

John Conrad
House Agricultural Committee
1301 Longworth House Office
  Building
Washington, DC 20515

Charles G. Cook
USDA/ARS
2413 E. Hwy 83
Weslaco, Texas 78596

Katrina Cornish
USDA/ARS/WRRC/PBT
800 Buchanan St
Albany, California 94710

Gordon M. Cragg
Natural Products Branch
National Cancer Institute
Frederick Cancer R&D Center
Frederick, Maryland 21702

Jonathan H. Crane
University of Florida IFAS
Tropical Research and Education
  Center
18905 S.W. 280 Street
Homestead, Florida 33031-3314

John S. Cundiff
Department of Horticulture
Saunders Hall
Virginia Polytechnic Institute
  and State University
Blacksburg, Virginia 24061

F.P. Cuperus
Agrotechnological Research Institute
ATO–DLO
P.O. Box 17, 6700 AA
Wageningen, The Netherlands

Lonni R. Davenport
Purdue University
1165 Horticulture Building
West Lafayette, Indiana 47907-1165

P. David
George Washington Carver
  Agricultural Experiment Station
Tuskegee University
Tuskegee, Alabama 36088

C.G. Davidson
Agriculture Canada Research Station
P.O. Box 3001
Morden, Manitoba R0G 1J0
Canada

H. Maelor Davies
CALGENE
1920 Fifth St
Davis, California 95616

Jeanine M. Davis
Department of Horticultural Science
North Carolina State University
2016 Fanning Bridge Rd.
Fletcher, North Carolina 28732

Bill B. Dean
Department of Plant and Soils
Washington State University
Pullman, Washington 99164-6420

Charles D. DeCourley
Department of Horticulture
1-40 Agriculture Building
University of Missouri
Columbia, Missouri 65211

Joseph DeFrank
Department of Horticulture–CTAHR
University of Hawaii
3190 Maile Way
Honolulu, Hawaii 96822

J.T.P. Derksen
Agrotechnological Research Institute
ATO–DLO
P.O. Box 17, 6700 AA
Wageningen, The Netherlands

David A. Dierig
USDA/ARS
Water Conservation Lab
4331 E. Broadway Rd.
Phoenix, Arizona 85040

James A. Douglas
MAP Technology
Ruakura Agricultural Centre
Private Bag
Hamilton, New Zealand

Robert J. Dufault
Clemson University
CREC
2865 Savannah Hwy
Charleston, South Carolina 29634

James A. Duke
USDA/ARS
Plant Science Institute
Bldg 001 Room 133 BARC-W
Beltsville, Maryland 20705-2350

J.L. Eckhoff
Southern Agricultural Research
 Station
Montana State University
748 Railroad Highway
Huntley, Montana 59037-9099

W. Hardy Eshbaugh
Department of Botany
Maimi University
Oxford, Ohio 45056-3624

Ali Estilai
Department of Botany and Plant
 Sciences
University of California
Riverside, California 92521

David W. Evans
Department of Crop and Soil
 Sciences IAREC
Washington State University
Prosser, Washington 99350-9687

Lowell C. Ewart
Michigan State University
Department of Horticulture
East Lansing, Michigan 48824

C. Fan
CALGENE
1920 Fifth St
Davis, California 95616

Erik B.G. Feibert
Malheur Experiment Station
Oregon State University
Ontario, Oregon 97914

L.A. Field
Center for Alternative Plant and
 Animal Products
University of Minnesota
Borlaug Hall
St. Paul, Minnesota 55108

Antonio Figueira
Purdue University
1165 Horticulture Building
West Lafayette, Indiana 47907-1165

Michael Foster
Texas Agricultural Experiment
 Station
Box 9000
Fort Stockton, Texas 79735

Cary Fowler
Rural Advancement Fund
 International
P.O. Box 655
Pittsboro, North Carolina 27312

James L. Fowler
Department of Agronomy and
 Horticulture
New Mexico State University
Box 30003/Department 3Q
Las Cruces, New Mexico 88003-0003

J. Friedman
Department of Botany
The George S. Wise Faculty of Life
 Sciences
Tel–Aviv University
Tel–Aviv, Israel

I-Mo Fu
Department of Horticulture
Saunders Hall
Virginia Polytechnic Institute
 and State University
Blacksburg, Virginia 24061

R.M. Gareau
Department of Plant, Soil and
 Entomological Science
University of Idaho
Moscow, Idaho 83843-4196

Karen L.B. Gast
Department of Horticulture and
 Forestry
Kansas State University
Manhattan, Kansas 66506-4002

A.C. Gathman
Biology Department
Southeast Missouri St. University
Cape Girardeau, Missouri 63701

Kenneth M. Gilbertson
Southern Agricultural Research
 Station
Montana State University
748 Railroad Highway
Huntley, Montana 59037-9099

G.C. Gilliland
Department of Crop and Soil
 Sciences IAREC
Washington State University
Prosser, Washington 99350-9687

Michael R. Grever
Natural Products Branch
National Cancer Institute
Frederick Cancer R&D Center
Frederick, Maryland 21702

Robert Griesbach
SDA/ARS/BARC-W
Bldg 004 Rm 208
Beltsville, Maryland 20705-2350

James T. Hall
USDA/ARS
Office of Cooperative Interactions
BARC-West, Building 005
Beltsville, Maryland 20705

An N. Hang
Department of Crop and Soil
 Sciences IAREC
Washington State University
Prosser, Washington 99350-9687

R.M. Hannan
USDA/ARS
59 Johnson Hall
Washington State University
Pullman, Washington 99164-6402

James Hanover
Department of Forestry
Michigan State University
East Lansing, Michigan 48824-1222

N. Haq
International Centre for
 Underutilised Crops
Wye College
Wye TN25 5AH, UK

Jack R. Harlan
1016 North Hagen Ave
New Orleans, Lousiana 70119

A. Hashemi
Department of Botany and Plant
 Sciences
University of California
Riverside, California 92521-0124

D.J. Hawkins
CALGENE
1920 Fifth St
Davis, California 95616

M.K. Heikkinen
Department of Plant, Soil and
 Entomological Science
University of Idaho
Moscow, Idaho 83843-4196

T.L. Henderson
Crop and Weed Sciences
 Department
North Dakota State University
Fargo, North Dakota 58105

W.M. Hess
Department of Botany and Range
 Science
Brigham Young University
Provo, Utah 84602

Errol Hewett
Department of Horticultural Science
Massey University
Palmerston North, New Zealand

Marcin Horbowicz
Department of Soil, Crop and
 Atmospheric Sciences
Cornell University
619 Bradfield Hall
Ithaca, New York 14853-1901

J. Huang
Department of Botany and Range
 Science
Brigham Young University
Provo, Utah 84602

S. Huyskens
Obst- und Gemüsebau Institut der
 Universität Bonn
Germany

Loren D. Israelsen
Murdock International
142 West 4600 North
Provo, Utah 84604

Philip Ito
Beaumont Research Center
University of Hawaii
Hilo, Hawaii 96720

Mary Jackson
Mt. Pleasant Sweetgrass
 Basketmakers Association
Mt. Pleasant, North Carolina 29464

Jules Janick
Purdue University
1165 Horticulture Building
West Lafayette, Indiana 47907-1165

Dianna Jasso de Rodriguez
Universidad Autónoma Agraria
 Antonio Narro
Buenavista
Saltillo, Coahuila, Mexico 25000

Casimir A. Jaworski
USDA/ARS
University of Georgia
P.O. Box 946
Tifton, Georgia 31793

Mitra N. Jha
Department of Agronomy
Colorado State University
Fort Collins, Colorado 80526

Duane L. Johnson
Department of Agronomy
Colorado State University
Fort Collins, Colorado 80526

George P. Johnson
Arkansas Technical University
Russelville, Arkansas 72801

R.C. Johnson
USDA/ARS
59 Johnson Hall
Washington State University
Pullman, Washington 99164-6402

Pablo S. Jourdan
Department of Horticulture
The Ohio State University
2001 Fyffe Court
Columbus, Ohio 43210

F.A Kiehn
Agriculture Canada Research Station
P.O. Box 3001
Morden, Manitoba R0G 1J0
Canada

Barnabas Kiula
Agronomy Department
University of Nebraska
Lincoln, Nebraska 68583-0915

Greg Kleine
Texas Agricultural Experiment
 Station
Box 9000
Fort Stockton, Texas 79735

Steven J. Knapp
Department of Crop Science
Oregon State University
Corvallis, Oregon 97331

Herbert Knudsen
Natural Fibers Corporation
P.O. Box 830
Searle Field
Ogallala, Nebraska 69153

J.C. Konovsky
East–West Seeds
120 State NE, Suite 1183
Olympia, Washington 98501

H. Koopowitz
UCI Arboretum
University of California
Irvine, California 92716

Michael J. Koziol
Latinreco S.A.
Centro Nestlé de Desarrollo de
 Alimentos en América Latina
Casilla Postal 17-110-6053
Quito, Ecuador

K. Anand Kumar
Agronomy Department
University of Nebraska
Lincoln, Nebraska 68583-0915

Ljerka Kunst
NRC Canada
Plant Biotechnology Institute
110 Gymnasium Rd
Saskatoon, Saskatchewan S7N 0W9
Canada

Sathyanarayanaiah Kuruvadi
Universidad Autónoma Agraria
　Antonio Narro
Buenavista
Saltillo, Coahuila, Mexico 25000

Mary Lamberts
University of Florida
18710 SW 288th Street
Homestead, Florida 33030

K.J. Larson
Department of Agronomy and Soils
Washington State University
Pullmanm Washington 99164-6420

Brian M. Lawrence
R.J. Reynolds Tobacco Company
Bowman Gary Technical Center
PO Box 2959
Winston-Salem, North Carolina
27102-2959

Wudeneh Letchamo
Institute of Plant Growing and
　Breeding
Justus Liebig University
Giessen
D-3557 Ebsdorfergrund-4, Germany

A. López Benitez
University Autónoma Agraria
　Antonio Narro
Saltillo, Coahuila, Mexico

Thomas A. Lumpkin
Department Agronomy and Soils
Washington State University
Pullman, Washington 99164-6420

Bruce Macdonald
University of British Columbia
　Botanical Garden
6504 SW Marine Drive
Vancouver, British Columbia V6T 1W5
Canada

Samuel L. MacKenzie
NRC Canada
Plant Biotechnology Institute
110 Gymnasium Rd
Saskatoon, Saskatchewan S7N 0W9
Canada

Richard Manshardt
Department of Horticulture–CTAHR
University of Hawaii
3190 Maile Way
Honolulu, Hawaii 96822

Dyremple B. Marsh
Lincoln University
900 Moreau Drive
Jefferson City, Missouri 65101

Paul L. Mask
Department of Agronomy and Soils
Auburn University
Auburn, Alabama 36849-5633

A. Matus
Crop Development Centre
University of Saskatchewan
Saskatoon, Saskatchewan S7N 0W0
Canada

G. Mazza
Agriculture Canada Research Station
P.O. Box 3001
Morden, Manitoba R0G 1J0
Canada

Richard McCain
Quail Mountain Farms
14310 Camagna Way
Watsonville, California 95076

Laura McCann
Center for Alternative Plant and
　Animal Products
University of Minnesota
411 Borlaug Hall
St. Paul, Minnesota 55108

Dean C. McClary
Department of Crop and Soil
　Sciences
Washington State University
Pullman, Washington 99164-6420

Jerry L. McLaughlin
Department of Medicinal Chemistry
　and Pharmacognosy
Purdue University
West Lafayette, Indiana 47907

Steven P. McLaughlin
Office of Arid Land Studies
University of Arizona
845 North Park Avenue
Tucson, Arizona 85719

Tesfai Mebrahtu
Department of Forestry
Michigan State University
126 N.R. Building
East Lansing, Michigan 48824

Ana L. Medina
Whistler Center for Carbohydrate
　Research
Purdue University
West Lafayette, Indiana 47907

S. Mendlinger
The Institutes for Applied Research
Ben-Gurion University of the Negev
P.O. Box 1025
Beer-Sheva 84110, Israel

P. Mendosa
Department of Biology
Pontificia Catholic University
Quito, Ecuador

F. Meyer
UCI Arboretum
University of California
Irvine, California 92716

Gregory Miller
Empire Chestnut Company
Carrollton, Ohio 44615

David Mills
The Institutes for Applied Research
Ben-Gurion University of the Negev
P.O. Box 1025
Beer-Sheva 84110, Israel

Yosef Mizrahi
Ben-Gurion University of the Negev
P.O. Box 1025
Beer-Sheva 84110, Israel

Jaroy Moore
Texas Agricultural Experiment
　Station
Box 9000
Fort Stockton, Texas 79735

K.J. Moore
USDA/ARS
Department of Agronomy
University of Nebraska
332 Keim Hall
Lincoln, Nebraska 68503-0915

Mario R. Morales
Purdue University
1165 Horticulture Building
West Lafayette, Indiana 47907-1165

Fredrick J. Muehlbauer
UDSA/ARS
Washington State University
215 Johnson Hall
Pullman, Washington 99164-6421

G.L. Mullins
Department of Agronomy and Soils
Auburn University
Auburn, Alabama 36849-5633

B.G. Muuse
Agrotechnological Research Institute ATO–DLO
P.O. Box 17, 6700 AA
Wageningen, The Netherlands

Robert L. Myers
216A Waters Hall
University of Missouri-Columbia
Columbia, Missouri 65211

Ram G. Nadimpalli
Department of Horticulture
University of Georgia
Tifton, Georgia 31793

S. Kristine Næss
Horticulture Department
University of Maryland
College Park, Maryland 20742

J.M. Nelson
Department of Plant Science
University of Arizona
Tucson, Arizona 85721

Avinoam Nerd
Ben–Gurion University of the Negev
P.O.B. 1025
Beer-Sheva, Israel

Timothy J. Ng
Department of Horticulture
University of Maryland
College Park, Maryland 20742-5611

Ralph L. Obendorf
Department of Soil, Crop and Atmospheric Sciences
Cornell University
619 Bradfield Hall
Ithaca, New York 14853-1901

Ervin A. Oelke
Department of Agronomy & Plant Genetics
University of Minnesota
411 Borlaug Hall
St. Paul, Minnesota 55108

A.G. Ogg
Department of Crop and Soil Sciences
Washington State University
Pullman, Washington 99164-6420

Edward S. Oplinger
Agronomy Department
University of Wisconsin
1575 Linden Drive
Madison, Wisconson 53706

Desmond A. O'Rourke
Department of Agronomy and Soils
Washington State University
Pullman, Washington 99164-6420

R. Martin O'Shea
Smithers Scientific Services, Inc.
425 West Market Street
Akron, Ohio 44303-2044

Richard H. Ozminkowski Jr
Department of Horticulture
The Ohio State University
2001 Fyffe Ct
Columbus, Ohio 43210

David A. Palzkill
Bioresources Research Facility
250 E Valencia Rd
Tucson, Arizona 85609

Zhiqang Pan
USDA/ARS/WRRC/PBT
800 Buchanan St
Albany, California 94710

Jerry A. Payne
USDA
Southeastern Fruit & Tree Nut Research Lab
P.O. Box 87
Byron, Georgia 31008

Sharad C. Phatak
Department of Horticulture
University of Georgia
Tifton, Georgia 31793

William M. Potter
Department of Medicinal Chemistry and Pharmacognosy
Purdue University
West Lafayette, Indiana 47907

Daniel H. Putnam
Center for Alternative Plant and Animal Products
University of Minnesota
411 Borlaug Hall
St. Paul, Minnesota 55108

Glen C. Rains
Department of Horticulture
Saunders Hall
Virginia Polytechnic Institute and State University
Blacksburg, Virginia 24061

John F. Rajewski
Agronomy Department
University of Nebraska
Lincoln, Nebraska 68583-0915

F. Ramirez
University Autónoma Agraria Antonio Narro
Saltillo, Coahuila, Mexico

Kåre Rapp
State Agricultural Research Station
Holt, 9001
Tromsø, Norway

Sunil Ratnayake
Department of Medicinal Chemistry and Pharmacognosy
Purdue University
West Lafayette, Indiana 47907

Eran Raveh
Ben–Gurion University of the Negev
P.O.B. 1025
Beer-Sheva, Israel

Damian A. Ravetta
Bioresources Research Facility
250 E Valencia Rd
Tucson, Arizona 85609

Dennis T. Ray
Department of Plant Sciences
University of Arizona
Tucson, Arizona 85721

D.W. Reeves
Department of Agronomy and Soils
Auburn University
Auburn, Alabama 36849-5633

William R. Reid
Pecan Experiment Field
Kansas State University
Chetopa, Kansas 67336-0247

William Reinert
Campbell Soup
28605 County Road 104
Davis, California 95616

E.G. Rhoden
George Washington Carver
 Agricultural Experiment Station
Tuskegee University
Tuskegee, Alabama 36088

M. Rios
Department of Biology
Pontifica Catholic University of
 Ecuador
Quito, Ecuador

N. Riveland
Crop and Weed Sciences
 Department
North Dakota State University
Fargo, North Dakota 58105

Frank E. Robinson
Imperial Valley Agricultural Center
University of California
1004 E Holton Road
El Centro, California 92243

Joseph C. Roethli
USDA/CSRS/SPSS
Office of Agricultural Materials
Aerospace Bldg. Rm. 342
14th and Independence Avenue S.W.
Washington, DC 20251-2200

J. Kent Rupprecht
Department of Medicinal Chemistry
 and Pharmacognosy
Purdue University
West Lafayette, Indiana 47907

Edward J. Ryder
USDA/ARS
1636 East Alisal St
Salinas, California 93905

Stephen K. Salvo
USDA/ARS
Raleigh, North Carolina 27609

Isaac Sanchez Valdez
Universidad Autónoma Agraria
 Antonio Narro
Buenavista
Saltillo, Coahuila, Mexico 25000

Blaine G. Schatz
Carrington Research Center
North Dakota State University
Box 219
Carrington, North Dakota 58421

A.A. Schneiter
Crop and Weed Sciences
 Department
North Dakota State University
Fargo, North Dakota 58105

Saul Schepartz
Natural Products Branch
National Cancer Institute
Frederick Cancer R&D Center
Frederick, Maryland 21702

J.R. Schulz-Schaeffer
Montana State University
Southern Agricultural Research
 Station
748 Railroad Hwy
Huntley, Montana 59037-9099

Andrew W. Scott Jr.
Rio Farms, Inc.
Rt. 1, Box 326
Monte Alto, Texas 78538

Ramsey L. Sealy
Austin Community College
712 Keasbey
Austin, Texas 78751

Rodney Serres
Department of Horticulture
University of Wisconsin-Madison
Madison, Wisconson 53706

Michael C. Shannon
Department of Botany and
 Plant Sciences
University of California
Riverside, California 92521

Carol Shennan
Department of Horticulture
Saunders Hall
Virginia Polytechnic Institute
 and State University
Blacksburg, Virginia 24061

Clinton C. Shock
Malheur Experiment Station
Oregon State University
Ontario, Oregon 97914

James E. Simon
Purdue University
1165 Horticulture Building
West Lafayette, Indiana 47907-1165

Bharat P. Singh
Agricultural Research Station
Fort Valley State College
Fort Valley, Georgia 31030-3298

A.E. Slinkard
Crop Development Centre
University of Saskatchewan
Saskatoon, Saskatchewan S7N 0W0
Canada

T. Small
George Washington Carver
 Agricultural Experiment Station
Tuskegee University
Tuskegee, Alabama 36088

Robin M. Smith
Malheur Experiment Station
Oregon State University
Ontario, Oregon 97914

Kenneth M. Snader
Natural Products Branch
National Cancer Institute
Frederick Cancer R&D Center
Frederick, Maryland 21702

Jacqueline A. Soule
Department of Botany
University of Texas at Austin
Austin, Texas 78713-7640

Matti Sovero
Ameri–Can Pedigree Seed Company
1 Calgene Drive
Memphis, Tennessee 38120

Stephen A. Spongberg
Arnold Arboretum of Harvard
 University
125 Arborway
Jamaica Plain, Massachusetts
02130-3519

Gilbert F. Stallknecht
Montana State University
Southern Agricultural Research
 Station
748 Railroad Hwy
Huntley, Montana 59037-9099

Elden J. Stang
University of Wisconsin
Department of Horticulture
1575 Linden Drive
Madison, Wisconson 53706-1597

D.M. Stout
USDA/ARS
59 Johnson Hall
Washington State University
Pullman, Washington 99164-6402

Matthew Suffness
Natural Products Branch
National Cancer Institute
Frederick Cancer R&D Center
Frederick, Maryland 21702

Glenn H. Sullivan
Purdue University
1165 Horticulture Building
West Lafayette, Indiana 47907-1165

Harry Jan Swartz
Horticulture Department
University of Maryland
College Park, Maryland 20742

L.K. Tanigoshi
Department of Crop and
 Soil Sciences
Washington State University
Pullman, Washington 99164-6420

Charles S. Taylor
Kenaf International Inc.
120 E. Jay Avenue
McAllen, Texas 78504

David C. Taylor
NRC Canada
Plant Biotechnology Institute
110 Gymnasium Road
Saskatoon, Saskatchewan S7N 0W9
Canada

Douglas P. Taylor
Department of Soil, Crop and
 Atmospheric Sciences
Cornell University
619 Bradfield Hall
Ithaca, New York 14853-1901

Anson E. Thompson
USDA/ARS US Water Conservation
4331 E Broadway Road
Phoenix, Arizona 85040

Maxine M. Thompson
Department of Horticulture
Oregon State University
Corvallis, Oregon 97333

Haji Tinggal
Universiti Brunei
Darussalam
Gadong 3186
Brunei

Robert Tinguely
Department of Agronomy and
 Horticulture
New Mexico State University
Box 30003, Department 3Q
Las Cruces, New Mexico 88003-0003

Suresh C. Tiwari
Alcorn State University
Lorman, Mississippi 39096

J.E.G. van Dam
Agrotechnological Research Institute
ATO–DLO
P.O. Box 17, 6700 AA
Wageningen, The Netherlands

A. Vandenberg
Crop Development Centre
University of Saskatchewan
Saskatoon, Saskatchewan S7N 0W0
Canada

Willem M.J. van Gelder
Agrotechnological Research Institute
ATO–DLO
P.O. Box 17, 6700 AA
Wageningen, The Netherlands

E. van Santen
Department of Agronomy and Soils
Auburn University
Auburn, Alabama 36849-5633

Louis J. M. van Soest
Center for Plant Breeding
and Reproduction Research
Post Bus 16, 6700 AA
Wageningen, The Netherlands

M. Ventura
The Institutes for Applied Research
Ben–Gurion University of the Negev
P.O. Box 1025
Beer–Sheva 84110, Israel

Nicolas Verlet
Ministry of Agriculture
CFPPA
26110 Nyons, France

Toni A. Voelker
CALGENE
1920 Fifth St
Davis, California 95616

Kenneth P. Vogel
USDA/ARS
Department of Agronomy
University of Nebraska
332 Keim Hall
Lincoln, Nebraska 68503-0915

Keith A. Walker
Agrigenetics Company
Centre Plaza North
35575 Curtis Boulevard, Suite 300
Eastlake, Ohio 44095

Sarah M. Ward
Department of Agronomy
Colorado State University
Fort Collins, Colorado 80526

William Waycott
USDA/ARS
1636 East Alisal St
Salinas, California 93905

Charles L. Webber III
USDA/ARS/SCARL
P.O. Box 159
Lane, Oklahoma 74555

D.J. Weber
Department of Botany and Range
  Science
Brigham Young University
Provo, Utah 84602

Julia Weiss
Ben–Gurion University of the Negev
P.O. Box 1025
Beer–Sheva 84110, Israel

Gregory E. Welbaum
Department of Horticulture
Saunders Hall
Virginia Polytechnic Institute
  and State University
Blacksburg, Virginia 24061

George A. White
USDA/ARS
Room 322-Bld 001-BARC West
Beltsville, Maryland 20705

Wayne F. Whitehead
Agricultural Research Station
Fort Valley State College
Fort Valley, Georgia 31030

Trevor Williams
International Fund for Agricultural
  Research
1611 N Kent St Suite 600
Arlington, Virginia 22209-2134

Merle D. Witt
Kansas State University
4500 E. Mary
Garden City, Kansas 67846

A.C. Worrell
CALGENE
1920 Fifth St
Davis, California 95616

Umedi L. Yadava
Agricultural Research Station
School of Agriculture
Fort Valley State College
Fort Valley, Georgia 31030-3298

Francis Zee
USDA/ARS
National Clonal Germplasm
  Repository
PO Box 4487
Hilo, Hawaii 96720

Richard D. Zeller
Natural Fibers Corporation
P.O. Box 830
Searle Field
Ogallala, Nebraska 69153

Preface

This volume is an outcome of the Second National Symposium (NEW CROPS: Exploration, Research, Commercialization) held October 6–9, 1991 in Indianapolis, Indiana. The objective of the symposium was to provide a national forum for leading authorities from industry, government, agricultural experiment stations, and academia to discuss and review the status and future of new crop development in North America. The contents include papers from invited speakers and scientists who presented their research as poster presentations during the meetings. The contributions include a diverse assortment of topics and views. Many papers extended information first presented at the first symposium but new topics, new crops, and new crop opportunities are also included. The topics of new crop exploration, new crop commercialization, and policy issues are covered in special sections. This volume along with its predecessor, *Advances in New Crops* (Proceedings of the First National Symposium *NEW CROPS; Research, Development, Economics*) published in 1990 by Timber Press, Portland, Oregon, provide a running commentary on new development in this emerging field. Because of the large inter-national input, we anticipate that this compilation will have reverberations outside of the United States.

As in the previous symposium. we encountered a wave of euphoria and good feeling about new crops and their potential for enriching the agriculture of the United States and other countries. The success of this endeavor is attributable to many people and organizations including speakers, participants, poster presenters, exhibitors, and sponsors. We thank the Honorable Richard Lugar, senior senator from Indiana, who addressed the group in the welcome reception and shared his views on the farm bill and the future of American agriculture. We gratefully acknowledge the sponsors listed on the title page, who backed up their belief in new crops with the tangible support necessary to make the symposium, and thus, this volume, a reality.

We especially acknowledge the expertise of Anna L. Whipkey who was in charge of all computer operations for the symposium and this book and who single-handedly transformed the manuscripts into camera-ready copy. Finally, we dedicate this work to Glenn W. Burton and Jack R. Harlan, two giants in the field of new crops.

Jules Janick   Henry L. Shands
James E. Simon   Anson E. Thompson
Symposium Organizers

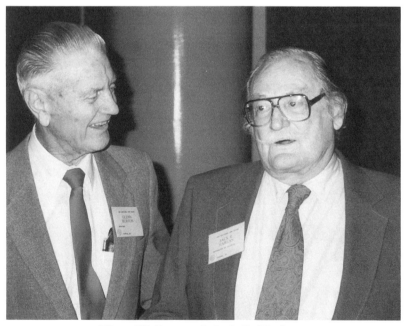

Glenn W. Burton & Jack R. Harlan

Foreword

Jules Janick

The United States, despite its large size, is a deficit area for native crop species. Interest in new crops has always been strong throughout its history as colonists imported potential new crops from both the New and Old Worlds. The agrarian history of this country in many ways is a chronicle of the rise and fall of new crop species. Our major grains including maize, wheat, rice, barley, and oats are all new crops introduced by native Americans or European colonists. There are also many new crop failures; historic examples include indigo and tea. The twentieth century, a period when crop patterns stabilized, still continued to witness the introduction and development of new crops. Successful examples included soybean, now one of the major crops of the United States and the world, blueberry and cranberry (native species improved by breeding efforts), avocado (in California and Florida), macadamia (in Hawaii), and pistachio (in California). A number of crops were also lost to the United States in this century; notable examples include tung and castorbean. Yet despite the successes of new crops, there had been no concerted national policy to accelerate their introduction and commercialization.

Recent interest in new crops has increased as a result of a number of interacting forces. One is the upsurge of interest in the last 20 years in germplasm conservation which developed after the late blight epidemic in maize in the 1970s, as a result of the susceptibility of a widely used male–sterile cytoplasm (Texas) to *Helminthesporium maydis*. Other contributing factors include low agricultural prices of major commodities over the last decade which have increased interest in diversification; the continued strength of the environmental movement which has spurred interest in crop diversity and alternate agriculture; increasing consumer demand for new culinary products; and the rise of ethnic foods due to changing demographic forces. Finally, economic forces continue to reward successful innovators which attracts entrepreneurs not deterred by high risk. Recently, this area has been vitalized by the development of a number of state programs and centers devoted to new and alternate crops in Indiana, Minnesota, Missouri, and Washington, as well as the creation of some national organizations (e.g., American Association of Industrial Crops, New Uses Council). Although national funding for new crops research has been erratic, the 1990 Farm Bill has made funding provisions available for an alternative Agricultural Research and Commercialization Center (AARC) which should play a growing role in new crop development.

Because of the complexity of new crop development, it is difficult to make rapid progress. In fact, the case can be made that we really do not know exactly how to get the job done. There are many reasons for this. For example, federal subsidies in the form of crop supports for basic crops limits the introduction of new feed grains. Similarly, the introduction of new crops generates antipathy from supporters of old crops. Finally, the development of crops is a process perfected by primitive peoples, most of them in prehistory during Neolithic times, a skill that, one might argue, has been lost.

The general consensus is that a number of new crops will make it; the winners will depend on a combination of market acceptability, research information, economic incentive, and enthusiastic and persistent crop champions. This volume along with its predecessor (*Advances in New Crops*, the Proceeding of the First National Symposium on New Crop) provides a passport to this fascinating expedition, a trip with unexpected vistas, turns, deadends, and detours. We can all agree, however, that it is an exciting journey and we proceed with anticipation. Welcome aboard.

NEW CROPS

PART I
POLICY & PROGRAMS

POLICY

National New Crops Policy

John W. Conrad III

As a close observer of our political system at some of its highest levels, it is my hope to share some of those observations in order to gain a better understanding of the purpose and ramifications of federal agricultural science policy. In particular, I wish to focus on the policy for new crops, the expectations which the House Agriculture Committee and the Congress have for the scientific establishment, and the goals set forth in legislation.

FEDERAL INVOLVEMENT IN AGRICULTURE AND SCIENCE

To fully understand and appreciate the role of the government, and particularly the Congress, in agricultural science today, it is necessary to place it into an historical context. The relationship between government and agriculture is basic and has existed for a long time. A happy people, content and not prone to revolution or overthrow of government, is a people who are well-fed, well-clothed, and well-housed. It is in the government's own best interest that these three conditions are met on a timely and continuous basis. The Constitution recognizes the role which science plays in helping to achieve these ends. Article I, Section 8 of this venerable document empowers the Congress "To promote the Progress of Science ..." As a fledgling nation in the midst of expansion and beginning a cruel and costly civil war, Justin Morrill and Abraham Lincoln recognized the importance of agriculture in our national life and proceeded to establish the structure for its continual improvement and modification. It became the official policy of the United States, by way of the Land Grant Colleges Act of 1862 and 1890 (the First and Second Morrill Acts) and subsequent legislation, that each State establish a college of agriculture and the means for the transmittal to the public of agricultural discoveries and related information. The 1890s institutions are, of course, the historically black colleges, including Tuskegee University.

The resulting Land Grant educational and research system of the United States is second to none. It has helped to establish the United States as a preeminent agricultural nation. Our production agriculture is the envy of the world. Our people, on the whole, have been among the best fed, best clothed, and best housed. Our over-production has helped to feed, cloth, and house many peoples in lands around the world.

The Land Grant system is recognized around the world as the best. Many come from foreign lands to receive their education here. The entire agricultural leadership of some foreign countries has been educated and trained within the United States Land Grant college system. Land Grant institutions are also expected by many to play a significant role in the redevelopment of agriculture and the promotion of economic stability in the emerging democracies and the Soviet Union.

NEW CROPS AND CONGRESS

The Congress has exercised its Constitutional responsibility by establishing an agriculture science framework and policy. From time-to-time that policy is revisited and revised, most recently in the 1990 Farm Bill. Much attention has been given to production agriculture. However, over the years, interest in new crops and new uses for agricultural commodities in the Congress has varied from intense to subdued. Congressional interest is once again intensifying due to national and world economic conditions. Those of you working on the development of new crops and new uses know that policy has not always been consistent in this area. Interest has depended, in part, upon funds availability, the viewpoint of the then-current Secretary of Agriculture and/or Congress, and the amount and duration of the surplus production from traditional commodities.

At times with high commodity surplus levels, the interest in alternative crops that farmers can profitably raise has been keen. Individual farmers, commodity groups, legislators and political appointees ask what is going on with research and how soon can we have an acceptable alternative to assist with farm income and to reduce farm program cost. They seem to conveniently forget that solutions to these problems take time. It takes years of hard and consistent work to develop a new crop or new use. It takes more years to develop farmer and general public acceptance of a new crop. And, it can take several years to develop the necessary seed stock so that it can be grown in sufficient quantities. Interest wanes at the point that traditional commodity surpluses dip, due to weather or other production shortfalls, and turn into scarcity. Surpluses cease to be surpluses and become strategic reserves. Interest in new crops, new uses and new markets also disappears.

Over the years, the Congress has tried to deal with new crops and new uses through a variety of legislation. Richard Wheaton (1990) summarized much of this legislation in his talk before the First National Symposium on New Crops in 1988. That legislation includes the Strategic and Critical Materials Stockpiling Act of 1979, the National Materials and Minerals Policy Research & Development Act of 1980, the Critical Materials Act of 1984, the Native Latex Act of 1979, and the Critical Agricultural Materials Act of 1984.

Since that time and in a continued effort to address the need for new crops and new uses, the Agriculture Committees and the Congress have passed legislation reauthorizing programs and creating new entities to further necessary research in this area. I am referring to the reauthorization of the Critical Agricultural Materials Act and to Subtitle G of the Farm Bill, which creates the Alternative Agriculture Research and Commercialization Center.

There is also the provision in the Farm Bill pertaining to the production of energy from biomass. In this area, feedstock improvements are of interest and hold promise. The substitution of renewable resources for depletable resources continues to capture the imagination of the Congress, the public, and the farming community. It is an important area for further development, an area which could affect the quality of life in both rural and urban areas of the United States.

During the debate on the 1990 Farm Bill, Members expressed concern about the state of United States agricultural commodity exports. Economic data shows that global trade in bulk commodities is increasing at approximately 1% per year. On the other hand, trade in value added products increased at about 5% per year during the 1980s. Consumer oriented food products account for 53% of world agricultural trade.

Recognizing the need to compete in world markets, the advantage of having one organization within the USDA whose sole duty would be to develop new uses for traditional and new agricultural commodities, and responding to advice from the scientific community, the 1990 Farm Bill established the Alternative Agriculture Research and Commercialization Center (AARCC). AARCC is directed to "(research and) commercialize new nonfood, nonfeed uses for traditional and new agricultural commodities in order to create jobs, enhance the economic development of the rural economy, and diversify markets for raw agricultural and forestry products."

Diversification could lead to a sounder agricultural sector in the next century. However, the strength of diversification will depend upon the markets found and developed for these new crops and new uses. It will do no good to have new surpluses of new crops and no new uses. An idea may be a good idea, a discovery may be great, a new crop or new use may fulfill a need, but no idea, no discovery, or no need is fulfilled without money. We can be altruistic about new crops and new uses, but the harsh reality everyone in all walks of life faces is the need for money. It takes adequate, consistent funding to discover, develop, and market new crops and new uses.

Funded at a level of $4.5 million for fiscal year 1992, it is hoped that AARCC will be able to provide adequate and consistent funding for this area. That is one of the fundamental, founding principles for its establishment. There is a strong desire to remove the peaks and valleys from funding efforts and provide continuity and stability for our new crops and new uses research establishment. The work you are doing is important every day of every year, not just when someone needs it.

In response to a strong call from the scientific community, the 1990 Farm Bill established the National Competitive Research Initiative (Section 1615), focused on basic research. Authorized funding for the initiative begins at $150 million for fiscal year 1991, increasing to $500 million in fiscal year 1995.

The AARCC and the National Initiative represent two sides of the same agricultural research coin. The focus of the AARC is more along the lines of applied and adaptive research, and the commercialization of agricultural research. On the other side, the National Initiative addresses the area of basic agricultural research. One hopes that these two great efforts will compliment each other.

There was considerable debate on the merits of these two areas, about what and how much of either was actually needed. The resulting consensus endorsed both. However, I would observe that applied and adaptive research with an eye toward commercialization continues to build momentum and catch the interest of Members.

There are, I believe, several reasons for this. One, Members interested in rural development are looking for new ways to improve the rural economy and way of life. They see scientific innovation, that which has not only been discovered, but which has also been applied, adapted, and commercialized, as a way to achieve some rural development goals. Two, Members are concerned about commodity surpluses and their affect on rural income. Three, with the tight budget situation, Members are looking for tangible, useful results for research dollars spent.

With the flag of caution raised on fiscal matters, I would observe that money is the bane of Washington at this time. There is not enough money to fund all of the programs that deserve funding. When asked to support new agricultural research projects or programs, Members can be frequently heard asking whether or not the proposal can be funded through the National Initiative or AARCC.

The budget agreement reached last year, which placed limits on military, domestic, and foreign aid spending, has everyone scrambling for the few dollars available for funding. Severe restraints have been placed on spending by the Congress. And the agreement is for three years. This has led to a high degree of frustration in the Congress over spending priorities. Agriculture is affected by this agreement. Commodity programs, nutrition programs and research are all in the same boat. Too many requests for spending, too little money to honor those requests.

Some of you may have read recent news accounts of an effort by some Members to modify and change the existing budget agreement. They believe that the changes in the international political situation, that is the breakup of the Soviet Union and changes in Eastern Europe, should be reflected in the United States budget. This would translate into less spending on defense and more spending for domestic programs. At this time, there is no renegotiation in progress. Should the Administration even agree to discuss the matter, that process could be as long, as tedious and as explosive as the previous negotiations were. Any potential new agreement would not take affect until the fiscal year 1993 budget, at the earliest.

CONCLUSION

There is a long history of Congressional interest and involvement in agricultural scientific research. This involvement is manifested in a Congressionally mandated agricultural scientific research structure and programs, which are from time-to-time revisited and revised.

The most recent debate, during the 1990 Farm Bill, reauthorized existing programs and established two new funding mechanisms: the AARCC and the National Research Initiative. AARCC concentrates on applied and adaptive research and commercialization of discoveries, while the National Initiative will fund basic research. The lack of funding for needy spending programs is a very real problem affecting the Congress and the Administration. Funding agricultural research is directly affected by this problem.

The need for new crops and new uses research continues to exist. The intent of the Congress is for the USDA to explore all possibilities for substituting renewable resources for depletable resources in order to reduce excess production capacity in American agriculture and the high cost of government farm programs.

REFERENCES

Wheaton, E.R. 1990. Industrial crops commercialization, p. 41–46. In: J. Janick and J.E. Simon (eds.). Advances in new crops. Timber Press, Portland, OR.

International New Crops Policy

J.T. Williams and N. Haq

In an era when funding for agricultural research, whether international or domestic, is decreasing and against a background of a substantial increase in agricultural production worldwide, it is difficult to capitalize on the scientific groundswell of support for new crops. Almost certainly, the major hope for any research program to be sustained is to build up its capacity for strategic planning. This involves the assessment of a number of policy options.

The discussion is complicated by issues of sustainability, environment, and loss of plant resources. None will be addressed by focusing narrowly on, for instance, small farmers, or on agricultural technology as an inefficient means of alleviating rural poverty, or on investment opportunities. Also, the issues differ between disparate economic and social systems of industrial and developing countries. Furthermore, the research areas associated with new crops span interest in alternative crops for crop diversification, in old crops for new purposes, and in new crops for new needs.

Although this symposium is oriented towards the interests of the United States, this paper will address the international complexities, since no country can afford to isolate itself from research elsewhere. In addition, funding sources stress the need to strengthen capacities to cooperate effectively, and this requires sound planning. It is also often forgotten that international research has evolved over the past two decades. The green revolution as a plant production instrument of development cooperation, conceived as a quick countermeasure to hunger, was quickly followed by efforts to strengthen national research systems. Lessons from the green revolution were taken into development cooperation philosophies so that the focus of rural development was on the small farmer and strategies for self-help and structural adjustments. The cultivation of indigenous food crops (many of them domesticates, which became recognized as having potential for wider use) was certainly in place before ecology and the preservation of natural resources became pivotal concerns of development policy.

INFORMATION

Perhaps the biggest gap which would enhance policy decisions is the lack of a specifically targeted information system on new crops. Despite a number of symposia, such as those of the American Association for the Advancement of Science in 1978 (Ritchie 1979), the United States National Symposium on New Crops in 1988 (Janick and Simon 1990), or special reports spanning the last 15 years of the National Research Council (NAS 1975; NRC 1979), FAO (1982), or the International Board for Plant Genetic Resources (IBPGR) (Arora 1985), there is no comprehensive database retrieval system for new crops. In 1987, at the first major international symposium on new crops, Williams (1989) proposed that decision making on new crops depended on the following factors: (a) Does the species need to be brought into cultivation, is potential production adequate without major breeding efforts, and will insurance against genetic vulnerability be made through active genetic resources programs? (b) What is known about domestication and the spectrum of diversity in the genepool? (c) What decisions on conservation need to be made to sustain research and availability of materials? Discussions later added the need for data on basic successes and failures of agronomic experiments, many not published widely.

A number of databases exist, such as that on a past program of USDA on new crops research (Princeton 1977), a specific comprehensive one on legumes (International Legume Database and Information Service), specific taxonomic ones at botanical gardens such as TROPICOS at Missouri Botanical Garden, a semi-arid lands one at Royal Botanical Gardens, Kew, and a palms one at New York Botanical Gardens. The needs have been translated into action for plant resources of regions (Lemmens et al. 1989, for Southeast Asia), proposals for economic plants databases (Smithsonian/IUCN proposal for the Americas, unpublished), and others. The International Center for Underutilised Crops has started to establish a database on underutilized crops which specifically focuses on potential and agronomic successes and failures.

Such a facility would provide the capacity to understand and analyze global, regional, and national needs in their economic, political, and technological environments. It would also provide the logical basis for cooperative and enhanced international attention to the problems of new crops. If it were to be organized fully as an international effort, it would provide three added advantages. First, it could positively link public and private sector research, and probably linkages between university scientists and those of the productive sector in developing countries. Second, it could highlight the needs of developing countries so that mutually beneficial cooperation could be forged despite the economic and social discrepancies between North and South. Third, it could help in developing policies based on priorities.

The idea of a comprehensive database is not new. It has been promulgated by botanic gardens since they are repositories of much unpublished information (Booth and Lucas 1989). FAO is discussing a global information system, and the Institut de la Vie has convened meetings of interested scientists to discuss genetic resources information systems and what gaps exist. New vision, avoiding vested interests, is urgently needed.

PRIORITIES

The need for priorities is essential at the present time, when the immediate goals of alternative agriculture, agribusiness, and securing food supply through the prudent use of the world's natural resources differ and often conflict with the preservation of indigenous nations and the rights of smallholders and the landless poor. The World Commission on Environment and Development (WCED 1987) and the forthcoming UN Conference on Environment and Development in 1992 have and will point out that we cannot afford to go for food security at any price. But crop diversification in the developed world or agricultural development elsewhere is not possible without research. It is essential to set priorities and take action, recognizing the constraints posed by bilateral and multilateral assistance agencies, national research systems, the lack of congruence between existing research budgets, and the economic importance of major commodities or commodity groupings (Ruttan 1988) and biodiversity imperatives or environmental rehabilitation (McNeely et al. 1990). Arguments for research support must be supported by the analysis of expected demand and input prices, types of technologies (managerial, biological, chemical, or other), and the public-good nature of research outputs. There must also be clear ideas as to whether the research outputs are pre-technology, prototype or usable technology (Evenson 1983), in order to evaluate the balance between public sector or private sector inputs.

Giving further thought to these criteria, a number of important possibilities come to light:

(a) There are substantial opportunities to develop sustainable production systems on a number of fragile resource areas (Ruttan 1991). These include the semi-arid tropics of Africa, the tropical rain forests of Latin America, and arid areas such as the southwestern United States. However, none are likely to become important components of the global food supply system.

(b) There are substantial opportunities to develop new crop production (especially woody species) on degraded lands marginal to food production in many parts of the world. These are low production lands where parallel generation of off-farm income can be a key social return. But allocation of scarce research resources has to be fully justifiable (Schuh 1990), and often new institutional arrangements are needed to give communities more control over their resources.

(c) Much of the sustainability and environmental issues will be addressed through sustainable production on the robust agricultural lands. Interests of environmentalists will only be partly met by concentrating on local marginal lands; the major issues of economic development and efficient ways of alleviating rural poverty will not be addressed at all. Hence, many new crops could well become parts of multiple cropping systems. This means that aside from new crop development, farming systems research will be needed. Most research on multiple cropping relates to improved food crop yields and sustainability, and substantial results have been obtained through cooperative network activities (Hoque 1986). There is interest in using plants capable of providing products and services in addition to fuelwood and food; and selection of the right germplasm for the system is critical (Turnbull and de la Cruz 1991).

(d) It is not possible to propose public sector/private sector partnerships in an empirical way. Outside the developed world private R&D is located primarily in Latin America and Asia and concentrated in a few large countries (Brazil, Mexico, Argentina, and India). Further, many less developed countries could increase national welfare by releasing constraints on private R&D (Pray and Echeverria 1991). Additionally, without patents and rights, investment is likely to be small.

(e) Most private sector interest is related to plantations, followed by plant breeding; pesticides and machinery rank much lower and food and feed processing lower still (Pray and Echeverria 1991). Historically, the private sector has made major contributions to the development of plantation crops, and new crops taken up by the plantation industry will have a much greater chance of success than those promoted unilaterally by scientists or aid donors (Corley 1989).

(f) Priority setting will probably fall within the framework of:
- enhancing supplies of deficit products in specific areas such as vegetable oils, although there have to be compelling reasons for use of new crops;
- using new crops to satisfy particular international trade requirements;
- using new crops to produce innovative products with a market potential;
- using old crops for new purposes of major trade significance or for local use;
- addressing stressed ecosystems by the use of new crops, e.g. on sloping lands, degraded lands or acid or saline soils.

This symposium provides examples of all of these, including information on the USDA/ARS reallocated funding to projects on non-food and industrial uses of farm commodities at the North Regional Research Center, Peoria, IL; Western Regional Research Center, Albany, CA; and the Southern Regional Research Center in New Orleans, LA.

(g) It has been eloquently pointed out recently that the paradigms of environmental management and economic development are evolving. The paradigm of resource management which developed in the 1970s is still the dominant way of thinking, where all major types of resources should be incorporated into calculations of national wealth. However, ecodevelopment is overtaking this as a paradigm (Mathews and Tunstall 1991), and the integration of ecology and economics is urgent and needs to be based on accurate, more timely, and more credible information. Since this information does not, in practice, exist for new crops, some recent diverse examples illustrate the varying criteria for priority setting.

India. In 1982 an All-India Coordinated Research Project on Under-Utilized and Under-Exploited Plants was initiated to include research on selected food crops (winged bean, rice bean, amaranth, buckwheat, chenopods), fodder plants (woody species), energy plants (sugarcane, bamboo, sweet potato), hydrocarbon and industrial plants (guayule, jojoba, and others), oil yielding plants, and some drug producing plants. All these were prioritized according to economic importance. In parallel, priorities were established for plants for extreme environmental and emergency situations in desert, arid, saline, and flooded areas.

The India program has been closely associated with a Commonwealth effort on life-support species, and a symposium for Asia and the Pacific was held in 1987 (Paroda et al. 1988), where the potential species for India, Nepal, Malaysia, Sri Lanka, Bangladesh, Thailand, Pakistan, and a number of other countries were itemized. Emphasis for priorities was laid on stress prone environments.

Europe. In recent years, as in other parts of the developed world, interest in new crops relates to alternative crops and new uses for existing crops, due to surplus production of major crops. A number of countries have assessed the potential of flax, plants which contain vegetable oils of specific composition, plants which produce essential oils, alkaloids and other chemical products, a limited number of ethnic salad and vegetable plants with potential in the health foods industry, and others. Buckwheat, borage, and evening primrose are among the new crops.

Whereas most priorities relate to reducing the need for imports through added-value products, some countries without the surpluses of the EEC are seriously examining new crop strategies, e.g. Poland. Maybe, for developed regions, the solution to surpluses is not so much alternative crops as the development of industrial uses for crop products, exploiting their value as continually renewable resources (Tayler 1989).

Africa. A milestone in priority setting was seen when a group of Nigerian scientists, along with colleagues from Cameroon and Ghana, discussed underutilized plants and their diversity and set priorities on the basis of genetic variability and erosion, economic potential and relevance to local communities, and itemized 22 species for 15 different products/purposes. Scientists are now formulating a research organization to take action in this area (Diversity 1990).

These efforts will become complementary to those proposed by the United Nations University Institute for Natural Resources in Africa, which will be a research and training center with a specific program on traditional plant resources (Okigbo 1991).

These three examples show priority setting for diverse purposes and against three diverse funding scenarios. In the first, there is commitment by the national government, in the second by industry, and in the third, international aid organizations have to be convinced.

DEVELOPMENT OF PRIORITIES

Priority setting has important implications for funding. We can ask the question, why are public funds not often available when priority species have been determined? Leaving aside the unusual examples of winged bean, kenaf, rosy periwinkle, vettiver grass, and other new crops which have received funding in the past, what about clear priorities, especially those where there are demonstrable benefits to be accrued? Clearly private funds will not be available until the crop is near commercial. Additionally, public funding, especially donor funding for development, is rarely available since priorities for their availability usually relate to major crops. We are left with the conundrum of mobilizing funding: the following comments might be helpful.

To a governing authority, new crops often appear to be very high risk ventures, largely because of research interests leading to a low rate of return in the short to medium term. Additionally, researchers often pay little attention to how to integrate new crops into existing or modified cropping patterns and farming systems. Few funding sources will take the risk of paying for domesticating and bringing a new species into production, because the cost is high and long-term funding is required.

Nonetheless, policies can be justified which introduce new crops into new areas and incorporate new species into farming systems, especially in view of sustainability and environmental concerns. In both of these areas the public sector is the logical focus (Smith 1988).

Policies relating to domestication and development of hitherto wild species will have to be related to lucrative markets, which might well be finite and temporary, and a risk analysis performed. In a limited number of cases, small, risky projects can indeed be justified, because they are diluted in the large pool of investments in agricultural or products research. But many opportunities exist for justification under the umbrella of conservation and protection of natural resources.

INTERNATIONALIZATION OF RESEARCH ON NEW CROPS

An international symposium was held in 1987, sponsored by the United Nations Environment Program (UNEP), IBPGR, International Foundation for Science (IFS), Commonwealth Development Corporation, EEC Technical Centre for Agricultural and Rural Cooperation, British Council, Federal Republic of Germany–GTZ, and Southampton University, UK. A recurring theme in the discussions was the need to network research and to include partnerships between developed and developing countries. As a result, the International Center for Underutilised Crops (ICUC) was established. The ICUC has temporary headquarters in England, but the trustees have agreed as a matter of policy that it should move to a developing country in the near future.

For the first time an organizational framework came into being, albeit recently, to establish networking, priorities, and to act as an information and training resource, the latter for the benefit of developing countries. Relevant policy decisions include priority attention to the following areas: new crops of wide applicability over whole regions or ecoclimatic zones, species not being researched by international agricultural research centers of the Consultative Group on International Agricultural Research (CGIAR), and technical assistance to developing countries as a major feature of the research and development.

Recently ICUC joined with the agricultural program of the Commonwealth Science Council (CSC) to establish a testing network for two underutilized species—lablab (*Dolichos lablab*) and carob (*Ceratonia siliqua*)—and is preparing a research strategy on small grains.

GERMPLASM ASPECTS

It is clear that all new crops research needs to tap the diversity of plants from all parts of the world. Although the information base is slender (see section II above), germplasm acquisition and testing need to be looked at with a clear distinction made between plant introduction and plant genetic resources programs. This is an area of great international misunderstanding and misinformation where supposed controversies rage. In practice, scientists and others view such plant resources as a global commons which forms a heritage valuable to all who can use it. This principle has been embodied in an International Undertaking promulgated by FAO. However, the lessons of the past, which often stemmed from exploitative situations, have impugned many unjustified ulterior motives to scientific activities of the present, especially in relation to North-South linkages. Also, global public interest requires management and cooperation between nations—something which often proves to be difficult, due to diversity in interests and values. The South sees international law and international organizations as instruments for change despite their own reluctance to make long term commitments to environmental and genetic resource conservation. International cooperation is based more on common human interests than rigid law, but the whole arena is an evolving one and not widely appreciated by those debating regulatory procedures for germplasm. Let us see if out of the morass of literature and the deliberations of the FAO Commission on Plant Genetic Resources we can arrive at some clear facts on which to develop policies.

First of all, plant introduction is a way of testing materials from elsewhere in the world; it was the basis of many agricultural operations of governments in the past. Many programs, depending on the materials, grew into plant breeding, which necessitated a much wider range of diversity and number of samples, or plant genetic resources, to sustain the breeding. From this grew the need for genetic conservation of primitive forms, mostly of domesticates, and for these to be available through international programs.

Many plants used for plant introduction represent very limited diversity, often in samples with high heterogeneity, but sufficient for testing and development of products or the development of forage and forest lands with species that are selected but not really bred. Only where the original habitats are being degraded will there be needs for genetic conservation programs, and much of the need for conservation will be addressed through nature reserves. Some exciting possibilities have been opened up through debt for development exchange. Whereas most of these have been for nature conservation, some have been brokered to enhance international agricultural research partnerships. Opportunities exist for those involved with plant introduction to broker similar mutually advantageous arrangements, both through the public and the private sectors.

Secondly, as already pointed out, attention to internationalization of research should forge partnerships between germplasm donors and germplasm users. The best example of this is the germplasm collection efforts related to major crops and forages where use of materials is balanced by effective aid packages, with CGIAR providing freely new derivatives as breeding materials. Even in a situation where plant variety rights are taken on developed materials, they and parental materials are still available for further research by anyone, including germplasm donors.

Third, the people who benefit from the plant introduction should attempt to see that the people from where the resource came also benefit, and plans for this should be built into the research proposals. The benefits can be tangible, such as provision of training and other mechanisms to strengthen weak programs in developing countries, or through material transfer agreements as developed by the US National Institute of Health, which screens plants. In the event of a company licensing a product, the NIH makes all efforts to negotiate the inclusion of royalties to the donor country. In what is said to be the first deal of its kind (Washington Post 1991), the world's largest pharmaceutical company has agreed to provide $1 million to the National Institute of Biodiversity (INBIO) in Costa Rica for the right to screen organisms for possible drug use and royalty payments if any become marketable, and for INBIO to help to protect natural resources. This is creating jobs in Costa Rica through the training of locals to assist INBIO.

Fourth, beneficial use of plant resources is often well down the road (10 to 15 years), and many resources may prove to be of no value.

Fifth, whereas there is focus through a number of programs for new crops research and development, there is no simple focus for coordinated international work on survey, collection, conservation, and documentation of the genetic resources. Current activities of IBPGR and FAO are limited by funding restraints, and in any event, genetic conservation of new crop genepools is so intimately linked to rural development and commercial interests that perhaps a new mechanism should be considered. Responsibility could be placed with the relevant international center, possibly in association with a number of externally evaluated, nongovernmental organizations with multiple constituencies, which could attract funding more readily than others associated mostly with public sector agencies.

Sixth, apart from the need for genetic conservation programs where there is clear evidence of genetic erosion, many underutilized crops are likely to remain in their agroecosystems where they have proved useful. Many such crops in developing countries are grown from propagules produced and saved by farmers, and they're likely to persist without sophisticated genetic resources programs. More advanced programs are only needed when germplasm enhancement is warranted and priorities for the crops have been established.

In conclusion, policy development requires the good will of all, whether researchers or authorities, and sensitivity to the issues we have outlined, which R&D on new crops will generate. However, quantum jumps in establishment of policy will emerge when attempts are made, on the one hand, to develop adequate information and data, and on the other, to effectively work together.

REFERENCES

Arora, R.K. 1985. Genetic resources of less known cultivated food plants. Natl. Bur. of Plant Genet. Resources, New Delhi, India.

Booth, F.E.M. and G.L.I. Lucas. 1989. The role of botanic gardens in economic botany, p. 452–470. In: M.S. Swaminathan and S.L. Kochhlar (eds.). Plants and society. Macmillan, London.

Corley, R.H.V. 1989. Assessment of new crops for plantations, p. 53–65. In: G.E. Wickens, N. Haq, and P. Day (eds.). New crops for food and industry. Chapman and Hall, London.

Diversity. 1990. New plant diversity research effort launched at Nigerian symposium. Diversity 6(3/4):7–8.

Evenson, R.E. 1983. Intellectual property rights, agribusiness research and development: Implications for the public agricultural research system. Amer. J. Agr. Econ. 65:967–975.

FAO. 1982. Fruit-bearing forest trees. FAO Forestry Paper 34. FAO, Rome, Italy.

Hoque, M.Z. (ed.). 1986. Cropping systems in Asia. International Rice Research Institute, Los Banos, Philippines.

Janick, J. and J.E. Simon (eds.). 1990. Advances in new crops. Timber Press, Portland, OR.

Lemmens, R.H.M.J, P.C.M. Jansen, J.S. Siemonsma, and F.M. Stavast (eds.). 1989. Plant resources of southeast Asia. Basic list of species and commodity grouping. Wageningen, Netherlands.

Mathews, J.T. and D.B. Tunstall. 1991. Moving toward eco-development: generating environmental information for decisionmakers. Issues and Ideas. World Resources Institute. Aug. 1991.

McNeely, J.A., K.R. Miller, W.V. Reid, R.A. Mittermeier, and T.B. Werner. 1990. Conserving the world's biological diversity. IUCN/WRI/CI/WWF-US/World Bank. Gland, Switzerland and Washington, DC.

NAS. 1975. Underexploited tropical plants with promising economic value. NAS, Washington, DC.

NRC. 1979. Tropical legumes: resources for the future. NAS, Washington, DC.

Okigbo, B. 1991. The Institute for Natural Resources in Africa (UNU/INRA) (mimeo.). UN Office Complex, Gigiri, P.O. Box 30592, Nairobi.

Paroda, R.S., P. Kapoor, R.K. Arora, and B. Mal (eds.). 1988. Life support plant species. Diversity and conservation. Natl. Bur. of Plant Genet. Resources, New Delhi, India.

Pray, C.E. and R.G. Echeverria. 1991. Private-sector agricultural research in less-developed countries, p. 343–364. In: P.G. Pardey, J. Roseboom, and J.R. Anderson (eds.). Agricultural research policy: international quantitative perspectives. Cambridge Univ. Press, Cambridge.

Princen, L.H. 1977. Potential wealth in new crops: research and development, p. 1–15. In: D.S. Seigler (ed.). Crop resources. Academic Press, New York.

Ritchie, G.A. (ed.). 1979. New agricultural crops. AAAS Selected Symposia 38. Westview Press, Boulder, CO.

Ruttan, V.W. 1988. Towards a global agricultural research system, p. 321–348. In: E. Javier and U. Renborg (eds.). The changing dynamics of global agriculture. ISNAR/DSE/CTA, The Hague, Netherlands.

Ruttan, V.W. 1991. Challenges to agricultural research in the 21st century, p. 399–411. In: P.G. Pardey, J. Roseboom, and J.R. Anderson (eds.). Agricultural research policy: international quantitative perspectives. Cambridge Univ. Press, Cambridge.

Schuh, G.E. 1990. Sustainability, marginal areas, and agricultural research. Development 1990(3/4):138–43.

Smith, R.W. 1988. The place of life support species in hostile or risk-prone environments: an overview, p. 14–19. In: R.S. Paroda, P. Kapoor, R.K. Arora, and B. Mal (eds.). Life support species: diversity and conservation. Natl. Bur. of Plant Genet. Resources, New Delhi, India.

Tayler, R.S. 1989. Alternative crops for Europe, p. 185–193. In: G.E. Wickens, N. Haq, and P. Day (eds.). New crops for food and industry. Chapman and Hall, London.

Turnbull, J.W. and de la Cruz, R.E. 1991. Tree technologies with potential to contribute to sustainability in marginal uplands of Southeast Asia, p. 107–113. In: G. Blair and R. Lefroy (eds.). Technologies for sustainable agriculture on marginal uplands in Southeast Asia. ACIAR, Canberra.

Washington Post. 1991. U.S. drug firm signs up to farm tropical forests, by William Booth, Sept. 21 1991.

World Commission on Environment and Development. 1987. Our common future. Oxford Univ. Press, Oxford.

Williams, J.T. 1989. Plant introduction and international responsibilities, p. 345–351. In: G.E. Wickens, N. Haq, and P. Day (eds.). New crops for food and industry. Chapman and Hall, London.

New Crops and the International Agricultural Research Centers

Robert B. Bertram

The image of the International Agricultural Research Centers (IARCs) is not one which immediately brings to mind new crops. As institutions, the Centers are best known for their contributions to crops which are distinctly "old" and established such as rice and wheat. To these crops that are familiar around the globe can be added commodities more restricted to the developing countries of the tropics and subtropics such as cassava, millet, or pigeonpea; some of this latter group may be considered new crops in areas where they have not traditionally been cultivated. In addition, in a few cases, IARCs carry out research on truly novel crops, developed or domesticated only recently.

Generally, each international Center is connected to a relatively few, "mandate" crops. This is not an accident—they have sought to target their limited resources on areas with highest potential payoff. Despite this focus on a limited number of major crops, the Centers have made significant contributions in the area of new crops. These include a truly new crop, triticale, as well as several ancient crops that are little known outside their region of origin, and thus can be considered as new. In other cases, international Centers have played key roles in introducing a new crop to a region. Breeding programs have in some cases broadened the adaptability of a crop to a point where it can be grown outside its area of traditional adaptation—tropical wheats or day length insensitive pigeonpeas are examples (Villareal and Klatt 1985). Other Center activities, such as genetic resources and farming systems programs frequently include work on minor or new crop species.

Some of the means by which Centers conduct their principle research programs (germplasm collections, international nurseries, collaborative networks) can be readily adapted to species that are new crops. They can serve as focal points for regional or international interest in a particular species, even if not conducting extensive research on the crop. Thus, in addition to actual research contributions, international Centers can provide some minor new crop species with an institutional home, through which interested workers can access germplasm and each others' contributions. Increased emphasis on natural resources (including genetic resources) and the environment, as well as the growing applicability of biotechnology, may offer expanded opportunities for international Center contributions in the area of new crops.

THE IARCS AS PART OF AN INTERNATIONAL NETWORK

The IARCs occupy a pivotal position in global agricultural research, a collective endeavor that is increasingly international in scope. Their principal responsibility is to improve, through research, the agricultural production systems of developing countries of Africa, Asia, and Latin America. This effort includes substantial involvement of scientists in developing countries, particularly those of the national agricultural research systems. The IARCs incorporate an array of disciplines to achieve their objectives, from agronomy to molecular genetics to economic policy and management. Centers conduct work on a wide array of crops, and are important nodes in the flow of germplasm around the world.

Most of these research Centers are supported by a group of donors known as the Consultative Group on International Agricultural Research (CGIAR). Founded in 1971, by donor countries and international organizations, the CGIAR provides a forum for supporters of international agricultural research to jointly consider and fund research on food production, hunger alleviation and natural resource conservation. Over time, the group has grown to include nearly 40 organizations, including multilateral development banks, United Nations agencies, several foundations and the international development agencies of many European, North American, and Pacific countries (CGIAR 1992). Several developing countries are also donors (e.g., Philippines, India, Brazil, Mexico). In addition to the donors themselves, the CGIAR system draws on two Secretariats (located at the UN Food and Agricultural Organization and the World Bank) and a Technical Advisory Committee made up of scientists from around the world.

Center Mandates

By 1992, some twenty years after the CGIAR was established (some Centers predate the CGIAR), the system has grown to include 17 research institutions. Most of these remain oriented to commodities, although increasingly the focus is on important production ecologies and natural resource management.

The largest single activity of the IARCs is crop breeding. This is an activity where the comparative advantage of transnational genetic improvement programs is clear. The product, improved seed, is an example of a discrete technology package that can be adopted easily by national researchers or farmers. The CGIAR efforts have been most successful for wheat and rice (Dalrymple 1986a,b), where the striking advances are known as the "green revolution." There has historically been a recognition that impact depends on well targeted efforts. This targeting of each Center's program is expressed in its mandate from the CGIAR system.

As noted above, the IARCs are hardly synonymous with new crops. Their crop focus lies on improvement of major, staple crops which constitute important dietary components for low-income producers and consumers in the developing world. This has been a successful strategy, as it is now estimated that gains in wheat and rice production associated with the IARCs provide enough additional food for more than one-half billion people (Anderson et al. 1988). There is general consensus that the IARCs should remain highly focussed institutions, and their mandates provide for this. The Center mandates, which can be at either the global or regional level, are

Table 1. IARC mandates as an expression of research priorities and strategies in roughly chronological order—1960s to the present.

Criteria	Focus
Number of people fed	Cereals
Improved nutrition, esp. protein	Grain legumes
Regional, "safety-net" crops	Roots/tubers
Mixed-farming, drier zones	Livestock
Equity	Farming systems/food policy
Research capacity	Research management
Environment	Natural resource management
Deforestation	Forestry/agroforestry

the subject of considerable and on-going study expressed through a variety of criteria and the resulting program emphasis. Table 1 presents a general scheme for the development of mandates.

During the 1960s, the IARCs concentrated on cereal crops (rice, wheat, maize) seen as holding the best promise of quickly increasing food production; these commodities offered the best opportunities for preventing food shortages, especially in Asia where widespread famine was predicted. After initial successes, the IARC system expanded through the 1970s to include legumes, to provide better nutrition, and roots and tubers (potato, sweet potato, cassava, and aroids), which were particularly important foods in many poorer, rural areas. Livestock were added for their critical role in areas of Africa, and forage work was undertaken in support of animal agriculture in Africa and Latin America. By the early 1980s, increased attention was given to food policy and research management and natural resources. Most recently, several new Centers have been added emphasizing natural resource management, forestry, and agroforestry.

INTERNATIONAL BOARD FOR PLANT GENETIC RESOURCES (IBPGR)

Of all the international Centers, only the IBPGR is broadly identified with new crops and economic botany. Established in 1974, the IBPGR has a unique role in fostering collection, characterization, and conservation of plant genetic resources. From its inception, it has worked with many researchers on all kinds of lesser-known crops, both woody and herbaceous. An excellent discussion of IBPGR's activity in relation to new crops is given in Mark Perry's paper in the first symposium in this series (Perry 1988). IBPGR work in this area has many direct linkages to the work on new crops at other IARCs and in other research programs around the world.

Four areas of IBPGR activity can be emphasized in relation to new crops. First, is their support of germplasm collecting and conservation; many of the species included in IBPGR register of genebank collections can be considered new crops. Some examples, to name a few, are amaranth, lupin, and a number of cucurbits (*Luffa, Momordica, Tricosanthes*, and others). IBPGR has also collaborated extensively with the IARCs in collecting the germplasm of minor species related to principal mandate crops of the Centers. In recent years, the collection emphasis on wild relatives has increased. For example, by 1986, 16% of collections made in IBPGR sponsored trips were wild materials (IBPGR 1988). The number of forage collections, which are essentially wild material, increased to more than one-fourth of all collected samples by the late 1980s. In some cases, groups of wild relatives have received special attention, for example wheat relatives of the tribe Triticeae. Such efforts involve on-going planning, sponsoring of symposia and other activities in support of broad-based research on crop relatives.

Another important contribution of the IBPGR has been through the development of taxonomic descriptors; these are especially important in collecting and exchanging germplasm. A few examples of note are descriptor lists for kodo millet, winged bean, quinoa, and bambarra groundnut. In line with growing interest in wild relatives, in 1990 IBPGR published descriptors for wild species of *Arachis, Brassica, Raphanus*, and eggplant (IBPGR 1991).

A third important contribution of the IBPGR is its publication, jointly with the UN Food and Agricultural Organization, of the *Plant Genetic Resources Newsletter*. The newsletter contains articles and brief notes on a wide array of economically important species and their genepools. This is an excellent and important forum for those interested in lesser known species, where opportunities for information exchange and publication may be more limited.

In recent years, the IBPGR has initiated a series of eco-geographic genepool surveys based on review of herbarium materials and supplemented with field work. Some of these are directly relevant to new crops. For example, in 1991, IBPGR published *The Distribution of Hibiscus L. section Furcaria in Tropical East Africa* (Edmonds 1991). This group includes two important new crops, kenaf and rosella. Kenaf in particular has generated a good deal of interest and was the subject of several papers in the first and second symposium in this series. IBPGR initiated this work in cooperation with the International Jute Organization and several international donor agencies interested in alternative fiber crops.

IBPGR, although holding no materials of its own, and for the most part, working through other national and international research organizations, has had an important and stimulating effect within the CGIAR Centers. Over time, the large commodity-oriented IARCs have given increasing attention to minor species and wild materials related to their mandate crops (Table 2). IBPGR activity has directly supported the efforts of other IARCS, often providing a base for larger and later involvement by an IARC. A good example is the recent decision by the International Potato Center (CIP) to increase its effort on several Andean roots and tubers (CIP 1991); IBPGR has for some time carried out germplasm collecting and conservation efforts for these crops. Both IBPGR and

Table 2. Germplasm holdings of IARCs (source: various CGIAR and IARC reports).

Center (Host countries)	Species	Number of accessions
CIAT (Colombia)	Common bean (*Phaseolus vulgaris*)	35,950
	other beans (*Phaseolus* spp.)	5,111
	Cassava (*Manihot esculenta*)	4,600
	Cassava wild relatives (*Manihot* spp.)	48
	Forage legumes	17,982
	Forage grasses	2,514
CIMMYT (Mexico)	Maize (*Zea mays, Tripscum, Teosinte*)	10,500
	Cereals (*Triticum aestivum, T. durum, Triticale, Hordeum*)	62,000
CIP (Peru)	Potato (*Solanum tuberosum*)	5,000
	Potato wild relatives (*Solanum* spp.)	1,500
	Sweet Potato (*Ipomea batatus*)	5,200
ICARDA (Syria)	Cereals (*Hordeum* spp., *Triticum* spp., *Triticale*)	49,749
	Food legumes (*Vicia, Lens, Cicer*)	16,890
	Forages	19,952
ICRISAT (India)	Sorghum (*Sorghum bicolor*)	31,030
	Pearl millet (*Pennisetum glaucum*)	19,796
	Minor millets (*Pennisetum* spp.)	6,610
	Groundnut (*Arachis* spp.)	12,160
	Pigeonpea (*Cajanus cajan*)	11,040
	Chickpea (*Cicer arietinum*)	15,564
IITA (Nigeria)	Cassava (*Manihot esculenta*)	2,000
	Plantain and banana (*Musa* spp.)	250
	Cowpea (*Vigna unguiculata*)	15,100
	Cowpea relatives (*Vigna* spp.)	810
	Rice (*Oryza* spp.)	12,000
	Soybean (*Glycine max*)	1,500
	Yam (*Dioscorea* spp.)	1,000
	Maize (*Zea mays*)	500
	Bombara groundnut (*Voandezia* spp.)	2,000
ILCA (Ethiopia)	Forage grasses	1,524
	Forage legumes	6,443
	Browse species	1,429
IRRI (Philippines)	Rice (*Oryza sativa*)	78,420
	African rice (*O. glaberrima*)	2,408
	Wild relatives (*Oryza* spp.)	2,214
	Other rices	21
WARDA (Ivory Coast)	Rice (African and Asian)	5,600
AVRDC (Taiwan)	Vegetables (tomato, mungbean, pepper, cabbage, amaranth, soybean, etc.)	32,200

(Originally compiled by Bertram for National Plant Genetic Resource Program Report to Congress 1991.)

CIP conduct these efforts jointly with national programs of the Andean countries.

RESEARCH AVENUES FOR NEW CROPS AT IARCS

Despite the pressures to have a narrowly focused research program, the IARCs developed a number of activities in support of their program objectives which directly relate to the subject of new crops. Two aspects of Centers' programs have been of particular importance: genetic resources conservation and farming systems research. A third case is unique. The International Maize and Wheat Improvement Center has a new crop, triticale, fully within its research mandate. This third avenue might be categorized as new crops representing special, significant research opportunities. In some respects, the inclusion of triticale could be done at very modest cost because the new crop program could be operated in tandem with the much larger, existing wheat program—in a sense offering a "research economy of scale." These three areas can overlap; when they do, the decision to allocate research resources to a new crop is more likely. Each of these three principal avenues for Center involvement is discussed below.

Mandate Crops

Triticale. Probably no other example of a new crop is as associated with the international Centers as triticale. Though dating as a crop from the 1920s and 1930s, the International Maize and Wheat Improvement Center (CIMMYT) began working with the crop in the 1960s. The work was initially a joint program with Canadian scientists who had been improving the crop since the early 1950s. There were several reasons behind the decision to allocate research resources to the new crop. Triticale had excellent potential for adaptability to a number of the environments for which CIMMYT was breeding wheat, particularly due to its tolerance of adverse soil and climatic conditions. Although grain quality at the time was poor, it contained high levels of protein and the amino acid lysine. These attributes generated considerable support for research on the crop, as protein was of considered the most significant nutritional deficiency by the wider research and development communities. Another significant factor was CIMMYT's ability to conduct a global triticale improvement program built on the its large, well-established wheat program.

The story of triticale at CIMMYT, detailed in the 1988 National Research Council Report (1988), is an exciting one, filled with hard work and some luck (Vietmeyer 1989). When work first began, the crop was plagued by lodging, poor seed set, and shriveled seed. A major breakthrough occurred when the accidental pollination of a triticale by a semidwarf bread wheat gave rise to significantly improved triticales. From that breakthrough, the progress made over the last 25 years has been very impressive. Yields of triticales now vie with the best breadwheats (Rowe pers. commun.), and test weight and grain quality for most uses has been greatly improved. The crop has been adopted widely, and is now grown on about 1.7 million ha worldwide. Most of the area lies outside the developing countries.

This concentration of tritcale area and interest in the more developed temperate areas presents a major policy dilemma for a Center like CIMMYT, where the main objective is to meet the needs of developing countries. CIMMYT breeders and leadership continue to believe that triticale has a great deal of relevance to many areas of the developing world. However, the extent to which a major program can be justified without sufficient interest from client groups is a problem, especially during a period of declining real funding. Triticale is not the only example of a fine product of research that has yet to find a strong constituency—the high quality protein maizes have also been greatly improved, but have yet to find a demand among national program researchers or farmers in developing countries.

Pearl millet. Pearl millet is a highly nutritious cereal crop for millions of people in the semi-arid regions of the Indian subcontinent and Africa, especially in the Sahel. As a major staple in developing countries, particularly among low income producers and consumers, it received attention from the CGIAR donors in the establishment of the International Crops Research Institute for the Semi-Arid Tropics (ICRISAT). Its particular strengths include good stand establishment and drought resistance in highly stressful environments. Outside the tropics, most interest in pearl millet has been as a forage crop (Burton 1990). More recently, interest has increased in pearl millet as a grain crop. An excellent discussion of progress in pearl millet breeding and its potential as new crop is presented by Andrews et al. (1993), elsewhere in this symposium. ICRISAT's breeding and genetic resources programs are an important source of genetic variability for researchers interested in pearl millet, and are good examples of how IARCs can contribute to work on new crops outside the regions where they normally work.

Pigeonpea. Also an ICRISAT crop, pigeonpea (*Cajanus cajan*) is a semi-woody shrub, traditionally requiring a long season for pod production. In order to increase the crop's utility in a variety of farming systems, ICRISAT breeders have developed short-duration and extra-short duration lines with decreased photoperiod sensitivity. In addition to their allowing the crop to be grown in new ways in drier tropical regions, they appear to have potentially good adaptation outside the tropics. Trials conducted using ICRISAT materials between 32°N and 46° latitudes have given yields between 1 and 4 tonnes/ha (Nene 1992 pers. commun.). Thus, researchers in the United States, New Zealand, Korea, and elsewhere are experimenting with ICRISAT-bred pigeonpeas. Pigeonpea, with its many excellent attributes, may eventually be produced more widely in temperate areas. This would be an example of the way in which Centers can contribute in the area of new crops.

Forage crops. The CGIAR Centers have sought to strengthen animal production systems in two principal ways, by conducting research on animals themselves and through development of improved forage crops. Most of the latter are based on the use of wild species and can, in themselves, be considered new crops. In many cases, legume pastures are critical components of rotation systems and are important to sustaining long-term productivity. As in the case of other crops, a range of research activity takes place, from collecting and conservation to screening, seed production and in some cases, sophisticated breeding.

The largest CGIAR effort of this kind is the tropical pastures program at CIAT, which is focused on the lowland tropics of Latin America. A major thrust of the program has been to develop grasslegume mixes emphasizing African grasses and native South American legumes. The latter in particular tend to be poorly adapted to the highly acid soils of the llanos and cerrados, extensive savannas covering large areas of Venezuela, Colombia, and Brazil. Improved mixtures allow for increased sustainability and carrying capacity of pastures in the savannas. They are also seen as having significant promise for enhancing land fertility, and offering better opportunity for integration of crops in a rotation system. Materials are disseminated to national programs chiefly through the International Tropical Pastures Evaluation Network, which reaches 20 countries and over 300 researchers. Species thought to have the greatest potential in lowland pasture systems include several grasses: *Andropogon gayanus, Brachyaria brizantha, B. dictyoneura, B. humidicola*, and *Panicum maximum*. The most promising legume species include: *Arachis pintoi, Centrosema acutifolium, C. brasilianum, C. macrocarpum, C. pubescens, Desmodium ovalifolium, Stylosanthes capitata*, and *S. guianensis*.

For the cool, wet winter areas of North Africa and Southwest Asia, the International Center for Agricultural Research in the Dry Areas (ICARDA) conducts a program emphasizing the role of leguminous pastures and forage crops in cultivated areas and the more marginal grazing areas. Genera of importance include many legumes (e.g., *Pisum, Vicia, Trifolium, Medicago, Trigonella*, and *Lathyrus*) and several forage grasses. In addition to forage accessions in the above and many other species, the ICARDA germplasm collection also contains several hundred accessions of *Rhizobium* strains for nodulation and nitrogen fixation in various leguminous hosts.

The International Livestock Center for Africa (ILCA) conducts an animal feed resources program which includes extensive screening of species for pastures and fodder banks. The Center's programs are directed toward cooler, high altitude regions, through mid-altitude areas, to a range of lowland areas including humid, sub-humid, and semi-arid zones. The ILCA forage germplasm collection contains more than 10,000 accessions of grasses, legumes, and browse species. The program actively distributes germplasm for screening and selection by national researchers; in 1989, for example, nearly 7,000 accessions were sent out in response to 245 requests (ILCA 1989). The Center recently established its herbage seed unit in response to national requests for additional training and technology transfer in forage seed handling. In support of increased use of multi-purpose trees, where traditional field collection methods are difficult, ILCA is working on in-vitro cultures as a means to conserve, multiply, and distribute tree germplasm.

Agroforestry. The International Council for Research on Agroforestry (ICRAF) recently joined the CGIAR, changing its name to the International Center for Research on Agroforestry. Based in Kenya, the Center conducts a program of research and outreach on the integration of woody species into agricultural production systems. Like the other Centers, it distributes germplasm to national programs for screening and potential inclusion in national research and extension activities. A wide range of trees are evaluated for use in many different environments. Important genera include both legumes, e.g., *Leucaena, Sesbania, Cassia, Acacia*, and non-legumes, e.g., *Grevillea* and *Eucalyptus*. As part of its expanding research program, the Center is enlarging its efforts in genetics an germplasm conservation of multi-purpose trees.

Interest in agroforestry is increasing as a source not only for timber and fuelwood, but as a means to increase nutrient cycling and long-term sustainability of tropical production systems. Several other Centers also conduct research on multi-purpose trees; an example is IITA's longstanding alley cropping program which involves research and extension aimed towards developing sustainable, economic alternatives to slash and burn agriculture, and resulting deforestation. At present, a new CGIAR tropical forestry research institution is being set up in Southeast Asia which will focus on sustainable tropical forestry.

Genetic Resources

In connection with their plant breeding activity, most Centers have developed comprehensive, well-run genetic resource programs. In the early years, these were tied closely to the commodity breeding programs, but over time, as interest in plant genetic resources has grown, the scope of their work has broadened to include entire genepools for their mandate crops. Thus, land races, related crops and wild relatives are generally included in the germplasm collections of the IARCS. Table 2 presents a summary of genetic resources conserved in the genebanks located at international Centers.

The bulk of the holdings are accessions of the staple crops of the Center mandates. Some, such as pigeonpea and pearl millet, mandate crops of the International Crops Research Institute for the Semi-Arid Tropics, may be considered new crops in the United States (as witnessed by papers in both the current and previous symposia). In such cases, Centers' genetic resources and breeding programs may be important sources of genetic variability to workers in countries where the crops have not been traditionally grown.

Wild materials in cultivated or related species are increasingly included in genetic resources collections at Centers. New research techniques such as embryo rescue, tissue culture, or the use of molecular markers may make the rich genetic diversity of such materials increasingly accessible. Generally, it would be expected that the principle use of tertiary genetic resource would be in the improvement of current crops. However, the development of novel, interspecific, or even intergeneric combinations cannot be ruled out, with triticale being an excellent example of the last.

New Crops as Genetic Resources

Tepary bean. A case in point is *Phaseolus acutifolius* or tepary bean. The International Center for Tropical Agriculture (CIAT), located in Colombia, conducts a common bean (*P. vulgaris*) breeding program under a global mandate from the CGIAR. As part of the Center's breeding strategy, it has sought to explore the genepools of related species—both cultivated and wild materials.

In addition to over 30,000 accessions of *P. vulgaris*, the CIAT collection has some four thousand accessions of three cultivated and eleven wild species of *Phaseolus* (Hidalgo 1988). Tepary is of particular interest because of its adaptation to dry climates. CIAT has amassed a collection of 271 accessions of which 126 are cultivated and 145 are wild (M. Iwanaga pers. commun.). Sixty percent are Mexican in origin and 26% are from the southwestern United States. As always, these materials are collected or obtained in collaboration with researchers in the country of origin, and duplicate accessions remain in that country. Collected materials are subsequently made available to any researcher.

This germplasm has been evaluated at CIAT for some 24 plant descriptors and 5 seed characters. The cultivated types have been screened for response to disease resistance and three insect pests of beans: *Empoasca, Zabrotes,* and *Acanthoscelides*. Wild forms have been collected more recently and are just beginning to be evaluated. CIAT scientists have used embryo rescue techniques and backcrosses in attempts to introduce tepary traits into common bean. They are now seeking to do this using DNA markers; the specific objectives of this work are bacterial blight resistance and drought tolerance. CIAT maintains close links with researchers interested in tepary at the the University of California at Riverside and elsewhere.

Minor millets. As part of its responsibilities for crops grown in the semi-arid tropics, ICRISAT has since 1976 conducted collection, conservation, and distribution of the minor millet species, in addition to pearl millet, one of its mandate crops (Table 3). Until recently, most of the activity on these crops was confined to collecting, conserving, and distributing their genetic resources. The collection continues to grow, and is actively used. In 1990, 164 new accessions from India, the Maldives, Pakistan, Taiwan, and Zimbabwe were added, and over 2,500 samples were distributed to research and plant germplasm programs in India, Kenya, Korea, Nepal, Sudan, the United States, Zambia, and Zimbabwe (ICRISAT 1990).

ICRISAT scientists have targeted three of the minor millets for increased research attention: finger millet, foxtail millet, and proso millet. The Indian national program conducts research program on the latter two. In response to interest from researchers in eastern and southern Africa, ICRISAT in 1987, began to expand its work on finger millet to include screening and genetic improvement in, primarily focused on blast resistance. This decision was subsequently confirmed in the Center's strategic planning and the crop was formally added to ICRISAT's mandate. This increased emphasis on a wider range of components important in regional production systems—termed by the CGIAR Technical Advisory Committee as the "eco-regional" approach—is leading to a greater role for new crops at the IARCs (see discussion of Andean tubers, below).

Vegetables. Although not a CGIAR-sponsored Center, the Asian Vegetable Research and Develpment Centre (AVRDC), located in Taiwan, pursue similar objectives for the vegetable crops in its mandate, and is supported by many of the same donor agencies. A significant challenge in defining the AVRDC program has been the great diversity of vegetable crops used around the world. The Center conducts research on the most important vegetable crops for Asia (vegetable soybean, tomato, mungbean, pepper, Chinese cabbage, and recently added eggplant and onion), and is currently developing regional programs of collaborative research with national programs on priority species for other areas, some of which can be considered new crops (Okigbo 1990). For example, Philippine and Indonesian researchers will provide leadership for research on yardlong bean (*Vigna unguiculata*), a regional favorite (Javier 1991 pers. commun.). Tanzania and other African countries are working with the Center to develop collaborative efforts on important African vegetables, including amaranth and okra (*Abelmoschus esculentus*).

In addition to research, AVRDC also operates a genetic resources program for conservation of vegetable species from around the world (total number of accessions, 35,948), many of which can be considered new crops. Table 4 lists some of the lesser-known species conserved by the Center's genetic resources program. In addition to the genebank, the Center, like IBPGR, conducts collaborative collecting expeditions with many national programs, fostering interest and support for work with lesser-known species as well as the Center's mandate species. Many of the IARCs provide an institutional base for developing country scientist interested in collecting or accessing germplasm of minor species.

Farming Systems Research

During the 1970s, there was a growing interest in devising agricultural technologies that were sensitive to prevailing farming systems and farmers' needs. Researchers paid increasing attention to the larger system of

Table 3. ICRISAT minor millet collection (1988 figures).

Species	No. of accessions
Eleusine coracana (finger millet)	2848
Setaria italica (foxtail millet)	1404
Panicum miliaceium (proso millet)	831
Panicum sumatrense (little millet)	401
Echinochloa spp. (barnyard millet)	582
Paspalum scrobiculatum (kodo millet)	544
Total	6610

Source: ICRISAT 1988 Annual Report

production within which they were working. Within the CGIAR Centers, one result of this effort was consideration of non-mandate crops which were nevertheless integral components of production systems. Centers began to experiment with a wide variety of crops which grow side by side maize, cassava, and other mandate crops. Even single crop Centers like the International Rice Research Institute (IRRI) began small programs covering integration of a variety of species in trials devoted to crop rotation or farm diversification in rice-based farming systems. Another program at IRRI studied the integration of Azolla, a blue-green algae and itself a new crop, as a source of added nitrogen in paddy rice. Farming systems programs were instituted at a number of Centers, and several of these became important sites for information and planting materials for what were essentially lesser known or new crops.

International Institute for Tropical Agriculture (IITA). A Center for which this trend was particularly relevant to new crops is the IITA, located in Nigeria. When the Center, inaugurated in 1969, came under the CGIAR umbrella in 1972, its trustees explicitly included the following in a statement of research emphasis: "Conduct exploratory studies with crops' potential usefulness in the humid tropics. Examples are lima, Jack, winged and yam beans, and Asian grams among the grain legumes, and potatoes and cocoyam among the root and tuber crops" (IITA 1973).

Some of the crops that IITA researchers experimented with went on to be incorporated into the Center's mandate—plantain and aroids (*Colocasi, Xanthosoma*) are the chief examples. True yams (*Dioscorea* spp.), were included among the Center's principal commodities from its inception. Legumes attracted considerable interest because of their potential for fixing nitrogen fixation and contributing to improved nutrition. Under the leadership of Dr. K.O. Rachie, The International Grain Legumes Information Centre was established as a clearinghouse for information and, in many cases, planting material for a wide array of legume crops. Thus, crops of local importance such as Bambarra groundnut (*Voandezia subterranea*) and Kersting's groundnut (*Kerstingiella geocarpa*), could both be integrated in farming system's research at the Center and distributed to researchers outside the Center.

Table 4. Germplasm conserved by AVRDC: lesser-known crops (partial listing).

Genus	Species	Common name	No. of accessions
Abelmoschus	*esculentus, manihot*	okra, aibika	53
Amaranthus	spp.	amaranths	127
Basella	*alba*	Malabar spinach	3
Benincasa	*hispida*	wax gourd	29
Cajanus	*cajan*	pigeon pea	16
Clitoria	*ternatea*	butterfly pea	3
Dolichos	*lablab*	hyacinth bean	101
Ipomea	*aquatica*	kangkong	4
Lagenaria	*siceraria*	gourd	34
Luffa	spp.	sponge gourd	64
Momordica	*charantia*	bitter gourd	34
Mucuna	*pruriens*	velvet bean	4
Pachyrhizus	*erosus*	yambean	12
Psophocaryus	*tetragonolobus*	winged bean	40
Sauropus	*androgynus*	chekkurmanis	4
Trichosanthes	*cucumerina*	snake gourd	2
Vigna	*angularis*	adzuki bean	153
	mungo	black bean	747
	radiata	mungbean	5,359
	umbellata	rice bean	295
	unguiculata	yardlong bean	335

Source: AVRDC Genetic Resources Unit, 1991.

In the 1980s, there was considerable pressure to narrow the mandates of the Centers—at least in terms of crop breeding—and at IITA, the scope of its efforts on new crops was reduced. Responsibility for the aroids in its mandate was turned over to national research programs in Nigeria and cameroon, and the emphasis on the lesser known legumes shifted towards germplasm conservation and away from experimentation. Current germplasm holdings at the Center are listed in Table 2; the Center's genetic resources unit continues to distribute materials on request. Studies on Bambarra groundnut have been undertaken, focusing on yield potential and ecogeographic differentiation. And now, with increasing interest in "ecoregional" approaches to production systems, the role of the crop in Nigerian farming systems is being evaluated by IITA researchers (Brader, pers. commun.). A resurgence of interest in agricultural and biolgical diversity may lead to increased IARC interest in minor species and new crops.

International Potato Center (CIP). In considering the ecoregional approach, the CIP, Lima, Peru, will undertake an integrated program to improve the productivity and sustainablity of Andean agricultural systems. One aspect of this effort will be the addition of several lesser-known Andean roots and tubers to its research and genetic resources programs. They include three tubers: oca (*Oxalis tuberosa*), ulluco (*Ullucus tuberosus*), and mashua (*Tropaeolum tuberosum*); and three root crops: arracacha (*Arracacia xanthorrhiza*), yacon (*Polymnia sonchifolia*), and maca (*Lepidium meyenii*). As a group, they are uniquely adapted to highland environments and associated physical stresses; several have high yield potential and would be good candidates for plant breeding. Maca is noteworthy as one of the highest growing cultivated food plants in the world, reaching elevations of 4,000 m. It also has the distinction of being the sole Brassicaceae domesticate in the New World; in addition, it has a specialty market as an aphrodaisiac in Peru!

The new effort has grown out of a regional program involving CIP, IBPGR, and the national programs of the Andean countries. CIP has the advantage of being located in the Center of diversity, and has strong links to researchers in Ecuador, Colombia, Peru, and Bolivia, who share an interest in these little-known crops. In addition, many of the approaches that have been useful in the Center's potato and sweet potato research efforts can also be adapted to working with the Andean crops. And, in line with CGIAR system objectives, these crops are important to the livelihood of poorer farmers.

Despite the efforts of researchers, genetic diversity of these crops is being lost, and collections have been less comprehensive than desired. Some field collections have been lost due to pests but also due to lack of support and civil upheaval. Thus, a top priority for CIP will be collecting and safeguarding germplasm representing the range of environments where the commodities are grown. In addition to field collections duplicated at national and CIP research sites, the Center will develop an in vitro germplasm collection for more secure storage. Other possibilities include development of long-term cryogenic storage. As is the case with most vegetatively propagated crops, viral diseases are confirmed or suspected problems.

Initial CIP efforts indicate that tissue culture and thermotherapy can be used to generate virus-free planting material which can give increased yields. In addition, development of "clean" propagative materials is critical for germplasm exchange among countries within the region and beyond. For example, many of these species adapted to altitudes over 2,000 m may be adaptable to highland tropical and subtropical areas and some temperate regions. of all the crops native to the high Andes, only potato really took hold outside the region; many scientists believe that others could have wider appeal in the Andean region and beyond.

WIDE CROSSES AND BIOTECHNOLOGY

Improving techniques for successfully crossing species that are otherwise reproductively isolated are increasingly available to plant researchers; embryo rescue, for example, has been used to succesfully incorporate gones of wild *Arachis* spp. into cultivated groundut. At the IARCs, interest in wild species has generally been as a source of new resistance to pests and diseases. An example of the latter is the very successful efforts by IITA breeders to transfer genes for resistance to African Cassava Mosaic virus and bacterial blight into cassava from *M. glaziovii* (Beck 1982). Increasingly, breeders have been interested in more complex quantitative traits. K.B. Singh, in a joint ICARDA–ICRISAT program is developing lentils with much greater resistance to frost, based on the incorporation of genes from wild species of *Lens* which come from areas with severe winters.

The availability of new markers to track specific genes or traits in segregating populations, for example, RFLP markers for quantitative trait loci are enhancing the ability of researchers to select traits where specific types of introgression are desired. In many cases, the new genetic variability will result in relatively minor, though still significant changes in a crop. But it is also possible that wider combination of genepools will lead to novel developments similar to triticale. With their broad collections of germplasm of both cultivated and minor species, the international centers will be poised both to break new ground and to assist other researchers in doing so.

CONCLUSION

New crops will probably not be a major area of endeavor for the international agricultural research centers for the foreseeable future. Centers will, however, remain important sites for those interested in new crops, especially with regard to their roles in developing countries. Just as with more major crops such as rice, wheat, and maize, collaborative efforts between scientists and others interested in improving or adapting commodities for improved production will be a major feature of progress in breeding and other research efforts. Scientists in developing and developed countries will collaborate, with mutual benefit, and centers will be an active participant and conduit in the process. Genetic resources activities of the centers on wild species and other novel crops are increasing. Scientific techniques for both the storage and access of new types of variability is increasing in many crops. And consumer interest in both developing and developed countries may help to stimulate activity in new crop species on the part of both researchers and farmers.

Centers will continue their efforts to assist national programs in supporting and strengthening sustainable, productive and economically viable farming systems in developing countries. For the most part, this effort will maintain a tight focus on the "pile of rice," helping to ensure that hunger is alleviated and famine prevented. But diversity will also remain an important concept, in both its genetic and economic implications, and as such a broader concept of farming systems and the scope of their components may evolve. New crops will certainly have a role in the development of robust agricultural economies, and the international agricultural research centers will continue to play an important part in both research and especially research support as new crops continue to develop and take hold.

REFERENCES

Anderson, J.R., R.W. Herdt, and G.M. Scobie. 1988. Science and food: the CGIAR and its partners. The World Bank, Washington, DC.

Beck, B.D.A. 1982. Historical perspectectives of cassava breeding in Africa, p. 13–18. In: S.K. Hahn and A.D.R. Kerr, (eds.). Root Crops in Eastern Africa. International Development Research Centre, Ottawa, Canada.

CIAT Annual Report. 1990. International Center for Tropical Agriculture. Cali, Colombia.

CGIAR Annual Report 1991. 1992. CGIAR, Washington, DC.

Dalrymple, D.G. 1986a. Development and spread of high-yielding rice varieties in developing countries. U.S. Agency for International Development, Washington, DC.

Dalrymple, D.G. 1986b. Development and spread of high-yielding wheat varieties in developing countries. U.S. Agency for International Development, Washington, DC.

Edmonds, J.M. 1991. The distribution of *Hibiscus* L. section *Furcaria* in tropical east Africa. International Board for Plant Genetic Resources, Rome, Italy

Hidalho, R. 1988. The *Phaseolus* world collection, p. 67–90. In: P. Gepts (ed.). Genetic resources of *Phaseolus* beans. Kluwer, Dordrecht, Holland.

ICRISAT Annual Report. 1990. International Crops Research Center for the Semi-arid Tropics, Hyderabad, India.

IBPGR Annual Report. 1988. International Board for Plant Genetic Resources, Rome, Italy.

IBPGR Annual Report. 1991. International Board for Plant Genetic Resources, Rome, Italy.

IITA Report. 1973. International Institute of Tropical Agriculture, Ibadan, Nigeria.

ILCA Annual Report 1988. International Livestock Center fdor Africa, Addis Abba, Ethiopia.

International Potato Center (CIP). 1991. Meeting the challenge: The International Potato Center's strategy for the 1990s and beyond. CIP, Lima, Peru.

Okigbo, B.N. 1990. Vegetables in tropical Africa. In: Vegetable research and development in SADCC countries. Asian Vegetable Research and Development Center, Tainan, Taiwan.

Plucknett, D.L., N.J.H. Smith, J.T. Williams, and N.M. Anishetty. 1987. Genebanks and the worlds food. Princeton University Press, Princeton, NJ.

Vietmeyer, N.D. (ed.). 1989. Triticale—a promising addition to the world's cereal grains. Report of an Ad Hoc Panel, Board on Science and Technology for International Development, National Research Council. National Academy Press, Washington, DC.

Vietmeyer, N.D. (ed.). 1979. Tropical legumes: Resources for the future. National Academy of Sciences, Washington, DC.

Villareal, R.L. and A.R. Klatt (eds.). 1985. Wheats for more tropical environments. International Maize and Wheat Improvement Center, Mexico, D.F., Mexico.

1990 Progress Report. Asian Vegetable Research and Development Center, Tainan, Taiwan.

International Conflicts in New Crops Policy

Cary Fowler

The year, 1992, is the 500th anniversary of the "discovery" of the New World by Columbus. This voyage marked the beginning of the "Columbian Exchange," the first systematic and massive transfer and diffusion of plants between continents.

To be sure, people had been moving domesticated and other valuable plants about for thousands of years. Some primitive agricultural crops spread slowly as populations of the earliest "farmers" grew and as hunter/gatherers migrated. Other crops were "captured" as the fruits of war. Murals on the walls of Egyptian temples depict the botanical booty won in battle over 3,400 years ago. From these days onwards, it was not just gold and silver but plants and plant products which helped create and shape the world's nascent geopolitics, affecting everything from the fate of kingdoms to the daily bread of their most ordinary citizens.

Columbus and those who followed him brought maize, potatoes, squash, cassava, peanuts, common beans, and other crops back to Europe. The seeds of the hevea rubber tree were shipped from Brazil to Kew Gardens and seedlings sent to botanical gardens in Singapore where controlled distribution established the rubber industry of Southeast Asia. Asian production brought ruin to the rubber industry of Brazil. The economy of northeast Brazil collapsed and hundreds of thousands of people perished of famine.

In "exchange," many crops including coffee, bananas, and sugar were introduced to the New World. The boom and bust cycles of these crops, and the association of sugar with slavery and deforestation are well known. Colonial powers attempted to control certain biological materials by force. The French threatened anyone taking indigo out of Antigua with the guillotine. The Spanish outlawed the production of amaranth due to its association with "pagan" religions. The Dutch decreed that production of cloves and nutmeg be limited to three islands in the Moluccas.

In Europe, great wealth was generated from the control over the production and marketing of such crops. The many conflicts and controversies which arose over the acquisition, control, and transfer of plants largely escape our attention today and are of little to concern to us. But, these transfers were not solely altruistic or scientific. Rather, they had a great deal to do with both the creation of wealth and power and its loss or lack of realization.

During the first century of the Columbian Exchange, fewer than 100 new plants were introduced into England. Some 1,000 plants were introduced in the 17th century and 9,000 were brought in during the 18th century (Lemmon 1968). These were the plants which were to form the basis of European dye, chemical, and pharmaceutical industries. Imagine how different our modern world would be had these botanical acquisitions and transfers not taken place!

The United States itself benefitted tremendously from imported genetic materials. From the early days of the 19th century, prior to the establishment of a viable commercial seed trade, the Patent Office oversaw the collection of seeds from all over the world. These seeds were distributed to American farmers for experimentation and adaptation. By 1878, a third of the budget of the young United States Department of Agriculture was being spent on germplasm collection and distribution (Klose 1950). Tens of millions of packages of seeds (including those of many "new crops" discussed in this conference) were sent annually to farmers by the end of the century. Such germplasm importations facilitated the spread of American agriculture and the rise of the United States seed industry.

The value of genetic resources of plants and plant products has long been appreciated and has been at the center of many of the fundamental events in economic and political history for literally thousands of years. Conflicts over the ownership, control, use, distribution, and benefits of genetic resources are just as old. They are a common feature of this history. When we speak of "international conflicts in new crops policy," we must keep in mind that today's conflicts have roots which sink deep in history. Indeed, certain elements of these conflicts have remained remarkably consistent throughout the ages.

MODERN-DAY CONFLICTS

In this century, awareness of the importance of genetic resources increased with their more intensified use following the rediscovery of Mendel's paper on heredity. As modern agriculture with its scientifically-bred crop cultivars made inroads in areas of great genetic diversity (principally in the Third World), awareness of the value of these resources was highlighted by the realization that these resources were being lost at an alarming rate. Modern cultivars were replacing traditional "farmer-bred" cultivars and in the process much diversity was being lost. Valuable breeding material was disappearing and becoming extinct. In this context it could be argued that the perceived value of this material was increasing as a consequence of its scarcity.

As in colonial days, donors of this material had no formal recognized mechanism for realizing value from "their" genetic resources. These resources, the ownership of which had long been determined through sheer force and physical possession, were now deemed by many to part of the "common heritage" of mankind.

Transfers of genetic material continued. Major collections were made and placed in the twentieth century version of the botanical garden—the gene bank. Emphasis was shifting from the collecting of interesting new species to the collection of "varieties" (landraces) with interesting and useful characteristics.

It is tempting to think of this as a period devoid of serious conflict over genetic resources. One need not look far to uncover the conflict. In the Third World, economic disruptions and social tensions associated with the introduction of modern cultivars during the "Green Revolution" have been amply documented (Griffin 1972; Lappe' 1977; Perelman 1977). In the United States, the struggle over questions of ownership and control moved into the political and legal arenas. The seed and nursery trades waged campaigns of nearly a century to establish the patent and patent-like rights over new cultivars of crops (Berg et al. 1991). Viewed historically, these laws were intended to establish a legal system of rules over ownership of biological material to replace previous systems based simply on physical control—a difficult form of control to maintain. Beginning in the late 1800s and continuing at least until the late 1960s, the industry faced serious internal divisions plus the opposition of public sector scientists, the United States Department of Agriculture, and farmer organizations. Intellectual property proposals suffered defeats in Congress on a number of occasions throughout the century (Kloppenburg 1988).

From the 1970s, concerns and conflict have centered on "equity" and "environmental" issues. Significantly, these issues were recognized as such and addressed by virtually all participants in this field in one form or another. These were not simply the concerns of a single individual or organization.

Concerns about the environment were manifested in questions about the loss of genetic diversity and the ability of conservation systems to conserve that diversity. Individual scientists (notably Jack Harlan and his father Harry Harlan, Otto Frankel, Erna Bennett, and Garrison Wilkes) and organizations such as the National Research Council of the National Academy of Sciences issued passionate statements about the on-going loss of genetic diversity (Harlan and Martini 1936; Harlan 1972; Frankel and Bennett 1970; Wilkes 1977; National Research Council 1972). Many criticized the American government and others for inadequate collection and storage efforts. Funding levels for this work were, in fact, woefully inadequate and they remain so largely because the message of the importance of genetic resource conservation has still not reached Washington, 50 years later.

Concerns about equity were manifested in, we might say, a renewed debate over the Columbian Exchange. Have, for example, the "grain rich" countries benefitted disproportionately from the acquisition of genetic resources from the "gene rich" countries? Since the world had moved beyond the gunboat style of settling ownership questions, conflicts arose over emerging forms of legal ownership including patents as cited above. These issues were debated in different arenas such as the United States Congress and the UN's Food and Agriculture Organization (FAO)—largely depending on where the different actors (corporations, governments, advocacy groups, etc.) thought they could get their best and most effective hearing.

At the FAO, a series of proposals were introduced by Third World governments led principally by Mexico. Over a period of a decade, the following initiatives were approved:

1. FAO Commission on Plant Genetic Resources. This body was established in 1983. It is an intergovernmental body with over 110 member nations. Prior to its existence, there had been no forum where governments—as governments—could meet to discuss issues concerning genetic resources. The Commission meets every two years. Its working group meets in interim years.

2. The FAO Undertaking on Plant Genetic Resources. This low-level, non-binding statement sets standards and rules for the conservation and exchange of genetic resources. It calls for all categories of genetic resources to be fully exchanged as the common heritage of mankind. However, by pointedly refusing to exclude patented materials and breeders' lines from its definition of genetic resources, FAO angered industrialized countries and a number refused to join the Commission or sign the Undertaking as a result. Recently, an "agreed interpretation" of this section has been accepted resolving this problem and membership in the Commission has grown.

3. International Network of Gene Banks. FAO established—on paper—a network of gene banks whose material would be considered to be held under the auspices of the FAO and subject to the guidelines on exchange set out in the Undertaking. This network was seen as a form of reassurance that genetic resources would remain in the public domain and that their availability would not be subject to political considerations. However, much material is still held outside of this network.

4. International Gene Fund. This fund was established to support genetic conservation and utilization programs. Politically, this fund was seen as a mechanism for the recognition of farmers' contributions to the generation and conservation of genetic diversity. Plant breeders receive their reward through royalties and profits obtained with the help of intellectual property laws. Farmers' efforts would be rewarded indirectly through this fund in the form of support for various conservation and breeding programs. Contributions to this fund are voluntary.

Each of these four initiatives was extremely controversial. Debates were highly contentious and often personal. Adversaries' motives as well as their views were routinely questioned. This was both sad and ironic, because most individuals obviously shared a real and deep commitment to conservation of genetic diversity.

As the debate raged in the United States Congress over patenting and in the FAO over the above issues, the media finally took notice. The *Wall Street Journal* coined the term "seed wars" to describe the controversy (Paul 1984). Criticism—at times unjust—was met by defensiveness and counter-attack. Views became more and more polarized. Third World governments and a number of advocacy organizations supported the FAO initiatives. Industrialized countries (with the exception of Spain) opposed them. Corporations pushed for intellectual property legislation and were opposed by farmers, church, and advocacy groups. Very real differences in politics or approach to the various issues were exacerbated by overly-simplified and sensationalized press reports and by the lack of direct communication between adversaries.

The controversy, which was both engaged in and widely deplored by the scientific community, accomplished something which had eluded all prior to the beginning of the fireworks in the early 1980s. It placed the topic of genetic resources before the public. It generated editorials and front-page coverage in the *New York Times* and the *Washington Post*. Newspaper features on seed savers and "heirloom" vegetables and fruits became commonplace. There were NOVA, Donahue, NPR, and MacNeil-Lehrer programs. Books and dissertations were written. Studies were undertaken. Congressional hearings were held. Citizens groups like the Seed Savers Exchange and the American Minor Breeds Conservancy organized to promote and facilitate their members active participation in conservation activities. New seed companies sprung up to satisfy consumer demand for "heirloom" varieties. This increased public awareness and attention was a major factor contributing to improved funding for federal conservation programs.

It was not consensus but conflict which brought about increased public awareness and additional support for conservation programs. But, these benefits came with costs and risks. International polarization threatened to impede the exchange of genetic resources and harm breeding and conservation programs. While some individuals (in the corporations, government service, and non-government organizations) maintained a hard-line approach to the debate, others began to see the need for a conciliatory effort.

The late William Brown of Pioneer Hi-Bred, John Pino of the National Research Council and others approached the Keystone Center in Colorado. After a number of planning meetings, the Keystone Center agreed to act as a "neutral facilitator" in an international dialogue on plant genetic resources. The first plenary meeting focusing on ex situ conservation took place in Colorado in 1988. Subsequent plenary meetings were convened in Madras, India, and Oslo, Norway. Working group and steering committee meetings were held in Leningrad, Ottawa, Rome, and Uppsala. These meetings brought together many of the most prominent individuals involved in genetic conservation. Heads of the United States, Soviet Union, Chinese, Indian, Brazilian, Ethiopian, Nordic, and Dutch genetic resources programs participated. Prominent corporate officials from North America, South America, and Europe attended. Government, FAO, World Bank, and Consultative Group on International Agricultural Research (CGIAR) officials were involved. And members of grass-roots farm organizations and advocacy groups as well as distinguished individual scientists participated. Virtually all major points of view and constituencies were represented (Keystone 1988, 1990, 1991).

The informal and off-the-record style of the meetings helped dissolve many encrusted views and personal antagonisms which had built up over the years. The trust and indeed friendships which grew out of the meetings facilitated some rather remarkable policy breakthroughs. The dialogue recognized that questions of ownership, control, and the realization of value from genetic resources were linked with the problem of the conservation of those resources. Effective utilization of genetic resources and an equitable sharing of the benefits from these resources are an important, perhaps necessary part of effective conservation. The dialogue recognized the right of plant breeders to be rewarded for their labors, but noted that presently the world's farmers have no system which would reward them for past, present, and future contributions as plant selectors, breeders, and conservers. Participants realized that genetic resources are not simply "raw materials" used by scientists. They are materials which have already been altered and improved by the often conscious, knowledgeable, and creative efforts of farmers. To deny the intellectual contribution and thus, the intellectual property of these farmers was deemed unjust. Nevertheless, the dialogue participants realized that such innovation takes place in an informal, community setting which renders Western-styled patent laws with their emphasis on identifying the individual inventor (out of any social context) inapplicable.

Dialogue participants endorsed the establishment of a Fund which would recognize what has been termed "farmers' rights" and would support genetic conservation and utilization. The Fund would not attempt the impossible and inappropriate—to identify and reward or compensate individuals—but would assist farmers as a class through conservation and utilization programs. Subsidizing conservation alone is not enough. Different countries have different capacities to use genetic resources. Some have almost no capacity and must thus be assisted if conservation is to be beneficial. This is why the "progressive" collection etiquette of always leaving a duplicate sample in a donor country is inadequate—it ignores and does little to improve that country's ability to use materials which can be taken out and utilized profitably by others.

The dialogue calls for a new structure or remolding of existing institutions to administer this work. The Government of Norway has asked that these proposals, adopted as a consensus by the Keystone Dialogue, be considered formally by the UN Conference on Environment and Development in 1992. Outlined in detail in the three Keystone plenary documents (Keystone 1988, 1990, 1991), the recommendations may serve as an "action agenda" inside various UN bodies and international institutions during the 1990s.

The improved communication and cooperation gained as a byproduct of the Keystone process is already bearing some fruit. An innovative breeding and conservation program is being developed cooperatively by the Dutch and Ethiopian gene banks together with the Norwegian Centre for International Agricultural Development, and various non-government organizations (NGOs). Discussions on cooperative work between the CGIAR and NGOs are under way. And several controversies have been avoided by behind-the-scenes work by Keystone participants of divergent views.

The direction set by Keystone will not eliminate the millenia-old conflict or controversy over the handling of genetic resources. Threats to the delicate current alliance are already visible. United States initiatives at the General Agreement on Tariffs and Trade (GATT) may force Third World countries to adopt and recognize Western-style intellectual property laws for biological materials. If so, a serious imbalance will be created, because these laws were not designed for recognizing the creative contributions of the "informal" (farmer-community) sector and effectively exclude many in the Third World from benefiting from the resources they have identified, developed, and nurtured for years. In Europe and North America, attempts to circumscribe or eliminate the right of farmers to save seed of protected cultivars will generate more controversy.

If Keystone-style initiatives fail or if proposals such as those under debate at GATT succeed, "seed wars" may well break out again. Restrictions on access to genetic resources and tough codes of conduct on biotechnology, germplasm collection, and germplasm utilization can be expected. Some countries may push to create legal forms of protection for landraces or "folk varieties." Conservation and breeding programs may suffer in the short-term.

Those who work with "new crops" will need to be mindful of the context within which that work is done. That context includes an increased awareness of the value of genetic resources in both the public and private sectors and an increased sensitivity to questions about the socioeconomic and legal implications of collection and transfer of and access to genetic resources, particularly in the Third World. That context also involves an increasingly sophisticated discussion about the nature of intellectual property—a discussion which includes forceful assertions that scientists and their employers are not the only rightful claimants of intellectual property rights over or credit for new crop cultivars. Collectors and users of genetic resources will have to respect and work with donors and conservers of these resources at all levels—from the farm to the gene bank—to retain access to these materials and foster much needed goodwill. These steps will be taken more easily if all understand that the question of conservation of and access to genetic resources cannot be separated from the larger question of utilization and development. In the future, it will be more and more difficult to say that the science of plant genetic resources has nothing to do with the politics and economics of plant genetic resources. Students of history should understand that the distinction so frequently drawn is often convenient yet almost always false.

REFERENCES

Berg, T., Aa. Bjornstad, C. Fowler, and T. Skroppa. 1991. Technology options and the gene struggle. Agr. Univ. of Norway, Aas, Norway.

Frankel, O.H. and E. Bennett. 1970. Genetic resources in plants. Int. Biol. Prog., London.

Griffin, K. 1972. The green revolution: an economic analysis. UN Res. Inst. for Soc. Dev., Geneva.

Harlan, H.V. and M.L. Martini. 1936. Problems and results in barley breeding. Yearbook of agriculture. USDA, Washington, DC.

Harlan, J. 1972. Genetics of disaster. J. Environ. Quality 1(3).

Keystone Center. 1988. Final report of the Keystone international dialogue on plant genetic resources, session I: ex situ conservation of plant genetic resources. Keystone Center, Keystone, CO.

Keystone Center. 1990. Final consensus report of the Keystone international dialogue series on plant genetic resources: Madras plenary session. Keystone Center, Keystone, CO.

Keystone Center. 1991. Keystone international dialogue series on plant genetic resources final consensus report: global initiative for the security and sustainable use of plant genetic resources. Keystone Center, Keystone, CO.

Kloppenburg, J. 1988. First the seed: The political economy of plant biotechnology, 1492–2000. Cambridge Univ. Press, Cambridge, MA.

Klose, N. 1950. America's crop heritage: the history of foreign plant introduction by the federal government. Iowa State College Press, Ames.

Lappe, F.M., J. Collins, and C. Fowler. 1977. Food first: beyond the myth of scarcity. Houghton Mifflin, New York.

Lemmon, K. 1968. Golden age of plant hunters. Barnes, Cranbury, UK.

National Research Council. 1972. Genetic vulnerability of major crops. NAS, Washington, DC.

Paul, B. 1984. Third world battles for fruit of its seed stocks. Wall Street Journal. June 15, 1984.

Perelman, M. 1977. Farming for profit in a hungry world. Allanheld Osmun, Montclair, NJ.

Wilkes, G. 1977. The world's crop plant germplasm: An endangered resource. Bul. Atomic Scientists. February. 33(2):8–16.

INTERNATIONAL DEVELOPMENTS

New Crop Development in Europe

Louis J.M. van Soest

This paper summarizes the present activities on new crop development, particularly industrial crops in Europe. As Europe consists of more than 25 countries, this overview only briefly summarizes some of the continents new crops activities. The paper will mainly concentrate on plant exploration and primary production considerations of potential industrial crops, in the European Communities. The new crop programs in The Netherlands will receive special attention. Although several East European countries have a long history in industrial crop research, this paper will only deal briefly with developments in this part of Europe.

The surpluses of the major agricultural food crops in Europe have increased interest in new directions for the utilization of agricultural land. Options which have been taken in consideration and partly realized are: set aside programs, reforestation, biomass production for energy, land for recreation and nature preservation, and the production of agricultural feedstocks for industrial utilization. Since the second part of the 1980s, the Commission of the European Communities (EC) and several European governments, have stimulated research programs to develop crops for the production of renewable resources for industrial application (EC 1990; Raymond and Larvor 1985; von Wüllerstorff 1990). In The Netherlands, the narrow crop rotation and the intensive high input farming has caused large pressures of pests and diseases, particularly soil born pests like cyst nematodes and fungal diseases. New crops could reduce this pressure and broaden the present rotation.

Private breeding firms in most of the EC countries are responsible for the cultivar development of established crops. Cultivar development of new crops is considered a risk investment and therefore governmental institutes in Europe are responsible for both genetic research and cultivar development.

RESEARCH AND DEVELOPMENT PROGRAMS

There are four types of new crop development programs in Europe:

Agro-industrial Programs, established and co-financed by the EC, are "pre-competitive" research programs in the areas of agro-industry (EC 1990). Participation is required by two or more countries, including research in the field of primary production, industrial processing, transformations and utilization of biological feedstocks. Participation of private enterprises is sometimes required. Some of the EC programs include development of new potential crops, such as: *Cuphea*, jojoba, crambe, meadowfoam, castor bean, coriander, *Dimorphotheca pluvialis* (L.) Moench, *Euphorbia lagascae* Spreng., high erucic rape, high oleic sunflower, flax, *Miscanthus*, sweet sorghum, Jerusalem artichoke, and lupines.

Bilateral Programs are not common but are carried out on an informal basis between countries. These include exchange of information and germplasm.

National Programs have been established in several European countries in which universities and agricultural research institutes are working on new crops. Several new crop research programs with a duration of four years have been developed in the Netherlands (Table 1). In the Federal Republic of Germany programs are carried out on new oilseed crops such as coriander, marigold, *Euphorbia* spp., high erucic rape, and honesty (Röbbelen 1987; Wittmeyer 1990). Other new crops under investigation in Germany include Jerusalem artichoke, root chicory, sweet sorghum, and *Miscanthus*. In the United Kingdom, a new national program for the development of *Chenopodium quinoa* Willd. was initiated. An overview of a number of potential new crops investigated in Europe is illustrated in Fig. 1. Several countries in South Europe (France, Italy, Spain, Greece, and Portugal) are exploring the possibilities to introduce new crops, such as kenaf, castor bean, jojoba, *Cuphea*, and guayule, for the Mediterranean basin.

Industrial Programs are carried out by the private sector. Some industries are looking into the possibilities to develop new crops for the production of pharmaceutical, aromatic, and bioactive compounds. Research in this area is sometimes conducted with private breeding firms (e.g. evening primrose) but also on contract basis with governmental institutes. Information on these programs is often difficult to obtain.

Plant exploration and primary production is presently receiving high emphasis in European new crop programs, although several programs also involve characterization and processing of the desirable compounds (Tables 2, 3, 5, and 6). Programs within the framework of the EC–ECLAIR (European Collaborative Linkage of Agriculture and Industry through Research) need to have industrial partners where research on processing and application of potential products forms an integral part of the program. These EC research programs are aiming to improve the interface between agriculture and industry (EC 1990). In 1992, the EC will start a new research and technological development program in the field of Agriculture and Agro-Industry. This program with a duration of three of four years encompasses crop diversification, particularly for non-food production.

Table 1. National programs on new crops in The Netherlands (research conducted over 4 years).

Crops	R&D categories	Starting year	Industrial participation	Man-power (per year)	No. participants	Coordination
Hemp	I to III	1989	some	25	12	Agrotechnological Research Institute, ATO–DLO
Caraway	I to III	1990	some	15	7	Centre for Agribiological Research, CABO–DLO
Oilseeds	I to IV	1990	yes	17	9	Centre for Plant Breeding and Reproduction Research, CPRO–DLO
Quinoa	I and II	1992	yes	2	4	Research Station for Arable Farming and Field Production of Vegetables, PAGV–DAT

Agricultural Research Department of The Netherlands
Research and Development categories (R&D)
   I = Plant exploration and evaluation
   II = Crop improvement including plant breeding and agronomy
   III = Processing and application research
   IV = Marketing, commercialization, and utilization

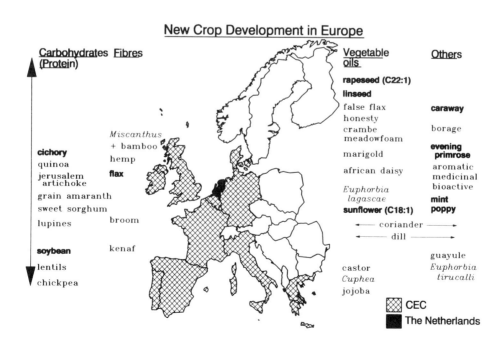

Fig. 1. Industrial crops under investigation in Europe. (Crops in bold print are already commercialized, others need to be further domesticated.)

Several new crops for industrial use have considerable of interest for Europe. The status of development varies from crop to crop and the opportunities to commercialize them depends particularly on the degree of domestication of the crop, the economic perspective of cultivation for farmers, and the interest of industries in the raw materials. Crops producing vegetable oils for industrial use, fibers for paper production as well as cellulose, and carbohydrates for industrial sugars and starches have been selected for further domestication. A number of pharmaceutical, aromatic, and medicinal crops are under investigation.

OILSEED CROPS FOR INDUSTRIAL UTILIZATION

Most of the oilseed crops under investigation in Europe produce special fatty acids. These include more or less domesticated crops like high erucic rapeseed and high oleic sunflower as well as those which need further domestication (Table 2, 3). The common feature of these oilseed crops is that the unique fatty acids in the oil are present in high amounts, sometimes up to 80%.

The production of bio-diesel from oilseed crops, particularly rapeseed, has been under discussion in several countries in Europe.

Domesticated or Partly Domesticated Oilseeds

High erucic rape seed (*Brassica napus* L.) and high oleic sunflower (*Helianthus annuus* L.) are now commercially grown in some European countries. The area of these crops, however, does not exceed 10,000 ha. Breeding programs have been established to enhance the erucic acid level of rapeseed above 50% and to increase the percentage oil of high oleic sunflower.

Linseed production in Europe, particularly Great Britain, increased tremendously from 20,000 ha in 1989 to more than 120,000 ha in 1991.

Castor bean (*Rinus communis* L.) and jojoba [*Simmondsia chinensis* (Link) Schneid.] are not sufficiently domesticated for commercial cultivation in Europe, but research continues in several South European countries. According to Mignoni (1991) the first crop of jojoba was harvested in 1989 in Sicily, Italy. Coriander (*Coriander sativum* L.) is presently cultivated in Europe for aromatic, medicinal, and cosmetic purposes, however the seed-oil which contains about 80% petroselenic acid, has potential for the production of oleochemicals (Röbbelen 1987). The EC (Directorate General for Science, Research and Development-DG XII) is supporting demonstration projects of most of these more or less domesticated oilcrops particularly those with promising market possibilities such as erucic rapeseed, oleic sunflower, and castor bean (von Wüllerstorff 1990).

Oilseed Crops

Numerous new potential oilseed crops have been introduced and evaluated, particularly in Germany and The Netherlands (Meier zu Beerentrup and Röbbelen 1987; Röbbelen 1987; van Soest 1990; Mulder et al. 1991). Many produce unique fatty acids with functional groups or double bonds, but they need to be further domesticated to achieve commercialization. In The Netherlands some 40 different potential oilseed crops were introduced and evaluated in the period 1986–1989 (van Soest 1990). Meier zu Beerentrup (1986) tested nearly 50 potential vegetable oilcrops with unusual fatty acids in Germany. Breeding research in Germany concentrates now on *Calendula officinalis* L., *Coriandrum sativum* L., *Cuphea* spp., and *Euphorbia* spp. Similar programs with a limited and selected number of species which are based on experience in Germany and The Netherlands, are being conducted in Norway and the United Kingdom. Breeding research on these crops, however, is concentrated presently only on a selected group (Table 4). Data obtained in The Netherlands of some promising new oilseed crops are presented in Table 4.

Breeding Research

There are major agricultural constraints related to the domestication of the novel oilseed crops:
- slow initial growth and development (*Euphorbia lathyris* L. and *Limnanthes alba* Benth.)
- poor competition with weeds (*L. alba* and *E. lathyris*)
- asynchronous flowering and seed ripening [*C. officinalis*, *Dimorphotheca pluvialis* (L.) Moench, *Euphorbia lagascae* Spreng. and *L. alba*]

- insufficient seed retention (*D. pluvialis*, *E. lagascae*, and *L. alba*).
- difficulties with incorporation in existing crop rotations because of pests and diseases (*Crambe abyssinica*, *C. officinalis*, and *D. pluvialis*)
- difficulties with mechanical harvesting (*L. alba*, *E. lagascae*, and *Cuphea* spp.).

Current research in Europe is aimed at finding solutions to these constraints. Our breeding research at the Center for Plant Breeding and Reproduction Research (CPRO-DLO), Wageningen, concentrates on further domestication of crops such as *C. abyssinica*, *D. pluvialis*, *E. lagascae*, and *L. alba*. One of the major problems is to locate sufficient variation in the available genepools for some of the constraints mentioned above. In general, the world-wide available germplasm of most of these new oilcrops is limited. Additional collection in the centers of origin is needed. Further domestication and genetic enhancement in the near future will obviously create new variation and broaden the available genepool. In *C. abyssinica*, a few new cultivars and lines have been developed during the last decades.

CARBOHYDRATE CROPS

Potential new crops being explored in Europe include both starch and sugar producing crops for industrial use. Some of these crops are often also considered to have potential for the production of biomass for renewable energy production.

Table 2. Domesticated or partly domesticated industrial oilseed crops in Europe.

Crop	Potential use	R&D categories[z]	Cultivation (status)	Countries
Coriander	Oleochemicals, cosmetics	I to III	Trials-demo*	Germany, UK, Netherlands, Norway, Eastern Europe
Crambe	Erucamides, plastics (nylon), lubricants	I to III	Trials-demo	Bulgaria, Germany, UK, Italy Netherlands, Norway, Sweden, USSR
Rapeseed (erucic)	Erucamides, lubricants, nylon 13	I to IV	Medium scale	Germany, Eastern Europe
Sunflower (oleic)	Coatings, detergents, lubricants, cosmetics	I to IV	Medium scale	France, Germany, Italy
Linseed	Coatings, lino	I to IV	Large scale	Northwest, Eastern Europe
Castor	Lubricants	I to III	Trials-demo	Spain, France, Italy, Portugal
Jojoba	Cosmetics, lubricants	I to III	Trials-demo	Spain, France, Italy, Portugal

[z]See Table 1.

Table 3. Industrial oilseeds under development in Europe.

Crop	Principal fatty acid	R&D categories[z]	Cultivation (status)	Countries
Calendula spp.	Calendic	I to II	Trials	Germany, UK, Netherlands
Cuphea spp.	Short chain	I to II	Trials	Germany, Portugal, Spain
Dimorphotheca spp.	Dimorphecolic	I to III	Trials-demo	Netherlands
Euphorbia lagascae	Vernolic	I to III	Trials-demo	Germany, Netherlands, Spain
Euphorbia lathyris	Oleic	I to III	Trials-demo	Germany, Eastern Europe
Limnanthes spp.	Long chain	I to III	Trials-demo	France, UK, Netherlands

Some exploration work on *Camelina sativa*, *Eruca sativa*, *Lesquerella* spp., and *Lunaria annua*.
[z]See Table 1.

Starch

Some research is underway on the pseudograin amaranth (*Amaranthus* spp.), but quinoa (*Chenopodium quinoa* Willd.) has received the most attention (Galwey 1989; Risi 1986; van Soest 1987). Quinoa is considered a multipurpose agro-industrial crop. The grain may be utilized for human food ("health sector" and low diet flour products) and animal feedstocks because of its high nutritional value. The starch with its uniformly small granules has several potential industrial applications. Breeding for genetic adaptation is presently a major research objective in Europe. According to Risi and Galwey (1989), plant characters required for temperate agriculture are present to a large extent in the accessions from near sea level in southern-central Chile, but the seed characteristics are scattered throughout the germplasm. Further breeding of quinoa in Europe needs to concentrate on earliness, uniformity, higher yields and quality aspects of the protein, and physico-chemical properties of the starch. An advantage of quinoa in Europe is that the crop is not very susceptible to soil-born nematodes like beet cyst and root-knot nematodes. As such, it may be of great importance in narrow crop rotations as presently practiced in The Netherlands.

Sugars

Two crops, Jerusalem artichoke (*Helianthus tuberosus* L.) and root chicory (*Cichorium intybus* L.) are sources of inulin which are stored in the tuber or root. Inulin can be transformed into fructose syrups by means of hydrolysis. Inulin can be used in food products as a low calory agent, whereas the fructose syrups can be used as a sweetener in beverages. Meanwhile application research is conducted to utilize inulin and possible derivates (furan chemistry) as industrial feedstock (Fuchs 1989). During the last 10 years breeding and crop improvement of *H. tuberosus* has intensified in Europe (Schittenhelm 1987; Spitters 1987; Mesken 1989). Meyer et al. (1991) studied the inulin production of both crops over a two-year period in The Netherlands and calculated inulin yields of Jerusalem artichoke from 4.5 to 8.3 t/ha, whereas root chicory produced 9.8 to 16.1 t/ha. Breeding of *H. tuberosus* in The Netherlands (CPRO–DLO) resulted in some 10 clones with inulin yields of 16 t/ha in 1989, but in the very dry year of 1990 only 7 t/ha (Toxopeus et al. 1991). Sugar industries in The Netherlands and Belgium recently selected root chicory as inulin-producing crop, and about 5,000 ha are expected to be cultivated in 1992 in both countries.

Sweet sorghum (*Sorghum bicolor* L.) is considered as an alternative low input crop for the Mediterranean areas and has also been tested in Germany (Anderlei et al. 1987). The crop can be used for syrup production, soft drinks, and confectionery, but also has potential for the production of renewable raw materials such as citric acid, and molasses for fermentation (Anderlei et al. 1987).

The production of ethanol from carbohydrate crops has been under discussion and several countries in Europe have conducted agronomic tests. The average yield of raw sugar of sweet sorghum cultivars tested in Germany from 1982 to 1986 was 8 t/ha. Anderlei et al. (1987) calculated that in Germany ethanol production of 5,770 liter/ha was feasible with sweet sorghum.

Table 4. Seed and yield characteristics of some promising new oilseed crops in Dutch trials, 1988–1990.

Species	Principal fatty acid	Principal fatty acid (%)	Oil (%)	Seed yield (kg/ha)	Protein (%)
Calendula officinalis	Calendic	58	17–20	1500–2500	18
Coriandrum sativum	Petroselenic	80	16–25	1500–2500	14
Crambe abyssinica	Erucic	58	26–39	2000–3000	26
Dimorphotheca pluvialis	Dimorphecolic	63	15–25	1500–1800	21
Euphorbia lagascae	Vernolic	61	45–52	1000–2000	25
Limnanthes alba	Long chain	94	17–29	200–1000	26

FIBER CROPS

A number of fiber crops are cultivated or under development in Europe (Table 6). Flax (*Linum usitatissimum* L.) has been cultivated for thousands of years in Europe. During the last two decades the cultivation of fiber flax for linen declined substantially in several countries of Europe (Riensema et al. 1990). Meanwhile research is underway for alternative utilization of flax fibers such as composite panels, geotextiles, and reinforced plastics (Riensema et al. 1990). The research on flax in Europe concentrates on processing and application aspects for non-traditional outlets, but breeding is conducted to improve fiber yield and quality related characters (Marshall 1989).

Hemp (*Cannabis sativa* L.) and kenaf (*Hibiscus cannabinus* L.) are both considered as alternative fiber crops, particularly for paper pulp production. The development of kenaf is concentrated in the Mediterranean region in areas with subtropical climates, and focus on primary production (e.g. cultivar testing). Hemp is grown commercially in some East European countries, particularly for the production of textiles and rope, whereas a small area is cultivated in France for paper production. In Hungary, hemp hybrids have been developed with higher stem yield. In 1989, a large multidisciplinary research program to develop hemp as alternative fiber crop for paper pulp production started in The Netherlands. Besides disciplines dealing with primary production, studies on economic perspectives and processing research are included in this program. At CPRO-DLO, breeding research on hemp concentrates on developing efficient selection methods to increase stem yield and stem quality related properties such as bark (phloem fibers) content. Furthermore the development of genetic stocks with low

Table 5. Crops producing carbohydrates (starch–sugars) under development in Europe.

Crop	Potential use	R&D categories[z]	Cultivation (status)	Countries
Quinoa	Industrial, starch, food	I to III	Trials-demo	Denmark, UK, Netherlands
Amaranth	Industrial, starch, food	I and II	Trials	Denmark, UK
Root chicory	Fructose syrup (inulin)	I to IV	Small scale	Belgium, Germany, France, Netherlands
Jerusalem artichoke	Fructose syrup (inulin)	I to III	Trials-demo	Austria, Denmark, Germany, Spain, France, Italy, Hungary, Netherlands, USSR
Sweet sorghum	Syrup, acids, solvents	I to III	Trials-demo	Germany, Spain, Italy, Hungary, USSR

[z]See Table 1.

Table 6. Fiber crops under development in Europe.

Crop	Potential use	R&D catagories[z]	Cultivation (status)	Countries
Flax	Linen, geotextiles, composites	I to IV	Large scale cultivation	Northwest Europe, Eastern Europe
Hemp	Textiles, rope, paperpulp	I to III	Small scale cultivation	France, Hungary, Netherlands, Rumania, USSR
Kenaf	Paperpulp, composites	I to III	Trials/demo	Italy, France, Portugal
Miscanthus	High quality paper, energy	I to III	Trials	Denmark, Germany, Netherlands
Fiber sorghum	Special paper	I to III	Trials	Spain, France, Italy

[z]See Table 1.

levels of cannabinols, particularly Δ-9-THC and CBD is of importance for commercial cultivation as is work on optimizing growing and harvest techniques and pulping processes.

The perennial grass *Miscanthus sinensis* 'Giganteus' and the annual sorghum *Sorghum vulgare* var. *technica* (broomcorn or fiber sorghum) are also evaluated in Europe as potential fiber crops (Nielsen 1987; Nimz and Pilz 1991). Total dry matter production of *Miscanthus* can reach 35 to 40 t/ha annually once the crops has been established (Frerichs 1991). Several research groups in northwest Europe are considering *Miscanthus* as possible energy crop (Knoblauch 1991; Rupp et al. 1991). The EC is developing demonstration projects of many fiber crops (Table 6).

OTHER POTENTIAL CROPS

A very large and diverse group of more or less domesticated crops are under investigation in Europe. This group can be divided in a number of subcategories:
- aromatic plants containing essential oils and flavonoids; caraway, mint, coriander, lavender, fennel, thyme, and rose are of some importance;
- pharmaceutical/medicinal plants; crops like poppy, hemp, evening primrose, borage, foxglove, and valerian;
- other crops producing special compounds such as for the production of dyes (madder), latex (*Euphorbia* spp.), or repellents (caraway).

Some of these crops are already cultivated, particularly in East Europe. All these specialty crops have limited acreage which can fluctuate tremendously due to uncertain markets. Most of these crops are of interest to individual farmers, but can however, only partly solve the structural problems of European Agriculture (Franz 1987).

Evening primrose (*Oenothera* spp.) was introduced in the UK some 15 years ago (Lapinskas 1989). In The Netherlands, the area of evening primrose was approximately 700 ha in the mid-1980s, declined to about 50 ha by the end of the decade, and now in 1991 about 1,000 ha were grown.

Caraway (*Carum carvi* L.) has grown in The Netherlands for the past 200 years on an area fluctuating from 100 to 10,000 ha. The seeds are mainly used in the bakery trade, and its essential oil for cosmetic products. A national Dutch R&D program started in 1990 to create new markets for carvone as the most important bioactive compound of the essential oil. Potentially, carvone can be used for the inhibition of sprouting of potatoes, as an insect repellant, and for the inhibition of fungal growth in cereals.

CONCLUSIONS

Over 100 potential new crops are presently being explored in Europe. Some of these crops are cultivated to a limited extent whereas others are only grown in the framework of demonstration projects. Interest in new crop development has increased tremendously in Europe during the last five years. The EC and national governments are stimulating and increasingly funding research programs to create alternatives for the surpluses of the major agricultural food crops.

Although expectations of the farmers are high, it will take years before a real breakthrough can be expected. Only a few crops have reached the stage that would permit commercialization in the next 5 or 10 years. Most of the crops discussed need to be further domesticated. Plant breeding for adaptation and particularly increase of yield stability should be given high priority in future research activities, as well as product development and marketing. After years of plant exploration and evaluation in several European countries, it is now time to select the most promising new crops and concentrate further research and commercialization on these species.

REFERENCES

Anderlei, J., W. Mechelke, J.F. Seitzer, H. Schiweck, and G. Steinle. 1987. Sweet sorghum (*Sorghum bicolor* L.), a renewable energy source? Results of first experiments in Southern Germany, p. 255–258. In: Proc. Workshop on Evaluation of Genetic Resources for Industrial Crops. Eucarpia. FAL, Braunschweig, Germany.

EC. 1990. ECLAIR–European Collaborative Linkage of Agriculture and Industry through Research. 1988–1993. Commission of European Communities DG XII. Brussels, Belgium.

Franz, Ch. 1987. Evaluation of genetic resources of medicinal and aromatic plants, p. 167–184. In: Proc. Workshop on Evaluation of Genetic Resources for Industrial Crops. Eucarpia. FAL, Braunschweig, Germany.

Frerichs, L. 1991. Ernte und Aufbereitung von *Miscanthus sinensis*, p. 46–57. In: *Miscanthus sinensis*, KTBL-Arbeitspapier 158. Darmstadt, Germany.

Fuchs, A. 1989. Perspectives of inulin and inulin-containing crops in the Netherlands and in Europe, p. 80–102. In: A. Fuchs (ed.). Proc. Third Seminar on Inulin. NRLO report nr. 90/28. Wageningen, The Netherlands.

Galwey, N.W. 1989. Quinoa-exploited plants. Biologist 36:267–274.

Knoblauch, F. 1991. *Miscanthus sinensis* 'Giganteus' als nachwachsender Energie- und Industrierohstoff in Dänemark, p. 79–83. In: *Miscanthus sinensis* KTBL-Arbeitspapier 158. Darmstadt, Germany.

Lapinskas, P. 1989. Commercial exploitation of alternative crops, with special reference to evening primrose, p. 216–221. In: G.E. Wickens, N. Haq, and P. Day (eds.). New crops for food and industry. Chapman and Hall, London, England.

Marshall, G. 1989. Flax: Breeding and utilization. Kluwer Academic, Dordrecht, The Netherlands.

Meier zu Beerentrup, H. 1986. Identifizierung, erzeugung und verbesserung von einheimischen ölsaaten mit ungewöhnlichen fettsäuren. Thesis Universität Göttingen, Germany.

Meier zu Beerentrup, H. and G. Röbbelen. 1987. Screening for European productions of oilseed with unusual fatty acids. Angewandte Botanik 61:287–303.

Meyer, W.J.M., E.W.J.M. Mathijssen, and G.E.L. Borm. 1992. Crop characteristics and inulin production of Jerusalem artichoke and chichory, In: A. Fuchs (ed.). Inulin and inulin-containing crops. Elseviers, Amsterdam (in press), The Netherlands.

Mesken, M. 1989. Induction of flowering, seed production, and evaluation of seedlings and clones of Jerusalem artichoke (*Helianthus tuberosus* L.), p. 137–143. In: G. Grassi and G. Gosse (eds.). Topinambour (Jerusalem artichoke). Proc. Jerusalem artichoke CEC Workshop, 1987. Madrid, Spain.

Mignoni, G. 1991. The Jesuits and the jojoba. Agro-food-Industry Hi-Tech 1:9–15.

Mulder, F., L.J.M. van Soest, E.P.M. de Meyer, and S.C. Wallenburg. 1992. Current Dutch research on new oilseed crops. In: Proc. First Int. Conf. New Ind. Crops and Products. Riverside, CA. (in press).

Nielsen, P.N. 1987. Produktiviteten af elefantgræs, *Miscanthus sinensis* 'Giganteus' på forskellige jordtyper. (The productivity of *Miscanthus sinensis* 'Giganteus' on different soil types). Tidsskrift for Platenavl 91:275–281.

Nimz, H.H. and A. Pilz. 1991. Zellstoffgewinnung aus *Miscanthus sinensis* 'Giganteus', p. 105–113. In: *Miscanthus sinensis*, KTBL-Arbeitspapier 158. Darmstadt, Germany.

Raymond, W. and P. Larvor. 1985. Alternative uses for agricultural surpluses. Proc. Seminar on Research and the Problems of Agricultural Science in Europe of CEC. Elsevier Applied Science, London, England.

Riensema, C.J., R.A.C. Koster, and T.J.H.M. Hutten. 1990. Vlas 2000 (Flax 2000). Onderzoekverslag LEI, Den Haag, The Netherlands.

Risi, C.J. 1986. Adaptation of the Andean grain crop quinoa (*Chenopodium quinoa* Willd.) for cultivation in Britain. PhD thesis, University of Cambridge, England.

Risi, C.J. and N.W. Galwey. 1989. The pattern of genetic diversity in the Andean grain crop quinoa (*Chenopodium quinoa* Willd.). I. Associations between characteristics. Euphytica 41:147–162.

Röbbelen, G. 1987. Development of new industrial oil crops. Fat Sci. Technol. 89:563–570.

Rupp, M., A. Stulgies, and F. Jondanski. 1991. Energetische Nutzung von Miscanthus-Stroh durch Vergassung, p. 90–98. In: *Miscanthus sinensis*. KTBL-Arbeitspapier 158. Darmstadt, Germany.

Schittenhelm, S. 1987. Preliminary results of a breeding programme with Jerusalem artichoke (*Helianthus tuberosus* L.), p. 209–220. In: Proc. Workshop on Evaluation of Genetic Resources for Industrial Crops. Eucarpia. FAL, Braunschweig, Germany.

Soest, L.J.M. van. 1987. Introduction and preliminary evaluation of some potential industrial crops, p. 19–28. In: Proc. Workshop on Evaluation of Genetic Resources for Industrial Crops. Eucarpia. FAL, Braunschweig, Germany.

Soest, L.J.M. van. 1990. Introduction and breeding of new oil crops, p. 36–44. In: Biotechnology and fatty acids: new perspectives for agricultural production? Pudoc, Wageningen, The Netherlands.

Spitters, C.J.T. 1987. Genetic variation in growth pattern and tuber yield in *Helianthus tuberosus* L., p. 221–235. In: Proc. Workshop on Evaluation of Genetic Resources for Industrial Crops. Eucarpia. FAL, Braunschweig, Germany.

Toxopeus, H., J. Dieleman, and M. Mesken. 1991. Breeding techniques and genetic improvement of productivity in Topinambour (*Helianthus tuberosus* L.). Book of Abstracts of Int. Congress on Inulin and Inulin-containing Crops. Wageningen, The Netherlands.

Wittmeyer, D. 1990. Coordination of an industry-orientated agriculture in the Federal Republic of Germany, p. 5–15. In: Biotechnology and fatty acids: new perspectives for agricultural production? Pudoc, Wageningen, The Netherlands.

Wüllerstorf, B. von. 1990. Outlook for oleochemicals in Europe, p. 1–4. In: Biotechnology and fatty acids: new perspectives for agricultural production? Pudoc, Wageningen, The Netherlands.

Characterization and Processing Research for Increased Industrial Applicability of New and Traditional Crops: A European Perspective

W.M.J. van Gelder, F.P. Cuperus, J.T.P. Derksen, B.G. Muuse, and J.E.G. van Dam

The surpluses of agricultural commodities have generated an increasingly growing interest in novel applications of agricultural produce. As crops are currently grown almost entirely for food and feed applications, a basic element of the policy within the European Community (EC) is increasing the use of traditional crops, and developing new crops for industrial applications (Rexen 1991). An encompassing R&D strategy is needed for achieving this goal.

R&D must be market oriented and the most promising technologies and products, selected after thorough evaluation for market potentials, should be commercialized. In research programs the entire production chain should be studied including primary production, harvesting, storage and processing technologies, product development and evaluation, marketing studies and economics.

Hence, a multidisciplinary approach is needed and both the public and private sector must participate. Introduction of agricultural commodities as industrial raw products is often hampered because the current raw materials used by industry are inexpensive, readily available and of acceptable quality. Thus, the specific advantageous properties of agricultural raw materials must be identified and exploited. Process technologies enabling exploitation of such preferential properties need also to be developed.

This paper presents a brief description of the background of the EC-surplus situation and of proposed measures for surplus reduction, especially by non-food applications of crops. This includes relevant R&D programs within the EC in general and in the Netherlands in particular. Some examples of research on new/industrial crops directed to exploiting preferential properties for technical applications are presented in more detail.

EC SURPLUS POLICY

History

After World War II, the agricultural production capacity in Europe was mainly employed to produce food and feed. After the EC had been founded, the agricultural policy of the community was to increase agricultural productivity to provide a reasonable and stable income for farmers and to ensure a stable food supply to consumers at reasonable prices. An important aim was to achieve a good balance between production and the market. In the 1960s and 1970s, this policy proved very successful. Afterwards, the EC-countries appeared unable to slow down increases in productivity, in order to keep supply and demand in balance. Moreover, as a result of its success in producing commodities for food and feed applications, agriculture had neglected entirely the opportunities of raw material production for the non-food industry, although agricultural products had been used for non-food applications for a long time. Among the traditional applications were natural fibers for ropes, cords, and textile, starch and proteins for glues, natural pigments for dyes, medicinal plants for pharmaceutics, and vegetable oils and fats for paints, linoleum, soaps, lubricants, and fuels. Due to their increasing prices, many of these raw materials became replaced by mineral- or petrochemical-based materials produced by the chemical industry. In addition, the chemical industry developed superior technologies and products after the second world war, while agriculture was focussing on producing commodities for food and feed.

EC Price System

The EC guarantees farmers a minimum price for their products—which is often (much) higher than the world-market price—even in the situation of excess production and within the frame-work of open-end intervention. As a result, the subsidies the EC has to pay to her farmers have now become an intolerable burden. Moreover, important trade-partners of the EC strongly object to the EC price system. For these reasons, the EC is changing the policy which will affect many farmers, especially the small family farms, resulting in a dramatic loss of income. As this situation leads to enormous political problems, the EC and its individual member-states are diligently looking for solutions for the surplus problem.

Reducing the Surpluses

A number of options for reducing the surpluses in the EC have been proposed: set-aside programs (laying agricultural areas fallow); increased land for recreation and nature preservation; afforestation; planting "fast-growing wood," such as popular and spruce, for pulp and paper production; and biological feedstocks for industry. Set-aside programs and afforestation have already been put into practice and much attention is being directed to finding industrial market-outlets for agricultural (annual) crops, especially for non-food/non-feed applications. On the longer term, diversifying agriculture to produce industrial feedstocks could reduce on a structural base the excess production and strengthen the agricultural economy. However, for many potential applications, agricultural raw materials must compete with mineral products which are often, but not always, cheaper and sometimes superior. Advantages of agricultural raw materials that can contribute to achieving a durable society will appear very important on the longer term. Compared to fossil raw materials those of agriculture are renewable, environmental friendly, and enable gradually growing to a closed carbon-dioxide cycle.

Although plants contain many unique valuable components that cannot, or only at very high costs, be produced by the chemical industry, it will be very difficult to introduce plant materials as replacement for current synthetic products. This is largely due to the relative primitiveness of many agricultural non-food processing technologies. Little investments have been made in this area in the last five decades, while the chemical industry invested billions of dollars in R&D. Thus, for the development of the raw products for industry based on agricultural materials new processing technologies have often to be developed.

In the proposed strategy, cooperation is essential between agriculture as the raw material supplier, the agricultural research field, and industry. As little is known on the specific characteristics of agricultural materials for modern technical applications, it is difficult to compare characteristics of most plant materials with the technical specifications demanded by industries. For this reason, the EC-countries direct much agricultural R&D effort in the coming years to characterize potential raw materials. In cooperation with industry, non-food process technologies and intermediate and consumer products will be developed. As the agricultural sellers market has changed into a buyers market, agriculture can only profit from the interesting opportunities that exist at the expense of very large investments in R&D.

Research Programs within the EC

EC programs. The EC Directorates General VI (Agriculture) and XII (Science, Research and Development) at Brussels, initiate and support research on creating new market-outlets for agricultural crops. Important programs which are (partly) directed to this field are: ECLAIR and FLAIR (Agro-industrial Technologies), total budget 105 million ECU (equivalent to US$ 130 million), 1988–1993; CAMAR (Adapting Agriculture to the New Situation and Market Policy), total budget 55 million ECU (US$ 68 million), 1989–1993; AIR (Agricultural and Agro-industrial Research), total budget 330 million ECU (US$ 410 million), 1991–1994; and a number of smaller programs and demonstration projects or studies.

Recently, the non-food uses have been assigned a key-area for EC-research (Rexen 1991). Especially within ECLAIR, CAMAR, and AIR, much emphasis is put to this area. To obtain support from the EC AIR-program, research projects must show a strategic approach and be market oriented. This means that the entire production chain must be represented in the project including pilot plants on a near reality scale for economic evaluation and participation of the industry. Additional conditions are amongst others, that processes and products to be developed must be "environmental and energy friendly" (Rexen 1991).

National research programs. In a number of EC countries, e.g. Germany, France, and The Netherlands, substantial research programs on increasing the non-food applicability of agricultural crops are or have been initiated. In The Netherlands, the research programs are initiated by the Ministry of Agriculture, Nature Management and Fisheries, some of them in cooperation with the Ministry of Economic Affairs. The total budget that has been allocated until now exceeds the equivalent to US$ 30 million. The Dutch programs focus on (increased) industrial application of carbohydrates, oils, fibers, and secondary metabolites from arable crops and proteins from plant and animal origin.

In addition to organizing and/or subsidizing these programs, in 1989, the Agrotechnological Research Institute (ATO–DLO) was founded in Wageningen, by the Ministry of Agriculture, Nature Management and Fisheries of the Netherlands. ATO–DLO consists of seven research divisions and now has 270 employees. The division Industrial Crops, Products and Process Technologies employs over 65 research workers involved in research on new and traditional crops for industrial utilization. The topics concur in general with those of the ministries. Research programs are multidisciplinary between scientists trained in plant physiology, organic chemistry, and biochemistry, biotechnology, processing technology, polymer and materials science, (molecular) physics, and the development of appropriate agrologistic systems.

In several programs, the entire production chain is studied including crop harvesting, storage, extraction, pre-processing, processing, product evaluation, and economics. Cooperation with plant breeders and agronomists is critical for improving the yield potential of the desired raw material. Close contacts/cooperation with chemical or non-food processing industries exist for developing economically feasible applications for agricultural raw materials.

Important topics within each research program are: (1) characterization of the agricultural raw material from an industrial perspective; (2) development of extraction, preprocessing, and processing techniques that can be applied by industries willing to use agricultural raw materials as an alternative to current raw materials; (3) development of required (bio)reactor systems; and (4) development of intermediate and/or other products.

New Crops

In addition to developing new applications for traditional crops, four groups of new crops are under evaluation:

Fiber crops. Fiber hemp (*Cannabis sativa* L.), fiber flax (*Linum usitatissimum* L.) and elephant grass (*Miscanthus sinensis* L.) are being studied for chemical, physical, and morphological characteristics that determine fiber quality. The relationship between fiber quality and harvesting date and processing conditions are under evaluation. Process technologies and products are being developed. Applications include fibers for reinforced composites, building and construction materials, and geotextiles (see hereafter) and pulp and cellulose for the paper industry.

Oilseed crops. The oil content and triglyceride and fatty acid compositions of a large number of oil seed crops and the yield of the desired fatty acids in relation to sowing and harvesting dates are being evaluated. Advanced techniques are being developed for enzymatic hydrolysis of specific fatty acids such as labile fatty acids or technical fatty acids on the 1,3 positions of the triglycerides. Development of bioreactor and enzymatic transesterification technologies for modification of triglycerides of new oil crops is in progress.

Carbohydrate crops. Inulin, a linear ß2-1 polyfructoside from root chicory (*Cichorium intybus* L.) and

Jerusalem artichoke (*Helianthus tuberosus* L.), showing a degree of polymerization of DP 3 to DP > 70, is used as a sweetener after hydrolysis. Applications which exploit the polymeric nature of inulins are a novel approach and deserve much attention. The 3-D molecular structure of inulin is being studied and selective oxidation and cross-linking techniques are studied for valorization of the inulins.

Protein crops. The proteins of new or underutilized crops such as faba beans (*Vicia faba* L.), peas (*Pisum sativum* L.), lupins (*Lupinus albus* L.), and quinoa (*Chenopodium quinoa* Willd) are being isolated and characterized. The physical properties are being evaluated such as solubility, viscosity, elasticity, gel-forming, foaming and emulsifying properties, and coating characteristics. Chemical and enzymatic modification procedures are being developed for use by the food and non-food processing industries.

EXPLOITING ADVANTAGEOUS PROPERTIES OF CROPS FOR INDUSTRIAL APPLICATION

Some examples of research at ATO–DLO are presented below. These include studies on characterization and exploitation of specific properties of arable crops including development of necessary processing technologies; research in the application of agrofibers from "new" crops in composite and construction materials; and the primary production and processing of technical oils from new oil seed crops.

Agrofibers for Composites and Construction Materials

Crops such as fiber flax and fiber hemp are very interesting for diversifying agriculture as they require less pesticides and fertilizers than potato and sugar beet, which are the most important crops in The Netherlands. In order to introduce such agrofiber crops into the rotation scheme or to increase their area, novel non-textile applications must be developed. Potential and interesting applications of agrofibers are: agrofiber reinforced synthetic composite materials (thermoplastics and thermoset resins); fiber and particle boards; asbestos replacement in cement boards; insulating fiber mats (thermal and acoustic); filter materials; geotextiles.

Development of such innovative products is encouraging as the industry is interested in certain specific properties of these fibers. For instance, agrofibers show some advantages in the reinforcement of composites over glass fibers which are currently used. The low wear factor, low brittleness and low irritation factor are of interest to operator and production equipment, the high elasticity modulus and the low brittleness allow the composite to be moulded after the production process, which is usually not feasible with glass-fiber reinforced composites. Biodegradability and incinerability of agrofibers enables easy disposal of wastes or used-up composites; glass-fiber reinforced composites are more and more causing problems in this respect. Agrofibers may be price-competitive with glass-fiber. The prices of short and long flax fibers and hemp bast fibers vary between 0.2 and 3 US$/kg, the price of E-glass-fiber is 3 to 4 US$/kg. This shows that a margin for improvement/modification of the agrofibers may even exist.

Multidisciplinary (basic) research that is carried out in order to realize the novel applications includes the following topics:
1. Characterization of quality parameters from an industrial perspective. Agrofibers must meet the technical specifications demanded by industries. Standardized quality assessments are needed for enabling a guaranteed supply of constant quality and uniform batches of raw materials (Kessler et al. 1988). Important technical parameters for processing and end-use appear to be aspect ratio, tensile strength, and elasticity modulus (Table 1). The processing and compounding conditions are dependent on compatibility of fibers with the matrix, moisture content, and thermal stability. Among the performance demands of end products are durability (UV, chemical, and wear resistance), insulating capacity, dyeability and color fastness. These quality characteristics are dependent on the gross chemical composition (Table 2), especially the lignin content, and on the structures of the agrofibers, especially the crystallinity of the cellulose, and can be adapted to a certain extent, to meet the industrial demands.
2. Identification of preferences for different agrofiber crops is essential for estimating market potentials. For instance, aspect ratio (L/D) of fibers is important for final product quality of fiber reinforced composite materials. Table 1 shows that natural fibers from different crops vary strongly in their aspect ratios. Fiber flax and hemp show favorable ratios and are the more interesting fibers for advanced composites.

3. Physical and/or chemical modification of agrofibers. The performance of the fibers must sometimes be improved; examples include durability, water resistance, or compatibility with the synthetic (often hydrophobic) matrix. For efficiently developing modification methods, detailed studies on the chemical compositions and the structures have to be conducted. Table 3 shows the carbohydrate composition of fiber flax and fiber hemp. The glucose originates almost entirely from cellulose and the other monosaccharides from hemicellulose. Studies on the structure of the lignocellulose complex and the crystallinity of the cellulose are in progress.
4. Development or adaptation of process technologies for manufacturing agrofiber-reinforced products are carried out in close cooperation with industries; the latter are responsible for the economics and the marketing.

Primary Production and Processing of Oils from New Seed Crops

Yield potential of desired fatty acids. Crambe abyssinica Hochst, *Euphorbia lagascae* Spreng., *Limnanthes alba* Benth., and *Calendula officinalis* L. are potential new oilseed crops for which an increasing industrial interest exists (Haumann 1991; Hirsinger 1989; Sonntag 1991; Purdy and Craig 1987; Burg and Kleiman 1991). The oils contain valuable fatty acids and possess a number of other interesting chemical and physical properties (Muuse et al. 1992). However, as very little information was available on the optimization of the yield from these crops of the unusual primary fatty acids, studies were undertaken on the effect of sowing and harvesting dates on the yield of the primary fatty acids of these new oilseeds. For each new oilseed crop, three sowing dates with one month intervals were chosen starting at the end of March 1990 (Fig. 1). Seeds were harvested at early, medium, and late stages of seed development (expressed as thermal time after start of flowering) and analyzed for fatty acid composition and oil content.

Table 1. Dimensions and physical properties of technical and individual (ultimate cells) fibers from fiber flax, fiber hemp, jute, and sisal.

Characteristic	Fiber flax	Fiber hemp	Jute	Sisal
Length (mm)	200–1400	1000–3000	1500–3600	600–100
Diameter (mm)	0.4–062	---	0.03–0.14	0.1–0.46
Cell length [L](mm)	4–77	5–55	0.8–6	0.8–8
Cell width [D](mm)	0.005–0.076	0.01–0.051	0.005–0.025	0.007–0.047
Aspect ratio [L/D]	1000–2500	1000–1600	65–380	50–500
Specific gravity (kg/m^3)	1500	1500	1500	1450
Tensile strength (GN/m^2)	1.0	0.7	1.0	0.53
Elasticity modules (GN/m^2)	60	32	59	36
Break elongation (%)	2.5	2.2	1.5	2.0

Table 2. Gross chemical composition of fibers from fiber flax, fiber hemp, jute, sisal.

Fiber	Composition (% w/w)				
	Cellulose	Hemicellulose	Pectin	Lignin	Fats, wax
Flax	65–80	15–20	2–5	1–3	2–3
Hemp bast	60–75	12–18	---	1–4	2–4
Jute	64	12–16	1	12	0.4
Sisal	60–70	12–16	1	10	0.3

Within each sowing date, only slight differences were found in the contents of the primary fatty acids with respect to harvest time (Fig. 2). This means that fatty acid yield is not dependent on harvest time. On the contrary, when thermal times after start of flowering were compared, differences of up to 20% in seed fatty acid content were observed between the various sowing dates. The date of sowing is much more critical than the date of harvest to maximize primary fatty acid yield. The relatively low effect of harvest date on primary fatty acid yield is agronomically important for growing these crops in climatologically unstable countries such as The Netherlands. Consequently, the yield of seeds can be considered as an important and easy harvest criterion.

Dedicated down-stream processing of specific fatty acids. The seed oil of *Dimorphotheca pluvalis* L. contains over 60% of the interesting, but highly reactive, dimorphophecolic acid (C 18:2, 9-OH) (Muuse et al. 1992). This fatty acid can be used in the production of polymers and coatings. Conventional production of fatty acids (by Colgate-Emery or Twitchell processes) will lead to impure products and/or a high degree of degradation and loss of reactive groups, especially in case of the labile dimorphecolic acid. Therefore, a method is needed to specifically and mildly isolate the desired fatty acid from the oil. Since the fatty acid was shown to be primarily located on the α-positions of the triglycerides, the use of bioreactors containing immobilized 1,3-specific lipases will show many advantages in processing such new industrial oils (Derksen et al. 1991; Muuse et al. 1992). A prudent choice of membrane in bioreactor construction may enable simultaneous hydrolysis of triglycerides and extraction of the desired reaction products, thus promoting favorable reaction kinetics as well as easy down-stream processing.

Table 3. Carbohydrate composition of fibers from fiber flax (retted) and fiber hemp.

Fiber	Composition (% w/w)					
	Arabinose	Xylose	Mannose	Galactose	Rhamnose	Glucose
Flax	0.9	1.0	3.8	2.5	0.7	71.9
Hemp	0.7	1.5	2.3	1.7	0.4	66.7

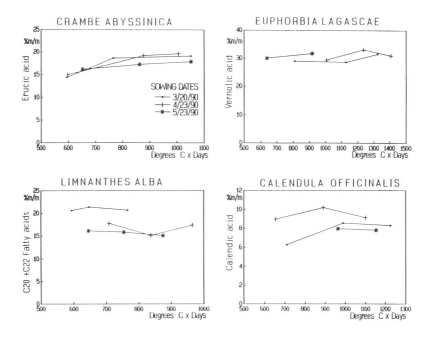

Fig. 1. Effect of sowing and harvest time on the yield of major (technical) fatty acids (% of dry seed weight) of four new oilseed crops: *Crambe abyssinica*, *Euphorbia lagascae*, *Limnanthes alba*, and *Calendula officinalis*. Time of seed development expressed as thermal time after start of flowering in degree (C) days.

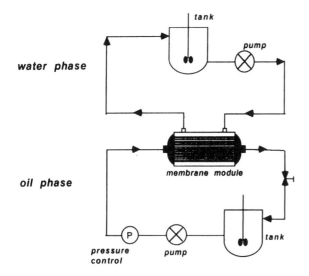

Fig. 2. Laboratory-scale hollow-fiber membrane bioreactor. Lipase (500 mg) immobilized on 1 m² of cellulose hollow-fiber membrane. Reaction temperature 25°C.

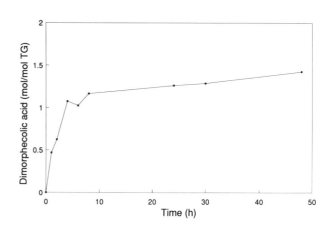

Fig. 3. Production of dimorphecolic acid (mol/mol triglyceride) from *Dimorphoteca* oil by enzymatic hydrolysis in a membrane bioreactor using *Rhizopus javanicus* lipase.

Fig. 2 schematically shows a membrane bioreactor system dedicated to processing *Dimorphoteca* oil. In the membrane module, *Rhizopus javanicus* lipase is immobilized on the lumen side of hydrophilic cellulose hollow-fibers, separating a water phase from an organic phase, as described by Pronk et al. (1988). Dilute *Dimorphotheca* oil (20% in hexane) is recirculated through the lumen of the reactor at 25°C. Triglycerides and liberated fatty acids mono-, and diglycerides were quantified (Muuse et al. 1992) by high-temperature capillary gas chromatography using octacosane and triheptadecanoin as internal standards. Dimorphecolic acid is liberated upon hydrolysis of *Dimorphoteca* oil in this membrane bioreactor system (Fig. 3). The initial reaction rate is high, but after 5 h the reaction rate decreases and hydrolysis runs at an equilibrium. As the lipases are immobilized onto the membrane and can remain active during a considerable period of time (reaction periods of over 300 h have been realized) multiple reuse of the enzyme is allowed.

The results show that lipases with 1,3-positional specificity can be employed for the production at mild conditions of unstable oxygenated fatty acids from new oil seed crops in pure form. Therefore, research is in progress to simultaneously hydrolyse the oil and recover the liberated dimorphecolic acid, thereby driving the hydrolysis reaction to completion. Such a system enables continuous processing of *Dimorphoteca* oil.

SUMMARY

The surpluses of agricultural commodities have generated a strongly growing interest in increasing the use of traditional crops and developing new crops for industrial applications. The EC has initiated large research programs directed to increasing the application of agricultural feedstocks in the (non-food) industry. In the Netherlands, the scope of research programs in this field includes the application of carbohydrates, oils, fibers, proteins, and secondary metabolites from arable crops. Strategies for finding and realizing new market-outlets for agriculture must include characterizing and exploiting the preferential properties of traditional and new industrial crops. Advantageous technical characteristics are being explored for fiber crops (flax and hemp) and new oilseed crops *Crambe abyssinica*, *Euphorbia lagascae*, *Limnanthes alba*, and *Calendula officinalis*, and new processing technologies are being developed.

REFERENCES

Burg, D.A. and R. Kleiman. 1991. Preparation of meadowfoam dimer acids and dimer esters, and their use as lubricants. J. Amer. Oil Chem. Soc. 68:600–603.

Derksen, J.T.P., G. Boswinkel, and W.M.J. Van Gelder. 1991. Lipase-catalyzed hydrolysis of triglycerides from new oil crops for oleochemical industries, p. 377–380. In: L. Alberghina, R.D. Schmid, and R. Verger (eds.). Lipases, structure, mechanism and genetic engineering. VCH Publishers, New York.

Haumann, B.F. 1991. Work continues on new oils for industrial use. Inform 2:678–692.

Hissinger, F. 1989. New annual oil crops, p. 518–532. In: G. Röbbelen, R.K. Downey, and A. Ashri (eds.). Oil crops of the world. McGraw-Hill, New York.

Kessler, R.W., A. Blum, and G. Werner. 1988. Entwiklung objektiver. Qualitätskriterien für Flachs Teil 1: Chemische und Morfologische Untersuchungen. Melliand Textilberichte 12:854–858.

Muuse, B.G., F.P. Cuperus, and J.T.P. Derksen. 1992. Composition and technical properties of oils from new oilseed crops. Ind. Crops. Prod. 1:(in press).

Pronk, W., P.J.A.M. Kerkhof, C. Van Helden, and K. Van 't Riet. 1988. Biotechnol. Bioengin. 32:512–518.

Purdy, R.H. and C.D. Craig. 1987. Meadowfoam: New source of long-chain fatty acids. J. Amer. Oil Chem. Soc. 64:1493–1498.

Rexen, F. 1991. Industrial crops—EC research strategies, p. 12. In: Abstract book First European Symposium on industrial crops and products. Maastricht, 25–27 Nov. 1991.

Sonntag, N.O.V. 1991. Erucic, bekenic: feedstocks of the 21st century. Inform 2:449–463.

Potential New Specialty Crops from Asia: Azuki Bean, Edamame Soybean, and Astragalus

T.A. Lumpkin, J.C. Konovsky, K.J. Larson, and D.C. McClary

Agricultural exports help to maximize the utilization of United States agricultural potential, strengthen the overall economy, and improve the balance of trade. For example, Japan imports about $23 billion worth of agricultural commodities each year, about $8 billion from the United States. Major agricultural exports like wheat and soybeans, which are in surplus on the world market, comprise only a small portion of the value of Japan's agricultural imports. About 60% of Japan's $23 billion in food imports are niche market commodities, many having potential for development as new crops and value-added exports from the United States. Niche markets for agricultural commodities common in Pacific Rim countries (e.g. Japan, Korea, Taiwan), but not important on a worldwide basis, have received relatively little attention from United States researchers or food corporations. This paper presents information on two of the numerous East Asian crops that have niche market export potential. In addition, many East Asian crops have potential for use as forage, fodder, and soil reclamation within the United States. The East Asian Crop Development Program of the IMPACT Center at Washington State University studies some of these East Asian crops, including azuki bean, edamame vegetable soybean, and *Astragalus adsurgens* Pall.

AZUKI BEAN

Botany

Azuki seeds are subcylindric with subtruncated ends with a length of 5.0 to 9.1 mm, width of 4.0 to 6.3 mm, thickness of 4.1 to 6.0 mm, and weight of 50 to 250 mg/seed (McClary 1990). Much of the size variability among cultivars can be attributed to the development of two distinct market classes in Japan, regular-sized (>4.2 mm length) and a larger dainagon type (>4.8 mm length) (Hoshikawa 1985). The seed has a smooth seed coat, a strongly defined cotyledonary ridge, and an elevated micropyle. The white azuki hilum is 2.4 to 3.3 mm long and 0.6 to 0.8 mm wide. Seed colors range from a common solid maroon to solid black, blue-black, grey, brown, straw, white, and various mottled combinations of these.

Seedlings emergence is hypogeal; seed leaves are cordate, long-petioled, and simple. The plant is a bushy, usually erect and slightly pubescent annual that grows from 27 to 90 cm high. Some azuki cultivars exhibit viney growth and can climb from 1 to 3 m. Stem color is normally green but some cultivars are purplish. Branching occurs between the 4th to 9th main stem nodes (Hoshikawa 1985) and secondary branching does not occur under normal planting densities.

Stipules are small, entire or faintly 3-lobed, peltate, lanceolate, acuminate, and have basal appendages. The leaf is pinnately trifoliate with the middle leaflet being broadly ovate and attached to the petiole by a long petiolule; leaflets are 5 to 8 cm wide and 5 to 10 cm long. Some cultivars produce lanceolate-shaped leaflets (Hoshikawa 1985).

Azuki has a taproot type of root system that can extend in a sphere 40 to 50 cm from the point of seed germination; secondary branch development occurs later in the season and can reach 40 cm. Root nodules resulting from cowpea group rhizobium infections are spherical, 4 to 10 mm in diameter, and begin developing when primary leaves start to unfold (Hoshikawa 1985).

Azuki flowers are bright yellow, have hairy styles, flattened stigmas, and an asymmetrical keel that curves to the left and has a hornlike appendage on one side. Inflorescence and flower primordium start developing 23 and 21 days before anthesis, respectively; anthesis normally starts in the morning and can continue for up to 40 days (Hoshikawa 1985). Racemes are axillary, borne on long pedicels on higher parts of the plant and short-subsessile pedicels on the lower parts, and consist of from 6 to 20 flowers. Floral development progresses upward with anthesis beginning on lower main stem nodes and branches first.

Azuki pods are smooth, cylindrical, thin-walled, and green turning white to grey as they mature. Pods hang down and are restricted between seeds when mature. They are 6 to 13 cm long, 0.5 cm in diameter, with 2 to 14 seeds/pod, 2 to 6 pods/pedicel, and 5 to 40 pods/plant. Maturation is indeterminate but, 85% of all pods mature at about the same time. Pod shatter during seed ripening and harvesting is a problem under certain conditions. Components of yield were reported by Nakaseko (1983) to range from 53.4 to 81.2 pods/plant, 1.0 to 1.67 pods/node, 5.1 to 7.5 seeds/pod, and 31.8 to 74.4 g dry seed yield/plant for six cultivars.

Production

Azuki is or could be grown in ecosystems with between 530 to 1730 mm of annual precipitation, a 7.8° to 27.8°C range in mean annual air temperature, a soil pH between 5.0 to 7.5 and up to 48°N latitude (Duke 1981). However, current sites of major azuki production are between 40 to 45°N.

Almost all production of azuki occurs in four countries: Japan, China, Taiwan, and South Korea. Other past or present azuki producing countries include Australia, the Philippines, Japan, the Republic of Congo, Thailand, India, Italy, New Zealand, USSR, China, Belgium, United States, Brazil, Argentina, Malaysia, Kenya, Zaire, and Angola.

Japan produces about 90,000 t of azuki each year on about 64,000 ha, of which 60% is on the island prefecture of Hokkaido. Yields average about 1,500 kg/ha in Japan but can vary widely, especially on Hokkaido, depending mostly upon the length of the growing season, accumulated degree days and weather conditions.

The main site of Chinese production occurs in Wuging county, Hebei province, with 4,000 to 5,000 ha annually. Other azuki producing areas are western Jilin province, Tai Lai county of Heilongjiang province, north of the Huaihe River and near Qinling. In Taiwan, azuki is an important winter crop grown in rice paddies, especially in Pingtung and Kaohsiung provinces which account for 98% of all Taiwanese production. Azuki is one of the four most important grain legumes produced in South Korea in terms of planted area and production. Production is scattered throughout the country, usually on hill-side land in rotation with wheat and barley or some in converted paddy fields.

Azuki is believed to have been introduced into the United States by the Perry expedition in 1854. Piper and Morse (1914) provided a list of early introductions of azuki into the United States. The United States has never been a major world producer of azuki although the crop has been grown experimentally and/or on a limited production scale in several states over the past 130 years. Early adaptation experiments were conducted in Kansas, Virginia, and North Carolina, and it was used as a green fodder crop in some southern sections of the country (Hoshikawa 1985; Sacks 1977).

Uses

Azuki has been consumed in East Asia for over 2,000 years in a myriad of ways that take advantage of the seed's maroon color and delicate flavor; it is traditionally served on festive days such as weddings, birthdays, or New Year parties (McClary et al. 1989). Azuki is made into a sweet confectionery paste (*an*), candied whole beans (*amanatto*), a component of sweet soups (*zenzai* and *sarashi ame*), a mixture with rice (*azuki-mochi* and *sekihan*), sprouts (*moyashi*), or flour.

The most common use of azuki is the sweetened paste form called *an*. Azuki *an*, either in a smooth or chunky form, is used in numerous East Asian foods and desserts such as cakes, *manju* (steamed *an*-filled buns), *yokan* (cold gelatinized *an* slices), *taiyaki* (*an*-filled waffle), ice cream, snow cone toppings, and as a base for a beverage served hot from vending machines (*Shiruko*). About 30% of all *an* is used by the Japanese and Korea ice cream industries. *An* can also be flavored with soy sauce or with sweet syrups. A white seeded azuki is also used to make high quality white *an* for specialty Japanese bakery products (Narikawa 1972).

Azuki *an* is produced from seed by the following generalized steps: soaking, boiling, rinsing with water to remove antidigestive compounds, crushing, removal of seed coats, drying, and then combined with sugar and various stabilizing ingredients such as agar agar (Duke 1981). Traditional *an* is composed of equal parts azuki paste and sugar. Rice beans and various common beans are occasionally substituted for azuki in Japanese *an* production, but azuki is the preferred seed for high quality *an* (McClary et al. 1989). *An* can substitute for other traditional Western-style fillings and flavorings in sweet rolls, donuts, and ice cream. Japanese azuki consumption is currently broken down into the following categories: *an* paste (68.9%), candied seeds (12.8%), boiled seeds (2.4%) and other (15.9%) (Japan Bean Fund Assoc. 1987). In the mid 1970s, 85% of Japanese domestic production and imports of azuki were being used in the production of *an*.

EDAMAME SOYBEAN

Botany

Edamame is a specialty soybean [*Glycine max* (L.) Merrill] harvested as a vegetable when the seeds are at the immature R6 stage and have expanded to fill 80 to 90% of the pod width. The botany of edamame is similar to the field soybean except for minor morphological and physiological differences (Konovsky et al. 1992).

Production

Immature soybean seeds are consumed as vegetables in almost every country that produces soybeans. In Japan, China, Korea, and Taiwan special cultivars of soybeans were selected for the eating quality of their immature seeds. These edamame cultivars of soybean can be transplanted or direct seeded. In Japan, transplants are used in forced and early production systems (Kono 1986). Forced production occurs in CO_2 enriched, heated greenhouses. Planting starts in November and production ends with the last harvest in July. Early spring field production starts in February with the planting of seedling nurseries. Seedlings are transplanted in to small plastic tunnels 25 to 30 days later and harvested by the end of July. Regular field production begins in March and ends by October. Early summer demand pressures farmers to harvest as early as possible to obtain higher prices, therefore the onset of harvest is being continually advanced through improved crop management and cultivar development.

Most edamame is harvested by hand. When edamame is sold on the stem, plants are hand cut or pulled out with roots intact, unacceptable pods and lower leaves are culled, and branches are tied together in small, aesthetically pleasing bundles. For sale of harvested pods, plants are cut and pods stripped off, sorted, and packaged. In Japan, electrical powered, stationary pod strippers are available and in Taiwan, an Italian single row bean picker is being tested (Konovsky et al. 1992). Initial studies on mechanical harvesting have been conducted in Tennessee (Collins and McCarty 1969) and at INTSOY (1987). For frozen product, standard methods for processing have been described (Liu and Shanmugasundaram 1982).

Japan is the largest commercial producer, nearly 105,000 t in 1988 (MAFF 1990), and the largest importer, over 33,000 t in 1989 (JTA 1989). Taiwan supplies over 99% of those imports as frozen edamame. Almost all Japanese production is consumed as fresh product during the summer months (Kono 1986). Other countries which have produced commercial quantities of edamame include Argentina, Australia, Israel, Mongolia, New Zealand, Taiwan, and Thailand. Home gardeners are known to produce it in Bhutan, Brazil, Britain, Chile, France, Germany, Indonesia, Malaysia, Nepal, Philippines, Singapore, and Sri Lanka (after Wang et al. 1979).

Uses

In most of East Asia, vegetable soybeans are harvested and sold as pods-on-stems, loose pods, or shelled beans (*mao dou* in China, *edamame* in Japan, and *poot kong* in Korea). The pods-on-stems form is no longer commonly consumed in China or Korea, but is still a popular form in Japan, partially because appearance and flavor factors decline more slowly after harvest while pods remain attached to the stem. In China, vegetable soybeans are usually cooked as shelled immature seeds, but sold in the pod or shelled; they are used primarily as an ingredient in stir fry dishes. In Korea, the beans are added to rice and cooked together (*pub mi kong*). In Japan, vegetable soybeans are usually sold as loose pods, occasionally on the stem, and rarely shelled, although shelled forms have been used to make a sweetened paste (*zunda*) and edamame tofu.

Edamame is consumed mainly as a snack, but is also used as a vegetable, an addition to soups, or processed into sweets. As a snack, the pods are lightly cooked in salted, boiling water and then consumed by pushing the seeds directly from the pods into the mouth with the fingers. As a vegetable, the beans are mixed into salads, stir fried, or combined with mixed vegetables. In soup (*gojiru* in Japanese), the beans are ground into a paste with miso and is used to form a thick broth. Confectionery products such as sticky rice topped with sweetened edamame paste are occasionally prepared (*zunda mochi* in Japanese). For marketing, edamame pods are sold fresh on the stem with leaves and roots, or stripped from the stem and packaged fresh or frozen as either pods or beans.

In North America, edamame is usually called vegetable soybean, but also beer bean, edible soybean, fresh green soybean, garden soybean, green soybean, green vegetable soybean, immature soybean, large-seeded soybean, vegetable-type soybean, and the Japanese name, edamame (Shurtleff pers. commun.). The use of the word green is confusing because mature soybean seeds with a green seed coat or cotyledons are also called green soybeans.

Edamame research as been conducted in the United States for over 50 years. Dorsett and Morse collected extensive germplasm from 1929 to 1931, and Morse used it to develop 49 cultivars of edamame (Hymowitz 1984). Research flourished during the 1930s and 1940s because of a protein shortage (Smith and Van Duyne 1951). A second surge of research began with the interest in organic farming in the 1970s. The Rodale Research Center focused edamame research on adaptability and quality (Hass et al. 1982). Basic agronomic research was begun at Cornell (Kline 1980) and seed companies developed new cultivars, e.g. 'Butterbeans'. Today, some home gardeners grow edamame, but there is little commercial production. Asian-Americans seeking edamame are usually limited to frozen imports in specialty supermarkets.

ASTRAGALUS

Botany

Astragalus adsurgens Pall, Fabaceae (upstanding milkvetch, green great wall astragalus, or *sha da wang* which means flourishes in sand storms, in Chinese) is a perennial plant distributed throughout northern and southwestern China and northern North America. It is very cold tolerant and well suited for high temperature, arid to semi-arid regions with poor or saline soils, previously considered wastelands. Its deep tap root system can access water from deep within the soil profile. In sandy, arid areas of China, it is cultivated for fodder, green manure and is used for soil conservation.

Plants have several stems which grow to a height of 1.5 to 2.0 m, and are covered with compound pinnate leaves having T-shaped soft hairs. The primary root is thick and long with many lateral roots. The secondary root system begins 20 to 30 cm below the soil surface and can attain 150 cm in width. Rhizobium nodules develop on the upper portions of the roots near the soil surface.

Seedlings grow slowly, averaging 0.5 cm daily, the first year. Once established, its growth exceeds that of competing weeds. Rapid growth continues from the second to fourth year, primarily in May and June (1 cm daily).

Plants will reach a height of 70+ cm and tiller during July and August, reaching a final height of 105 to 110 cm with 20 to 25 tillers.

Flowers bloom throughout August. Some racemes are apical, but most are axillary. Inflorescences are indeterminate and have 17 to 79 small blue, purple or blue-purple papilionaceous flowers. Pod development is evident 2 or 3 days following bloom and pods are square in cross-section, consisting of two chambers with 10 dark brown seeds per chamber and are 6 to 13 mm long with a bent beak-shaped top. Seed development begins 7 days post-anthesis (Barneby 1964).

Production

An estimated 670,000 ha of potential grasslands were aerially sown between 1979 and 1986 with *A. adsurgens* seed in China (Ning et al. 1984b). The seed is pelletized along with Rhizobium in a peat medium. The pelleted seed is then aerial sown in sandy, semi-arid regions to promote vegetative growth. These pastures of mixed forbes traditionally feed camels, sheep, and goats.

Studies on forage yield and quality, along with seed production have shown that *A. adsurgens* is capable of producing 75 t/ha of coarse, fresh fodder. The crop can be harvested 2 or 3 times yearly beginning the second year. Crude protein values range from 12 to 14% and crude fiber range from 27 to 30%. Profuse seed production continued even under semi-arid growing conditions. The *A. adsurgens* planted at Pullman, Washington has been growing successfully for five years under 500 mm mean annual rainfall.

A superior Rhizobium strain, CA 8116, was identified for *A. adsurgens* (Ning et al. 1984a,b). Plants inoculated with CA 8116 increased nodulation from 27 to 47% at the first leaf stage, while, total biomass increased by 81%.

Uses

Chinese research focuses on soil conservation and livestock feeding trials. Feeding trials have included but are not limited to pigs (Chen et al. 1987) and broiler chickens (Lei et al. 1987). Studies have shown comparable growth on pigs and chickens when fed limited quantities (4% for broilers and 20% for pigs) of *A. adsurgens* meal incorporated in daily diet rations as compared to alfalfa meal. No signs of toxicity were noted in the liver and kidney or blood glucose levels. These studies are significant, as both species are non-ruminant animals and require greater care in daily diets as compared to sheep and cattle, both ruminants.

CONCLUSIONS

Both edamame and azuki share a common challenge to their development as viable new crops: the lack of adequate information about the cultivation and processing required to produce products that satisfy the quality conscious Japanese market. Edamame production is similar to soybean production, but there are unique cultivars and management practices used in Japan that enhance its quality. The management practices are not well documented in English-language journals. A small literature review on azuki was prepared by Sacks (1977), but left many questions concerning cultivation and processing unanswered. There is an extensive body of literature in Japanese about azuki that has been reviewed in a book (Lumpkin and McClary 1992). By drawing on Japanese research, the development of these two Japanese crops as new crops in the United States can be hastened.

Edamame and azuki each face other issues related to quality. Japanese consumers show a strong preference for the taste and other qualities of Japanese cultivars of edamame over those from Taiwan or the United States. The edamame germplasm collection of 600 accessions at Washington State University (WSU) will be used to develop cultivars well suited to the Pacific Northwest climate with the qualities the Japanese desire.

For azuki, there are no industry standards for the quality of *an* paste in the United States and a very poor understanding of Japanese quality standards. While a rudimentary understanding of the general process and technology required for paste production was obtained on a tour of azuki facilities, quality issues are being studied at WSU to find quantifiable characters. Future United States *an* paste production will depend upon our understanding and meeting Japanese quality standards.

The introduction of two new crops to the Pacific Northwest will further diversify United States agricultural exports away from surplus commodities. With proper research, the potential exists for United States producers to capture a large share of the Japanese and Korean market for imported azuki and edamame. Market analyses for both commodities indicate a consistent opportunity for export of high quality raw and processed products to Japan (Cook 1988). A market study by our research group on azuki has just been completed and is available from the IMPACT Center at Washington State University (McClary et al. 1989). Several East Asian countries cannot meet their own needs for many niche crops and the long-term demand in the marketplace is stable, thus the United States has the opportunity to export products needed in foreign markets if they are of higher quality and more competitively priced than current imported.

New East Asian crops should also be considered for solving environmental problems within the United States Chinese selections of *A. adsurgens* were recently introduced into the United States. Although limited research has been conducted within the United States thus far, the plant holds great potential for restoration and conservation in cold arid regions where soil erosion is a problem.

REFERENCES

Barneby, R. 1964. Atlas of North American astragalus part II. Mem. New York Bot. Gard. Vol. 13.

Chen, W.Z., M. Ni, F. Li, and H. Liu. 1987. Feeding effects of various ratio of ground fodder from alfalfa, *Astragalus adsurgens* Pall, and *Sesbania cannabina* in pig's daily rations. China Grassland 4(4):12–16.

Collins, J.L. and I.E. McCarty. 1969. Handling of vegetable soybeans mechanically. Soybean Dig. 12:20–21.

Cook, A.K. 1988. The evolution of Japanese food spending patterns: 1963–1984. Washington State University, IMPACT Center Rpt 26. Pullman.

Duke, J.A. 1981. *Vigna angularis* (Willd.) Ohwi & Ohashi, p. 288–293. In: Handbook of legumes of world economic importance. Plenum Press, New York.

Haas, P.W., L.C. Gilbert, and A.D. Edwards. 1982. Fresh green soybeans: analysis of field performance and sensory qualities. Rodale, Emmaus.

Hoshikawa, K. 1985. Azuki beans (in Japanese), p. 460–471. In: Edible crops. Yokendo Publisher, Tokyo.

Hymowitz, T. 1984. Dorsett-Morse soybean collection trip to East Asia: A 50 year perspective. Econ. Bot. 38:378–88.

INTSOY. 1987. INTSOY research focuses on green soybeans as commercial frozen vegetable. INTSOY Newsletter 37:1–2.

Japan Bean Fund Association. 1987. Information on miscellaneous beans (in Japanese). (July) Tokyo.

Japan Tariff Association (JTA). 1989. Japan exports and imports. Tokyo.

Kline, W.L. 1980. The effect of intra and interrow spacing on yield components of vegetable soybeans. MS Thesis, Cornell Univ., Ithaca, NY.

Kono, S. 1986. Edamame, p. 195–243. In: K. Tanaka, E. Ishida, S. Kono, and M. Kohata (eds.). Methods of bean production (Sakukei o Ikasu Mamerui no Tsukurikata). Nosangyoson Bunka Kyokai, Tokyo.

Konovsky, J., T.A. Lumpkin, S. Shanmugasundaram, and T.S.C. Tsou. 1992. Edamame: the vegetable soybean. Asian Vegetable Research and Development Center, Tainan, Taiwan.

Lei, Z.Y., Z. Zhang, X. Feng, and J. Wang. 1987. The effects of feeding diets containing *Astragalus adsurgens* Pall. and *Coronilla varia* L. on broiler chickens. Acta Veterinaria Zootechnica Sinica. 18(3):157–162

Liu, C. and S. Shanmugasundaram. 1982. Frozen vegetable soybean industry in Taiwan, p. 199–212. In: M.C. Ali and L.E. Siong (eds.). Vegetables and ornamentals in the tropics. Univ. Pertanian Malaysia, Serdang.

Lumpkin, T.A. and D.C. McClary. 1992. Azuki bean: botany, production and uses. Commonwealth Agr. Bureau Int., Oxon, UK.

McClary, D.C. 1990. Azuki, *Vigna angularis* (Willd.) Ohwi & Ohashi: A literature review and agronomic evaluations for production in the Columbia Basin. MS Thesis, Washington State Univ., Pullman.

McClary, D.C., T.L. Raney, and T.A. Lumpkin. 1989. Japanese food marketing channels: a case study of azuki beans and azuki products. Washington State Univ., IMPACT Center Rpt. 29. Pullman.

Ministry of Agriculture, Forestry, and Fisheries (MAFF). 1990. Statistical handbook. Norinsuisansho, Tokyo.

Nakaseko, K. 1983. Studies on dry matter production, plant type, and productivity in grain legumes (in Japanese, English summary). Ann. Hokkaido Univ. Agr. Dept. 14(2):103–158.

Narikawa, T. 1972. Kidney bean and azuki bean in Japan with reference to breeding in Hokkaido, p. 179–188. In: Symposium on food legumes: Proc. Symposium on Tropical Agriculture Researches, 12–14 September 1972. Trop.Agr. Res. Ser. 6.

Ning, G.Z., Y. Li, Y. Wu, Y. Huang, and D. Yu. 1984a. Selection and application of rhizobium astragalus. J. Soil Fert. 6:35–36. Inst. Soil Fert., Chinese Acad. Agr. Sci., Beijing.

Ning, G.Z., Y. Li, Y. Wu, Y. Huang, and D. Yu. 1984b. Study on the characterization and application of rhizobium strain CA 8116 (*Astragalus adsurgens* Pall). J. Soil Fert. 6:37–38. Inst. Soil Fert., Chinese Acad. Agr. Sci., Beijing.

Piper, C.V. and W.J. Morse. 1914. Five oriental species of beans. U.S. Dept. Agr. Bul. 119:1–32.

Sacks, F.M. 1977. A literature review of *Phaseolus angularis*—the adzuki bean. Econ. Bot. 31:9-15.

Smith, J.M. and F.O. Van Duyne. 1951. Other soybean products, p. 1055–1078. In: K.S. Markley (ed.). Soybeans and soybean products. Vol. 2. Interscience, New York.

Wang, H.L., G.C. Mustakas, W.J. Wolf, L.C. Wang, C.W. Hesseltine, and E.B. Bagley. 1979. Soybeans as human food—unprocessed and simply processed. U.S. Dept. Agr. Utilization Rpt. 5.

New Crop Development in New Zealand

James A. Douglas*

New Zealand lies between the 33° to 53° south latitudes in the South Pacific about 1,600 km east of Australia. It consists of two main islands similar in size to Japan or the British Isles. The climate is temperate and dominated by a westerly wind flow within an oceanic environment that gives a weather pattern which is changeable over short periods. In the southern main island a mountain chain exceeding 3,000 m in height modifies the weather pattern. The country as a whole is subject to extremes of wind and rain with annual rainfall varying from below 400 mm to over 12,000 mm in the Southern alps. Summer droughts are common in many areas and all regions of the country experience frost except the northern part of the North Island.

New Zealand has been settled by Europeans for 170 years with the total population now 3.3 million. About 18 million hectares are occupied with pastoral farming being the major form of land use. In 1988, New Zealand had 65 million sheep, 8 million beef and dairy cattle, 1.3 million goats, and 0.6 million farmed deer. Primary products from these stock, forestry products, fruit and vegetables, and fish make up 64% of the New Zealand export trade of $NZ15 billion ($NZ = 0.59 US$, 1991). The important point about this trade is that, with the exception of fish, it is based on animals and plants which have been introduced into New Zealand over the past 150 years. The pastoral industry is based on the European pasture species perennial ryegrass (*Lolium perenne* L.) and white clover (*Trifolium repens* L.), the forestry industry on the Monterey pine (*Pinus radiata* D. Don) from coastal California, and the fruit industry on the Eurasian apple (*Malus* ×*domestica* Borkh.) and the kiwifruit [*Actinidia deliciosa* (A. Chev.) C.F. Liang & A.R. Ferg.] from China.

NEW CROP PROGRAM

The wide range of climatic variation in New Zealand from low to high rainfall, cool temperate to marginally subtropical gives a capacity to grow a very wide range of crops. The difficulty has been to narrow down the number of potential crops from those which are environmentally feasible to those which are profitable. To do this, the focus has been moved from examining what crops will grow in New Zealand to using market intelligence to identify crops with defined international or niche market opportunities and then working back to the feasibility of production in New Zealand. Published information about target markets has been used to identify growth areas

---

*I thank M.H. Douglas, J.M. Follett, I.R. Hall, A. Richardson, and B.M. Smallfield for providing information from their individual programs.

within markets but often this information is too generalized to identify specific crops. Consequently, these desk studies have been followed up by commissioned within market investigations to gather the detailed information required to identify crops which have established markets but which are not currently grown in New Zealand. Available literature has been collected on each crop to characterize their environmental requirements and assess the likely adaptation to New Zealand conditions. Target crops are sourced, plant material imported, and grown in preliminary trials to assess their local environmental adaptation and their ability to produce the product required by the market place. Crop samples are sent to the target markets to assess the quality standard and market acceptability. Crops which exhibit potential proceed to more sophisticated trials with a greater selection of cultivars to determine their specific environmental, agronomic, and postharvest requirements to optimize yield and quality parameters.

The new crops program is carried out at a number of research stations which span the major island environments (Fig. 1). Climatic recordings from these research stations or close by, listed in Table 1, indicate the temperate nature of the New Zealand environment. In summer, temperatures above 30°C are uncommon and in winter, snow is normally only a one or two day phenomena in the southern regions. There are six programs: new export vegetable crops; European and Asian medicinal herbs; culinary herbs and essential oils; edible fungi; fruit; nuts; and ornamentals.

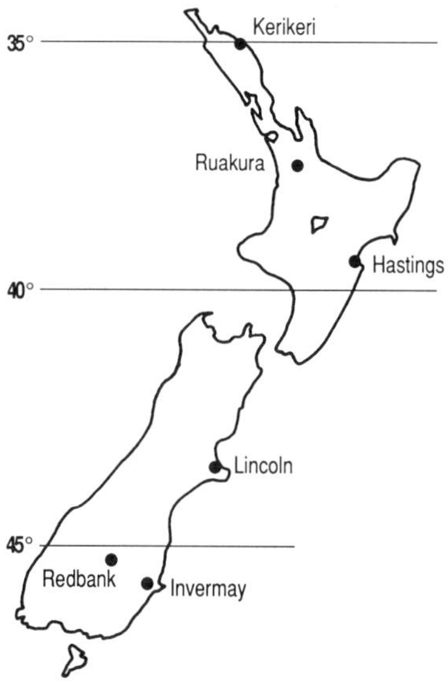

Fig. 1. Location of research stations involved in the New Zealand new crop program.

Table 1. Climatic observations relevant to each research station shown on Fig. 1.

Research station	Rainfall (mm)	Mean air temp. (°C)	Avg. daily range (°C)	Mean Jan. air temp. (°C)	Mean July air temp. (°C)	No. degree days above 10°C	No. air frost free days
Redbank	360	10.1	13.4	16.5	2.5	889	112
Invermay	691	10.2	10.7	14.7	5.0	791	195
Lincoln	666	11.4	10.5	16.5	5.8	1067	206
Hastings	764	13.9	10.5	19.1	8.4	1317	189
Ruakura	1201	13.3	11.2	17.8	8.3	1376	228
Kerikeri	1682	15.1	10.1	18.9	10.8	1912	603

NEW EXPORT VEGETABLES

Research on new export vegetables has concentrated on investigating the requirements of the Japanese market. Already, New Zealand exports significant volumes of squash, asparagus, and onions to Japan. Traditional Japanese vegetables, which are not widely known outside Japan, have strong internal demand. The possibility of growing such vegetables in New Zealand and exporting them to Japan provide the basis of this program. New Zealand has many climatic features similar to Japan and is environmentally suitable to produce Japanese vegetables. The major constraint is the need to choose vegetables which have sufficient shelf life so that they can be freighted to Japan in good condition.

Subsequent to an examination of Japanese market information, two crops, wasabi [*Wasabia japonica* (Miq.) Matsumara] and myoga ginger (*Zingiber mioga* Roscoe), were identified as having strong market potential. Research began on wasabi in 1982 and myoga in 1983.

Wasabi

Wasabi or Japanese horseradish is a native perennial crucifer of Japan which is used as a traditional condiment of Japanese food. It requires specific conditions of light and water to thrive. In Japan, the highest quality fresh product is grown on tree shaded, terraced gravel beds covered by a thin layer of cool running water from mountain streams or on artificially shaded mounded gravel ridges formed in larger river beds (Hodge 1974; Follett 1986). Lower quality wasabi for processing is grown in soil.

Wasabi plants grow poorly in New Zealand in full sunlight and artificial shading is required to keep the light levels below 700 μmol m^{-2} s^{-1} otherwise the plant is liable to wilt. Japanese recommendations of using 50% shade cloth were inadequate under New Zealand conditions and a further 30% shade cloth was required during the summer. Further research on the shade requirement of wasabi is needed.

The initial New Zealand trials on wasabi were established in large concrete troughs filled with rock and gravel similar to the tatami ishi wasabi beds of Shizuoka, Japan. Spring water of 13° to 14°C was flowed over the beds at about 160 liters/min. Unrooted cuttings were planted at 25 cm centers and the crop grown for two years. Sequential harvests from 15 months indicated that there was a need to leave the crop at least 18 months before harvest to achieve a reasonable production of stems over 50 g (Table 2).

Wasabi has a number of major pests and diseases and is known to suffer from various mosaic viruses which can cause rapid crop decline if successive crops are grown from infected sideshoot cuttings. Regular spraying is required to control aphids and white cabbage butterfly caterpillars. Leaf diseases such as white rust (*Albugo* sp.) are also controlled by foliar sprays but the more difficult diseases to control include the stem and root fungal diseases, *Phoma* and *Botrytis* and bacterial softrot, *Erwinia*. Control of these diseases is largely unresolved in the natural running water systems.

Considerable progress has been made in New Zealand in the past 5 years on how to grow wasabi to produce a marketable crop, but it is only the beginning. A greater understanding of the physiology of the crop in relation to its environmental requirements, improved cultivars, and better disease control should all allow higher yields and more efficient production methods to be developed. Research in these areas is underway.

Table 2. The effect of crop age on the stem yield of wasabi.

Harvest time (mo.)	Mean stem wt (g)	Total stem wt/plant (g)	Stems/plant >50 g	Stem yield (t/ha)		
				<20 g	20-50 g	>50 g
15	14	192	0.44	8	11	3
18	20	266	1.38	7	8	10
22	22	296	1.41	5	8	7

Myoga Ginger

Myoga ginger (*Zingiber mioga* Roscoe), a cold tolerant member of the ginger family (Zingiberaceae), is a native perennial of Japan grown as a traditional Japanese vegetable for its spring shoots or its summer/autumn flower buds. The production of flower buds is highly seasonal and consequently there is an opportunity for a southern hemisphere producer such as New Zealand to supply myoga to Japan when their supplies are low.

Preliminary research on myoga was conducted in New Zealand by Palmer (1984) and following an investigation of Japanese production systems (Follett 1986) further plants were introduced. The plant is established vegetatively from rhizome sections with faster and more even plant emergence from coolstored rhizomes (Follett 1991). The plant is frost sensitive and dies down in winter but the dormant rhizomes have proved to be quite winter hardy (Palmer 1984). Myoga is vigorous and largely disease and pest free when grown on free draining soils, although rhizome rotting from *Fusarium* and *Pythium* species has been noted on poorer drained soils. Under New Zealand conditions, myoga topgrowth sunburns and becomes chlorotic without shading and consequently trials have been established under 50% shade cloth. A comparison is presently being made between artificial shade and natural shade given by spaced Paulownia (*Paulownia elongata* S.Y. Hu) trees.

Myoga production beds established with 30 cm between rhizomes and 1 m between rows have yielded 6.75 t/ha of flower buds in the second year. This is comparable to Japanese production levels. The flower buds develop from underground stems on the edge of the plant mass and to achieve top quality produce, the buds should be picked before they emerge and turn green. To facilitate this, a 10 cm layer of sawdust was applied so that the buds could be located by fossicking and picked. Picking was carried out every 2 to 3 days over a 2 month period.

Myoga is a very new crop in New Zealand with little grown commercially. There remains considerable research to be undertaken in defining its agronomic management but research results to date and the successful test marketing of New Zealand grown myoga indicate that it is likely to be a successful new crop for New Zealand.

Medicinal Herbs

There is a large and expanding international market for medicinal herbs and plants for the manufacture of pharmaceuticals (Principe 1989). New Zealand has no significant production of these products although in the late 1970s commercial extraction of solasodine from the native *Solanum* species (*S. aviculare* Forst., *S. laciniatum* Ait.) was begun but later abandoned (Mann 1978; Mann et al. 1985). Nevertheless, the New Zealand environment provides good conditions for the growth of a wide range of medicinal herbs and in many instances they are familiar as weeds. Examples include dandelion (*Taraxacum officinale* G. Weber), St John's wort (*Hypericum perforatum* L.), horehound (*Marrubium vulgare* L.), burdock (*Arctium lappa* L.), Variegated thistle [*Silybum marianum* (L.) Gaertner], briar rose (*Rosa rugosa* Thunb.), and hawthorn (*Crataegus monogyna* Jacq.).

The current research program is focussed on understanding the agronomic requirements of seven medicinal herbs: coneflower [*Echinacea purpurea* (L.) Moench], valerian (*Valeriana officinalis* L.), *Arnica montana* L., dandelion, feverfew (*Chrysanthemum parthenium* Pers.), goldenseal (*Hydrastis canadensis* L.), and ginseng (*Panax ginseng* C.A. Mey., *P. quinquefolius* L.). Test marketing of samples from preliminary research on valerian, dandelion, rosehips, and chamomile [*Chamomilla recutita* (L.) Rauschert] has already shown that these crops can be produced to international market standards. Collections of a wide range of European and Asian medicinal herbs are being assembled for preliminary evaluation of both their growth potential and quality assessment before proceeding to more sophisticated agronomic programs. A Plant Extracts Research Unit provides the quality assessment of the medicinal herbs and also produces plant extracts for examination of their biological activity. This research program is in its infancy and although few results are available, the initial indication is that a wide range of medicinal herbs should be able to be grown successfully in New Zealand.

Culinary Herbs

A wide range of culinary herbs are grown by home gardeners and herb enthusiasts in New Zealand and the more common ones are supplied fresh to local markets with a small export industry based on fresh herbs. There is however no significant industry growing herbs to supply the international dried herb market. Preliminary research has already shown that lemon balm (*Melissa officinalis* L.), lemon verbena [*Aloysia triphylla* (L'Her.)

Britton], sage (*Salvia officinalis* L.), and thyme (*Thymus vulgaris* L.) have all produced good quality herbage which meets international market standards. Research has been planned on these crops as well as oregano (*Origanum vulgare* L.), peppermint (*Mentha xpiperita* L.), and spearmint (*M. spicata* L.), to examine the environmental and agronomic requirements to produce high quality produce. It is expected that as a greater understanding of each crop is developed more emphasis will be placed on growing these crops organically.

Essential Oils

New Zealand has the potential to grow a wide range of essential oil crops but no major industry has yet developed. Considerable research has been conducted describing the essential oil content of New Zealand native species and a small industry extracts manool from the native pink pine [*Halocarpus biformis* (Hook.) Quin] (Brooker et al. 1988). Research on peppermint begun in 1968, led to some commercial planting but this industry did not persist due to the difficulties with mint rust (*Puccinea menthae* pers. commun.) (Lammerink and Manning 1971, 1973).

The current research program seeks to systematically define the oil yield, composition analysis, and international quality assessments of a number of species (Table 3). The results have been very encouraging from this research and commercial extraction of essential oil and sclareol from clary sage is currently under investigation. Agronomic trials have been established to examine the influence of cultivars, environment, weed control, time of harvest, and distillation on oil yield and quality.

Edible Fungi

New Zealand has an industry based on the cultivation of the button mushroom [*Agaricus bisporus* (Lange) Sing.] and a growing interest in the cultivation of shiitake [*Lentinus edodes* (Berk.) Sing.]. In the past, a small industry has been based on the collection of the jelly fungus *Auricularia polytricha* (Mont.) Sacc. to supply the Chinese market (Brooker et al. 1988).

The current research program is directed at developing techniques to establish and produce the sought after mycorrhizal fungi, black truffle (*Tuber melanosporum* Vitt.), white truffle (*T. magnatum* Pico.), matsutake [*Tricholoma matsutake* (S. Ito & Imai) Sing.], and cep (*Boletus edulis* Bull.). Research has successfully devised techniques to inoculate black truffle onto oaks and hazels and although the fungus is evident in the field no truffle production has yet occurred (Hall and Brown 1989).

Table 3. Essential oil crops under evaluation.

Scientific name	Common name	Favorable yield estimates of essential oils (liters/ha)	International market assessment on essential oils
Artemisia dracunculus L.	French tarragon	40	
Carum carvi L.	Caraway seed	100	
Coriandrum sativum L.	Coriander seed	16	yes
Hyssopus officinalis L.	Hyssop	---	yes
Lavandula angustifolia Mill.	Lavender	30	
Lavandula xintermedia Emeric ex Loisel.	Lavandin	50	
Lavandula latifolia Medik.	Spike lavender	35	yes
Mentha xpiperita L.	Peppermint	50	
Mentha spicata L.	Spearmint	---	
Origanum vulgare L.	Oregano	110	
Rosa damascena Mill.	Rose	---	
Salvia officinalis L.	Sage	60	yes
Salvia sclarea L.	Clary sage	50	yes
Thymus vulgaris L.	Thyme	40	yes

Fruit, Nuts, and Ornamentals

Research on new fruits is directed at identifying appropriate cherimoya (*Annona cherimola* Mill.) cultivars for the northern regions of New Zealand. There are now over 60 named cherimoya cultivars in New Zealand and evaluation continues to seek a fruit which has the attributes of high yield, smooth skin, low seed number, good flavor, and a reasonable shelf life (Anderson and Richardson 1990). At the present time, there is no cherimoya industry in New Zealand.

There is a small and developing industry on macadamia (*Macadamia integrifolia* Maiden & Betche, *M. tetraphylla* L.A.S. Johnson) nuts in New Zealand but low yields limit the commercial success (Richardson and Dawson 1991). Research is continuing on evaluation of cultivars from mainly Australian and Hawaiian sources and investigating the effect of pollination and nutrition on crop yields to highlight possible ways to increase yields.

Preliminary research has begun to better define pollination of chestnuts (*Castanea sativa* Mill., *C. crenata* Siebold & Zucc.) and identification and control of fungal pathogens which spoil stored nuts. Small commercial plantings of chestnut have taken place based mainly on superior selected trees from local seedlings and there is a need for further cultivar evaluation.

Biogeographic principles are being used to pinpoint sources of appropriate plant material for new plant introductions into New Zealand where there are perceived market potentials not currently being addressed. Particular emphasis is being directed towards sourcing plants from the enormous germplasm resource of South America. Species collected are fed into the herb, essential oil, fruit, and ornamental programs. New ornamentals obtained in South America such as some *Begonia, Ennealophus, Fuchsia*, and *Tibouchina* species which are new to New Zealand are evaluated for growth habit, flowering behavior, and postharvest shelf life to estimate their potential as cut flowers or potted plants.

CONCLUSION

The emphasis in this research program is to identify and develop new export trade opportunities for New Zealand. The focus is on what the marketplace demands both in terms of type and quality of product. To reach this endpoint the new crops program is built around an approach of identifying the market opportunity, evaluating the adaptability and productivity of the new crop, and test marketing samples of the crop to be assured the product reaches market specifications. In this way, the New Zealand new crops program has a clear focus and clearly defined goals. The program is new and open-ended in relation to identifying new opportunities and although many of the crops under investigation have not been previously grown in New Zealand, we believe the approach will see many of them become established industries in the future.

REFERENCES

Anderson, P. and A. Richardson. 1990. Which cherimoya cultivar is best? Orchard New Zeal. 63(11):17–19.

Brooker, S.G., R.C. Cambie, and R.C. Cooper. 1988. Economic native plants of New Zealand. Botany Division DSIR Christchurch, NZ.

Follett, J.M. 1986. Production of four traditional Japanese vegetables in Japan. Ruakura Agr. Centre, Hamilton, NZ.

Follett, J.M. 1991. Propagation notes for new and novel crops introduced into New Zealand. Proc. Int. Plant Prop. Conf. 41 (in press).

Hall, I.R. and G. Brown. 1989. The black truffle, its history, uses and cultivation. Ministry of Agr. and Fisheries, Wellington, NZ.

Hodge, W.H. 1974. Wasabi: Native condiment plant of Japan. Econ. Bot. 28:118–129.

Lammerink, J. and T.D.R. Manning. 1971. Yields and composition of oil from peppermint grown at Lincoln, New Zealand. New Zeal. J. Agr. Res. 14:745–51.

Lammerink, J. and T.D.R. Manning. 1973. Peppermint oil composition and yield, flowering time, and morphological characters of four naturalised South Island clones and the Mitcham strain of *Mentha piperita*. New Zeal. J. Agr. Res. 16:181–184.

Mann, J.D. 1978. Production of solasodine for the pharmaceutical industry. Adv. Agron. 30:207–245.

Mann, J.D., J.E. Lancaster, J.A. Douglas, G.J. Goold, and N.S. Brown. 1985. Preliminary investigation into the solasodine yield from *Solanum aviculare* and *Solanum laciniatum* at 5 sites in the North Island, New Zealand. New Zeal. J. Expt. Agr. 13:67–70.

Palmer, J.A. 1984. Myoga, a possible ginger crop for New Zealand. New Zealand Inst. Hort. J. 12:105–108.

Principe, P.P. 1989. Economic significance of plants and their constituents as drugs. Econ. Med. Plant Res. 3:1–17.

Richardson, A. and T. Dawson. 1991. New Zealand macadamias: the industry and its research needs. Orchard New Zeal. 64(6):30–33.

New Horticultural Crops in New Zealand

Errol W. Hewett

New Zealand, a small country located in the South Pacific (latitude between 35° and 47°S and longitude 167° and 178°E) has a population of 3.3 million. Horticulture is a small but important contributor to the national economy having NZ$1.2 billion export earnings in 1991, 7.4% of total exports (NZ$1 = US$0.54, 1992). Four new fruit crops have been successfully introduced to international trade during the 20th century: avocado, blueberry, kiwifruit, and macadamia (Janick 1991). Of these, kiwifruit has arguably made the largest and most dramatic impact over the last 20 years.

The kiwifruit is a unique fruit with unusual visual (a brown, hairy skin with a spectacular green translucent flesh containing an attractive circle of black seeds around a white pith), nutritive (low calories, high fiber, high potassium, and vitamin C content), and storage (quality can be maintained for up to 12 months in air or controlled atmosphere storage) characteristics. It has successfully captured the imagination of traders and consumers who have paid high prices to purchase this new fruit. Associated profitability has seen kiwifruit planted in large numbers throughout the world during the 1980s.

ESTABLISHED FRUIT CROPS

New Zealand grows a wide range of temperate fruit crops, but only contributes significantly to world trade with kiwifruit and apples. Major efforts are currently underway to improve the existing range of cultivars to exploit consumer demand for new taste and visual sensations.

Largely as a result of the foresight, dedication, perseverance, and skill of the late D.W. McKenzie, major breeding and plant improvement programs are being undertaken by the Department of Scientific Research (DSIR) on a range of crops including kiwifruit, apples, pears, apricots, and a range of subtropical fruits.

Kiwifruit [*Actinidia deliciosa* (A. Chev.) C.F. Liang & A.R. Ferguson] var deliciosa, Actinidiaceae

Commercial plantings of kiwifruit in New Zealand are known to have derived from one seed acquisition brought from China in about 1903 by Miss Isabel Fraser, sister of Miss Katie Fraser, a missionary in Xichang. It is possible that the majority of kiwifruit grown in New Zealand (and to a large extent elsewhere especially France, Italy, and Australia) originated from seed from one fruit, certainly from only a few fruit collected from the wild by E.H. Wilson from one region in China (Ferguson 1990). Hence, the present genetic base of existing kiwifruit plantings is extremely limited.

The genus *Actinidia* is known to have more than 50 species and more than 100 taxa (Liang and Ferguson 1986, Ferguson 1990). The cultivar 'Hayward', which accounts for more than 95% of the current kiwifruit plantings in New Zealand today, was selected by Hayward Wright, a nurseryman who has been called "the Luther Burbank of New Zealand horticulture." In the period from 1903 to 1946, when kiwifruit were grown mainly as an ornamental plant, many enthusiastic nurserymen were involved in the propagation, improvement and sale of these novel plants; in particular Bruno Just, Alexander Allison, James McGregor, and Hugh Gorton, made significant contributions (Ferguson and Bollard 1990).

Scientists in DSIR recognized the inherent danger of relying on such a narrow genetic base for the development and continued success of an important new crop. They were also well aware of the diverse range of species, indigenous in China, which while providing fruit for a range of products (jam, pastes, medicines) had not been subject to any concerted or deliberative screening programme for improving size or quality. Since the 1970s there has been a joint effort by DSIR and Chinese scientists to obtain seed material from a broad range of *Actinidia* species, to grow them together under uniform conditions of cultivation and training for comparison of fruiting characteristics and to obtain diverse material to be used in breeding programmes by traditional or novel molecular biology means.

The genus *Actinidia* is characterized by having a wide range of growth habits, fruit size, shape, color, and nutritive qualities. Some species are cross compatible and interspecific crosses are easily achieved, while others are incompatible, and interspecific hybrids may only be possible by using recently developed embryo transfer techniques. Three major thrusts are being adopted by scientists involved in the current breeding program:

1. to obtain improved or different selections from existing plantings or "Hayward lookalikes." Selections already made and under evaluation include: more uniform fruit shape, earlier fruit maturation, hermaphrodite as distinct from diecious plants, more productive plants than 'Hayward', higher vitamin C, and reduced flats and fans.
2. to develop vigor controlling rootstocks which will also offer better flowering after mild winters, produce high export yields, enhance precocity from young vines, and reduce flats and fans.
3. to crossbreed with other *Actinidia* species, in particular from *A. chinensis* Planchon, to produce fruit with smooth skins like a peach or pear, maybe with different colored skins and/or flesh. *A. chinensis* vines are precocious and high yielding, some are early maturing with good flavor. A range of flesh colors from green through yellow to pink are available, and fruit store for 2 to 3 months. Successful hybridization between *A. deliciosa* and *A. chinensis* is likely to produce fruit combining the desirable features of both species. *A. arguta* (Seibold & Zuccarini) Planchon ex Miquel, marketed as a home garden vine in North America, produces fruit about grape-size, very sweet, with red or green flesh. A green skinned hairless fruit from a highly productive vine has already been produced.

Results from these different approaches already indicate that there is a major potential for a dramatic increase in the range of cultivars of kiwifruit of commercial potential. Even more exciting is the possibility of the emergence of "new" fruits based on the genetic diversity of the *Actinidia* species. These long term strategic plant improvement programs are financially supported by the kiwifruit industry which recognizes the commercial necessity and opportunities which accrue from successful new cultivar development.

Apples (*Malus* x *domestica* Borkh., Rosaceae)

One of the main reasons for the success of the New Zealand apple industry is the ability to provide customers with a range of 5 to 9 distinct cultivars over a 4 to 6 month marketing period. This contrasts with some other apple producing countries which tend to produce only two or three major cultivars. In addition, the New Zealand Apple and Pear Marketing Board has successfully introduced several highly acceptable new cultivars to international trade in recent years. The cultivars 'Braeburn', 'Gala', and 'Royal Gala' have had a major impact in apple markets highlighting New Zealand's reputation of being able to develop and market appealing new fruit sensations.

The late D.W. McKenzie, working for DSIR, with great perspicacity, foresaw the need for a concentrated and directed breeding program to ensure a continuous release of new apple cultivars onto major markets. With perseverance and dedication, he overcame serious opposition in New Zealand, and acting against prevailing international trends, initiated a program to produce a bright red, late maturing highly flavored apple to have a market slot after 'Granny Smith'.

While none of his original selections are likely to achieve major success, subsequent releases from his work, together with hybrids from current programs, are likely to have a substantial impact in the next decade. 'Splendour' x 'Gala' crosses are undergoing commercial evaluation and two are being focussed on by the New Zealand Apple and Pear Marketing Board for test marketing. In particular, GS2085, looks promising. It is a rosy pink cultivar which ripens late in the season with 'Granny Smith'; it has an extremely crisp and crunchy texture with a sweet flavor and a good acid balance. The trees are precocious, like a 'Golden Delicious' in openness and vigor, having good branch angles and carrying good fruit loads on young branches. GS2085 has tolerance to black spot and is less susceptible to mildew than existing cultivars.

Later crosses, including selections from a collaborative program with Japanese plant breeders, are equally, if not more exciting. It is anticipated that a portfolio of selections will be produced which will provide quite different taste and texture sensation for consumers contrasting markedly with major cultivars available today. Enhanced pest and disease tolerance/resistance is another major objective in the ongoing pome fruit breeding program in an attempt to reduce the importance of pesticides in producing high quality fruit. A pear breeding program is also underway in DSIR, but this is less advanced than the apple projects. Recognition of the strategic importance of providing new apple cultivars has resulted in considerable financial input from the New Zealand apple industry to this program.

THE SOUTH AMERICAN CONNECTION

In tropical South American countries, at altitudes between 2,000 and 3,000 m, there occur endemic fruiting plants that are really warm temperate species. Many of these appear to be well adapted to warmer parts of New Zealand. Over the past 20 years, both private and Government sponsored expeditions have visited a number of countries, including Colombia, Ecuador, Peru, Chile, and Brazil to obtain propagating material for evaluation under New Zealand conditions. The rapid destruction of natural rainforest vegetation in several of these countries is placing many precious food plants at risk of extinction; there is an urgent need to collect and preserve as many of these plants as soon as possible if they are not to be lost forever. New Zealand has been fortunate in being recipients of some most interesting fruit and vegetable crops from South America, many of which were common foods of the Incas (Veitmeyer 1991).

Tree Tomato [*Cyphomandra betacea* (Cav.) Sendtn., Solanaceae]

The tree tomato [renamed the tamarillo in New Zealand, not to be confused with the tomatillo (*Physalis ixocorpa* Brot.)] is an egg shaped/sized, bright red fruit developed in New Zealand from seed thought to have been obtained from a missionary in Ecuador early this century. In the wild, the fruit is generally small, splotchy and yellow or pale red in color (Veitmeyer 1991). Large red-fruited strains were developed by nurserymen in New Zealand, and recently large golden colored cultivars have been produced.

Tamarillos are rapidly growing trees which produce good crops after 18 months. They are frost tender which limits their distribution. Fruit is highly attractive, but some people find the skin and flesh too astringent to make it a popular fresh fruit. While the fruit has a high vitamin C content, it has a limited storage life, suffering from chilling injury and postharvest pathogens if maintained below 5°C for any sustained period of time. Fruit processes extremely well. They can be frozen or canned and can be used for a range of products including jam, pulp, puree, chutney, and juice; there is considerable potential for combining with milk products such as yogurt.

Unfortunately, tamarillo trees are easily infected with tamarillo mosaic virus, which results in production of blotchy, streaked unattractive fruit. Until disease resistant stock can be obtained, opportunities for existing tamarillo cultivars are limited. A wide range of seeds have been collected from indigenous tamarillo plants in South America and these are currently under evaluation.

Feijoa (*Feijoa sellowiana* Berg, Myrtaceae)

Originating in the plateau lands of southeast Brazil, the feijoa, known as pineapple guava in California, has been grown in New Zealand for many years. It has a shrub-like growth habit producing attractive flowers. It is more hardy than tamarillo, being able to tolerate mild winter frosts. In California, it is grown mainly as an ornamental hedge, while in southern Russia and Israel, it has been grown as a commercial fruit crop. Until recently, most plantings in New Zealand have been with seedlings, resulting in extreme variation in fruit size, shape, flavor, and keeping quality. Over the last decade, a number of improved selections have been made and the availability of grafted plants is ensuring consistency in fruiting.

The ovoid green skinned fruit with vanilla-colored flesh has a very sweet and aromatic taste when eaten fresh. Flesh has to be scooped as the skin is bitter. No satisfactory maturity index has been developed so it is difficult to determine optimum harvest maturity. Fruit catching structures are placed under trees by the serious feijoa growers in order to prevent fruit dropping to the ground when ripe; if this occurs fruit is likely to be damaged and become infected with postharvest pathogens. Recent research has produced cultivars with large fruit having thin smooth dark green skins, strong aromatic flavor, good sugar/acid balance, smooth texture with a minimum of grittiness, and a moderate storage life. Fruit may be canned to create a pleasing product.

Pepino (*Solanum muricatum* Ait., Solanaceae)

The pepino is a small, shrubby plant which produces large (up to 15 cm diameter) fruit with a sweet smell, subtle flavor, and attractive yellow/golden skin color often with purple stripes. It is grown widely in the north of South America and cultivated extensively in Chile. Seed material, introduced to New Zealand in 1973, produced extremely variable fruit with a range of shapes and flavors. It grows well in New Zealand, generally in the same climate as tomato. Early sales of seedling fruit by entrepreneur growers wanting to cash in on this new crop, created serious market problems, as fruit was often small, bitter, unattractive to both the eye and the palate.

A selection and breeding programme by DSIR scientists in conjunction with a committed and enthusiastic grower, has led to the production of several outstanding cultivars. However, best crops seem to be produced under protected cultivation and many management problems involving nutrition temperature, light, and maturity indices have still to be solved.

In spite of an apparently receptive market in Japan for high quality pepinos, this industry has virtually lapsed for want of necessary research input.

Babaco [*Carica xheilbornii* Badillo m. pentagona (Heilborn) Caricaceae]

The babaco is native of Ecuador and is a hybrid between two Andean papayas, producing more and larger fruit than the mountain papayas. It was introduced to New Zealand in 1973, but popularized by an ardent nurseryman who made numerous visits to Ecuador to collect this and other exotic fruit material.

Babaco is extremely productive, producing large (2 kg) green, torpedo shaped fruit hanging in clusters around the trunk. The fruit has a subtle flavor when ripe; it is very refreshing to eat and make an acceptable and healthy juice. Although difficult to propagate initially, many plants were sold to real and "would-be" horticulturists during the boom times of the early 1980s. However, this crop has not been a commercial success either locally or for export, possible because of their novelty (and lack of promotion) and their large size (they are too expensive for the consumer wanting to try something new).

Cape gooseberry (*Physalis peruviana* L., Solanaceae)

These plants grow all over the Andes and were fruit of the Incas (Veitmeyer 1991). Cape gooseberries (which are neither gooseberries nor from the Cape; seeds were obtained from the Cape of Good Hope late last century) are grown on a few small properties in New Zealand. Production is small and fruit is supplied mainly to the local market. Removed from the paper-like husks, the attractive yellow marble-sized fruit makes an extremely tasty jam. Fruit has a high vitamin A, B, and C content, is a rich source of carotene, phosphorous, and iron, and also contains vitamin P. It may be eaten fresh, in salads or in cocktails. No research effort is being made in New Zealand to improve this crop.

Cherimoya (*Annona cherimola* Mill., Annonaceae)

Considerable interest is currently being shown for this green-skinned, softball-sized fruit sometimes called "the queen of subtropical fruits." A range of cultivars have been introduced from Ecuador, Chile, and Peru for evaluation in warmer climates in New Zealand and several commercial orchards have been planted. A reasonable market potential seems to exist for this very tasty fruit (enhanced by the recent freeze in California which destroyed a major production area). However, selection of cultivars for good production of high quality fruit in marginal New Zealand climatic conditions is still necessary; fruit with fewer seeds and extended shelf life are also required before this fruit could become a substantial export earner from New Zealand.

Oca or "Yam" (*Oxalis tuberosa* Mol., Oxalidaceae)

The oca (or yam as it is called in New Zealand) is a small, red, waxy, crinkled tuber was probably a staple food item of the Andean Indians (Veitmeyer 1991). They are grown on a very small scale in a localized area in New Zealand and sold only on the local market. The tubers have a tangy, acid nutty flavor and are eaten mainly with roast dinners. The original planting material probably came from Chile to New Zealand in the late 1800s with immigrants. Oca does not seem to be widely grown outside of South American countries and so appears to qualify as "one of the lost crops of the Incas" (Veitmeyer 1991).

Other Crops

A range of other unusual and exotic South American food crops are being grown in New Zealand, generally by enthusiastic horticulturalists. These include: naranjilla (*Solanum quitoense* Lam., Solanaceae), which produces an orange hairy fruit which makes a green frothy drink, and has a flavor reminiscent of pineapple and strawberry; capulin cherry (*Prunus capuli* Cav., Rosaceae) a red skinned, green fleshed fruit with excellent flavor; yacon (*Polymnia sonchifolia* Poepp. & Endl., Asteraceae) a root vegetable, which when eaten uncooked, is very crunchy, watery to translucent, and sweet. Any attempt to improve or develop these plants further is being undertaken by private individuals.

Another fruit vegetable that has received some interest in recent years is the kiwano or African Horned Melon (*Cucumis metuliferus* E.H. Mey. ex Schrad., Cucurbitaceae). It grows on the fringes of the Kalahari Desert in Africa and was introduced to New Zealand during the 1970s. The orange spiny fruit with intensely green flesh is extremely attractive. The fruit has many seeds, a subtle flavor, and has an excellent storage life at room temperature. However, it is more of a novelty crop and has not undergone commercial development.

NEW FLOWER CROPS

New Zealand is a very small producer of flowers by international standards. Orchids are the most important flower in terms of exports. However, there are a few new flower types that have been developed which are poised to make a contribution in the near future. Private breeders are also producing international prize winning cultivars with traditional flowers.

Calla (*Zantedeschia* spp., Araceae)

Originating in Southern Africa, several New Zealand nurserymen have specialized in developing an extensive range of new brightly colored callas. These are versatile plants and can be used as bedding plants, pot plants, and cut flowers. A considerable amount of basic research has been undertaken at Massey University to understand the factors controlling the growth cycle of these plants, including flowering, dormancy, and productivity, with a view to producing a production management blueprint for purchasers of the export tubers and plants (Funnell et al. 1988). A recent innovation has been to develop a miniature potted version of the white arum lily (*Z. aethiopica* cv. Childsiana) which holds considerable potential as a decorative or commemorative living momento.

Nerine (*Nerine* spp., Amaryllidaceae)

In recent years, New Zealand has obtained ownership of probably the most extensive collection of nerine species and cultivars in cultivation in the world. A very limited number of growers are involved in evaluating this collection in New Zealand conditions, with a view to exporting both bulbs and a range of diversely colored cultivars.

Sandersonia (*Sandersonia auriantiaca* Hook., Liliaceae)

A protected genera now in South Africa, Sandersonia stock was obtained by a New Zealand nurseryman over 70 years ago, but commercial development has been very slow. Grown from tubers, the plants produce beautiful, orange, bell-like granny's bonnet shaped flowers which have a reasonable shelf life. Both tubers and cut flowers are grown for export.

Other flowers

New Zealand has some highly accomplished private flower breeders who are making major advances in new cultivars. Prominent among these are: Keith Hammett who has gained international awards for his outstanding new selections of dahlias, sweet peas, and carnations; Sam McGredy, originally from Ireland, who now resides in New Zealand and continues to produce world class roses with infinite shape, color, and aroma; Bill Doreen who has been producing a wide range of colorful and exciting lilies for many years.

A number of other flower crops are being grown by committed enthusiasts; these include peony, leucodendrons, limonium, and gypsophila. A recent novel development has been the production of miniature flower plants of *Leptospermum* spp. (Myrtaceae) and kowhai [*Sophora* spp., Leguminosae (subfamily Faboideae)].

NATIVE PLANTS FROM NEW ZEALAND

New Zealand has a unique flora. Many indigenous shrubs and trees are not well-known in other parts of the world. Some of these have potential for pot plants or foliage. While some have been developed by nurserymen for local sale, most of the range of foliage and flower types available have not been utilized as commercial products.

A number of *Cordyline* spp. and *Phormium* spp. (both Agavaceae) have been selected; these include dwarf species, and selections with a range of foliage from deep reds through yellow to green, as well as a range of variegated types.

One tree with considerable potential is the pohutakawa or New Zealand Christmas tree (*Meterosideros* spp., Myrtaceae). In the wild, it grows as a huge gnarled tree, often protruding precariously from high cliffs overlooking the sea. Trees have brilliant crimson red flowers which cover the whole tree in December in New Zealand. It is possible to produce trees in pots and to induce flowering within two years of planting. Further research is required to manipulate growth and flowering with more precision before a successful export industry can develop, but there is considerable potential for this spectacular specimen.

Hebe spp. (Scrophulariaceae) are common throughout New Zealand. Many have been developed as garden and potted plants, as much for their varied foliage as for their range of flower types. Increasingly, these Hebes are being developed in countries other than New Zealand, (Denmark) as successful commercial nursery plants.

CONCLUSION

Possingham (1990) identified two contrasting influences at work in horticultural industries in developed countries. On the one hand there is a strong move to develop new and exotic crops, often drawn from diverse species growing in the wild, which have the potential to produce good profits for growers and others involved in horticultural trade. On the other hand, there is a reduction in the number of cultivars being grown as market requirements define apparently narrower quality characteristics.

New Zealand horticulture generally follows the first trend. While Maoris, the original inhabitants of New Zealand, brought several vegetable crops, notably the sweet potato, with them from the Pacific, the majority of new plant introductions occurred with the arrival of English settlers in the late 19th century.

Most of the traditional horticultural crops grown in New Zealand are well known in other fruit growing countries in temperate climates. Introductions of apples, pears, stonefruit, berryfruit, citrus, flowers, and ornamental plants continue to this day from diverse international sources.

However, there has been a large element of serendipity in the introduction of new or different plants. Missionaries, travellers, explorers, and visitors have all had an influence on the introduction of new and unusual plants. The kiwifruit from China and the range of species from South America exemplify this fact.

Highly skilled, observant, and entrepreneurial nurserymen probably had the major role in transforming wild growing species into potential commercial cultivars. Many of these nurserymen were very talented plantsmen who initiated plant improvement programs themselves by selection and breeding. The seminal influence of Alexander Allison, Bruno Just, and Hayward Wright in the initial development of the kiwifruit has been well documented (Ferguson and Bollard 1990). The influence of nurserymen on the development of other crops mentioned in this article is not documented.

Invariably, success depended on the efforts of a "champion" of the crop. Whether this champion was a nurseryman, a grower, a scientist, or a marketer, almost without exception, any product which has achieved any economic significance in New Zealand can be identified with an enthusiastic, committed, and skillful plantsman who are unabashed advocates for their particular crop.

A more recent feature of new crop development in New Zealand has been the involvement of Government scientists, mainly from DSIR, but also from the Ministry of Agriculture and Fisheries and from Universities. The Government has funded a number of plant improvement programs, both in selection and breeding in major and minor crops, and the scientists involved have worked closely with growers and nurserymen. This collaboration has accelerated in the last two decades, particularly but not exclusively with the major crops such as apples and kiwifruit.

Both of these industries have well developed infrastructures and a strong marketing role. Industry personnel have agreed with scientists on the strategic importance of developing an extended range of cultivars which should provide a market advantage for this country in the future. Input from marketing experts to the scientists breeding program is an important characteristic of today's efforts which are underpinned by both Government and industry funding.

While many other groups have developed to represent the collective interests of those producing or marketing particular products, they lack the organizational structure and the financial success of the major product groups. Consequently less "seed" money has been available for attracting subsequent Government research effort.

Recent structural and philosophical changes have occurred in science organization in New Zealand which is impacting on research carried out on minor horticultural crops. The 1980s have seen the introduction of "user pays;" that is research perceived to bring direct benefit to an individual or an industry is expected to be increasingly funded by that individual or industry. Therefore, while the apple and kiwifruit industries currently contribute nearly $6 million to research, and as a consequence still receive substantial Government support, minor industries are in no position to provide enough funding to attract significant Government support. In spite of the fact that there is potential for commercial success from one or more of a range of "sunrise" crops, (i.e. crops at early stages of development and perceived to have potential for growth), the Government policy of not picking winners and not funding research on crops/sectors that do not provide research funds, means that the effort being directed into minor crops has diminished drastically over the past eight years.

New Zealand has turned a complete circle. Successful development of new and exotic crops in the future will come again from the private nurseryman, the enthusiastic amateur horticulturist, the perceptive grower, and from the non-institutional groups such as the Tree Crops Society. Either individually or collectively they will collect, import, select, and develop horticultural crops which they will champion. Only when an individual crop can be demonstrated to have commercial success will the Government research scientists be in a position to lend their considerable expertise to further improvement. New Zealand will continue to have an international reputation for producing a diverse range of new and exciting horticultural crops. New apples and kiwifruit, diverse and colorful plants and flowers, and exotic fruits sourced from South America will be traded successfully in world fruit markets during future decades.

REFERENCES

Ferguson, A.R. 1990. Botanical nomenclature: *Actinidia chinensis*, *Actinidia deliciosa* and *Actinidia setosa*, p.36–57. In: I.J. Warrington and G.C. Weston (eds.). Kiwifruit science and management. Ray Richards, Auckland, New Zealand.

Ferguson, A.R. and E.G. Bollard. 1990. Domestication of the kiwifruit, p.165–246. In: I.J. Warrington and G.L. Weston (eds.). Kiwifruit science and management. Ray Richards, Auckland, New Zealand.

Funnell, K.A., B.O. Tjia, C.J. Stanley, D. Cohen, and J.R. Sedcote. 1988. Effect of storage temperature, duration, and gibberellic acid on the flowering of *Zantedeschia elliotiana* and *Z*. 'Pink Satin'. J. Amer. Soc. Hort. Sci. 113:860–863.

Janick, J. 1991. New fruits from old genes. Acta Hort. 297:25–42.

Liang, C.F. and A.R. Ferguson. 1986. The botanical nomenclature of the kiwifruit and related taxa. New Zealand J. Bot. 24:183–184.

Possingham, J.V. 1990. Under-exploited wild species that have potential for horticulture, p. 49–55. In: 23 I.H.C. Lectures. Special publication of the International Society for Horticultural Science from the XXIII Int. Hort. Cong., Firenze, Italy.

Vietmeyer, N. 1991. Lost crops of the Incas. New Zealand Geographic 10:49–67.

Genetic Resources in Africa

Jack R. Harlan

Indigenous African crops that have made an impact on the world scene include: coffee (*Coffea arabica*), sorghum (*Sorghum* spp.), pearl millet (*Pennisetum glaucum*), finger millet (*Eleucine corocana*), watermelon (*Citrullus lanatus*), oil palm (*Elaeis guineensis*), cowpea (*Vigna sinensis*), and at least some date germplasm (*Pheonix dactylifera*). These crops are established in suitable regions around the world and have their own special interest groups. They cannot be considered new crops in any sense of the term. But, Africa has other genetic resources, not new in a temporal sense, but new to the American experience.

CEREALS

First, let me call attention to some of the other cereals, both wild and tame. Fonio or acha, *Digitaria exilis* (Kipp.) Stapf, has been given the misnomer "hungry rice" by English colonials. It is not grown to relieve hunger but because of its quality. It is a chief's food, a gourmet item, and couscous made of fonio is better than couscous made from wheat. Tef, *Eragrostis tef* Trott, is the noble grain of Ethiopia, and enjera, the bread made from it, is the food of the upper classes. There are now Ethiopian restaurants in the United States that are flourishing because of the demand and interest in ethnic foods, enjera and watt (a spicy stew). These are first class foods. It should not be difficult to develop considerable markets for them, not just because they are ethnic and exotic, but because both fonio and tef are genuinely superior cereals. As whole grains, they are nourishing, and enjera is vitamin enriched by yeast from a short fermentation of the dough.

Less well known are the grains of wild cereals that were harvested on a huge scale in the 19th and early 20th centuries. Again, the colonials, both French and English, spoke of them in contemptuous terms ("scarcity foods," "céréales de disette") without ever giving them a fair trial. Anyone reduced to eating wild grass seeds must be on the verge of starvation. The fact is that these, too, were luxury items. They were harvested, not for food for the harvesters, but for sale and export. The harvesters probably reserved some seed for special occasions and ceremonies, but wild grass seeds brought higher prices in the market than the staples, sorghum, pearl millet, and rice, and in the Sahara, even more than wheat. The prejudice of European colonizers closed their mind to the potential. Wild grass seeds are still harvested, but not on the scale of a century ago (Harlan 1989a,b). It has been suggested that a return to wild grass harvests on a substantial scale could stop the trend toward desertification brought on by the destructive method of livestock rearing now practiced (Vietmeyer in press).

In the desert proper, *Aristida pungens* Desf. and *Panicum turgidum* Forsek., are the most important, the former in the north and the latter in central and south. But, we do not expect much production from a desert. In the Sahel and southern desert fringes, *Cenchrus biflorus* Roxb. is the main grass, but it is a sandbur with spines that can torment. In the broadleaved savanna, a group of grasses collectively called kreb(s) over a considerable region from Mali to Kordofan in Sudan is still harvested. The mixture varies in species composition from place to place and probably from year to year and includes species of *Panicum*, *Eragrostis*, *Dactyloctenium*, *Brachiaria*, and others. *Panicum laetum* Kunth is one of the most common, and *E. pilosa* Beauv., one of the components, is probably the progenitor of tef (Harlan 1989a,b).

LEGUMES AND OILSEEDS

Voandzeia subterranea (L.) Thouars is a legume that produces seed underground, like a peanut, except the seeds are much larger, usually one to the pod. A number of tests in Africa have indicated that this legume can yield as well or better than peanuts, and it is a common experience that a crop removed from its native territory without a normal suite of diseases and pests can perform much better than in its homeland. The crop, sometimes called Bambara groundnut, is actually widespread in Africa and not especially tied to the Bambara tribe. It is more of a garden crop than a field crop and important in subsistence agriculture, primarily in the broadleaved savannas from west Africa to east Africa and southward to southern Africa. Realistic figures on production are not available. A longer shot is *Kerstingiella geocarpa* Harms, another "groundnut," but not nearly so widespread and probably with less potential. It has not been especially important in Africa, and that suggests limited value elsewhere. Still, have either of these plants been adequately tested as a potential "new crop?" The wild forms of both species are found in eastern Nigeria and in Cameroon.

Noog, *Guizotia abyssinica* Cass., Asteraceae, an oilseed crop, is the most important edible oil in Ethiopia. It is much kinder to the grower than safflower, lacking spines and the crop would be easy to mechanize. Extensive trials on noog have not been conducted.

Telfairia occidentalis Hook. f., Cucurbitaceae, produces a course vine with rather large gourd-like fruits. Oil is extracted from the seeds. It is a garden plant of West Africa and is grown from the broadleaved savanna into the forest zone. While we have plenty of oil seed crops, there could well be a place for this plant in tropical subsistence agriculture outside of Africa. I have seen it, for example, in Jamaica.

OTHER CROP RESOURCES

There appears to be several forms of *Solanum* grown for their fruits and often lumped together as "garden eggs" by English speakers. A serious study might reveal some potentially useful vegetables. Africa has, of course, wild races of coffee, sorghum, the millets, rice, cotton, cowpea, cola, and watermelon. These might have some useful genes, and wild races of most crops are poorly collected. African rice is not likely to replace Asian rice, but some useful genes have been found, and for Africa, at least, it has what the French call "rusticité," or the ability to yield something no matter what calamities it may suffer. The most useful forage grasses for tropical pastures come from Africa, but this subject is treated elsewhere in the Proceedings of the symposium.

Finally, attention is called to plants with medicinal potential. Herbal medicine is well developed in Africa and intimately interlaced with witchcraft, voodoo, and various occult arts. I can find few serious studies of either the remedies or the witchcraft in which they are embedded. Both should be studied as R.E. Schultes has done in Amazonia (Schultes 1990). While lacking experience in these matters, I sense that such field studies should be done by Africans. Who knows what potential there might be for cures or the arrest of cancer, AIDs, or even the common cold? We have not yet investigated.

REFERENCES

Harlan, J. 1989. Wild grass seeds as food in the Sahara and Sub-sahara. Sahara 2:69–74.

Harlan, J.R. 1989. Wild grass-seed harvesting in the Sahara and Sub-sahara of Africa, p.79–98. In: D.R. Harris and G.C. Hillman (eds.). Foraging and farming: the evolution of plant exploitation. Unwin Hyman, London.

Schultes, R.E. and R.F. Raffauf. 1990. The healing forest: Medicinal and toxic plants of the Northwest Amazonia. Dioscorides Press, Portland, OR.

Vietmeyer, N.D. The lost crops of Africa. Natl. Res. Council, Natl. Academy Press, Wasington. DC. (in press).

REGIONAL DEVELOPMENT

New Crops Research: Northeastern Region and National Federal Efforts

George A. White*

The objective of this paper is to provide a broad overview of new crops research in the Northeastern Region of the United States as well as the National federal efforts. This paper is mainly limited to species not yet established commercially or recently commercialized on a small scale. This limitation would exclude crops such as guar, hops, and sunflowers. An electronic search of the CRIS projects that were active from October 1, 1989 onward plus a few non-CRIS projects are included in this review. An excellent review of new industrial crops that covers a wide range of species and includes germplasm status has been published by Thompson et al. (1992).

STATE RESEARCH ON NEW CROPS—NORTHEASTERN REGION

Most of the new crops efforts in the Northeast Region are directed toward the introduction of exotic, ethnic vegetables, and crops or new cultivars of crops that are grown in other regions of the United States (Table 1).

Table 1. State research on new crops, Northeastern Region.

State	Crop plant/group	Nature of research
Connecticut	Globe artichoke, witloof chicory, Chinese cabbage, pak choi, herbs	Culture, quality, germplasm evaluation
Delaware	Kenaf	Enhancement of chicken litter, bulking agent in peat-based growth media
Maine	*Lupinus albus*	Selection, adaptability, culture
Maryland	Duckweed	Concentrate fresh duck weed into a dry storable animal feedstuff
Massachusetts	Witloof chicory	Yield and quality
	Easter cactus	Control of vegetative and reproductive development
New Hampshire	*Cucurbita pepo*	Breeding, culture; hull-less seed as a food snack
	Alternative floriculture species	Production schedules for various species
New Jersey	Natural insecticides	Assess production potential, emphasis on pyrethrum
	Chicory, longan, lychee, passion fruit, etc.	Clearance of chemicals/biologics for minor/special uses
New York	Canola, lupine	Adaptability of protein and oil crops

Connecticut

Hill and Maynard (1989) reported results of trials with 29 foreign and domestic cultivars of globe artichoke (*Cynara scolymus*) where this normally biennial species was grown as an annual through vernalization of seeds and application of gibberellic acid to young plants. The potential for producing commercial quality artichokes from annual culture in Connecticut appears promising. Encouraging results were obtained with trials on witloof and radicchio chicories (*Cichorium intybus*), Chinese cabbage (*Brassica pekinensis*), and pak choi (*B. chinensis*) (Hill 1989, 1991).

Delaware

Kenaf (*Hibiscus cannabinus*) research has concentrated more on the utility of the stems and the two main stem components than on production of the crop. Some studies were conducted on the use of chopped stems as

---

*I thank those many researchers who contributed information and photographs and reviewed the manuscript. A special note of appreciation goes to John Meyers and Shawn Conrad for several Current Research Information Service (CRIS) project retrievals.

a sewage sludge filler. The chopped stems have appeared promising as a bulking agent in peat-based growth media (W.G. Pill pers. commun.). The outer-stem bast (phloem) fibers when separated from the short-fibered inner core (xylem) can command premium prices for use in specialty papers and other high quality products. This fact has prompted research on uses for the core. The magnitude of the broiler industry in the Delmarva Peninsula requires large quantities of litter for which kenaf stem core might be suitable. Studies by Malone et al. (1989) showed no difference on weight gain, feed efficiency, or mortality rate of broilers raised on kenaf stem core as compared to pine sawdust. The quality of used core is being evaluated for feed after enhancement with feed grains. Fiber Kore, Inc. of Delaware is cooperating with the chicken litter studies in Delaware and with Natural Fibers of Louisiana in the separation of kenaf bast and core fibers and in identifying markets for them (Kugler 1991).

Maine

Since 1987, researchers have been studying the effects of crop rotation and tillage practices of crops grown in rotation with potato. White lupine (*Lupinus albus*) uniquely fits the niche as a soil improving plant and as a source of protein rich seeds (Merrick 1990). According to G.A. Porter (pers. commun.), white lupine is being grown experimentally for grain and for green manure in comparison to grain (oats) and green manure (clover) in rotation with potatoes. The main limiting factors for production in Maine are slow maturation, limited seed availability and cost, and weed control. Progress in selecting for determinate, early maturing types has been good.

Massachusetts

The objectives of research on Easter cactus (*Rhipsalidopsis gaertneri*) are to determine the environmental requirements for vegetative and reproductive growth. Different light, temperature, and fertilizer regimes have been tested to determine optimum environmental conditions for maximizing number of flowers with minimum fertilizer and extended warm temperatures. Boyle and Stimart (1989) have published a grower's guide based on their research results. A reduction in the night temperature from 18° to 10°C for 6 to 8 weeks before flowering increased the number of buds but did not affect flowering time appreciably on 'Crimson Giant' Easter cactus (Boyle 1991). Fuel savings from the temperature change would be beneficial to commercial growers.

Research on Witloof chicory (*Cichorium intybus*) is based on forcing development of the floral axis and basal leaves with subsequent formation of chicons. Corey et al. (1990) reported that marketing factors may limit the crop more than production constraints. The use of weights on the crown at the start of forcing resulted in improved yields and quality of chicons (Tan and Corey 1990). The length:diameter ratios of the chicons decreased, a quality indicator, with increasing weight.

New Hampshire

Research on *Cucurbita pepo* hybrids comparing bush and vine types with the hull-less seed trait (Fig. 1) has given promising results and could lead to commercialization of the seeds as a snackseed (J.B. Loy pers.

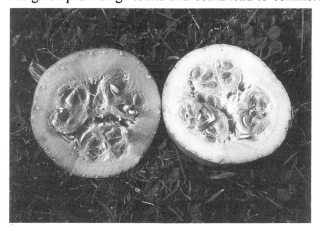
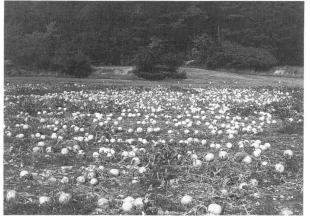

Fig 1. (a) Cross-section of pumpkin (*Curcurbita pepo*) hybrid showing abundance of hull-less seeds and (b) a productive field of hull-less seeded pumpkins in New Hampshire (Photo by J.B. Loy, Univ. of New Hampshire).

commun.). Seed yields up to 2,400 kg/ha have been obtained from small-fruited, bush or intermediate selections (Loy 1990).

The alternative floricultural crops project includes work on production schedules for *Lisianthus*, *Gerbera*, *Anigozanthos*, and other species.

New Jersey

Chrysanthemum cinerariaefolium frequently referred to as pyrethrum has been known for many years as a source of the natural insecticide, pyrethrin. Most of the world's production of pyrethrum is concentrated in Kenya. However, pyrethrum could be produced successfully in New Jersey and other states (Sievers and Lowman 1941). According to C.C. Still (pers. commun.), the perennial plants have persisted for more than five years at the College of Agriculture farm. The focus of the pyrethrum project includes selection for increased cold hardiness, repellency trials, pyrethrin content, and vegetative propagation, and production for on-farm use.

FEDERAL RESEARCH ON NEW CROPS

State projects that are funded through Hatch Act funds administered by the Cooperative State Research Service (CSRS) of USDA are not directly discussed. This compilation includes ARS research, projects supported through special CSRS funds (such as Natural Latex, 1890, and Special Grants), and Cooperative Agreements funded in part or wholly by ARS.

NORTHEASTERN REGION

Research in this Region is quite limited with the exception of service activities relative to new crops germplasm. Projects are summarized in Table 2.

Maryland

A research program carried out at the Beltsville Agricultural Research Center on new species of florist/nursery crops includes species direct from the wild; species commercialized in other countries but not in the United States; improved form of existing cultivars such as from tall cut flowers to short potted plants; new production technology to reduce cropping time; and developing year-round forcing for species with unpredictable flowering (Roh and Lawson 1990). *Eucrosia*, native to Ecuador and Peru, is an example of a beautiful wild species under study (Fig. 2).

While research at Beltsville on *Stokesia laevis* as an oilseed seed source of epoxy fatty acid has ceased, Campbell (1981) appraised its agronomic potential and released four improved lines (Fig. 3).

Crotalaria juncea (sunn hemp) is under investigation as a potential new annual source of paper pulp. This species, immune to root knot nematodes, is being tested as a rotation crop with kenaf. At the Frederick Plant Disease Laboratory, Leather and Forrence (1990) have found that the seeds of sunn hemp contain a potent phytotoxin that inhibited growth of leafy spurge. These same researchers have shown that artemisinin extracted from *Artemisia annua*, a potential new crop for medicinal and pesticide purposes, inhibited root induction in duckweed (CRIS progress report).

Table 2. Federal research on new crops, Northeastern Region.

State	Crop plant/group	Nature of research
Maryland, Beltsville	*Aeschynanthus*, *Anigozanthus*, *Eustoma*, *Lachenallia*, *Ornithogalum*	Collection, evaluation, genetics, management of new florist/nursery species
	Guayule	Break seed & seedling dormancy, develop super propagules
Frederick	*Crotalaria juncea* and *Artemisia annua*	Biological control with natural product chemicals
Pakistan, Peshawar[z]	Medicinal plants	Propagation, culture, harvest, processing

[z]Grant between the Pakistan Forest Institute and the National Germplasm Resources Laboratory, USDA/ARS.

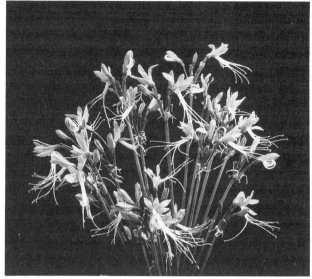

Fig 2. *Eucrosia*, an attractive new ornamental (Photo by M. Roh, USDA/ARS).

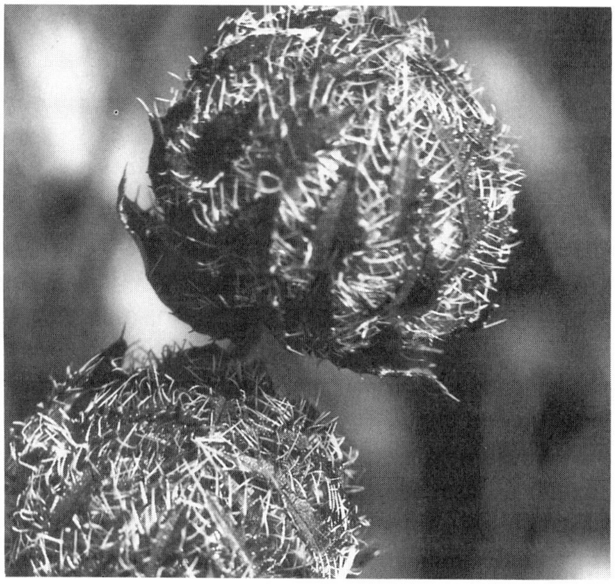

Fig 3. Heads of Stokes aster (*Stokesia laevis*) with inflexed bracts that contribute to seed retention.

NORTH CENTRAL REGION

Most of the Federal new crops efforts in the region are concentrated on industrial use oilseeds with minor efforts on *Amaranthus* and *Chenopodium* for applications in the food industry. Semi-technical updates on new sources of industrial oils including rapeseed, crambe, jojoba, *Lesquerella*, meadowfoam, *Cuphea*, *Vernonia*, and chia (*Salvia hispanica*) appear in INFORM, a news publication of the American Oil Chemist's Society (Anon. 1991a). In reviewing the status of the industrial feedstocks and products from high erucic acid oils extracted from crambe and rapeseed, Van Dyne et al. (1990) covered aspects of production, products and usage, seed composition, processing, economics, and oil outlook. Articles by Vignolo and Naughton (1991) and by Browning (1991) suggest that efforts on the one time new crop castor (*Ricinus communis*) should be revived because of the diversity and approved uses of its seedoil and the high volume of imports.

A number of special projects referred to as High Erucic Acid Development Effort (HEADE) on *Crambe* and *Brassica* have been funded by USDA/CSRS and were established to accelerate commercialization of these crops. There are six of these projects in the North Central region. The major portion of direct federal research on the chemistry, processing, and end-use products from potential new crops with emphasis on oilseeds is conducted at the Northern Regional Research Center, Peoria, Illinois (Table 3). There researchers identified in the 1960s and 1970s many species having unique seed oils and recently described some of the fatty acids and the crop status of the species involved (Kleiman and Princen 1991). This Center also funds Cooperative Agreements at other locations. Research results on sources of critical materials and chemicals have been reported on the new oilseed crops *Limnanthes* (Erhan and Kleiman 1990a,b), *Lesquerella* (Carlson et al. 1990; Chaudhry et al. 1990), and jojoba (Abbott et al. 1990). A high boiling point, non-dimer product from *Limnanthes* oil may become a unique lubricant (Erhan and Kleiman 1990a).

Illinois

Research at Urbana is concentrated on crambe meal for use in chicken rations and glucosinolates in the meal as possible cancer deterrents.

Iowa

The HEADE project at Ames consists of three parts: (1) Crambe breeding and cultural practices. Efforts include evaluation of breeder lines for yield, seed retention, and oil and fatty acid content. Cooperative efforts are underway to obtain approval for use of the herbicide Treflan (R), (2) Improved processing of crambe. Studies

Table 3. Federal research on new crops in the North Central, Southern, and Western Regions

Location	Crop plants/group	Nature of research
NORTH CENTRAL		
Iowa, Ames	Cuphea and others	Germplasm collection, evaluation, and enhancement
	Crambe, rapeseed[z]	Market development, production and utilization of high erucic acid oil
	Cuphea[z]	Evaluation of oil for support of health, reproduction, and longevity
Illinois, Peoria	Jojoba	Jojobin isolation
	Cuphea, Lesquerella, Limnanthes, jojoba	Chemically evaluate germplasm/breeding lines for oil and fatty acid content
	Cuphea, Lesquerella, Limnanthes, jojoba	New crop and product development for production of critical materials and chemicals
	Guayule	Infrastructural evaluation of the natural rubber
Illinois, Urbana	Canola	Weed control measures and herbicide residues in harvested crop
	Crambe	Meal and glucosinolates
Michigan, East Lansing	Black locust	Evaluation, improvement through breeding to expand usage
Wisconsin, Madison	Kenaf	Evaluate kenaf pulps for linerboard and coated papers
SOUTHERN		
Arkansas, Booneville	Amaranth	Yield, quality, economics of vegetable and grain types on hill-lands of the mid-south
Arkansas, Pine Bluff	Forage legumes, new/minor crops	Evaluate for adaptability on acid soils, feed, and insect pests
Florida, Miami	Carambola, other tropical/ subtropical fruits	Selection & breeding
Georgia, Tifton	Pearl millet	Evaluation of landraces, germplasm enhancement
	Cuphea	Screen germplasm for desirable traits and adaptability
Mississippi, Hattiesburg	Guayule	Develop products from plant by-products after rubber extraction
Mississippi State	Kenaf[y]	Agronomic & economic potential in the Midsouth
Stoneville	Kenaf	Develop germplasm, improve cultural practices
Oklahoma, Lane	Kenaf	Production practices, managing nematodes & root diseases
Stillwater	Kenaf[x]	Organic matter & N digestibility of forage. Economics of adding forage to a wheat-livestock system
Puerto Rico, Mayaguez	Tanier (*Xanthosoma*)	Improvement through breeding and management
Texas, College Station	Kenaf	Control of nematodes
	Kenaf[x]	Seed increases
Edcouch	Kenaf[w]	Cultural practices for production in South Texas
McAllen	Kenaf[v]	Demonstration for harvest system & new products
Pecos	Guayule	Integrate agronomic, processing, and product development research
Weslaco	Kenaf	Improved cultivars/cultural practices, evaluate pesticides to support registration
	Guayule	Production practices in South Texas
Virginia, Petersburg	Lesquerella, Limnanthes, Vernonia	Biochemical & nutritional studies
WESTERN		
Arizona, Phoenix	*Guayule, Lesquerella, Vernonia*, others	Germplasm improvement and cultural methods
	Guayule	Establishment, breeding, genetics, rubber quality & quantity
	Lesquerella	Assess commercialization prospects
Tempe	Guayule	Isolation & characterization of rubber transferase and associated genes

Table 3. Continued.

Tucson	Guayule[u]	Establishment by direct seeding
	Guayule, *Lesquerella* *Vernonia*, others[w]	Germplasm and cultural development
California, Albany	Guayule, *Hevea, Ficus*	Biotechnological production of natural rubber
Pasadena	Guayule	Mechanism of bioregulation of plant responses
Riverside	Guayule	Breeding and development
Idaho, Moscow	Winter rapeseed[t] (*Brassica napus*)	Energy source for agriculture production
New Mexico, Las Cruces	*Crambe, Brassica*, other alternative crops	Introduction and breeding
	Guayule	Germplasm evaluation and seed increase
Oregon, Corvallis	*Cuphea* spp.[s]	Development as a source of medium chain triglycerides
	Meadowfoam[z]	Improvement through breeding and cultural practices

[z]Cooperative Agreement with USDA/ARS, Peoria, IL
[y]Cooperative Agreement with USDA/ARS, Stoneville, MS
[x]Cooperative Agreement with USDA/ARS, College Station, TX
[w]Cooperative Agreement with USDA/ARS, Weslaco, TX
[v]Cooperative Agreement with USDA/ARS, Washington, DC
[u]Cooperative Agreement with USDA/ARS, Phoenix, AZ
[t]Cooperative Agreement with USDA/ARS, Tifton, GA
[s]Cooperative Agreement with USDA/ARS, Ames, IA

include evaluation of solvents for extracting oil and glucosinolates, water extraction of glucosinolate from defatted meal, and reverse osmosis to improve oil extraction, and (3) Economics of crambe and rapeseed production. Studies are underway in cooperation with Idaho, Missouri, and North Dakota to determine the areas where crambe, industrial rapeseed (high in erucic acid), and canola can compete with other crops, the areas that are the best economical sources of erucic acid, and the cost comparisons with international markets.

Research to reduce or eliminate extended postharvest seed dormancy in *Cuphea wrightii* and *C. laminuligera* is underway at the Plant Introduction Station, Ames. The best results on germination and seedling survival of these sources of medium-chain-length fatty acids were obtained from excised seeds on agar medium (Roath and Widrlechner 1988).

Kansas

The HEADE project at Manhattan concentrates on selection, improvement of cultural practices, and evaluation of meal quality for rapeseed. Variety selection emphases are concentrated on winter hardiness, pest resistance, and yield. Feeding studies to evaluate performance, carcass quality, and protein supplement efficacy when feeding rapeseed meal are underway. Extrusion technology as a possible means of deactivating the enzyme in rapeseed meal that breaks glucosinolates into anti-nutritional compounds is also being evaluated.

Michigan

Continuing research at Michigan State University on Black locust (*Robinia pseudoacacia*), a fast-growing leguminous tree indicates excellent potential for expanded production of this species because of a variety of uses (Barrett et al. 1990). Black locust is an excellent forage crop under proper management with high biomass yields. For black locust to become more important as a lumber source in the United States, trees are needed with straight stems and resistance to borer insects.

Missouri

As part of a HEADE project at Columbia three facets of high erucic acid crop development are under study: (1) Crop production—evaluating rapeseed cultivars for forage adaptability, and seed yield as well as herbicidal, disease, and date of planting studies, (2) Product development/marketing—nylon 1313 and other products from high erucic acid oils are under evaluation, and (3) Economics—production costs as well as the economic feasibility of biodiesel fuel from rapeseed oil are under evaluation.

Nebraska
The HEADE project at Lincoln concentrates on the uses of high erucic acid oils and includes the development of an engineering properties database.

North Dakota
The HEADE project at Fargo features research on cultural practices, product development, and economics. Cooperation with National Sun Industries in generating interest among farmers to grow crambe and to provide technical assistance to the growers, has been successful. In 1990, most of the 890 ha of commercially grown crambe was in North Dakota (Anon. 1991a). Of the 1,800 ha contracted for 1991, about 1,560 ha were harvested and, the projected crop for 1992 is 8,100 ha (J.C. Gardner pers. commun.).

Wisconsin
The Forest Products Laboratory at Madison, USDA/Forest Service, has a research agreement with the Northern Regional Research center, USDA/ARS, Peoria, Illinois to evaluate kenaf pulps as major fibrous furnish components for linerboard and light weight coated papers.

SOUTHERN REGION
Federal new crops research in the Southern Region covers a wide range of species including fruits, vegetables, cereals, forages, oilseeds, and paper pulp sources (Table 3). However, the most projects and greatest financial support relate to kenaf as a source of paper pulp and forage.

Arkansas
Research at the Booneville South Central Family Farms Center, is underway on *Amaranthus* both as a vegetable (greens) and a grain. United States consumption exceeds 150 mt yearly and should increase in the future (Makus 1990a). Studies are underway on nutrition including aluminum accumulation (Makus 1989) and response to nitrogen (Makus 1990b).

Florida
At least 16 subtropical and tropical fruits are grown commercially in Florida and 20 additional fruit and nut species are grown as roadside and dooryard crops (Knight 1988) with 9,246 ha in commercial production (Campbell 1988). Carambola (*Averrhoa carambola*) is an example of a new fruit crop (Fig 4) with promise for increasing production (Knight 1989).

Georgia
Recent interest in *Cuphea* spp. at Athens is directed toward agronomic improvement as a seedoil source of short chain fatty acids but *Cuphea* especially *C. ignea* has long been used on a limited basis as an ornamental. Three superior selections of *C. glutinosa* were made on the basis of overwintering and other desirable characteristics and 'Lavender Lady' was formally released (Jaworski and Phatak 1990a,b).

Pearl millet has excellent potential to become a new feed grain crop in Georgia and elsewhere (W.W. Hanna pers. commun.). Hybrids grown at the Tifton Coastal Plain Station (Fig. 5) have shown excellent productivity, drought tolerance, and adaptability to pH levels of 4.5 to 8.0. Inbred parental lines for hybrid production are being formally released by USDA/ARS.

Mississippi
A feasibility study for a 100,000 ton fiber separation and chemical pulp mill is underway (Kugler 1991).

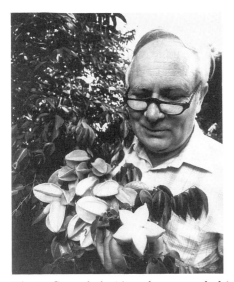

Fig 4. Carambola (*Averrhoa carambola*) an expanding new fruit crop in Florida (Photo by R.J. Knight, USDA/ARS).

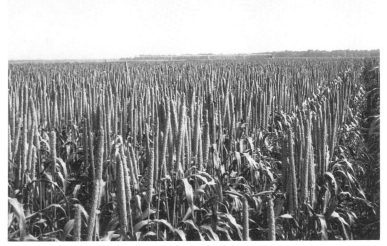

Fig 5. A field planting of a hybrid pearl millet (*Pennisetum glaucum*), Tifton, Georgia (Photo by W.W. Hanna, USDA/ARS).

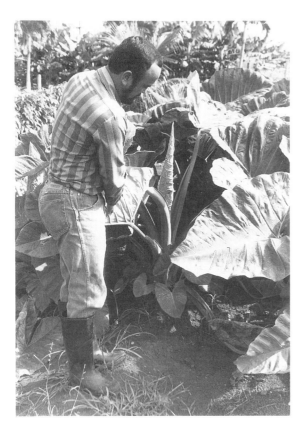

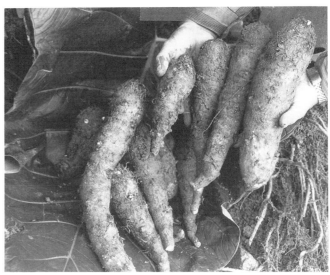

Fig 6. (a) A robust, disease-free hybrid tetraploid of tanier (*Xanthosoma sagittifolium*) and (b) cormels in Puerto Rico (Photo by A. Rivera, USDA/ARS).

Oklahoma

Kenaf research at Lane includes cultural aspects for both fiber production and use as livestock feed. Harvest dates significantly affected harvest index (Webber 1991a). Other studies compared the effects of locations and cultivars on yield, leaf to stem ratios, and percentage of bast and core fibers (Ching et al. 1991; Webber 1991b).

Puerto Rico

Studies at Mayaguez are underway on root and tuber crops such as tanier (*Xanthosoma sagittifolium*) whose cormels are consumed much like potatoes. Tanier hectarage has been steadily declining primarily because of dry root-rot syndrome (Rivera et al. 1990). Diploid commercial cultivars are susceptible to the syndrome but tetraploids and pentaploids are resistant. Resistant hybrid tetraploids (Fig. 6) resulting from crosses between natural tetraploids and colchicine-induced tetraploids of diploid cultivars have been produced.

Texas

Kenaf is a suitable host for all four races of *Meloidogyne incognita* and all four races can significantly reduce stem yields (J.A. Veech pers. commun.) but some variability in sensitivity among kenaf cultivars was observed. At College Station, a quick method for evaluating kenaf cultivars and breeding lines for resistance to nematodes has been developed (Veech 1990).

Resistance to *Phymatotrichopsis omnivora* (root rot), has been explored in Weslaco in kenaf and sunn hemp (Cook and Hickman 1990). Sunn hemp was considerably more resistant than kenaf; but of the kenaf cultivars, 'Tainung No. 1' appeared to be more resistant than 'Everglades 41'. According to Kugler (1991), Texas researchers concluded that kenaf stem core is comparable to wood shavings for poultry litter.

Guayule has been evaluated as a crop on dryland in south Texas, (Gonzalez 1988). The highest plant densities gave the highest yields. Harvesting the whole plant (including roots) every three years was recommended rather than harvesting tops and regrowth after one or two years. Nitrogen and potassium increased dry weight of guayule plants but decreased the accumulation of resin and rubber (Thomas and Hickman 1989). Nitrogen stress actually increased the percentage of resin and rubber; however a marked reduction in biomass because of N stress reduced total rubber production.

WESTERN REGION

Federal research on new crops in the Region (Table 3) is concentrated on industrial-use crops especially guayule, bladderpod (*Lesquerella* spp.), and meadowfoam (*Limnanthes* spp.). Lesser efforts are being expended on crambe/rapeseed, jojoba, Cuphea, and Vernonia.

Arizona

Guayule. Numerous research papers have been published on plant development, production, breeding, harvesting, and processing. Results of the Second Guayule Uniform Yield trials indicate that three new test entries performed well with AZ101 having the highest biomass and resin yields, and Cal-6 and Cal-7 ranking first and second in rubber yield. Evaluations of Arizona selections showed improvement over a standard variety as rubber content and yields were consistently high and regeneration after harvests was good (Ray et al. 1989; Dierig et al. 1992). Rubber content ranged from 4.5 to 7.5%. Several of the tested selections are included in trials in other states.

In evaluation studies with 42 selected lines, Dierig et al. (1989a,b) found that the variables of plant height, width, volume, and dry weight accounted for 85% of the rubber yield and that considerable variation occurred among some lines for various characters. Even though guayule plants are drought tolerant, they responded positively for biomass production with irrigation (Nakayama et al. 1991). Studies of postharvest storage of guayule plant material prior to processing for natural rubber showed that the degree of rubber degradation varied among test entries (Dierig et al. 1991). Studies on guayule in cooperation with the Botany Dept., Arizona State Univ., Tempe, include photoperiodic induction of flowering (Backhaus and Higgins 1989) and the effects of Morphactin and DCPTA on growth and rubber induction (Dierig and Backhaus 1990).

Bladderpod. Of the various species of *Lesquerella*, *L. fendleri* has long been considered as a good candidate for new crop status as a seedoil source of hydroxy fatty acids. Interest in developing bladderpod into a viable new crop for arid lands has recently been revitalized. Since extensive wild populations exist over wide areas, genetic diversity should be easily obtainable for use in breeding and crop improvement. Seed yields of *L. fendleri* obtained from unselected bulked populations and improvement after one selection cycle appear sufficient to justify major efforts on crop development (Thompson et al. 1989). An excellent assessment of the industrial potential of bladderpod that covers production, seed crushing and processing, products, and economics has recently been published (Anon. 1991b).

Cuphea. Species of *Cuphea* have not been adaptable in Phoenix, therefore research efforts have been shifted primarily to Iowa and Oregon where *Cuphea* is more easily grown. Nevertheless, considerable research has been conducted in Arizona. For example, Thompson et al. (1990) reported variation for lauric acid (12:0) and capric acid (10:0) and seed weight within self-pollinating accessions of *C. lutea*, *C. tolucana*, and *C. wrightii*. Ronis et al. (1990) used isozymes to verify interspecific hybrids of *Cuphea*.

Idaho

In Moscow, rapeseed has been evaluated as a potential source of "biodiesel" (methyl ester of rapeseed oil). Spring types are preferred in the northern states because of severe winters (Auld et al. 1991). Adapted winter types with good cold tolerance, low vernalization requirements, and pest resistance could greatly enhance production in the Southeast. Engine endurance tests with biodiesel gave equivalent performance and durability to diesel. Rapeseed crops could produce vast quantities of vegetable oil for processing and use as biodiesel, a renewable resource. Gareau et al. (1990), evaluated six species of *Brassica* and one of *Eruca* to determine their adaptability to the Northwest. Under Idaho conditions, *B. hirta* and *B. juncea* showed the most promise. Considerable effort on improvement of *B. hirta* through breeding is being expended under a HEADE project and economic evaluations are underway as part of the project in cooperation with other state universities.

Oregon

Studies in Corvallis with *Limnanthes alba* have included reproductive physiology (Jahns and Jollif 1990). Multiple bee visits to flowers will be necessary to increase seed set per flower and hence increase seed yields in field production.

Research on *Cuphea* include genetics of allozyme variation in *C. lanceolata* (Knapp and Tagliani 1989a) and in *C. laminuligera* and *C. lutea* (Krueger and Knapp 1990); seed dormancy in *C. laminuligera* and *C. lanceolata* (Knapp and Tagliani 1989b; Knapp 1990); mating systems of *C. laminuligera* (Krueger and Knapp 1991) and outcrossing in *C. lanceolata* (Knapp et al. 1991a); fatty acid mutants (Knapp and Tagliani 1991) and oil diversity (Knapp et al. 1991b) of *C. viscosissima*; and finally genetic parameters for oil yield in *C. lanceolata* (Webb and Knapp 1991).

NATIONAL SERVICES IN SUPPORT OF NEW CROPS RESEARCH

Several groups provide services in support of new crop researchers (Table 4). The USDA's Plant Introduction Office (PIO) coordinates the international exchange of new crop germplasm, facilitates movement of plant materials through quarantine, and provides documentation of passport data through PI (plant introduction) number assignments. This office frequently introduces new crop germplasm and coordinates the quarantine and initial distribution in the United States of new crop accessions collected abroad.

Table 4. National services for new crops research.

Service group	Location	Activities
Plant Introduction Office, NGRL	Beltsville, MD	Introduction, quarantine, passport data documentation
Plant Exploration Office, NGRL	Beltsville, MD	Field collection of new crop germplasm, determine collection gaps
Database Management Unit, NGRL	Beltsville, MD	Maintain database information
Research Leader, NGRL	Beltsville, MD	Facilitate Crop Advisory Committees
Curators (Seed and Clonal)	Various	Increase, evaluate, maintain, distribute document information, collect germplasm
National Seed Storage Laboratory	Ft. Collins, CO	Long term seed storage

The Plant Exploration Office (PEO) plans, participates, and assists with field collections in the United States and abroad. This office determines germplasm gaps in collections and pinpoints areas where collecting is needed. Good locality and use data are obtained routinely.

The Germplasm Resources Information Network (GRIN) contains the national database for new crop germplasm that resides in NPGS collections. The Database Management Unit (DBMU) is responsible to maintain the integrity of data and assist researchers in accessing data in support of their research. Crop Advisory Committees (CAC) are important because of the technical knowledge imparted relative to the needs of the crops involved. A New Crops CAC was formed in 1990. The CAC activities are facilitated by the Research Leader of the National Germplasm Resources Laboratory (NGRL).

Many services relative to new crops are provided by crop germplasm curators and their staffs. Most of the germplasm of new crop species are maintained at the Regional Plant Introduction Stations (RPIS) that are responsible for the increase, evaluation, maintenance, distribution, and information documentation for all new crop species assigned to their location. Staff members may also be directly involved in research and plant exploration efforts such as efforts on Cuphea at Ames, Iowa, the curatorial site. Germplasm collection sites in NPGS for selected new crops are as follows:

Use	Site	Crop
Industrial	RPIS, Griffin, GA	Kenaf, roselle, Stokes aster, sunn hemp
	RPIS, Ames, IA	Crambe, *Cuphea*, rapeseed, *Vernonia*, aromatic plants
	RPIS, Pullman, WA	Guayule, jojoba, *Lesquerella*, *Limnanthes*
Food/feed	RPIS, Griffin, GA	Pearl millet
	Horticulture Research Station, Miami, FL	Carambola, other fruits
	RPIS, Ames, IA	Amaranth, quinoa, herbs, spices
	NCGR, Mayaguez, PR	Tanier

Long term storage and associated research for new crops germplasm in the NPGS is provided by the staff of the National Seed Storage Laboratory (NSSL) in Colorado. The crop curators at the working collections are responsible for submitting good quality seed to NSSL for storage.

Other groups such as inspectors of the Animal Plant Health Inspection Service (APHIS), USDA and State Department of Agriculture inspectors are involved in the exchange of new crop germplasm. Chemists at the Northern Regional Research Laboratory, Peoria, Illinois may run limited chemical analysis of new crop seeds in support of production research.

The history and operation of NPGS has been described (White et al. 1989) and various activities summarized in some detail (Janick 1989).

SUMMARY

In the Northeastern Region, most of the State effort is devoted to assessing the potential for production of exotic, specialty or ethnic vegetables, new ornamentals, herbs, natural insecticides, and green manure crops. The potential for commercialization of globe artichoke, hull-less seeded pumpkin, lupine, and canola is being explored. Other research includes two possible commercial applications for kenaf and clearance of chemicals for pest control.

The National federal effort is largely aimed at the production and end-uses of industrial new crops especially oilseeds such as crambe, rapeseed, meadowfoam, *Cuphea*, bladderpod, and jojoba; the natural rubber source guayule; and fibers from kenaf. The research is heavily concentrated in Arizona, Florida (subtropical fruits), Illinois, Iowa, Oklahoma, Oregon, and Texas. In addition to in-house research by the USDA/ARS, demonstration/pilot processing runs, and rather specific research projects are funded by the ARS and the CSRS of the USDA. The CSRS has funded eight special HEADE projects to promote the commercialization of the high erucic acid oilseeds of crambe and rape (mostly winter type). The commercialization prospects for pearl millet as a feed grain and the likely expansion of carambola acreage appear very favorable.

Supportive service activities are provided by curators of crop germplasm collections, elements of the National Germplasm Resources Laboratory, and others through the enlargement, documentation, and maintenance of new crop germplasm.

REFERENCES

Abbott, T.P., W.A. Phillips, J.L. Swezey, G.A. Bennett, and R. Kleiman. 1990. Large-scale detoxification of jojoba meal for cattle feed. Proc. Eighth Int. Conf. on Jojoba and Its Uses. p. 1–13.

Anon. 1991a. Work continues on new oils for industrial use. INFORM 2(8):678–692.

Anon. 1991b. Lesquerella as a source of hydroxy fatty acids for industrial products. USDA/CSRS Growing Industrial Materials Series.

Auld, D.L., C.L. Peterson, and R.A. Korus. 1991. Winter rapeseed as a renewable fuel for the United States. Proc. Natl. Bioenergy Conf., Coeur d'Alene, ID. p. 117–122.

Backhaus, R.A. and R.R. Higgins. 1989. Photoperiodic induction of flowering in guayule. HortScience 24:939–941.

Barrett, R.P., T. Mebrahtu, and J.W. Hanover. 1990. Black Locust: A multi-purpose tree species for temperature climates, p. 278–283. In: J. Janick and J.E. Simon (eds.). Advances in new crops. Timber Press, Portland, OR.

Boyle, T.H. 1991. Temperature and photoperiodic regulation of flowering in the cultivar 'Crimson Giant' of Easter cactus. J. Amer. Soc. Hort. Sci. 16:618–622.

Boyle, T.H. and D.P. Stimart. 1989. A grower's guide to commercial production of Easter cactus. Grower Talks 53(7):50–52.

Browning, J. 1991. Outlook for U.S. castor production is positive. INFORM 2(8):700–701.

Campbell, C.W. 1988. Tropical fruits produced and marketed in Florida. HortScience 23:247.

Campbell, T.A. 1981. Agronomic potential of Stokes aster. 20:287–295. In: E.H. Pryde, L.H. Princen, and K.D. Mukherjee (eds.). New sources of fats and oils. Amer. Oil Chem. Soc. Monograph 9. Champaign, IL.

Carlson, K.D., R. Kleiman, L.R. Watkins, and W.H. Johnson, Jr. 1990. Pilot-scale extrusion processing/solvent extraction of *Lesquerella* seed. Proc. First Int. Conf. on New Ind. Crops and Prod.

Chaudhry, A., R. Kleiman, and K.D. Carlson. 1990. Minor components of *Lesquerella fendleri* seed oil. J. Amer. Oil Chem. Soc. 67:863–866.

Ching, A., C.L. Webber III, and S.W. Neill. 1992. The effect of location and cultivar on kenaf yield components. J. Ind. Crops and Prod. (in press).

Cook, C.G. and M.V. Hickman. 1990. Response of kenaf and sunn crotalaria to *Phymatotrichopsis omnivora*. El Guayulero 12(3–4):4–9.

Corey, K.A., D.J. Marchant, and L.F. Whitney. 1990. Witloof chicory: a new vegetable crop in the United States, p. 414–418. In: J. Janick and J.E. Simon (eds.). Advances in new crops. Timber Press, Portland, OR.

Dierig, D.A. and R.A. Backhaus. 1990. Effects of Morphactin and DCPTA on stem growth and bioinduction of rubber in guayule. HortScience 25:531–533.

Dierig, D.A., D.T. Ray, and A.E. Thompson. 1989a. Variation of agronomic characters among and between guayule lines. Euphytica 44:265–271.

Dierig, D.A., A.E. Thompson, and D.T. Ray. 1989b. Relationship of morphological variables to rubber production in guayule. Euphytica 44:259–264.

Dierig, D.A., A.E. Thompson, and D.T. Ray. 1991. Effects of field storage on guayule rubber quantity and quality. Rubber Chem. Technol. 64:211–217.

Dierig, D.A., A.E. Thompson, and D.T. Ray. 1992. Yield evaluation of new Arizona guayule selections. Proc. First Int. Conf. on New Ind. Crops and Prod., Oct. 8–12, 1990. Riverside, California (In press).

Erhan, S.M. and R. Kleiman. 1990a. Vulcanized meadowfoam oil. J. Amer. Oil Chem. Soc. 67:670.

Erhan, S.M. and R. Kleiman. 1990b. Meadowfoam oil factice and its performance in natural rubber mixes. Rubber World 203:33–36.

Gareau, R.M., D.L. Auld, and M.K. Heikkinen. 1990. Evaluation of seven species of oilseeds as spring planted crops for the Pacific Northwest. Univ. Idaho Prog. Rpt. 277.

Gonzalez, C.L. 1988. Effects of plant density and harvesting methods of guayule on rubber and resin production under dryland conditions. J. Rio Grande Valley Hort. Soc. 41:51–57.

Hill, D.E. 1989. Witloof chicory (Belgian endive) and radicchio trials—1987-1988. Conn. Agr. Expt. Sta. Bul. 871.

Hill, D.E. 1991. Chinese cabbage and pak-choi trials 1990. Conn. Agr. Expt. Sta. Bul. 887.

Hill, D.E. and A.A. Maynard. 1989. Globe artichoke trials—1987–1988. Conn. Agr. Expt. Sta. Bul. 867.

Jahns, T.R. and G.D. Jollif. 1990. Pollen desposition rate effects on seed set in meadowfoam. Crop Sci. 30:850–853.

Janick, J. (ed.). 1989. The national plant germplasm system of the United States. Plant Breed. Rev. 7:1–230.

Jaworski, C.A. and S.C. Phatak. 1990a. *Cuphea glutinosa* selections for flowering ornamental ground cover in Southeast United States, p. 467–469. In: J. Janick and J.E. Simon (eds.). Advances in new crops. Timber Press, Portland, OR.

Jaworski, C.A. and S.C. Phatak. 1990b. Release of ornamental *Cuphea glutinosa* cultivar Lavender Lady. USDA/ARS and Univ. of Georgia.

Kleiman, R. and L.H. Princen. 1991. New industrial oilseed crops. Proc. World Conf. on oleochemicals: Into the 21st century. p. 127–132.

Knapp, S.J. 1990. Recurrent mass selection for reduced seed dormancy in *Cuphea laminuligera* and *Cuphea lanceolata*. Plant Breed. 104:46–52.

Knapp, S.J. and L.A. Tagliani. 1989a. Genetics of allozyme variation in *Cuphea lanceolata* Ait. Genome 32:57–63.

Knapp, S.J. and L.A. Tagliani. 1989b. Genetic variation for seed dormancy in *Cuphea laminuligera* and *Cuphea lanceolata*. Euphytica 47:65–70.

Knapp, S.J. and L.A. Tagliani. 1991. Two medium-chain fatty acid mutants of *C. viscosissimi*. Plant Breed. 106:338–341.

Knapp, S.J., L.A. Tagliani, and B.H. Liu. 1991a. Outcrossing rates of experimental populations of *Cuphea lanceolata*. Plant Breed. 106:334–337.

Knapp, S.J., L.A. Tagliani, and W.R. Roath. 1991b. Fatty acid and oil diversity of *Cuphea viscosissima*: A source of medium-chain fatty acids. J. Amer. Oil Chem. Soc. 68:515–517.

Knight, Jr., R.J. 1988. Miscellaneous tropical fruits grown and marketed in Florida. Proc. Interamer. Soc. Trop. Hort. 32:34–41.

Knight, Jr., R.J. 1989. Carambola cultivars and improvement programs. Proc. Interamer Soc. Trop. Hort. 33:72–78.

Krueger, S. and S.J. Knapp. 1990. Genetics of allozyme variation in *Cuphea laminuligera* and *Cuphea lutea*. J. Hered. 81:351–358.

Krueger, S.K. and S.J. Knapp. 1991. Mating systems of *Cuphea laminuligera* and *Cuphea lutea*. Theor. Appl. Genet. 82:221–226.

Kugler, D.E. 1991. Product and business prospects for kenaf in 1991. Proc. Third Annu. Int. Kenaf Assn. Conf., Tulsa, OK, February 28–March 2, 1991.

Leather, G.R. and L.E. Forrence. 1990. *Crotalaria juncea* seeds contain a potent phytotoxin. Int. Soc. Chem. Ecol. p. 32. (Abstr.).

Loy, J.B. 1990. Hull-less seeded pumpkins: a new edible snackseed crop, p. 403–407. In: J. Janick and J.E. Simon (eds.). Advances in new crops. Timber Press, Portland, OR.

Makus, D.J. 1989. Aluminum accumulation in vegetable amaranth grown in a soil with adjusted pH values. HortScience 24:460–463.

Makus, D.J. 1990a. Composition and nutritive value of vegetable amaranth as affected by stage of growth, environment, and method of preparation. Proc. Fourth Natl. Amaranth Symp. Minneapolis, MN. p. 35–46.

Makus, D.J. 1990b. Applied nitrogen affects vegetable and grain amaranth seed yield and quality. Proc. Fourth Natl. Amaranth Symp. Minneapolis, MN. p 187–188. (Abstr.)

Malone, G.W., H.D. Tilmon, and R.W. Taylor. 1989. Evaluation of kenaf core for broiler litter. Poultry Sci. 68:88.

Merrick, L.C. 1990. White lupin: an example of new crop development in Maine, p. 171. In: J. Janick and J.E. Simon (eds.). Advances in new crops. Timber Press, Portland, OR.

Nakayama, F.S., D.A. Bucks, R.L. Roth, and B.R. Gardner. 1991. Guayule biomass production under irrigation. Bioresource Technol. 35:173–178.

Ray, D.T. and State Cooperators. 1989. The second guayule uniform regional yield trials. El Guayulero 11(3–4):46–54.

Rivera, E., A. Sotomayor-Rios, R. Goenaga, and P. Hepperly. 1990. New advances in the search for resistance to the dry-root-rot syndrome of tanier (*Xanthosoma* spp.) in Puerto Rico. Proc. XXXVI Annu. Mtg. PPCMCA, San Salvador.

Roath, W.W. and M.P. Widrlechner. 1988. Inducing germination of dormant *Cuphea* seed and the effects of various induction methods on seedling survival. Seed Sci. Tech. 16:699–703.

Roh, M.S. and R.H. Lawson. 1990. New floricultural crops, p. 448–453. In: J. Janick and J.E. Simon (eds.). Advances in new crops. Timber Press, Portland, OR.

Ronis, D.H., A.E. Thompson, D.A. Dierig, and E.R. Johnson. 1990. Isozyme verification of interspecific hybrids of *Cuphea*. HortScience 25:1431–1434.

Sievers, A.F. and M.S. Lowman. 1941. Harvesting pyrethrum. USDA Cir. 581.

Tan, Z.Y. and K.A. Corey. 1990. Technique for improving marketable yield and quality of hydroponically forced Witloof chicory. HortScience 25:1396–1398.

Thomas, J.R. and M.V. Hickman. 1989. Effect of N,P,K on growth, mineral composition, resin, and rubber accumulation in guayule [*Parthenium argentatum* (Gray)]. El Guayulero 11(3&4):25–35.

Thompson, A.E., D.A. Dierig, and E.R. Johnson. 1989. Yield potential of *Lesquerella fendleri* (Gray) Wats., a new desert plant resource for hydroxy fatty acids. J. Arid Environ. 16:331–336.

Thompson, A.E., D.A. Dierig, S.J. Knapp, and R. Kleiman. 1990. Variation in fatty acid content and seed weight in some lauric acid rich *Cuphea* species. J. Amer. Oil Chem. Soc. 67:611-617.

Thompson, A.E., D.A. Dierig, and G.A. White. 1992. Use of plant introductions to develop new industrial crop cultivars. Use of plant introductions in cultivar development, Part 2, CSSA Special Publication 20. p. 9–48.

Van Dyne, D.L., M.G. Blase, and K.D. Carlson. 1990. Industrial feedstocks and products from high erucic oil: crambe and mustard seed. Printing Services, Univ. of Missouri, Columbia.

Veech, J.A. 1990. Evaluating root-knot nematode resistance in kenaf. Proc. Second Annu. Conf. Intl. Kenaf Assoc. p. 6.

Vignolo, R. and F. Naughton. 1991. Castor: a new sense of direction. INFORM 2:692–699.

Webb, D.M. and S.J. Knapp. 1991. Estimates of genetic parameters for oil yield of a *Cuphea lanceolata* population. Crop Sci. 31:621–624.

Webber, C.L. III. 1991a. The effects of kenaf cultivars and harvest dates on plant growth, protein content, and dry matter yields. Proc. First Int. Conf. on New Crops and Prod. Oct. 8–12, 1990. Riverside, CA (In press).

Webber, C.L. III. 1991b. Yield components of kenaf, p 219–222. Proc. TAPPI Pulping Conf.

White, G.A., H.L. Shands, and G.R. Lovell. 1989. History and operation of the National Plant Germplasm System. Plant Breed. Rev. 7:5–56.

New Horticultural Crops for the Southeastern United States

Mary Lamberts

There are many reasons for the upsurge in interest in new horticultural crops. One industry expert (Cook 1990) reported that during the period between 1978 and 1989, consumption of fresh produce in the United States expanded 23%. The retail produce industry is now worth $32 billion. While the aging of American consumers also is a factor which can lead to overall reduced food purchases, it also has the potential for proportional increases in fresh fruit and vegetable consumption. Americans between the ages of 55 and 64 consume 39% more fresh fruit and 34% more fresh vegetables than the national average. As consumers move into their peak income-earning years, they purchase more high-value products and look for greater diversity.

According to Manning (1990), the American produce industry has been riding the crest of a powerful demographic wave which will flatten by the year 2000. Manning predicts that although the nutritional appeal of fresh fruits and vegetables will continue, health options for consumers will increase; growers will need to create more demand and retailers will need to be convinced that consumers will pay more for produce before raising wholesale prices.

Cook (1990) reports that the growth in ethnic populations also contributes to demand for product diversity within the produce department. Foods previously considered ethnic or regional in nature increasingly are being consumed by a broader portion of the population. This helps explain why shipments of Oriental, Mexican, tropical, and exotic produce accounted for about 5% of fresh vegetable shipments in 1988, whereas in previous years the volumes had been too low to track. Some of the states with large populations, such as California, expect to have minority ethnic groups make up almost half the population by the year 2000. This will lead to an increase in fresh produce consumption and will continue to broaden the product mix within the produce category.

One of the challenges that will come with meeting these demands is the need for information on production, packaging, temperature management, storage, merchandising, preparation, and other handling requirements. These require changes, not only for researchers and on the farm, but also in the distribution chain since there is a lack of knowledge about proper handling of specialty products.

With these in mind, this paper will examine steps the Southeastern states have taken in meeting these projected needs for new horticultural crops. The paper has been divided into sections on fruit crops, vegetable crops, and ornamentals. A table summarizing the new crops within each category follows the state by state discussion. Work within each section has been separated by state. Studies carried out in a particular state are based on information supplied by state extension specialists and other researchers. Some of the information was obtained through telephone conversations, with the remainder gathered through correspondence and a survey.

FRUIT CROPS

Alabama

An active breeding, evaluation, and development program is underway for Chinese chestnuts, a potential new nut crop for the South. Research is needed on mechanical harvesting and on postharvest handling. Other fruits which are part of active evaluation programs in Alabama are kiwifruit, Asian and American pears, Oriental persimmon, and pomegranate. Researchers report the need to identify adapted seedlings.

Other new fruit crops which are in the experimental stage include mayhaws, and pineapple guava, or feijoa. Of these, mayhaw seems to have some promise, while pineapple guava or feijoa has problems at present since it sustains winter injury and has no known pollinators in Alabama.

Florida

Most of the new fruit crops being grown in Florida are discussed in much greater detail elsewhere in this volume by J. Crane (1993). They include carambola (240 ha), atemoya (80 ha), passion fruit (40 ha), and sugar apple (30 ha). All are commercially important. Hectareage is increasing for all but sugar apple, though demand for this fruit is still good. For carambola, current research includes field trials on fertilizer, pruning, and cultivar evaluation. 'Arkin' is the dominant carambola cultivar; 'Gefner' is the dominant atemoya cultivar. Current research includes field trials on tree training and pruning and laboratory trials on seed germination. For passion fruit, purples and reds are the most popular types. Research efforts are directed towards pesticide clearance trials. Research on sugar apples is limited to laboratory trials on seed germination.

Georgia

There are about 40 ha of Asian pears being grown on an experimental basis. Mayhaws are also part of an active research program (Krewer et al. 1990; Payne and Krewer 1990; Payne et al. 1990). Some plants are wild, others are cultivated, but interest is increasing on the part of both researchers and industry. Oriental persimmons are being screened, with some success, for cold hardiness. Georgia currently has 65,000 bushes of Southern highbush blueberry, and this number is increasing. Florida bunch grapes, figs, jujubes, pawpaw, plums, and pomegranate are other potential new fruit crops that we may see in the future in Georgia (Krewer et al. 1990; G.W. Krewer pers. commun.).

Both feijoa and kiwifruit have been tried, but neither shows much promise in Georgia (Krewer et al. 1986). There are currently about 5 ha of commercial kiwifruit, but this is declining since it is difficult to grow commercially.

Table 1. New fruit crops for the Southeastern United States.

Crop	Scientific name[z]	State(s) examining the new crop
American pear	*Pyrus communis* L.	Alabama
Apricot	*Prunus armeniaca* L.	Virginia
Asian pear	*Pyrus pyrifolia* (Burm. f.)	Alabama, Georgia,
Sand pear	Nakai	Kentucky, Maryland,
Chinese pear	*P. serotina* Rehd.	South Carolina, Virginia
Atemoya	*Annona cherimola* Mill. x *A. squamosa* L.	Florida
Brambles	*Rubus* spp.	Kentucky
Bunch grapes	*Vitis aestivalis* Michx.	Georgia
Carambola	*Averrhoa carambola* L.	Florida
Chinese chestnut	*Castanea mollissima* Bl.	Alabama
Feijoa	*Feijoa sellowiana* Berg.	Alabama, Georgia
Figs	*Ficus carica* L.	Georgia, Louisiana
Jujubes	*Zizyphus* spp.	Georgia
Kiwifruit	*Actinidia chinensis* Planch.	Alabama,
	A. deliciosa	Georgia, South Carolina
Mayhaw	*Craetaegus aestivalis* (Walt.) Torrey & Gray	Alabama, Georgia, Louisiana
Oriental persimmon	*Diospyros kaki* L.f.	Alabama, Louisiana
Passion fruit	*Passiflora* spp.	Florida
Pawpaw	*Asimina triloba* (L.) Dunal.	Georgia, Kentucky, South Carolina
Persimmons	*Diospyros lotus* L.	Louisiana
Pineapple guava	*Feijoa sellowiana* Berg.	Alabama, Georgia
Plums	*Prunus* spp.	Georgia
Pomegranate	*Punica granatum* L.	Alabama, Georgia
Rabbiteye blueberry	*Vaccinium ashei* Reade	Tennessee
Southern highbush blueberry	*Vaccinium corymbosum*	Georgia, Kentucky, Louisiana, Tennessee
Sugar apple, Sweetsop	*Annona squamosa* L.	Florida

[z]Scientific names and authorities listed in Hortus Third.

Kentucky
There is interest in Southern highbush blueberries, brambles, and Asian pears. Trials are underway with pawpaws.

Louisiana
Studies are underway with Southern highbush blueberries (La. Coop. Ext. Serv. 1992) and mayhaw. There are currently 4 to 10 ha in mayhaws with an increase likely; some wild plants are being harvested as well. Mayhaws are currently being considered for processing. Trials are underway with figs and persimmons.

Maryland
Only Asian pears are under trial.

South Carolina
Potential new fruit crops include kiwifruit, Asian pears, and pawpaws. Of these, kiwifruit appear marginal.

Tennessee
New fruit crops include brambles and both Southern highbush and rabbiteye blueberries (A. Rutledge pers. commun.).

Virginia
Cultivar trials are underway with Asian pear and apricots. There are currently 24 to 30 ha of Asian pears, but less than 4 ha of apricots (R. Marini pers. commun.).

VEGETABLE CROPS

Florida
Trials are underway with calabaza, seedless watermelon, asparagus, bulb onions, Japanese muskmelons, rhubarb, and leeks (D. Maynard pers. commun.). Florida growers are producing several Oriental vegetables commercially. These include Chinese okra or angled luffa, lauki or bottle gourd, smooth luffa, tindora or ivy gourd, very small amounts of parvar or pointed gourd, guar or cluster bean as a green shell bean, hyacinth or lablab bean, yard-long or asparagus beans, winged bean, and pea and Thai eggplants (Lamberts 1990). There is very little research on these latter commodities except for limited surveys of diseases and insects. Most of the initiative for these new vegetables comes from the growers themselves.

Georgia
Several new vegetable crops have been tried with varying degrees of success. The main new vegetable produced today is collards, which is now at 3,645 ha and expanding. It is grown as a second crop after peanuts and so is a specialty crop for those growers. Green onion area has also expanded, with 81 to 101 ha planted in recent years. The third most popular new vegetable is hot peppers, primarily 'Piquin' and jalapeño types; the different colored bell peppers are also being grown. The fourth most popular is English peas, grown as an early crop which can take advantage of a market window (W. McLauren pers. commun.).

There is limited production of pumpkins of various types for roadside stands and pick-your-own. There is limited area in beets, some Oriental vegetables, including lemon grass, and asparagus. Other new vegetable crops for Georgia include ginseng, fresh cut herbs, green peanuts for the early market, and husk tomatoes for the Mexican market in Atlanta. Radicchio was tried, but problems with marketing have resulted in declining production; a recovery is not anticipated (W. McLauren pers. commun.).

Kentucky
Commercial production of Oriental vegetables such as napa, bok choy, and daikons is underway and expected to increase with a growing ethnic population. Other new vegetables under trial include staked and

processing tomatoes and sugar enhanced and super-sweet sweet corn. Various mushrooms are currently being tried. The mushroom industry is very competitive and in a state of flux (D. Ingram pers. commun.).

Louisiana

The early phase of domestication of apios is underway (Reynolds et al. 1990). Researchers think it will be productive for home gardens, but there is a need to commercialize this crop, which will require work on marketing. Apios will most likely be used as a processed product, and could also be developed as a high protein food, possibly for developing countries, or as a health food. Apios is highly productive and harvesting can be mechanized. The tubers have a taste similar to a combination of boiled potatoes and boiled peanuts. Apios is mealier than potato and chips well. Other new vegetables being tried some on a commercial basis, include Shiitake and oyster (pleurotis) mushrooms, tomatillo, and greenhouse cucumbers (Koske 1989; W. Blackmon pers. commun.).

Maryland

An increase in Oriental vegetable production is underway (B. Quebedeaux pers. commun.).

Mississippi

Little is being done with new vegetables. There is interest in two cultivars of hot pepper, 'Mississippi hot' and 'Passion', the latter from Japan, and 'Little Fingers' eggplant. There is some commercial mushroom production of shiitake and pleurotis types. Paste tomatoes are a new crop for Mississippi (M. Burnham pers. commun.).

North Carolina

Several new vegetables are being tried, including intermediate day dry bulb onions. Researchers have evaluated 90 to 100 cultivars for bolt tolerance and winter survival with some success. Onions are planted in October and harvested June or July; there were 120 ha in 1990–91. Broccoli is usually planted in August–September as a fall crop and harvested from mid-September through Christmas. Spring plantings are sown in late February–March and harvested in May. This is seen as an alternative to a potential increase in California production.

Production of ethnic vegetables is increasing, especially for Oriental vegetables such as Chinese cabbage (napa and bok choy), melons, greens, and daikon; and ethnic peppers such as jalapeño, ancho, Anaheim, and other chiles. The major problem for scientists working with these items is the lack of published literature in English. This is one of the reasons the same item may be marketed under a variety of different ethnic names. There have been some changes in specialty lettuce cultivars which allow for an extra day or two of shelf life (D. Sanders pers. commun.). There is some herb production, including ginseng, in the mountainous areas of North Carolina, Georgia, and Tennessee. Shiitake mushrooms are also being evaluated.

Tennessee

Limited cultivar evaluation trials have been carried out with Chinese cabbage for spring and fall production since 1989. Researchers have recommended fall production since many cultivars, especially from Group Pekinensis bolt under spring conditions. Some cultivars from Group Chinensis are quite susceptible to *Fusarium* spp. Yield and quality for both Groups have generally been acceptable (D. Coffey pers. commun.).

Some domestic and some wild ginseng is being produced; nitrogen and copper evaluations on farm have been carried out for this crop. Both cherry and paste tomatoes are being produced (A. Rutledge pers. commun.).

Virginia

Broccoli is a small, but growing industry with a bright future. Cauliflower appears to have excellent potential for mountainous areas at elevations of 1,800 m, but it is not yet grown commercially (C. O'Dell pers. commun.). Other vegetables include storage cabbage, Belgian endive, elephant garlic, heat tolerant head lettuce, exotic mushrooms, Brussels sprouts, Chinese cabbage, medicinal herbs such as American ginseng and goldenseal, golden-fleshed potatoes, and commercial production of organic vegetables (G. Welbaum pers. commun.).

Table 2. New vegetable crops for the Southeastern United States.

Crop	Scientific name[z]	State(s) examining the new crop
Apios	*Apios americana* Medic.	Louisiana
Asparagus	*Asparagus officinalis* L.	Florida, Georgia
Asparagus bean	*Vigna unguiculata* ssp. *sesquipedalis* (L.) Verdc.	Florida
Belgian endive, witloof chicory	*Chicorium intybus* L.	Virginia
Bottle gourd	*Lagenaria siceraria* (Molina) Standl.	Florida
Broccoli	*Brassica oleraceae* L., Botrytis Group	North Carolina, Virginia
Brussels sprouts	*Brassica oleraceae* L., Gemmifera Group	Virginia
Cabbage	*Brassica oleraceae* L., Botrytis Group	Virginia
Calabaza	*Cucurbita moschata* (Duch. ex. Lam.) Duch. ex. Poir	Florida
Chinese cabbage	*Brassica rapa* L. Chinensis Group Pekinensis Group	Kentucky, North Carolina, Tennessee
Chinese okra, angled luffa	*Luffa acutangula* (L.) Roxb.	Florida
Cluster bean	*Cyamopsis tetragonolobus* (L.) Taub.	Florida
Collards	*Brassica oleracea* L. Acephala Group	Georgia
Cucumbers, greenhouse	*Cucumis sativus* L.	Louisiana
Daikon	*Raphanus sativum* L. var. *Longipinnatus* Bailey	Kentucky, North Carolina
Garlic, elephant	*Allium* spp.	Virginia
Ginseng	*Panax quinquefolium* L. Wallich	North Carolina, Tennessee, Virginia
Goldenseal	*Hydrastis canadensis* L.	Virginia
Guar	*Cyamopsis tetragonolobus* (L.) Taub.	Florida
Herbs, fresh	various	Georgia, North Carolina
Husk tomato	*Physalis ixocarpa* Brot.	Georgia, Louisiana
Hyacinth bean	*Dolichos lablab* L.	Florida
Ivy gourd	*Coccinea grandis* (L.) Voigt	Florida
Lablab bean	*Dolichos lablab* L.	Florida
Lauki	*Lagenaria siceraria* (Mol.) Standl.	Florida
Leeks	*Allium ampeloprasum* L. Porrum Group	Florida
Lemongrass	*Cymbopogon citratis* DC. ex. Ness	Georgia
Lettuce, specialty	*Lactuca sativa* L.	North Carolina, Virginia
Luffa, smooth, sponge gourd	*Luffa aegyptiaca* Mill.	Florida
Mushrooms	*Agaricus* spp. *Disparus* spp., and others	Kentucky, Louisiana, Mississippi, North Carolina, Virginia
Muskmelons, Japanese	*Cucumis melo* L.	Florida
Onions, bulb	*Allium cepa* L.	Florida, North Carolina
Onions, green	*Allium cepa* L.	Georgia
Organic vegetables	various	Virginia
Oriental vegetables	various	Georgia, Maryland, North Carolina
Parvar	*Trichosanthes dioica* Roxb.	Florida
Peanuts, green	*Arachis hypogaea* L.	Georgia
Peas, English	*Pisum sativum* L.	Georgia
Pepper, hot	*Capsicum* spp.	Georgia, Mississippi, North Carolina
Pepper, bell (colored)	*Capsicum annuum* L.	Georgia
Pea eggplant	*Solanum torvum* L.	Florida
Pointed gourd	*Trichosanthes dioica* Roxb.	Florida
Potatoes, golden-fleshed	*Solanum tuberosum* L.	Virginia

Table 2. Continued.

Pumpkin	*Cucurbita* spp.	Georgia
Radicchio	*Chicorium intybus* L.	Georgia
Rhubarb	*Rheum rhababarum* L.	Florida
Sweetcorn, super-sweet	*Zea mays* L.	Kentucky
Thai eggplant	*Solanum macrocarpon* L.	Florida
Tindora	*Coccinea grandis* (L.) Voigt	Florida
Tomatillo	Physalis ixocarpa Brot.	Georgia, Louisiana
Tomatoes	*Lycopersicon lycopersicum* (L.) Karst	Kentucky, Tennessee
Yard-long bean	*Vigna unguiculata* ssp. *sesquipedalis* (L.) Verdc.	Florida
Watermelon, seedless	*Citrullus lanatus* (Thunb.) Matsum. & Nakai	Florida
Winged bean	*Psophocarpus tetragonolobus* (L.) DC	Florida

[z]Scientific names and authorities listed in Hortus Third (1976).

ORNAMENTALS

Alabama

The focus of work on new ornamental crops is primarily on means of adapting woody plants from the temperate zone for interior environments (Keever et al. 1986, 1988).

Florida

New crops include anthuriums for foliage and flowering and new cut foliage and bedding plants, and *Calathea* spp., amaryllis, and caladium (R. Henley pers. commun.).

Georgia

Various verbenas such as native moss verbena, are under investigation for roadside plantings in southern and coastal Georgia and for commercial landscapes. Flower colors range from white, pink, and pale lilac to darker shades. Verbena is drought tolerant and requires low maintenance. Vervain, another native, has primarily dark royal purple flowers and can be used for roadsides. It has been in cultivation for some time. The cultivar in the trade is 'Polaris' with pale lilac-blue flowers. Rose verbena or creeping vervain, an old species, is widely used in landscapes because of its hardiness and drought tolerance. The most common cultivar is 'Rosea' or 'Roseum' which has pinkish rose flowers; additional colors are available. Various vincas are now heavily used in landscaping as well. Use of gomphrena, a tough, hardy plant, is increasing in landscapes (J. Lewis pers. commun.)

Kentucky

Research is underway in godetia or satin flower, including trials on field production and greenhouse trials (Anderson 1990a,b,c; Anderson and Hartley 1990; Anderson et al. 1991). This crop requires cool, high light conditions and so probably will not be a major cutflower in the Southeastern United States. Greenhouse trials are continuing with velvet sage which shows good potential as a greenhouse cutflower grown under the same conditions as a 7-week chrysanthemum. Other greenhouse trials are being conducted with yarrow, which has good potential as a greenhouse cutflower. It requires three weeks in propagation plus six weeks in the greenhouse under 6 h supplemental high intensity daylight (R. Anderson pers. commun.).

Maryland

Ornamentals are the fastest growing part of the agricultural industry in Maryland, with a 10% increase annually over the past 5 years. In the metropolitan areas, there has been an increase in direct marketing of cut flowers through roadside stand, farmers markets, and as an add-on at pick-your-own operations. Cut flowers is a generic term which is applied to any dried material such as everlastings, yarrow, and statice, and to anything that can be cut which will last 5 days.

There is a new market for bedding plant material from 4 July to the first frost. Some of the production now includes greenhouse production of containerized annuals which are sold in various pot sizes throughout the season. Flowering cabbage and flowering kale are used for fall color.

The market for woody ornamentals is exploding, particularly with specialty trees and shrubs and clonal selection of unique cultivars such as Japanese maple, but anything unusual is being sought (Healy 1986, 1989; Healy and Aker 1988a,b; Healy and Espinosa 1988a,b; Healy and Graper 1987, 1989; Healy and Wilkins 1985; Healy et al. 1990).

North Carolina

Research on flowering plants is focused on orange browallia, pink trumpet vine, and blue daze. Orange browallia shows excellent potential as a flowering potted plant and a hanging basket. Pink trumpet vine has potential as a flowering hanging basket; it has very fragrant pink flowers. The major problem with this crop is bud and leaf drop with sudden changes in environment. Blue daze is a newly introduced bedding plant and hanging basket plant which has blue flowers (D. Bailey pers. commun.).

Table 3. New ornamental crops for the Southeastern United States.

Crop	Scientific name[z]	State(s) examining the new crop
Amaryllis	*Amaryllis* spp.	Florida
Anthuriums for foliage & flowering	*Anthurium* spp.	Florida
Bedding plants	various	Maryland
Blue daze	*Evolvulus glomeratus grandiflorus*	North Carolina
Bulbs	various	Virginia
Caladium	*Caladium* spp.	Florida
Calathea	*Calathea* spp.	Florida
Containerized annuals	various	Maryland
Crape-myrtle	*Lagerstroemia* spp.	South Carolina
Cut flowers, dried	various	Maryland
Dried flowers	various	Virginia
Flowering cabbage	*Brassica oleraceae* L. Acephala Group	Maryland
Flowering kale	*Brassica oleraceae* L. Acephala Group	Maryland
Godetia	*Clarkia amoena* ssp. *Whitneyi* ('Grace' series)	Kentucky
Holly	*Ilex* spp.	South Carolina
Nursery crops	various	Virginia
Orange browallia, firebush	*Streptosolen jamesonii* (Benth.) Miers.	North Carolina
Pink trumpet vine	*Podranea ricasoliana* (Tanfani) T. Sprague	North Carolina
Satin flower	*Clarkia amoena* ssp. *Whitneyi* ('Grace' series)	Kentucky
Specialty trees & shrubs	various	Maryland
Velvet sage	*Salvia leucantha*	Kentucky
Verbenas:		
Moss verbena	*Verbena tenuisecta* Briq.	Georgia
Rose verbena, creeping vervain	*Verbena canadiensis* (L.) Britt.	Georgia
Vervain	*Verbena rigida* K. Spreng.	Georgia
Woody ornamentals	various	Maryland
Woody plants for interior use	various	Alabama
Yarrow	*Achillea millifolium*, German hybrids	Maryland

[z]Scientific names and authorities listed in Hortus Third (1976).

South Carolina

Studies are underway with new cultivars of holly and crape myrtle and heat tolerant shade trees (A. King pers. commun.).

Virginia

Research is being carried out on bulbs such as tulips and daffodils, on nursery crops, and on dried flowers (G. Welbaum pers. commun.).

CONCLUSIONS

The new fruit crop being tried in the greatest number of states was the Asian pear (Georgia, Kentucky, Maryland, South Carolina, and Virginia). Southern highbush blueberry was second in importance (Georgia, Kentucky, Louisiana, and Tennessee). Four fruit crops are being evaluated in at least three states: mayhaw and persimmons (Alabama, Georgia, and Louisiana), kiwifruit (Alabama, South Carolina, and Georgia), and pawpaw (Georgia, Kentucky, and South Carolina). Brambles are being tested in Kentucky and Tennessee; passion fruit is under trial in Alabama and Florida.

Oriental vegetables are being grown in six states (Florida, Georgia, Kentucky, Maryland, North Carolina, and Virginia). Ginseng is being grown in five states (Georgia, Kentucky, North Carolina, Tennessee, and Virginia). Mushrooms (shiitake, oyster, and various types) are being tried in Florida, Kentucky, Louisiana, and Mississippi. Four states are growing either hot or colored bell peppers (Florida, Georgia, Mississippi, and North Carolina). Onions and herbs are being evaluated in Florida, Georgia, and North Carolina; tomatoes in Kentucky, Mississippi, and Tennessee. Broccoli, lettuce, sugar enhanced and super-sweet sweet corn, asparagus, pumpkin/calabaza, and husk tomato (tomatillo) are being evaluated in at least two states each.

In contrast, there is little commonality for ornamentals where unique crops are being evaluated in each state. At present, there is no one single crop which shows promise to become the South's kiwifruit. For fruits, a number of crops such as Asian pear, Southern highbush blueberry, mayhaw, persimmon, pawpaw, and the subtropical fruits of Southern Florida all have potential, though most likely as combined enterprises rather than as sole crops. For vegetables, this same trend of a combination of crops is more likely than any one single crop. Oriental vegetables, which is a very broad area, are becoming more popular. Other crops with promise include ginseng, various mushrooms, and peppers, both hot types and colored bells. With few exceptions, state programs or local growers or a combination of the two, are interested in expanding the horticultural horizons of the South beyond the crops for which this area has traditionally been known.

REFERENCES

Anderson, R.G. 1990a. Gotta get Godetia. Greenhouse Grower, Oct.

Anderson, R.G. 1990b. Gotta pot Godetia. Greenhouse Grower, Nov.

Anderson, R.G. 1990c. Satin flower. GrowerTalks, May.

Anderson, R.G. and G. Hartley. 1990. Use of growth retardants on satin flower, godetia, for pot plant production. Acta Hort. 272:285–292.

Anderson, R.G., L. Utami, and R.L. Geneve. 1991. Gotta cut Godetia. Greenhouse Grower, Jan.

Armitage, A.M. 1990. New herbaceous ornamental crops research, p. 453–456. In: J. Janick and J.E. Simon (eds.). Advances in new crops. Timber Press, Portland, OR.

Blanchet, P. 1985. Les degats de gels sur kiwi. L'Aboriculture Fruitière 370:43–49.

Blight, H.C. 1981. The climatic requirements for the successful cultivation of kiwi fruit. Citrus Subtrop. Fruit J. 6–7.

Boudreaux, J.E. 1991. Commercial vegetable production recommendations. Louisiana Coop. Ext. Serv. Pub. 2433. Baton Rouge.

Caldwell, J. 1989. Kiwifruit performance in South Carolina and effect of winter chilling. Proc. 10th Annu. Meeting and Shortcourse Ala. Fruit and Veg. Growers Assoc. p. 127–129.

Callaway, M.B. 1991. Germplasm collection using public contests: The *Asimina triloba* example. HortScience 26:692. (Abstr.)

Callaway, M.B. 1990. The pawpaw (*Asimina triloba*). Kentucky State Univ., Pub. CRS-Hort 1-901T., Frankfort.

Cook, R. 1990. Catering to the American consumer. Fresh trends '91, The Packer, 54:12,14,16,18,20,22,24,26.

Crane, J.H. 1989. Acreage and plant densities of commercial carambola, mamey sapote, lychee, longan, sugar apple, atemoya, and passion fruit plantings in South Florida. Proc. Fla. State Hort. Soc. 102:239–242.

Crane, J.H. 1993. Commercialization of carambola, atemoya, and other tropical fruits in South Florida. In: J. Janick and J.E. Simon (eds.). Progress in new crops. Wiley, New York.

Crane, J.H., C.F. Balerdi, and C.W. Campbell. 1991. The avocado. Univ. of Florida, Fruit Crops Fact Sheet FC-3, Gainesville.

Crane, J.H. and R.M. Baranowski. 1990. Planning grower funded tropical fruits research in Florida. Proc. Interamer. Soc. Trop. Hort. 34:19–23.

Crane, J.H. and C.W. Campbell. 1991. The mango. Univ. of Florida, Fruit Crops Fact Sheet FC-2, Gainesville.

Crane, J.H., C.W. Campbell, and R. Olszack. 1989. Current statistics for commercial carambola groves in South Florida. Proc. Interamer. Soc. Trop. Hort. 33:94–99.

Ferguson, A.R. 1990. Kiwifruit management, p. 472–503. In: G.J. Galletta and D.G. Himelrick (eds.). Small fruit management. Prentice Hall, Englewood Cliffs, NJ.

Ferguson, J.J., J.H. Crane, and R. Olszack. 1988. Growth of young carambola trees using standard and controlled-release fertilizers. Proc. Interamer. Soc. Trop. Hort. 32:20–24.

Ferree, M.E., R.M. Crassweller, and G.W. Krewer. 1983. Commercial muscadine grape culture. Univ. of Georgia, Coop. Ext. Serv. Bul. 739. Athens.

Gremminger, U., A. Huistein, and A. Aeppli. 1982. Reaction of young *Actinidia chinensis* plants to frost. Schweizerische Z. für Obstund Weinbav. 118:110–115.

Harris, H., J.D. Norton, and J.C. Moore. 1980. 3 new Chinese chestnuts AU-Cropper, AU-Leader, and AU-Homestead: Their history and production. Auburn Univ., Agr. Expt. Sta. Cir. 247, Auburn.

Healy, W. 1986. Currently produced outdoor cut flowers. Univ. of Maryland, Hort. Dept. Mimeo HE 143-86, updated 1989, College Park.

Healy, W. 1989. Chrysanthemum cultivars for fall sales. Univ. of Maryland, Hort. Dept. Mimeo HE 157-89, College Park.

Healy, W. and S. Aker. 1988a. Cut flower field studies—1988. Univ. of Maryland, Hort. Dept. Mimeo HE 155-88, College Park.

Healy, W. and S. Aker. 1988b. Producing cut flowers—general field crop management. Univ. of Maryland, Coop. Ext. Serv. Fact Sheet 468, College Park.

Healy, W., S. Aker, and S. Klick. 1990. Cut flower field studies—1989. Univ. of Maryland, Hort. Dept. Mimeo HE 157-89, College Park.

Healy, W. and I. Espinosa. 1988a. Producing cut flowers—florist statice. Univ. of Maryland, Coop. Ext. Serv. Fact Sheet 469, College Park.

Healy, W. and I. Espinosa. 1988b. Producing cut flowers—liatris. Univ. of Maryland, Coop. Ext. Serv. Fact Sheet 467, College Park.

Healy, W. and D. Graper, 1987. 1987 Cut flower production at the Wye Research Center. Univ. of Maryland, Hort. Dept. Mimeo HE 97-90, College Park.

Healy, W. and D. Graper. 1989. Flowering kale and cabbage. Univ. of Maryland, Hort. Dept. Mimeo HE 148-89, College Park.

Healy, W. and H.F. Wilkins. 1985. Alstroemeria culture. Univ. of Maryland, Hort. Dept. Mimeo HE 134-85, College Park.

Hewett, E.W. and K. Young. 1981. Critical freeze damage temperatures of flower buds of kiwifruit (*Actinidia chinensis* Planch.). New Zeal. J. Agr. Res. 24: 73–75.

Johnson, D.M., C.A. Hanson, and P.H. Thomson. 1988. Kiwifruit handbook. Bookcrafters Inc., Celsea, MI.

Keever, G.J. and G.S. Cobb. 1986. Temperate zone woody plants for interior environments. J. Environ. Hort. 4:16–18.

Keever, G.J., G.S. Cobb, and J.C. Stephenson. 1988. Interior performance of temperate zone landscape plants. J. Environ. Hort. 4: 16–18.

Koske, T.J. 1989. Sources of shiitake forest mushroom spawn. Louisiana Coop. Ext. Serv. Baton Rouge.

Krewer, G., P. Bertrand, S. Meyers, and D. Horton. 1986. Kiwi cold injury, other problems beset southeastern plantings. Fruit South. Aug.–Sept., p. 12–15.

Krewer, G.W., T.F. Crocker, S.C. Myers, P.F. Bertrand, and D.L. Horton. 1990. Minor fruits & nuts in Georgia. Univ. of Georgia, Coop. Ext. Serv. Bul. 992, Athens.

Krewer, G.W., S.C. Myers, P.F. Bertrand, and D.L. Horton. 1987. Commercial bramble culture. Univ. of Georgia, Coop. Ext. Serv. Bul. 964. Athens.

Krewer, G.W., S.C. Myers, P.F. Bertrand, D.L. Horton, S. Brown, and M. Austin. 1989. Commercial blueberry culture. Univ. of Georgia, Coop. Ext. Serv. Cir. 713, Athens.

Krewer, G., P. Sumner, and T. Hall. 1988. Trunk protection for reducing cold injury of kiwifruit. Vol. 3. Proc. Southeaster Professional Fruit Workers Conf. Paper 13.

Lamberts, M. 1990. Latin American vegetables, p. 378–387. In: J. Janick and J.E. Simon (eds.). Advances in new crops. Timber Press, Portland, OR.

Louisiana Cooperative Extension Service. Commercial blueberry production. Ext. Serv. Pub. 2363, Baton Rouge.

Louisiana Cooperative Extension Service. 1989. Figs for commercial and home orchards in Louisiana. Ext. Serv. Pub. 1529 (rev), Baton Rouge.

Louisiana Cooperative Extension Service. 1991. The Louisiana home orchard. La. Coop. Ext. Serv. Pub. 1884 (rev), Baton Rouge.

Louisiana Cooperative Extension Service. 1992. Growing rabbiteye blueberries in Louisiana. Ext. Serv. Pub. 1978 (rev), Baton Rouge.

Lu, S. and M. Rieger. 1990. Cold acclimation of young kiwifruit vines under artificial hardening conditions. HortScience 25:1628–1630.

Manning, J. 1990. Riding the produce wave. Fresh trends '91. The Packer 54:8,10.

Midcap, J.T. and K.D. Coder. New trees and shrubs for Georgia. Univ. of Georgia, Coop. Ext. Serv. Bul. 1063, Athens.

Moriconi, D.N., M.C. Rush, and H. Flores. 1990. Tomatillo: A potential vegetable crop for Louisiana, p. 407–413. In: J. Janick and J.E. Simon (eds.). Advances in new crops. Timber Press, Portland, OR.

Norton, J.D., A.G. Hunter, and H. Harris. Research with Chinese chestnut in Alabama. 74th Annu. Rpt. Northern Nut Growers Assoc.

O'Dell, C.R., S.B. Sterrett, B.M. Young, and A.M. Borowski. 1989. A procedure for evaluating production potentials and developing extension recommendations for new horticultural crops. Va. Coop. Ext. Serv. Pub. 438-015, Blacksburg.

O'Dell, C.R., S.B. Sterrett, B.M. Young, and A.M. Borowski. 1990. Evaluating production potentials and developing extension recommendations for new vegetable crops, p. 57–61. In: J. Janick and J.E. Simon (eds.). Advances in new crops. Timber Press, Portland, OR.

Payne, J.A. and G.W. Krewer. 1990. Mayhaw: A new crop for the south, p. 317–321. In: J. Janick and J.E. Simon (eds.). Advances in new crops. Timber Press, Portland, OR.

Payne, J.A., G.W. Krewer, and R.R. Fitenmiller. 1990. Mayhaws: trees of pomological and ornamental interest. HortScience 25:246,375.

Puls, E.E., Jr. 1967. Nematode resistance in figs. Louisiana Agr. 10(4).

Puls, E., Jr. 1991. Commercial mayhaw culture. Louisiana Coop. Ext. Serv. Pub. 2429, Baton Rouge.

Reynolds, B.D., W.J. Blackmon, E. Wickremesinhe, M.H. Well, and J. Constantin. 1990. Domestication of *Apios americana*, p. 436–442. In: J. Janick and J.E. Simon (eds.). Advances in new crops. Timber Press. Portland, OR.

Roh, M.S. and R.H. Lawson. 1990. New floricultural crops. p. 448–453. In: J. Janick and J.E. Simon (eds.). Advances in new crops. Timber Press. Portland, OR.

Sale, P.R. 1985. Kiwifruit culture. V.R. Ward Gov. Printer, Wellington, New Zealand.

Southern Rural Development Center. 1990. Inventory of non-traditional agricultural commodity activities in the southern region. Southern Rural Development Center, Mississippi State.

University of Kentucky. Cultivating ginseng in Kentucky. ID-60, Lexington.

University of Kentucky. Ginseng seed and root sources for planting in Kentucky. HO 73, Lexington.

Warrington, I.J. and G.C. Weston. 1990. Kiwifruit science and management. Massey Univ., Palmerston North, New Zealand.

Weet, C.S. 1979. Frost damage to kiwifruit vines. Avocado Grower. April: 26–29. 59.

Welbaum, G. (compiler). A survey of public sponsored alternative crops research and development projects in Virginia. Dept. of Hort. VPI&SU, Blacksburg.

Wickremesinhe, E.R.M, W.J. Blackmon, and B.D. Reynolds. 1990. Adventitious shoot regeneration and plant production from *Apios americana*. HortScience 25:1436–1438.

Wickremesinhe, E.R.M, W.J. Blackmon, and B.D. Reynolds. 1990. In vitro propagation of *Apios americana*. HortScience 25:1439–1440.

Widrlechner, M.P. 1990. Trends influencing the introduction of new landscape plants, p. 460–467. In: J. Janick and J.E. Simon (eds.). Advances in new crops. Timber Press, Portland, OR.

Development of New Agronomic Crops in the Midwest

Edward S. Oplinger

Development of new or "alternative" agronomic crops in the Midwest (Fig. 1) has occurred primarily in four areas: agronomic and economic research; utilization research; development and dissemination of information; and commercial production and marketing. This review and summary is limited to agronomic crops which are new to the Midwest.

AGRONOMIC & ECONOMIC RESEARCH

A telephone survey conducted by the author indicated that there was some research activity on a few new crops in all states in the Midwest in 1990 and 1991. Agronomists from all states reported field studies were being conducted on canola and/or oilseed rape, *Brassica napus* and *Brassica campestris*. The studies ranged from cultivar evaluations, to planting practices, fertility requirements, and harvesting techniques. Almost all of these states also reported some commercial production of these crops.

At least four states, Indiana, Minnesota, Missouri, and North Dakota, now have research centers receiving state and/or federal funding and have full-time personnel working on new or alternative crops. The descriptions of their research activity are described elsewhere in these proceedings.

UTILIZATION RESEARCH

The extent of the research activity on new crop utilization is more difficult to identify. Much of the new uses or value added research is being conducted on more traditional crops, especially maize (*Zea mays*), soybean (*Glycine max* L. Merr.), and small grains. Recent research at Wisconsin has demonstrated the value of feeding unprocessed soybeans to dairy cows. This resulted in a 25% increase in the state's hectarage and production in 1991, with the majority of the increase being grown by first time producers. Thus, for some producers, soybean is a new or alternative crop in Wisconsin. Development of soybean cultivars with reduced levels of trypsin inhibitors is creating expanded feed uses for the crop. Waxy hulless barley (*Hordeum vulgare* L.) is currently being developed as a highly soluble fiber source.

INFORMATION DEVELOPMENT AND DISSEMINATION

As recent as two years ago, alternative crops were not delineated in defining commodity responsibilities. This has changed and the most recent Extension Personnel Directory lists seven of the 14 midwestern states with one or more individuals identified with alternative crop responsibilities (Fig. 1). The remaining seven states also have at least one extension individual that answers questions and provides information on alternative crops.

Several states have developed fact sheets and extension bulletins on the agronomic and economic potential of specific alternative crops. Wisconsin and Minnesota have developed and distributed an Alternative Field Crops Manual (Oplinger and Oelke 1991) which describes 48 crops and their potential for production in the Upper Midwest. Each chapter (crop) is divided into eight sections covering: History, Uses, Growth Habits, Environmental Requirements, Cultural Practices, Yield Potential and Performance Results, Economics of Production and Markets, and Information Sources. Over 500 copies of the manual have been sold and distributed to educators, farmers, agribusinesses, and government personnel. It was used as a resource on the National Satellite Extension Program on the "Flex" opportunities in the 1990 Farm Bill.

COMMERCIAL PRODUCTION AND MARKETING

All states in the Midwest report that some commercial production of canola and/or rapeseed has occurred during the past five years (Fig. 2). For most areas, hectarage of this new crop has increased significantly in the past two years. In addition to its value as a high quality oil source, canola has been stimulated by the provisions of the Farm Bill which encourage planting of alternative oil crops. White Lupin (*Lupinus albus* L.) production has occurred on over three thousand hectares in Minnesota, Wisconsin, and Michigan. This cool-season crop is being produced primarily for a source of livestock protein in areas of these states where soybean is not competitive. Food and industrial uses for lupin products are also being developed.

Amaranth (*Amaranthus cruentus* L. and *A. hyprochondriaxus* L.) is being produced on a commercial scale in Minnesota, Nebraska, Wisconsin and perhaps other states. The principle use of crop as grain is flour which is mixed with other cereal flours to enhance the nutritive quality. Two other cereals which have seen increased use by some farmers as forage and grain for livestock are triticale (*Triticale hexaploide* Lart.) and spelt (*Triticum aestivum* L. var. *spelta*).

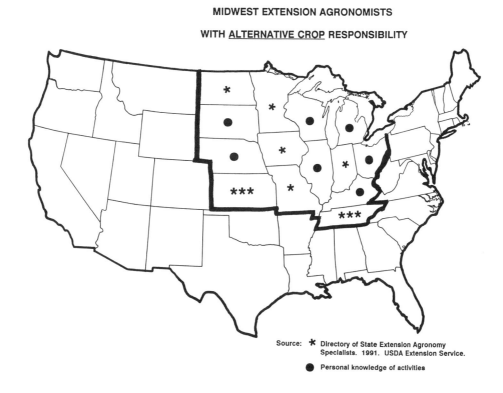

Fig. 1. Midwest extension agronomists with alternative crop responsibilities for new agronomic crops, 1991

After several years of research in the Midwest, the first successful field-scale production, processing and marketing of crambe (*Crambe abyssincia* Hochst) an industrial oilseed crop occurred in North Dakota (Gardner et al. 1991). Over 2,000 ha were produced and processed in 1991, with an anticipated expansion to 8,000 ha in 1992. Wild rice (*Zizania palustris* L.) represents a recent effort to domesticate a native cereal grain. Prior to 1960, all of the wild rice was harvested from natural stands in lakes and rivers. Today, 95% of the grain in commerce comes from cultivated fields primarily through research efforts in Minnesota. Perhaps one of the most unique new crops commercialized in recent years has been milkweed in Nebraska. Milkweed floss has commercial potential as a substitute for down, as a component of pulp and paper products and as a blending fiber in natural yarns (Knudson 1993).

OPPORTUNITIES FOR NEW CROP DEVELOPMENT IN THE MIDWEST

The Midwest has several distinct advantages for new crop development. Soil resources, fertility, water, and sunlight in the Midwest are generally not a limitation for most potential new crops. The Midwest is close to high population centers, thus transportation costs to get new food products to market should not be excessive. There are relatively large animal numbers in the Midwest for potential utilization of feed and forage from new crops. There is a considerable potential market in the Midwest which may also provide some resources for new crop development.

With the majority of the crop area in the Midwest in maize, soybean, and wheat, there is mounting evidence to support expanding the traditional grain crop rotations with new or additional crops. In some cases, the economic incentive for considering an additional rotational crop will be because of the improved yields and lower production costs of the traditional crop. Finally, the Midwest has a considerable "flex acres" affected by the 1990 Farm Bill which can be planted to alternatives like canola, rapeseed, sunflower, and flax.

LIMITATIONS TO NEW CROP DEVELOPMENT IN THE MIDWEST

The Midwest also has some unique characteristics which will limit the introduction and planting of sizeable area of new crops. Dominance from maize, soybean, wheat, and sorghum is an impediment. These crops are well adapted to the Midwest, and support from government programs for maize and wheat will make them difficult

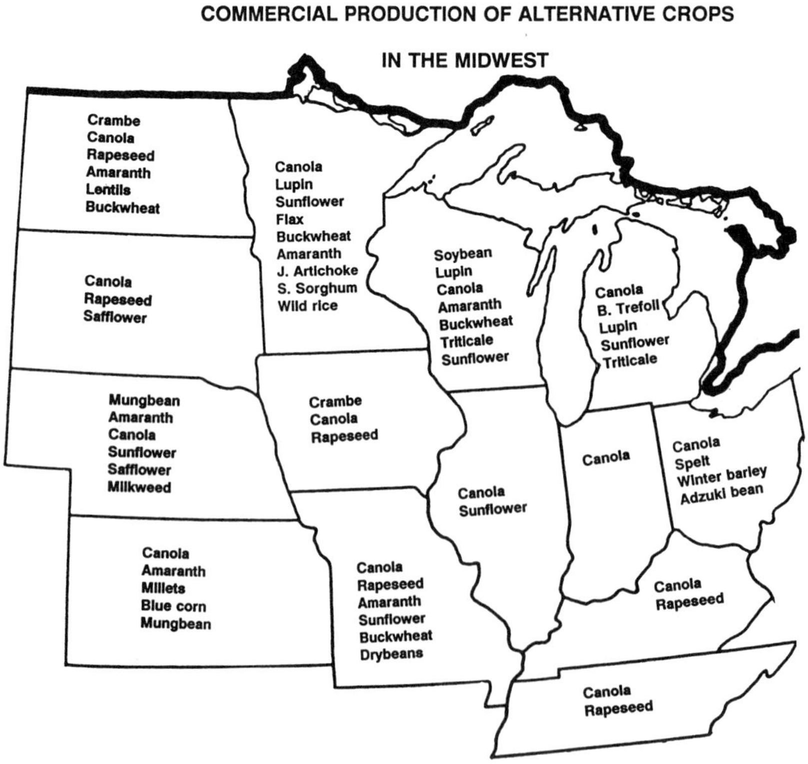

Fig. 2. Commercial production of alternative agronomic crops in the Midwest, 1991.

to replace. In some cases, growers in the Midwest have a limited amount of planting and harvesting equipment due to specialization.

Additional limitations to new crop development resulted from crop area being removed from active crop production resulting from federal programs such as the Conservation Reserve Program. Fluctuations in the exchange rate and the strength of the American dollar has resulted in shifts in production areas for some minor and alternative crops. Mustard production in North Dakota has recently shifted across the border to Canada as a result of the exchange rate.

SUMMARY

Significant advances in the development of new agronomic crops in the Midwest during the past three to five years have occurred primarily with canola, white lupin, amaranth, crambe, spelt, triticale, and wild rice. In certain areas, production and utilization of these crops has increased to a level that some producers consider them as alternatives to their traditional crops. These new crops are being used as a source of protein for livestock, forage and grain for livestock, food for human consumption, or oil for food or industrial purposes. In some cases, new uses for traditional crops have altered traditional cropping systems.

REFERENCES

Gardner, J.C., B.G. Schatz, P.M. Carr, D. Klinkebeil, S.F. Swinger, and M. Hollatz. 1991. Field-scale evaluation of crambe as an alternative crop. In: Alternative crop and alternative crop production research: A progress report. North Dakota State Univ., Fargo, ND.

Knudson, H.D. 1993. The milkweed business. In: J. Janick and J.E. Simon (eds.). Progress in new crops. Wiley, New York.

Oplinger, E.S. and O.E. Oelke. 1991. Alternative Field Crops Manual. A3532. Univ. of Wisconsin and Minnesota Cooperative Extension Services. Madison, WI.

Development of New Crops in the Western United States

Dick L. Auld

Introducing new crops into the 11 western states of the continental United States holds unique challenges (Auld et al. 1986). Since less than 10% of the total land area is suitable for crop production, most agricultural commodities are grown on relatively small production areas that are geographically diverse (USDA 1989). The broad dispersal of agricultural lands in this region make it difficult to concentrate sufficient production of specific crops, such as oilseeds, to allow economic transportation and processing. The limited rainfall and semi-arid conditions of the western states limit crop productivity while irrigation greatly increases the cost of production (U.S. Environmental Data Service 1989). The extremely high altitudes and low relative humidities found in the West combine to produce very short growing seasons that limit the adaptation of crops originally introduced from tropical regions such as cotton and soybeans. Poorly developed transportation systems and long distances to both domestic and export markets for agricultural commodities also contribute to the difficulty of introducing economically competitive new crops. To be effective in introducing new crops into this region, research and commercialization programs must answer each of these challenges.

Of the 304.3 million ha of land mass found in these eleven western states, only 23.9 million (7.8%) are currently used for crop production (Table 1) (USDA 1989). The percentage of land dedicated to crop production ranges from only 0.9% in Nevada to a high of 17.8% in Washington. This region has over 100 million ha used for pasture and nearly one million ha (4% of total crop land) classified as conserved. Slightly over 56% (9.7 million ha) of the crop land is irrigated. Some states such as Washington have less than 20% irrigated crop land while other states such as Nevada have 133% irrigated crop land indicating that some improved pasture is also irrigated.

Table 1. Land utilization of 11 states in the western United States which could support production of new crops (USDA 1989).

State	Total area (M ha)	Total farm (M ha)	Crop land (M ha)	Crop % of total	Irrigated area (M ha)	Cropland irrigated (%)	Conserved area (M ha)	Wheat area (M ha)
Arizona	29.4	14.6	0.5	1.7	0.4	52.9	0.06	0.04
California	40.5	12.7	3.9	9.6	3.1	79.2	0.08	0.20
Colorado	26.9	13.6	3.8	14.2	1.2	31.9	0.11	1.10
Idaho	21.3	5.5	2.3	10.6	1.2	57.1	0.09	0.49
Montana	37.7	24.5	6.2	16.3	0.8	13.2	0.16	1.90
Nevada	28.5	3.6	0.2	0.9	0.3	133.3	0.03	0.08
New Mexico	31.4	18.0	0.7	2.2	0.3	41.2	0.19	0.20
Oregon	24.9	7.2	1.7	7.0	0.7	37.2	0.06	0.32
Utah	21.3	4.8	0.6	2.7	0.5	85.7	0.07	0.08
Washington	17.3	6.5	3.1	17.8	0.6	19.7	0.06	0.85
Wyoming	25.2	14.1	0.9	3.7	0.6	65.2	0.04	0.12
Total	304.3	125.12	3.9	7.9	9.7	56.1	0.93	5.4

There are 5.4 million ha of wheat grown in the western states each year, indicating that nearly one of four cultivated ha is dedicated to the production of an agricultural commodity that is in surplus and supported by federal programs.

The production climates found in the western states vary almost as much within a single state as between states (Table 2). Even the warmer states such as California and Arizona have crop production regions that have less than 60 frost free days while other regions in the same state can expect more than a 300 day growing season. Even the longest growing seasons in the colder states such as Montana and Wyoming are less than 170 days. Several crop production zones in the arid Southwest receive less than 250 mm of annual precipitation while some areas of Oregon and Washington receive in excess of 1,900 mm of annual rainfall.

Generally, most agricultural production regions where new crops would be most economically competitive have only 120 to 150 day growing seasons and receive less than 450 mm of annual precipitation (U.S. Environmental Data Service 1989). Often what limited moisture can be expected, is the result of intense thunderstorms or is reasonably distributed so the crops can still experience severe moisture stress in the middle and late summer months. In regions with Mediterranean climates, winter annuals and very short season summer annuals are often most competitive under dryland conditions. To compete on irrigated lands, a new crop must have a value equivalent to or greater than existing crops. These climatic and land allocation factors make successful commercialization of new crops in the western states very difficult.

A telephone survey was conducted in June and July of 1991 to profile 22 new crops research programs in the western states (Table 3). A series of questions were asked to determine which crops were being investigated; the area of research being addressed; sources of funding for the new crops research; what factors limited additional production of the new crops; and what total production area of new crops are currently being grown and will be grown by the year 2000 in their specific region.

The projects were working at average altitude of 866 m (but ranged from 15 to 1,800 m) and had been active for an average of 11 years (1 to 40 yrs). The researchers indicated that the crops on which they were now working were grown on an average of 3,320 ha (but ranged from 0 to 122,000 ha) and had the potential to be grown on an average of 92,000 ha the turn of the century. The survey indicated that the potential impact of specific new crops during this period ranged from no commercial production to as much as one million ha of an individual crop.

Over 50% of the projects were working on legumes, cereals, or oilseed crops (Table 4). Less than a third of the projects were actively searching for new forage crops, condiments, or vegetables. These results have been biased since primarily projects supported by the Department of Agronomy at land grant institutions were surveyed. The specific crops listed by the researchers included five legume species, four species of oilseed and

Table 2. Average climatic factors of 11 states in the western United States which could influence adaptation of new crops. (U.S. Environmental Data Service 1989).

State	No. climatic zones	Range in frost free days, 1989 Minimum	Range in frost free days, 1989 Maximum	Range in avg. temp (°C)	Range in avg. rainfall (mm)
Arizona	7	6–286	308–339	16–22	107–325
California	7	1–172	145–322	7–18	185–1047
Colorado	5	1–129	136–208	4–10	297–409
Idaho	10	2–111	110–239	6–11	252–706
Montana	7	3–101	132–168	6–7	333–508
Nevada	4	1–184	131–305	7–17	135–277
New Mexico	8	60–156	170–225	8–16	224–384
Oregon	9	1–137	127–290	6–11	254–1996
Utah	7	5–184	163–237	6–15	203–480
Washington	10	3–181	177–282	6–11	244–2479
Wyoming	10	1–88	81–170	3–8	239–546

Table 3. Results of a telephone survey on introducing new crops into the western United States.

Name	Location	Firm	Selected crops
Hal Purcell	Tucson, AZ	Private Farm	Jojoba
Gene Aksland	Fresno, CA	Goldsmith Seeds	Lupine, triticale
Ali Estilal	Riverside, CA	UC-Riverside	Guayule
Steve Schaffer	Sacramento, CA	Calif. Dept. Agr	Kenaf, lupine
Duane Johnson	Fort Collins, CO	Colorado State Univ.	Amaranth, quiona
Stephen Guy	Moscow, ID	Univ. of Idaho	Canola, mustard
Joe McCaffrey	Moscow, ID	Univ. of Idaho	Canola, rapeseed
Grant Jackson	Conrad, MT	Montana State Univ.	Canola
Gil Stallknecht	Huntley, MT	Montana State Univ.	Teffy amaranth
Leon Welty	Kalispell, MT	Montana State Univ.	Canola, legumes
Mel Westcott	Corvallis, MT	Montana State Univ.	Mints, vegetables
Dave Whichman	Mocasin, MT	Montana State Univ.	Canola, forages
Charlie Glover	Las Cruces, NM	New Mexico State Univ.	Vegetables, chiles
Koert Lessman	Las Cruces, NM	New Mexico State Univ.	Crambe
Clyde Florenson	Reno, NV	Univ. of Nevada	Alfalfa
Gary Jolliff	Corvallis, OR	Oklahoma State Univ.	Meadowfoam
R.S. Albrechtsen	Logan, UT	Utah State Univ.	Wheat, barley
An Hang	Prosser, WA	Washington State Univ.	Canola, rapeseed
Tom Lumpkin	Pullman, WA	Washington State Univ.	Legumes, condiments
Baird Miller	Pullman, WA	Washington State Univ.	Canola
Joe Lauer	Powell, WY	Univ. of Wyoming	Canola, crambe
Jim Krall	Torrington, WY	Univ. of Wyoming	Legumes, canola

industrial chemical crops, four species of new cereals, four species of forage/fiber crops, three species of condiments, and five species of vegetable crops.

A large majority of the projects were interdisciplinary (86%) and vertically integrated to include growers, processors, and agricultural distribution firms (68%). Nearly all of the researchers indicated that introduction of new crops required application of nearly all disciplines of modern agricultural research as well as the direct cooperation of growers and processors to achieve final commercialization of any new crop.

Every researcher surveyed was working in some aspect of new crop production and 77% were screening one or more species of new crops for adaptation to the climate of their agricultural producing region (Table 4). There was less activity in the areas of the impact of new crops on crop rotations (18%), marketing (32%), crop processing and utilization (45%), and economics (41%). Most researchers felt that marketing and economics were important but did not agree when it was best to include these activities in programs to introduce new crops. Some researchers indicated that economic assessments should be delayed until the biological adaptation and agronomic potential of a crop species had been established.

All of the researchers indicated that lack of research funding has limited the efforts to develop new crops for the western states. Private and state funds provided financial support to over 70% of the projects while federal funds were available to only 55% of the projects (Table 4). Only 27% of the projects obtained their funding from a single sector while 71% obtained funds from private industry, state funds, and federal support. Most private funding came from fees charged for varietal adaptation trials.

When asked to define those factors which most directly limited the development of new crops in the western states, several were identified (Table 4). Lack of research funds was the most common factor (45%), followed by Farm and Government Policy (15%), and lack of developed markets (15%). Transportation costs, failure of grower to accept new crops, and the economic uncompetitiveness of new crops were also identified as factors which currently limit production. Although not included in the survey, some research indicated that lack of registered pesticides had also limited the production of new crops recently introduced into the United States.

Based on the results of this telephone survey it was apparent that the introduction of new crops will require a consistent source of research funding as well as the inclusion and encouragement of new crop production as a stated goal of American farm policy. It is unfortunate that one of the single largest deterrents to introducing new crops is the federal government's policies. The farm program has historically penalized a grower's production base when hectares were diverted from protected crops to production of new crops. Federal subsidies of selected crops create an artificial economic climate in which unsubsidized new crops often cannot compete.

Researchers developing crops for irrigated areas should concentrate on crops with high value to help defer the cost of irrigation and transportation to domestic and export markets. There is a desperate need to develop additional crops which can be grown on the arid and semi-arid regions typical of dryland production areas. Identification of species of new crops adapted to the 255 million ha of pasture, rangeland, and forests of the western

Table 4. Responses of 22 researchers conducting new crops research in the western United States in 1991.

Category / Examples	Response distribution (%)	Category / Examples	Response distribution (%)
Classes of crops in research program		Source of research support	
Oilseeds	82	Private companies	77
Cereals	50	State funds	72
Legumes	50	Federal funds	55
Forages	27	Number of sources of research support	
Condiments	18	One	27
Vegetable	14	Two	41
Area of research		Three	32
Production	100	Factors limiting introducing new crops	
Adaptation	77	Research funds	45
Processing and utilization	45	Market development	15
Economics	41	U.S. farm policy	15
Marketing	32	Transport to market	9
Crop rotation	18	Grower acceptance	6
		Economic competitiveness	6

states should also be initiated. Even a moderate increase in carrying capacity or timber yields across such a vast area would have tremendous economic impact. Finally, researchers working on new crops both in the United States and globally should more actively communicate and exchange scientific information. With limited financial support and only a few scientific personnel working in such a critical area it is important to encourage cooperation and avoid duplication.

REFERENCES

Auld, D.L., G.A. Murray, and F.V. Pumphrey. 1986. Alternate crops in conservation tillage system. Proc. STEEP Symp. Spokane, WA. p 137–156.

U.S. Department of Agriculture. 1989. Agricultural statistics. Government Printing Office, Washington, DC.

U.S. Environmental Data Service. 1989. Climatological data, annual summary. National Climatic Center, Ashville, NC. Vol. 94.

The Western Regional Plant Introduction Station: A Source of Germplasm for New Crop Development

V.L. Bradley, R.C. Johnson, R.M. Hannan, D.M. Stout, and R.L. Clark

The mission of the Western Regional Plant Introduction Station (WRPIS) at Pullman, Washington is to maintain the diversity and the accessibility of plant germplasm resources. This is accomplished by implementing a multi-faceted program (Fig. 1). Current trends indicate that diversification by the agricultural and industrial communities will benefit both producers and consumers. Reasons for diversification include (Anon. 1989): growing interest in crops that are less demanding on renewable resources; crop diversification may reduce farmer's financial risk; growing interest in alternative and sustainable agricultural systems; demands for new and exotic varieties of food from consumers; plants can supply raw materials for industry.

The agronomic community is encouraging diversification by the growth and development of new crops. Once a plant has been identified as having the potential to become a new crop, it must be developed into a marketable commodity. Desirable traits may be transferred to the crop from germplasm available in accessions which are preserved at Plant Introduction stations.

The WRPIS currently utilizes two Washington state locations in the regeneration program. A third environment at Maricopa, Arizona will soon be operating and will allow seed increase of accessions of *Parthenium*

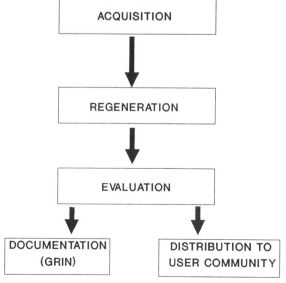

Fig. 1. Germplasm maintenance program.

argentatum Gray (guayule), *Simmondsia chinensis* (Link) C. Schneider (jojoba), *Lesquerella* S. Watson, and other species which are adapted to the southwest desert climate.

The WRPIS germplasm collection is a plant materials resource for new crops, underexploited crops, herbs, medicinal, and ornamental plants. Samples of available accessions, usually 50 to 100 seeds, are sent upon request to researchers worldwide.

NEW CROPS

Eragrostis tef (Zucc.) Trotter, Poaceae, commonly referred to as tef (also t'ef and teff), is an annual C-4 grass (Kebede et al. 1989) native to Ethiopia which is grown in Australia, India, and South Africa as forage (Costanza et al. 1979). Tef flour is used by Ethiopians to make an unleavened sourdough bread called "injera." Tef seed has a good balance of essential amino acids, except lysine (Ebba 1969). The great diversity within the species is evident in seed color differences; there are reports of purple, white, brown, and red-seeded types (Mengesha 1966; Costanza et al. 1979). The diversity also enables tef to be grown in a variety of environments. There are 366 *Eragrostis tef* accessions at the WRPIS, some of which are cultivars that were developed in Ethiopia. The accessions are regenerated at the Central Ferry Research Farm, located on the Snake River, 45 miles southwest of Pullman, Washington.

Lesquerella, Lamiaceae, is also known as bladderpod. Many of the species within this genus are native to the arid southwestern United States. *Lesquerella* is considered a prime candidate to be used as an oil seed crop because of the presence of three new hydroxy fatty acids which are similar to a primary component in castor oil. Castor oil is a main ingredient in the production of lubricants, plastics, and drying agents (Purseglove 1974). *Lesquerella* seed meals were found to be relatively high in lysine, indicating potential for use as a protein supplement in feed grains (Thompson and Dierig 1988). The 53 accessions maintained by the WRPIS will be increased at a new off-station site located at Maricopa, Arizona.

Lactuca sativa L., Asteraceae, or lettuce, is not normally considered a new crop. In recent years, the practice of offering only 'iceberg' lettuce in American supermarkets has declined, and in most produce sections, one can now find selections of red, leaf, romaine, and other types of lettuce. Germplasm for developing new types of lettuce with potential consumer appeal is abundant in the 742 accessions managed by the WRPIS.

Lupinus L., Fabaceae, the "legume" family, have been a useful crop for both human consumption and livestock feed for centuries (Forrest 1991). *Lupinus albus* L. (white lupin), and *L. mutabilis* Sweet (pearl lupin or tarwi) have been the subject of several studies. In both species, lines with low levels of alkaloids have been found. These lines are desirable as food for livestock and humans due to the high protein, up to 50%, and oil content, up to 24% (Langer and Hill 1982). A wide assortment of germplasm is present in the 743 accessions of *Lupinus* which the WRPIS maintains and regenerates at the Soil Conservation Service Plant Materials Center at Pullman, Washington. Lupins vary in such phenotypic characters as growth habit, flower color, seed color, and height.

Parthenium argentatum Gray, Asteraceae, commonly called guayule, is a drought tolerant shrub that is a good source of natural rubber. It was cultivated in the southwestern United States during World War II when *Hevea* rubber was not available from Southeast Asia (Princen 1977). Although direct seeded stand establishment has been a factor limiting the development of guayule as a crop, researchers have recently developed techniques to alleviate this problem (Foster and Moore 1989). The 27 guayule accessions at the WRPIS will be regenerated at the Maricopa Research facility.

UNDEREXPLOITED CROPS

Carthamus tinctorius L., Asteraceae, or safflower, is an annual crop that has been grown since about 1600 BC (Langer and Hill 1982). Major cultivation of this crop in the United States began about 1950 (Purseglove 1974). Safflower is primarily grown for use as a low saturated fat cooking oil. One type, oleic safflower oil, is a result of a mutation discovered at the University of California, Davis (Smith 1985). In the mutated seed, the normal ratio of linoleic to oleic fatty acids (usually 77 to 15%) is reversed. The mutation produces an oil that is monounsaturated instead of polyunsaturated. After the oil is pressed out, the seed is valued as a high protein (approximately 43%) livestock feed (Langer and Hill 1982). The 1,706 accessions held at the WRPIS vary in oil content and quality, spininess, leaf shape, flower size, height, and flower color.

Lens culinaris Medikus, Fabaceae, also known as lentil, has been cultivated since ancient times in Egypt, southern Europe, and western Asia (Purseglove 1974). Lentils are highly branched annual legumes that grow to a height of about 40 cm. They are grown mostly in Pakistan and north India (Langer and Hill 1982). The WRPIS is located in the Palouse Region of Washington, where 98% of the lentils produced in the United States are grown. The American Dry Pea and Lentil Association estimated that in 1991, 76,000 t of lentils were grown on the Palouse. A national lentil festival is held in Pullman, Washington every September to promote lentils and lentil cuisine. The WRPIS lentil collection consists of 2251 accessions. Many accessions have been used extensively in lentil cultivar development programs.

Cicer arietinum L., Fabaceae, commonly referred to as chickpea or garbanzo bean, is an annual legume that is thought to have originated in western Asia. Chickpea seed has approximately 20% protein, 5% oil, and 60% carbohydrate. The whole or ground seed is used in many ways by Mediterranean cultures and is also a favorite ingredient in the American salad bar. Livestock are fed crop residues (Langer and Hill 1982). The 3,741 accessions of chickpea managed by the WRPIS are grown at the Pullman site. The WRPIS and the USDA Grain Legume Genetics and Physiology Research Project are collaborating on a project to screen for resistance to *Ascochyta* blight, a major disease of chickpea, to develop large-seeded, blight resistant cultivars. To date, 400 WRPIS accessions have been screened for resistance to blight.

The WRPIS is also responsible for the preservation of other new and interesting crops. *Cucurbita foetidissima* Kunth (buffalo gourd), *Limnanthes* R. Br. (meadowfoam), and *Simmondsia chinensis* (Link) C. Schneider (jojoba) as well as many herbs, ornamental, and medicinal plants (Table 1) are of potential interest to those working to introduce or improve new crops.

CONCLUSION

Crop diversification has become a major goal in the agronomic community. For developing new crops, researchers may utilize germplasm from the Western Regional Plant Introduction Station. Accessions of *Lesquerella*, *Parthenium argentatum*, and *Eragrostis tef* are among the new crops maintained in the WRPIS collection. Accessions of underexploited crops such as *Cicer arietinum*, *Lens culinaris*, and *Carthamus tinctorius*, are also maintained at Pullman. These and other new and underexploited species maintained at the WRPIS are a valuable germplasm resource for individuals and groups working to improve nontraditional crops.

Table 1. Selected herbs, ornamental, and medicinal plant accessions preserved at the Western Regional Plant Introduction Station.

Scientific name	Common name	Use
Achillea millefolium L.	Yarrow, milfoil	Ornamental, an ingredient in mead (Adams 1987)
Aquilegia L.	Columbine	Ornamental
Artemisia absinthium L.	Wormwood	Aromatic, ornamental (Adams 1987)
Borago officinalis L.	Borage	Culinary herb with cucumber flavor, source of γ-linolenic acid (Fletcher 1972)
Papaver somniferum L.	Opium poppy	Source of codeine and morphine (Fletcher 1972)
Plantago ovata L.	Psyllium	Laxative, stabilizer in ice cream (Morton 1977)
Salvia officinalis L.	Sage	Culinary herb used as pork and poultry seasoning (Prakash 1990); source of antioxidants
Sanguisorba minor Scop.	Salad burnet	Culinary herb (Prakash 1990)
Satureja hortensis L.	Summer savory	Culinary herb (Adams 1987)
Trigonella foenum-graecum L.	Fenugreek	Culinary herb, sprouts for salad, imitation maple syrup from seed, used in salves and poultices (Adams 1987)

REFERENCES

Adams, J. 1987. Landscaping with herbs. Timber Press, Portland, OR.

Anonymous. 1989. New crops researchers explore varied topics at first symposium. Diversity 5:41.

Costanza, S.H., J.M.J. DeWet, and J.R. Harlan. 1979. Literature review and numerical taxonomy of *Eragrostis tef* (T'ef). Econ. Bot. 33:413–424.

Ebba, T. 1969. T'ef (*Eragrostis tef*)—The cultivation, usage, and some of the known diseases and insect pests. Haile Selassie I Univ., College of Agr., Dire Dawa, Expt. Sta. Bul. 60. Ethiopia.

Fletcher, H.L.V. 1972. Herbs. Drake Publishing, New York.

Forrest, R.E. 1991. Experiences and prospects for lupins in Canada, p. 11–17. In: Prospects for lupins in North America: A Symposium sponsored by the Center for Alternative Plant and Animal Products. Univ. of Minnesota, St. Paul, March 21–22, 1991. Ext. Special Prog., St. Paul, MN.

Foster, M.A. and J. Moore. 1989. Direct seeding guayule in west Texas. Abstracts of the First annual conference of the Association for the Advancement of Industrial Crops, October 2–6, 1989. Peoria, IL.

Kebede, H., R.C. Johnson, and D.M. Ferris. 1989. Photosynthetic response of *Eragrostis tef* to temperature. Physiol. Plant. 77:262–266.

Langer, R.H.M. and G.D. Hill. 1982. Agricultural plants. Cambridge Univ. Press, Cambridge, UK.

Mengesha, M.H. 1966. Chemical composition of teff (*Eragrostis tef*) compared with that of wheat, barley and grain sorghum. Econ. Bot. 20:268–273.

Morton, J.F. 1977. Major medicinal plants: Botany, culture and uses. Charles C. Thomas, Springfield, IL.

Prakash, V. 1990. Leafy spices. CRC Press, Boca Raton, FL.

Princen, L.H. 1977. Potential wealth in new crops: research and development, p. 1–15. Crop resources. Academic Press, New York.

Purseglove, J.W. 1974. Tropical crops, dicotyledons. 3rd ed. Wiley, New York.

Smith, J.R. 1985. Safflower: due for a rebound? J. Amer. Oil Chem. Soc. 62:1286-1291.

Thompson, A.E. and D.A. Dierig. 1988. *Lesquerella*—A new arid land industrial oil seed crop. El Guayulero 10:16–18.

Determining Amaranth and Canola Suitability in Missouri Through Geographic Information Systems Analysis

Robert L. Myers

Missouri currently produces relatively few grain crops, with maize, soybeans, wheat, and sorghum occupying most of the grain crop area. The lack of grain crop diversification within the state has reduced the economic stability of both individual farms and the overall state agricultural economy. Alternative crops have been evaluated in a limited way at a few sites around the state in the past, but there has never been a systematic evaluation of Missouri's resources in regard to alternative crop requirements.

Geographic information systems (GIS) provide an increasingly utilized approach for systematically evaluating a set of site-specific resources for their relationship to a given problem domain (Bjerklie 1989). In a GIS project, the spatial relationships of several parameters are analyzed using compiled databases, and visualized in the form of digitized maps. This approach has been used to identify new school locations, target ambulance services, and make wildlife and fisheries management decisions (Peuquet and Marble 1990).

GIS analysis has yet to see extensive use in agriculture, but is well suited to the site-specific nature of agricultural production decisions. For example, GIS was recently used to identify suitable vegetable growing regions in Tennessee (Brooker and Gray 1990). Decisions about crop choice typically depend on soil characteristics, climatic conditions, distance to markets, equipment availability, and relation of labor needs to labor availability, factors which all have a geographical dimension. In the past, it has been difficult to relate these geographic factors due to limited computer hardware and software capabilities, but new computer tools now make it possible for much more sophisticated consideration of geographically-based resource use (Tomlinson 1990). For example, although the unions of different soil and climate polygons could be visually determined from transparency overlays, it would not be possible to mathematically weight the relative importance of each of those factors in developing a new polygon without GIS software (Environmental Systems Research Institute 1990).

An alternative crop GIS can allow an innovative farmer to more accurately determine appropriate alternative crops for his or her farm, without necessarily having to wait for field research to be conducted in his or her region. Maps indicating the most suitable regions for selected alternative crops can also be useful for siting field research studies, or for assisting businesses that want to be involved with an alternative crop.

The specific objective in this project was to utilize GIS analysis to generate prototype suitability maps for canola/rapeseed and amaranth production in Missouri. Canola and rapeseed are being grown on increasing acreages in Missouri, and have generated tremendous interest. Amaranth is not currently grown commercially in Missouri, but appears to be adaptable to Missouri and has good long term potential as a grain crop alternative.

METHODS

Data Collection

The data used in the final maps consisted of soil classification, area and yields of selected traditional crops, probability of disease incidence, and in the case of amaranth, rainfall averages and labor data. Soils information was based on a general soils map of Missouri that provides eight regional soil classifications groups (USDA Soil Conservation Service 1979). Crop areas and yield were taken from the Missouri Agricultural Statistics Office annual agricultural statistical summary. Estimates of disease incidence, by region, were made by J. Mihail, Deptartment of Plant Pathology, University of Missouri. Climatic information was obtained from the University of Missouri Atmospheric Sciences Department. Labor information was collected from the U.S. Census county unemployment data.

Computer Tools

Once the appropriate data was collected, it was entered into an ARC/INFO GIS database running on a Dec Station 5000 minicomputer system (ARC/INFO, Environmental Systems Research Institute, 380 New York St., Redlands, CA 92373; version 5.0.1). Most data was collected in tabular format and entered with geographic tags. Soil maps, township boundaries, and regional pathogen ratings were digitized using a graphics tablet. Once entered into the database, data was handled through a vector-based approach which generated new polygon coverages when factors were combined.

Factors Used

Amaranth is grown in Missouri as a summer annual, and is more likely to substitute for sorghum than other Missouri crops. Sorghum is a drought hardy crop, like amaranth, that is planted fairly late (late May through late June), and harvested in October. Since the growth cycle and soil needs of amaranth are similar to sorghum, it was felt that sorghum production areas might be likely candidates for amaranth production. However, there is no data on how amaranth yields compare to sorghum yields on different soil types, so sorghum yields were not included as a factor. Areas with historically high rainfall during fall harvest were rated lower, due to possible harvest loss. An assumption was made that amaranth would require more labor than traditional crops, so labor availability was a factor. The following factors were used in the pilot project, with weighting shown in parentheses: soil classification (20%); percent of sorghum grown as a percentage of all row crops in the county (15%); estimated probability of amaranth disease (10%); 30 year rainfall averages during fall harvest period (15%); and labor availability based on unemployment data (10%).

Canola and rapeseed are grown in Missouri as winter annuals, and are more likely to substitute for wheat than other Missouri crops. This alternative crop does not do well on poorly drained soils, or soils likely to flood in the spring. Winter kill is a serious problem, yet efforts to use historical climatic data as a factor proved impossible without knowing more about the exact conditions that can lead to plant death. The following factors were used in the pilot project, with weighting shown in parentheses: soil classification (35%); wheat yields (15%); percent of wheat grown as a percentage of all row crops in the county (35%); and estimated probability of canola or rapeseed disease (15%).

Wheat is the crop most likely to be substituted for by canola or rapeseed, since it is the only widely grown winter annual crop in Missouri. The growing season for canola is very similar to that of wheat, except that canola is planted a few weeks earlier. Canola typically yields well in the same areas as wheat. It was expected that canola would either be grown in rotation with wheat, or could substitute for wheat provided that the wheat is not normally preceded by full season summer annual crop varieties.

RESULTS

The Missouri maps generated by the GIS software provided eight different levels of suitability for each crop. For amaranth, the most suitable regions were shown to be in southeast Missouri, with other well suited areas indicated across central Missouri and along the western edge of the state (Fig. 1). For canola and rapeseed, the most suitable areas appeared to be in the west central portion of the state, and other well suited areas were identified along the Mississippi and Missouri river valleys (Fig. 2). The least suitable region for both crops is a large region taking up most of the south central portion of the state, which is an area of shallow, rocky Ozark soils that are almost exclusively forest or permanent pasture land.

Although no extension validation of these results was undertaken in this pilot project, some review of the results was done by experts. H. Minor and T. Ballman, both individuals with several years of canola production experience in Missouri, felt that the canola and rapeseed suitability map was a reasonable match with their experience and intuition. I have evaluated amaranth at seven locations in Missouri, and found that the amaranth suitability map corresponded well to the limited production experience, except for the high ratings received in the southeast portion of Missouri. That area received relatively high ratings due to extensive sorghum production and productive soil types, even though a factor not considered, which is the late onset of fall frost in the area, could have a detrimental impact on harvest (successful harvest normally requires a killing fall frost to dry down green stems and leaves of amaranth).

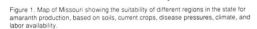
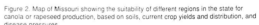
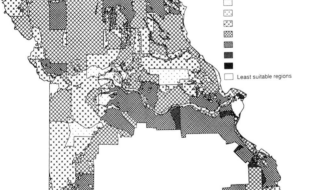
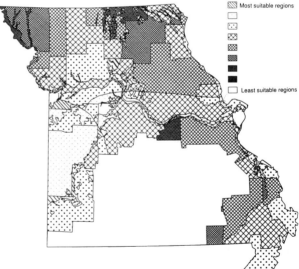

Fig. 1. Map of Missouri showing the suitability of different regions in the state for amaranth production, based on soils, current crops, disease pressures, climate, and labor availability.

Fig. 2. Map of Missouri showing the suitability of different regions in the state for canola or rapeseed production, based on soils, current crop yields and distribution, and disease pressures.

DISCUSSION

Although the prototype suitability maps appear to provide useful information on the most favorable parts of the Missouri for the crops under consideration, there are unquestionably other factors that should be considered. For both amaranth and rapeseed, the following factors will need to be incorporated into the GIS systems for better evaluation of suitability regions: the role of transportation; factors influencing part-time and full-time labor available for farms; regional differences in weeds and insects; and, potential on-farm use for livestock feed.

For canola and rapeseed, it will be particularly important in future GIS iterations to understand the sequence of weather events that are most likely to contribute to winter kill. A major effort was made during this project to identify a way that climatic information for locations around the state could be used to avoid areas more likely to have winter kill problems. Thirty year averages on weekly temperature were examined with a focus on three separate time periods: a period near the beginning of the winter (Julian week 50; the two weeks that typically approximate the onset of spring conditions (Julian weeks 10 to 11); and, the coldest average week during the winter (Julian week 2). This information led to suitability maps based on climate that were not easily reconciled with maps based on other factors. Also, average weather conditions are not satisfactory for predicting what the extreme weather conditions might be in a specific region.

CONCLUSION

A GIS approach provides a sophisticated way of handling relationships between site-specific factors affecting alternative crop production. In this project, the suitability maps generated will be used to site future field research with rapeseed and amaranth, and to help industries determine the best areas for canola and rapeseed production. However, suitability ratings generated for different regions by GIS techniques need some form of validation that goes beyond a logical construction procedure and intuitive reactions to the final maps by project members. The best validation would involve multiple sites of long term trials, plus actual observance of where the crop gets grown by producers, but part of the purpose of GIS in this case is to avoid such long, costly field work. Agroclimatic characteristics and pest incidence for different regions are only part of what will influence adoption of alternative crops. Other factors affecting the adoption of these crops, such as labor, transportation, markets, and relevant farmer experience must also be considered. Finally, GIS analysis, like simulation modeling, can identify components of a system needing research, such as the need for a better understanding of the weather events that will contribute to winter kill in canola or rapeseed.

REFERENCES

Bjerklie, D. 1989. The electronic transformation of maps. April, 1989, MIT Technol. Rev.

Brooker, J.R. and M.D. Gray. 1990. Identification of vegetable growing areas in Tennessee from computer-generated maps based on geographic information systems. Tennessee Farm and Home Science, Number 153, Winter 1990, Univ. Tennessee Agr. Expt. Sta.

Environmental Systems Research Institute. 1990. Understanding GIS: The ARC/INFO method. ESRI, Inc., Redlands, CA.

Peuquet, D.J. and D.F. Marble. 1990. ARC/INFO: an example of a contemporary geographic information system. In: Introductory readings in geographic information systems. Taylor and Francis, New York.

Tomlinson, R.F. 1990. Geographic information systems—a new frontier. In: D.J. Peuquet and D.F. Marble (eds.). Introductory readings in geographic information systems. Taylor and Francis, New York.

USDA Soil Conservation Service. 1979. Missouri general soil map and soil association descriptions. USDA/SCS, Columbia, MO.

Preliminary Agronomic Evaluation of New Crops for North Dakota

Marisol T. Berti and A.A. Schneiter

The evaluation of new crops is an important ongoing process. Any crop that can be profitably produced in an area where it was not previously grown provides the producer an opportunity to diversify agricultural production. This is especially important in areas, such as the northern great plains where environmental conditions greatly restrict the crop species that can be grown. Preliminary studies have been initiated to identify and evaluate new crops with potential adaptation to North Dakota environments.

Twelve annual crops were evaluated but limited genetic diversity was tested within each species. Studies were conducted at Langdon, Carrington, Prosper, and Fargo, North Dakota and Breckenridge, Minnesota.

CROPS WITH GOOD AGRONOMIC POTENTIAL

Fenugreek

Trigonella foenum-graecum L., Fabaceae, is an annual that originated in Mediterranean regions and the near East and is used for imitation maple syrup flavoring, condiments, and for synthesis of hormones (Duke 1981). Fenugreek seeds contains 0.1 to 0.2% of diosgenin which is used for cortisone preparations and synthesis of other hormones (Jorgensen 1988). Fenugreekine a C_{27}-steroidal sapogenin-peptide ester is present in plants and its hydrolysis gives diosgenin, yamogenin, and other products (Ghosal et al. 1974). Stand establishment and vigor were excellent at all locations and planting dates. No major shattering problems were observed. Several diseases, which have not been identified at this time, could be a limiting production factor.

Coriander

Coriandrum sativum L., Apiaceae, is an annual native of the Mediterranean region (Purseglove et al. 1981). The seed is used as a spice and the oil which is rich in petroselinic fatty acid may have potential in industrial uses, although its cleavage to lauric acid remains expensive (Placek 1963; Kleiman 1990). Stand establishment and seedling vigor were excellent. Seed set was good although yields were reduced by lodging and shattering caused by strong winds.

CROPS WITH SOME AGRONOMIC POTENTIAL

Borage

Borago officinalis L., Boraginaceae, is an annual native to Europe, North Africa, and Asia Minor (Beaubaire and Simon 1987). Borage seeds contain γ-linolenic acid (GLA) which is a precursor of prostaglandins in the human body (Cutting 1985; Jorgensen 1988; Kernoff 1977). Excellent stands and seed vigor were observed at all locations and planting dates. Average seed yield was 200 kg/ha which may have been limited by the lack of native pollinators. This observation must be confirmed by further research. High seed shatter (60 to 80%) may also have limited seed yield.

Calendula

Calendula officinalis L., Asteraceae, is an annual native to Mediterranean regions. Calendula seeds are an important source of fatty acids with conjugated double bonds and could be used as an industrial oil (Beerentrup and Robbelen 1987b). Excellent stand and seed vigor were observed at all locations and planting dates. Seed yield was limited by ash blister beetles (*Lytta sphaericollis* Say), seed shattering, and seed cleaning difficulties.

Camelina

Camelina sativa L., Brassicaceae, is an annual oilseed crop which originated in southwest and central

Europe and is well adapted to Minnesota (Robinson 1987). Stand establishment was a problem due in part to the small seed size. Camelina flowered, set seed quickly and yielded acceptable amounts of seed (600 kg/ha) at Prosper, North Dakota. Shattering was a problem at some locations.

Quinoa

Chenopodium quinoa Willd., Chenopodiaceae, is a native of Andean regions in South America. The grain is used for human food in breakfast cereals, snack food, toasted, puffed, and flour products (Vietmeyer 1989). Good stands were obtained at the three southern locations. Several serious insect problems including leafhoppers, stem borers, leafminers, and lygus bugs (species have not been identified) significantly reduced yield. Insect control methods need to be developed in order to evaluate the potential of this crop in North Dakota.

Sesame

Sesamum indicum L., Pedaliaceae, is a herbaceous annual that probably originated in Africa. The oil extracted from the seed is used for cooking and confectionary products. Dehulled whole seeds are used by the baking industry (Seegeler 1983). Stands were excellent at the three southern locations (Prosper and Fargo, North Dakota, and Breckenridge, Minnesota). Only one of the two cultivars tested reached physiological maturity before first frost.

CROPS WITH LIMITED AGRONOMIC POTENTIAL

Euphorbia

Euphorbia lagascae Spreng, Euphorbiaceae, is an herbaceous annual plant native to Spain. Plants flower indeterminately, reach a height of 60 to 100 cm (White et al. 1973) and have potential as a source of epoxy acid which is present in the seed oil. Epoxy acid is used for adhesives, plasticizers, industrial coatings, varnishes, and paints (Kleiman et al. 1965; Beerentrup and Robbelen 1987a; Krewson and Scott 1966; Earle 1970). The eight lines tested were all late maturing, although some seed was obtained. Seed shattering was extensive. Lines with slightly earlier maturity may have potential in North Dakota.

Fennel

Foeniculum vulgare var *dulce* (Mill.), Apiaceae, is a perennial plant grown as an annual, and has been exploited for its seed, leaves, and bulb (enlarged base of the stalk) (Simon 1989, 1990). Fruits (known as fennel seed) are used as condiments for food flavoring. Seeds are rich in petroselinic acid (Moreau et al. 1966) which can be used to form lauric and adipic acids, although this cleavage remains too expensive for commercial purposes (Kleiman 1990). The volatile oil extracted from fruits of fennel exhibits fungistatic toxicity (Shukla and Tripathi 1987). Although stand establishment and vigor was good at all locations, plants failed to produce viable seed prior to the first frost (Sept. 26).

Gumweed

Grindelia camporum (Greene), Asteraceae, is a perennial plant native to North America. Gumweed is a potential source of diterpene resin acids, which are extracted from the stem, leaves, and involucres (Mclaughlin 1986). Diterpene resin acids are used in inks, adhesives, and as a substitute or complement for pine rosin (a type of resin) (Hoffmann and McLaughlin 1986). Although a perennial plant, gumweed was grown in North Dakota to determine the potential biomass, yield, and resin production per hectare in one growing season. Poor stand establishment and slow rate of growth were the major agronomic deficiencies. Biomass yield was low. Anthesis did not occur prior to frost.

Niger

Guizotia abyssinica Cass., Asteraceae, is an annual plant believed to be native to Ethiopia. The crop is grown for its high quality oil which is extracted from the seed. Niger oil is used for human consumption and in the manufacture of soap and paints. Niger is also grown for bird food (Seegeler 1983). The five lines tested were all late maturing and seed set was low. Early maturing lines need to be developed in order for this crop to be productive in North Dakota. Severe root rot diseases (not identified) were observed.

Psyllium

Plantago ovata Forsk., Plantaginaceae, is an annual of west Asian origin (Dastur 1962). The seed contains about 30% mucilage (Mital and Bhagat 1979). The mucilage is the major use for the plant which is being grown mainly in India (Gupta 1982). It has medicinal uses (Costa et al. 1989; Zara and Mehta 1988) and has been incorporated into breakfast cereals, ice cream, instant beverages, bakery products, and dietary products (Chan and Wypiszyk 1988; Kalyanasundaram et al. 1984). Poor stand establishment and low seed set occurred at all locations and planting dates. The few plants established were very short (20 cm).

REFERENCES

Beaubaire, N.A. and J.E. Simon. 1987. Production potential of (*Borago officinalis* L.). Acta Hort. 208:101–113.

Beerentrup, H.M. Zu, and G. Robbelen. 1987a. Screening for European productions of oilseed with unusual fatty acids. Angew. Botanik 61:287–303.

Beerentrup, H.M. Zu, and G. Robbelen. 1987b. Calendula and coriandrum—new potential oil crops for industrial uses. Fett. Wiss. Technol. 89:227–230.

Chan, J.K.C. and V. Wypiszyk. 1988. A forgotten natural dietary fiber: *Psyllium mucilloid*. Cereal Food World 33:919–922.

Costa, M.A., T. Mehta, and J.R. Males. 1989. Effects of dietary cellulose, psyllium husk and cholesterol level on fecal and colonic microbial metabolism in monkeys. J. Nutr. 119:986–992.

Cutting, O. 1985. Borage calls for a high level of management. Arable Farming 12:30–33.

Dastur, J.F. 1962. Medicinal plants of India and Pakistan, p. 133–134. Taraporeval Sons & Co., Bombay, India.

Duke, J.A. 1981. *Trigonella foenum-graecum* L., p. 268–271. In: Handbook of legumes of world economic importance. Plenum Press, New York.

Earle, F.R. 1970. Epoxy oils from plant seeds. J. Amer. Oil Chem. Soc. 47:510–513.

Gupta, R. 1982. Recent advances in cultivation of Ibsagol (*Plantago ovata* Forsk) in India, p. 406–480. In: C.K. Atal and B.M. Kapur (eds.). Cultivation and utilization of medicinal plants. Reg. Res. Lab. Council of Sci. and Ind. Res. Jammu-Tawi.

Hoffmann, J.J. and S.P. McLaughlin. 1986. *Grindelia camporum*: potential cash crop for the arid southwest. Econ. Bot. 40:162–169.

Jorgensen, I. 1988. Experiment in alternative crops. Ugeskrift for Jordburg. 133:731–735.

Kalyanasundaram, N.K., S. Sriram, B.R. Patel, R.B. Patel, D.H. Patel, K.C. Dalal, and R. Gupta. 1984. Psyllium: a monopoly of Gujarat. Gujarat Agr. Univ., India.

Kernoff, P.B.A., A.L. Willis, K.J. Stone, J.A. Davies, and G.P. McNichols. 1977. Antithrombotic potential of dihomo-gamma-linolenic acid in man. Brit. Med. J. 3:1441–1444.

Kleiman, R. 1990. Chemistry of new industrial oilseed crops, p. 196–203. In: J. Janick and J.E. Simon (eds.). Advances in new crops. Timber Press, Portland, OR.

Kleiman, R., C.R. Smith, Jr., S.G. Yates, and Q. Jones. 1965. Search for new industrial oils. XII Fifty eight Euphorbiaceae oils, including one rich in vernolic acid. J. Amer. Oil Chem. Soc. 42:169–172.

Krewson, C.F. and W.E. Scott. 1966. *Euphorbia lagascae* Spreng, an abundant source of epoxy oleic acid: seed extraction and oil composition. J. Amer. Oil Chem. Soc. 43:171–174.

McLaughlin, S.P. 1986. Differentiation among populations of tetraploid *Grindelia camporum*. Amer. J. Bot. 73:1748–1754.

Mital, S.P. and N.R. Bhagat. 1979. Studies in floral biology in *Plantago ovata* Forsk in northern Australia. Trop. Agr. 66(1):61–64.

Moreau, J.P., R.L. Holmes, T.L. Ward, and J.H. Williams. 1966. Evaluation of yield and chemical composition of fennel seed from different planting dates and row spacings. J. Amer. Oil Chem. Soc. 43:352–354.

Placek, L.L. 1963. A review on petroselinic acid and its derivatives. J. Amer. Oil Chem. Soc. 40:319–329.

Purseglove, J.W., E.G. Brown, C.L. Green, and S.R.J. Robbins. 1981. Spices. Vol. 2. Longman Inc., New York. p. 736–813.

Robinson, R.G. 1987. Camelina: A useful research crop and a potential oilseed crop. Minnesota Agr. Expt. Sta. Bul. 579. St. Paul.

Seegeler, C.J.P. 1983. Oil plants in Ethiopia, their taxonomy and agricultural significance. Agr. Res. Rpt. 921. Wageningen, Netherlands.

Simon, J.E. 1989. Fennel: new specialty vegetable. Herb. Spice Med. Plant Dig. 7(4):5.

Simon, J.E. 1990. Essential oils and culinary herbs, p. 472–483. In: J. Janick and J.E. Simon (eds.). Advances in new crops. Timber Press, Portland, OR.

Shukla, H.S. and S.C. Tripathi. 1987. Studies on physico-chemical, phytotoxic and fungitoxic properties of essential oil of *Foeniculum vulgare* Mill. Beitrage Biologie Pflanzen. 62(1):149–158.

Vietmeyer, N.D. 1989. Lost crops of the Incas. National Academy Press, Washington, DC.

White, G.A., B.C. Willingham, W.H. Skrdla, J.H. Massey, J.J. Higgins, W. Calhoun, A.M. Davis, D.D. Dolan, and F.R. Earle. 1973. Agronomic evaluation of prospective new crop species. Econ. Bot. 25:25–43.

Zara, D.A. and T. Mehta. 1988. Tree-week psyllium-husk supplementation: effect on plasma cholesterol concentrations, fecal steroid excretion, and carbohydrate absorption in men. Amer. J. Clin. Nutr. 47:67–74

Public Sponsored New Crops Research and Development Projects in Virginia

Gregory E. Welbaum

A survey of new crops research and development projects in Virginia was conducted to summarize the publicly funded projects ongoing in the state, to identify unnecessary duplication of research efforts, and to provide information for the planning of future research and extension programs. Input for the survey was solicited from the Virginia Cooperative Extension Service, departments in the College of Agriculture and Life Sciences at the Virginia Polytechnic Institute and State University (VPI&SU), and new crops researchers at Virginia State University (VSU).

SURVEY RESULTS

The survey identified 32 individuals who are involved to varying degrees with 24 projects covering the following crops: organically grown apples, broccoli, Brussels sprouts, flower bulbs, Chinese cabbage, storage cabbage, rapeseed, cauliflower, Belgian endive, dried flowers, elephant garlic, American ginseng, goldenseal, medicinal herbs, head lettuce, exotic mushrooms, nursery, yellow-fleshed Irish potatoes, grain sorghum, and sweet sorghum. Four projects dealt with new agronomic crops, three with ornamental, one with fruit, and 16 with vegetable crops. Twenty-two of the projects were under the direction of research and extension faculty from VPI&SU and VSU, while only two were done solely by county extension agents without university assistance. The majority of the projects were supported by the state of Virginia through annual operating budgets and not funds earmarked specifically for alternative crops research. Of these programs, 24% received at least partial funding from the federal government and 20% received support from private industry. Five of the projects were more than five years old. One of the primary objectives in 15 of the projects was to assess market demand and profitability of the crop. Another important objective stated for most studies was to develop production recommendations. Fifteen of the projects involved adapting production of existing agronomic or horticultural crops from other areas of the United States to Virginia. Only nine projects involved research with exotic plant species. Two projects addressed the growing need for information about organically grown apples and vegetables, even though both of these commodities are already major crops in Virginia.

DISCUSSION

The results of the survey were unexpected. Cotton, one of the most successful new crops in Virginia, is not supported by a publicly funded development program. The area of cotton grown in Virginia has risen steadily over the past several years, and over 2,146 ha of cotton were grown in southeastern Virginia in 1990 (Anon. 1991). Although two projects dealing with rapeseed research were identified, both are primarily cultivar trials. Only in the last year have researchers and extension specialists at VPI&SU and VSU promoted rapeseed as a viable alternative crop for Virginia. Yet in 1991, an estimated 405 ha of rapeseed were grown in Virginia (D. Starner pers. commun.).

It is interesting to compare the success of pickling cucumbers, cotton, and rapeseed with broccoli which has been the focus of a large research and extension program in the College of Agriculture at VPI&SU over the past 10 years, but has not lived up to its potential as an alternative crop. In the early 1980s when prices were severely depressed, a group of tobacco growers from southern Virginia asked the College of Agriculture at VPI&SU for assistance in developing alternative crops for their region. A USDA marketing study showed that there was a strong demand for fall broccoli in the eastern United States. Since broccoli produces a high return per unit area, as does tobacco, and because of the long growing season in southern Virginia, researchers at VPI&SU developed production recommendations and encouraged growers to produce fall broccoli. Extension specialists enthusiastically provided on site production demonstrations for interested growers. The state government helped finance a modern vegetable cooperative in Halifax to market broccoli. Yet in spite of this massive effort, today less than 40 ha of broccoli are produced in the tobacco belt of southern Virginia, only a fraction of the area that was originally envisioned.

Broccoli has failed to become an important crop in southern Virginia for several reasons. The tobacco market which had been depressed in the early 1980s rebounded dramatically, largely due to tobacco exports. Today, there is a near record high 21,457 ha of tobacco grown in Virginia (Anon. 1991). Broccoli is a delicate crop and requires more precise management than tobacco, making it a more difficult crop for farmers to produce. Unlike tobacco, broccoli is a very perishable crop that must be harvested and transported to market in a timely manner. Most of the farmers who tried growing broccoli continued raising tobacco as well. Often planting dates for broccoli, irrigation schedules, and fertilizer applications conflicted with the tobacco harvest, and as a result the broccoli crop was often neglected. Stand establishment was also a problem because of the high late summer temperatures during planting season. One of the most important factors working against the successful development of broccoli as an alternative crop was the fact that tobacco had been a staple crop and a part of the local culture for many generations. Consequently, farmers were reluctant to abandon tobacco in favor of an another crop, despite the economic potential it offered.

Approximately 80 ha of pickling cucumbers are grown in southern Virginia by tobacco growers for a pickle packer in North Carolina who has encouraged production in the area (P. Ramsey pers. commun.). Pickling cucumbers only return about $1,225 per ha, much less than broccoli or tobacco. However, pickling cucumber production is much more compatible with tobacco than broccoli because the cucumber harvest coincides with the slack period before tobacco harvest. This allows growers to maximize the use of farm laborers throughout the entire summer.

Cotton has become a successful alternative crop for several reasons. Cotton offers growers a higher return per hectare when compared with other traditional agronomic crops grown in southeastern Virginia. The production practices, although some what different, were similar to those used for other crops. New and used harvesting equipment was available in nearby North Carolina. Although no research and extension work had been done in Virginia on cotton, production recommendations developed at North Carolina State University were successfully used by growers in southeastern Virginia.

Rapeseed is a crop that could also be grown using existing farm equipment. Rapeseed production is compatible with other crop rotations and provides a comparable or higher return compared with other winter annuals. Grain dealers set up collection points in northern Virginia which made marketing easier. In addition, grain dealers and a farm supply company distributed a video cassette on rapeseed production to growers throughout the state which stimulated interest in the crop.

While the results of this study show that the agriculture universities in Virginia are very actively involved in new crop development, the role of the private sector in the process should not be discounted. In times of reduced public funding for agricultural programs, private industry should be looked upon to provide funding and markets for new commodities. The successful development of alternative crops in Virginia involves many complex factors that may make the success of a project difficult to predict. Grower interest in all aspects of the production and marketing of a given crop is essential. The results of this study suggest that grower interest in alternative crops involves other considerations besides profitability.

REFERENCES

Anon. 1991. Virginia crops and livestock report. Virginia Agr. Statistics Serv. and the U.S. Dept. of Agr. 63(2):2.

CENTERS

Center for Alternative Plant and Animal Products: Programs in Information Exchange and Research

Daniel H. Putnam, Ervin A. Oelke, and Laura McCann

The mid-1980s brought with it economic and environmental conditions which convinced many in the agricultural community that changes were necessary to maintain the viability of modern agriculture. The resounding successes in productivity of the American agricultural system since World War II seemed dampened by a severe depression in prices and lower farm incomes. The burden of farm debt and frequent farm auctions forced angry farmers to descend upon state and national capitals demanding change. Although the "farm crisis" was many-faceted, the 1990 Farm Bill, with its emphasis on "flexibility" in crop choice, was a recognition of the negative effect that overproduction of major crops had on the farm community, and a confirmation of the desirability of crop and livestock enterprise diversification.

This economic turmoil and dislocation of rural communities presented a challenge to University State Experiment Stations, Departments of Agriculture and Natural Resources, Extension, and Educational institutions. Perceived as bureaucratic in nature, slow to change, and often difficult to access, these entities nevertheless had tremendous resources which could be brought to bear on these issues. Recognition of these possibilities led University of Minnesota Horticulture Professors Luther Waters and David Davis to form the Center for Alternative Plant and Animal Products in 1986. It was visualized not as a new department within the College of Agriculture, but as a means to focus energies from several departments on the area of crop diversification and utilization. It arose not by legislative mandate or from large grants, but from faculty discussions exploring ways to achieve cooperation between disciplines to increase crop diversity. Part of the impetus for the Center came from experience implementing integrated production-to-market horticultural projects in the early 1980s (Waters 1991).

New crop development is not new to Minnesota. Wild rice (*Zizania aquatica* L.) once a very minor gourmet specialty crop, is now widely marketed nationwide, and was born in the swamps, lakes, and streams of northern Minnesota. It was aided in its development by entrepreneurial farmers and University of Minnesota researchers. Sunflower (*Helianthus annuus* L.), an underutilized native-American crop (until the Russians proved its viability), developed rapidly in Minnesota in the 1970s, partly due to agronomic research at the University of Minnesota. Fieldbean (*Phaseolus vulgaris* L.) was at first a failure in Minnesota and the Dakotas, but subsequently succeeded when a change in technology (herbicides) made it an economically viable crop (Robinson 1987).

DEFINITIONS

Since alternative agricultural enterprises could include everything from developing bed and breakfast operations to roadside vegetable stands, the Center narrowed its focus to diversification of plant and animal production and marketing. An alternative crop or animal is simply one different from crops or animals currently being cultivated. Obviously, this concept yields a universe of possibilities, each with its own series of limitations (Vietmeyer 1986). Sources of alternative plants or animals include: (1) newly developed species (e.g. triticale); (2) new commodities developed from existing crops or animals (canola, dairy sheep); (3) domestication of wild plants or animals (crown vetch, wild rice, red deer); and (4) previously domesticated crops or animals newly introduced into a region (lupin, llama). For example, the introduction of cold-tolerant soybean into northern Minnesota, Oregon, or Canada (where farmers are largely unfamiliar with it), is an extension of the crop-introduction process. All the factors important to the introduction of a new crop impact this process, even if the crop is familiar elsewhere. Undoubtedly, this is the most common form of species introduction or new crop development.

Alternative crops could include (1) *lower risk* crops for which significant portions of the Production-Utilization-Marketing matrix are known (e.g., canola); or (2) *higher risk* options for which significant knowledge of production, utilization, and marketing does not widely exist (e.g., milkweed, quinoa). Alternative crops could include (1) commodity crops, the product of value of which is largely generic and enters into a broad market, such as protein or oil (examples are oilseed sunflower or lupin for protein), or (2) specialty crops or animals, where the uses and markets are limited (e.g., mustard or Belgian endive).

PHILOSOPHY

The Center was created as an entity to (1) generate, receive, and evaluate new crop or product ideas; (2) facilitate research on alternative plant or animal production or products; and (3) disseminate information to the public on alternative plant and animal products.

Value of Diversity

A central point of agreement among Center participants is that agricultural and natural resource diversification is desirable. It is recognized that diversification of plant or animal enterprises may be important sources of economic development, contribute to the utilization of marginal lands, help in fighting erosion, enhance nutrition, provide new industries, or spread out economic risk for farmers (CAST 1984). Crop diversity has the potential to contribute sustainability or stability from either an environmental or economic perspective. It is recognized that not all new or alternative plants or animals will do all of these things (indeed some are less desirable from several perspectives than our traditional crops and livestock), but simply that biodiversity is an untapped resource that deserves attention. The end result of our efforts should be the creation of an agricultural or natural resource option where none previously existed.

Importance of Markets

New plant or animal enterprises must be market-driven to be successful. Although there are many ideas for alternative plant and animal product development, the Center has recognized that a plausible scenario should be developed which would tie each idea to an economically viable outcome. Each new crop or animal should be considered from a whole-system, "production-utilization-marketing" perspective, recognizing the opportunities and limitations of each component. This approach has been widely recognized nationwide as being critical to the success of new crop efforts (Knox and Theisen 1981; Thompson 1988).

An Open Forum

New ideas (even outlandish ones) deserve a reasonable hearing. Too often, new crop ideas are rejected (in a knee-jerk fashion), or embraced (in a knee-jerk fashion) due to lack of an in-depth hearing or careful analysis. Some new crop or product ideas just might be "crazy" enough to work (e.g., kiwi fruit or alfalfa sprouts), and an environment should be provided where creativity is enhanced.

Importance of Information

This is the "Information Age," and we believe that agriculture provides no exception to the value of information to the modern economy. It is first necessary to develop in-depth knowledge of the biology of unconventional crops as well as potential markets and utilization patterns for that crop option. However, knowledge by itself may not benefit a new crop option. Information often exists in various forms but is poorly distributed and largely unavailable. When farmers, researchers, food processors and entrepreneurs have access to information, the value of that information is multiplied manyfold. It is probably in the area of information exchange that the Center has proved to be most valuable.

Long-term Orientation

A final point is that new crops and products require sustained long-term efforts. *All* new crop, animal, and product options have problems or limitations. Minor crops are minor, largely because there is something wrong with them! Humanity has selected the crops we grow over millennia of trial and error, a force which we shouldn't ignore (Robinson 1987). What were the reasons that the plants we now call new or minor crops are *not* more widely grown? Many of the plants under consideration today previously were rejected by older civilizations. Are there significant changes or potential changes in technology or markets to justify their viability today? The answers to these questions are not easily provided (as the history of any new crop will attest) and require sustained efforts to elucidate (CAST 1984).

STRUCTURE

The Center staff consists of a director (half-time faculty), a full-time coordinator, a part-time accountant, a steering committee and advisory board, and students and others hired on a part-time basis. Luther Waters served as co-founder and director until 1990, and Laura McCann has been program coordinator with the Center since its inception. The steering committee sets direction and policy in cooperation with the director and consists of individuals from the departments of Agricultural and Applied Economics, Agricultural Engineering, Agronomy and Plant Genetics, Animal Science, Entomology, Food Science and Nutrition, Horticultural Science, Forest Resources, Plant Biology, Plant Pathology, and Soil Science.

The Center has an administrative board (department heads, deans and directors) and an advisory board. The latter has proven to be especially valuable to the Center, helping to set direction and policy. The advisory board currently consists of state senators and representatives, individuals from the Minnesota Department of Agriculture, agricultural and product-based corporations and cooperatives, as well as legislators, farmers, county extension agents, and people from commodity groups and the banking industry.

FUNCTIONS AND ACCOMPLISHMENTS

Idea Evaluation

One role of the Center is to provide a forum for fielding and evaluating new crop ideas. At the outset, a legitimate focus for debate was realized as a need. The Center has served as a central point of access for outside groups and individuals interested in alternative crops and animals. Within the University, the Center provides an important incentive and a catalyst for interdisciplinary work. The Center has held several structured "brainstorming" sessions to address specific research needs. Outside groups have requested better access to the resources of the University to answer specific questions or develop specific ideas. Extension and research faculty have received many inquiries asking essentially, "What else can I grow?" Although individual faculty still get many questions like this, the Center has functioned as a central point of access to more efficiently field questions on alternative plant and animal enterprises. This is especially important given the wide range of expertise required. The Center has developed a "Registry of Expertise" within the University to help channel ideas and questions to the right resource personnel.

Research Coordination

A second function is to provide structure and incentives for conducting interdisciplinary research on new plant and animal products. Several projects of the Center have been completed recently and others are currently underway (Table 1). Ideas for research have come from the steering committee, advisory board, other faculty, producers, farm groups, or even funding agencies, who perceive a need. The major contribution of the Center to this process was to write grants, assemble teams, administer grant funds, help write reports, communicate results to the public, and negotiate between various participants in a research project. This role provides a significant incentive for faculty to tackle sometimes difficult and time-consuming interdisciplinary projects. The very existence of the Center has helped to develop linkages between researchers from different disciplines and with private sector groups who otherwise would not have been in contact.

Symposia

The Center has sponsored in-depth symposia on many different alternative agricultural enterprises, ranging from dairy sheep to amaranth (Table 2). These have provided in-depth educational and networking opportunities for researchers, extension agents, farmers, entrepreneurs, and agribusinesses, and have several benefits: (1) they create public awareness of the existence of an opportunity; (2) they assemble expertise from a wide geographic area; (3) they result in a publication which has value into the future; and (4) they may lead to further research or termination of an idea (Waters 1991). These symposia have been largely self-supporting or supported with small

Table 1. Research projects conducted through the Center for Alternative Plant and Animal Products.

Project	Funding source[z]
Amaranth Feasibility Study (1988-89)	Minnesota Department of Agriculture
Belgian Endive Development (1990-91)	Agricultural Utilization Research Institute
Canola Task Force (1990-91)	Agricultural Utilization Research Institute
Risk Assessment of Lupin (1988-91)	Central Minnesota Initiative Fund
	Agricultural Utilization Research Institute
	Bremer Foundation
Production of Native Wildflowers (91-92)	Legislative Committee on Minnesota Resources

[z]All of these funding sources operate primarily in the state of Minnesota.

Table 2. Symposia sponsored and co-sponsored by the Center for Alternative Plant and Animal Products[z].

Subject	Date
Symposia Sponsored by the Center:	
Grain Legumes as Alternative Crops	July 1987
Soybean Utilization Alternatives	Feb. 1988
Cut and Dried Flowers	Dec. 1988
Shiitake Mushrooms	May 1989
North American Dairy Sheep	July 1989
Deer Farming	Sept. 1989
Wood-Based Economic Development	Apr. 1990
Alternative Agric. Opportunities Workshop	June 1990
Organic Meat	June 1990
Grain Amaranth: Perspectives in Production, Processing and Marketing	Aug. 1990
Prospects for Lupins in North America	Mar. 1991
Cosponsored Symposia:	
First National Symposium on New Crops	Oct. 1988
Strategies for New Crop Development (Amer. Soc. Agron.)	Nov. 1988
Herbs 91—International Herb Growers and Marketers Association	July 1991
Second National Symposium on New Crops	Oct. 1991

[z]All of these symposia have resulted in the publication of proceedings which are available from the Center or cooperating agencies.

grants. The research and educational value of such symposia should not be underestimated. In some cases, more could be learned in several days by bringing together "experts" in a field than by years of dogged individual efforts.

Information Exchange

The fourth role that the Center has played is in the area of information exchange, publications, and database assembly. Symposia are a form of information exchange and a source of publications, but other publications have also been developed (Table 3). The Center has helped in creating, under the leadership of Ed Oplinger, University of Wisconsin and Erv Oelke, University of Minnesota, a comprehensive Alternative Field Crops Manual. This consists of chapters on a wide range of about 50 alternative field crops, from adzuki bean to vernonia. Little may be known of many of these crops, but in other cases, information was available, but poorly assembled and distributed. The goal was to make information on minor crops more widely available. This project began in 1989 and is now virtually complete. The Alternative Field Crops Manual has been distributed to over 30 states and

Table 3. Publications and audio-visuals produced primarily by the Center for Alternative Plant and Animal Products (October, 1991).

Symposia Proceedings (see Table 2)
Prospects for Canola in Minnesota—A White Paper
Lupin Production and Utilization Guide
Alternative Crops for Minnesota
Alternative Field Crops Manual (with Univ. of Wisconsin)
Lesser Known and Grown Field Crops Slide Set
"Flex Crop Opportunities in the 1990 Farm Bill"
National Video-teleconference (with USDA)
Alternative Agricultural Opportunities Database (with USDA)
Joint US–USSR Lupin Database (citations and abstracts)
"BioOptions" Newsletter (quarterly)

---

7 provinces, and to all county agents in 4 states. This project is an excellent example of successful inter-state cooperation towards a defined goal.

The Center helped to produce a video teleconference "Flex-Crop Acreage Opportunities in the 1990 Farm Bill" (February, 1991), which was downlinked to many communities nationwide. This teleconference featured Center Steering Committee members, economists, national farm bill experts, USDA personnel, and the opportunity for call-in questions on minor crop options available under the bill.

Several research reports and production guides have been developed on specific crops or products (Table 3). A "white paper" on canola, which analyzed the prospects for this crop in Minnesota was published early in 1991.

The Center personnel have made presentations at University of Minnesota Branch Station Field Days, agricultural fairs, field plot demonstrations, and public meetings to inform the public about minor crops. One effort was the production of a "Biodiversity Dinner" which was conducted at the St. Paul campus of the College of Agriculture. This was designed to spark the imagination of faculty, students, and staff as to the potential culinary offerings from minor species. Dishes included buffalo meat, buckwheat, quinoa, amaranth crackers, adzuki bean pastries, apios vegetables, lupin pasta, multi-grain breads, soybean dishes, and wild rice soup.

One information-exchange effort is the development of minor crop databases. The Center has made some progress in this area, but there is much room for expansion in the future. The Center has created an "Alternative Agricultural Opportunities Database," an assemblage of over 1,500 fact sheets, experiment station and extension publications from all over the United States and Canada on many different alternative crops and enterprises. Many of these publications are out of print or difficult to locate. This database has been made available to the National Agricultural Library (Beltsville, MD) and has recently been published.

A database on lupin was developed in cooperation with researchers in Russia and Ukraine, where considerable work on lupin has been conducted. Nearly finished, this database has over 4,500 entries of titles and/or abstracts on all aspects of lupin from both Slavic-language and English-language sources. This database contains many articles not previously available in the west and is one early fruit of glasnost. We have had excellent cooperation with our (formerly Soviet) cooperators, in spite of many logistical difficulties in working between the two cultures and over great distances.

Developing Linkages

The Center has been quite successful at attracting many individuals with diverse interests to contribute to a combined effort. In addition, linkages with other states, federal, and industrial sectors are critical to the success of new crop efforts (Thompson 1988) and the Center has begun to make these connections. All of these projects have been highly interdisciplinary in nature, with excellent cooperation from many quarters. More recently linkages with "Sustainable Agriculture" efforts within the University are underway.

It is our view that one of the most valuable and powerful tools we have in agriculture and natural resources today is the free flow of information. One need only visit a (previously) closed society to realize the value of information as a stimulus for progress in agricultural research as well as economic development, and the penalties which are incurred by curtailing free exchange of ideas and information. The same should be said of flow of germplasm, as the development of a new crop is closely related to the quality of the plant germplasm research system (Thompson 1988). It is perhaps in this way that a center such as the Center for Alternative Plant and Animal Products can be most valuable: in creating new knowledge of opportunities, and providing a forum for collection and dissemination of information, with the aim of creating agricultural options where none previously existed.

CONCLUSIONS

The Center for Alternative Plant and Animal Products, University of Minnesota, developed largely on the volunteerism of its steering committee and without large funding, has proved to be a valuable structure in the area of information exchange, research management, and dissemination of knowledge relating to alternative plant and animal enterprises. Most participants in sponsored activities and projects have provided positive comments. However, these efforts are small in relation to what is required to fully tackle the development of new crops, and recurring support for this long-term type of activity is difficult to find. Interest often fluctuates depending upon the prices of major commodities and size of state budgets. However, it is our feeling that if research and information dissemination dollars are to help *create* agriculture importance, rather than *follow* agriculture importance (which has been largely the case with our established crops), then larger sustained investments are required to accomplish this goal.

REFERENCES

Council for Agricultural Science and Technology (CAST). 1984. Development of new crops: needs, procedures, strategies and options. Rpt. 102. Ames, IA.

Jolliff, G.D. and S.S. Snapp. 1988. New crop development: Opportunity and challenges. J. Prod. Agr. 1:83–89.

Knox, E.G. and A.A. Theisen (eds.). 1981. Feasibility of introducing new crops: production-marketing consumption (PMC) systems. A report prepared for the National Science Foundation, Soil and Land Use Technology, Columbia, MD. Rodale Press, Emmaus, PA.

Robinson, R.G. 1987. New crops: Successes, failures, and why? In: Grain Legumes as Alternative Crops. Proc. Symp. 23–24 July, 1987. Center for Alternative Plant and Animal Products, Univ. of Minnesota, St. Paul.

Thompson, A.E. 1988. Alternative crop opportunities and constraints on development efforts. Strategies for Alternative Crop Development: Case Histories. Center for Alternative Plant and Animal Products, Univ. of Minnesota, St. Paul.

Vietmeyer, N.D. 1986. Lesser-known plants of potential use in agriculture and forestry. Science 232:1379–1384.

Waters, L. 1991. Alternative crop development efforts in Minnesota. HortScience 26:1129–1131.

Interdisciplinary Teamwork for New Crop Development in Missouri

Robert L. Myers

The components of the effort with new or alternative crops at the University of Missouri include both research and extension efforts. Field research and informal coordination of new crop research are carried out by the Alternative Crops Project, which is part of the interdisciplinary Foods, Feeds, and Products Cluster. The Cluster is one of several cooperative research groups in the College of Agriculture, Food, and Natural Resources that receive Food for the 21st Century funding from the Missouri legislature. The extension efforts with new crops are carried out primarily by faculty in agronomy and agricultural economics, and also through the Missouri Alternatives Center.

The Foods, Feeds, and Products Cluster consists of 20 faculty from the Departments of Agricultural Economics, Agricultural Engineering, Agronomy, Animal Science, Biological Sciences, Chemical Engineering, Food Science and Human Nutrition, and Plant Pathology. The general goal of the cluster is to "...increase the profitability, diversity, and sustainability of Missouri's agricultural industry." Cluster members are interested in accelerating the process of converting raw materials from new or traditional crops into new or improved products. Emphasis areas corresponding to different parts of this product development process include "economic evaluation," "agronomic evaluation," "processing," and "utilization."

Economic evaluation includes identifying market needs, marketing of by-products, and assessing profitability of new crop enterprises. Both improved food and feed products and new industrial product opportunities are explored. The possibility of using agricultural resources to replace nonrenewable resources is considered particularly critical by scientists in the cluster. Success in market expansion of food, feed, and industrial products depends not only on fully utilizing farm level resources, but also human and capital resources in small communities.

Agronomic evaluation is a comprehensive effort involving several steps, such as determining plant adaptability, evaluating performance of germplasm, and developing production practices. Among the diverse species of plants with potentially valuable products, relatively few have been utilized. Agronomists and plant scientists are conducting field and laboratory trials with a significant number of these underutilized plants. This research has already shown that canola and industrial rapeseed are excellent options for the region, and thus several investigators are involved in agronomic research with canola/rapeseed. Replicated field studies are underway with several other promising crops, such as sunflower, buckwheat, crambe, amaranth, dry beans, and sesame. In an attempt to identify regions of the state most suited for amaranth and canola/rapeseed production, agroclimatic and economic factors have been incorporated into geographic information system databases, and used to generate maps showing most suitable areas.

Processing efforts are centered around extrusion process to create new or improved food and feed products, and fermentation processing that can be used for conversion of starches or other conversions. Extrusion processing of foods and feeds is a process of exposing raw ingredients to high temperature in combination with mixing, kneading, cooking, shearing, and forming processes to produce cereals, snacks, pet foods, texturized meat substitutes, modified starches, and other products. Fermentation processing involves use of anaerobic and aerobic microorganisms to convert starting materials into intermediate or end-use products.

Utilization research is focused on adding value to by-products and wastes. By-products such as rapeseed meal are evaluated for their nutritional value for livestock, while other products are subjected to fermentation processing. These efforts not only hold the potential for adding value to low value or waste materials, but also keep those materials out of the waste stream, potentially reducing certain environmental problems.

A current focus of the Foods, Feeds, and Products Cluster is to develop the rapeseed and canola industry in the Missouri region. This includes research on production methods and utilization studies, as described above. It also involves investigation into some of the more fundamental questions about the crops and their potential. Perhaps most uniquely, the Cluster includes among its activities efforts to generate markets for the crops and their products, in part by raising consumer awareness, and in part by direct interaction with industry. For example, members of the agricultural economics faculty have met with several different processors and utilization experts in agricultural corporations to pursue market development for canola and rapeseed.

The work the Cluster carries out with rapeseed is part of a multi-state effort called the High Erucic Acid Development Effort (HEADE). This interstate collaboration allows better research support and evaluation within and across disciplines. Missouri's role is a central one due to the involvement of university personnel in the administration and research of the HEADE program.

The alternative crops emphasis within the Cluster was catalyzed with the addition of the Alternative Crops Project in 1989. This project, one of four F21C supported positions/projects in the Cluster, has the responsibility of evaluating diverse crop species for potential in Missouri. The work ranges from established alternatives, such as canola, to less well known grains such as amaranth. Crops grown elsewhere in the world, but not in Missouri, are receiving attention, such as sesame, while certain native, undomesticated, Midwestern species are also being examined, particularly those which were once cultured by indigenous Midwestern groups for their grain production, such as goosefoot, marsh elder, and knotweed. Research with these crops includes agronomic characterization, development of production practices and cropping system strategies, and investigation into the physiology and ecology of more promising species. The most promising "grains" to date are canola and sunflowers, while other options may be feasible in a few to several years, such as sesame, amaranth, and grain-type pearl millet.

The Alternative Crops Project provides the lead on interdisciplinary research with alternative crops carried out by the F21C Cluster. Cooperators from agricultural economics, agricultural engineering, agronomy, animal science, anthropology, biological sciences, entomology, food science and human nutrition, geography, horticulture, and plant pathology all contribute to the research effort with alternative crops.

Research is not the only action needed to increase the adoption of alternative crops. Efforts in educating both consumers and producers about alternative crops and products are essential to the long term success of these crops. Extension programs are carried out by personnel in both agronomy and agricultural economics. Information is provided not only through traditional media such as grower meetings and extension publications, and interviews with print and broadcast journalists, but also through computer-based multi-media systems. Alternative crops currently covered by extension guides include canola, sunflowers, and buckwheat. Other guides are planned for the future.

Individuals who contact the University of Missouri for information related to crop alternatives are usually directed to either the Alternative Crops Project or to the Missouri Alternatives Center. The Missouri Alternatives Center is an extension effort that handles a large volume of phone and mail requests about unusual or exotic plants and animals. The Center maintains a large collection of reference materials on an assortment of plant and animal species, and sends out photocopies of information relevant to a particular request. Information files at the Center are maintained and supported by Center staff, by an independent consultant, and by campus research projects such as the Alternative Crops Project. The Alternative Crops Project maintains information files on approximately 100 different crops or potential crops, with the focus on plants that would be harvested primarily for their seeds.

Efforts on new or alternative crop research and extension are also being carried on at other Missouri institutions. At Lincoln University, a program in horticulture focused on ethnic food markets has generated much interest (primarily specialty vegetables). Northwest Missouri State University staff have stimulated farmers into growing horticultural and industrial crops as part of cooperative on-farm research and demonstration efforts. The programs at University of Missouri, Lincoln University, and Northwest Missouri State University combine to provide the state's farmers with good technical support for looking at a wide array of alternatives.

In sum, key elements of the new crops programs at University of Missouri include interdisciplinary cooperation, long term commitment from the University administration, and base funding provided by the state. Although various individuals have promoted or researched selected new or alternative crops during the past few decades in Missouri, the current comprehensive initiative was initiated only in 1989. The early focus with canola and rapeseed has and will continue to have immediate impact in the state. Efforts with many other alternative crops will take a number of years to achieve desired goals, but the enthusiasm, support, and participation of many individuals should greatly improve the chance of success.

IMPACT and the East Asian Crop Development Program

Thomas A. Lumpkin, Bill B. Dean, and Desmond A. O'Rourke

Traditional crops have become less profitable over the last two decades forcing the Washington State agricultural industry to search for alternatives. Appropriate alternatives could allow innovators to improve their economic situation and position themselves favorably for the future. Washington State is on the Pacific Rim, close to the rapidly growing and industrializing Asian countries such as Japan, which are markets for a wide range of products not familiar to Washington State producers. Washington State University (WSU) has established an international marketing center to assist our producers in the development and export of agricultural products to these markets.

HISTORY OF THE IMPACT CENTER

The origin of the International Marketing Program for Agricultural Commodities and Trade (IMPACT) Center can be traced to early 1983, when James Ozbun, the previous Dean of the College of Agriculture and Home Economics at WSU, set up a committee to examine a possible international marketing institute. This idea was inspired by Ozbun's earlier visit to the Food and Feed Grain Institute (FFGI) in Kansas. The envisioned institute was to incorporate many of FFGI's features and apply them to a broader spectrum of ideas. The President of WSU and the University Provost requested an initial budget of $49,500 from the state legislature, which was approved in March, 1984, and matched by WSU. This money was provided on a provisional basis to test the concept of the IMPACT Center. In 1985, the IMPACT Center was finally established within the University based on an October 1, 1985 amendment to the federal National Agricultural Research, Extension, and Teaching Policy Act of 1977, which provided the legislative basis for this action. From the 1988 fiscal year until this year, IMPACT has been receiving federal matching funds.

IMPACT is a separate administrative unit of the College of Agriculture and Home Economics at WSU (Fig. 1) in Pullman, Washington (affiliated scientists are also located at other sites in the state, and over-seas in export markets), and is devoted to studies that ultimately assist in the export marketing of agricultural commodities (Day 1985; Steury 1990; Tacoma 1987; USDA 1990). IMPACT is also responsible for assembling, analyzing, and disseminating relevant market information to producers, producer associations, commodity commissions, processors, packers, shippers, brokers, transporters, financiers, and other agencies engaged in the marketing of Washington State's agricultural products.

IMPACT supports teams of scientists to address problems in the export marketing of agricultural products. This approach utilizes WSU's collective knowledge and capacity for research and extension. IMPACT's guidance and funding allow university scientists to concentrate on problems without being subject to short-term time and profit constraints faced by individual firms. Thus, the IMPACT Center has become a hub for innovative scientific research and information that promotes Washington State's agricultural exports. This comprehensive and systematic approach is not available to the state's agricultural industry from any other source.

Washington's legislature intended for the IMPACT Center to be problem oriented and able to rapidly respond to issues arising in international markets. However, in order to solve such problems, some fundamental or basic research has been required before applying the solution or application. IMPACT has attempted to keep a balance by funding projects that provide rapid results as the state legislature envisioned and those projects requiring longer research periods which may eventually yield greater net benefits to the state.

FUNDING

IMPACT obtains funds from state, federal, and private industry (O'Rourke 1989) (Table 1). State funds support functions such as basic staffing, attendance at trade shows, and development of curricula. Federal funds matched with state funds are used to pay for research projects selected by the IMPACT Review Committee. In addition, researchers may receive financial assistance from commodity groups and private sources.

IMPACT uses federal and state funds to support research on a range of large and small commodities and new products. Federal grants and private contributions are occasionally obtained for specific projects which are not funded by IMPACT.

Table 1. IMPACT Center's sources of funding, 1985–86 and 1990–91.

Year	Funding ($)				Non-state (%)
	State match	Federal	Other[z]	Total	
1985–86	549,500	0	228,800	778,300	29.4
1990–91	596,500	522,705	550,000	1,699,205	64.9

[z]Other funds include grants from federal and private sources, as well as contributions from producer organizations and domestic and foreign businesses.

Uses of State Funds

State funds are allocated for permanent faculty in the departments of Agricultural Economics, Food Science and Human Nutrition, Horticulture, and core staff; an annual grant to the College of Business and Home Economics for the development of curricula related to international agricultural marketing; an annual grant to the Wood Materials and Engineering Laboratory of the College of Engineering for attending and sponsoring seminars, and participating in trade shows; and limited funding to competitively bid projects.

Uses of Federal Matching Funds

Federal requirements state that funds be used for agricultural research and that an equal (matching) amount be obtained from non-federal sources. Non-federal sources include contributions made by the state, private companies, and agricultural groups. Federal grants for individual research projects do not count toward matching funds. IMPACT has used virtually all federal matching funds for competitively bid projects. However, because of a change in federal policy, beginning FY 1992, all matching funds are to be terminated, and replaced by special allocations.

Uses of *Other* Funds

Other funds are obtained from private industry (domestic and foreign), agricultural groups, and federal grants other than federal matching funds. All funds generated in the *other* category are earmarked for specific projects as specified by the contributors. In many instances, these funds are contributed because the donors support specific IMPACT projects. Occasionally *other* funds support projects which are not selected by the IMPACT review board. For example, IMPACT is currently conducting research on potato black spot bruising which is being financed by the potato industry.

Commodity Commissions and the USDA/ARS support research on large scale crops. IMPACT balances these activities and projects by funding research on smaller crops. Alternative crops research is also financed by state and federal funds. Maintaining a balance between the international competitiveness of Washington State's large exporters and developing new products for market niches is a goal of IMPACT. Less-established and alternative crop groups must rely heavily on state and federal funding, and cooperation and financial support from foreign market representatives.

Challenges

In it's sixth year, IMPACT has increasingly focused on major challenges which compliment WSU's scientific talents, as well as those which benefit the agricultural and forest products of Washington. These challenges include: (1) determining worldwide market opportunities for Washington's agricultural products; (2) improving the competitiveness of Washington's agricultural products in yield, quality, price, and service; (3) solving specific technical problems faced by Washington's agricultural exporters; (4) developing nondestructive tests for quality; (5) developing new products or processes; and (6) putting scientific findings to work in real world marketing situations.

Since IMPACT's establishment in 1985, studies funded through IMPACT have revealed information that has increased our understanding of world markets (Cook and Kullberg 1986; McClary et al. 1989), changing consumer tastes in Japan (Jussaume 1989), Asian quality preferences, and improved marketing strategies. Information collected and generated by the IMPACT center enhances agricultural market opportunities for Washington, as well as reducing risks for certain agricultural products in a rapidly diversifying and integrated international market. IMPACT's challenges can be illustrated by it's effort to develop new products to meet opportunities arising from access to the world's consumers. Many opportunities exist for research and development of new specialized agricultural products, and major priority is given to new products and processes that are likely to generate additional exports. Japanese markets exist for products such as wagyu beef, chicory for artificial sugar production (Dean 1990), edamame vegetable soybeans, and azuki beans. These commodities are currently being tested at WSU for marketing in Asia and in the United States. Development of these commodities requires specialized expertise in agricultural, social and cultural aspects of international trade in addition to agroeconomic knowledge.

Specific Approaches to Alternative Crops

Traditional crops grown in Washington State, face declining prices and over-capacity. Major commodities like apples, wheat, and potatoes have seen production grow and prices decline over the last twenty years. High value new crops have the potential to displace some of these traditional crops. When high value new crops are shipped to export markets they are more likely to contribute to the profitability of the agricultural economy rather than just substituting one low value crop for another.

Previous efforts to commercialize many alternative crops have failed for a number of reasons. In 1987, the IMPACT Center organized a conference, to examine previous attempts at developing alternative crops in Washington State over the previous fifty years. Conclusions from the conference indicated that most efforts failed because of a lack of an integrated effort. In some cases crops failed because of inadequate processing facilities. In other cases crops failed because a market did not exist, or from the unwillingness of growers to commit the needed hectarage. Many potential crops, such as sunflower, failed because they could not yield profitably under local conditions. A major exception in the last fifty years has been the Washington wine industry, which after thirty years of ineffective growth, put together an integrated effort combining research, extension, government regulation and industry support to achieve the development of a successful industry.

THE EAST ASIAN CROP DEVELOPMENT PROGRAM.

The IMPACT Center has been using federal matching funds to support the study of alternative crops via the East Asian Crop Development Program in the Department of Crop and Soil Sciences (Fig. 1). Initial successes have been achieved by this program in the development of azuki beans and edamame soybeans (discussed in detail in a companion paper), although several agronomic and processing problems restrain full development until new varieties and processes are approved for release. These products have a ready market as raw commodities in Asia, and have the potential for added value in processing.

The three part approach of the East Asian Crop Development Program is: (1) identification of East Asian alternative crops for the domestic and export market; (2) comprehensive coordination of efforts to commercialize these alternative crops from the planting of its seed to final consumption; and (3) formulation of a generalized model for development and commercialization of alternative crops.

This generalized approach has numerous sequential but overlapping stages. The early stages involve studying the import statistics of targeted countries. A list of imported agronomic commodities is developed and a cursory analysis is made for their potential production in the state based on environmental considerations. Next, sample cultivars of potential crops are located, grown in an East Asian observation garden, and a simple review of Washington State, national, and international research publications is undertaken. If a new crop grows well in the garden, simple yield plots are established and basic production, processing and marketing requirements are established. When yield is found to be reasonable and constraints not prohibitive, a graduate student is assigned to the crop. Next, an exhaustive effort is made to select cultivars, collect research literature, and identify cooperating producers, processors, marketers, and a multi-disciplinary research team. At this stage, the graduate student, cooperators, and the research team undergo an intensive process of education on all aspects of the crop via literature review, observation plot results, test processing, and visits to the Asian market. In addition, the

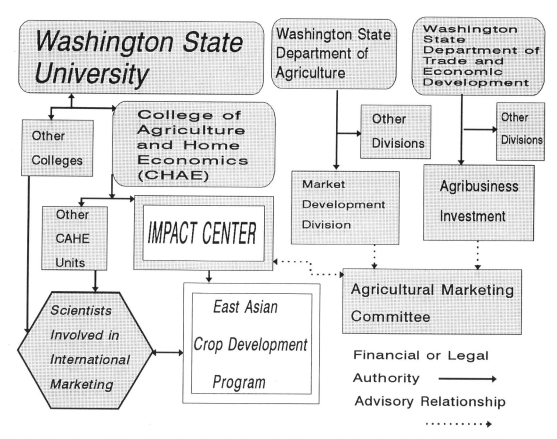

Fig. 1. Flow chart of financial or legal authority and advisory relationships for the IMPACT Center and the East Asian Crop Development Program.

graduate student is placed on the farm of an Asian producer for the growing season and/or at an Asian university or research institute that studies the crop. As a prerequisite, graduate students are selected for interest in Asia and trained in an Asian language and culture. These students tend to be highly motivated older students. As graduates, they are viewed as a form of technology transfer from the program to the state's agricultural industry.

At any stage in this process, efforts on a selected crop can be terminated if commercial production seems impossible or requiring an excessive investment in time or research support. If the crop shows promise, a package of management practices is established, an internal bulletin of production guidelines is prepared and training workshops are provided to producers. Also, foreign importers are provided samples of various cultivars for quality and taste testing. The research team is provided feed-back from producers, test trials and importers, and sub-groups are assigned to overcome identified constraining factors. If the team and cooperators feel comfortable with agronomic progress, preliminary studies on processing are undertaken. Since the ultimate goal of the IMPACT center is to generate revenue in the State and create jobs, adding value through processing is a high priority. Concurrent with processing efforts, breeding, commercial scale-up and test marketing are undertaken.

The East Asian Crop Development program is involved in the coordination of research and marketing activities, in addition to education and promotion. At the point of commercialization, the director must occasionally convene and mediate negotiations between cooperating producers, processors, and importers on prices and responsibilities. An understanding of cultural and political sensitivities is crucial at this stage. Once full commercialization occurs, a commodity commission can be established to takeover many of IMPACTS' responsibilities for further development of the crop.

CONCLUSION

The success of the IMPACT Center, the East Asian Crop Development Program, and other institutes such as the Center for Alternative Plant and Animal Products at the University of Minnesota, suggest that they can serve as models for the creation of similar institutions in other states and at the national level. Success of these efforts has come from their comprehensive approach, their ability to understand and serve the needs of the consumer (Steury 1990), and to bridge the gap between academics and business. Success has also come from the recognition of regional strengths and weakness, especially, for Washington, the opportunities in Asia that lie hidden because of cultural differences. The comprehensive system developed by the East Asian Crop Development Program for identification, evaluation, development, and promotion of new East Asian crops has many useful features for other alternative product programs, especially its use of graduate students. This system is successfully producing and marketing new crops within the United States and to Asia, where other less comprehensive approaches have failed.

REFERENCES

Cook, A. and V. Kullberg. 1986. A demographic profile with implications for marketing agricultural products. An IMPACT Center Report: Information Series 8, IMPACT Center, Washington State Univ., Pullman.

Day, T. 1985. WSU could IMPACT port business, p. 11-12. Port of Seattle U.S.A. Tradelines, Jan./Feb.

Dean, W. 1990. Research on marketing quality vegetables. Special report, IMPACT Center, Washington State Univ., Pullman.

Jussaume, R.A. 1989. Food consumption in Seattle, WA and Kobe, Japan. An IMPACT Center Report: Information Series 28. Washington State Univ., Pullman.

McClary, D.C., T.L. Raney, and T.A. Lumpkin. 1989. Japanese food marketing channels: A case study of Azuki beans and Azuki products. An IMPACT Center Report: Information Series 29. Washington State Univ., Pullman.

O'Rourke, D. 1989. IMPACT biennial report 1989-91. IMPACT Center, Washington State Univ., Pullman.

Steury, T. 1990. Giving the world what it wants. Universe. 3(1):12-18.

Tacoma, Port of. 1987. Research centers make an IMPACT on State's marketing efforts, p. 5-7. Pacific Gateway, Summer.

United States Department of Agriculture. 1990. Washington's IMPACT Center makes research pay off for exporters. AgExporter April 2(4):13.

Indiana Center for New Crops and Plant Products

Jules Janick

Indiana agriculture is based on crops that were once considered new. Though a process of introduction, trial and error, Indiana agricultural systems have been stabilized into a narrow group of crop species based on maize (2.4 million ha), soybeans (2.0 million ha), traditional grasses and legumes for hay and pasture (0.8 million ha), and small grains (0.4 million ha) with only about 20,000 ha in horticultural crops. As a result of the concentration of crop species, the majority of Indiana growers have relatively few alternatives, so that low prices on major commodities have a disastrous impact on Indiana agriculture.

New crops offer alternatives to increase farm income, improve diets, lower costs, expand markets, diversify products, and increase exports. However, there is a dilemma to new crops developments. Processors and other entiities in the production chain are not interested in establishing facilities for new crops unless volume and markets are assured, while farmers will not plant without assured markets. This is the weak link in the chain of new crop development. Successful development of new crops and plant products requires a working partnership between scientist, farmers, industry, and government.

THE CENTER

To encourage crop diversity, Purdue University initiated a New Crops and Plant Products Center in 1990 with the hope that a coordinated effort can overcome obstacles to new crop development. The broad mandate of the Center is to establish and promote a cooperative, synergistic relationship between farmers, scientists, processors, and state and federal government in order to promote new opportunities for Indiana agriculture. The specific objectives are as follows:
1. Identify, adapt and commercialize new crops for growers and processors.
2. Create new plant based industries based on new crops products.
    The following four-stage plan was proposed to accomplish these objectives:
    a. Researchers, growers, and processors, and growers would be surveyed for their interest and activities to identify promising ideas and projects. New crop candidates would be identified by the Center. The Center would coordinate new crop activities with interested researchers, growers, and processors to develop working partnerships.
    b. Field trials of targeted crops would be carried out on University Research Farms and commercial farms to evaluate performance and market potential. Where possible, risks incurred would be shared between the center, growers, and processors to establish a strong proactive relationship among interested parties.
    c. Successful candidates would undergo crop commercialization research, product development, and market evaluation on the basis of a "seed" grants program.
    d. Separate grower/market organizations would be initiated for new crops that show economic promise.

The Center was officially approved by the the Purdue University School of Agriculture in 1990 with Jules Janick, Department of Horticulture, as Director. Support was solicited and received for a New Crops Initiative from the Indiana Corporation for Science and Technology (later renamed the Indiana Business Modernization and Technology Corporation or BMT) for 1990 and the grant was renewed in 1991 involving the Departments of Agronomy, Agricultural Economics, Horticulture, and Forestry and Natural Resources, to support three major projects: Expansion of Canola Production; Commercialization of Specialty Crops; and Development of Edible Soybean. Funding for 1992–1993 was approved. Projects and personnel are listed in Table 1.

CENTER ACHIEVEMENTS

By the second year of funding, the research initiative was able to demonstrate substantial results. The 1990-91 Indiana canola crop was approximately 2,800 ha harvest in early summer of 1991. Efforts of the New Crop Center project concentrated on providing Indiana growers with research information on planting dates, fertilization practices, appropriate cultivars, and alternative tilling methods. Preliminary research with pearl

Table 1. Projects funded for New Crop Iniative, 1990–1992.

Title	Personnel	Department
1990–92		
Development of Edible Soybeans	N.C. Nielsen	Agronomy
	J.R. Wilcox	Agronomy
Expansion of Winter Canola and	E. Christmas	Agronomy
Pearl Millet Production	J. Axtell	Agronomy
	H. Doster	Agricultural Economics
	J. Rogler	Animal Science
	S. Weller	Horticulture
Commercialization of Specialty Crops for	J.E. Simon	Horticulture
Processing and Fresh Market	J. Janick	Horticulture
	G. Sullivan	Horticulture
	P.B. Brown	Forestry & Natural Resources
1992–1993		
Development of Alternative Double Crops in Indiana		
A. Introduction of Pearl Millet to	J. Axtell	Agronomy
Indiana Agriculture	R. Nielsen	Agronomy
	G. Brown	Agronomy
	E. Christmas	Agronomy
B. Development of Weed Management Strategies for Pearl Millet	S. Weller	Horticulture
C. Evaluation of the Nutritional Value of	L. Adeola	Animal Science
Pearl Millet in Pig Diets	J.C. Rogler	Animal Science
D. Expansion of Winter Canola Production	E. Christmas	Agronomy
	H. Doster	Agricultural Economics
E. Introduction of Annual Medics into Indiana	K.D. Johnson	Agronomy
Agriculture	J.J. Volnec	Agronomy
Development of New Specialty Crops		
A. Commercializing New Essential Oil Crops	J.E. Simon	Horticulture
	J. Janick	Horticulture
	D.J. Charles	Horticulture
	M.R. Morales	Horticulture
B. Commercialization of Specialty Melons	J.E. Simon	Horticulture
	J. Janick	Horticulture
	M.R. Morales	Horticulture
	D.J. Charles	Horticulture
	G.H. Sullivan	Horticulture
	D. Scott	Horticulture
C. Development of Integrated Production and Marketing Strategies for Commercial Expansion in the Fresh Melon Industry	G.H. Sullivan	Horticulture
D. Evaluation of New Fruit Crops	B. Bordelon	Horticulture
	R.H. Hayden	Horticulture
	J. Janick	Horticulture
E. Soft-Shell Crayfish Expansion	P.B. Brown	Forestry & Natural Resources
F. Evaluation of Transgenic High-solid Tomatoes	A.K. Handa	Horticulture

millet in Indiana have indicated that this African crop could find a place as a potential double crop after wheat on as many as 30,000 acres for the northern third of Indiana. Research on edible soybeans has been aimed at exploiting specialty markets for export. Progress has been obtained in characterizing lines with altered oil content as well as improved flavor for tofu production, a major component of the Japanese market. Research with a number of specialty crops including essential oil crops such as basil and artemisia, new melon crops, dry beans, and crayfish have demonstrated promising opportunities for Indiana farmers throughout the state. The 1992 proposal has expanded the number of crops through direct Center support as well as alternative funding opportunities.

OUTREACH

National outreach of the Center has been achieved through symposia to determine the status and future of new crops research and development; to explore the potential of new crops, to identify new uses for existing and underexploited crops; and to develop strategies for establishing partnerships among state, federal, and industrial organizations. Two national symposia have been held in Indianapolis, Indiana. The proceedings of the first symposium held on October 23–36, 1988 (*NEW CROPS: Research, Development, Economics*) was published by Timber Press in a 560 page book entitled *Advances in New Crops*. The proceedings of the second national symposium (*Progress in New Crops*) held Oct. 6–9, 1992 is the subject of the present volume. The Purdue New Crops Center has agreed to host a third national symposium in conjunction with the AAIC in 1995 or 1996.

The Center has developed a newsletter (*New Crops News*) which is distributed to the New Crops community. Symposia featuring individual new crops are planned; the first on Crayfish production was held in July 1992. Internally, the New Crops Center has served as a focal point to engender cooperation among disparate researchers interested in various aspects of new crops. A seminar program in new crops has been helpful for this purpose.

The outreach program has had a national and international impact. For example the American Association of Industrial Crops (AAIC) was organized at the first symposium and was a co-organizer of the second national symposium. Following our lead, international new crops symposia have been held in London in 1989 and in Jerusalem in 1992. Finally the Alternative Agricultural Research and Commercializaetion Center (AARC) based on a $4.5 million federal appropriation represents national support for new crop efforts.

FUTURE PLANS

Future Center activities will depend on the flow of funding support which will depend largely on the success of present programs. It is difficult to predict which of the current programs will be successful, but we are confident that a few of them will reward our early enthusiasm with solid accomplishments that will translate to a more diversified Indiana agriculture.

REFERENCES

Janick, J. and J.E. Simon (eds.). 1990. Advances in new crops. Timber Press, Portland, OR.

PART II
RESEARCH & DEVELOPMENT

EXPLORATION

Peppers: History and Exploitation of a Serendipitous New Crop Discovery*

W. Hardy Eshbaugh

Few could have imagined the impact of Columbus' discovery of a spice so pungent that it rivaled the better known black pepper from the East Indies. Nonetheless, some 500 years later, on the quincentennial anniversary of the discovery of the New World, chili peppers (*Capsicum*) have come to dominate the world hot spice trade and are grown everywhere in the tropics as well as in many temperate regions of the globe. Not only have hot peppers come to command the world's spice trade but a genetic recessive non-pungent form has become an important "green" vegetable crop on a global scale especially in temperate regions.

The New World genus *Capsicum* is a member of the Solanaceae, a large tropical family. Various authors ascribe some 25 species to the genus but this is only an estimate with anticipated new species to be discovered and named as exploration of the New World tropics expands. Exploration and plant collecting throughout the New World have given us a general but false impression of speciation in the genus. Humans unconsciously selected several taxa and in moving them toward domestication selected for the same morphological shapes, size, and colors in at least three distinct species. Without the advantage of genetic insight these early collectors and taxonomists named these many size, shape, and color forms as distinct taxa giving us a plethora of plant names that have only recently been sorted out reducing a long list of synonymy to four domesticated species. The early explorations in Latin America were designed to sample the flora of a particular region. Thus, any collection of *Capsicum* was a matter of chance and usually yielded a very limited sample of peppers from that area. Only with the advent of collecting trips designed to investigate a particular taxon did the range of variation within a species begin to be understood. One needs only to borrow specimens from the international network of herbaria to appreciate what a limited sample exists for most taxa, particularly for collections made prior to 1950. The domesticate *Capsicum pubescens*, for example, that is widespread in the mid-elevation Andes from Colombia to Bolivia, is barely represented in the herbarium collections of the world. Most herbarium collections of *Capsicum*, with the exception of *Capsicum annuum* holdings, are woefully inadequate. Furthermore, besides *Capsicum annuum*, very little attention has been paid to the many cultivars of each of the domesticated species. Often material is unusable because it was collected only in fruit neglecting the most important and critical characters associated with floral anatomy and morphology. With the advent of germplasm collecting programs during the past three decades, and concomitant improvement in herbarium collections we have come to better understand the nature of variation in the genus *Capsicum*. The increasing number of *Capsicum* herbarium specimens permits renewed interest and debate on the proper species classification.

TAXONOMY

One of the more perplexing questions regarding the taxonomy of *Capsicum* is defining the genus (Eshbaugh 1977, 1980b; Hunziker 1979). The taxonomy of the genus *Capsicum* is confounded within certain species complexes, e.g. *C. baccatum sensu lato*. Major taxonomic difficulties below the species level in other taxa, e.g. *C. annuum*, also exist. Armando T. Hunziker (unpublished) is currently working on a revision of the genus. What taxa are ultimately included in *Capsicum* may indeed change if the concept of the genus is broadened to include taxa with non-pungent fruits but with other common morphological and anatomical traits such as the nature of the anther, the structure of nectaries, and the presence of giant cells on the inner surface of the fruit (Pickersgill 1984).

---

*The investigations cited and drawn upon in this paper were supported most recently by a grant from the National Science Foundation (BSR 8411136). I am indebted to many colleagues for their thoughts and comments regarding the evolution of the genus *Capsicum*, although I accept sole responsibility for the comments in this paper. I especially acknowledge Charles B. Heiser, Jr. who started me on a course of study into the evolution of the genus *Capsicum* that has lasted more than 30 years. My wife, Barbara, has been with me on every step of this journey and deserves a special thanks for all her support, patience, and understanding.

Capsicum, as presently perceived, includes at least 25 species, four of which have been domesticated (Table 1). An understanding of each of these domesticates is instructive when trying to appreciate their origin and evolution. The data from plant breeding and cytogenetics confirm that the domesticated species belong to three distinct and separate genetic lineages. Earlier studies suggested two distinct lineages based upon white and purple flowered groupings (Ballard et al. 1970) but an evaluation of more recent data argues for the recognition of three distinct genetic lineages. Although the barriers between these gene pools may be broken down this rarely, if ever, occurs in nature.

CAPSICUM PUBESCENS

Capsicum pubescens forms a distinct genetic lineage. This pepper, first described by Ruiz and Pavon (1794) never received wide attention from taxonomists until recently (Eshbaugh 1979, 1982). Morphologically, it is unlike any other domesticated pepper having large purple or white flowers infused with purple and fruits with brown/black seeds. Genetically, it belongs to a tightly knit group of wild taxa including *C. eximium* (Bolivia and northern Argentina), *C. cardenasii* (Bolivia), and *C. tovarii* (Peru). *Capsicum pubescens* is unique among the

Table 1. Synopsis of the genus *Capsicum* (Solanaceae)[z,y].

Capsicum	New world distribution
annuum L.	Colombia north to southern United States
baccatum L.	Argentina, Bolivia, Brazil, Paraguay, Peru
buforum Hunz.	Brazil
campylopodium Sendt.	South Brazil
cardenasii Heiser & Smith	Bolivia
chacoense Hunz.	Argentina, Bolivia, Paraguay
chinense Jacq.	Latin and South America
coccineum (Rusby) Hunz.	Bolivia, Peru
cornutum (Hiern) Hunz.	South Brazil
dimorphum (Miers) O.K.	Colombia
dusenii Bitter	Southeast Brazil
eximium Hunz.	Argentina, Bolivia
glapagoensis Hunz.	Ecuador
geminifolium (Dammer) Hunz.	Colombia, Ecuador
hookerianum (Miers) O.K.	Ecuador
lanceolatum (Greenm.) Morton & Standley	Mexico, Guatemala,
leptopodum (Dunal) O.K.	Brazil
minutiflorum (Rusby) Hunz.	Argentina, Bolivia, Paraguay
mirabile Mart ex. Sendt	South Brazil
parvifolium Sendt.	Colombia, Northeast Brazil, Venezuela
praetermissum Heiser & Smith	South Brazil
pubescens Ruiz & Pav.	Latin and South America
scolnikianum Hunz.	Peru
schottianum Sendt.	Argentina, South Brazil, Southeast Paraguay
tovarii Eshbaugh, Smith & Nickrent	Peru
villosum Sendt.	South Brazil

[z]The following *Capsicum* species have been omitted: *C. anomalum*, *C. breviflorum*, and *C. ciliatum* following the earlier suggestion of Eshbaugh (1983). Also, *C. flexuosum* Sendt. has been treated as a variety of *C. schottianum* by Hunziker. The treatment of *C. frutescens* L. remains to be resolved and some may choose to retain it as a distinct species of *Capsicum* while others submerge it into *C. chinense*, as suggested in this paper. Finally, *C. eximium* var. *tomentosum* Eshbaugh & Smith is so distinctive that it may deserve species status.

[y]This table has been developed, adapted, and modified from Hunziker 1956; Eshbaugh 1977, 1980b; and Pickersgill 1984.

domesticates as a mid-elevation Andean species. *Capsicum pubescens* is still primarily cultivated in South America although small amounts are grown in Guatemala and southern Mexico, especially Chiapas. This species remains virtually unknown to the rest of the world. A small export market seems to have reached southern California. Two of the major difficulties in transferring this species to other regions include (1) its growth requirements for a cool, freeze free environment and long growing season and (2) the fleshy nature of the fruit that leads to rapid deterioration and spoilage.

CAPSICUM BACCATUM VAR. *PENDULUM*

Capsicum baccatum var. *pendulum* represents another discrete domesticated genetic line. Eshbaugh (1968, 1970) notes that this distinct South American species is characterized by cream colored flowers with gold/green corolla markings. Typically, fruits are elongated with cream colored seeds. The wild gene pool, tightly linked to the domesticate, is designated *C. baccatum* var. *baccatum* and is most common in Bolivia with outlier populations in Peru (rare) and Paraguay, northern Argentina, and southern Brazil. This lowland to mid-elevation species is widespread throughout South America particularly adjacent to the Andes. Known as aji, it is popular not only as a hot spice but for the subtle bouquet and distinct flavors of its many cultivars. This pepper is little known outside South America, although it has reached Latin America (Mexico), the Old World (India), and the United States (Hawaii). It is a mystery as to why it has not become much more wide spread, although the dominance of the *Capsicum annuum* lineage throughout the world at an early date may be responsible.

CAPSICUM ANNUUM VAR. *ANNUUM—CAPSICUM CHINENSE*

Pickersgill (1988) has stated that "the status of *Capsicum annuum, C. chinense*, and *C. frutescens* as distinct species could legitimately be questioned." Several authors have previously raised this issue culminating in the observation that "at a more primitive level one cannot distinguish between the three species. On the one hand we treat the three domesticated taxa as separate while the corresponding wild forms intergrade to such an extent that it is impractical if not impossible to give them distinct taxonomic names" (Eshbaugh et al. 1983). McLeod et al. (1979, 1983) have argued that isoenzyme data make it impossible to distinguish between these three taxa. From an extensive isoenzyme study of these three taxa and several other species, Loaiza-Figueroa et al. (1989) argue that "thus far, this substitution of alleles constitutes a good argument against the proposal that these species form an allozymically indistinguishable association of a single polytypic species" as advanced by Mcleod et al. (1982, 1983) and Eshbaugh et al. (1983) in their published studies. Nonetheless, Pickersgill (1984) has pointed out that "each domesticate intergrades with morphologically wild accessions by way of partially improved semidomesticates. Any subdivision of the wild complex into three taxa, each ancestral to one of the domesticates, becomes decidedly arbitrary, although clusters corresponding to wild *C. annuum, C. chinense*, and wild *C. frutescens* can be detected." Clearly, Loaiza-Figueroa et al. missed the point of these earlier papers which argue for the complexity of the problem noting that the real difficulty comes as one approaches the more primitive forms of these taxa. Furthermore, the Loaiza-Figueroa et al. (1989) dendrogram (p. 183) suggests that the number of *C. chinense* and *C. frutescens* taxa included in their study is insufficient to reach any definitive conclusion regarding the status of these three taxa. There is a very close relationship of these three taxa based on crossing data from several studies (Smith and Heiser 1957; Pickersgill 1980). Stuessy (1990) has observed that "the ability to cross does not just deal with a primitive genetic background; it deals with the degree of genetic compatibility developed in a particular evolutionary line." As Stuessy (1990) has inferred there can be no stronger argument for relationship than the data obtained from plant breeding. Regardless of one's viewpoint, it is clear that the *C. annuum—C. chinense—C. frutescens* complex has been and continues to be a most difficult taxonomic morass. Some preliminary information from the studies of Gounaris et al. (1986) and Mitchell et al. (1989) suggest that molecular data may be useful in resolving this and other taxonomic questions. For the present, I have chosen to recognize the *Capsicum annuum* complex and the *Capsicum chinense* complex as two distinct domesticated species. Where *C. frutescens* fits into this scenario remains to be resolved. William G. D'Arcy, A.T. Hunziker, and others may solve the problem by merging the three taxa under a single taxonomic entity. Taxonomists and formal taxonomy are having a very difficult time coping with what is a complex and dynamic evolutionary process.

The problem is heightened by the economic importance of *Capsicum* and the requirement that not only the domesticated species be named properly but that the several cultivars receive taxonomic recognition.

Capsicum annuum is the best known domesticated species in the world. Since the time of Columbus, it has spread to every part of the globe. The non-pungent form, bell pepper, is widely used as a green vegetable. Another non-pungent form, "pimento," is also present throughout much of the globe. The hot spicy forms of this species have come to dominate the spicy foods within Latin America and the rest of the world. *Capsicum annuum* probably became the dominant pepper globally in part because it was the first pepper discovered by Columbus and other New World explorers (Andrews in press). This taxon was the first *Capsicum* species taken to Europe and quickly spread to other regions.

Capsicum chinense was also discovered at an early date and spread globally but to a lesser extent than *C. annuum*. The more limited global expansion of this species is most probably related to its later discovery in South America and the competitive edge enjoyed by *C. annuum* which was firmly established in the Old World before *C. chinense* was introduced there.

ORIGIN

A discussion of the geography of *Capsicum* touches on two questions. The first relates to the origin of the genus *Capsicum* and the second to the origin of the domesticated taxa. The area of origin of *Capsicum* cannot be resolved until we understand the nature of the genus. If we accept the genus as currently circumscribed and limited to pungent taxa, then a clear center of diversity is to be found ranging from southern Brazil to Bolivia (McLeod et al. 1982; Eshbaugh et al. 1983; Pickersgill 1984). However, if the genus is reconstituted to include other non-pungent taxa, another center of diversity may be recognized in Central America and southern Mexico. Ultimately, our definition of the genus *Capsicum* and what species it includes will determine our view of its center of origins and whether the genus is monophyletic or polyphyletic. The emerging molecular studies of J.D. Palmer and R.G. Olmstead should give us a better sense of where *Capsicum* belongs within the framework of the Solanaceae.

Determining the place of origin of the genus and each of the domesticated species is at best a problematic exercise. In 1983, I stated that "it appears that the domesticated peppers had their center of origin in south-central Bolivia with subsequent migration and differentiation into the Andes and Amazonia." This is a condensation of a highly speculative hypothesis (McLeod et al. 1982). From that hypothesis Pickersgill (1989) later suggested that I (Eshbaugh 1983) argued that all the domesticated taxa arose in Bolivia. Without question, I could have stated this idea more clearly. We (McLeod et al. 1982) have speculatively hypothesized that Bolivia is a nuclear center of the genus *Capsicum* and that the origin of the domesticated taxa can ultimately be traced back to this area. That does not imply that each of the domesticated species arose in Bolivia. Clearly, evidence supports a Mexican origin of domesticated *C. annuum* while the other domesticated species arose in South America. Nonetheless, the ancestry of the domesticates can be traced to South America. While McLeod et al. (1982) have hypothesized a Bolivian center of origin for *Capsicum* there is no evidence for a polyphyletic origin of the genus as now understood.

Evidence suggests that *C. annuum* originally occurred in northern Latin America and *C. chinense* in tropical northern Amazonia (Pickersgill 1971). *Capsicum pubescens* and *C. baccatum* appear to be more prevalent in lower South America (Fig. 1). Thus, at the time of discovery, the former two species were exploited while the later two species awaited a later discovery and remain largely unexploited outside South America today.

In considering the question of origin of each particular domesticated species two issues must be considered. First, what wild progenitor is the most likely ancestor of each domesticated species and second, where is the most probable site of domestication?

Capsicum pubescens ranges throughout mid-Andean South America. An analysis of fruit size of this domesticate indicates that fruits of a statistically smaller size occur in Bolivia, while fruits from accessions outside Bolivia on the average are somewhat larger suggesting that Bolivian material approaches a more primitive size (Eshbaugh 1979).

Eshbaugh (1979, 1982) has argued that the origin of this domesticate can be found in the "ulupicas," *C. eximium* and *C. cardenasii*. Clearly, these two taxa are genetically closely related to each other and *C. pubescens*.

Natural hybrids between these taxa have been reported and evaluated (Eshbaugh 1979, 1982). Furthermore, the two species that show the highest isoenzyme correlation with *C. pubescens*, *C. eximium* and *C. cardenasii*, occur primarily in Bolivia (Eshbaugh 1982; McLeod et al. 1983; Jensen et al. 1979). All three of these taxa form a closely knit breeding unit with the two wild taxa hybridizing to give fertile progeny with viable pollen above the ninety percent level. Crosses between the wild taxa *C. eximium* and *C. cardenasii* and the domesticate *C. pubescens* most often show hybrid pollen viability greater than 55%. These factors lend to the conclusion that domesticated *C. pubescens* originated in Bolivia and that *C. eximium*—*C. cardenasii* is the probable ancestral gene pool. This does not prove that these two taxa are the ancestors of *C. pubescens* but of the extant pepper taxa they represent the most logical choice. One perplexing question remains to be investigated and that is the origin of the brown/black seed coat in domesticated *C. pubescens*, a color unknown in any of the other pepper species.

Capsicum baccatum var. *pendulum* is widespread throughout lowland tropical regions in South America. It ranges from coastal Peru to Coastal, Brazil. The wild form, recognized as *C. baccatum* var. *baccatum*, has a much more localized distribution but still ranges from Peru to Brazil. These two taxa have identical flavonoid (Ballard et al. 1970; Eshbaugh 1975) and isoenzyme profiles (McLeod et al. 1979, 1983; Jensen et al. 1979) and are morphologically indistinguishable except for the overall associated size differences found in the various organ systems of the domesticated taxon (Eshbaugh 1970). The wild form of *Capsicum baccatum* exhibits a high crossability index with domesticated *C. baccatum* var. *pendulum* with the progeny typically exhibiting pollen viability in excess of 55 percent (Eshbaugh 1970). The greatest center of diversity of wild *C. baccatum* var. baccatum is in Bolivia leading to the conclusion that this is the center of origin for this domesticate.

Can we ever unscramble questions about the origin and evolution of the *C. annuum*—*C. chinense*—*C. frutescens* species complex? Pickersgill (1989) states that there is an "overwhelming likelihood of at least two independent domestications of the chile peppers of this complex." She also notes that one "may ... argue about whether wild forms of this complex should really be assigned to different species, and indeed whether domesticated *C. annuum* and domesticated *C. chinense* are really conspecific." I would agree that the evolutionary lineage of *C. annuum*—*C. chinense*—*C. frutescens* complex is intimately linked but I would further emphasize that when,

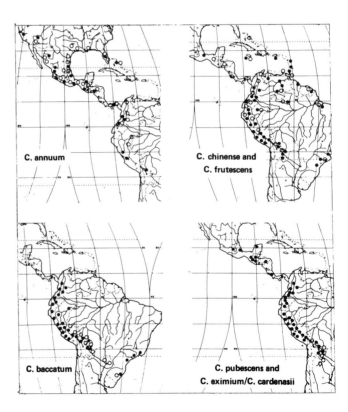

Fig. 1. Distribution of domesticated species of *Capsicum* (solid circles) and wild progenitor taxa (open circles). *Capsicum chinense* and *C. frutescens* are combined together because they may represent the same taxon. Copyright Bul. Torrey Bot. Club, 1975.

where, and how they diverged is obscured in antiquity and that the extant wild forms of these three taxa are so similar as to make them very difficult to separate. One might well ask whether, at a minimum, *C. chinense* and *C. frutescens* are conspecific or grades within the same species.

In contrast, a reasonably clear picture emerges on origin and progenitor of *C. annuum*. *Capsicum annuum* has its center of diversity in Mexico and northern Central America with a local, and more recent distribution in parts of South America. The wild bird pepper, *Capsicum annuum* var. *aviculare*, ranges from northern South America (Colombia) into the southern United States and Caribbean. Crossing studies indicate that the wild bird pepper is genetically the most closely related taxon to domesticated *C. annuum* (Emboden 1961; Smith and Heiser 1957; Pickersgill 1971). Pickersgill (1971), using karyotype analysis, suggests that the origin of domesticated *C. annuum* is to be found in southern Mexico. Pickersgill et al. (1979) also provided a detailed phenetic analysis of the *C. annuum—C. chinense—C. frutescens* complex and the difficulty of separating these taxa at the most primitive level is apparent.

Capsicum chinense remains the least understood of the four domesticated taxa with respect to center of origin and probable progenitor. If one maps the range of forms in *C. chinense*, it is clear that amazonian South America is the center of diversity of this species. Furthermore, *C. chinense* does occur sporadically throughout the Caribbean. It is likely that *C. chinense* spread into the Caribbean at a later date since the diversity of taxa is more limited in that region than in amazonian South America. In considering the progenitor of *C. chinense*, one is bewildered by the evidence. It has been suggested that *C. frutescens*, in its primitive form, may be the ancestor of *C. chinense* (Eshbaugh et al. 1983). However, one needs to ask whether *C. frutescens* is merely a weedy offshoot of *C. chinense* or *C. annuum*. It is clear that the three species, *C. annuum*, *C. frutescens*, and *C. chinense*, hybridize with each other. They form a morphological continuum especially at a primitive level (McLeod et al. 1979). Genetic evidence from isoenzymes also confirms the close relationship of these three taxa (McLeod et al. 1983; Jensen et al. 1979).

EXPLOITATION

The spread of domesticated peppers throughout the world during the 500 years since discovery is truly a phenomenon. Two of the domesticated species, *C. annuum* var. *annuum* and *C. chinense* have been widely utilized on a global scale. Both *C. baccatum* var. *pendulum* and *C. pubescens* have been extensively exploited in South America but remain largely confined to that market. Given both the unique qualities and flavors of these later two species they each represent a potential source for future development.

Of special interest to those working with peppers is the use and exploitation of the wild species. Wherever wild taxa of *Capsicum* occur, humans use them for their hot properties. In a few cases, exploitation of wild species has reached a commercial level. *Capsicum praetermissum* is collected and sold commercially in parts of Brazil (reported by correspondents). *Capsicum chacoense* and *C. eximium* are collected and bottled and marketed throughout southern Bolivia (pers. observ.). Fresh *C. cardenasii* is harvested and transported to the La Paz, Bolivia market for sale (pers. observ.). In Mexico and the southwestern United States wild *C. annuum* var. *aviculare*, the chiltepin, has been locally used for many years (Nabhan et al. 1989). More recently, a commercial market has developed for chiltepin. A large amount of this wild species is now harvested and sold to the gourmet food market. Nabhan et al. (1989) indicate that "currently chiltepin is almost completely wild harvested." They note that "as much as 12 tons of chiltepines may be harvested from a single Sonoran municipio in a good year, but total harvest may vary from perhaps 8 to as high as 50 tons."

While the quantity of *C. eximium*, ulupica, being harvested in southern Bolivia is unknown, there is an extensive commercial trade in bottled whole peppers. Bolivians have not attempted to commercially plant wild plants of *C. eximium*, but Nabhan et al. (1989) indicate that incipient cultivation of *C. annuum* var. *aviculare* was initiated with extensive planting of the chiltepin by Sonoran farmers in the 1980s. The manipulation of these two wild species in each setting has led to some significant changes for the wild species. In both the case of *C. annuum* var. *aviculare* and *C. eximium*, larger fruit size has been selected for in the incipient area of cultivation and manipulation. Sonoran farmers are selecting for larger fruit size in the wild chiltepin. In *C. eximium*, there is a statistically significant larger fruit form of this ulupica in the zone of exploitation when compared to regions where the fruit is not widely collected (Eshbaugh 1979, 1982). In both cases we are witnessing incipient or semi-domestication of the wild species.

Apparently, a market exists for the exploitation of peppers for the medicinal properties of capsaicin and several companies are pursuing such investigations. Two of the more interesting products to come to market in the last five years are the prescription drug Zostrix (Genderm registered trade mark), an analgesic cream, containing 0.025% capsaicin that is used topically to treat shingles and to provide enhanced pain relief for arthritis patients and Axsain (GalenPharma registered trade mark) that contains 0.075% capsaicin and is used for relief of neuralgias, diabetic neuropathy, and postsurgical pain. Both products are believed to work by action on a pain transmitting compound called substance P.

Several pepper species, because of their unique fruit shapes and bright fruit colors, have been widely used as ornamentals. The presence of capsaicin, however is a potential hazard.

GERMPLASM

In August, 1980, an expert consultative group, under the auspices of the IBPGR (International Board for Plant Genetic Resources), met at CATIE (Centro Agronomico Tropical de Investigacion y Ensenanza) in Turrialba, Costa Rica, to discuss the status of *Capsicum* germplasm collections and to map a strategy for future collecting and management of these resources (Genetic Resources of Capsicum 1983). The discussions led to a plan to systematically collect *Capsicum* throughout New World paying particular attention to the wild species most closely related to the domesticated taxa. The efforts of the past decade have resulted in a significant accumulation of pepper germplasm (seeds) that is now stored in various collections. Eshbaugh (1980a, 1981, 1988) has detailed the history of *Capsicum* germplasm collecting prior to 1980 and discussed the collecting efforts of peppers in Bolivia. Capsicum germplasm collections are now maintained in a number of facilities in the United States, as well as Mexico, Costa Rica, Bolivia, and Brazil.

REFERENCES

Andrews, J. In Press. Good and hot. Macmillan, New York.

Ballard, R.E., J.W. McClure, W.H. Eshbaugh, and K.G. Wilson. 1970. A chemosystematic study of selected taxa of *Capsicum*. Amer. J. Bot. 57:225–233.

Emboden, W.A., Jr. 1961. A preliminary study of the crossing relationships of *Capsicum baccatum*. Butler Univ. Bot. Studies 14:1–5.

Eshbaugh, W.H. 1968. A nomenclatural note on the genus *Capsicum*. Taxon 17:51–52.

Eshbaugh, W.H. 1970. A biosystematic and evolutionary study of *Capsicum baccatum* (Solanaceae). Brittonia 22:31–43.

Eshbaugh, W.H. 1975. Genetic and biochemical systematic studies of chili peppers (*Capsicum*—Solanaceae). Bul. Torrey Bot. Club 102:396–403.

Eshbaugh, W.H. 1977. The taxonomy of the genus *Capsicum*—Solanaceae, p. 13–26. In: E. Pochard (ed.). Capsicum 77. Comptes Rendus 3me Congres EUCARPIA Piment, Avignon–Montfavet, France.

Eshbaugh, W.H. 1979. Biosystematic and evolutionary study of the *Capsicum pubescens* complex, p. 143–162. In: National Geographic Society research reports, 1970 Projects. National Geographic Society, Washington, DC.

Eshbaugh, W.H. 1980a. Chili peppers in Bolivia. Plant Genet. Resources Nwsl. 43:17–19.

Eshbaugh, W.H. 1980b. The taxonomy of the genus *Capsicum* (Solanaceae)—1980. Phytologia 47:153–166.

Eshbaugh, W.H. 1981. Search for chili peppers in Bolivia. Explorers J. 58:126–129.

Eshbaugh, W.H. 1982. Variation and evolution in *Capsicum eximium* Hunz. Baileya 21:193–198.

Eshbaugh, W.H. 1983. The genus *Capsicum* in Africa. Bothalia 14:845–848.

Eshbaugh, W.H. 1988. *Capsicum* germplasm collecting trip—Bolivia 1987. Capsicum Nwsl. 7:24–26.

Eshbaugh, W.H., S.I. Guttman, and M.J. McLeod. 1983. The origin and evolution of domesticated *Capsicum* species. J. Ethnobiol. 3:49–54.

Genetic Resources of Capsicum. 1983. International Board for Plant Genetic Resources (IBPGR). Rome, Italy.

Gounaris, I., C.B. Michalowski, H.J. Bohnert, and C.A. Price. 1986. Restriction and gene maps of plastid DNA from *Capsicum annuum*. Curr. Genet. 11:7–16.

Hunziker, A.T. 1956. Synopsis of the genus *Capsicum*. Huit. Congr. Int. de Bot., Paris 1954, Compt. Rend. des Seanc. et Communic. desposes lors du Congres dans Sec. 3,4,5, et 6. Sec. 4:73–74.

Hunziker, A.T. 1979. South American Solanaceae: a synoptic survey, p. 49–85. In; J.G. Hawkes, R.N. Lester, and A.D. Skelding (eds.). The biology and taxonomy of the Solanaceae. Academic Press, London.

Jensen, R.J., M.J. McLeod, W.H. Eshbaugh, and S.I. Guttman. 1979. Numerical taxonomic analyses of allozymic variation in *Capsicum* (Solanaceae). Taxon 28:315–327.

Loaiza-Figueroa, F., K. Ritland, J.A. Laborde Cancino, and S.D. Tanksley. 1989. Patterns of genetic variation of the genus *Capsicum* (Solanaceae) in Mexico. Plant Syst. Evol. 165:159–188.

McLeod, M.J., W.H. Eshbaugh, and S.I. Guttman. 1979. A preliminary biochemical systematic study of the genus *Capsicum*—Solanaceae, p. 701–714. In: J.G. Hawkes, R.N. Lester, and A.D. Skelding (eds.). The biology and taxonomy of the Solanaceae. Academic Press, London.

McLeod, M.J., S.I. Guttman, and W.H. Eshbaugh. 1982. Early evolution of chili peppers (*Capsicum*). Econ. Bot. 36:361–368.

McLeod, M.J., S.I. Guttman, W.H. Eshbaugh, and R.E. Rayle. 1983. An electrophoretic study of the evolution in *Capsicum* (Solanaceae). Evolution 37:562–574.

Mitchell, C.D., W.H. Eshbaugh, K.G. Wilson, and B.K. Pittman. 1989. Patterns of chloroplast DNA variation in *Capsicum* (Solanaceae): A preliminary study. Int. Organization of Plant Biosystematics Nwsl. 12:3–11.

Nabhan, G.P., M. Slater, and L. Yarger. 1989. New crops for small farmers in marginal lands? Wild chiles as a case study, p. 19–26. In: M.A. Altieri and S.B. Hecht (eds.). Agroecology and small farm development. CRC Press, Boston.

Pickersgill, B. 1971. Relationships between weedy and cultivated forms in some species of chili peppers (genus *Capsicum*). Evolution 25:683–691.

Pickersgill, B. 1980. Some aspects of interspecific hybridization. In: *Capsicum*. Unpublished and preliminary report at the IVth Eucarpia Capsicum working group meetings in Wageningen, The Netherlands.

Pickersgill, B. 1984. Migrations of chili peppers, *Capsicum* spp., in the Americas, p. 105–123. In: D. Stone (ed.). Pre-Columbian plant migration. Papers of the Peabody Museum of Archeology and Ethnology. vol. 76. Harvard Univ. Press, Cambridge, MA.

Pickersgill, B. 1988. The genus *Capsicum*: a multidisciplinary approach to the taxonomy of cultivated and wild plants. Biol. Zent. 107:381–389.

Pickersgill, B. 1989. Cytological and genetical evidence on the domestication and diffusion of crops within the Americas, p. 426–439. In: D.R. Harris and G.C. Hillman (eds.). Foraging and farming: The evolution of plant exploitation. Unwin Hyman, London.

Pickersgill, B., C.B. Heiser, Jr., and J. McNeill. 1979. Numerical taxonomic studies on variation and domestication in some species of *Capsicum*, p. 679–700. In: J.G. Hawkes, R.N. Lester, and A.D. Skelding (eds.). The biology and taxonomy of the Solanaceae. Academic Press, London.

Ruiz, Don Hipoito and Don Joseph Pavon. 1794. Florae peruvianae, et chilensis prodromus. Madrid (en la imprenta de sancha).

Smith, P.G. and C.B. Heiser, Jr. 1957. Breeding behavior of cultivated peppers. Proc. Amer. Soc. Hort. Sci. 70:286–290.

Stuessy, T. 1990. Plant taxonomy. Columbia Univ. Press, New York.

Exploration and Introduction of Ornamental and Landscape Plants from Eastern Asia

Stephen A. Spongberg

FIRST INTRODUCTIONS

While there is no doubt that a limited number of woody plants were carried from eastern Asia into Europe before the 18th century—some credited to Marco Polo—only scant, often anecdotal records document these early peregrinations of plants from East to West. Ironically, one of the first woody ornamentals to be introduced from eastern Asia into Europe in the 18th century was a plant now considered to be extinct in nature and a "living fossil" to boot! By the middle of the 1730s, *Ginkgo biloba* L., the maidenhair tree or ginkgo, was established and growing in the botanical garden at Utrecht, the species having been brought back to the Netherlands on board a Dutch East India Company ship that had called at their Japanese outpost on the island of Deshima in Nagasaki harbor. While other plants were ultimately to follow from Japan in ginkgo's wake, a handful of species were to arrive in Europe from China before the Japanese flora and the many plants of horticultural importance included in that flora were to become known in the West.

While Chinese merchants were able to limit their business with western traders at Canton and at the Portuguese-held port of Macau, by the middle of the 18th century Jesuit missionaries had been able to penetrate the Chinese Empire to a limited degree. As a consequence, a mission had been established in the imperial city of Peking. It was there that one French Jesuit Father, Pierre Nicholas le Chéron d'Incarville, began collecting the seeds of a number of the more notable trees and shrubs cultivated in the environs of that great city. Sometime before 1747, d'Incarville entrusted a few of his collections to a member of a Russian caravan that visited the Chinese metropolis every three years. As a consequence, the seeds of two Chinese species—*Koelreuteria paniculata* Laxmann, the golden rain-tree, and *Sophora japonica* L., the pagoda tree or scholar's tree—found their way to Europe and eventually to the Jardin des Plantes in Paris. The seeds of these two species germinated in French soil and were soon being cultivated on a limited basis in other European botanical gardens. By 1753, for example, the pagoda tree was growing in England, and in 1811 it was being grown in a glasshouse at the Elgin Botanical Garden in Manhattan, New York City.

On occasion, d'Incarville was able to make additional shipments of seeds to European correspondents, and Philip Miller received seeds of *Ailanthus altissima* (Miller) Swingle, the tree of heaven, at the Chelsea Physic Garden in London in 1751. Eventually, plants raised from this seedlot were shared with plantsmen throughout Europe and with William Hamilton, who later introduced the species into North America when he planted the tree of heaven on the grounds of "The Woodlands," his Philadelphia estate. Little did Hamilton or other enthusiastic plantsmen of 18th century America realize that by the end of the twentieth century the tree of heaven would have invaded native American woodlands and have become synonymous with the city environments and the urban sprawl of present-day America.

ROBERT FORTUNE AND THE EDWARDIAN CASE

While the first introductions of trees and shrubs from China and Japan arrived in European ports during the 18th century, it is not known how many seedlots failed to germinate after prolonged sea voyages or being carried on the long overland routes that connected Europe with eastern Asia. Coupled with the fact that both China and Japan were essentially closed to the western world, would-be plantsmen and horticultural explorers were greatly restricted and so had little access to Asian germplasm. It was not until the Opium War of 1840 had been waged and won by the British and the Treaty of Nanjing signed in 1842 that China was forced to relax her grip on trade with western nations, and foreigners were allowed to travel more freely within the confines of eastern China.

Shortly after the Treaty of Nanjing had been signed and the so-called treaty ports had been opened along China's eastern seaboard, the Horticultural Society of London decided that the time was ripe to send a plant collector to the Celestial Empire with the express purpose of introducing horticultural novelties into cultivation in England. The Horticultural Society selected Robert Fortune as their agent, a Scotsman with little previous training, and Fortune sailed for China aboard the *Emu* early in 1843.

All told, Robert Fortune (Fig. 1) was to visit China and other eastern Asian countries on four occasions between 1843 and 1859, first for the Horticultural Society and on subsequent trips as a representative of the English East India Company and the government of the United States. And, on all of his trips, Fortune was extremely successful in introducing plants that would become extremely popular in cultivation in the West and would begin the transformation of European and American garden landscapes to those which we know today.

Included among the plants with which Fortune's name is associated are many of the now widely-grown cultivars of the tree peony or moutan (*Paeonia suffruticosa* Andrews) and an even larger number of cultivars of the camellia (*Camellia reticulata* Lindley and *C. japonica* L.), cultivars which had been selected and grown by generations of Chinese horticulturists. The golden larch [*Pseudolarix amabilis* (Nelson) Rehder] ranks as one of the unique, deciduous conifers introduced by Fortune, as does the equally ornamental lacebark pine (*Pinus bungeanus* Endlicher), mature specimens of which develop an exfoliating bark that is mottled white and gray. Fortune was also the first to send the cryptomeria [*Cryptomeria japonica* (L. f.) D. Don] directly to both Europe and North America in 1844. Likewise, Fortune sent plants of the Chinese fringe tree (*Chionanthis retusus* Lindley), an outstanding ornamental shrub or sometimes a small tree, which is closely related to the American fringetree (*Chionanthus virginicus* L.) of the southeastern United States. A third species (*Chionanthus pygmaeus* Small) of this small genus in the olive family has yet to enter the horticultural marketplace on a large scale, but is endemic to Florida.

Still other woody plants introduced by Fortune include such horticultural favorites as the double-file viburnum (*Viburnum plicatum* Thunberg), the old-fashioned weigela of Victorian gardens [*Weigela florida* (Bunge) A. DC.], the greenstem forsythia (*Forsythia viridissima* Lindley) one of the first species of this exclusively Asian genus to reach the West, and the winter honeysuckle (*Lonicera fragrantissima* Lindley & Paxton). Also included in the list of Fortune introductions are the common pearlbush [*Exochorda racemosa* (Lindley) Rehder] an extremely floriferous shrub in the Rosaceae which has been recently neglected in cultivation but which is deserving of far greater popularity, the Chinese abelia (*Abelia chinensis* R. Brown), and fortune rhododendron (*Rhododendron fortunei* Lindley), the first of the evergreen type, as opposed to species of the azalea group, to be sent from China. Last, but certainly not least in this abbreviated catalogue of Fortune's woody plant introductions, mention must be made of the white-flowered Chinese wisteria [*Wisteria sinensis* (Sims) Sweet 'Alba']. Lastly, it should be remembered that the old-fashioned bleeding heart [*Dicentra spectabilis* (L.) Lemaire] and balloon flower [*Platycodon grandiflorus* (Jacquin) A. DC.] number among his herbaceous introductions.

During his travels in eastern Asia, Fortune set the standards for future plant hunters who were to follow in his footsteps. Because travel was highly restricted, he was unable to penetrate very far westward into the vast Chinese Empire to any great extent but was limited to travel on the highly populated eastern seaboard. As a consequence, Fortune was able to sample the garden flora of China, and it is to this subset of the overall Chinese flora that the majority of his introductions relate. His success in sending living plants to Europe and North America, moreover, was greatly increased by his use of the Wardian case, which had been invented by a London physician, Nathaniel Ward, shortly before Fortune's departure for China in 1843.

PHILIPP VON SIEBOLD AND GEORGE ROGERS HALL IN JAPAN

While Robert Fortune was busily searching for and collecting Chinese plants for shipment to England in Wardian cases, a German Physician in the employ of the Dutch East India Company was actively soliciting living plants and plant specimens from an adoring circle of Japanese friends at the Dutch outpost on the man-made island of Deshima in Nagasaki harbor. Philipp Franz Balthasar von Siebold's opportunities for travel in Japan were even more limited that those of Fortune in China. None-the-less, and largely due to his skill in performing successful cataract operations on sight-impaired Japanese, von Siebold was able to establish a network of Japanese friends who were willing to repay the adept physician by responding to his requests for specimens, living individuals, and seeds of Japanese plants. The living plants were sometimes established in the small botanical garden on Deshima, but other plants and their seeds were more often than not smuggled onboard Dutch ships for transport to Europe. Thus, the first large consignments of Japanese plants followed in the wake of the ginkgo and were destined to be added to the garden floras of Europe, and eventually, North America.

It was not until the Treaty of Kamagawa had been signed in 1854—as the result of an early example of gunboat diplomacy by Commodore Matthew Perry—that Japan, like China, was forced to open her long-closed doors to foreigners. But unlike their continental neighbors, the Japanese adapted far more quickly to the presence of foreigners, even adopting many western customs and technological advances. As a consequence, travel bans were less rigidly enforced, and the country became open to general foreign travel at an earlier date than in China.

While Phillipp von Siebold turned these circumstances to his advantage, he was joined in Japan in 1859 by an American physician, George Rogers Hall (Fig. 2), who had left the hospital he had helped to establish in Shanghai a decade earlier to join the lucrative trade that had already been established between Japan and the United States. A native of Bristol, Rhode Island, Hall had maintained contacts with friends in New England, and in 1861, Hall entrusted several Wardian cases filled with Japanese plants to F. Gordon Dexter, who was returning to Boston. Once in Boston after the long sea voyage from Yokohama, Dexter delivered the plants into the care of Francis Parkman, widely noted for his historical studies but also one of Boston's leading horticulturists.

Many of the plants introduced by Hall in his first shipment of Japanese plants as well as in subsequent shipments sent to the Parsons nursery company of Flushing, Long Island, were obtained from von Siebold, while

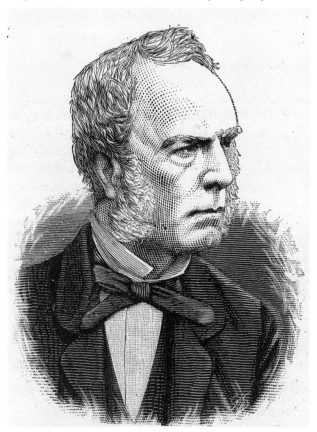

Fig. 1. Robert Fortune (1812–1880) represented the Horticultural Society of London (now the Royal Horticultural Society) as a collector in China shortly after the Treaty of Nanjing had brought the Opium War to a close. Through his use of the Wardian case, Fortune was able to introduce many of the best-known Chinese garden plants into cultivation in Europe and North America. (Photographic Archives of the Arnold Arboretum.)

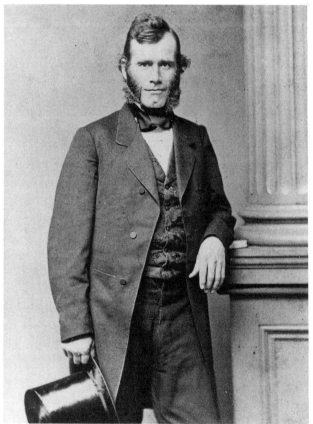

Fig. 2. George Rogers Hall (1826–1899) of Bristol, Rhode Island, the physician turned trader who first sent living plants in Wardian cases from Japan directly to New England. (Photographic Archives of the Arnold Arboretum.)

others had been collected by, or for, Hall himself. This was the first time that shipments of Asian plants came directly to New England, and a large proportion of the species included were or had been introduced simultaneously into Europe by von Siebold.

Included among the plants sent by von Siebold to Europe and Hall to North America were many Japanese species that have become commonplace ornamentals in western parks and gardens. An abbreviated listing would begin with the Japanese yew (*Taxus cuspidata* Siebold & Zuccarini), a conifer that has been utilized extensively as a landscape plant since its introduction into North America by George Rogers Hall. Other conifers introduced by Hall include the so-called umbrella pine [*Sciadopitys verticillata* (Thunberg) Siebold & Zuccarini], ten garden forms of the sawara cypress [*Chamaecyparis pisifera* (Siebold & Zuccarini Endlicher], and the beautiful hinoki cypress [*Chamaecyparis obtusa* (Siebold & Zuccarini) Endlicher], slow-growing forms of which are frequently trained as bonsai. The kobus magnolia (*Magnolia kobus* DC.), and the well-known star magnolia [*Magnolia stellata* (Siebold & Zuccarini) Maxim.] and Japanese crab apples (*Malus floribunda* Van Houtte and *M. halliana* Koehne f. *parkmanii* Rehder) now enliven North American landscapes in spring as does the Japanese wisteria [*Wisteria floribunda* (Willd.) DC.], while Japanese maples (*Acer palmatum* Thunberg and *A. japonicum* Thunberg) add color and interest to our gardens and parklands in summer and fall. The Japanese zelkova [*Zelkova serrata* (Thunberg) Makino], another Hall introduction that concludes this brief listing, is now widely cultivated as a replacement for native American elms ravaged by Dutch elm disease.

OPENING OF THE CELESTIAL EMPIRE

In 1860, while von Siebold and Hall were sampling the Japanese flora for horticultural novelties, the Chinese were forced to lessen the restrictions on foreign travel in the Celestial Empire. Under the terms of a new treaty, western missionaries were free to travel and establish missions anywhere they chose in the Chinese kingdom. Two years later, in 1862, a French Lazarist priest by the name of Armand David (Fig. 3) was to arrive at his order's mission in Peking and was subsequently to undertake three great journeys of exploration to inaccessible regions of China. The second of these trips, which occupied the years between 1868 and 1870, proved to be extraordinarily important botanically and ultimately led to the horticultural investigation of the western Chinese flora. On this second trip, David prepared dried botanical specimens of upwards of 1,500 species of plants that were new to science, and included among his haul was the astonishingly beautiful and botanically unique dove tree (*Davidia involucrata* Baillon). All in all, the specimens Abbé David forwarded to the natural history museum in Paris attested to a far richer flora in western China than anyone could have predicted.

Similar shipments of dried botanical specimens were to arrive at the herbarium at the Royal Botanical Gardens, Kew, beginning in 1885. In this instance, the plants had been gathered by Augustine Henry, a medical officer in the Imperial Chinese Maritime Customs Service based in Ichang on the Yangtze River in Hubei Province, a post one thousand miles inland from the east coast port of Nanking. Like David's specimens received in Paris, Henry's collections indicated a floristic richness that no one could have predicted. Upwards of five hundred new species, twenty-five new genera, and an entirely new family of plants were based on Henry's dried specimens. And included in his haul were specimens of the dove tree, the same species Abbé David had collected earlier from a location roughly one thousand miles to the west. So beautiful were the specimens of the *Davidia* that Daniel Oliver, a botanist at Kew, wrote "*Davidia* is a tree almost deserving a special mission to Western China with a view to its introduction to European gardens" (Oliver, 1891).

Reading these words prompted Sir James Veitch (Fig. 4), head of the Chelsea branch of the Veitch family's nursery empire in England, to travel to Kew to see the specimens for himself. He too, was beguiled by the beauty of the specimens and asked Kew's director, Sir William Turner Thiselton-Dyer, to recommend an individual to send to China with the specific purpose of introducing the dove tree into cultivation. Thiselton-Dyer recommended twenty-five year old Ernest Henry Wilson (Fig. 5), a recent graduate of the diploma course at Kew to undertake the task. Wilson was hired by the Veitch firm, and in 1899 he left England for China on what would be the first of two plant hunting expeditions for the Veitch nursery. Wilson's first expedition between the years 1899 and 1902 ended in complete success—seeds of the dove tree were collected in quantity—and the second trip between the years 1903 and 1905 was equally successful. On both trips, Wilson introduced an incredible number of horticulturally significant plants, many of which had been known in the West only as they were represented by the dried herbarium collections of David and Henry.

News of the collecting activities of David, Henry, and Wilson had not escaped the notice of Charles Sprague Sargent (Fig. 6), the first director of Harvard University's Arnold Arboretum. Sargent was keenly interested in the Asian flora, and he had personally inaugurated the Arboretum's botanical and horticultural exploration of Asia when he traveled to Japan in 1892. As a consequence of his four month sojourn, Sargent was able to author the *Forest Flora of Japan*, the first thorough scientific study of the woody plants of the island nation. Moreover, he was able to introduce a significant number of Japanese plants into American gardens. Notable Sargent introductions that have remained popular to the present day include the Sargent crab apple (*Malus sargentii* Rehder), Sargent cherry (*Prunus sargentii* Rehder), the long-stalk holly (*Ilex pedunculosa* Miquel) and the commonplace hill azalea (*Rhododendron kaempferi* Planchon), which was quickly christened the torch azalea once it was in cultivation in the West. Other introductions resulting from Sargent's 1892 trip include the Nikko maple (*Acer maximowiczianum* Miquel), one of the trifoliolate species, and one of the precocious flowering magnolias, the anise-leaved or willow-leaved magnolia [*Magnolia salicifolia* (Siebold & Zuccarini) Maximowicz].

While Sargent's Japanese exploits served to whet his appetite for additional Asian plants to be tested in the Arnold Arboretum, by 1900 he realized that due to his age—he turned 59 in 1900—he would be unable to undertake strenuous field work in China. As a consequence, Sargent turned his attention to locating another man who might serve as the Arboretum's agent in China, and the unparalleled success of Ernest Henry Wilson's trips for the Veitch nursery firm between 1899 and 1905 were uppermost in Sargent's mind.

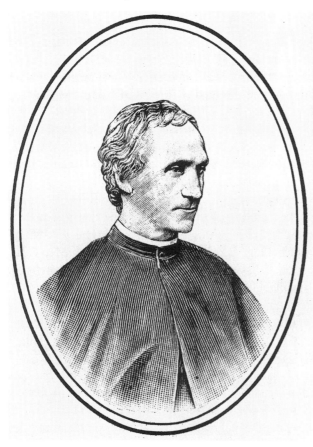

Fig. 3. The Abbé Armand David (1826–1900), the first naturalist to collect the dove tree (*Davidia involucrata*), which was named to honor his many contributions in making the natural history of China better known scientifically. (Photographic Archives of the Arnold Arboretum.)

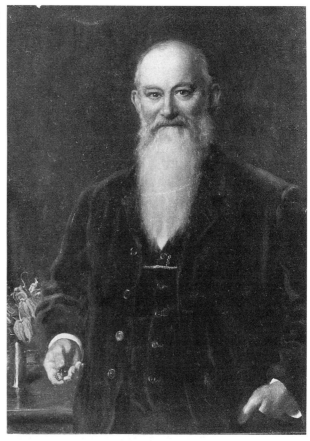

Fig. 4. Sir James Veitch (1840–1924), head of the famous Veitch nurseries of Chelsa and Coombe Wood, who first employed E.H. Wilson to go to China to introduce the dove tree into cultivation in western gardens. (Photographic Archives of the Arnold Arboretum.)

After hard-fought negotiations, Sargent was finally able to enlist the services of Wilson on behalf of the Arnold Arboretum. In late December of 1906, Wilson once again departed for China, returning to Boston in 1908. A fourth trip was begun in 1909 when Wilson undertook his second expedition under Arboretum auspices. This journey, unfortunately, ended in catastrophe when Wilson's leg was broken in two places when he was caught in a landslide in the valley of the Min River in northwestern Sichuan Province. Despite this crippling mishap, Wilson returned to the Arnold Arboretum, where he was given a permanent appointment, and he spent the better part of the second decade of the twentieth century collecting for the Arboretum in Japan, Korea, and Taiwan. Wilson's success as a plant hunter and in introducing new Asian species into western horticulture are well-known, Alfred Rehder, well-known taxonomist at the Arnold Arboretum, credited Wilson with having introduced over 1,000 species previously unknown to cultivation.

While space does not allow a complete listing of Wilson's introductions, mention will be made here of several of his more notable plants collected in eastern Asia. This list begins with the extremely popular beauty bush (*Kolkwitzia amabilis* Graebner), a shrub of easy propagation and one which became commonplace across North America in Wilson's lifetime. The paperbark maple [*Acer griseum* (Franchet) Pax], Schmidt's birch (*Betula schmidtii* Regel), and the Korean stewartia (*Stewartia koreana* Rehder), are three outstanding Wilson introductions that have year-round landscape appeal due to their interesting ornamental bark. Both the paperbark maple and the Korean stewartia produce exfoliating bark, that of the maple cinnamon colored, while that of the stewartia is mottled and gives a piebald appearance to the sinuous trunks of the small trees. The bark of the Schmidt birch, by contrast, is similar to that of our native shagbark hickory.

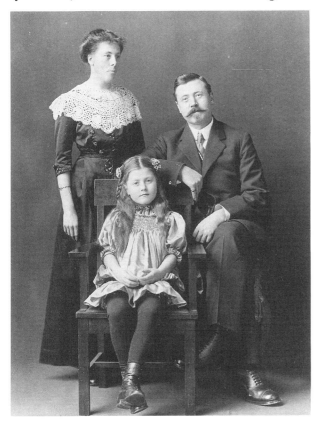

Fig. 5. Earnest Henry "Chinese" Wilson with his wife Helen (neé Ganderton) and their daughter Muriel Primrose in a photograph taken in Japan. Wilson undertook four major expeditions to China between 1899 and 1911 and spent much of the second decade of the present century exploring for plants in Japan, Korea, and Taiwan. (Photographic Archives of the Arnold Arboretum.)

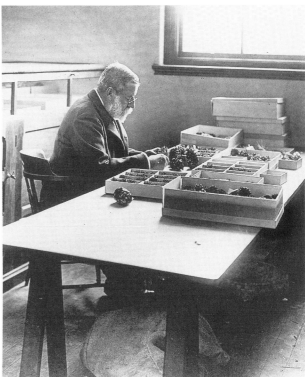

Fig. 6. Charles Sprague Sargent (1841–1927), first director of the Arnold Arboretum of Harvard University. Sargent inaugurated the Arboretum's interest in eastern Asia in 1892 when he personally visited Japan and introduced many new Japanese plants into American gardens. (Photographic Archives of the Arnold Arboretum.)

Other ornamental trees introduced by Wilson include several outstanding magnolias of the Yulana section, the most noteworthy being *Magnolia sprengeri* Pampanini in its cultivar 'Diva', while Sargent's magnolia (*Magnolia sargentiana* Rehder & Wilson), and Dawson's magnolia (*Magnolia dawsoniana* Rehder & Wilson) are also extremely beautiful ornamental species. Flowering crabs also number among Wilson's introductions, and the so-called tea crab [*Malus hupehensis* (Pampanini) Rehder] is one of the most notable, while the Chinese sand pear [*Pyrus pyrifolia* (Burman f.) Nakai] also ranks high as a spring-flowering ornamental. The evergreen *Viburnum rytidophyllum* Hemsley has been widely planted, and the Korean forsythia (*Forsythia ovata* Nakai), perhaps the hardiest of all species of forsythia, has played an important role in hybridization programs that have developed a series of hardier cultivars that have expanded the ornamental range of these early spring flowering ornamentals into regions with colder winter climates. Wilson was also the first to introduce the kiwi fruit or Chinese gooseberry (*Actinidia chinensis* Planchon), into cultivation in the West, and it was his material that ultimately led to the establishment of the kiwifruit industry in New Zealand. Certainly, any listing of Wilson introductions must include the regal lily (*Lilium regale* Wilson), and this brief catalogue will end with the hardy silk tree [*Albizia julibrissin* (Willd.) Durazz. 'Ernest Wilson'], which extended the ornamental use of this interesting summer-flowering tree into the northeastern United States. This was one of the very last plants Wilson introduced into cultivation during his long and productive career as a plant hunter in eastern Asia. Seeds from which this hardy strain of the silk tree were grown were collected in the garden of the Chosen Hotel in Seoul, Korea, in 1918, shortly before Wilson was to return to Boston at the conclusion of his final Asian excursion.

Few plants were introduced into North America from the temperate regions of eastern Asia between 1918 —when E.H. Wilson returned from the Orient for the last time—and the end of the Sino-Japanese and Second World Wars. Political upheaval and wartime conditions combined to make this period one in which horticultural and botanical pursuits in that geographical area were temporarily set aside. Yet, just as the bamboo curtain was falling around communist China, news of the discovery of a strange new, deciduous conifer came to the attention of Elmer D. Merrill, then director of the Arnold Arboretum. Collaborating with Chinese colleagues, Merrill was able to send a small sum of money that enabled the Chinese to mount an expedition to collect the seeds of the new tree, and the plant was successfully introduced into cultivation in the West early in 1948, before the species had even been named and described by Chinese botanists. Ironically, this tree, the last to be introduced before China became off-limits to American collectors, was, like the ginkgo, a living fossil that was on the edge of extinction in its native habitat. The dawn redwood (*Metasequoia glyptostroboides* Hu & Cheng) received great notoriety in the press shortly after its introduction, and the tree is widely cultivated across North America and Eurasia today.

RECENT RENEWED EXPLORATIONS

A new era in plant introduction from eastern Asia began in 1980 as a consequence of ping-pong diplomacy. In the late 1970s, American and Chinese botanists reestablished relationships through reciprocal exchanges of delegations to the People's Republic of China and the United States. In 1979, it was decided that future collaboration should include the participation of American botanists on field trips in China, while Chinese botanists would be invited to join American colleagues in field work in the United States, and invitations were forthcoming from the Academia Sinica for American participation in the first Sino-American Botanical Expedition in 1980. As a consequence of that inaugural undertaking, five American botanists were able to travel to western Hubei Province where collections of both botanical specimens and germplasm were made for a three month period. Several new ornamental species were introduced into American gardens as a result, and notable among these were the so-called seven-son-flower (*Heptacodium miconioides* Rehder), an interesting fall-flowering shrub in the honeysuckle family, the Zen magnolia (*Magnolia zennii* W.C. Cheng), a precocious flowering species from eastern China that had previously eluded collectors, and Yu's mountain ash (*Sorbus yuana* Spongberg), a simple-leaved species not previously known and described as new by an expedition participant.

Given the floristic richness of eastern Asia—the flora of China alone is estimated to consist of 30,000 species of vascular plants compared to an estimate of 10,000 species for all of North America north of Mexico—the future remains bright for further introductions of landscape trees and shrubs of great potential value in western landscapes. And the decade since 1980 has seen renewed participation by the American and European botanical and horticultural communities in collaboration with their Asian colleagues in realizing this potential. Previously little-known plants and totally new ones as well are destined to enter the horticultural marketplace as the twenty-first century approaches.

REFERENCES
Bretschneider, E. 1898. History of European botanical discoveries in China. Sampson Low Marston & Company, Ltd., London.
Oliver, D. 1891. *Davidia involucratta* Baill. Hooker's Icones Plantarum 20. translation 1961.
Spongberg, S.A. 1990. A reunion of trees: The discovery of exotic plants and their introduction into North American and European landscapes. Harvard University Press, Cambridge & London.

Plant Exploration for New Forage Grasses*

K.H. Asay

The first and probably most important phase of any plant breeding program is to assemble the genetic resources from which breeding populations can be developed. The most elaborate facilities and selection procedures will not compensate for an inadequate germplasm base. Plant exploration has been particularly instrumental in providing the genetic diversity for breeding programs involving forage and turf grasses. Most important temperate grasses in North America were introduced from other continents. Plant breeders and other scientists working to improve these species must, therefore, rely heavily on germplasm collected from their native habitats or centers of diversity. Although the principal objective of most plant exploration expeditions is to provide germplasm resources for existing breeding programs, insight must also be used to identify new species or those that have not been evaluated on this continent.

INTRODUCED FORAGE GRASSES

Introduction of forage grasses in North America began in earnest with the arrival of the first colonists. Seed of many species were carried to the new world in the ballasts of ships or in livestock feed. Introductions also were made intentionally by settlers and by plant explorers such as N.E. Hansen and F.N. Meyer (Asay 1991). Germplasm from these early introductions remains an important component of the National Plant Germplasm System (NPGS) and is included in the parentage of several modern cultivars. The number of accessions included in the NPGS sheds some light on the relative impact of plant exploration on important grass genera. For example in 1989, 1,928 accessions of *Panicum* and 1,612 accessions of *Festuca* were included (GRIN 1989).

Several instances could be cited to illustrate the impact of plant exploration for forage grasses on American agriculture. Tall fescue (*Festuca arundinacea* Schreb.) in North America began with the release of two cultivars, 'Ky-31' and 'Alta'. Although the exact origin of 'Ky-31' is somewhat obscure, the parentage of both cultivars trace to European introductions. Parental germplasm for 'Ky-31' was obtained from a naturalized ecotype found growing on a hillside on the W.M. Suiter farm in Menifee County, Kentucky. This ecotype had apparently been established on this site since 1887. Under the direction of E.N. Fergus, seed was collected and after extensive evaluation, the cultivar was released by the Kentucky Agriculture Experiment Station in 1931 (Buckner et al. 1979; Hanson 1972). The tall fescue cultivar 'Alta', which was developed in cooperation with the USDA/ARS and the Oregon Agricultural Experiment Station, traces to three introductions from Germany (PI 19728, 24838, and 25206). Subsequent evaluation and selection led to the release of the cultivar in 1940 (Hanson 1972).

---

*Cooperative investigations of the USDA/ARS and the Utah Agricultural Experiment Station, Logan. Paper no. 4260.

Since the release of these cultivars, the germplasm base of tall fescue has been expanded through plant exploration and hybridization (Asay et al. 1979) and it has become the predominant grass in the United States. It is estimated that the species occupies from 12 to 14 million ha in pure and mixed stands (Buckner 1985) and 44 cultivars have been registered by the Crop Science Society of America (CSSA) [Germplasm Resources Information Network (GRIN) 1991]. The turf potential of tall fescue is now being exploited by plant breeders. Selections have been made from products of plant exploration that are lower growing and have finer leaves and more dense tillers than typical tall fescue. Although the currently available tall fescue cultivars are somewhat coarser than Kentucky bluegrass, they have demonstrated more resistance to insects and diseases than typical Kentucky bluegrass cultivars.

The identification of an endophyte (*Acremonium coenophialum* Morgan-Jones & Gams) in tall fescue presents some interesting alternatives in plant exploration and breeding. From a negative perspective, the presence of the endophyte is associated with serious toxicity problems in livestock consuming the forage. On the other hand, alkaloids produced by the endophyte contribute to the vegetative vigor and resistance of the plant to pests and environmental stress (Bacon and Siegel 1988; Read and Camp 1986). Future plant exploration may contribute to research leading to the identification of an endophyte that will positively influence plant growth and persistence without the deleterious side effects.

Orchardgrass (*Dactylis glomerata* L.) was introduced over 200 years ago from central and western Europe, but its value was not fully recognized in the United States until about 1940. This productive and nutritious grass was first cultivated in Virginia and is now one of our most widely accepted forage grasses. According to GRIN (1991), 12 cultivars have been registered by CSSA. In his review of the parentage of 29 orchardgrass cultivars, Hanson (1972) found that 12 were developed from introduced accessions or PIs and five were introduced as cultivars developed in foreign countries. The remaining cultivars were derived from selections from existing cultivars, old pastures, and naturalized strains (Hanson 1972).

Smooth bromegrass (*Bromus inermis* Leyss.) was apparently first introduced into North America from Hungary in the late 1800s and was known early as Hungarian bromegrass. In 1898, N.E. Hansen obtained seed from the Penza Region of the USSR, which led to the predominance of the northern strains in the United States and Canada. Following the devastating drought of the 1930s, smooth bromegrass became a popular grass in the Midwest. Since then, naturalized southern strains and cultivars developed in breeding programs have become an important component of American seed trade (Carlson and Newell 1985). The cultivar 'Lincoln', which was derived from selections made from a productive stand in Nebraska, was the early standard (Barker and Kalton 1989) and according to GRIN, 17 additional cultivars have since been registered with CSSA.

Because it is so well adapted and widely distributed in the temperate regions of North America, Kentucky bluegrass (*Poa pratensis* L.) is often considered to be a native species. It is now known that this multipurpose grass is indigenous to Europe where it is called smooth meadow grass. It has been suggested that Kentucky bluegrass was introduced into North America through Labrador or Alaska; however, this has not been documented. The species was probably first introduced along the Atlantic Coast by the early immigrants and transported inland during the westward migration or indirectly by grazing animals. Plant exploration coupled with public and private breeding programs have led to development of several cultivars beginning with the release of 'Merion' in the early 1930s. Forty-five cultivars have been registered by CSSA (GRIN 1991) and the species is now found as a component of pastures in over 16 million ha and in some 40 million lawns throughout the United States and Canada (Duell 1985).

Like Kentucky bluegrass, Timothy (*Phleum pratense* L.) probably crossed the Atlantic with the early settlers in hay litter or ballast from ships. The colonists were convinced that the grass was native to North America because it was so well adapted; however, it was later shown to be introduced from Europe. It was originally called Herd grass after John Herd who is thought to have found it along the Piscataqua River near Portsmouth, New Hampshire about 1911 (Childers and Hanson 1985). The ultimate name sake for Timothy was Timothy Hanson, who promoted its use in Maryland, North Carolina, and Virginia. The name was first recorded in a letter from Benjamin Franklin to Jared Eliot in 1747 stating that the Herd grass he had received was "mere Timothy." The grass was so well accepted that in the early 1800s, it was considered to be the most important hay grass in America (Hoover et al. 1948; Childers and Hanson 1985). The genetic base of Timothy has since increased through plant exploration and in 1989, 573 accessions were included in the NPGS (GRIN 1989).

Crested wheatgrass (*Agropyron cristatum*, L., Gaertner and *Agropyron desertorum*, Fisch. ex Link, Schultes) has had a major impact on American grasslands. Since its introduction from USSR, this versatile grass has become the most widely used grass for revegetating depleted rangelands in western North America. During the "dust bowl" era of the middle 1930s, it was particularly instrumental in stabilizing abandoned wheatlands in the Northern Great Plains (Lorenz 1983).

Crested wheatgrass was first introduced into North America in 1898 by N.E. Hansen of the South Dakota Agricultural Experiment Station following an exploration trip to Russia and Siberia (Dillman 1946). He observed the grass in evaluation trials at the Valuiki Experiment Station on the Volga River near what is now Volgograd. Seed of five accessions were obtained and assigned PI numbers 835, 837, 838, 1010, and 1012. Seed from these accessions was distributed to Agricultural Experiment Stations in Alabama, Indiana, Michigan, Colorado, and Washington, and apparently to an experiment station in Highmore, South Dakota. No record is available regarding further increase or distribution of these introductions (Dillman 1946; Lorenz 1983).

In 1906, N.E. Hansen made a second importation of crested wheatgrass. This seed, which was obtained from the same source as the original introductions, consisted of five lots labeled *Agropyron desertorum* (Fisch.) Schult. These lots were assigned PI numbers 19537–19541. An additional lot, labeled *Agropyron cristatum* (L.) Gaertn. was assigned PI number 19536. Seed from one or more of these introductions was distributed to 15 experiment stations from 1907 to 1913. The greatest enthusiasm for crested wheatgrass was most evident in the northern Great Plains, particularly South and North Dakota. Nurseries established at the Belle Fourche Experiment Station, Newell, South Dakota, the Northern Great Plains Field Station, Mandan, North Dakota, and the Dickinson Substation, Dickinson, North Dakota were particularly noteworthy in the early evaluation and distribution of crested wheatgrass in North America. The planting of PI 19538 at Mandan, North Dakota has been maintained and is still productive.

Other introductions have since contributed to the crested wheatgrass gene pool in North America. In 1910, N.E. Hansen first introduced Siberian wheatgrass (*Agropyron fragile*, Roth, Candargy), which is native to the dry steppes of western European Russian and western Siberia. Several other explorations have since been made to USSR, China, Turkey, Iran, and other Asian countries (Lorenz 1983). More recently, D.R. Dewey and co-workers at the USDA/ARS Forage and Range Research Laboratory, Logan, Utah, have been actively involved in exploration for crested wheatgrass germplasm. Since 1972, 12 expeditions have been conducted by members of this research group to Europe and Asia to collect germplasm of crested wheatgrass and other species of interest.

The first documented introduction of crested wheatgrass into Canada occurred in 1911. Seed of PI 19536 (*A. cristatum*) and 19540 (*A. desertorum*) was received by John Bracken of the University of Saskatchewan at Saskatoon (Lorenz 1983; Rogler 1960). Nurseries were established from this seed in 1916 by L.E. Kirk, then a graduate student at the University. The cultivar 'Fairway', which has since become an important component of the Canadian grass seed trade, was derived from selected plants of PI 19536 in these nurseries. The release of 'Fairway' was delayed until 1927 by a fire that destroyed the building where the original "breeder" seed was stored. Fortunately, the parental clones were still in the field and new seed was produced the following season (Lorenz 1983). 'Fairway' was the first cultivar of crested wheatgrass to be released in North America (Elliott and Bolton 1970).

Cytological studies have determined that crested wheatgrass is essentially an autoploid series of diploid ($2n = 2x = 14$), tetraploid ($2n = 4x = 28$), and hexaploid ($2n = 6x = 42$) forms (Dewey 1966). The diploids are represented by the cultivar 'Fairway' and cultivars subsequently released, 'Parkway' and 'Ruff' (Hanson 1972; Asay and Knowles 1985). Prominent tetraploid cultivars include 'Nordan', 'Hycrest', 'Ephraim', and 'P-27'. 'Nordan' was developed by the USDA/ARS Northern Great Plains Research Center at Mandan, North Dakota from plants in an old seeding at Dickinson, North Dakota. It has been the dominant cultivar in the United States. 'Hycrest' was released in 1984 by the USDA/ARS in cooperation with the Utah Agricultural Experiment Station and the USDA/SCS. It was derived through hybridization between induced tetraploid *A. cristatum* and natural tetraploid *A. desertorum* (Asay et al. 1985b). This cultivar has demonstrated superior establishment characteristics on harsh range sites and is rapidly becoming a major component in seeding mixtures, particularly in the Intermountain Region (Asay et al. 1986).

Plant materials recently obtained through plant exploration have contributed to breeding efforts in crested wheatgrass. Species of the complex are normally caespitose (bunch type); however, accessions recently received from Turkey, Iran, and China develop extensive rhizomes. These plants also are shorter in stature and have finer leaves and greater tiller density than typical crested wheatgrass. Progeny lines selected from these populations have been entered in a breeding program to intensify these characteristics. The research objective is to develop cultivars that are adapted for lawns, along roadsides, soil stabilization, and similar applications in water-limited environments and other areas where water conservation is a major concern (Asay 1991).

Crested wheatgrass has been criticized for the rapid decline in the quality of its forage as plants approach maturity during the summer. Soon after anthesis, leaves normally wilt and die back leaving a preponderance of stems until later in the season when new tillers are developed. Promising hexaploid accessions, recently obtained from Kazakhstan in the USSR, may provide the genetic resources to alleviate this concern. One particular accession, designated in the NPGS as PI 406442, has exceptionally broad leaves. In addition, leaves of this accession remain on the plant and retain their green color longer in the growing season than typical crested wheatgrass. This hexaploid accession also has larger seeds and seedling vigor advantages that are often associated with this trait. Hexaploid breeding populations have been established from selections within the Soviet accession and hybridization with other hexaploids obtained from Iran.

A breeding program also has been initiated to combine the leafiness and seedling vigor attributes of the Soviet hexaploid accession with the positive attributes of tetraploid 'Hycrest'. Hybrids between the two ploidy levels were readily obtained and the pentaploid progenies were relatively fertile. Moreover, the broadleaf character was easily detected in hybrid plants. Pentaploid hybrids, selected largely on the basis of leaf width and length were crossed among themselves and successively backcrossed to Hycrest clones. Relatively fertile and genetically stable tetraploid and hexaploid forms have been identified in these breeding populations, indicating that it is feasible to combine the genetic resources from the three ploidy levels in crested wheatgrass at either the tetraploid or hexaploid level. It is also evident that interploidy breeding schemes are valuable tools for more effectively utilizing genetic resources obtained through plant exploration to improve the forage quality, seedling vigor, and other characteristics of this valuable range grass.

Russian wildrye [*Psathyrostachys juncea* (Fisch.) Nevski] is a cool-season perennial grass that is native to the steppe and desert regions of USSR and China. The species was introduced into the United States in 1927, but its value in reseeding depleted rangelands was not fully recognized until about 25 years later (Hanson 1972). Although it is particularly noted for its productivity of palatable and nutritious forage during the spring and early summer, its nutritive value is retained better during the late summer than many other cool-season grasses. Russian wildrye has been widely used in rangeland seeding programs; however, its acceptance has been somewhat impeded by problems associated with seedling establishment, particularly on harsh range sites. Accordingly, improved seedling vigor is a major objective of breeding programs with this species (Asay and Johnson 1980; Berdahl and Barker 1984; Lawrence 1979).

Plant exploration and associated breeding programs have led to the release of several Russian wildrye cultivars. The cultivar 'Vinall' set the early standard in the United States. It was developed by the USDA/ARS at Mandan, North Dakota from collections made in the USSR (PIs 75737, 108496, and 111549) and released in 1960 (Hanson 1972). In 1978, 'Swift' was released by Agriculture Canada at Swift Current, Saskatchewan. Improved establishment vigor was emphasized during its development. More recent releases include 'Bozoisky-Select' by the USDA/ARS at Logan, Utah (Asay et al. 1985a) and 'Mankota' by the USDA/ARS at Mandan, North Dakota (Berdahl and Barker 1991b). 'Bozoisky-Select' was derived from PI 440627, an introduction from the USSR. It is significantly more robust and productive than 'Vinall' in the seedling as well as the more advanced growth stages. It is rapidly establishing itself as the dominant Russian wildrye cultivar in the Intermountain West. The parental germplasm for Mankota was obtained from PIs 314675 and 272136 and an experimental breeding population. Its performance has been superior to other Russian wildrye cultivars adapted to the northern Great Plains.

Russian wildrye is normally a diploid; however, promising tetraploid accessions were obtained from Soviet scientists during a recent plant exploration in the republic of Kazakhstan. Tetraploid forms are typically characterized by larger seeds, better seedling vigor, and a more robust growth habit than their diploid counterparts (Berdahl and Barker 1991a; Lawrence et al. 1990). Breeding populations have been developed from these accessions through selection and hybridization with induced tetraploids from promising diploid cultivars.

NATIVE FORAGE GRASSES

Exploration for grasses native to North America has provided valuable germplasm to the NPGS. There is justifiable concern that in some instances, we may be in danger of losing valuable native germplasm to activities associated with population growth as well as industrial and agricultural development. Grass breeders, primarily in the public sector, have exploited genetic diversity in native populations and several improved cultivars have been released. A crusade exists, particularly in the Intermountain West, to use only native species in rangeland seeding mixtures. Although the controversy centers on public lands, other areas are affected as well. Multiple demands including those imposed by livestock, wildlife, and recreation, have significantly altered the environmental forces in the plant community. These environmental changes have a profound influence on the optimum vegetative climax associated with a particular range site. It is therefore, not always in the interest of good land management to restore the vegetative ecosystem to its native state or to what we presume it to have been a few hundred years ago. New combinations of native and introduced plant species will be essential if we are to enjoy the maximum benefits of our natural resources. It is regrettable that decisions of this nature are often made in the political arena, with little consideration of the complex biological interactions involved.

Introduced germplasm has had and will continue to have a major impact on American agriculture. Grasses indigenous to Asia, Europe, and Africa have for the most part been subjected to more intense grazing pressure than our native species. It is not surprising that natural selection under such conditions would generate germplasm that is better adapted to this type of management even when transported to another continent. This is not to imply that native species do not have a role to play in rangeland improvement. They most assuredly do, but we must utilize other sources as well. Adaptability to the environment or intended use should be a more valid criterion for evaluating plant materials than their nationality.

INTERSPECIFIC HYBRIDIZATION

Many of our native temperate grasses are closely related to European and Asian species. These introduced relatives can be valuable genetic donors to their native counterparts. Genetic introgression from introduced germplasm has been used to improve bluebunch wheatgrass [*Pseudoroegneria spicata* (Pursh) Löve]. Bluebunch wheatgrass is a cool-season native rangegrass. This caespitose species is drought resistant and produces nutritious forage; however, it is selectively grazed in mixtures with other species and stands are often depleted under heavy grazing (Hafenrichter et al. 1968; Mueggler 1975). Quackgrass [*Elytrigia repens* (L.) Nevski] has proven to be a valuable genetic donor in crosses with bluebunch wheatgrass in the USDA/ARS research program at Logan, Utah. The positive contribution of quackgrass in any breeding program may be surprising, as this aggressive species is often considered to be a noxious and troublesome weed. However, it has many desirable attributes and is considered to be a valuable forage in many temperate regions of the world. It is a productive, long-lived perennial grass, with moderate salinity tolerance, and because of its extensive rhizome development, it has excellent soil-binding characteristics.

The F_1 hybrid between hexaploid ($2n = 42$) quackgrass and the tetraploid form ($2n = 28$) of bluebunch wheatgrass was disappointing (Dewey 1967). It was a pentaploid ($2n = 35$), meiotically irregular, and largely sterile. The hybrid also was plagued with deleterious traits and in general had poor vegetative vigor. Selected plants from the hybrid population were included in a breeding program in 1974 with the objective of combining the caespitose growth habit, drought resistance, and forage quality of bluebunch wheatgrass with the persistence, durability, productivity, and salinity tolerance of quackgrass. Eight generations after the initial cross, a population (designated as RS hybrid) with relatively good fertility and a stable chromosome number of $2n = 42$

was obtained. Characteristics of both parental species were evident in the population, which was released as the cultivar 'NewHy' in 1989 (Asay et al. 1991). Other introduced relatives such as *Pseudoroegneria stipifolia* (Czern. ex Nevski) may be valuable sources of genetic diversity for improving bluebunch wheatgrass.

A promising accession of quackgrass (*Elytrigia repens*) was recently collected in Turkey. Most plants in this collection produced extensive rhizomes; however, genetic segregation for the caespitose growth was also evident. A recurrent selection program was initiated with this population and after four cycles, a caespitose form of quackgrass was obtained. This breeding population is productive and leafy, and has excellent salinity tolerance. The original parental germplasm may trace to a hybrid between quackgrass and an Asian form of bluebunch wheatgrass. As a result of plant exploration, a much better alternative is now available for revegetation of saline sites on semiarid rangelands.

Hybridization between introduced and native *Leymus* (wildrye) species is also a promising breeding approach. *Leymus* germplasm recently collected in the Soviet Union has been hybridized with a native relative, Great Basin wildrye [*Leymus cinereus* (Scrib. & Merr.) Löve]. The hybrid population is extremely robust and appears to be a promising source of germplasm for extending the grazing season during the late fall and winter on temperate rangeland.

WARM-SEASON FORAGE GRASSES

Although this review is concerned primarily with temperate grasses, it is evident that plant exploration has contributed to the improvement of warm-season grasses as well. Warm-season grasses can be divided into two groups, western and southern, based on their adaptation to soil and climatic factors. Pasture improvement in the southern states has relied heavily on introduced species, whereas in the West, several native warm-season species have merited substantial breeding effort (Burton 1989).

Domestic exploration and subsequent breeding has led to significant genetic advance in switchgrass (*Panicum virgatum* L.). The cultivar 'Pathfinder' was developed from collections made in the Midwest and released in 1967 by the USDA/ARS and the Nebraska Agricultural Experiment Station. Subsequent research led to the development of an improved cultivar 'Trailblazer'. This cultivar represents a significant advance in terms of animal performance (Vogel et al. 1991). The genetic base of switchgrass and other native western warm-season grasses continues to expand as a result of plant exploration. These include big bluestem (*Andropogon gerardii* Vitman var *gerardii*), sand bluestem (*A. gerardii* var paucipilus (Nash) Fern), and indiangrass [*Sorghastrum nutans* (L.) Nash] (K.P. Vogel pers. commun.).

Germplasm introduced from foreign countries has contributed in a significant way to the improvement of grasses adapted to the southern states. The most prevalent warm-season grass in the South is common bermudagrass [*Cynodon dactylon* (L.) Pers.]. Bermudagrass is native to Africa and was probably introduced to America in livestock feed by the Spaniards. Similar to quackgrass, this aggressive grass has been a troublesome weed, but it has provided germplasm for several improved forage and turf cultivars. The most notable of these is the cultivar 'Coastal' (Burton 1989). This cultivar was developed by the USDA/ARS at Tifton, Georgia from a hybrid between 'Tift' common bermudagrass and two introductions from South Africa (Burton 1947). Coastal has been vegetatively propagated on 5 million ha in the South and has served as a germplasm resource in the development of other cultivars including 'Midland', 'Tifton 44', 'Coastcross-1', and 'Tifton 78'. More recent introductions are being used in crosses to improve the winter hardiness and extend the range of bermudagrass further north (Burton 1989).

Other warm-season grasses that have reached American shores through plant introduction include bahiagrass (*Paspalum notatum* Flugge), which was first introduced from South America in 1913 by the Florida Agricultural Experiment Station (Watson and Burson 1985). Germplasm obtained from Africa has contributed to improved forage quality and disease resistance in pearl millet [*Pennisetum glaucum* (L.)] (Burton 1989). Buffelgrass (*Cenchrus ciliaris* L.) has significantly improved the productivity of 1 million ha of American grasslands. This apomictic species was introduced to south Texas from southern Africa in 1946 (Voigt and MacLauchlan 1985). Common dallisgrass (*Paspalum dilatatum* Poir), a native of South America, has become an important grass in the United States, although its popularity has declined somewhat in recent years (Watson and Burson 1985). Weeping lovegrass [*Eragrostis curvula* (Schrad.) Nees] was introduced from Africa in 1927 and introductions have contributed to its continued improvement since then (Voigt and MacLauchlan 1985; Voigt 1971; Hanson 1972). Tragic circumstances are associated with the introduction of centipedegrass [*Eromochloa ophiuroides* (Munro) Hack.]. Original seed of this species was found in the baggage of the prominent plant explorer, F.N. Meyer, who had been collecting in the Hunan Province in China. He apparently fell overboard from a steamer in the Yangtze River.

CONCLUSIONS

It is evident that plant exploration has and will continue to have a significant influence on the quality and productivity of American grasslands. Early introductions were often made by accident such as inclusion in the ballasts of ships or imported livestock feed. Limited exploration provided some genetic diversity, but most pasture and rangeland seedings were made with unimproved accessions that were often poorly suited for the particular environment or intended use. In some instances, adapted strains were generated through natural selection; however, the most meaningful genetic improvement was achieved through purposeful plant exploration and subsequent breeding. With more areas in the world opened to exploration and the scientific community more amenable to germplasm exchange, the outlook for continued improvement has never been better.

REFERENCES

Asay, K.H. 1991a. Breeding temperate rangeland grasses. Plant Breed. Abstr. 61:643–648.

Asay, K.H. 1991b. Contributions of introduced germplasm in the development of grass cultivars, p. 115–125. In: H.L. Shands and L.E. Wiesner (eds.). Contributions of introduced germplasm to cultivar development. CSSA Spec. Pub. 17. ASA, CSSA, and SSSA, Madison, WI.

Asay, K.H., D.R. Dewey, W.H. Horton, K.B. Jensen, P.O. Currie, N.J. Chatterton, W.T. Hansen II, and J.R. Carlson. 1991. Registration of 'NewHy' RS hybrid wheatgrass. Crop Sci. 31:1384–1385.

Asay, K.H., R.V. Frakes, and R.C. Buckner. 1979. Chapter 7, Breeding and cultivars. In: R.C. Buckner and L.P. Bush (eds.). Tall fescue. Agronomy 20:111–139. Amer. Soc. of Agron., Madison, WI.

Asay, K.H., D.R. Dewey, F.B. Gomm, D.A. Johnson, and J.R. Carlson. 1985a. Registration of 'Bozoisky-Select' Russian wildrye. Crop Sci. 25:575–576.

Asay, K.H., D.R. Dewey, F.B. Gomm, D.A. Johnson, and J.R. Carlson. 1985b. Registration of 'Hycrest' crested wheatgrass. Crop Sci. 25:368–369.

Asay, K.H., D.R. Dewey, F.B. Gomm, W.H. Horton, and K.B. Jensen. 1986. Genetic progress through hybridization of induced and natural tetraploids in crested wheatgrass. J. Range Manag. 39:261–263.

Asay, K.H. and D.A. Johnson. 1980. Screening for improved stand establishment in Russian wildrye grass. Can. J. Plant Sci. 60:1171–1177.

Asay, K.H. and R.P. Knowles. 1985. Wheatgrasses, p. 166–176. In: R.F. Barnes, D.S. Metcalfe, and M.E. Heath (eds.). Forages: the science of grassland agriculture. Iowa State Univ. Press, Ames.

Bacon, C.W. and M.R. Siegel. 1988. Endophyte parasitism of tall fescue. J. Prod. Agr. 1:45–55.

Barker, R.E. and R.R. Kalton. 1989. Cool-season forage grass breeding: progress, potentials, and benefits. In: D.A. Sleper, K.H. Asay, and J.F. Pedersen (eds.). Contributions from breeding forage and turf grasses. Spec. Pub. 15. Crop Sci. Soc. Amer. Madison, WI.

Berdahl, J.D. and R.E. Barker. 1984. Selection for improved seedling vigor in Russian wild ryegrass. Can. J. Plant Sci. 64:131–138.

Berdahl, J.D. and R.E. Barker. 1991a. Characterization of autotetraploid Russian wildrye produced with nitrous oxide. Crop Sci. 31:1153–1155.

Berdahl, J.D. and R.E. Barker. 1991b. Mankota Russian wildrye. Release Notice. USDA/ARS, USDA/SCS, and North Dakota Agr. Expt. Sta. Mandan.

Buckner, R.C. 1985. The fescues, p. 233–240. In: R.F. Barnes, D.S. Metcalfe, and M.E. Heath (eds.). Forages: the science of grassland agriculture. Iowa State Univ. Press, Ames.

Buckner, R.C., J.B. Powell, and R.V. Frakes. 1979. Historical development. In: R.C. Buckner and L.P. Bush (eds.). Tall fescue. Agronomy 20:111–139. Amer. Soc. Agron., Madison, WI.

Burton, G.W. 1947. Breeding bermudagrass for the southeastern United States. J. Amer. Soc. Agron. 39:551–569.

Burton, G.W. 1989. Progress and benefits to humanity from breeding warm-season forage grasses, p. 21–29. In: D.A. Sleper, K.H. Asay, and J.F. Pedersen (eds.). Contributions from breeding forage and turf grasses. Spec. Pub. 15. Crop Sci. Soci. Amer., Madison, WI.

Carlson, I.T., and L.C. Newell. 1985. Smooth bromegrass, p. 198–206. In: R.F. Barnes, D.S. Metcalfe, and M.E. Heath (eds.). Forages: the science of grassland agriculture. Iowa State Univ. Press, Ames.

Childers, W.R. and A.A. Hanson. 1985. Timothy, p. 217–223. In: R.F. Barnes, D.S. Metcalfe, and M.E. Heath (eds.). Forages: the science of grassland agriculture. Iowa State Univ. Press, Ames.

Dewey, D.R. 1966. Inbreeding depression in diploid, tetraploid, and hexaploid crested wheatgrass. Crop Sci. 6:144–147.

Dewey, D.R. 1967. Synthetic hybrids of new world and old world Agropyrons III. *Agropyron repens* xtetraploid *Agropyron spicatum*. Amer. J. Bot. 54:93–98.

Dillman, A.C. 1946. The beginnings of crested wheatgrass in North America. J. Amer. Soc. Agron. 38:237–250.

Duell, R.W. 1985. The bluegrasses, p. 188–197. In: R.F. Barnes, D.S. Metcalfe, and M.E. Heath (eds.). Forages: the science of grassland agriculture. Iowa State Univ. Press, Ames.

Elliott, C.R. and J.L. Bolton. 1970. Licensed varieties of cultivated grasses and legumes. Canada Dept. Agr. Pub. 1405.

Germplasm Resources Information (GRIN). 1991. USDA/ARS. Germplasm Services Laboratory. Database Management Unit. Beltsville MD.

Hafenrichter, A.L., J.L. Schwendiman, H.L. Harris, R.S. Mclauchlan, and H.W. Miller. 1968. Grasses and legumes for soil conservation in the Pacific Northwest and Great Basin. USDA Agr. Handb. 339.

Hanson, A.A. 1972. Grass varieties in the United States. USDA Agr. Handb. 170. U.S. Government Printing Office, Washington, DC.

Hoover, M.M., M.A. Hein, W.A. Dayton, and C.O. Erlanson. 1948. The main grasses for farm and home, p. 639–700. In: A. Stefferud (ed.). Grass: the yearbook of agriculture. U.S. Government Printing Office. Washington, DC.

Lawrence, T. 1979. Swift, Russian wild ryegrass. Can. J. Plant Sci. 59:515–518.

Lawrence, T., A.E. Slinkard, C.D. Ratzlaff, N.W. Holt, P.G. Jefferson. 1990. Tetracan, Russian wild ryegrass. Can. J. Plant Sci. 70:311–313.

Lorenz, R.J. 1983. Introduction and early use of crested wheatgrass in the Northern Great Plains, p. 9–20. In: K.L. Johnson (ed.). Crested wheatgrass: its values, problems and myths. Utah State Univ., Logan.

Mueggler, W.F. 1975. Rate and patterns of vigor recovery in Idaho fescue and bluebunch wheatgrass. J. Range Manag. 28:198–204.

Read, J.C. and B.J. Camp. 1986. The effect of the fungal endophyte in tall fescue on animal performance, toxicity and stand maintenace. Agron. J. 78:848–850.

Rogler, G.A. 1960. Crested wheatgrass—History, adaptation and importance. Western Grass Breeder's work Planning Conference. Conf. Proc. Univ. Sask., Saskatoon.

Vogel, K.P., F.A. Haskins, H.J. Gorz, B.A. Anderson, and J.K. Ward. 1991. Registration of 'Trailblazer' switchgrass. Crop Sci. 31:1388.

Voigt, P.W. 1971. Registration of Morpa weeping lovegrass (Reg. No. 20). Crop Sci. 11:312.

Voigt, P.W. and R.S. MacLauchlan. 1985. Native and other western grasses, p. 177–187. In: R.F. Barnes, D.S. Metcalfe, and M.E. Heath (eds.). Forages: the science of grassland agriculture. Iowa State Univ. Press, Ames.

Watson, V.H. and B.L. Burson. 1985. Bahiagrass, carpetgrass, and dallisgrass, p. 255–262. In: R.F. Barnes, D.S. Metcalfe, and M.E. Heath (eds.). Forages: the science of grassland agriculture. Iowa State Univ. Press, Ames.

Exploration and Exploitation of New Fruit and Nut Germplasm

Maxine M. Thompson

There is a critical need for exploration, introduction and exploitation of new and more diverse fruit and nut germplasm because of the extremely narrow genetic base that exists in our major crop species. Some United States fruit and nut industries are based primarily on one or two major cultivars, e.g. 'Montmorency sour cherry', 'Bing' and 'Royal Ann' sweet cherry, 'Tilton' and 'Blenheim' apricot, 'Bartlett' pear, 'Barcelona' hazelnut, 'Kerman' pistachio, and 'Hayward' kiwifruit. In other crops, such as blueberry, strawberry and peach, where breeding efforts have produced a greater number of commercial cultivars, levels of inbreeding, which have been documented recently, were found to be unacceptably high (Hancock and Siefker 1982; Sjulin 1987; and Scorza et al. 1985). Many breeding programs have reached the point where infusion of new and more diverse germplasm is essential for achieving modern objectives for new cultivars with more efficient fruit production and environmentally safer orchard operations and which will satisfy future consumer demands.

FACTORS LIMITING RAPID PROGRESS IN FRUIT BREEDING

In contrast to the marvelous progress achieved through breeding in major field crops over the past several decades, fruit breeding efforts have resulted in relatively few success stories. First, it is obvious that the length of each generation along with the large space and intensive labor necessary to grow even a limited number of progenies to reproductive age requires a huge investment of both time and money. Evaluation of replicated trial plots of advanced selections further extends by several years the time before a new cultivar can be released to the public. Thus, the minimum time from making the cross-pollination between the ideal parents until the release of a new cultivar is at least 20 years. It is not uncommon for fruit breeders to spend their entire careers making crosses and evaluating seedling populations only to have the next generation breeder release new cultivars resulting from crosses made 20 to 30, or more, years previously. The financial burden of such prolonged selection progress is a major factor in the decline of the number of publicly-funded fruit breeding programs (Brooks and Vest 1985). The paucity of short-term, publishable results may not only delay professional advancement of faculty but is a major obstacle to attracting would-be plant breeding graduate students.

Secondly, the lengthy quarantine process required for many fruit species has discouraged breeders from introducing new germplasm. Clones are usually retained for virus testing at the Quarantine Center at Glenn Dale, Maryland for 6 to 10 years. Many do not survive at the Center due either to propagation failures, cultural problems or, diseases such as fireblight on pears and apples. However, progress in facilitating movement of plants through quarantine is promised now that this facility is being managed jointly by the National Germplasm Resources Laboratory (NGRL) and the Animal and Plant Health Inspection Service of the USDA (APHIS) and more funds and staff are being allocated for this important facet of plant introduction.

A third major limiting factor for breeding progress, one not so obvious to the non-fruit scientist, is the limited sampling of the potential genetic diversity that has been available to American breeders. For historical reasons, much of the fruit and nut germplasm existing in the United States has been derived from introductions from Western Europe which, itself, is relatively poor in native populations of these species. Lack of access to the three major Asian centers of origin and diversity for temperate fruit and nut crop species has presented a formidable obstacle to obtaining and utilizing the great wealth of unexploited fruit germplasm found there. In the Soviet Union, the Caucasus Mountain region is one of the centers of diversity for apple, European pear, quince, sweet cherry, cherry plum, fig, pomegranate, walnut, hazelnut, chestnut, pistachio, and grape. The Central Asian region, including the Republics of Turkmenistan, Uzbekistan, Tadjikistan, and Kazakhstan, is another center for apple, apricot, cherry, plum, fig, pomegranate, almond, pistachio, walnut, and grape. China is well known as the center of diversity for peach, apricot, oriental plum, Asian pear, persimmon, citrus, litchi, Chinese chestnut, and kiwifruit. The multitude of diverse local cultivars, wild forms of cultivated species and many related species in the Soviet Union and China have been "off-limits" for about 70 years for political reasons. The recent opening of these two countries provides the heretofore unavailable opportunity to collect exciting new genetic traits unknown, or rare, in western collections. Exploration for fruit and nut germplasm in these newly opened regions is of primary importance in order to provide the much-needed genetic diversity. In this paper, I shall focus mainly on the potential value of new germplasm acquired through recent plant explorations for a few fruit and nut crops whose breeding progress has been particularly restricted by inadequate germplasm.

Exploration in Central Asia

In 1930, Nicolai Vavilov informed the western world about the wild populations of fruit species in the Soviet Union in a paper presented at the International Horticulture Congress in London entitled "Wild progenitors of the fruit trees of Turkistan and the Caucasus and the problem of the origin of fruit trees" (Vavilov 1930). Since that time, Soviet scientists have studied and written many publications describing the variability and distribution of various wild populations of fruit and nut species. They have established extensive collections of local cultivars and species, but these plant materials remained inaccessible to the West. Fortunately, in recent years, exchange of scientists and germplasm between the Soviet Union and Western countries, including the United States, has been escalating. In fact, a 5-year reciprocal exchange program for plant exploration is currently underway between the Vavilov Institute for Plant Industry (VIR) in St. Petersburg and the U.S. National Plant Germplasm System.

Apple exploration in the Soviet Union. In 1989, Calvin Sperling and Herbert Aldwinkle visited the wild apple forests near Alma Ata in Central Asia and observed an enormous range of diversity in such traits as fruit size, color, shape, and ripening time, from small wild-type to large-fruited types comparable to commercial cultivars. Prof. A.D. Djangaliev of the Kazakh Academy of Sciences has studied these wild apples and has propagated selections from the forests at the Botanical Garden in Alma Ata. There is sufficient regional variation in botanical characteristics that Soviet scientists have classified the apples there into three species: *Malus sierversii* (Ldb.) M. Roem, *M. kirghisorum*, Al. & An. Theod. and *M. niedzwetzkyana* Dieck. Among several hundreds of young seedlings already growing in Geneva, N.Y. from seeds collected in the mountains near Alma Ata, genetic resistance to three major apple diseases, apple scab [*Venturia inaequalis* (Cooke) Wint.], cedar apple rust (*Gymnosporangium juniperi virginianea* Schweim), and fireblight [*Erwinia amylovora* (Burr.) Winslow et al.], has been identified (H. Aldwinkle pers. commun.). These plants may provide distinctly different genetic sources of resistance from those currently available in the United States. Fruit of these seedlings and of the clonal selections introduced will be evaluated when trees reach reproductive age, and when the clonal germplasm is released from quarantine, it will become available for utilization.

Apricot exploration in the Soviet Union. In 1990, I was fortunate to join Calvin Sperling and David Ramming on a second official fruit exploration to Central Asia, this time for apricots. That year, among 633 apricot cultivars in the collection at the VIR Station in Tashkent, Uzbekistan, about 95% had lost their crop due to a late spring frost. Although we were disappointed not to see more fruit variability, this climatic event provided a natural screen for spring frost tolerance. We collected seeds and scions of several cultivars that bore some fruit in spite of adverse spring temperatures. The trait of late bloom, or frost tolerance, provides a genetic solution to the most limiting factor for expanding domestic apricot production beyond the very restricted climatic zone where our cultivars are adapted. At a period when most cultivars, if they had a crop, would have already been harvested, there was 'Zima Stoiki' (= winter hardy) with a heavy crop of very immature fruit, obviously late blooming as well as very late maturing. Late fruit maturity, also seen in the cultivar 'Oktoberski', will contribute to new cultivars with ripening periods extending far beyond the 5-week span in early summer of current American cultivars.

Several Central Asian cultivars, collectively called "luchak," have glabrous skins, a trait previously unobserved in American cultivars or germplasm collections. This glossy appearance, sometimes with a bright red blush, represents an entirely new, and especially attractive fruit type. Should this trait be determined by a single gene, as is the case for glabrous peaches (nectarines) it should be possible to repeat within a fairly short time period the successes achieved in nectarine breeding, i.e., the creation of a whole series of large-fruited, glabrous apricot cultivars with a wide span in ripening periods.

Another trait of interest was high soluble solids, a trait that greatly enhances the quality of both the fresh and dried product. By contrast to American cultivars whose soluble solids register about 12° Brix, Central Asian cultivars range above 20°. Historically, in Central Asia there has been strong selection pressure for very sweet fruit because there was no other source of sugar.

Also, sweet, edible seeds is a common trait which has been selected through the centuries by local people whose goal has been to maximize food production on a limited amount of tillable land. A unique trait that was said to occur in a local cultivar, one which we did not see or collect, is an endocarp (the hard part of the pit) that is so thin that it can be cracked with one's teeth. Incorporation of edible kernels in new duo-purpose domestic cultivars would certainly enhance orchard profits and provide a new nutritional product for American consumers.

In the Zailinsky mountains near Alma Ata, we had the opportunity to visit the wild apricot forests with Tatanya Nicolaievna Sulova, a botanist who has studied variation and made selections from among these trees. Wild apricot forests grow in some of the same general regions as the wild apples but at a somewhat lower elevation. At about 1,060 m, apricot trees merge into the lower limits of the range of apples. These wild populations occur at the northernmost range of this species and are clearly more cold hardy than Central Asian cultivars which can be grown only in milder climates farther south. In one extremely cold winter in Alma Ata, wild trees survived midwinter temperature of –43°C, whereas trees of cultivars perished. Most of the wild fruit have bitter seeds and is small, but size varies considerably as do all other traits such as color, time of ripening, and quality. This year when most trees were severely attacked by *Coryneum* blight [*Stigmina carpophila* (Lev.) M.B. Ellis], some of Tanya's selections were practically free of symptoms, a trait she has observed consistently over several years. This may be a valuable source of genetic disease resistance to incorporate in new domestic cultivars.

Walnut germplasm in the Soviet Union. There are vast forests of wild walnuts in the Tien Shan mountains in the Soviet Union which are located west of the province of Xinziang in China. While on the apricot expedition last year, we received information about the walnut collections and selection programs underway at various institutes in Kirghizia, Tajikistan, and Uzbekistan. Clones having clusters with 10 to 20 nuts, precocious trees, dwarf trees, and paper-shell nuts were mentioned. However, at that time, as we were unable to visit these Institutes, we obtained only some market samples of diverse, unknown origin. Hopefully, an expedition can be arranged soon to explore further this exceptionally rich Central Asian center of diversity for walnuts.

Apricot exploration in Northern Pakistan. In 1987, David Brenner and I studied and collected Central Asian apricots in another geographic region—the Karakoram and Himalayan mountains of Northern Pakistan. Among these extremely high, precipitous mountains, in very small river valleys, lie several former mini-kingdoms, each isolated from the other and from the outside world until very recently. One of these, Hunza, is famous for supposedly having exceptionally long-lived people. Through centuries, as peoples filtered into these mountain valleys from various regions in Central Asia they brought apricots which, for them, was a main staple food, providing fresh fruit throughout the summer, dried fruit and edible kernels for winter, oil from bitter seeds for lamps, and firewood in this relatively treeless land. The practice of planting seeds from the best trees over an extended period of time has resulted in an incredible amount of variation. Many years ago, they learned to graft so now, in each village, in addition to seedling trees, one finds many favorite local cultivars. While some exist in only one village, others are distributed more widely, but primarily within the confines of each former kingdom. In the several villages we visited, we encountered 180 different named cultivars which is only a sample of the variation that exists in the region as a whole. Overall, fruits are characterized by very high soluble solids, sweet seeds, and relatively small size. Fruit size is not important there. Selection has been for quality and total productivity.

In Hunza, one of the larger-fruited cultivars, 'Habiju', has outstanding quality for both fresh and dried usage, with high soluble solids (averaging about 23° Brix), pronounced aroma, and rich flavor. 'Alishah Kakas' was another favorite in Hunza because of its exceptionally high soluble solids (31° Brix), fine quality, and firm texture making it suitable for shipping fresh, as well as excellent for drying.

In Baltistan, 'Margulam' was prized as a fresh fruit for its juiciness, sweetness, and fine flavor, whereas 'Halmon' was the best for drying due to its high soluble solids (30° Brix) and rapid drying characteristic. 'Kachachuli' was unique in that, although the fruit has relatively high soluble solids (22° Brix), the flesh reaches a moderate degree of firmness but does not soften further with age. In fact, the local name actually means "apricot that doesn't ripen." It reminded me of the non-ripening trait in our shipping tomatoes. Locally, 'Kachachuli' is grown mainly for its large edible seed, but I envision this non-ripening trait incorporated, through breeding, into larger, high quality cultivars with remarkable storage and shipping characteristics. A local storage cultivar, 'Sharappa Margulam', was said to hold its quality until March if stored underground (the only method of temperature control available). The introduction of a longer storage life into new cultivars could greatly extend the apricot marketing period, as could a series of cultivars ripening successively. As in the Soviet Union, we found cultivars ripening over a 3-month period, from late June until late September. A useful trait for a home-garden fruit tree was found in 'Rangbuon' whose fruit ripens over a 5-week period on the same tree. Although a record of bloom time was not available, we were told that some were two weeks later than others and it is most likely that the late maturing cultivars do bloom considerable later.

In Haripur, the lowest elevation site (540 m), low chilling requirement may be found in the popular cultivars 'Nukap', 'Lala', 'Boi', and 'Safeda'.

Walnut exploration in Northern Pakistan. Diversification of walnut germplasm was increased by random sampling collections that we made in the mountains of Northern Pakistan and adjacent regions in Kashmir, India. In this region, there are walnut trees, all seedlings, in every village from about 1,000 to 3,000 m elevation, some of which are very ancient. In this region, both wild (with inedible nuts) and cultivated forms of *Juglans regia* L. are distinguished. While we did not study walnuts in depth there, we did observe an enormous amount of variation in nut size, shape, and shell thickness. From one tree, we collected nuts which had very thin, porous, incomplete shells and, in two different cases, we heard about a tree with nuts having no shell at all, merely a membranous covering around the shell. Loy Shreve has found resistance to walnut blight and leaf fungal diseases in a clone introduced earlier from Pakistan. The original tree was notable for heavy, regular bearing, freedom from diseases, and for having a large nut with good quality. Grown in southern Texas, it has proven to exhibit these desirable traits as well as the ability to retain an attractive light kernel color in the hot climate there. Several small plantations of this selection, termed 'Abbotabad' (from the city where it was found) are already growing in Texas and appear to show good potential (Loy Shreve pers. commun.).

Plant Exploration in China

Walnut germplasm in China. Three walnut exploration trips to China provide another example of recent success in securing much-needed, greatly expanded germplasm diversity. Abundant wild walnut forests are distributed throughout the Tien Shan mountain range, which lies mostly in the Central Asian Republics of the Soviet Union, but which extends into northwest Xinziang Province in The People's Republic of China. Walnuts are widely cultivated in several provinces, and there are several research programs directed towards improving cultural methods and selection of new cultivars (Ji 1980).

In 1986, Loy Shreve was the first horticulturist to visit Chinese walnut research stations from which he succeeded in obtaining about 20 selections, mostly from Xinziang, which are now under test in the warm climate of Texas. Two years later, in 1988, Bill Gustafson, Todd Morrissey, and C. Bish went to both Xinziang in Northwestern China and to Jilin and Inner Mongolia in the Northeast with the major goal of locating cold-hardy nut germplasm suitable for Nebraska. They were able to collect 78 seedlots of horticultural/forestry plant materials including walnuts, almonds, hazelnuts, pistachio, and several other genera. Additional scions and seeds were subsequently sent by the Chinese. Representative plants of these accessions are now under test in Nebraska and elsewhere.

In 1990, Gale McGranahan, Charles Leslie, and William Barnett visited Xinziang and the vicinity of Beijing with the objective of collecting more diverse germplasm for the California breeding program. Although several new walnut cultivars have been released from the California program over the past several years, all of these have been derived from a single parent, 'Payne'. Until now, this was the *only* clone available which has, and transmits to its progeny, the unique trait of bearing nuts on both lateral and terminal positions. This characteristic results in precocious bearing and much heavier yields than other walnuts whose nuts are borne only terminally. As walnut is one of the orchard crops most delayed in coming into full production, one of the most valuable finds in Xinziang was the extreme precocity of many selections. In the vicinity of Aksu, virtually all of the walnuts had the lateral bearing habit and many seedlings are so precocious that they set nuts in, or before, the third growing season, or during the first year after grafting. Another useful reproductive trait in some clones is the occurrence of two or more waves of flowering, which could be a valuable aid in avoiding spring frost damage. The trait of multiple-nut clusters, commonly 8 to 12 nuts on spikes, as compared to domestic cultivars with 2 to 3 per cluster, offers the potential for greatly increased yields. Among these clones bearing several flowers on spikes, some spikes bear only pistillate flowers, some only staminate flowers, and some bear both. Of even greater significance, in some clones, spikes had some perfect flowers. Strong selection pressure for perfect flowers has the potential of eliminating the need for planting two cultivars for cross-pollination in orchards, currently a necessary practice for this normally dichogamous species. Of particular importance, is that many of the Chinese selections are resistant to important diseases, e.g., walnut blight, anthracnose, and various leaf fungal diseases. Extreme early maturity, with nuts harvested in mid-August, was also observed. Scions of several selections with outstanding traits as well as large numbers of seeds representing a wide array of diversity have been introduced from both Xinziang and from the Qiong Long Shan Experiment Station near Beijing and have been propagated in Davis, California for future evaluation and exploitation.

Plant Exploration in Eastern Europe

Sour cherry exploration. The weaknesses of 'Montmorency', the 400-year-old French cultivar that comprises 99% of the United States sour cherry industry, and the extremely limited germplasm available in the United States made it imperative to acquire new germplasm in order to make any breeding progress. This moderate-sized tree species, *Prunus cerasus* L., which occurs wild and has been cultivated for a very long time in Eastern European countries, originated long ago from chance hybridization between the large-statured, cold-sensitive sweet cherry, *Prunus avium* L., whose native range includes Southeast Europe-Southwest Asia, and the shrubby, cold-hardy species, *Prunus fruticosa* Pall., whose distribution ranges farther north into the Soviet Union. The known sour cherry diversity found in regions surrounding the Caspian, Black, and Adriatic Seas suggests that this is the center of origin of this species. Since 1984, Amy Iezzoni has made five trips to seven Eastern European countries to study this variability and to collect germplasm (Iezzoni 1984). She found there a huge spectrum of variation ranging from plants that resemble the sweet cherry progenitor to those that are more similar to the other progenitor and all possible combinations of both. A wide variation was found in bloom time, fruit maturity, cold hardiness, important fruit qualities such as color, soluble solids, firmness, flavor, size, plant growth habit (from small dwarf trees to tall trees comparable to sweet cherry), and, of great significance, resistance to one of the most important diseases attacking our orchards, cherry leaf spot (*Coccomyces hiemalis* Higgins). She collected among the countless local cultivars that have been selected through centuries of cultivation, as well as acquired modern cultivars and selections from various Experiment Station breeding programs.

Iezzoni's methods of approach have greatly hastened the exploitation of this new germplasm and serve as a fine example for what can be done to circumvent the lengthy quarantine period as well as the long generation time of fruit tree crops. In addition to introducing clonal material to the Quarantine system, she has made the best possible use of seeds and pollen and currently has over 10 ha of seedling trees representing new germplasm from elite sources. Not only has she collected and planted open-pollinated seeds from select cultivars in Eastern Europe; she has introduced pollen from abroad and used it for crosses with her local selections. In addition, because of the on-going working relationships she established, her European collaborators have made crosses for her between their selected clones and sent the hybrid seed for growing out in Michigan. Already these seedling trees are being screened for disease resistance, growth characteristics and fruit characteristics (Hillig and Iezzoni 1988; Krahl et al 1991). This rapid progress was made possible by an extremely important component of plant exploration, and one which is too often overlooked; that is, the establishment of friendships and on-going collaboration with individual scientists in the host countries which has the potential for long-term benefits for both parties.

CONCLUSION

The dazzling diversity that has been collected in Central Asian apricots and walnuts, in Chinese walnuts, and in Eastern European sour cherries compared to the limited germplasm available to American breeders, provides examples of what may be in store for other fruit and nut species when explorers are able to search geographic centers of diversity. During the 1980s and 1990s we are experiencing a new "golden age" for fruit plant exploration, wherein we need to take advantage of all possible opportunities. Further, the establishment of the National Clonal Germplasm Repositories during the past decade provides the mechanism for securing long-term maintenance of newly introduced germplasm for future utilization. Because of quarantine and generational time constraints, we will be well into the 21st century before the benefits of this new germplasm will be realized in new cultivars. Only then will we be able to evaluate the full value of exploitation as we begin to see new cultivars which, (1) represent a greatly expanded germplasm base, thus reducing genetic vulnerability, (2) provide a wider range of climatic adaptation, (3) spread the harvest season, (4) have a modified plant architecture (e.g. dwarf, precocious walnut trees), (5) have improved fruit quality, (6) have longer storage life, (7) provide new products, and (8) exhibit greater resistance to pests and diseases.

REFERENCES

Brooks, H.J. and G. Vest. 1985. Public programs on genetics and breeding horticultural crops in the United States. HortScience 20:826–830.

Hancock, J.F. and J.H. Siefker. 1982. Levels of inbreeding in highbush blueberry cultivars. HortScience 17:363–366.

Hillig, K.W. and A.F. Iezzoni. 1988. Multivariate analysis of a sour cherry germplasm collection. J. Amer. Soc. Hort. Sci. 113:928–934.

Iezzoni, A.F. 1984. Sour cherry breeding in Eastern Europe. Fruit Vars. J. 38:121–125.

Ji, Bien. 1980. Walnut cultivation and utilization in China. Fruit Vars. J. 34:98–99.

Krahl, K.H., A. Lansari, and A.F. Iezzoni. 1991. Morphological variation within a sour cherry collection. Euphytica 52:47–55.

Scorza, R, S.A. Mehlenbacher, and G.W. Lightner. 1985. Inbreeding and coancestry of the freestone peach cultivars of the eastern United States and implications for peach germplasm improvement. J. Amer. Soc. Hort. Sci. 110:547–552.

Sjulin, T.M. 1987. Genetic diversity of North American strawberry cultivars. J. Amer. Soc. Hort. Sci. 112:375–385.

Vavilov, N.L. 1930. Wild progenitors of the fruit trees of Turkistan and the Caucasus and the problem of the origin of fruit trees. Rpt. and Proc. Int. Hort. Cong., London.

The Search for New Pharmaceutical Crops: Drug Discovery and Development at the National Cancer Institute

Gordon M. Cragg, Michael R. Boyd, John H. Cardellina II, Michael R. Grever, Saul Schepartz, Kenneth M. Snader, and Matthew Suffness

In 1937, the United States National Cancer Institute (NCI) was established with its mission being "to provide for, foster and aid in coordinating research related to cancer." In 1955, NCI set up the Cancer Chemotherapy National Service Center (CCNSC) to promote a cancer chemotherapy program, involving the procurement, screening, preclinical development, and clinical evaluation of new agents. All aspects of drug discovery and preclinical development are now the responsibility of the Developmental Therapeutics Program (DTP), a major component of the Division of Cancer Treatment (DCT). During the past 35 years, over 400,000 chemicals, both synthetic and natural products, submitted by investigators and organizations worldwide, have been screened for antitumor activity, and NCI has played a major role in the discovery and development of many of the available commercial and investigational anticancer agents (Driscoll 1984). Prior to 1960, the screening of natural products was concerned mainly with the testing of fermentation products, but the establishment of an interagency agreement with the United States Department of Agriculture in 1960 for the collection and screening of plants marked the start of a systematic program for the discovery and development of anticancer agents from plant sources. Initially, collections were made in the United States and Mexico, but were later expanded to about 60 countries through both field collections by USDA personnel and procurements from contract suppliers. Between 1960 and the termination of this particular collection program in 1982, some 114,000 extracts of an estimated 35,000 plants were tested for antitumor activity, mainly using the in vivo L1210 and P388 mouse leukemias as the primary screening models. The collection strategy, and the scope and achievements of this program, have been reviewed in depth in earlier reports (Perdue 1976; Suffness and Douros 1979, 1982), and will not be discussed in this paper.

Although a number of plant-derived antitumor compounds, such as taxol (Fig. 1) and camptothecin (Fig. 2), were discovered in the 1970s and subsequently have become of great interest at NCI in the 1990s, the program was discontinued in the early 1980s, since it was perceived that few novel active leads were being isolated from natural sources. Indeed, there was concern that natural products were failing to yield novel agents possessing activity against the more resistant solid tumors. This apparent failure might, however, be attributed more to the nature of the primary screens rather than a deficiency of nature. In 1985, development of a new in vitro human cancer cell line screen, incorporating panels of cell lines representing various solid tumor disease-types (e.g. colon, lung, ovarian), was initiated. This revision of the antitumor screening strategy also was accompanied by the implementation of a new NCI natural products program involving new procurement, extraction, and isolation

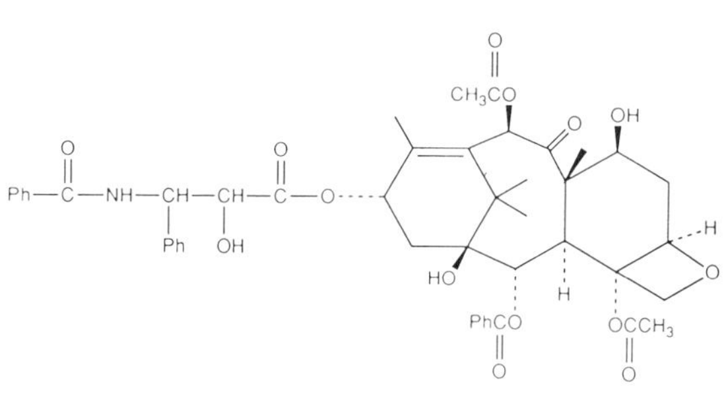

Fig. 1. Taxol.

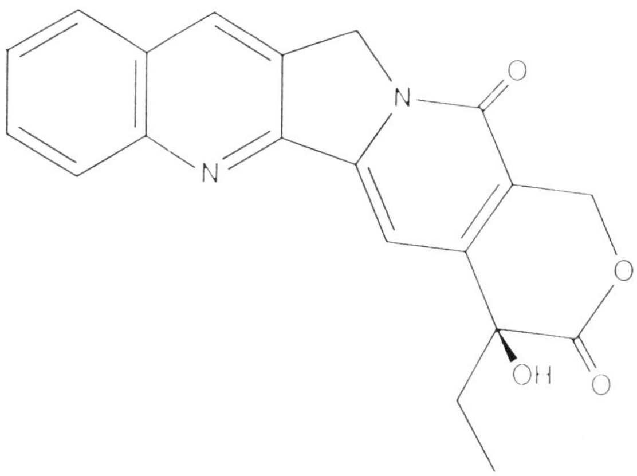

Fig. 2. Camptothecin.

components. Additionally, the initiation in 1987 of a major new program within NCI for the discovery and development of anti-HIV agents provided yet further impetus and resources for the renewed focus upon natural products.

PLANT ACQUISITION PROGRAM

In September, 1986, three five-year contracts were awarded for plant collections in tropical and sub-tropical regions worldwide. In awarding the contracts, NCI specified that collections should encompass a broad taxonomic diversity, but that emphasis should be given to reputed medicinal plants when reliable information was available. Each contract called for the collection of 1,500 samples of 0.3 to 1.0 kg (dry weight) per year, with different plant parts constituting separate, discreet samples. Each sample is assigned a unique NCI collection number, expressed in the form of a barcode label, which is attached to the cloth sample bag in the field. Detailed documentation of each sample is required, including taxonomy, plant part, date and location of collection, habitat, hazards (e.g. thorny), and, when available, any information concerning medicinal uses and preparations. At least five voucher specimens of each plant species are collected; one is donated to the national herbarium in the country of collection, and one is deposited with the Botany Department of the Museum of Natural History, Smithsonian Institution. Dried plant samples are shipped by air freight to the NCI Natural Products Repository (NPR) in Frederick, Maryland. An import permit has been provided to the contractor maintaining the repository (Program Resources, Inc.: PRI) by the Animal and Plant Health Inspection Service (APHIS) of the United States Department of Agriculture, which has provided excellent support to NCI in facilitating the import of thousands of plant samples. On arrival at the NPR, the samples are stored in large $-20°C$ walk-in freezers for at least 48 h; this freezing of samples is required by APHIS in order to minimize the survival of plant pests and pathogens.

The initial contracts were awarded to the Missouri Botanical Garden, the New York Botanical Garden, and the University of Illinois in Chicago (assisted by the Arnold Arboretum and the Bishop Museum) for collections in Africa and Madagascar, Central and South America, and Southeast Asia, respectively. These contracts were recompeted recently and awarded again to these same organizations for a further five years, beginning September, 1991. In investigating the natural resources of other countries, many of the latter in the developing world, NCI has recognized the need to develop substantive collaborations with the scientific community in countries participating in the collection programs. Measures aimed at promoting such collaborations, and establishing mechanisms for compensation of contributing organizations, groups, or individuals in these countries, have been formulated and incorporated in the NCI Letter of Intent. The Letter of Intent contains both short-term and long-term measures aimed at assuring countries participating in NCI-funded collections of NCI's good intentions (National Cancer Institute, unpublished). In the short-term, NCI periodically invites appropriate officials or scientists from local scientific organizations to visit the drug discovery facilities in Frederick, Maryland to discuss the goals of the drug discovery and development program. When laboratory space and resources permit, suitably-qualified scientists are invited to spend periods of up to a year working with scientists in NCI facilities on research topics of mutual interest to NCI and the collection country organizations. To date, scientists from 14 countries have visited NCI and United States Collection contractor facilities for periods of one to two weeks, while chemists from five countries are carrying out collaborative research projects with chemists in NCI facilities.

As screening test data become available, these are provided to collection contractors for dissemination to interested scientists in countries participating in their collection programs. Each country receives only data obtained from organisms collected within its own borders, and scientists are requested to keep data on active organisms confidential until NCI has had sufficient time to assess the potential for development of new agents from such organisms. The request for confidentiality is related to the possibility of obtaining patents on these new agents; in the event of a patent being licensed to a pharmaceutical company for development and eventual marketing of a drug, NCI will make its best effort to insure that a clause is included in the licensing agreement requiring the company to pay a percentage of the royalties, accruing from sale of the drug, to the country of origin of the organism yielding the drug. This form of compensation is regarded as a potential long-term benefit, since development of a drug to the stage of marketing can take 10 to 20 years from its time of discovery. Another potential benefit to the country of origin is the development of large-scale harvesting or cultivation programs to supply sufficient raw material for bulk production of the drug. In licensing a patent on a new drug to a pharmaceutical company, NCI will require the company to seek, as its first source of supply, the natural product produced in the country of origin. The Letter of Intent already has formed the basis for agreements between research organizations in Madagascar and Tanzania and NCI, and will also be used in establishing formal collaborations with research organizations in countries not formally participating in current NCI contract collections.

DRUG DISCOVERY AND DEVELOPMENT

Plant samples are transferred from the Natural Products Repository to the Extraction and Grinding Laboratory (EGL; also operated by PRI). Ground material is sequentially extracted at room temperature with a 1:1 mixture of methanol and methylene chloride and water to give organic solvent and aqueous extracts. Five 100 milligram samples of each extract are weighed out into small vials to give aliquots suitable for screening, while the remaining materials are kept as bulk samples suitable for subsequent fractionation and isolation studies, if necessary. All extract samples are assigned discreet NCI sample numbers, and are returned to the NPR for storage at –20°C until requested for screening and further investigation.

Extracts are tested in vitro for selective cytotoxicity against panels of human cancer cell lines representing major disease-types, such as lung, colon, melanoma, ovarian, renal, brain, and leukemia (Boyd 1989). Anti-HIV activity is also determined in vitro by measuring the survival of virus-infected human lymphoblastoid cells in the presence or absence of the extracts (Weislow et al. 1989). Extracts found to exhibit anti-HIV activity or a cytotoxicity profile of interest in the human tumor cell line screen are subjected to bioassay-guided fractionation by a team of NCI chemists and biologists to isolate the pure compounds responsible for the observed activity. In bioassay-guided fractionation, all fractions produced at each stage of the separation are tested for activity in the relevant bioassay, and the subsequent fractionations are performed only on the active fraction(s). This process of fractionation and testing is continued until the pure active component(s) is isolated. The initial plant collection sample (0.3 to 1.0 kg) will generally yield enough extract (10 to 40 g) to permit isolation of the pure, active constituent in sufficient quantity for complete structural elucidation. Subsequent secondary testing and preclinical studies (pharmacology, formulation, toxicology), however, might require gram or even kilogram quantities, depending on the degree of activity and toxicity of the active agent (Driscoll 1984).

As of September, 1991, approximately 26,000 plant samples had been collected, and over 14,000 had been extracted to yield over 28,000 extracts. More than 14,000 of these extracts had been tested in the anti-HIV screen, and about 1,300 had shown some activity. Of these, roughly 1,000 are aqueous extracts, many of which are likely to contain ubiquitous compound-types, such as polysaccharides or tannins, as the active constituents. Such compounds currently are not considered a priority for drug development, and typically are eliminated early in the process of fractionation. Amongst the agents which have been isolated and found to show interesting in vitro anti-HIV activity are prostratin (Fig. 3) from the Samoan medicinal plant, *Homalanthus acuminatus*, collected by

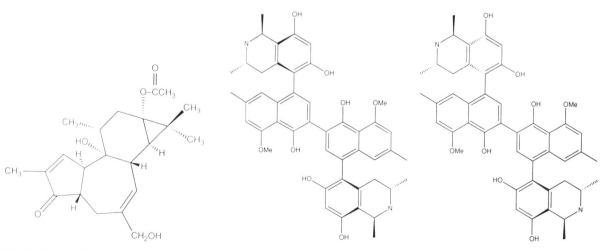

Fig. 3. Prostratin.   Fig. 4. Michellamines.

ethnobotanist, Paul Cox (Gustafson et al. 1991), and the michellamines (Fig. 4) from the Cameroon plant, *Ancistrocladus abbreviatus* (Manfredi et al. 1991).

In order to obtain sufficient quantities of an active agent for early preclinical development, recollections of 5 to 50 kg of the dried plant material are carried out, preferably from the original site of collection. Should the preclinical studies justify development of the agent towards clinical trials, considerably larger amounts of plant material would be required, and data on the distribution and abundance, as well as the drug content of the various plant parts, would need to be collected. In addition, the potential for mass cultivation of the plant would need to be assessed. If problems are encountered due to lack of abundance or inability to adapt the plant to cultivation, a search for alternative sources may be necessary. Other species of the same genus or of closely related genera can be analyzed for drug content, and techniques, such as plant tissue culture, can be investigated. While total synthesis must always be considered as a potential route for bulk production of the active agent, it should be noted that the structures of most bioactive natural products are extremely complex, and bench-scale syntheses generally are not readily adapted to economical large-scale production.

The large-scale production of taxol, which typifies the challenges and problems associated with this phase of drug development, is discussed in the next section.

LARGE-SCALE PRODUCTION OF TAXOL

Early Development of Taxol

Taxus brevifolia Nutt bark was first collected by the USDA in 1962, as part of the exploratory screening program of the NCI CCNSC. An extract was shown to be active in the KB cytotoxicity assay, and the isolation of taxol as the active constituent was reported by Wani et al. (1971). A survey of the various parts of *T. brevifolia* showed that extracts of the bark were consistently more active than those of other parts, and the bark was selected for further collections. Although taxol exhibited moderate in vivo activity against the P388 and L1210 murine leukemia models, there was little interest in developing it further. Observation of strong activity against the B16 melanoma system in 1974 to 1975, however, revived interest, and, in 1977, it was adopted by NCI as a candidate for preclinical development. In 1978, taxol was shown to exhibit significant activity against several human tumor xenograft systems, including the MX-1 mammary tumor, and, in 1979, Horwitz and Manfredi reported its unique mechanism of action in promoting tubulin polymerization and stabilizing microtubules against depolymerization (Manfredi and Horwitz 1984). Formulation studies were completed in 1980, and toxicology studies initiated. Following completion of toxicology in 1982, approval was granted for INDA filing, and Phase I trials were started in 1983.

Current Status of Taxol Development

Taxol has shown significant clinical activity against refractory ovarian cancer (Rowinsky et al. 1990), and recent clinical trial results indicate good activity against advanced breast cancer. Further trials against these disease-types are in progress using combinations of taxol with other agents, such as cisplatin, adriamycin, and granulocyte colony-stimulating factor (G-CSF). Other ongoing trials include small cell lung and non-small cell lung, colon, head and neck, prostate, and upper gastro-intestinal cancers.

Early preclinical and clinical development required only modest amounts of taxol, and, up to 1990, approximately 4 kg had been isolated. Discovery of its efficacy in the treatment of refractory ovarian cancer increased the demand to over 25 kg per year, which requires processing of 340,000 kg of *Taxus brevifolia* bark, equivalent to about 38,000 trees. In February, 1991, Bristo–Myers Squibb (BMS) entered into a Cooperative Research and Development Agreement (CRADA) with NCI after being selected in an open competition involving a number of pharmaceutical companies interested in collaborating with NCI in the development of taxol. Under the CRADA, BMS is responsible for the continued production of taxol. Bark collections are continuing in the Pacific Northwest, mainly under the direction of Hauser Northwest, a subsidiary company of Hauser Chemical Research of Boulder, Colorado. Harvesting is permitted only from areas designated for clear-cutting, and bark is not accepted from unauthorized sources. The projected harvest for 1991 is 340,000 kg, sufficient to meet the taxol needs for the treatment of 12,000 patients suffering from ovarian cancer. All the bark collected is designated for production of taxol for use in clinical trials, and is being processed by Hauser Chemical Research using procedures approved by the Food and Drug Administration (FDA).

The bulk production of taxol for clinical use will continue to rely on the bark source for the next 2 to 3 years and, in June, 1991, BMS entered into a cooperative agreement with the USDA Forest Service and the Bureau of Land Management whereby BMS will fund a comprehensive inventory of *Taxus brevifolia* on Government land. To date, no detailed inventory of this tree has been carried out, but estimates, based on stand information and satellite imagery, have indicated that up to 130 million yew trees occur on 720,000 ha of National Forest lands in Oregon and Washington.

Alternative Sources of Taxol

While the annual demand for taxol to treat patients with ovarian cancer exceeds 25 kg for the United States alone, the promise being shown in the treatment of breast cancer and other serious cancers could result in annual demands exceeding 200 to 300 kg. NCI, BMS and other organizations involved in taxol production fully realize that alternative sources of taxol need to be developed, and intensive studies are being directed to meet these needs. NCI and its Frederick-based Contractor, Program Resources, Inc. (PRI) are collaborating with various organizations in undertaking analytical surveys of *Taxus* species worldwide. Surveys of *T. brevifolia* have been completed, or are ongoing, in collaboration with Weyerhaeuser Company, USDAFS, and the Canadian Ministry of Forests. These surveys are identifying high-yielding trees which will be propagated in nurseries to use as seed stock for replanting and mass-cultivation programs.

Analyses of the needles of *T. brevifolia* have shown that the yield of taxol is generally 5 to 10 times lower than that from bark. Analyses of the needles of other *Taxus* species and cultivars, however, indicate that the taxol yield is often considerably higher than that from *T. brevifolia* bark, and, in addition, substantial amounts of key taxol precursors, such as 10-desacetylbaccatin III, are usually present. The ready conversion of these precursors to taxol or related active agents by relatively simple semi-synthetic methods has been achieved by several research groups (Denis et al. 1988; Holton 1990). The availability of millions of ornamental *Taxus* plants representing a variety of species and cultivars in United States nurseries, as well as the abundant supply of several other wild *Taxus* species in other countries, makes the isolation of taxol and key taxanes an attractive proposition for long-term bulk production from this renewable resource. The variation of content of these compounds in the needles of different commercial cultivars and wild species is being evaluated, as is the propagation of a number of high-yielding cultivars.

Analytical surveys of needles of a number of *Taxus* species are being undertaken by NCI and PRI in collaboration with various organizations (names in parentheses). They include *T. baccata* from the Black Sea-Caucasus region of the Soviet Union (T. Elias, Director, Rancho Santa Ana Botanic Garden), *T. canadensis* from the Gaspe Peninsula of Quebec (Canadian Ministry of Forests), *T. globosa* from Mexico (R. Nicholson, Arnold Arboretum), and various *Taxus* species from the USDA in Beltsville, Maryland (J. Duke). An investigation of *T. wallichiana* from Himalayan regions is in progress, while BMS is collaborating with Chinese groups in the study of *T. chinensis* and *T. yunnanensis*. The potential of nursery cultivars is being explored by Zelenka Nursery in collaboration with Ohio State University and the University of Mississippi; 16,000 kg of dried needles is to be supplied to NCI by this collaborative group through an interagency agreement between NCI and USDA signed in September, 1991. A research agreement was recently signed by BMS and Weyerhaeuser Company for the mass propagation of high-yielding *Taxus* cultivars, and Weyerhaeuser currently has 500,000 seedlings being grown in their nurseries as mother-stock for this project.

Thus, extensive efforts are well under way to develop the renewable needle resources, but various parameters first need to be established before this resource can totally replace the bark as a source of human-use taxol. Unlike the bark, the method and duration of drying of the needles appears to be critical to achieving optimum yields of taxol, and the drying and storage processes are being studied by a number of groups in collaboration with NCI and BMS. In addition, only taxol derived from the bark has the necessary approval by the Food and Drug Administration for human use. Use of a new source, such as needles, requires development of a new isolation procedure following good manufacturing practices (GMP) for FDA approval, and the new needle-derived taxol also requires FDA approval. While these development and approval processes are not viewed as major obstacles, they will nevertheless take some time to complete. Until then, reliance on the bark as the major source of clinical taxol will remain.

Another potential source receiving attention from research groups worldwide is plant cell culture. USDA has patented a process for production of taxol, and is collaborating with Phyton Catalytic in the development of this process. Success in this area has also been reported by Escagenetics Corporation, and both these efforts are receiving NCI grant support.

There is often the perception that, once the structure of a natural product has been determined, large-scale production will inevitably be achieved by total chemical synthesis. Natural product drugs are often very complex molecules with many chiral centers, and, as such, pose formidable synthetic challenges. Thus, the important plant-derived anticancer drugs, vinblastine and vincristine, are still isolated from the source plant, *Catharanthus roseus*, despite over 20 years of synthetic endeavor. Likewise, microbially-derived anticancer drugs, such as the bleomycins and daunorubicin, are still produced by fermentation rather than total synthesis. Taxol, with 11 chiral centers, and hence 2048 potential diastereomeric isomers, is no exception, and, while small-scale total syntheses will no doubt be achieved, the development of an economically viable process on the 100 kg scale is likely to present considerable problems. These synthetic endeavors could be productive in another sense, however, since some simpler intermediates might be discovered which are more amenable to large-scale synthesis and retain the desired anticancer properties. In addition, as noted earlier, semisynthetic procedures, involving plant-derived taxol precursors, have already contributed substantially to the ultimate long-term solution of the taxol and taxol analog supply problems.

NCI is playing a key role in all these research endeavors through grant support totaling over $2.5 million annually. In addition to studies of plant genetics and propagation, synthesis, and tissue culture, NCI is supporting research in the area of biosynthesis, formulation, metabolism, and tubulin-binding. BMS is also supporting research directed at improving the supply and production of taxol and key taxanes.

NCI has been criticized for not having addressed the taxol supply problem at a much earlier stage in its development. It should be noted, however, that it was only the observation of good activity against refractory ovarian cancer in 1989 that established confidence in the future of taxol as an efficacious clinical agent. With the future of taxol as a clinical agent now assured, NCI and its CRADA partner, BMS, are vigorously pursuing its development by all possible means.

REFERENCES

Boyd, M.R. 1989. Status of the NCI preclinical antitumor drug discovery screen. Principles and Practice of Oncology Updates 3(10):1–12. Lippincott, Philadelphia.

Denis, J-N., A.E. Greene, D. Guenard, F. Gueritte-Voegelein, L. Mangatal, and P. Potier. 1988. A highly efficient approach to natural taxol. J. Amer. Chem. Soc. 110:5917–5919.

Driscoll, J.S. 1984. The preclinical new drug research program of the National Cancer Institute. Cancer Treat. Rpt. 68:63–76.

Gustafson, K.R., J.H. Cardellina II, O.S. Weislow, J.A. Beutler, J.B. McMahon, J. Ishitoya, N.A. Sharkey, P.M. Blumberg, G.M. Cragg, P.A. Cox, and M.R. Boyd. 1991. Isolation and identification of a new AIDS-antiviral agent from a Samoan medicinal plant, *Homalanthus acuminatus*. J. Med. Chem. (in press).

Holton, R.A. 1990. Approaches to the total synthesis of taxol. Abstracts of Workshop on Taxol and *Taxus*: Current and Future Perspectives. J. Nat. Cancer Inst.

Manfredi, J.J. and S.B. Horwitz. 1984. Taxol: An antimitotic agent with a new mechanism of action. Pharmacol. Ther. 25:83–125.

Manfredi, K.P., J.W. Blunt, J.H. Cardellina II, J.B. McMahon, L.K. Pannell, G.M. Cragg, and M.R. Boyd. 1991. HIV inhibitory natural products. 4. Novel alkaloids from the tropical plant *Ancistrocladus abbreviatus* inhibit cell-killing by HIV-I and HIV-2. J. Med. Chem. (in press).

Perdue, R.E. Jr. 1976. Procurement of plant materials for antitumor screening. Cancer Treat. Rpt. 60:987–998.

Rowinsky, E.K., L.A. Cazenave, and R.C. Donehower. 1990. Taxol: A novel investigational antimicrotubule agent. J. Natl. Cancer Inst. 82:1247–1259.

Suffness, M. and J. Douros. 1979. Drugs of plant origin, p. 73–125. In: V.T. De Vita and H. Bush (eds.). Methods in cancer research. Vol XVI. New York Academic Press, New York.

Suffness M. and J. Douros. 1982. Current status of the NCI plant and animal product program. J. Nat. Prod. 45:1–14.

Wani, M.C., H.L. Taylor, and M.E. Wall. 1971. Plant antitumor agents. VI. The isolation and structure of taxol, a novel antileukemic and antitumor agent from *Taxus brevifolia*. J. Amer. Chem. Soc. 93:2325–2327.

Weislow, O.S., R. Kiser, D.L. Fine, J. Bader, R.H. Shoemaker, and M.R. Boyd. 1989. New soluble-formazan assay for HIV-1 cytopathic effects: Application to high-flux screening of synthetic and natural products for AIDS-antiviral activity. J. Natl. Cancer Inst. 81:577–586.

A Novel Method for Identification and Domestication of Indigenous Useful Plants in Amazonian Ecuador

J. Friedman, D. Bolotin, M. Rios, P. Mendosa, Y. Cohen, and M.J. Balick*

The Amazonia: an incalculable value, an untapped emporium of germplasm for new economic plants.
Richard Evans Schultes, 1979

In the rain forests in eastern Ecuador (Oriente), a considerable number of indigenous societies still rely on plant gathering, hunting, and fishing. Our aims have been to foster cultivation of indigenous useful plants among these tribal societies to help improve their economy, to preserve knowledge about and germplasm of some of their important useful plants, and to help strengthen their cultural identity. We assumed that indigenous useful plants which are highly rated by their consumers will be sufficiently attractive to foster plant adoption and that social change, from plant gathering to plant cultivation, will follow with the least constraints if traditional societies first employ their own indigenous useful plants, prior to receiving domesticated foreign crops.

To fulfil these aims, useful indigenous plant species have been identified and botanically classified, selected and propagated in nurseries. To increase attractiveness of adoption, efforts were concentrated on identification and reproduction of the most tasteful plants as well of those considered to be the most efficacious medicinals. Nurseries have been established within the communities and, subsequently, plantlets distributed free to families willing to grow them, to be planted in their gardens.

METHODOLOGY

The most common language along the Upper Napo river is Quichua. However, in each community there is always a number of people, particularly teachers, who also know Spanish. These people provided translation services for our project. Most people were acquainted with the edible plants in their surrounding forests. As information on useful plants had already disappeared, we first sought to interview and survey the few remaining highly knowledgeable people. For the identification of edible plants, we attempted to interview selected informants, including those people recommended by at least five independent people, as the best knowledgeable

---

*The authors are indebted to Dr. Naranjo Plutarcho, Health Minister of Ecuador for his encouragement and help, to Prof. Laura Arcos and Dr. Roberto Padilla, Dept. of Biological Sciences, Pontificia Catholic University, Ecuador. Thanks also to US–A.I.D. (CDR) for financial support of this project during 1989–1992 Grant C8-159; DHR-5544-G-SS-9064-0.

plantsmen in the region. However, for rating of the most popular edible plants, any person willing to cooperate were included in order to obtain the widest possible concensus.

Preliminary Evaluation of Edible Plants

During several excursions with knowledgeable guides (informants) in the rain forests in several localities, along the Upper Napo river (Campano Cocha, Santa Rosa, and Caspi Sapa, Fig. 1), a list of 41 species of common edible plants was compiled (Table 1). Since plants from different culinary categories are difficult to directly compare, plants were classified into the following three types: food plants (plantas para tomar), juicy plants (plantas para chupar), and herbs and spices. Lists in alphabetical order, of Quichua plant names were presented to each person interviewed. Forty-five people were interviewed, usually on Sundays in church. Interviewees were requested to rate the plants of each category, according to declining preference, based on their own taste. When the order of culinary grades corresponded to the alphabetical order of the plant names, data was excluded from the study. Although, each interviewee was literate, we provided a tutor for each.

Preliminary Evaluation of Medicinal Plants

To identify the most attractive medicinal plants for the indigenous communities studied, we used a quantitative ethnopharmacological method developed among Bedouins in Israel (Friedman et al. 1986). During an ethnopharmacological field survey in the Negev desert, it was noticed that informants, when independently interviewed, sometimes have different ideas as to the major purpose for which a given medicinal plant is used. Such disagreements appeared also when highly reputed informants with at least six independent recommendations, were interviewed. To analyze the efficacy of the plants which were applied to different ailments, we requested information on the major and the secondary applications of medicinal plants from each informant. However, to avoid the risk of memory failure, each informant was also requested to elaborate on the uses of each plant within a given list (Table 2).

Based on field experience, a list of 100 commonly used species of medicinal plants (Table 2) was compiled. This enabled us to detect information missed due to memory failure, as well as species unknown to individual informants.

The percentage of informants claiming the use of a certain plant for the same major purpose, also known as its Fidelity Level (FL), was calculated for each species. Thus, plants could be rated on the basis of their relative efficiency, as they appear in the eyes of their consumers. Since some plants which received high FL values were

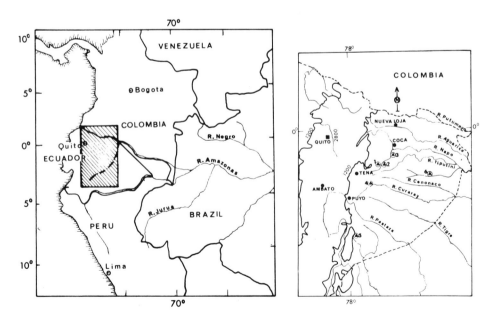

Fig. 1. Map of Ecuador and area under investigation.

Table 1. A list of edible plants from upper Napo river (Eastern Ecaudor).

Plant catagory / Family	Species	Plant part consumed[z]	Way of consumption
Food plants			
Araceae	*Colocasia esculenta*	T	Fresh
Arecaceae	*Bactris gasipaes*	F,S	Fermented or cooked for chicha
Arecaceae	*Jessenia bataua*	F	Cooked
Arecaceae	*Mauritia flexusa*	F	Fresh
Convolvulaceae	*Ipomea batatas*	T	Cooked or fermented for chicha
Cucurbitaceae	Ucsha (species unknown)	F	Fresh/cooked
Dioscoraceae	*Dioscorea trifida*	T	Cooked
Euphorbiaceae	*Caryodendron orinocense*	S	Fresh/dried
Euphorbiaceae	*Plukenetia volubilis*	S	Cooked
Fabaceae	*Phaseolus vulgaris*	S	Cooked
Lecythidaceae	*Grias neuberthii*	F	Fresh/cooked
Mimosaceae	*Inga* sp. (Ilta)	F,S	Fresh/cooked
Phytolaccaceae	*Phytolacca rivinoides*	L	Fresh/cooked
Sapotaceae	*Chrysophyllum venezuelanense*	F	Cooked/fried
Sapotaceae	*Pouteria* sp.	F	Fresh
Sterculiaceae	*Herrania* sp.	S	Cooked
Sterculiaceae	*Theobroma bicolor*	S	Cooked fried
unknown	Butum; Butio	n.d.	n.d.
unknown	Garabatu yuyu	n.d.	n.d.
unknown	Sani papa	T	Cooked
unknown	Shimbi	n.d	n.d.
Juicy plants			
Annonaceae	*Annona cherimolia*	F	Fresh
Apocynaceae	*Tabernaemontana sananho*	F	Fresh
Bombacaceae	*Matisia cordata*	F	Fresh
Cecropiaceae	*Pourouma cecropiaefolia*	F	Fresh
Malpighiaceae	*Bunchosia* sp.	F	Fresh
Mimosaceae	*Inga edulis*	F	Fresh
Mimosaceae	*Inga* sp. (Machitona)	F	Fresh
Passifloraceae	*Passiflora* sp. (Maracuya)	F	Fresh
Passifloraceae	*Passiflora* sp. (Granadilla)	F	Fresh
Sapotaceae	*Pouteria caimito*	F	Fresh
Solanaceae	*Solanum quitoense*	F	For juice
Sterculiaceae	*Herrania nitida*	F	Fresh
Theophrastaceae	*Calvija harlingii*	F	Fresh
Herbs and spices			
Apiaceae	*Eryngium foetidum*	L	Fresh for salad or soup (similar to coriander)
Bignoniaceae	*Mansoa standleyi*	L	Fresh/dried, soup
Bixaceae	*Bixa orellana*	S	Fried/soup
Lamiaceae	*Ocimum basilicum*	L	Fresh/soup or salad
Lauraceae	*Ocotea quixos*	L, Calyx	Fresh/dried
Liliaceae	*Allium* sp.	L	Fresh/salad or soup (similar to chives)
Moraceae	*Brosimum uleti*	Latex	Fresh

[z] F = fruit; L = leaf; n.d. = no documentation; R = root; S = seed; St = stem: T = tuber.

Table 2. A list of medicinal plants from the upper Napo river (Eastern Ecuador).

Family	Species or Quichua name	Plant part[z]	Major use
Acanthaceae	Quihui yuyu (species unknown)	L,P	Sprain
Apocynaceae	*Himatanthus lancifolius*	La	Anemia, strengthening
Apocynaceae	*Tabernaemontana sananho*	B,L	Stomachache
Aquifoliaceae	*Ilex guayuosa*	L	Stimulant
Araceae	*Colocasia* sp.	Rh	Cuts
Arecacea	Supai chunda (species unknown)	Apex	Tonic, strengthening
Asteraceae	*Clibaduim asperum*	L,St	Fish poisoning
Asteraceae	*Spilanthes* cf.	L	Cuts
Bignoniaceae	*Mansoa standleyi*	L	Grippe
Boraginaceae	*Corida nodosa*	L	Gangrens from snakebite
Brassicaceae	Amarun uchu (species unknown)	P	Skin problems (granos)
Caesalpiniaceae	*Senna ruiziana*		
Capparidaceae	*Capparis sola*	B	Skin problems (granos)
Cecropiaceae	*Cecropia* sp.	B	Strengthening
Celastraceae	*Maytenus krukovii*	B	Rheumatism, body pains
Commelinaceae	*Commelina erecta*	B	Blood pressure
Crassulaceae	*Bryophyllum ginnatum*	L,St	Cuts, wounds
Cyclanthaceae	*Carludovica palmata*		Rheumatism, swelling
Erythroxylaceae	*Erythroxylum gracilipes*	L	Tranquilliar, rheumatism
Euphorbiaceae	*Croton lechleri*	La	Panacea, gingivitis
Fabaceae	*Lonchocarpus nicou*	St	Fish poison
Fabaceae	*Myroxylon balsamum*	B	Grippe, fever
Fabaceae	*Swarzia simplex*	B	Strengthening
Flacourtiaceae	*Neosprucea* sp.	B	Tuberculosis
Gesneriaceae	*Columnea archidonae*	L	Menstruation set up
Lamiaceae	*Hyptis pectinata*	L	Kidney disorder
Lauraceae	*Persea americana*	S	Contraceptive
Lecythidaceae	*Grias neuberthii*	B	Vomiting, diarrhea
Loganiaceae	*Potalia amara*	L	Snakebite
Malpighiaceae	*Banisteriopsis caapi*	B	Hallucinogen, "insight drug"
Melastomaceae	*Blackea* cf. *rosea*	L	Cuts, wounds
Melastomaceae	Cana agria (unknown species)	St	Cuts
Meliaceae	Flor del sielo (unknown species)	L, Fl	Rabies
Meliaceae	*Guarea cinnamomea*	B	Asthma
Mimosaceae	*Piptademia pteroclada*	B	Diarrhea, vomiting
Moraceae	*Brosimum utile*	La	Purgative for children
Ochnaceae	*Ourateae* sp.	B	Diarrhea, stomachache
Orchidaceae	Rayu palanda (unknown species)	L	Skin problems (granos)
Piperaceae	*Piper veneralense*	L	Diarrhea
Piperaceae	*Piper* sp.	L	Gingivitis
Polypodiaceae	*Asplenium* sp.	L	Nervous disorders
Polypodiaceae	*Lomariopsis* sp.	L	Diarrhea, vomiting
Rubiaceae	*Duroia hirsuta*	B	Diarreha, stomachache
Rubiaceae	*Simira* sp.	B	Contraceptive, menstruation set up
Sapindaceae	*Paullinia* sp.	St, (Sap)	Intestinal parasites
Smilaceae	*Smilax* sp.	R	Skin problems (acne)
Solanaceae	*Brugmansia arborea*	L	Hallucinogen
Solanaceae	*Brunfelsia chiricaspi*	R	Body pains, grippe
Solanaceae	*Brunfelsia grandiflora*	R	Body pains, grippe
Solanaceae	*Solanum mamosum*	F	Skin parasites in chicken
Theophrastaceae	*Clavija harlingii*	R	Grippe

Table 2. Continued.

Family	Species	Part	Use
Urticaceae	*Urera caracasana*	L,St	Pains, rheumatism
Verbenaceae	*Verbena brasiliansis*	L	Stomach disorders
Zingiberaceae	*Zingiber officinale*	R	Grippe
unknown	Accha huasca	B	Antibaldness
unknown	Amiruca panga	L	Hallucinogen, "insight drug"
unknown	Andia paju (caspi)	B	Diarrhea with blood
unknown	Armangui	L	Chicken parasites
unknown	Ayacara	B	Stomachache
unknown	Bujiu panga	L	Aphrodiatsiac
unknown	Chiri panga	L,St	Clean the body from evil spirits
unknown	Chunchu	B	Skin problems (granos)
unknown	Cucu tsicta	L	Hair parasits
unknown	Cuilichi lulu	L, La	Wounds
unknown	Dumduma	T	Snakebite
unknown	Flur huasca	St	Syphylis, diarrhea
unknown	Gallu caspi	B	Skin problems
unknown	Huagra huanduj	St	Rheumatism
unknown	Huarangayura	B	Stomachache, diarrhea
unknown	Huiqui huasca	La	Stomachache
unkown	Icsa nanai yura	B	Stomachache
unknown	Ilia huanga lumu		Rheumatism
unknown	Isla vapa yura	Resin	Skin problems
unknown	Lustunda	F,B	Tuberculosis
unknown	Luta luta	P	Sprains
unknown	Machacui caparina		Snakebite
unknown	Machacui mandi	T	Snakebite
unknown	Machacui mishu	T	Snakebite
unknown	Machi manga		Cancer
unknown	Mati muyu caspi	B	Grippe
unknown	Munu chupa	L,R	Diarrhea
unknown	Pala panga	L	Gential cancer
unknown	Pinsha caliu	P	Bleeding
unknown	Piri piri panga	L	Aphrodisiac
unknown	Puma yuyu	Mer, L	Hallucinogen, strengthening
unknown	Pupa huasca	St	Grippe
unknown	Puru panga	L	Menstruation set up
unknown	Quihuin ambi	L,St	Fish poison
unknown	Rayu paju		Skin-problems (granos)
unknown	Sacha huanduj	L	Rheumatism
unknown	Sacha limon	F,L	Grippe
unknown	Santa maria panga	L	Bleeding
unknown	Sarsiliu	B	Tuberculosis
unknown	Shia huasca	R,B	Diarrhea, stomachache
unknown	Shiu panga	L	Diarrhea, stomachache strengthening
unknown	Sirlu panga	L	Heart disorders
unknown	Sitimu panga	L	Diarrhea
unknown	Sucuva	La	Skin tumors
unknown	Supai caspi		Hernia
unknown	Suru panga	L	Clean the body from evil spirits
unknown	Yacami panga	L	Strengthening children

B = bark; F = fruit; Fl = flower; L = leaf; La = latex; Mer = meristem; P = plant; R = root; Rh = rhizom; S = seed; T = tuber. "Insight drug"—taken by witch doctor for a better diagnosis.

known to only a fraction of the informants, an appropriate correction factor was introduced. The Relative Popularity Level (RPL) can be calculated for each plant from the relationship between the number of informants who know of a certain plant and the average number of uses per plant (Friedman et al. 1986). The corrected fidelity level, or Rank Order Priority (ROP) of a given plant is: ROP = FL × RPL. Therefore, the ROP value can be used to classify medicinal plants according to their efficiency as evaluated by their consumers.

Establishment of Nurseries

Nurseries were established within the communities, usually in the vicinity of a school, or near the house of a family that showed interest in maintaining the nursery. With the help of the local people, 10 × 20 m plots were cleared and black polyethylene sheets were stretched across the plats to prevent weeds. A germinating box (5.0 × 1.5 × 0.4 m) filled with sand from the river bank floored on the polyethylene. Usually seeds were planted, but, if plants of interest were encountered at a season when no seeds were available, cuttings were inserted after disinfection. In some cases, standard plant hormones (NAA) at 2,000 and 4,000 ppm were applied to enhance rooting

Two to three weeks after emergence, young plantlets were transplanted into 25 × 30 cm plastic bags filled with sand. Some fast germinating seeds were planted directly in plastic bags. A black polyethylene shading net, which intercepts 30% of the sunlight was stretched above the plants.

RESULTS AND DISCUSSION

Six informants from disparate localities were selected for interviews, and provided information on 191 species. Despite occasional difficulties in ascertaining whether a particular plant grows mainly in nature and gathered form the wild, or is cultivated, our data suggest that of 59 edible plants, 41 species are gathered and the other 18 are sporadically cultivated. We found that 132 species were used for medicinal purposes.

Edible Plants

The eight most popular species obtained within a strip of 100 km, between Misahaulli and Coca, in the Upper Napo river region, are presented in Table 3. From the eight plants with the highest culinary grade, five were found to be already cultivated by tribal societies, although on a very small scale and only in a few home gardens. These include: *Bactris gasipaes*, *Theobroma bicolor*, *Pouruma cecropiaefolia*, *Passiflora* sp. (maracuya), and *Matisia cordata*. The major herbs and spices were amongst the uncultivated plants, perhaps because only small quantities of these plants are consumed and they could be easily gathered. Although the relative culinary level among the plants in each of the three locales was different, the same species listed in Table 1 were at the top of the list in each locality. A survey of the literature suggests that some of the highly regarded edible plants in various Latin American states are already at different stages of domestication, e.g. *Bactris gasipaes* (chontaduro, pejibaye),

Table 3. Preferred edible plants in the Upper Napo river, Ecuador. The primary eight of 41 species in each of three culinary categories arranged according to their culinary grades.

Plant category	Preliminary idenfication	Quichua name	Collected (CO) or Cultivated (Cu)	Culinary grade^z ±SD
Food plants	*Caryodendron orinocense*, Euphorbiaceae	Achansu	Co	9.4±0.7
	Bactris gasipaes, Arecaceae	Chontaduro	CoCu	7.3±3.1
	Theobroma bicolor, Sterculiaceae	Patas	CoCu	6.9±3.4
Juicy fruit	*Purouma cecropiaefolia*, Cecropiaceae	Uvilla	CoCu	8.7±1.1
	Passiflora sp., Passifloraceae	Maracuya	CoCu	8.1±1.6
	Matisia cordata, Bombacaceae	Sapote	CoCu	8.1±1.7
Herbs & spices	*Ocotea quixos*, Lauraceae	Ishpingo	Co	8.3±1.8
	Eryngium foetidum, Apiaceae	Culantro	Co	7.8±2.8

^{z}An average of 30 informants, 0 = least tasty, 10 = most tasty.

(Popenoe and Jimenez 1921; Johnanessen 1966; Balick 1985; Clement and Arkcoll 1989), or *Pourouma cecropiaefolia* (National Academy of Sciences 1975).

In the same area, we found one plant with only a single squash like fruit. Locally it is called *Ucsha* in Quichua and the plant has not yet been botanically identified. Two old people claimed that it is very tasty when cooked and so *Ucsha* was included in our list. Nevertheless, most of those interviewed were young and were not acquainted with this plant and thus, it obtained a very low culinary grade. Only older people, who liked it very much were familiar with this species. A search for more plants or fruits for propagation was unsuccessful, possibly because villagers who were unaware of its possibilities for propagation had overexploited the disappearing species. The seeds of this one and only fruit were planted and the resultant seedlings grew extremely fast. At present, a few hundred plants are being cultivated. Other highly regarded species, unknown to the majority of the interviewees may also have been overlooked and not included among our top quality edible plants. Interviewing a considerable number of young people who can read, may provide in a rather short time, a concensus on the culinary level of common edible plants. However, we feel that those who are educated may be the least knowledgeable about native plants. Thus, plants that were once commonly used and eventually disappeared in part due to over exploitation will be unknown and ignored. The transition from wandering communities of food gatherers in the rainforest into settled communities that preserve the habits of plant gathering, imposed increasing constrains on those highly regarded edible plants. Highly-exploited species which were not adopted for cultivation in their home gardens, were gradually eliminated from around the village. Special efforts must be directed to detect such species and propagate them in large numbers. In order to uncover these valuable species, which are at the point of extinction, special efforts to work with wandering communities of food gatherers, as well as with highly knowledgeable informants should be made. We recommend that the eight species identified in this study should be given top priority for further propagation and distribution.

Medicinal Plants

Although conventional medicines are gradually expanding into the rainforests either through missionary activities or through small scale trading, most people continue to use traditional systems of health care including medicinal plants alone or in combination with modern pharmaceuticals. Nevertheless, it was a difficult task to interview highly reputed informants, who were independently recommended by different people as very knowledgeable. Those few authorities who still practice traditional healing usually join small remote communities and arrive only intermittently in more crowded settlements. During the first year of our activities, we approached six informants (Table 4). Interviews were conducted only after a period of acquaintance after residing for a few nights in the community, sharing food and carefully explaining our aims. Because of the numerous medicinal plants in the region, and the practical limits of time for an interview, each interview was combined with a field excursion for identification and collection of specimens. Verification of plant names was maintained through field

Table 4. Most preferable medicinal plants and their major therapeutical uses in the Upper Napo River region together with their relative grades (0 = the least, 100 = the highest efficiency).

Preliminary identification	Quichua name	Therapeutical uses	Fidelity level (FL)[z]
Maytenus krukowii, Celestraceae	Chu chu huasu	Anemia, rehumatism, grippe, headache	100
Potalia amara, Loganiaceae	Curarina	Snakebite	100
Species not identified	Machaqui mandi	Snake or scorpion bites	100
Paullinia sp., Sapindaceae	Pacai huasca	Intestinal parasites diarrhea	76
Mansoa standlevi	Sacha aju (Bignoniaceae)	Grippe, fever, headache	76
Ourateae sp., Ochnaceae	Tacu caspi or Amaron caspi	Diarrhea	61

[z]Average of 6 selected informants.

excursions, but when rainstorms occurred, we used colored pictures. Since objects shown in pictures appear at a smaller scale and are two-dimensional, interviewees must be given time to interpret these illustrations. In general, pictures were found to be more efficient for verification of edible than of medicinal plants, perhaps because these were more widely and commonly known.

It became apparent that, maximum information was obtained from any informant, when interviews were repeated at three to four different times. Only on the third meeting, could we present our arbitrary list of 100 species of medicinal plants and enquire specifically about each plant.

The limited number of informants employed in this part of the study did not allow us to draw concrete conclusions as to the rank order priority (ROP) or the relative efficiency of the medicinal plants. However, these informants were very carefully selected and their authenticity was high. Some of these species have already been noted as important medicinal plants of the Northwestern Amazonian region, e.g. *Maytenus krukowii*, *Potalia amara*, *Paullinia* sp., and *Mansoa standleyi* (Schultes and Raffauf 1990). Therefore, the list in Table 2 must be considered a preliminary guide-line for selection of so-called "attractive" indigenous medicinal plants for cultivation.

Establishment of Plants in the Nurseries

Three nurseries were established in the Upper Napo river, in Campano Cocha, Santa Rosa, and in Caspi Sapa, among Quichuas, and a fourth one in Tonianpari on the Curary river amongst Waorhanis. During 1990-1991, the nurseries included about 4,000 plants comprising about 50 species of which half were edible and half were medicinals. After germination or rooting, growth rate was rapid and the response to slow release nitrogen articles was good. About 600 propagates were distributed to local people. Prior to distribution, detailed instructions for planting and plant care were provided. Each distribution was followed with a detailed registration in order to follow the level of plant adoption, and to study ways to encourage cultivation. Those receiving planting material appeared to be enthusiastic.

These findings, which were obtained during a period of two years work has led to increased documentation of traditional knowledge of plant utilization and enhancement of plant cultivation of little known useful plants. The third year of the project will be dedicated to enlarging the scale of production and following the rates of plant adoption. During this period we hope, to ensure that the original owners maintain intellectual property rights over these plants so that they will be the first to benefit from their heritage. We are concerned however that additional effort requiring at least three to five years, will minimally be needed to ensure the success of this program.

REFERENCES

Balick, M.J. 1985. Useful plants of Amazonia: a resource of glocal importance. In: G.T. Prance and T.E. Lovejoy (eds.). Key environments: Amazonia. Pergamon Press, The New York Botanical Garden, New York.

Clement, C.R. and D.B. Arkcoll. 1989. The pejibaye palm: Economic potential and research priorities, p. 304–322. In: G.E. Wickens, N. Haq, and P. Day (eds.). New crops for food and industry. Chapman and Hall, London.

Friedman, J., Z. Yaniv, A. Dafni, and D. Palewitch. 1986. A preliminary classification of the healing potential of medicinal plants based on a rational analysis of an ethnopharmacological field survey among Bedouins in the Negev deserts, Israel. J. Ethnopharamcology 16:275–287.

Johanessen, C.L. 1967. Pejibaye palm: physical and chemical analysis of the fruit. Econ. Bot. 21:371–378.

National Academy of Sciences. 1975. Underexploited tropical plants with promising economic value. National Academy of Sciences, Washington, DC.

Popenoe, W. and Jimenez. 1921. The pejibaye, a neglected food plant of tropical America. J. Hered. 12:154–166.

Schultes, R.E. and R.F. Raffauf. 1990. The healing forest. Dioscorides Press, Portland, OR.

Schultes, R.E. 1979. The Amazonia a source of new economic plants. Econ. Bot. 33: 259–266.

BIOTECHNOLOGY

Fatty Acid Synthesis Genes: Engineering the Production of Medium-chain Fatty Acids

H. Maelor Davies, L. Anderson, J. Bleibaum, D.J. Hawkins, C. Fan, A.C. Worrell, and Toni A. Voelker

Certain plant species uniquely accumulate "medium-chain" acyl groups in their seed triacylglycerols (Hilditch and Williams 1964), and many of these fatty acids are important commercially. For example, coconut oil is a major source of laurate (12:0) for use in detergent formulations. The genus *Cuphea*, is particularly noteworthy for the considerable diversity of medium-chain compositions among its many species (Graham and Kleiman 1985). Such unusual acyl compositions have attracted the attention of lipid biochemists, not only because of their commercial relevance but also because they pose the challenge of understanding an uncommon variation in fatty acid biosynthesis. A number of theoretical explanations have been suggested (Stumpf 1987), but until recently neither measurements of metabolism in vitro (Deerberg et al. 1990), nor direct assays for hypothetical enzymes (Oo and Stumpf 1979), have provided any conclusive evidence to support them.

At Calgene, we are interested in isolating the genes involved in many areas of lipid biosynthesis, with a view to increasing the range of fats and oils that can be produced commercially in domestic rapeseed crops. Our interests include the medium-chain fatty acids, especially those such as 8:0, 10:0, and 14:0 that are not readily obtained from natural, renewable resources. We therefore began an investigation of medium-chain fatty acid biosynthesis, hoping that only one or two genes would have to be isolated and transferred to rapeseed in order to "re-program" the fatty acid biosynthesis pathway of that oilseed for medium-chain production.

IMPLICATION OF A MEDIUM-CHAIN THIOESTERASE

The choice of species for these investigations was determined by practical convenience. The Lauraceae contains several species that accumulate medium-chain fatty acyl groups in their seed triglycerides. One species is native to northern California and abundant, namely the California bay (*Umbellularia californica*). The seeds of this tree contain large embryos (2 to 2.5 g fresh weight before desiccation) whose oil content (55%) comprises almost entirely 10:0 (36%) and 12:0 (58%). To our knowledge, the mechanism of medium-chain biosynthesis in these embryos had never previously been investigated.

Ammonium sulfate fractions of immature oilseed embryos can synthesize fatty acids in vitro when supplied with the necessary substrates and co-factors. The requirement for acyl-carrier protein (ACP) is usually satisfied by providing *E. coli* ACP. Such an in vitro fatty acid synthesis (FAS) system from, for example, safflower seeds produces long-chain fatty acids de novo from acetyl-CoA and malonyl-CoA (Pollard and Singh 1987). An analogous system prepared from immature California bay (bay) cotyledons produced chiefly 10:0 and 12:0, in approximately a 1:2 ratio as in the intact seeds (Pollard et al. 1991). This suggested that the mechanism of medium-chain fatty acid formation continued to operate in vitro much as it did in vivo, and that the in vitro system could be used to investigate it.

The in vitro FAS system from bay cotyledons accumulated pools of acyl-thioesters as well as free fatty acids. Whereas the latter were chiefly 10:0 and 12:0, the acyl groups in the thioester pools were primarily 8:0 and 10:0 (Table 1). There was no detectable pool of 12:0 thioester. Taking the thioester pools to be acyl-ACPs (for which some evidence was obtained), this suggested to us that normal fatty acid biosynthesis was being modulated for medium-chain production by specific hydrolysis of 10:0-ACP and 12:0-ACP. Thus, although 8:0-thioester was accumulated it was not hydrolyzed to release free 8:0 in any appreciable amount. But 12:0-ACP was hydrolyzed so effectively that none of the thioester could be detected. The situation with 10:0-ACP was intermediate between these two extremes, resulting in some 10:0 production and 10:0-ACP remaining for extension to 12:0-ACP by the normal FAS pathway.

The simplest model to explain these results invoked a medium-chain specific acyl-ACP thioesterase, acting on 12:0-ACP and (to a lesser extent) on 10:0-ACP. By detaching these acyl groups from ACP the thioesterase would prevent their further extension to long-chain fatty acids and cause them to accumulate. Direct assay of bay cotyledon preparations showed the presence of such an enzyme activity (Pollard et al. 1991; Fig. 1). The usual long-chain thioesterase activity was also present, acting on 16:0-ACP, 18:1-ACP etc. (Fig. 1). Surprisingly, the medium-chain enzyme was primarily active on 12:0-ACP. It showed low activity on 14:0-ACP, but only a trace of activity was ever observed with 10:0-ACP as substrate. This apparent lack of an activity to account for the considerable 10:0 content of the bay seeds remains puzzling. One possible explanation is that the thioesterase interacts in some way with the FAS enzymes for more efficient interception of acyl-ACPs (in a manner perhaps analogous to the medium-chain acyl-ACP thioesterases of animal systems: deRenobales et al. 1980; Smith 1980), and that its specificity is a little different when working in this way. We hope to shed more light on this enigma when we have the bay 12:0-ACP thioesterase expressed in plants which normally produce long-chain fatty acids. Meanwhile, additional evidence was obtained to show that the 12:0-ACP thioesterase is involved in medium-chain production in vivo. For example, its activity is very low in young embryos that are not accumulating medium chains, and then it rises coincidentally with the onset of medium-chain deposition (Fig. 2).

ISOLATION OF THE THIOESTERASE GENE

The 12:0-ACP thioesterase was substantially purified from immature bay cotyledons by the scheme shown in Fig. 3 (Davies et al. 1991). The ACP affinity column not only contributed considerable purification, but also separated the activity from long-chain thioesterase (assayed with 18:1-ACP) and a 12:0-CoA hydrolase that was present (Fig. 4). The latter separation indicated that the 12:0-ACP thioesterase was much more active on 12:0-ACP than on 12:0-CoA, as expected for an enzyme involved in plastid-localized fatty acid biosynthesis. In spite of the effectiveness of this affinity chromatography step, the resulting preparation still contained several protein species as seen by SDS-PAGE and silver-staining. This preparation was subjected to additional chromatography and electrophoresis (examples shown in Fig. 3). We identified the proteins whose behavior in these experiments most closely matched the behavior of enzyme activity, and thereby prioritized the proteins as "candidates" for the thioesterase. The best candidates were a group of proteins (a single one in some preparations) of approximately 34 kDa molecular weight.

These proteins are quite "rare" in bay cotyledons, perhaps because the enzyme has a very high specific activity. Several kilograms of cotyledons had to be processed through the purification scheme to yield a few tens of µg of 34 kDa proteins for sequencing. Sequence of one of the candidates was obtained from several tryptic

Table 1. Products of in vitro fatty acid synthesizing system prepared from developing *Umbellularia californica* cotyledons[z].

Product	Chain length			
	8	10	12	18
Free fatty acids (pmol)	0	4.1	15.5	0
	0	3.6	11.9	0.8
Thioester acyl groups (pmol)	6.9	3.1	0	0
	5.7	1.4	0.3	0.5

[z]An ammonium sulfate fraction from developing cotyledons was supplied with *E. coli* ACP (0.2 mg/ml), acetyl-CoA, radiolabeled malonyl-CoA, reduced pyridine nucleotide and other typical requirements. Duplicate incubations are shown. Free fatty acids were extracted from the incubation mixture with hexane saturated with isopropanol and water. Acyl groups in the remaining aqueous fraction were considered to derive from thioesters. In a separate experiment it was confirmed that acyl-ACPs were present in this aqueous fraction, having the proportions of acyl groups shown above, i.e. $C_8 > C_{10}$ and very little C_{12} or C_9.

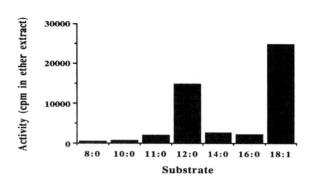

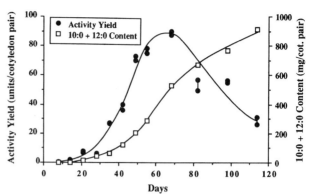

Fig. 1. Hydrolysis of acyl-ACP substrates by crude extract of developing *Umbellularia californica* cotyledons. Substrates were prepared from *E. coli* ACP and [1-^{14}C]-fatty acids. Incubation was with 4.5 μM substrate for 30 min at 30°C in 50 mM Na phosphate buffer pH 7.5. The radioactive products were extracted in ether, and in the case of laurate verified to be fatty acid by TLC.

Fig. 2. Extractable 12:0-ACP thioesterase activity and medium-chain fatty acyl contents of *Umbellularia californica* cotyledons at different stages in development. Seeds were harvested periodically from the same tree at the times indicated from an arbitrary starting date (plotted as day 8). At least 5 cotyledon pairs were combined and powdered at each sampling time for enzyme extraction and fatty acyl analysis. The activity results are duplicate assays of simple, crude extracts. Total fatty acyl compositions were determined singly, by acidic methanolysis of the powdered cotyledonary tissue.

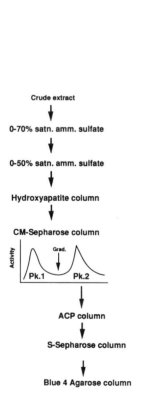

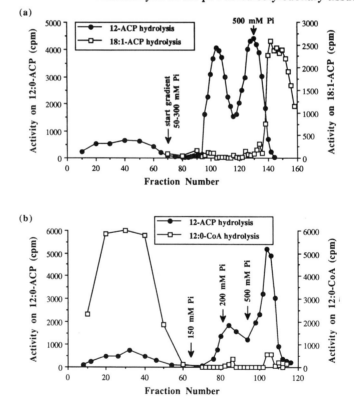

Fig. 3. Scheme for purification of 12:0-ACP thioesterase from immature cotyledons of *Umbellularia californica*.

Fig. 4. Chromatography of partially purified 12:0-ACP thioesterase and (a) the accompanying 18:1-ACP hydrolysis activity, or (b) the accompanying 12:0-CoA hydrolysis activity, on immobilized *E. coli* ACP. Experiments (a) and (b) were performed with different thioesterase preparations.

peptides and from the N-terminus. To generate a partial cDNA probe for use in gene isolation, we followed the strategy of mixed oligonucleotide primed amplification of cDNA. Poly(A) RNA was isolated from developing bay cotyledons, and reverse-transcribed to provide a single-strand cDNA to act as template in polymerase chain reactions (PCR). Sense and antisense degenerate oligonucleotides corresponding to the sequenced peptides were used as primers. The PCR procedure amplified a 0.8 kb DNA fragment, which was subsequently used to screen a plasmid cDNA library, resulting in the isolation of several clones.

The longest clone that was isolated contains an 1,163 bp open reading frame, within which is located an ATG surrounded by sequences which match the "rules" for plant initiation of translation (Fig. 5). This translation start predicts a 382 amino acid polypeptide, and the available N-terminal sequence indicates an 83-residue transit

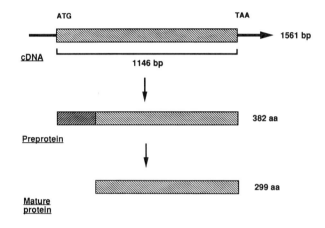

Fig. 5. Relative sizes of *Umbellularia californica* 12:0-ACP thioesterase cDNA, preprotein, and mature protein

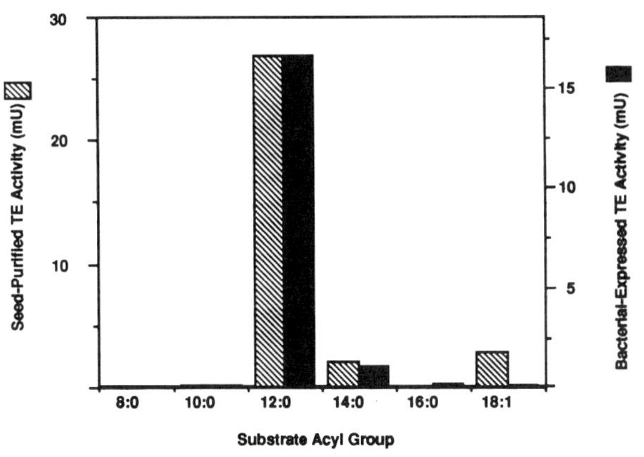

Fig. 6. Substrate specificities of thioesterases purified from *Umbellularia californica* seeds, and expressed in *E. coli*. The activity axes have been set so that the 12:0-ACP activity columns are of equal height, in order to show clearly the plant/bacterial comparisons for the other substrates. Background *E. coli* acyl-ACP hydrolysis activities were negligible at the dilutions required to maintain the introduced 12:0-ACP thioesterase within the linear range of the assay. The small amount of activity shown by the plant preparation towards 18:1-ACP resulted from incomplete separation of the medium- and long-chain thioesters during purification.

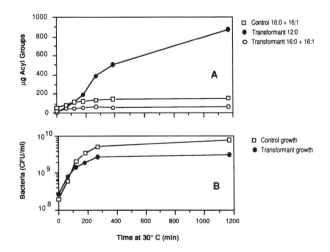

Fig. 7. Laurate accumulation (A), and growth curves (B), of control and transformed *fad*D *E. coli* cultures. Bacterial colonies were resuspended in growth medium and grown under continuous shaking at 30°C for 2 h in order to enter logarithmic growth (time zero). At the indicated times 10 ml samples were removed for fatty acyl analysis (A). The sum of 16:0 and 16:1 served as a measure of the endogenous bacterial fatty acyl content, comprising 66% of the total fatty acyl groups of control *E. coli* cultures. Laurate (12:0) levels are shown only for the *E. coli* transformed with *Umbellularia californica* 12:0-ACP thioesterase, the control 12:0 level being below the detection limit in this experiment.

sequence and 299-residue mature protein. The transit sequence contains typically conserved features of plastid transit peptides, and its presence is consistent with the protein being involved in fatty acid biosynthesis.

EXPRESSION OF THE THIOESTERASE GENE IN *E. COLI*

We tested the identity of this cDNA, and the correctness of the original protein identification, by expression in *E. coli*. A translational fusion was created using the "mature" bay sequence and the modified N-terminal coding sequence of the bacterial *lacZ* gene on a plasmid. *E. coli* cells containing this plasmid produced very high 12:0-ACP thioesterase activity, approximately 1,000-fold greater than the cells' own acyl-ACP hydrolysis activities (Fig. 6). The acyl-group specificity of this additional activity corresponded exactly with that of the seed-purified enzyme, confirming that the correct protein had been identified and the correct cDNA isolated.

Liquid cultures of *E. coli* transformants expressing the bay thioesterase cDNA had approximately twice the 12:0 content of control cultures. The absolute amount of 12:0 in the cultures was still small however (6.5% of the total fatty acids), which is surprising considering the very high thioesterase activity that was present. To ascertain whether a large amount of laurate was being produced and then catabolized, we transformed *E. coli* strains that were defective in fatty acid breakdown. The resulting 12:0 accumulation was considerable. For example, *fad*D mutants (lacking medium-chain acyl-CoA synthetase) accumulated sufficient 12:0 over a 20 h growth period to comprise 90% of the culture fatty acid content, a mass of 12:0 approximately equal to the total dry weight of the cells themselves (Fig. 7). The other fatty acids were accumulated to only 50% of their levels in *fad*D control cultures, and the transformed *fad*D cells reached stationary phase at a lower cell density (Fig. 7).

The growth rate of transformed *E. coli fad*D colonies on agar at 25°C was comparable to that of untransformed controls (results not shown). After several days' incubation, crystals formed on the plates of transformed colonies, both in the colonies themselves and on the agar surface. We identified these crystals as the potassium salt of 12:0.

CONCLUDING REMARKS

These results show that bay 12:0-ACP thioesterase is capable of interacting with the FAS system of *E. coli* in vivo to effect medium-chain fatty acid production. The products were what would be expected from the in vitro specificity of the enzyme, only very small amounts of 10:0 being formed. At present, it is unclear whether this particular thioesterase is responsible for both 10:0 and 12:0 formation, or only 12:0 production, in bay seeds. Experiments are underway to introduce the gene into rapeseed, under the control of embryo-specific promoters such as napin. These experiments will test (a) the efficiency of medium-chain production when this enzyme encounters a heterologous plant system; (b) the question of whether this thioesterase can effect 10:0 as well as 12:0 production in vivo; and (c) the efficiency with which medium-chains can be transported from the plastid to the cytoplasm and incorporated into triacylglycerols in a species that does not normally contain them.

REFERENCES

Davies, H.M., L. Anderson, C. Fan, and D.J. Hawkins. 1991. Developmental induction, purification, and further characterization of 12:0-ACP thioesterase from immature cotyledons of *Umbellularia californica*. Arch. Biochem. Biophys. 290: 37–45.

Deerberg, S., J.v. Twickel, H.-H. Forster, T. Cole, J. Fuhrmann, and K.-P. Heise. 1990. Synthesis of medium-chain fatty acids and their incorporation into triacylglycerols by cell-free fractions from *Cuphea* embryos. Planta 180:440–444.

de Renobales, M., L. Rogers, and P.E. Kolattukudy. 1980. Involvement of a thioesterase in the production of short-chain fatty acids in the uropygial glands of mallard ducks. Arch. Biochem. Biophys. 205:464–477.

Graham, S.A. and R. Kleiman. 1985. Fatty acid composition in *Cuphea* seed oils from Brazil and Nicaragua. J. Amer. Oil Chem. Soc. 62:81–82.

Hilditch, T.P. and P.N. Williams. 1964. p. 332–343. In: P.A. Siegenthaler (ed.). The chemical constitution of natural fats. Wiley, New York.

Oo, K.C. and P.K. Stumpf. 1979. Fatty acid biosynthesis in the developing endosperm of *Cocos nucifera*. Lipids 14:132–143.

Pollard M.R., L. Anderson, C. Fan, D.J. Hawkins, and H.M. Davies. 1991. A specific acyl-ACP thioesterase implicated in medium-chain fatty acid production in immature cotyledons of *Umbellularia californica*. Arch. Biochem. Biophys. 284:306–312.

Pollard, M.R. and S.S. Singh. 1987. p. 455–463. In: P.K. Stumpf, J.B. Mudd, and W.D. Ness (eds.). The metabolism, structure, and function of plant lipids. Plenum Press.

Smith, S. 1980. Mechanism of chain length determination in biosynthesis of milk fatty acids. J. Dairy Sci. 63:337–352.

Stumpf, P.K. 1987. p. 121–136. In: P.K. Stumpf, and E. Conn (eds.). The biochemistry of plants. Academic Press.

Bioassembly of Storage Lipids in Oilseed Crops; Target: Trierucin*

David C. Taylor, Ljerka Kunst, and Samuel L. MacKenzie

The long-range goal of the Plant Biotechnology Institute's Seed Oil Modification Project is the development, through recombinant DNA technology, of new plant cultivars capable of producing specifically-designed seed oils not attainable by conventional breeding methods. As a model, we intend to genetically modify *Brassica napus* L. to produce seed oils rich in erucic acid (22:1, *cis*-13-docosenoic acid) and other very long chain fatty acids (VLCFAs). VLCFAs are valued as industrial feedstocks for the production of surfactants, plasticizers, and surface coatings, while trierucin is an excellent high temperature lubricant (Princen and Rothfus 1984) and can also be used as a novel treatment for adrenoleukodystrophy (Van Dyne et al. 1990). While the primary use of high erucic oils is currently for the production of erucamide, employed as a slip and anti-block agent in the manufacture of plastic films, the expanded utilization of such seed oils for industrial applications has been forecast to increase with the advent of the USDA-sponsored High Erucic Acid Oil Project (USDA Co-operative State Research Service 1990; Van Dyne et al. 1990). Indeed, more than 200 patented applications have been catalogued for the C22 oleochemicals erucic acid, behenic acid (22:0, docosanoic acid) and their derivatives, and such compounds have been cited as strategic industrial feedstocks for the 21st century (Sonntag 1991). Some of these potential applications are listed in Table 1.

The scientific rationale for our model study to manipulate the bioassembly of triacylglycerols (TAGs) containing VLCFAs is as follows: (1) VLCFAs, such as erucic acid, are confined almost exclusively to the neutral lipid (chiefly triacylglycerol) fraction in developing oilseeds and are not components of membrane (phospho- or glyco-) lipids (Roughan and Slack 1982; Griffiths et al. 1988); (2) 22:1 is an excellent seed storage lipid marker for studying biochemical mechanisms specific to TAG assembly (Taylor et al. 1991); (3) Molecular-genetic modification of seed oils to enhance levels of VLCFAs will be TAG-specific, and should avoid any potentially-lethal interference with membrane lipid metabolism.

This report describes the combined biochemical and molecular-genetic approaches we have utilized to identify two target genes from oilseeds which, when isolated and transgenically (over) expressed in *B. napus*, might lead to seed oils high in strategic VLCFAs (e.g. trierucin). The first challenge lies in the fact that the lyso-phosphatidic acid acyltransferase or LPAT in *Brassica* species cannot insert erucic acid at the middle (*sn*-2) position on the glycerol backbone. However, other plant species do possess this function and therefore constitute targets for gene retrieval and transgenic expression to give *B. napus* this capability. It may also be necessary

---

* National Research Council of Canada 33534. The authors gratefully acknowledge the contributions of Drs. M.K. Pomeroy, N. Weber and R.J. Weselake and the technical assistance of D. Barton, M. Giblin, L. Hogge, J. Magus, D. Olson, and D. Reed.

to increase the capacity for VLCFA biosynthesis to provide adequate levels of these fatty acids for incorporation into storage oils. Thus, our second target is the "elongase" system, which creates VLCFAs by sequentially elongating C18 fatty acyl precursors.

BIOASSEMBLY OF TAGS CONTAINING VLCFAS IN *BRASSICA NAPUS* L.: THE MICROSPORE-DERIVED EMBRYO MODEL SYSTEM

The TAGs found in *B. napus* L. and other oilseeds of the Brassicaceae have an acyl composition typical of that shown in Fig. 1. VLCFAs such as eicosenoic (20:1) and erucic (22:1) acids are esterified to the *sn*-1 and *sn*-3 positions, but not the *sn*-2 position (Brockerhoff 1971; Norton and Harris 1983). Rather, the latter position is usually esterified with C_{18} fatty acids such as oleic (18:1) acid. While it is generally accepted that in higher plants, C_{16} and C_{18} fatty acyl moieties are incorporated into TAGs via the G-3-P pathway according to Kennedy (Barron and Stumpf 1962; Stymne and Stobart 1987) (Fig. 2), until recently, the mechanism involved in the biosynthesis of TAGs containing VLCFAs was not fully understood, despite a number of studies which attempted to elucidate the pathway in developing oilseeds (Pollard and Stumpf 1980a,b; Mukherjee 1986; Sun et al. 1988; Battey and Ohlrogge 1989; Bernerth and Frentzen 1990; Fehling and Mukherjee 1990). Primarily, the difficulty was due to the fact that, in typical metabolism studies, radiolabeled erucic acid or erucoyl-CoA were very poorly metabolized by developing zygotic embryo preparations in vitro.

In contrast to zygotic embryos, microspore-derived (MD) embryos are haploid and derived, as the name implies, from immature male microspores. Via techniques of tissue culture, the microspores can be "reprogrammed" to undergo embryogenesis in a manner similar to developing zygotic embryos in a fertilized seed (Fan et al. 1988; Pechan and Keller 1988). In particular, MD embryos developed in the high erucic acid cultivar Reston have been shown to accumulate VLCFAs such as 22:1 in TAGs in a manner similar to developing zygotic embryos of the same cultivar (Table 2) (Taylor et al. 1990b; Pomeroy et al. 1991; Taylor et al. 1991; Weber et al. 1992). More importantly, recent studies performed in this laboratory have demonstrated that, in comparison to its zygotic counterpart, the Reston MD embryo system actively metabolizes and incorporates radiolabeled erucoyl moieties into TAGs in vitro (Table 3). We have shown that the MD embryo system possesses all of the enzymes necessary for TAG bioassembly (Taylor et al. 1990b, 1991, 1992a).

We have exploited this model system to demonstrate for the first time, that TAGs containing erucoyl moieties at both the *sn*-1 and *sn*-3 positions in *B. napus* are bioassembled via the Kennedy Pathway, with G-3-P as the initial acceptor and erucoyl-CoA as the acyl donor (Fig. 3) (Taylor et al. 1992a). Furthermore, this mechanism is intimately linked, possibly via metabolite channeling, to de novo VLCFA biosynthesis from oleoyl-CoA via two-carbon extensions in the presence of malonyl-CoA and reducing equivalents. As the ^{14}C very long chain acyl-CoAs are synthesized in vitro, they are incorporated onto the glycerol backbone of G-3-P, into the Kennedy pathway intermediates LPA, PA, DAG and PC, and accumulate in TAGs (Fig 3). In the absence of exogenous G-3-P, there is a dramatic decrease in the incorporation of newly-synthesized VLCFAs into all glycerolipids but especially

Table 1. Industrial uses of trierucin, erucic acid, and derivatives[z].

Trierucin	Pharmaceuticals, lubricants, waxes, heat transfer fluids, dielectric fluids
Erucic acid	Erucamide: slip agent, plasticizers
	Amines: surfactants, antistats, flotation agents, corrosion inhibitors
Behenic acid	Antifriction coatings, mold release agents, flow improvers, mixing and processing aids
Erucyl alcohol	Surfactants, slip and coating agents
Behenyl alcohol	Surfactants, slip and coating agents
Wax esters	Lubricants, cosmetics
Brassylic Acid	Nylons, perfumes, plasticizers, polyesters, synthetic lubricants, paints and coatings
Pelargonic Acid	Plasticizers, plastics, coatings, flavors, perfumes, cosmetics

[z]Modified from Van Dyne et al. (1990).

TRIACYLGLYCEROL

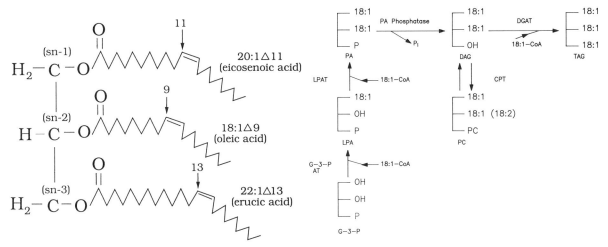

Fig. 1. Structure of a triacylglycerol typical of that found in the Brassicaceae (e.g. *B. napus*), indicating the stereo-chemically-distinct *sn*-1, *sn*-2 and *sn*-3 positions. Erucic acid (22:1) can be esterified at both the *sn*-1 and -3 positions, but is virtually excluded from the *sn*-2 position.

Fig. 2. Scheme for triacylglycerol bioassembly (Kennedy) pathway in developing oilseeds. 18:1-CoA, oleoyl-coenzyme A; 18:2, linoleic acid; G-3-P, glycerol-3-phosphate; G-3-P AT, glycerol-3-phosphate acyltransferase; LPA, lyso-phosphatidic acid; LPAT, lyso-phosphatidic acid acyltransferase; PA, phosphatidic acid; PA phosphatase, phosphatidic acid phosphatase; PC, phosphatidylcholine; DAG, diacylglycerol; DGAT, diacylglycerol acyltransferase; TAG, triacylglycerol; CPT, *sn*-1,2-diacylglycerol cholinephosphotransferase. After desaturation on the PC backbone, polyunsaturated C_{18} fatty acids can enter the acyl-CoA pool via the enzyme acyl-CoA:lyso-phosphatidylcholine acyltransferase (not shown). (Modified from Stymne and Stobart 1987).

Table 2. Proportions of very long chain fatty acids in total lipids from microspore-derived (MD) and zygotic (Z) embryos of *B. napus* cv Reston at different stages of development[z].

Developmental stage	Embryo source	Wt % fatty acid			
		20:0	20:1	22:0	22:1
Microspores		1.4	0.9	1.0	---[y]
Heart	MD	1.9	---	2.0	---
	Z	---	---	---	---
Torpedo	MD	1.8	0.7	1.1	---
	Z	1.3	1.0	1.2	1.2
Early cotyledonary	MD	1.7	2.6	0.3	1.0
	Z	1.3	1.8	0.2	0.6
Mid- cotyledonary	MD	0.9	6.9	0.3	5.0
	Z	1.5	4.0	0.6	2.3
Late cotyledonary	MD	0.8	8.2	0.4	11.1
	Z	1.0	11.9	0.2	13.0
Very late cotyledonary	MD	0.8	11.8	0.3	21.8
	Z	0.7	12.2	0.3	26.4
Seed		0.9	11.2	0.4	32.7

[z]Proportions (wt %) data for other fatty acids not shown.
[y]---not detected. Modified from Pomeroy et al. (1991).

Table 3. Comparison of in vivo and in vitro rates of TAG biosynthesis in developing zygotic and MD embryos of *B. napus* cv. Reston.

	Rate of triacylglycerol biosynthesis (pmol·min⁻¹·mg protein⁻¹)		
	in vivo[z]	in vitro[y]	
Embryo system		homogenate	microsomes
Zygotic	75	6 (8%)[x]	12 (16%)
Microspore-derived	142	166 (117%)	333 (234%)

[z]In vivo rate estimated from measurements of TAG and total protein in developing mid-late cotyledonary stage embryos during the rapid phase of TAG accumulation.

[y]In vitro rate measured in homogenates or microsomal preparations from mid-late cotyledonary stage embryos using the reaction system: G-3-P + 14C 22:1-CoA, and assuming one erucoyl moiety incorporated per TAG (18:1/18:1/14C 22:1) synthesized.

[x]Values in parentheses express the in vitro rate as a percentage of the estimated in vivo rate. Modified from Taylor et al. (1991).

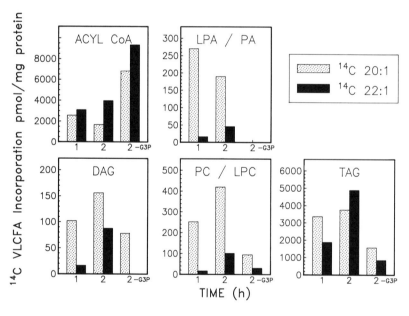

Fig. 3. Incorporation of newly-synthesized very long chain acyl-CoAs into glycerolipids via the Kennedy pathway in *B. napus* cv Reston MD embryos. A 15,000×g particulate fraction prepared from mid-cotlyedonary embryos was incubated with 40 μM ¹⁴C 18:1-CoA and 1 mM malonyl-CoA in the presence of 200 μM G-3-P, 0.5 mM NADH and 0.5 mM NADPH. 2 hour incubations were also conducted under identical conditions except that G-3-P was ommitted from the reaction mixtures (2 -G3P). At each time point, 14C-labeled acyl-CoAs and 14C glycerolipid species containing newly-synthesized VLCFA moieties (▒¹⁴C 20:1; ■¹⁴C 22:1) were isolated and analyzed as described by Taylor et al. (1992a). ¹⁴C 18:1-CoA incorporation data not shown. Modified from Taylor et al. (1992a).

TAGs, and a concomitant build-up of newly-synthesized very long chain acyl-CoAs (Fig. 3, 2 -G-3-P), a finding which strongly supports the key role of G-3-P as the initial acyl acceptor. The Kennedy pathway as the mechanism for the bioassembly of TAGs containing VLCFAs has also been confirmed in zygotic embryos of *B. napus* cv. Reston (Taylor et al. 1992a) and is supported by studies in other cruciferous oilseeds (Fehling et al. 1990). Stereospecific analyses of TAGs biosynthesized in vitro by the Reston MD embryo system following de novo VLCFA biosynthesis from ^{14}C oleoyl-CoA or ^{14}C 20:1-CoA, show that radiolabeled erucoyl moieties are incorporated into the *sn*-1 and *sn*-3 positions, but not the *sn*-2 position (Table 4). This pattern is similar to that found in endogenous TAGs of both MD and zygotic Reston embryos (Taylor et al. 1991). Furthermore, this finding confirms that *B. napus* lacks the enzymic capacity for placing erucoyl moieties into the *sn*-2 position, and indicates that the theoretical breeding limit for erucic acid content in *B. napus* is 2/3 or 66 mole %. Recent breeding efforts at the University of Manitoba have yielded a high erucic acid variety, Hero (Scarth et al. 1991), with an upper limit of about 56% 22:1 (Dr. Rachel Scarth pers. commun.).

ENZYME TARGETS FOR MANIPULATION OF VLCFA LEVELS IN *B. NAPUS*

Lyso-Phosphatidic Acid Acyltransferase (LPAT)

High erucic acid *B. napus* does not have erucoyl moieties at the *sn*-2 position in its seed oil (Brockerhoff 1971), and does not contain trierucin (Fig. 4A). However, within nature there exist examples of species which do have significant proportions of erucic acid at the *sn*-2 position (Table 5). Nasturtium (*Tropaeolum majus*) seed oil contains about 75% erucic acid of which about one third is esterified to the *sn*-2 position (Mattson and Volpenhein 1961). Furthermore, trierucin is the major TAG species in nasturtium, as confirmed in our laboratory by direct probe mass spectrometry of the TAG fraction isolated from mature seed (Fig. 4B). This is encouraging as it indicates that there is no stereochemical constraint preventing the biosynthesis of this triacylglycerol by developing plant embryos. Perhaps the best example of apparent *sn*-2 erucoyl specificity is meadowfoam (*Limnanthes douglasii*) which inserts about two thirds of its erucic acid into this position (Phillips et al. 1971) (Table 5).

Studies in this laboratory (Taylor et al. 1990a) (Table 6) and others (Cao et al. 1990; Löhden et al. 1990) have demonstrated that the accumulation of erucic acid at the *sn*-2 position of TAGs in meadowfoam species is

Table 4. Stereospecific distribution of radioactive acyl moieties in TAGs formed by homogenates of *B. napus* cv. Reston MD embryos[z].

Reaction tested	^{14}C acyl species	Distribution of Radioactivity (%)[y]			
		Position on the glycerol backbone			
		sn-1	*sn*-2	*sn*-3	Total
^{14}C 18:1-CoA +	18:1	31	65	4	100
Malonyl-CoA	20:1	17	10	73	100
	22:1	12	---	88	100
^{14}C 20:1-CoA +	20:1	8	9	83	100
Malonyl-CoA	22:1	13	---	87	100

[z]Homogenates prepared from developing MD embryos of *B. napus* cv. Reston were incubated with G-3-P and either ^{14}C 18:1-CoA or ^{14}C 20:1-CoA in the presence of malonyl-CoA and reducing equivalents. The radiolabeled TAG fraction was isolated and stereospecific analyses performed as described by Taylor et al. (1992a).

[y]Data is expressed as % distribution of each ^{14}C fatty acyl moiety over all three *sn*- positions on the glycerol backbone. Modified from Taylor et al. (1992a).

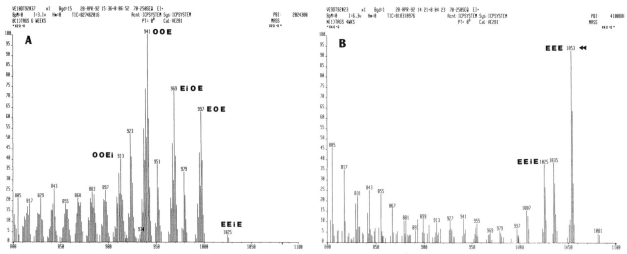

Fig. 4. Direct-probe electron impact mass spectrometry of triacylglycerol (TAG) fractions isolated from developing seed of (A) high erucic acid *B. napus*, cv Reston at 6 weeks post-anthesis; (B) *Tropaeolum majus* (nasturtium), cv dwarf cherry rose at 4 weeks post-anthesis. Mass spectrometry was performed as described by Taylor et al. (1991). Only the molecular ion (M⁺) region is shown. Acyl group assignments were confirmed by MS/MS daughter ion analyses (not shown). The major TAG species are designated as EOE, EiOE etc. for TAGs containing E=erucoyl, Ei=eicosenoyl, and O=oleoyl moieties. Each molecular ion cluster represents TAGs containing combinations of VLCFAs with 18:1, 18:2 or 18:3 on the glycerol backbone. *B. napus* (A) contains molecular ions for monoeicosenoyl (M^+=913), monoerucoyl, (M^+=941), monoeicosenoyl, monoerucoyl (M^+=969), dierucoyl (M^+=997) and dierucoyl, monoeicosenoyl (M^+=1025) TAG species. Trierucin (M^+=1053) is not detected. In contrast, trierucin (EEE, M^+=1053), is the major TAG species detected in *T. majus* (B). All major TAG species display characteristic [M-18]⁺ fragmentation.

Table 5. Content of erucic acid and its *sn*-2 distribution in various oilseeds.

Species	Common name	Total mol % 22:1 in TAGs	Mol % 22:1 at *sn*-2 position	Reference
B. napus	H.E.A. Rapeseed	40-57	Tr-2	Brockerhoff (1971); Norton and Harris (1983); Taylor et al. (1991)
C. abyss.	Abyssinian kale	51	3	Mattson and Volpenhein (1961)
T. majus	Nasturtium	70-75	34	Mattson and Volpenhein (1961)
L. dougl.	Meadowfoam	14-17	67	Phillips et al. (1971)

due to the high erucoyl-CoA specificity of the lyso-phosphatidic acid acyltransferase (LPAT). Based on relative specific activity, the 22:1-CoA:LPAT activity in homogenates or microsomal fractions from meadowfoam was 50 to 100-fold greater than the corresponding activity in *B. napus*. However, the 18:1-CoA:LPAT activities of meadowfoam and rapeseed were essentially identical (Table 6), suggesting that an LPAT highly specific for erucoyl moieties is present in meadowfoam. It is perhaps surprising that the in vitro erucoyl specificity of the nasturtium LPAT was not much higher than that observed in *B. napus* and about an order of magnitude lower than that present in meadowfoam (Taylor et al. 1990a).

We are currently taking two approaches to isolate and characterize the gene encoding the erucoyl-specific LPAT from meadowfoam. The first is a biochemical approach involving the isolation and purification of LPATs from various developing oilseeds followed by the use of either an antibody or oligonucleotide probe (designed after microsequencing) to screen a cDNA library from developing *Limnanthes douglasii* seed. The first step in purifying the enzyme was to find a subcellular fraction enriched in the protein of interest. The erucoyl-CoA specific LPAT from meadowfoam, while probably extra-plastidic, was found to be enriched in a 10,000xg pellet

Table 6. Comparison of relative LPAT activities in vitro in preparations from developing seed of meadowfoam, nasturtium and rapeseed (*B. napus*)[z].

Seed	Relative 22:1-CoA:LPAT activity[z]		Relative 18:1-CoA:LPAT activity[x]
	Homogenate	Microsomal fraction	Homogenate
Meadowfoam	100 (45)[y]	100	100
Nasturtium	12	7	nd[w]
Rapeseed	2 (0)[y]	1	95

[z]Unless otherwise indicated, 22:1-CoA:LPAT reactions were assayed in the presence of 15 μM ^{14}C 22:1-CoA + 45 μM 18:1-LPA; 100% activity for homogenate preparation = 30 pmol/min/mg protein; 100% activity for microsomal fraction = 103 pmol/min/mg protein.

[y]Numbers in brackets indicate activity assayed in the presence of 15 μM ^{14}C 22:1-CoA + 45 μM 22:1-LPA, relative to activity measured in the 15 μM ^{14}C 22:1-CoA + 45 μM 18:1-LPA reaction system.

[x]18:1-CoA:LPAT activity was assayed in the presence of 15 μM ^{14}C 18:1-CoA + 45 μM 18:1-LPA; 100% activity = 185 pmol/min/mg protein.

[w]Not determined. Modified from Taylor et al. (1990a).

fraction, which contained 95% of the total activity originally measured in a homogenate. While the specific activity of this fraction was somewhat lower than that found in a 100,000×g fraction, the overall recovery of total activity in the 10,000×g pellet made it the obvious choice as an enriched fraction for beginning enzyme purification. Thus far, the general protocol shown in Fig. 5 has been used to purify LPATs from developing embryos of meadowfoam and safflower and has yielded enzyme preparations which are purified nearly 1000-fold compared to the crude homogenates. The key factor in the protocol has been the "selective solubilization" of the 10,000×g pellet activity into a 10,000×g supernatant fraction using a combination of detergent treatment and physical dispersion methods. This step alone has yielded an apparent purification, based on specific activity, of >300-fold and has enabled further purification by gel filtration and ion exchange chromotographies. We are now approaching homogeneity with our LPAT preparations.

The second, more recent approach, is a molecular one, in which we hope to functionally complement an LPAT-deficient mutant of *E. coli* (Coleman 1990) with an oilseed gene encoding LPAT. This might be accomplished by direct transformation of competent cells of the mutant microbial host with a plasmid cDNA library, or by infection of the microbial mutant with specialized plant cDNA expression libraries (e.g. λYES *Arabidopsis* library, Elledge et al. 1991).

Once we acquire the meadowfoam LPAT gene, our goal is then to transform *B. napus* to allow the production of trierucin (Fig. 6). Two recent pieces of biochemical evidence from our laboratory are encouraging in this regard: (1) The meadowfoam LPAT will recognize 22:1-*lyso*-phosphatidic acid (22:1-LPA) and can insert erucic acid into the *sn*-2 position (Table 6). As we have shown, 22:1-LPA is an intermediate in the bioassembly of TAGs containing VLCFAs in *B. napus* (Fig. 3). (2) An in vitro experiment designed to simulate transformation of *B. napus* with the meadowfoam LPAT was conducted, in which homogenates or microsomal fractions from *B. napus* MD embryos were supplied with ^{14}C erucoyl-CoA and the non-indigenous 1,2-dierucin. Under these conditions, ^{14}C-labeled trierucin was produced by the *B. napus* system, proving that the 1,2-diacylglycerol acyltransferase (DGAT) was capable of utilizing diacylglycerol with 22:1 at both the *sn*-1 and *sn*-2 positions (Taylor et al. 1992b). Furthermore, the DGAT in MD embryos of *Brassica napus* exhibits a greater specificity for erucoyl-CoA over oleoyl-CoA at concentrations above 5 μM in vitro (Weselake et al. 1991).

Elongase

If the supply of erucic acid for TAG bioassembly is limiting, the targeted transformation of *B. napus* with meadowfoam LPAT as depicted in Fig. 6, may primarily result in a redistribution of existing erucoyl moieties, rather than an accumulation of sufficient trierucin. Thus, in order to be able to manipulate VLCFA levels in transgenic *B. napus*, our second target is the gene encoding the elongase responsible for VLCFA biosynthesis from oleoyl-CoA.

The approach to obtaining this gene is a molecular-genetic one. It involves the isolation of mutants in a small crucifer *Arabidopsis thaliana* deficient in VLCFA biosynthesis, characterization of the mutants to determine whether the elongase gene is marked by a mutation, and if so, cloning this gene using the technique of chromosome walking (Kunst and Underhill 1990). This technique takes advantage of the fact that *A. thaliana* has the smallest known higher plant genome (ca. 100,000 Kb) and possesses very little repetitive DNA (Meyerowitz 1989).

An EMS-mutagenized population of *A. thaliana* seed has been screened by GC and six mutant lines have been isolated with stably-inherited changes in the VLCFA content of seed lipids. Of these, four mutants contained less than 1% 20:1 (wild-type seed contains 18% 20:1), a reduced level of 20:0 and no detectable 22:1 (Kunst and Underhill 1990). Genetic analyses have shown that all the described changes in fatty acid composition of these four mutants are caused by a mutation at the same nuclear locus, *FAE1* (Lemieux et al. 1990). In addition, reciprocal crosses between one of these VLCFA mutants, designated AC56 (Kunst et al. 1992), and wild type have shown that F_1 progeny have VLCFA levels which are intermediate between the wild-type and mutant (Table 7). This incomplete dominance suggests that the amount of available gene product, i.e. "elongase," limits elongation, i.e. VLCFA biosynthesis. In vitro biochemical characterization of AC56, has revealed that, relative to wild-type, seeds of the mutant are deficient in the capacity to biosynthesize ^{14}C labeled 20:1 from ^{14}C 18:1-CoA, ^{14}C 22:1 from ^{14}C 20:1-CoA, and ^{14}C 20:0 from ^{14}C 18:0-CoA, in the presence of malonyl-CoA and reducing equivalents (Table 8) (Kunst et al. 1992).

Since the *FAE1* gene product is involved in the synthesis of all the VLCFAs in *A. thaliana*, we have chosen the *FAE1* gene as the target for isolation by chromosome walking. In preparing to chromosome walk to the *FAE1* locus, its postion has been mapped to chromosome 4 in the region encompassed by the *cer2* and *ap2* morphological markers (Kunst and Underhill 1990). The next step, high resolution mapping relative to appropriate RFLP markers, is currently underway. The RFLP closest to the elongase gene will serve as the starting site for the chromosome walk.

Once the elongase gene from *Arabidopsis* has been isolated, we intend to use it as a probe to isolate the corresponding gene in *B. napus*. Overexpression of the elongase function responsible for VLCFA biosynthesis may be required to produce sufficient trierucin in a transgenic *B. napus* housing the meadowfoam LPAT.

LPAT PURIFICATION

Dissected embryos (meadowfoam, safflower)

Crude homogenate

Centrifuge 10,000 x g, 15 min

Pellet dispersed by detergent + physical methods

Recentrifuged 10,000 x g, 15 min

LPAT "selectively solubilized" into supernatant

Superose 6 (gel filtration); est M_R > 600 - 800 kD

Q Sepharose HP (anion exchange)

Assess purity by PAGE

Fig. 5. General protocol for the purification of lyso-phosphatidic acid acyltransferase (LPAT) from developing oilseeds.

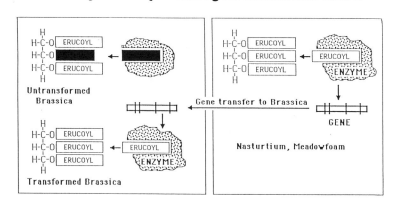

Fig. 6. Scheme for transformation of *B. napus* (breeding limit 66 mol % erucic acid) with a gene for meadowfoam LPAT expressing a high degree of erucoyl specificity, to produce a new ultra-high erucic acid cultivar capable of making trierucin. From National Research Council of Canada Plant Biotechnology Institute Annual Report, 1989–1990.

Table 7. Very long chain fatty acid composition of total lipids of wild type (WT), mutant (AC56), and F_1 (WT x AC56) seeds of *A. thaliana* grown at 22°C[z].

Fatty acid	Content (mol %±SD)[y]		
	Wild type	F_1	AC56
20:0	1.8±0.2	1.1±0.2	0.5±0.2
20:1	18.2±1.2	9.7±1.2	0.8±0.1
22:1	1.6±0.2	0.7±0.1	0.0±0.0

[z]Data for other fatty acids not shown. Modify from Kunst et al. (1992).
[y]n = 5

Table 8. Elongase activities in cell-free extracts of developing seed from wild type (WT) and mutant (AC56) *A. thaliana*[z].

Reaction tested seed line	Activity (nmol ^{14}C acyl product h^{-1} mg protein^{-1})	Relative activity (% of WT)
^{14}C 18:1-CoA elongation		
WT	12.9	100
AC56	0.2	1.6
^{14}C 20:1-CoA elongation		
WT	2.0	100
AC56	0	0
^{14}C 18:0-CoA elongation		
WT	6.8	100
AC56	0.5	7.4

[z]Aliquots of filtered seed homogenate (50 to 200 µg protein) were incubated at 30°C for 1 hour. Values are the means of 2 to 3 replicates in 2 to 4 independent experiments. ^{14}C 20:1, ^{14}C 22:1 and ^{14}C 20:0 were the products of ^{14}C 18:1-CoA, ^{14}C 20:1-CoA and ^{14}C 18:0-CoA elongation reactions, respectively, conducted in the presence of malonyl-CoA and reductant.

CONCLUDING REMARKS

Using the Reston MD embryo model system, we have established a biochemical baseline for the mechanism by which TAGs containing VLCFAs are made in high erucic acid *B. napus*. Modification of rapeseed through biotechnology would offer the opportunity to produce ultra-high erucic acid seed oils which can provide renewable, biodegradable industrial feedstocks and allow agricultural diversification for the Canadian farmer. A number of strategies combining techniques in biochemistry, genetics, and molecular biology are being exploited to achieve this goal in a program focused on the isolation and transgenic expression of genes encoding two target enzymes: meadowfoam LPAT and *B. napus* elongase. Clearly, the *B. napus* germplasm of choice for transformation with these target genes will be cultivars already optimized for the maximum erucic acid content (approaching 66 mol %) through plant breeding efforts.

REFERENCES

Barron, E.J. and P.K. Stumpf. 1962. The biosynthesis of triglycerides by avocado mesocarp enzymes. Biochim. Biophys. Acta 60:329–337.

Battey, J.F. and J.B. Ohlrogge. 1989. A comparison of the metabolic fate of fatty acids of different chain lengths in developing oilseeds. Plant Physiol. 90:835–840.

Bernerth, R. and M. Frentzen. 1990. Utilization of erucoyl-CoA by acyltransferases from developing seeds of *Brassica napus* (L.) involved in triacylglycerol biosynthesis. Plant Sci. 67:21–28.

Brockerhoff, H. 1971. Stereospecific analysis of triacylglycerides. Lipids 6:942–956.

Cao, Y-Z., K-C. Oo, and A.H.C. Huang. 1990. Lysophosphatidate acyltransferase in the microsomes from maturing seeds of meadowfoam (*Limnanthes alba*). Plant Physiol. 94:1199–1206.

Coleman, J. 1990. Characterization of *Escherichia coli* cells deficient in 1-acyl-*sn*-glycerol-3-phosphate acyltransferase activity. J. Biol. Chem. 265:17215–17221.

Elledge, S.J., J.T.Mulligan, S.W. Ramer, M. Spottswood, and R.W. Davis. 1991. λYes: A multifunctional cDNA expression vector for the isolation of genes by complementation of yeast and *Escherichia coli* mutations. Proc. Natl. Acad. Sci. (USA) 88:1731–1735.

Fan, Z., K.C. Armstrong, and W.A. Keller. 1988. Development of microspores in vivo and in vitro in *Brassica napus* L. Protoplasma 147:191–199.

Fehling. E. and K.D. Mukherjee. 1990. Biosynthesis of triacylglycerols containing very long chain monounsaturated fatty acids in seeds of *Lunaria annua*. Phytochemistry 29:1525–1527.

Fehling. E., D.J. Murphy, and K.D. Mukherjee. 1990. Biosynthesis of triacylglycerols containing very long chain monounsaturated acyl moieties in developing seeds. Plant Physiol. 94:492–498.

Griffiths, G., S. Stymne, and K. Stobart. 1988. Biosynthesis of triglycerides in plant storage tissue, p 23–29. In: T.H. Applewhite (ed.). Proceedings of the world conference on biotechnology for the fats and oil industry. Amer. Oil Chem. Soc., Champaign, IL.

Kunst, L. and E.W. Underhill. 1990. Cloning *FAE1*, a gene which controls fatty acid elongation in seeds of *Arabidopsis thaliana*, by chromosome walking, p 28. In: J.R. McFerson, S. Kresovich, and S.G. Dwyer (eds.). Sixth crucifer genetics workshop proceedings, 6–9 October, 1990. USDA/ARS Plant Genetic Resources Unit, Cornell University, Geneva, NY.

Kunst, L., D.C. Taylor, and E.W. Underhill. 1992. Fatty acid elongation in developing seeds of *Arabidopsis thaliana*. Plant Physiol. and Biochem. 30(4):425–434.

Lemieux, B., M. Miquel, C. Somerville, and J. Browse. 1990. Mutants of *Arabidopsis* with alterations in seed lipid fatty acid composition. Theor. Appl. Genet. 80:234–240.

Löhden, I., R. Bernerth, and M. Frentzen. 1990. Acyl-CoA:1-acylglycerol-3-phosphate acyltransferase from developing seeds of *Limnanthes douglasii* (R.Br.) and *Brassica napus* (L.), p 175–177. In: P.J. Quinn and J.L. Harwood (eds.). Plant lipid biochemistry, structure and utilization. Portland Press Ltd., London.

Mattson, F.H. and R.A. Volpenhein. 1961. The specific distribution of fatty acids in the glycerides of vegetable fats. J. Biol. Chem. 236:1891–1894.

Meyerowitz, E.M. 1989. *Arabidopsis*, a useful weed. Cell 56:265–269.

Mukherjee, K.D. 1986. Glycerolipid synthesis by homogenate and oil bodies from developing mustard (*Sinapis alba* L.) seed. Planta 167:279–283.

Norton, G. and J.F. Harris. 1983. Triacylglycerols in oilseed rape during seed development. Phytochemistry 12:2703–2707.

Pechan, P.M. and W.A. Keller. 1988. Identification of potentially embryogenic microspores in *Brassica napus*. Physiol. Plant. 74:377–384.

Phillips, B.E., C.R. Smith Jr., and W.H. Tallent. 1971. Glycerides of *Limnanthes douglasii* seed oil. Lipids 6:93–99.

Pollard, M.R. and P.K. Stumpf. 1980a. Long chain (C_{20} and C_{22}) fatty acid biosynthesis in developing seeds of *Tropaeolum majus*. An in vivo study. Plant Physiol. 66:641–648.

Pollard, M.R., and P.K. Stumpf. 1980b. Biosynthesis of C_{20} and C_{22} fatty acids in developing seeds of *Limnanthes alba*. Chain elongation and Δ 5 desaturation. Plant Physiol. 66:649–655.

Pomeroy, M.K., J.K.G. Kramer, D.J. Hunt, and W.A. Keller. 1991. Fatty acid changes during development of zygotic and microspore-derived embryos of *Brassica napus*. Physiol. Plant. 81:447–454.

Princen, L.H. and J.A. Rothfus. 1984. Development of new crops for industrial raw materials. J. Amer. Oil Chem. Soc. 61:281–289.

Roughan, P.G. and C.R. Slack. 1982. Cellular organization of glycerolipid metabolism. Annu. Rev. Plant Physiol. 33:97–132.

Scarth, R., P.B.E. McVetty, S.R. Rimmer, and B.R. Stefansson. 1991. Hero summer rape. Can. J. Plant Sci. 71:865–866.

Sonntag, N.O.V. 1991. Erucic, behenic: Feedstocks of the 21st century. Inform 2:449–463.

Stymne, S. and A.K. Stobart. 1987. Triacylglycerol biosynthesis, p 175–214. In: P.K. Stumpf and E.E. Conn (eds.). The biochemistry of plants: Lipids, Vol. 9. Academic Press, New York.

Sun, C., Y-Z. Cao, and A.H.C. Huang. 1988. Acyl coenzyme A preference of the glycerol phosphate pathway in the microsomes from the maturing seeds of palm, maize and rapeseed. Plant Physiol. 88:56–60.

Taylor, D.C., L.W. Thomson, S.L. MacKenzie, M.K. Pomeroy, and R.J. Weselake. 1990a. Target enzymes for modification of seed storage lipids, p 38–39. In: J.R. McFerson, S. Kresovich, and S.G. Dwyer (eds.). Sixth crucifer genetics workshop proceedings, 6–9 October, 1990. USDA/ARS Plant Genet. Resources Unit, Cornell University, Geneva, NY.

Taylor, D.C., N. Weber, E.W. Underhill, M.K. Pomeroy, W.A. Keller, W.R. Scowcroft, R. W. Wilen, M.M. Moloney, and L.A. Holbrook. 1990b. Storage protein regulation and lipid accumulation in microspore embryos of *Brassica napus* L. Planta 181:18–26.

Taylor, D.C., N. Weber, D.L. Barton, E.W. Underhill, L.R. Hogge, R.J. Weselake, and M.K. Pomeroy. 1991. Triacylglycerol bioassembly in microspore-derived embryos of *Brassica napus* L. cv. Reston. Plant Physiol. 97:65–79.

Taylor, D.C., D.L. Barton, K.P. Rioux, S.L. MacKenzie, D.W. Reed, E.W. Underhill, M.K. Pomeroy, and N. Weber. 1992a. Biosynthesis of acyl lipids containing very long chain fatty acids in microspore-derived and zygotic embryos of *Brassica napus* L. cv. Reston. Plant Physiol. 99:1609–1618.

Taylor, D.C., N. Weber, L.R. Hogge, E.W. Underhill, and M.K. Pomeroy. 1992b. Formation of trierucoylglycerol (trierucin) from 1,2-dierucoylglycerol by a homogenate of microspore-derived embryos of *Brassica napus* L. J. Amer. Oil Chem. Soc. 69:355–358.

United States Department of Agriculture Co-operative State Research Service. 1990. High erucic acid oil: from farm to factory. United States Department of Agriculture, Washington, DC.

Van Dyne, D.L., M.G. Blase, and K.D. Carlson. 1990. Industrial feedstocks and products from high erucic acid oil: Crambe and industrial rapeseed. Dept. of Agricultural Economics, Univ. of Missouri–Columbia Printing Services.

Weber, N., D.C. Taylor, and E.W. Underhill. 1992. Biosynthesis of storage lipids in plant cell and embryo cultures, p 99–131. In: A. Feichter (ed.). Advances in biochemical engineering /biotechnology, Vol. 45. Springer-Verlag, Berlin.

Weselake, R.J., D.C. Taylor, M.K. Pomeroy, S.L. Lawson, and E.W. Underhill. 1991. Properties of diacylglycerol acyltransferase from microspore-derived embryos of *Brassica napus*. Phytochemistry 30:3533–3538.

Engineering New Domestic Sources of Natural Rubber

Katrina Cornish, Zhiqang Pan, and Ralph A. Backhaus

Natural rubber is considered a vital raw material by developed countries and is valued for its high performance characteristics. Synthetic rubber, derived from petroleum, is not as elastic or resilient and does not have the heat transfer properties of natural rubber. Although synthetic rubber is often blended with natural rubber, various products, such as airplane tires, cannot be made without the natural form. Also, synthetic rubber is a non-renewable resource whereas natural rubber should be available indefinitely from renewable plant sources. The only commercial source of natural rubber, at the moment, is the Brazilian rubber tree [*Hevea brasiliensis* (A. Juss.) Mill. Arg.]. The rubber is harvested by tapping into the pipe-like network of latex-containing laticifers that run beneath the bark, a labor-intensive procedure. The expense of tapping and the tree's tropical growth requirements make *H. brasiliensis* unsuitable for cultivation within the United States. However, because natural rubber is the second most costly raw material imported into the United States after petroleum, there is strong commercial incentive to develop a domestic rubber crop. Moreover, as plantation-grown *H. brasiliensis* is derived from clonal material grafted onto seedling root stocks all plants of a commercial line are genetically identical to each other. Thus, *H. brasiliensis* is vulnerable to crop failure should a particularly virulent disease arise. An alternative rubber crop capable of rapid scale up, using fast-growing annual plants or fermentation in a bioreactor, could furnish a protective buffer in the event of an import shortfall. Even if the crop was not profitable initially, the commercial competitiveness of domestic rubber should steadily improve if natural rubber prices increase as anticipated (Greek 1992).

We are attempting to develop a domestic source of natural rubber using a biotechnological approach. To this end, we intend to clarify the biochemistry of rubber formation and identify and isolate the enzymes and genes responsible for the *cis*-1,4-polymerization of isoprene unique to rubber producing plants. Once accomplished, it should be possible to isolate, then insert and express the appropriate genes into annual plants and/or microorganisms. These systems would then be optimized to produce large amounts of high quality rubber.

A considerable body of information exists on the biological mechanism of rubber biosynthesis and on the adjacent portions of the isoprenoid pathway. This includes the isolation and cloning of genes for enzymes involved in the production of allylic pyrophosphate initiators for new rubber molecules (Anderson et al. 1989a,b). However, before transformation experiments on potential domestic rubber-producing species can be realistically begun, a definitive isolation of the rubber transferase enzyme responsible for rubber molecule elongation, and then its gene, is required.

Parthenium argentatum Gray (guayule) is a promising candidate for a domestic commercial source as it produces high quality rubber in its bark. Unlike, *H. brasiliensis*, which has the complex laticiferous anatomy to support its rubber production (d'Auzac et al. 1989), *P. argentatum* simply produces rubber in generalized parenchyma cells in its bark tissue (Backhaus 1985). Furthermore, *P. argentatum* is native to the warm arid regions of the southwestern United States and is being cultivated there in various preliminary trials. Disadvantages exist in obtaining the rubber from this perennial species as the destructive harvest of mature plants is required. Woody shrubs, at least three years old, must be ground up before the rubber can be extracted. Also, high yields only result when the crop is irrigated and fertilized, and *P. argentatum* cannot tolerate the severe winters of the northern United States. These characteristics of the crop make it unsuitable for an emergency supply as it could not be rapidly scaled up. Nonetheless, this species is a good model system for studying rubber biosynthesis, and provides a source of genes that may be useful in increasing its own rubber yield and/or for transformation of other species.

NATURAL RUBBER BIOSYNTHESIS

Natural rubber biosynthesis is a side-branch of the ubiquitous isoprenoid pathway (Fig. 1). Natural rubber is made almost entirely of isoprene units derived from the precursor isopentenyl pyrophosphate (IPP). Also, *trans*-allylic pyrophosphates are essential for rubber formation as they are used to initiate all new rubber molecules. The elongation of the rubber molecule is catalyzed by the enzyme *rubber transferase* (RuT) (EC 2.5.1.20)

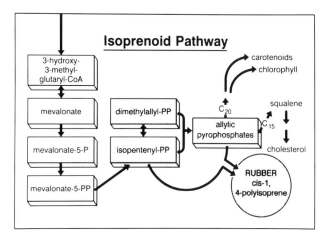 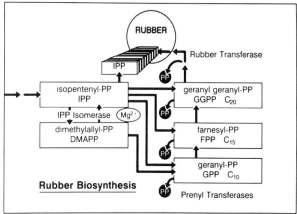

Fig. 1. A section of the isoprenoid pathway illustrating the position of natural rubber biosynthesis.

Fig. 2. The biosynthesis of natural rubber from isopentenyl pyrophosphate. Each new molecule of *cis*-1,4-polyisoprene requires an allylic pyrophosphate initiator before the isoprene units from IPP can be polymerized.

(Backhaus 1985). We do not know where the rate-limiting steps in rubber biosynthesis are located. Simply adding more RuT to a rubber-producing plant may not enhance its yield. We may need to overexpress earlier portions of the isoprenoid pathway to supply adequate substrate levels to support an increased level of rubber biosynthesis. It will also be necessary to ensure that the vital downstream portions of the isoprenoid pathway are not made substrate deficient by increased activity of the rubber biosynthesis branch.

The first biochemical step essential for, though not unique to, rubber biosynthesis is the isomerization of the C_5 IPP to dimethylallyl pyrophosphate (DMAPP) by the enzyme IPP-isomerase (Fig. 2). This is followed by prenyl transferase-catalyzed synthesis of the C_{10} (geranyl pyrophosphate, GPP), C_{15} (farnesyl pyrophosphate, FPP) and C_{20} (geranyl geranyl pyrophosphate, GGPP) allylic pyrophosphates by a series of additions of IPP (nonallylic pyrophosphate) in the *trans* configuration, to DMAPP. The prenyl transferases and the IPP-isomerase are soluble cytosolic or chloroplastic enzymes. In vivo, RuT appears to use FPP or GGPP to initiate rubber molecule formation (Tanaka 1989) although all the allylic pyrophosphates, from the C_5 DMAPP to the C_{20} GGPP, can initiate rubber molecule formation in vitro (Archer and Audley 1987; Berndt 1963; Cornish 1992; Madhaven et al. 1989). Once the initiator is in place, RuT can then begin the *cis*-elongation of isoprene units from IPP. Simply put, the longer the rubber chain, the greater the quality of the finished product. The highest quality rubber has a molecular weight of around 1.5 million.

There are over 2,000 species of plants from about 300 genera as well as at least two fungal genera (Archer et al. 1963; Backhaus 1985) that are known to make natural rubber but most make a short-chain form. A termination step, probably independent of RuT itself, may well govern chain length. Thus, a biological system transformed with the RuT gene from a high molecular weight species, may still generate short chain (poor quality) rubber unless termination is regulated.

LOCALIZATION OF RUBBER TRANSFERASE

In order to isolate the RuT enzyme, it is first necessary to determine the location of the enzymatic reaction. Rubber is compartmentalized into cytosolic rubber particles both in laticiferous species such as *H. brasiliensis* (d'Auzac et al. 1989), and in species that produce rubber in parenchyma cells such as in the bark of *P. argentatum* (Backhaus 1985). These two species are unusual among rubber-producers as they both can make commercial-grade rubber. During rubber biosynthesis, isopentenyl pyrophosphate is obtained from the aqueous environment outside the rubber particles and is dephosphorylated and polymerized by the RuT enzyme. The developing isoprene polymers extend into the particle interior. This process can be assayed by following the incorporation of labeled isoprene from ^{14}C-IPP into the newly-synthesized rubber chains (e.g. Archer and Audley 1987; Cornish and Backhaus 1990).

The nature of the reaction intimates that it takes place at the surface of the rubber particles. However, RuT may be cytosolic and associated only loosely with the particle or it may be particle-bound. This question was addressed experimentally using isolated rubber particles. Particles were prepared from both *H. brasiliensis* and from *P. argentatum* using a centrifugation/flotation procedure (Cornish and Backhaus 1990). Repeated washes, using this procedure, allowed the removal of soluble cytoplasmic components from the latex or bark homogenate. The isolated particles were then assayed for their RuT activity by incubating them in the presence of IPP and an allylic pyrophosphate initiator. When *P. argentatum* rubber particles were incubated with IPP and FPP no reduction of RuT activity was observed with washing, demonstrating the presence of a highly active bound RuT (Cornish and Backhaus 1990). Similar experiments demonstrated a bound RuT on *H. brasiliensis* rubber particles (K. Cornish unpubl. data), as has previously been reported (Archer et al. 1963; Berndt 1963). The bound RuT accounts for most, if not all, of the RuT activity in *H. brasiliensis* latex (K. Cornish unpubl. data). As no reduction of RuT activity with increasing purification of rubber particles was observed for either species, the RuT molecules are firmly associated with rubber particles in both *H. brasiliensis* (Archer et al. 1963; Berndt 1963) and *P. argentatum* (Benedict et al. 1990; Cornish and Backhaus 1990).

H. brasiliensis latex contains the prenyl transferases and IPP-isomerase necessary (Fig. 2) for initiator synthesis and some incorporation of label was observed when ^{14}C-IPP was added to the latex. However, washing the particles to remove the cytoplasmic components of the latex completely eliminates this activity. Without the control treatment, where allylic pyrophosphate added back to the washed rubber particles more than restored the original whole latex level of rubber biosynthesis (K. Cornish unpubl. data), it would be easy to misinterpret the results as meaning that the washing procedure had removed RuT itself, instead of the initiator system. An overview of this aspect of rubber biochemistry and a discussion of possible misinterpretations in the published literature, has been presented in detail (Cornish 1992).

PARTICLE-BOUND RUBBER TRANSFERASE

Although these biochemical assays of rubber biosynthesis were obtained using intact rubber particles, instead of a purified RuT enzyme, the bound-RuT activity does behave as a single enzyme system. The dependence of RuT activity upon substrate concentration, in both *P. argentatum* and *H. brasiliensis* and for several different allylic pyrophosphate initiators, IPP and various cofactors, has simple enzyme kinetics, giving rise to linear Eadie-Hofstee plots (Cornish and Backhaus 1990; K. Cornish unpubl. data). If a multicomponent system was present, these plots of V against V/[S] would generate curved instead of straight lines. The experiments also showed that the substrate binding characteristics of RuT from both species are extremely similar, suggesting that the active site of the two RuT enzymes may also be closely related (Cornish 1992). The RuT catalytic site is probably contained within a single enzyme or enzyme complex because two spatially separate active sites would be unlikely to permit the two different initiation and elongation substrates to be attached to each other.

Protein analysis of isolated rubber particles has been attempted in efforts to distinguish the RuT enzyme from the other particle-bound proteins (Benedict et al. 1990; Backhaus et al. 1991). Despite the biochemical similarity of the *P. argentatum* and *H. brasiliensis* rubber biosynthetic systems, the particle-bound protein profiles proved quite distinct. Silver-stained one-dimensional SDS-PAGE analysis of washed rubber particles revealed at least 20 distinct proteins associated with *H. brasiliensis* particles (K. Cornish unpubl. data) but only 4 to 8 in *P. argentatum* (Backhaus et al. 1991). As it has proved difficult to obtain solubilized RuT activity from the particles it should prove much easier to isolate RuT from amongst the 4 to 8 *P. argentatum* proteins than from amongst the much larger number of *H. brasiliensis* particle-bound proteins.

A PARTICLE-BOUND 48.5 KD PROTEIN FROM GUAYULE

The *P. argentatum* particle-bound 48.5 kD glycoprotein (RPP) is of most interest at present for several reasons. This protein is located largely within the particle but at the surface with the glycosylated moiety protruding into the cytoplasm (Backhaus et al. 1991). This is an appropriate locale for RuT, which must polymerize a hydrophobic molecule to the particle interior while obtaining hydrophilic substrates from the cytosol.

It is also the most abundant particle-bound protein and is present in all ages and lines of *P. argentatum* examined so far (Backhaus et al. 1991; Cornish and Backhaus 1990). Furthermore, other workers have reported solubilized RuT activity associated with this protein (Benedict et al. 1990).

MOLECULAR CLONING OF THE RPP GENE.

The RPP protein was purified to homogeneity from washed rubber particles using preparative SDS-PAGE and electroelution. The purified RPP was then sent to the University of California, Davis, Sequencing Laboratory for analysis. The amino acid composition was consistent with RPP being a membrane protein, and the calculated pI of 6.17 matched the pI of 6.2 determined earlier with isoelectric focusing (Backhaus et al. 1991). As the N-terminus of intact RPP was blocked, the protein was cleaved with cyanogen bromide at its five methionine residues and the resulting six peptide fragments were sequenced. Oligonucleotides corresponding to sequences determined were synthesized and used to prime plus and minus strand amplification of *P. argentatum* bark cDNA, using the polymerase chain reaction (PCR). The longest clone, c18, so far obtained from a *P. argentatum* stembark lambda ZAP cDNA library, accounts for 70% of the RPP gene and includes 4 out of the six peptide fragments obtained from the CNBr digests (Z. Pan and R.A. Backhaus unpubl. data).

Once the full-length gene has been obtained transformation experiments using *P. argentatum* and other species will be performed in attempts to increase rubber yield and to determine, conclusively, the role of RPP. This should be possible because *P. argentatum* has been successfully transformed with GUS and kanamycin resistance using *Agrobacteria* (Backhaus et al. in press).

CONCLUSIONS

In conclusion, RuT is bound to the rubber particle in both species examined, and this may prove to be true for all rubber-producing species. Rubber biosynthesis is biochemically indistinguishable in *P. argentatum* and *H. brasiliensis*. This suggests that the RuT may be alike in these two species and that their RuT genes may be readily interchangeable. The most abundant protein bound to *P. argentatum* rubber particles is a 48.5 kD glycoprotein positioned just beneath the particle surface. Evidence suggests that this protein is RuT, and 70% of its gene has now been isolated.

REFERENCES

Anderson, M.S., M. Muehlbacher, I.P. Street, J. Proffitt, and C.D. Poulter. 1989a. Isopentenyl diphosphate:dimethylallyl diphosphate isomerase. An improved purification of the enzyme and isolation of the gene from *Saccharomyces cerevisiae*. J. Biol. Chem. 264:19169–19175.

Anderson, M.S., J.G. Yarger, C.L. Burck, and C.D. Poulter. 1989b. Farnesyl diphosphate synthetase. Molecular cloning, sequence, and expression of an essential gene from *Saccharomyces cerevisiae*. J. Biol. Chem. 264:19176–19184.

d'Auzac, J., J.L. Jacob, and H. Chrestin. 1989. Physiology of rubber tree latex. CRC Press, Boca Raton, FL.

Archer, B.L. and B.G. Audley. 1987. New aspects of rubber biosynthesis. Bot. J. Linn. Soc. 94:181–196.

Archer, B.L., B.G. Audley, E.G. Cockbain, and G.P. McSweeney. 1963. The biosynthesis of rubber. Biochem. J. 89:565–574.

Backhaus, R.A. 1985. Rubber formation in plants—a mini-review. Israel J. Bot. 34:283–293.

Backhaus, R.A., K. Cornish, S-F Chen, D-S Huang, and V.H. Bess. 1991. Purification and characterization of an abundant rubber particle protein from guayule. Phytochemistry 30:2493–2497.

Backhaus, R.A., J. Ho, Z. Pan, and D-S Huang. 1992. Agrobacterium-mediated transformation of guayule (*Parthenium argentatum*) and regeneration of transgenic plants. Plant Cell Rpt. (in press).

Benedict, C.R., S. Madahavan, G.A. Greenblatt, K.V. Venekatachalam, and M.A. Foster. 1990. The enzymatic synthesis of rubber polymer in *Parthenium argentatum* Gray. Plant Physiol. 92:816–821.

Berndt, J. 1963. The biosynthesis of rubber. U.S. Government Res. Rpt. AD-601729.

Cornish, K. 1992. Natural rubber biosynthesis: a branch of the isoprenoid pathway in plants. In: W.D. Nes, E.J. Parish, and J.M. Trzaskos (eds.). Regulation of isopentenoid metabolism. ACS Symposium series, Vol. X.

Cornish, K. and R.A. Backhaus. 1990. Rubber transferase activity in rubber particles of guayule. Phytochemistry 29:3809–3813.

Greek, B.F. 1992. Rubber demand is expected to grow after 1991. Chem. Eng. News 69:37–54.

Madhavan, S., G.A. Greenblatt, M.A. Foster, and C.R. Benedict 1989. Stimulation of isopentenyl pyrophosphate incorporation into polyisoprene in extracts from guayule plants (*Parthenium argentatum* Gray) by low temperature and 2-(3,4-dichloro-phenoxy)triethylamine. Plant Physiol. 89:506–511.

Tanaka, Y. 1989. Structure and biosynthesis mechanism of natural polyisoprene. Prog. Polym. Sci. 14:339–371

CEREALS AND PSEUDOCEREALS

Pearl Millet: New Feed Grain Crop*

David J. Andrews, John F. Rajewski, and K. Anand Kumar

Pearl millet, [*Pennisetum glaucum* (L.) R. Br.] also known as bulrush or cattail millet, is the most important of a number of unrelated millet species grown for food worldwide on a total of 40 million ha (FAO 1986). Though figures are not available for separate species in all countries, pearl millet is grown on about 26 million ha in the warm tropics divided equally between Africa, particularly in the West African Sahel region, and the Indian subcontinent. In these areas, pearl millet is grown almost exclusively as human food, and indeed is the staple cereal of 90 million people who live in agroclimatic zones where there are severe stress limitations to crop production due mainly to heat, low and erratic rainfall, and soil type. Since fertilizers are not used and cultivation is by hand or animals, actual grain yields are low in these regions (~500 to 600 kg/ha), yet they are higher and more reliably obtained than from other possible tropical dryland cereal crops such as sorghum or maize. Grain is always the principal object of cultivation, but the stover is secondarily important as animal fodder, and stems can be used as fuel, fencing, and roofing.

CLASSIFICATION AND DOMESTICATION

Pearl millet is a cereal belonging to the genus *Pennisetum* which contains about 140 grassy tropical species. Previous names have been *P. typhoides* (Burm) Stapf. & Hubb., *P. typhoideum* (L.) Rich., and *P. americanum* (L.) Leeke, possibly because Clusius, in 1601, thought the type specimen he obtained from southern Spain had come from the Americas.

It is generally agreed that pearl millet was domesticated in Africa, probably on the southern edge of the Sahara, west of the Nile, some 3,000 to 5,000 years ago and subsequently spread to southern Asia (Harlan 1975; Brunken et al. 1977). The gene flow from probable progenitor wild species [spp. *monodii* (syn. *P. violaceum* Maire)] still occurs in West Africa, where weedy segregates (spp. *stenostachyum* Klotzsch) are common in cultivated varieties. The frequency of occurrence of these segregates declines through eastern to southern Africa, and they are absent in Asia.

BIOLOGY AND ADAPTATION

Pearl millet is a highly tillering, cross-pollinating diploid tropical C_4 cereal with grain on the surface of erect candle shaped terminal spikes. Grain size varies from 0.5 to over 2.0 g/100, and, depending on head size, grain number per head ranges from 500 to 3,000. Pearl millet tillers freely, compensating well for stand irregularities, and produces 2 or 3 times more heads per plant than sorghum at similar plant populations.

Three germplasm pools are recognized in respect of cultivated pearl millet (Harlan and de Wet 1971). The primary pool contains all cultivated, weedy, and wild diploid ($2n = 14$) pearl millets which are freely cross-fertile. The secondary pool is solely *P. purpureum* (Shum.) ($2n = 28$), elephant or Napier grass, a vigorous perennial species also from Africa. The cross between pearl millet and elephant grass is easily made (but is sterile unless the chromosome number is artificially doubled) and is widely used as a forage propagated by cuttings. Hanna (1990, 1991b) has demonstrated that part of the *purpureum* genome can be usefully transferred to pearl millet. The tertiary pool contains numerous more distantly related *Pennisetum* species of various ploidy levels which do not naturally interbreed with the primary pool, but can potentially be accessed through various wide crosses (Dujardin and Hanna 1989, 1990).

The cultivated gene pool in pearl millet contains a truly enormous range of genetic variability with no incompatibility and few linkage problems. Many important physiological and morphological traits essential for breeding a crop suitable for combine harvesting are readily available. These are reduced plant height and early maturity—independent of photoperiodic control, synchrony of tiller flowering, angle of tillering, stem and

---

*Joint contribution of the Department of Agronomy, University of Nebraska, research in part supported by USAID S&T Grant No. DAN-1254-00-0021-00 to INTSORMIL, and International Crops Research Institute for the Semi-Arid Tropics (ICRISAT).

peduncle thickness, peduncle length, grain color (white or cream simply dominant over gray), and mesocotyl length. Ample variation exists for head size (length × diameter) and grain number and size though, as expected, correlations between yield components are large and negative.

In areas where frost-kill can occur before harvest, standability is crucial. Both peduncle and stem lodging resistance are evident in inbred stocks, but most material is susceptible and this is one trait which will require much breeding attention. Differences in tolerance to some herbicides (propachlor and atrazine) have been noted and incorporated in selection and breeding strategies.

BREEDING

The floral morphology, breeding behavior and the structure of grain yield in pearl millet make it one of the most flexible and responsive crop species to breed. It appears possible to access genetic variability both from the secondary and tertiary germplasm pools (Hanna 1990; Dujardin and Hanna 1989, 1990). Pearl millet has relatively few large chromosomes and RFLP and RAPD techniques can be used (R.L. Smith pers. commun.).

Pearl millet is a naturally cross-pollinating species, which is achieved through protogyny, since all the sessile flowers on each head are perfect (i.e. both male and female fertile). On any one head, all flowers first exert stigmas over a 1 to 3 day period progressing from the mid-top to the bottom of the head. Anthesis occurs one to as many as 4 days later, in the same sequence from the same flowers, and sometimes, later from the pedicellate flowers. Thus, there is a period for each head, when flowers can only be fertilized by external pollen which is freely wind-born. Stigmas wither about 8 h after pollination. Self-pollination can occur when stigma emergence on later flowering tillers overlaps with the anthesis of earlier heads on the same plant. In random-mating situations (as in landrace cultivar populations or breeder created populations—synthetics or composites), the amount of self-pollination (considerations of common parentage and effective population size apart) is influenced by the degree of tillering, relative size and flowering relationships of tillers, and whether all or only primary tillers are harvested. As a generality, about 20% selfing is normal (Burton 1974; Chirwa 1991).

Selfed seed in pearl millet can be produced simply by placing a bag over a head prior to stigma emergence. If the stigmas are not short lived, 100% selfed seed set will then occur. Similarly, 100% hybrid seed can be made by pollinating a previously bagged head once at full protogyny prior to anther emergence. The breeding opportunities in pearl millet can be illustrated by the following: each of 3 heads on one plant in a population (tillering can be promoted by planting at reduced density) can be used for different objectives—one can be selfed, one crossed (full-sib, testcross, topcross) and one left to random-mate. Seed from each head will be sufficient to plant 20 plots each of 7.5 m^2.

At least four cytoplasmic-genic systems causing male sterility (CMS) are available in pearl millet (Kumar and Andrews 1984; Hanna 1989). The first and currently most widely used source (now termed A_1) was discovered by Burton (1958) in Tifton, Georgia, and released as Tift 23A in 1965 (Burton 1965). All forage hybrids in the United States are made with this CMS system. Its most extensive use, however, has been in grain hybrids in India, where an average of over 2 million ha have been grown annually over the last 23 years.

New lines in which male sterility is stable in all environments are difficult to breed in the A_1 system and have never been obtained with A_2 and A_3. The A_m source (Hanna 1989) using *monodii* cytoplasm is more stable and appears easier to breed, but restorers are scarce and hybrids have not been widely tested. An additional source of CMS has been reported by Marchais and Pernes (1985) but its relationship with others has not been established.

Pearl millet resembles maize in many respects in regard to gene action in performance traits. In general, additive effects are larger than non-additive effects, which can however be significant. Inbreeding depression is large—some 30% from one generation of selfing in populations (Khadr and El-Rouby 1978; Rai et al. 1984); however, vigorous inbred lines yielding 60 to 70% of open-pollinated cultivars of comparable maturity can be selected. As a generality, good hybrids will yield 20 to 30% more than the best open-pollinated cultivars of comparable maturity (Table 1) (Andrews and Rajewski 1990, 1991; Dave 1986).

With the correct selection of parent lines in regard to phenotype and relative maturity, hybrids can also be made in pearl millet by utilizing the natural period of protogyny. This method allows quicker hybrid development, greatly increases the range of possible parent combinations, and avoids diseases which are associated, particularly

Table 1. Mean grain yields in 1990 pearl millet regional grain yield trial.

Entry	Mean grain yield (kg/ha)					
	Georgia Tifton	Indiana Lafayette	Kansas Hays	Nebraska Mead	Sidney	North Dakota Carrington
MLS variety	2640	2990	2340	3120	3540	3090
68A x MLS[z]	2300	3790	3120	4130	4440	3670
EDS variety[y]	2600	3120	2190	2360	3320	2580
68A x EDS[z]	2980	3780	3070	3610	4360	3670
90PV0046 x 0049[y]	2640	3060	1920	2670	3190	1510
90PV0003 x 0005[y]	4790	2570	2460	4010	3480	790
90PV0016 x 0017[y]	3690	2980	2320	2900	2560	2730
90PV0016 x 0015[y]	3220	3330	2840	4050	3770	2190
H23DA1E x 77[x]	2950	1930	1260	3720	2510	810
RR23DAE x 77[x]	4950	2320	1180	4020	2590	1380
1163 x 86-7907[x]	2670	3960	3130	3330	3670	3810
2068 x 87-8025[x]	4610	2930	1990	3830	3030	2220
DK 39 sorghum[x]	5650	---	4860	6090	4170	1210
F 2233 sorghum[x]	5840	---	3660	5660	5220	2720
Mean	3680	3060	2590	3820	3560	2310
CV	24	20	13	14	13	28
LSD 0.05	1509	1064	551	934	787	1088

[z]cms topcross
[x]pro-hybrid single cross
[y]cms single cross

in Africa, with the use of CMS seed parents. These pro-hybrids, as they are termed, appear to have the most utility for developing countries where existing or reselected leading open-pollinated cultivars could be directly used as male parents for topcross hybrids.

Heterotic effects in pearl millet are large and most completely expressed in single crosses, though yields from topcross hybrids are similar in all but the highest yielding situations. Topcross hybrids have several advantages including stability and durability of performance and ease of production (Andrews 1986).

Yield Potential

Landrace open-pollinated cultivars of pearl millet exhibit high levels of vegetative vigor and a very high biomass production. These are necessary adaptive features for the crop to survive stressful low fertility conditions, pests, diseases, weed competition, yet take advantage of brief periods favorable for growth and still yield consistently. As a result, the harvest index of these traditional cultivars which are tall, is only 15 to 20%. A crop of a local variety of pearl millet, cv. ex Bornu, grown under high fertility conditions without irrigation, in northern Nigeria produced 22 t/ha of above ground dry matter 90 days after sowing, but only 3.2 tons of this (14.5%) was grain (Kassam and Kowal 1975). In contrast, grain yields on a field basis of over 5 t/ha were produced by semi-dwarf hybrids maturing in 85 days in India (Rachie and Majmudar 1980) where experimental yields of up to 8 t/ha have been reported (Burton et al. 1972). The harvest index in these genotypes has been improved to over 40%. The Indian hybrids, however, though their yield potential is high, do not possess the persistent stem strength needed for mechanical harvesting and are still partly photosensitive and thus mature too late when planted more than about 30° latitude from the equator. New phenotypes are required for Midwestern United States which should be non-photoperiod sensitive, early to very early, with sufficient stalk and peduncle strength, and an upright tiller habit to give effective lodging resistance following frost. There have been relatively few notable breeding achievements in the improvement of grain production in pearl millet. The first was the breeding of high yielding early maturing semi-dwarf hybrids in India in the 1960s, mentioned above, which was made possible by the crucial discovery of cytoplasmic male sterility and its incorporation of it into a semi-dwarf line of high combining ability (Burton 1965). The second was that when successive early hybrids broke down to the downy mildew disease [*Sclerospora graminicola* (Sacc.) Schroet] in India, open-pollinated cultivars were then bred in the late 1970s that combined durable disease resistance with yield levels nearly equivalent to the hybrids (Andrews et al. 1985). Currently, these high yielding cultivars occupy about the same area in India as newer hybrids, now with better disease resistance (ICRISAT 1990). The third achievement, which was slow to develop and has had less impact due to limited seed multiplication and extension efforts, was the generation in the early 1970s of widely adapted varieties from Serere, Uganda, with Iniati/Koupela parentage. These proved superior in tests and have been released in countries from Sudan to Botswana.

Breeding in the USA

The foundation for breeding pearl millet grain hybrids in both India and more recently in the United States traces directly back to the pioneering research done by Glenn Burton in the forage crops program at Tifton, Georgia, which commenced in 1936. Besides CMS, dwarf stocks with early maturity and other valuable information about pearl millet breeding and genetics have been produced from Tifton. The development of forage cultivars in the United States in the past 50 years, mostly due to research at Tifton, has progressed from open-pollinated cultivars, through synthetic cultivars, poly-cross F_1s to single-cross hybrids. Advances have been made in both biomass productivity and digestibility, the latter largely through the use of dwarfing genes to increase leaf/stem ratio. Tolerance to nematodes and diseases have been incorporated (see review by Andrews and Kumar 1992).

Why breeding grain hybrids in pearl millet did not immediately commence in the United States in the 1960s to parallel hybrid development in grain sorghum is not clear. Contributing factors may have been that grain production in sorghum was already established using dwarf and semi-dwarf inbred varieties that mostly had sufficient stalk strength to be combine harvested; and there was a relatively much larger germplasm base of adapted sorghum stocks from which to breed whereas the initial stocks from the Tifton program were phenotypes primarily intended for use in forage production. Also in the 1950s and 1960s, the relative nutritional advantage of pearl millet grain compared to sorghum was not widely appreciated.

In 1969, Kansas State University began a grain breeding program in pearl millet at Manhattan, Kansas, which grew partly out of the USDA/OAU joint Cereals Research Project 26 in Africa, which supported genetic research in pearl millet at Serere, Uganda. The millet breeding program at the Fort Hays Experiment Station started in 1971. Early sources of germplasm for the Hays program came from both East and West Africa; India; Tifton, Georgia; and the USDA Plant Introduction Station pearl millet germplasm collection, Experiment, Georgia. While the Tift A_1 cytoplasm has been the basis for the development of seed parents at Kansas State University, another accession (PI 185642) from the Ghana/Togo landrace called Iniati/Koupela, has been a parent of fundamental importance in transmitting the character associations of large (12 to 16 g/1000), round, slate-gray or yellow grain, relatively large head width/length ratio, good combining ability, and earliness uninfluenced by photoperiod response. Dwarf derivatives of another Togo type cultivar (Serere 3A) have contributed early maturity, large seed size, and high grain yield potential to numerous imported accessions, inbred lines, and populations used as sources of pollen parents of experimental hybrids. The breeding value of the Iniati/Koupela germplasm was independently recognized in breeding programs in India, East and now West and Southern Africa. Seed parents from Hays lines have been released via ICRISAT in India, and are used extensively in hybrid production in northwest Indian states.

Work at Hays, Kansas, now supported by INTSORMIL, is focused on improving stand establishment, fertility restoration, and lodging resistance—characteristics necessary for mechanized production of hybrid millet. Large seed size and ability to emerge from deep (7.5 to 10 cm) field plantings have been selected at Hays to overcome establishment difficulties (Stegmeier 1990). These materials emerge from normal planting depths up to one day earlier than unselected lines, which is advantageous when weather conditions cause either crusting or rapid drying of seedbeds.

Fertility restoration of the A_1 cytoplasm has been difficult to stabilize within the variable environment of the central Great Plains, but inbred lines have been identified that have consistently produced fertile hybrids in 20 or more tests during the past five years.

Severe stalk lodging and breaking of stem internodes occurs within all germplasm sources, lines, and hybrids selected for improved grain yield. Two sources of improved stalk quality have been found that reduce the incidence of lodging and are being incorporated into elite inbred lines.

Grain yield levels of up to 5.3 t/ha have been recorded (Christensen et al. 1984). Grain yield comparisons of sorghum and pearl millet hybrids of similar maturities (W.D. Stegmeier unpubl. data) indicate millet yields are to 60 to 90% as large as sorghum when grown on silty clay loam soils, 85 to 100% on silt loams, and will often exceed the yield of sorghum on sandy soils. On sandy soils in southcentral Kansas, Stegmeier (1990) reported pearl millet hybrids producing up to 76% more grain than the commercial sorghum hybrid check yield of 2.4 t/ha.

Research on grain production started as an adjunct to the on-going pearl millet forage breeding and wide crossing program at Tifton, Georgia, in the early 1980s. Dominant resistance to pearl millet rust (*Puccinia substriata* Ell. & Barth. var. *indica* Ramachar & Cumm) and blast (*Piricularia setariae* Nisikado) has been incorporated into A_1 seed parents (Hanna 1991a), while pollen parents have been obtained from crossing the doubled (6*x*) pearl millet × elephant grass cross back to pearl millet (Hanna 1991b). A hybrid (Tift 90DAE × 8677), with these parents has been released under an exclusive license and is being grown on a pilot scale of a few hundred hectares in 1991 on the sandy soils of Georgia and South Carolina.

The breeding program for grain pearl millet commenced at the University of Nebraska–Lincoln and High Plains Agricultural Station at Sidney in 1984 with the support of INTSORMIL. Germplasm introduced earlier had been random-mated into a population early enough to mature in western Nebraska. Breeding material was extensively introduced from India and Africa. Both population and pedigree breeding are being used to produce adapted inbreds for use as hybrid parents, in synthetics, and to make new populations. New seed parents have been produced in A_1 cytoplasm with improved seed set and lodging resistance. Seed and pollen parents are also being produced with the A_m (*monodii*) cytoplasm.

The possibility of producing hybrids by using the species natural protogyny, which would increase potential hybrid combinations and greatly reduce hybrid development time, is currently being investigated (Andrews 1990). Tests with mechanical mixtures of "seed parent" lines and pro-hybrid seed have been conducted to estimate the effect on hybrid performance of any self-pollination that might occur in the pro-hybrid seed parent during hybrid seed production. Provided the hybrid has a dominant phenotype, no significant loss in hybrid yields was found in three different hybrids when 20% inbred seed of the female parent was added (Andrews 1990). Actual losses were from 4 to 6% (for detailed results see Andrews et al. 1993 in this vol.). Much less than 20% selfing would be expected in a well managed seed plot. Protogynous hybrids, therefore, seem feasible to produce and may be particularly useful in African situations.

Pearl millet regional grain yield trials testing initial experimental hybrids and other entries from ARS/USDA, Tifton, Georgia; Kansas State University, Hays; and University of Nebraska, Lincoln; have been grown cooperatively at 5 locations in the United States since 1988 (Fig. 1). The 1990 results shown in Table 1 are typical. Across locations the best pearl millet hybrids averaged 85% of the grain yield of the sorghum hybrid checks. Only where the season was short as in North Dakota, and in double cropping after wheat in Indiana (sorghum failed to mature) did millet yields exceed sorghum. Considerations of maturity, height, lodging, leaf disease occurrence, and relative genotype yields suggest that there are at least two contrasting adaptation areas within the region in which the tests have been conducted. These are the Midwest High Plains and the Southeast. Cultivars from the Southeast are too late maturing in the Midwest (will mature in Kansas but require more moisture), tend to be tall, and have little resistance to lodging following frost. Conversely, Midwest cultivars are too early in the South, and have little resistance to leaf diseases.

GRAIN QUALITY AND FEED VALUE

Results from feed experiments involving pearl millet with maize or sorghum from literature reviewed by Hoseney et al. (1987), Rooney and McDonough (1987), Serna-Saldivar et al. (1990), Sullivan et al. (1990), and Bramel-Cox et al. (1992) indicate that pearl millet is at least equivalent to maize and generally superior to sorghum in protein content and quality, protein efficiency ratio (PER) values, and metabolizable energy (MEn) levels. Pearl millet does not contain any condensed polyphenols such as the tannins in sorghum that can interfere with or slow down digestibility.

Recent chick feeding experiments, Sullivan et al. (1990) (Table 2) and Hancock et al. (1990) (Table 3) show that weight gains and feed/gain ratios obtained in pearl millet based diets are equal to that of maize and some sorghums. Smith et al. (1989) similarly report that pearl millet can replace maize in chick diets without affecting weight gain or feed efficiency. Both the gross energy and MEn values of pearl millet tend to be higher then those of maize and many have been previously underestimated by 20% (Fancher et al. 1987). Tribble et al. (1986) reported that they were also able to substitute pearl millet for sorghum in sorghum based diets for growing pigs without affecting performance. Calder (1955, 1961) had previously concluded that pearl millet was suitable for pig feeding.

Studies on the comparative value of pearl millet with sorghum or corn for cattle are few. When millet and sorghum grain were compared in high-silage growing rations for steers adjusted to equal protein intake, the results suggested millet protein had a high biological value as the addition of Rumensin to the rations gave millet grain a 10% advantage over sorghum grain (Brethour 1982) (Table 4). With finishing steers, Brethour and Stegmeier (1984) comparing rations where 25% of the sorghum component was replaced with pearl millet, reported that average daily gains were 1.40 and 1.20 kg, and feed/gain ratios were 7.53 and 8.03, respectively, for millet based

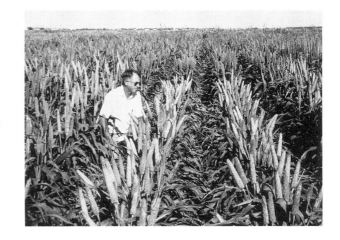

Fig. 1. Dwarf pearl millet grain hybrid (protogyny type), 1990 Pearl Millet Regional test, Hays, Kansas (2-row plots).

Table 2. Performance of broiler chicks fed pearl millet, maize, high (HT) and low (LT) tannin sorghum based diets[z].

Grain[y]	Added fat (%)[x]	Weight gain (g) d 1 to 42	Gain:feed d 1 to 42
Pearl millet	9.0/9.8	1466a[w]	0.472a
Maize	4.0/3.8	1372ab	0.469a
Sorghum, HT	9.6/9.8	1384ab	0.426b
Sorghum, LT	5.7/6.0	1329b	0.448ab

[z]Sullivan et al. (1990).
[y]Diets were isocaloric and iso-N; five replications of 60 birds/treatment.
[x]Fat levels in the starter/grower diets.
[w]Mean separation by Duncan's Multiple Range Test, 5% level.

versus sorghum based diets. Estimated net energy value of pearl millet was 4% higher than for sorghum. In both experiments, the amounts of soybean meal and/or urea needed for iso-N rations were less when pearl millet was used.

In a metabolism trial with steers, Hill and Hanna (1990) compared a diet with 79% pearl millet (PM) to diets of 76% sorghum + 2.8% soybean meal (GS) with a control (C) of 73% maize + 6% soybean meal. Ether extract and crude protein digestibilities were higher for C and PM than GS while retained N was similar for all. In an accompanying growth trial with yearling heifers, diet C gave a higher daily gain than PM, but feed:gain ratios were similar for all diets (8.5, 9.1, and 8.2 kg feed/kg gain^{-1}, respectively, for PM, GS, and C).

Table 3. Nutrient content of pearl millet, sorghum, and maize and growth performance of broiler chicks[z].

Crop	Crude protein (%)	Lysine (%)[y]	MEn (kcal/kg)[y]	Gain d 7 to 21 (g)	Gain/ feed
Pearl millet	10.3	0.35	3459	475	0.656
Sorghum	11.0	0.27	3397	467	0.638
Maize	10.1	0.30	3288	479	0.654

[z]Adapted from Hancock et al. (1990).
[y]Corrected to 90% dry matter.

Table 4. Rolled pearl millet compared to rolled sorghum in high silage steer growing rations[z].

Ration	Avg daily ration (kg)						Avg. daily gain (kg)	Kg feed/ 45.4 kg gain
	Sorghum silage	Rolled sorghum	Rolled pearl millet	Soybean meal	Premix	Air dry total		
Control								
Pearl millet	18.0	---	2.1	0.26	0.14	8.6	1.08	359
Sorghum	18.9	1.8	---	0.56	0.14	8.8	1.11	368
Rumensin[y]								
Pearl millet	17.5	---	2.1	0.26	0.18	8.4	1.18	337
Sorghum	17.8	1.8	---	0.56	0.18	8.5	1.07	364

[z]Adapted from Brethour (1982).
[y]No endorsement is intended, nor is any criticism implied of any similar product not mentioned.

Table 5. Percent anatomical grain composition and protein content of pearl millet and sorghum grain fractions.

Grain fraction	Pearl millet[z]		Sorghum[y]	
	% of grain	Protein	% of grain	Protein
Endosperm	75	10.9	82.3	12.3
Germ	17	24.5	9.8	18.9
Bran	8	17.1	7.9	6.7
Whole grain	100	13.3	100	12.3

[z]Abdelrahman and Hoseney (1984).
[y]Hubbard et al. (1950).

In general, feeding test results support data from biochemical analyses which indicate that pearl millet is similar to maize and superior to sorghum as a feed grain. A number of factors are thought to be responsible. Pearl millet grain generally has a higher crude protein level by 1 to 2 percentage points relative to sorghum grown with similar cultural practices. Pearl millet is still deficient in essential amino acids, but averages 35% more lysine than sorghum (Rooney and McDonough 1987). Pearl millet grain has 5 to 6% oil and a lower proportion of the less digestible cross-linked prolamins (Jambunathan and Subramanian 1988). These differences can be partly attributed to the different structure of the kernel. The proportion of germ in pearl millet grain (17%) is about double that of sorghum, while the endosperm accounts for 75% as against 82% in sorghum (Table 5). Amounts of bran are similar.

Major recessive genes that strongly influence grain protein lysine levels, as discovered in sorghum and maize, have not been found in pearl millet, despite an extensive survey of the world collection. However, selection for grain protein level in pearl millet has resulted in inbreds where crude protein levels (and consequently higher levels of lysine per sample) are 4 to 6 percentage points higher than normal, without affecting endosperm development (Singh et al. 1987). Hybrids made between these high protein inbreds and normal parents gave normal yield levels but with some elevation in grain protein, indicating partial dominance for the expression of grain protein content (ICRISAT 1984). It would appear possible to breed for moderately higher protein grain content levels (and higher lysine/sample) in pearl millet without the use of a high lysine gene that adversely affects endosperm development.

CULTIVATION

Cultivating, harvesting, and handling a pearl millet crop for grain with existing equipment and in ways similar to current farming practices, will be important for its successful adoption. Hybrid plant types are being bred with this in mind. Existing hybrids can be grown as a row crop like grain sorghum with some adjustments. Pearl millet establishes best when sown slightly shallower than sorghum in well prepared warmer seed beds on well-drained soils. It tolerates many of the post-emergence broad-leaf herbicides (bentazon, bromoxynil, and 2,4-D), but so far among the pre-emergence herbicides that control grassy weeds, only half rate atrazine is tolerated. (Selection is underway for propachlor resistance—see below). Plant densities should be similar or slightly higher (100,000 to 175,000 plants/ha) than for sorghum. The grain is tougher and more dense than sorghum and can be easily combined when well dry using higher cylinder speeds, more air and adjusting the screens for the smaller seed size. The point at which pearl millet is dry enough for harvesting can be easily judged in the field. When the crop is ripe and dry, grains will pop out cleanly when the head is pinched. The grain flows easily and trucks and grain bins do need to be completely grain-tight.

More agronomic research is needed now that new hybrids are available, particularly on seedling establishment and control of grassy weeds. Preliminary observations at UN–L indicate that the choice of hybrid phenotype (medium maturity, 120 to 130 cm height, elongated, and closed canopy), planting date (delay sufficient to allow germination and removal of some grass seed), and row spacing (mechanical cultivation of wide rows vs non-cultivated narrow rows) are important in reducing competition effects of foxtail and fall panicum grasses. Pearl millet seed protectants and safeners are not available for use with the amide family of herbicides (metolachlor and alachlor). We have made good progress at the University of Nebraska, Lincoln on selecting for propachlor tolerance and the tolerance is not limited to one source of germplasm. Selection for large seed size and long mesocotyl at Kansas State University, Hays has identified genotypes with better seedling establishment and early growth which thus can be planted a little deeper into assured moisture.

Apart from the rust and leaf blast in the South, no major diseases have so far been identified on pearl millet in the Midwest. Bacterial leaf spotting caused by (*Psuedomonas syringae* pv. *syringae* van Hall) (Odrody and Vidaver 1980) has occasionally occurred in July in pearl millet forage crops, but subsides later in the season. Increased stalk lodging can occur in high nitrogen soils (>112 kg N/ha) with some hybrids. As with sorghum, some peduncle attack of the European corn borer [*Ostrinia nubilalis* (Hübner)] can occur and cinch bugs [*Blissus leucopterus leucopterus* (Say)] can spread to pearl millet from adjacent wheat to increase head and stalk lodging or kill plants during the growing season. Pearl millet has two distinct advantages over sorghum or proso—its seed will not over-winter in moist soil, and there are no wild relatives in the United States to which it will naturally outcross, so it would not become a weed in subsequent crops.

CONCLUSION

Pearl millet is a widely grown Old World tropical food cereal well adapted to the hot drought prone areas of Africa and the Indian subcontinent where about 26 million ha (about 7 times the United States grain sorghum area) is grown. A very wide range of genetic variability is available in the primary germplasm pool for improvement of this species where genetic manipulation is facilitated by its tillering protogynous habit and high seed number per head. Sustained advances have been made in the United States since the 1940s on breeding pearl millet forage cultivars. The resulting genetic information and the discovery of CMS has been vital for breeding for grain yield.

Following the demonstration of the yield potential of early maturing hybrids in India, breeding commenced in the early 1970s on grain pearl millet in the United States at Kansas State University, Hays and was joined in the 1980s by USDA/ARS Tifton and the University of Nebraska-Lincoln and Sidney. Fully dwarf experimental hybrids which can be grown like sorghum have been produced and tested regionally since 1988, giving yields averaging 2.3 to 3.8 t/ha. Highest yields on a field basis (5.3 t/ha) were recorded in Kansas. Two adaptation zones, the Southeast and Midwest High Plains are evident from these tests.

Feeding tests on cattle, swine, and particularly chickens have shown pearl millet is at least equivalent to maize and often superior to sorghum in feed rations, generally because of high energy and grain protein levels.

Initial breeding efforts and utilization tests have given encouraging results. Further cultivar improvements can be expected. Opportunities for production will be dependent on a number of factors including marketing possibilities, which may first be by specific contracts. Clearly, more agronomic research is needed on determining optimum cultivation practices, but pearl millet crops can presently be grown well with existing row crop equipment and practices. Potential production areas are those where pearl millet will have a relative advantage over other summer cereals, such as in the Southeast coastal sands, in the drier or short-season parts of the Midwest High Plains, and possibly in double-cropping after wheat in the central Midwest.

REFERENCES

Abdelrahman, A.A. and R.C. Hoseney. 1984. Basis for hardness in pearl millet, grain sorghum, and corn. Cereal Chem. 61:232–235.

Andrews, D.J. 1986. Breeding pearl millet grain hybrids, p. 83–109. In: W.P. Feistritzer and A.F. Kelly (eds.) FAO/DANIDA regional seminar on breeding and producing hybrid varieties. Nov. 11–13, Surabaya, Indonesia. FAO Rome.

Andrews, D.J. 1990. Breeding pearl millet for developing countries. INTSORMIL Annual Report, Univ. of Nebraska–Lincoln. p. 114–118.

Andrews, D.J., B. Kiula, and J.F. Rajewski. 1993. The use of protogyny to make hybrids in pearl millet. In: J. Janick and J.E. Simon (eds.). Progress in new crops. Wiley, New York.

Andrews, D.J. and K.A. Kumar. 1992. Pearl millet for food, feed, and forage. Adv. in Agron. 48:90–128.

Andrews, D.J. and J.F. Rajewski. 1990. 1988 and 1989 pearl millet regional grain yield trials. Dept. of Agron., Univ. of Nebraska–Lincoln. (mimeo).

Andrews, D.J. and J.F. Rajewski. 1991. 1990 pearl millet regional grain yield trials. Dept. of Agron., Univ. of Nebraska–Lincoln. (mimeo).

Andrews, D.J., S.B. King, J.R. Witcombe, S.D. Singh, K.N. Rai, R.P. Thakur, B.S. Talukdar, S.B. Chavan, and P. Singh. 1985. Breeding for disease resistance and yield in pearl millet. Field Crops Res. 11:241–258.

Bramel-Cox, P.J., K. Anand Kumar, J.H. Hancock, and D.J. Andrews. 1992. Sorghum and millets for forage and feed. In: D.A.V. Dendy (ed.). Sorghum and the millets, chemistry and technology. Amer. Assoc. Cereal Chem. (in press).

Brethour, J.R. 1982. Beef cattle investigations, 1981–82. Kansas State Univ. Agr. Expt. Sta. Rpt. of Progress 417.

Brethour, J.R. and W.D. Stegmeier. 1984. Pearl millet for beef cattle, p. 13. In: Fort Hays Roundup, Kansas Expt. Sta. Bul. 71.

Brunken, J.N., J.M.J. de Wet, and J.R. Harlan. 1977. The morphology and domestication of pearl millet. Econ. Bot. 31:163–174.

Burton, G.W. 1958. Cytoplasmic male-sterility in pearl millet *Pennisetum glaucum* (L.) R. Br. Agron. J. 50:230.

Burton, G.W. 1965. Pearl millet Tift 23A released. Crops & Soils 17:19.

Burton, G.W. 1974. Factors affecting pollen movement and natural crossing in pearl millet. Crop Sci. 14:802–805.

Burton, G.W., A.T. Wallace, and K.O. Rachie. 1972. Chemical composition and nutritive value of pearl millet. Crop Sci. 12:187–188.

Calder, A. 1955. Value of munga (millet) for pig feeding. Rhodesia Agr. J. 52:161–170.

Calder, A. 1961. The production of pork pigs comparing maize, munga (millet) and pollards. Rhodesia Agr. J. 56:363–364.

Chirwa, R.M. 1991. Estimation of synthetic variety yields in pearl millet through parental line evaluation per se and in tester combinations. Ph.D. Diss., Univ. of Nebraska–Lincoln.

Christensen, N.B., J.C. Palmer, H.A. Praeger, Jr., W.D. Stegmeier, and R.L. Vanderlip. 1984. Pearl millet: a potential crop for Kansas. Keeping Up With Research No. 77, Kansas Agr. Expt. Sta., Manhattan.

Dave, H.R. 1986. Pearl millet hybrids, p. 121–137. In: J.R. Witcombe and S.R. Beckerman (eds.). Proc. Int. Pearl Millet Workshop. ICRISAT, Patancheru, India.

Dujardin, M. and W.W. Hanna. 1989. Developing apomictic pearl millet—characterization of a BC_3 plant. J. Genet. Breed. 43:145–151.

Dujardin, M. and W.W. Hanna. 1990. Cytogenetics and reproductive behavior of 48 chromosome pearl millet × *Pennisetum squamulatum* derivatives. Crop Sci. 30:1015–1016.

FAO. 1986. Production yearbook. Vol. 40. FAO, United Nations, Rome.

Fancher, B.I., L.S. Jensen, and R.L. Smith. 1987. Metabolizable energy content of pearl millet [*Pennisetum americanum* (L.) Leeke]. Poultry Sci. 66:1693–1696.

Hancock, J.D., P.J. Bramel-Cox, K.R. Smith, B.J. Healy, C.F. Klopfenstein, and M.D. Witt. 1990. Selection for increased in vitro digestibility improves the feeding value of sorghum grain. J. Anim. Sci. 90(Suppl. 1):320 (Abstr.).

Hanna, W.W. 1989. Characteristics and stability of a new cytoplasmic nuclear male-sterile source in pearl millet. Crop Sci. 29:1457–1459.

Hanna, W.W. 1990. Transfer of germplasm from the secondary to the primary gene pool in *Pennisetum*. Theor. Appl. Genet. 80:200–204.

Hanna, W.W. 1991a. Release of pearl millet seed parent Tift $90D_2A_1E_1$ (cms) inbred lines. Release notice, USDA/ARS–Georgia Expt. Sta. Tifton

Hanna, W.W. 1991b. Release of pearl millet cms restorer Tift 8677 inbred line. Release notice, USDA/ARS–Georgia Expt. Sta. Tifton

Harlan, J.R. 1975. Crops and man. Amer. Soc. Agron., Madison, WI.

Harlan, J.R. and J.M.J. de Wet. 1971. Toward a rational classification of cultivated plants. Taxonomy 20:509–517.

Hill, G.M. and W.W. Hanna. 1990. Nutritive characteristics of pearl millet grain in beef cattle diets. J. Anim. Sci. 68:2061–2066.

Hoseney, R.C., D.J. Andrews, and H. Clark. 1987. Sorghum and pearl millet, p. 397–456. In: R.A. Olson and K.J. Frey (eds.). Nutritional quality of cereal grains: Genetic and agronomic improvement. Agron. Monog. 28. ASA, Madison, WI.

Hubbard, J.E., H.H. Hall, and F.R. Earle. 1950. Composition of the component parts of the sorghum kernel. Cereal Chem. 27:415–420.

ICRISAT. 1984. Pearl millet high protein hybrids. ICRISAT 1983 Annual Report, Patancheru, India.

ICRISAT. 1990. ICRISAT's contribution to pearl millet production. ICRISAT, Patancheru, India.

Jambunathan, R. and V. Subramanian. 1988. Grain quality and utilization in sorghum and pearl millet. Proc. Workshop on Biotechnology for Tropical Crop Improvement, ICRISAT, Patancheru, India. p. 1330–1339.

Kassam, A.H. and J.M. Kowal. 1975. Water use, energy balance and growth of gero millet at Samaru, Northern Nigeria. Agr. Met. 15:333–342.

Khadr, F.H. and M.M. El-Rouby. 1978. Inbreeding in quantitative traits of pearl millet (*Pennisetum typhoides*). Z. Pflanzenzuch. 80:149–157.

Kumar, K.A. and D.J. Andrews. 1984. Cytoplasmic male sterility in pearl millet [*Pennisetum americanum* (L.) Leeke]: A review. Adv. Applied Biol. 10:113–143.

Marchais, L. and J. Pernes. 1985. Genetic divergence between wild and cultivated pearl millets (*Pennisetum typhoides*). I. Male sterility. Z. Pflanzenzuch. 95:103–112.

Odvody, G.N. and A.K. Vidaver. 1980. *Pseudomonas springae* on pearl millet in Texas and Nebraska. Sorghum Newsletter 23:134.

Rachie, K.O. and J.V.M. Majmudar. 1980. Pearl millet. Pennsylvania Univ. Press, University Park.

Rai, K.N., D.J. Andrews, and S. Babu. 1984. Inbreeding depression in pearl millet composites. Z. Pflanzenzuch. 94:201–207.

Rooney, L.W. and C.M. McDonough. 1987. Food quality and consumer acceptance in pearl millet, p. 43–61. In: J.R. Witcombe and S.R. Beckerman (eds.). Proc. international pearl millet workshop. ICRISAT, Patancheru, India.

Serna-Saldivar, S.O., C.M. McDonough, and L.W. Rooney. 1990. The millets, p. 271–300. In: K.J. Lorenz and K. Kulp (eds.). Handbook of cereal science technology. Markel Dekker, New York.

Singh, P., U. Singh, B.O. Eggum, K.A. Kumar, and D.J. Andrews. 1987. Nutritional evaluation of high protein genotypes in pearl millet. J. Food Sci. Agr. 38:41–48.

Smith, R.L., L.S. Jensen, C.S. Hoveland, and W.W. Hanna. 1989. Use of pearl millet, sorghum, and triticale grain in broiler diets. J. Prod. Agr. 2:78–82.

Stegmeier, W.D. 1990. Pearl millet breeding. INTSORMIL Annual Report, Univ. of Nebraska–Lincoln, p. 48–51.

Sullivan, T.W., J.H. Douglas, D.J. Andrews, P.L. Bond, J.D. Hancock, P.J. Bramel-Cox, W.D. Stegmeier, and J.R. Brethour. 1990. Nutritional value of pearl millet for food and feed. Proc. Int. Conf. in Sorghum Nutritional Quality, Purdue Univ., Lafayette, IN. p. 83–94.

Tribble, L.F., W.F. Stansbury, and J.J. McGlone. 1986. Value of pearl millet as a feed grain for swine. J. Anim. Sci. 63 (Suppl. 1):284 (Abstr.).

The Use of Protogyny to Make Hybrids in Pearl Millet

David J. Andrews, Barnabas Kiula, and John F. Rajewski

While cytoplasmic male sterility (CMS) facilitates hybrid seed production, the necessity of breeding CMS seed and restorer pollen parents which combine specifically, lengthens hybrid development time and restricts the possible combinations. In maize, these restrictions can be overcome by making hybrids by detasselling. In pearl millet [*Pennisetum glaucum* (L.) R. Br.], the protogynous nature of flowering can be used to make hybrids, termed pro-hybrids to distinguish them from CMS hybrids. The duration of complete stigma emergence, the protogyny period (see Fig. 1A) before anthesis (Fig. 1B) on pearl millet heads may vary between genotypes from 1 to 5 days. While choice of parent lines and careful management of pro-hybrid production fields will reduce self pollination in the chosen "seed parent," some may still occur. Prior research in hybrid/inbred mixtures in tall forage hybrids (Burton 1948, 1989) showed that up to 50% inbred line seed did not significantly reduce hybrid performance. Tall grain hybrids made in West Africa by protogyny using dwarf populations as females with tall varieties as pollinators showed as much as 45% heterosis over check variety and less than 5% female selfing (Lambert 1982). Our research investigated, using one top-cross (TC) and 3 single-cross (SC) hybrids, what effect various levels of simulated "seed parent" selfing would have on dwarf pro-hybrid performance.

METHODOLOGY

Experiments 1 [68A x MLS (TC)] and 2 [554 x 556 (SC)] were grown in 1989 and repeated in 1990. Experiments 3 [68A x 60051 (SC)] and 4 [205 x 319 (SC)] were added in 1990. All were grown at the UN–L

Farm, Mead, Nebraska, in experiments with 4 or 5 replications, 4 m plots, 2 row or single row plots. Treatments were hybrid seed mixed with 0, 20, 40, and 60% inbred seed and both parents. Seeds were mixed on the basis of live seed number, and no thinning was done. In Experiment 1, seed of 68B was used in mixtures while in Experiment 3 only late parent line 60015 was used. In Experiments 2 and 4, mixture treatments were made separately with both parents.

RESULTS AND DISCUSSION

Yields of the 80:20 hybrid/inbred mixtures were not significantly different from the control (100% hybrid) in either the TC (Fig. 2) or two out of three SC hybrid tests (Tables 1 and 2). Actual yield reductions were 4.4, 4.1, and 6.3%, respectively. In the remaining SC hybrid (Table 3), the yield of 60:40 mixtures were not significantly different (–14%) from the control but, for no discernable reasons, the 80:20 mixtures (–22%) were significantly lower yielding. Heterosis levels were 20% in the TC hybrid over the open-pollinated cultivar parent, and 275, 70, and 260% over the best inbred in the respective SC hybrids. Experiments are underway with marker traits to determine the actual hybrid/self seed percentages occurring in pro-hybrid seed production plots, but selfing is expected to be less than 20%.

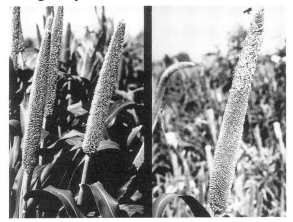

Fig. 1. (left). Pearl millet heads. (A) Protogynous heads with stigmas fully exerted prior to anthesis; (B) Anthesis following the period of protogyny.

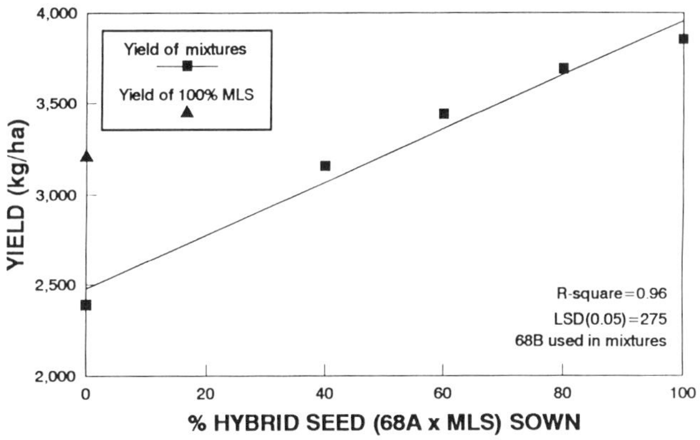

Fig. 2. Experiment 1. pearl millet top cross hybrid 68A x MLS. Grain yields (2 year means) of hybrid/seed parent mixtures.

Table 1. Grain yields and plant height of hybrid parents and mixtures of SC hybrid 554 x 556 (Expt. 2, Mead, Nebraska, 1989)[z].

Treatments (% mixtures)			Yield		Plant height (cm)
Hybrid 554 x 556	Inbred 1 554	Inbred 2 556	(kg/ha)	(% of pure hybrid)	
100	0	0	3330	100	83
80	20	0	3130	94	85
80	0	20	3120	94	84
60	40	0	2890	87	86
60	0	40	2860	86	80
40	60	0	2230	67	80
40	0	60	2180	65	82
0	100	0	1210	36	69
0	0	100	1150	35	83
LSD .05			406		6.6

[z]Expt. 2 in 1990 was discarded following chinch bug damage.

Table 2. Grain yields and plant height of hybrids, parents and mixtures of SC hybrid 68A ×60015 (Expt. 3, Mead, Nebraska, 1990).

Treatments (% mixtures)		Yield		Plant height (cm)
Hybrid 68A ×60015	Inbred 60015	(kg/ha)	(% of pure hybrid)	
100	0	3220	100	93
80	20	3090	96	90
60	40	2550	79	86
40	60	2390	74	87
0	100	1890	59	77
0	100 (68B)	1820	57	90
LSD .05		671		1.1

Table 3. Grain yields and plant height of hybrids, parents and mixtures of SC hybrid 205 ×319 (Expt. 4, Mead, Nebraska, 1990).

Treatments (% mixtures)			Yield		Plant height (cm)
Hybrid 205 ×319	Inbred 1 205	Inbred 2 319	(kg/ha)	(% of pure hybrid)	
100	0	0	2730	100	84
80	20	0	2080	76	87
80	0	20	2180	80	81
60	40	0	2410	88	82
60	0	40	2240	82	76
40	60	0	1830	67	86
40	0	60	1840	67	83
0	100	0	630	23	67
0	0	100	1040	38	74
LSD .05			520		1.8

CONCLUSION

The use of protogyny in pearl millet appears to have potential for making hybrids, thus permitting more rapid hybrid development and a wider choice of parent combinations compared to CMS systems. The presence of up to 20% inbred parent seed reduced grain yields only 4 to 6% in top-cross or 2 out of 3 single-cross hybrids, probably because inbred plants offered little competition to hybrid plants. The use of parent combinations which produce a dominant hybrid phenotype compared to that of the "seed parent" will reduce the effect of any possible selfing.

This research was conducted using dwarf hybrids. Where tall grain cultivars are preferred, as in Africa were 12 million ha of pearl millet are grown for food, and where susceptibility to ergot is associated with hybrids made with CMS seed parents, this method of hybrid seed production provides opportunities for the rapid development of top cross hybrids using existing tall cultivars as males and adapted semi-dwarf or dwarf lines as protogyny seed parents.

REFERENCES

Burton, G.W. 1948. The performance of various mixtures of hybrids and parent inbred pearl millet. J. Amer. Soc. Agron. 40:908–815.

Burton, G.W. 1989. Composition and forage yield of hybrid-inbred mixtures of pearl millet. Crop Sci. 29:252–255.

Lambert, C. 1982. IRAT and pearl millet improvement (in French). Agron. Tropicale 38:78–88.

Amaranth Rediscovered

G.F. Stallknecht and J.R. Schulz-Schaeffer

Amaranthus species were grown as the principle grain crop by the Aztecs 5,000 to 7,000 years ago, prior to the disruption of the South American civilization by the Spanish Conquistadors. Synonyms such as "mystical grains of the Aztecs," "super grain of the Aztecs," and the "golden grain of the Gods" were used to describe the nutritious amaranth grain. The grain was noted to be nourishing to infants and to provide energy and strength to soldiers on extended trips. While the early civilizations were aware of these nutrient factors by experience, it would take six centuries for modern biochemistry to confirm these facts. While the grain amaranths were the principle species used on the South American continent, amaranth have been cultivated as a vegetable crop by early civilizations over 2,000 years ago, and continue to be used essentially world-wide even at the present day (NAC 1985). Vegetable *Amaranthus* spp. were and are presently utilized for food from such diverse geographic areas as southwestern United States, China, India, Africa, Nepal, South Pacific Islands, Caribbean, Greece, Italy, and Russia. While various species of grain and vegetable types can be distinguished, often both the grain and leaves are utilized from individual types for use as both human and animal food (Saunders and Becker 1984; Tucker 1986). Present American production is estimated to be between 2,000 to 3,000 ha with the largest production in the Great Plains area, particularly Nebraska, with numerous smaller production areas throughout the Midwest. The stimulus for the present American production and marketing was initiated by the Rodale Foundation and the Rodale Research Center in the mid-1970s. The interest stimulated by the Rodale Foundation led to the establishment of the American Amaranth Institute in Bricelyn, Minnesota, and numerous Amaranth marketing companies, several of which deal exclusively in the purchase, milling, and distribution of amaranth products. In approximately only 15 years, American amaranth has gone from an obscure plant to a recognized grain.

Though quite small in comparison to other grains, amaranth has been extensively studied. There exists a surprisingly large volume of literature available, particularly on the nutritional qualities of amaranth. The strong interest in amaranth within the United States has been promoted by four National Amaranth Symposia and working group meetings by the American Amaranth Institute, and the first International Congress on Amaranth met in Oaxtepec, Mexico in 1991. Although amaranth is considered under new crop status, with minor production areas in the United States, unlike other "new crop candidates" there is an extensive literature and research base. Therefore, we will cite primary review papers in this paper; an overall review of amaranth was presented during the First National Symposium of New Crops (Kauffman and Weber 1990).

Since the historical, taxonomical, genetical, nutritional, processing, and marketing aspects of amaranth have been extensively reviewed, our objective is to focus primarily on production agronomics. Cultivar development and successful cropping management for economic production returns now hold the key to the future of the amaranth industry in the United States.

BOTANY

Taxonomy

The genus *Amaranthus* consists of approximately 60 species, however, only a limited number are of the cultivated types, while most are considered weedy species. *Amaranthus* germplasm is available in 11 countries (Sauer 1967; Toll and von Sloten 1982). Several thousand germplasm accessions are available in the United States at either the Rodale Research Institute, or the USDA North Central Regional Plant Introduction Station at Iowa State Univ., Ames. A taxonomic key for the cultivated species of *Amaranthus* has been developed by Feine-Dudley (Grubben and von Sloten 1981).

There is no distinct separation between the vegetable and grain type since the leaves of young grain type plants can be eaten as greens. The three principal species considered for grain production include: *A. hypochondriacus*, *A. cruentus*, and *A. caudatus*. The species grown as vegetables are represented primarily by *A. tricolor*, *A. dubius*, *A. lividus*, and *A. creuntus*. *Amaranthus palmeri* and *A. hybridus* were utilized by natives of early civilizations in the southwestern part of the United States. The weed amaranth, comes from *A. retroflexus* and is considered one of the worlds worst weeds (NAC 1984). The genetic and plant breeding characteristics among the cultivated *Amaranthus* spp. has been considered elsewhere (Kulakaw and Jain 1991; Weber and Kauffman 1990). The *Amaranthus* species have been separated into principally four groups: cultivated, wild and weedy, racial (based on geographic and morphological patterns), and landrace (populations from specific locations).

Physiology

Amaranth, a C_4 plant, is one of a few dicots in which the first product of photosynthesis is a four carbon compound. The combination of anatomical features in amaranth and C_4 metabolism, results in increased efficiency to use CO_2 under a wide range of both temperature and moisture stress environments, and contribute to the plant's wide geographic adaptability to diverse environmental conditions.

Morphology

Grain type amaranth plants have a main stem axis that terminates in an apical large branched inflorescence. The flowers are unisexual, purple, orange, red or gold in color, and are developed on branched flower clusters (glomerules). A glomerule is described as a diachsial cyme that forms large flowering panicles. Vegetable types are generally smooth leafed, with an indeterminate growth habit which produces new succulent axillary growth. The floral buds arise directly in the leaf axils. Amaranth seeds are borne in a utricle, which are classified as dehiscent, semi-dehiscent, or indehiscent types (Brenner and Hauptli 1990). The amaranth seed is quite small (0.9 to 1.7 mm diam) and seed weights vary from 1,000 to 3,000 seeds/g. Seed colors can vary from cream to gold and pink to black. Actual stature of the amaranth plant will vary significantly dependent upon species and environment. In Montana, individual cultivars can vary in height from 91 to 274 cm in height and have stem diameters from 2.54 to 15 cm, dependent upon plant stand density and available soil moisture. Likewise, seed heads have varied from 30 to 112 cm in diameter at the base and varied in height from 13 to 61 cm.

AGRONOMY

Amaranth grain entry into the marketing distribution arena has confronted numerous challenges. In contrast to many other established agricultural commodities, crop production challenges are even greater than marketing to the success of an amaranth industry. In regard to crop production, amaranth certainly is a specialty crop, since every aspect of production, from planting to harvest and storage requires special attention and consideration. Twentieth century amaranth production is vastly different from that of early civilizations or even from primitive agriculture systems present today. In the case of both early civilization and present day primitive agricultural systems, amaranth crop production is grown essentially all by hand in small plots intercropped with numerous other crops or at the very most, small isolated monocultural plots. Crop production under these systems can utilize marginal soils, and disease and insect pressures are often low due to the sparse cropping practices. In contrast, modern day agronomic practices of mechanization and extensive crop monoculture require competitive economic crop returns, and special considerations to integrated plant pest control. Producer production guidelines have been published for several states including Minnesota (Myers and Putnam 1988), Montana (Schulz-Schaeffer et al. 1988), Wisconsin (Putnam et al. 1989), and Nebraska (Baltensperger et al. 1991). A series of comprehensive production guides has been published by the Rodale Research Institute (Kauffman et al. 1983; Weber et al. 1988, 1989, 1990).

To initiate amaranth production, the producer should select and prepare a seed bed similar to that for small seeded vegetables or legumes, preferably on soils having a pH above 6.0 (Schulte et al. 1991). The seedbed should be well worked and firmed by a packer prior to planting. A firm moist seed bed with soil temperatures above 15°C is required to establish a good plant stand. Seeding rates of 1.2 to 3.5 kg seed/ha planted to an average depth of 1.3 cm is recommended. The most accurate commercial seeding rates have been achieved by using vegetable seeders which use seed plates of various sizes to meter the seed. Planting depth needs to be controlled. However, many producers have successfully planted amaranth with either a standard grain drill, or by using the insecticide boxes commonly found on row crop planters for beets, beans, or corn. While seeding rates are less accurate using grain drills, growers drill the seed by either shutting down the openings and seeding heavier rates, or by diluting the amaranth seed with cracked corn or vermiculite. Row widths can be controlled on grain drills by merely taping over selected drill openings to achieve the desired row spacing. Regardless of the type of drill used it is important to firm the seed row with a press wheel which will firm the contact between the amaranth seeds and the soil.

Fertility studies results in Arkansas, Minnesota, Montana, and Tennessee have been quite variable, for both vegetable and grain amaranth types (Walters et al. 1988; Elbehri et al. 1990; Makus 1990b; Putnam 1990; Schaeffer et al. 1990a). A generally suggested fertility guide for amaranth would be 112 to 135 kg/ha of total available N, with a soil test of 15 to 30 ppm P and 80 to 120 ppm K. Fertility needs will vary significantly, depending upon soil type, prior cropping, and fertilizer history. Higher applications of nitrogen would be applied in the high rainfall areas of the Midwest and under irrigated management as compared to the low rainfall production areas in the Great Plains. As the interest in amaranth production increases, additional fertility studies will be needed for economic production practices.

Presently, there are no herbicides labeled for weed control in amaranth, and it is unlikely that any chemicals will become cleared for commercial use. Weed control in amaranth is achieved by cultivation, hand weeding, delayed planting, and by manipulation of plant populations using narrow row spacings. Late planting to avoid spring frosts (as the plant is very susceptible to frost) can aid in weed control, since early spring emerged weeds can be mechanically controlled. Planting amaranth on narrow row spacings of 18 cm or less may aid in weed control, by the shading effect of the amaranth plants.

Harvesting of amaranth is difficult. When plant populations of amaranth are low, the seed heads become extremely large and do not properly dry. When amaranth is harvested prior to a killing frost, plant moisture levels will complicate the harvest. Adequate plant population and a killing frost to dry down the plants prior to harvest is necessary for an effective efficient harvest. Amaranth can then be effectively harvested by grain combines which are seed tight, and by reducing the cylinder speed just high enough to effectively thresh the seed heads. Since amaranth grain must have 12% moisture or lower for storage, the producer must be prepared to dry the harvested seed prior to storage. Storage methods must be sanitary if the seed is to be processed for human consumption.

Amaranth grain yields are extremely variable dependent upon cultivar selection and the growing season, particularly with regard to available soil moisture. Grain yields have ranged from a high of over 5,000 kg/ha in irrigated cultivar trials of the Montana State University Southern Agricultural Research Center at Huntley, to below 112 kg/ha in dryland trials. Yields of 450 to 700 kg/ha dryland and 900 to 2,000 kg/ha under irrigated or high rainfall would be considered reasonable using the better cultivars available to producers.

Nutritive Value

The nutritive composition of both grain and vegetable amaranth has been extensively studied (Becker et al. 1981; Teutonico and Knorr 1985; Pedersen et al. 1987; Bressani 1990). Amaranth grain is considered to have a unique composition of protein, carbohydrates, and lipids. The unique protein composition with regard to quality and quantity has been studied and reviewed (Bressani 1989; Lehman 1989). Grain amaranth has higher protein (12 to 18%) than other cereal grains and has a significantly higher lysine content. The high lysine content of amaranth grain makes it particularly attractive for use as a blending food source to increase the biological value of processed foods (Pedersen et al. 1987). The protein value of amaranth grains is highlighted when amaranth flour is mixed with other cereal grain flours. When amaranth flour is mixed 30:70 with either rice, maize, or wheat flour, the protein quality (based on casein) rises from 72 to 90, 58 to 81, and 32 to 52, respectively (Bressani 1989). Amaranth seed protein also differs from other cereal grains by the fact that 65% is found in the germ and 35% in the endosperm, as compared to an average of 15% in the germ and 85% in the endosperm for other cereals.

The carbohydrates in amaranth grain consist primarily of starch made up of both glutinous and non-glutinous fractions. The unique aspect of amaranth grain starch is that the size of the starch granules (1 to 3 μm) are much smaller than found in other cereal grains. Due to the unique size and composition of amaranth starch, it has been suggested that the starch may posses unique gelatinization and freeze/thaw characteristics which could be of benefit to the food industry (Becker et al. 1981; Lehman 1988). Several considerations for the use of amaranth starch in food preparation of custards, pastes, and salad dressing have been published in three papers (Singhal and Kulkarni 1990a,b,c).

Amaranth grain consists of approximately 5 to 9% oil which is generally higher than other cereals. The lipid fraction of amaranth grain is similar to other cereals, being approximately 77% unsaturated, with linoleic acid being the predominant fatty acid. The lipid fraction is unique however, due to the unusually high squalene content (5 to 8%) of the total oil fraction. Also present in the amaranth oil fractions were tocotrienols (forms of vitamin E) which are known to effect lower cholesterol levels in mammalian systems. Detailed studies and a review on amaranth grain oil have been published (Lyon and Becker 1987; Becker 1989; Lehman 1991). In addition to the unique characteristics of the major components of proteins, carbohydrates, and lipids, amaranth grain also contains high levels of calcium, iron, and sodium when compared to cereal grains (Becker et al. 1981).

In contrast to grain amaranth, vegetable amaranth has received significantly less research attention. While vegetable amaranth is used as a delicacy or a food staple in many parts of the world, use in the United States is limited to canned imports for ethnic uses, primarily in the New York City area. Vegetable amaranth has been rated equal to or superior in taste to spinach and is considerably higher in calcium, iron, and phosphorous (Makus 1984; Makus and Davis 1984; Igbokwe et al. 1988; Makus 1990a). Agronomic practices for vegetable production have also been published (Makus 1989, 1990b). The use of amaranth leaves and grain in feedstuffs has been reviewed (Cheeke and Bronson 1980; Sanders and Becker 1984; Teutonico and Knorr 1985; Pedersen et al. 1990; Wittaker and Ologunde 1990; Breene 1991; Pond et al. 1991). Results indicate that the amaranth used for human food should be heated for maximum nutritional benefit, while gains of lambs fed amaranth fodder, were similar to alfalfa (Pond and Lehman 1989). For uses of amaranth as livestock feed, see the review by Sanchez (1990).

Diseases and Pests

The most common insect and disease problems of amaranth have been described in 1990 Amaranth Grain Production Guide and the 4th National Amaranth Conference (Weber et al. 1990; Wilson 1990). A principle insect pest is the lygus bug, *Lygus lineolarius* (Polisot de Beauvois), which can extensively damage the flowering head. Amaranth can also suffer injury from the Fall armyworm, *Spodoptera frugiperda* (J.E. Smith), cabbage looper, *Trichoplusia ni* (Huebner), corn ear worm, *Heliothis zea* (Boddie), cowpea aphid, *Aphis craccavora* (Koch), and the blister beetle, *Epicuata vittata* (Fab.). The amaranth weevil, *Conotrachelus seniculus* (le Cont) can cause severe damage to the roots resulting in lodging and predisposition to root diseases.

In Montana, we have observed extensive damage to young seedlings caused from the potato flea beetle, *Epitrix cucumeris*. We have also identified serious problems induced by the curly top virus disease which is transmitted by the beet leafhopper, *Circulifer temellus* (Stallknecht et al. 1990). Both insect problems appear to be associated with large areas of sugar beets grown in south-central Montana, which is a host to these insects. The only chemical which has been approved for insecticidal use on grain amaranth is Pyrenone Crop Spray (Wilson 1990). Fungal pests of amaranth have been documented as *Pythium, Rhizoctonia* and *Aphanomyces sp.* causing seedling damping off, and stem cankers caused by either *Phoma* or *Rhizoctonia sp.* (Weber 1990). *Alternaria* leaf spot appears to be the most serious foliar pathogen (NARC 1985).

Cultivars

The first line of amaranth registered by The Crop Science Society of America was Montana-3 (MT-3) (Schulz-Schaeffer et al. 1989a). MT-3 is an *A. cruentus* from a selection of RRC-1041 obtained from the Rodale Research Center, Emmaus, PA. MT-3 is light green flowered, produces white seeds, and was selected for uniform height and high yields. Also registered in 1989, was Montana-5 (MT-5) an *A. cruentus* from a single selection of RRC-425 (Schulz-Schaeffer et al. 1989b). MT-5 is green flowered and has white seeds. MT-5 was selected for advanced dry-down characteristics, with the seed head dry down simultaneous to stalk dry down. The third amaranth selection released by Montana State University was named 'Amont' (Schulz-Schaeffer et al. 1991). 'Amont' is a selection taken from MT-3 (Fig. 1). 'Amont' is green flowered and has white seeds, and has resistance to lodging. The plant height of 'Amont' can vary from 91 to 244 cm dependent upon the moisture available through the season, and plant population. A semi-dwarf selection from RRC, K432 grows to 92 cm under irrigation, and

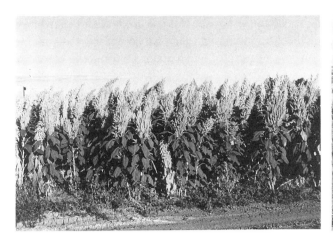

Fig. 1. 'Amont' amaranth growing under irrigation, Montana State University, Southern Agr. Res. Center, Huntley.

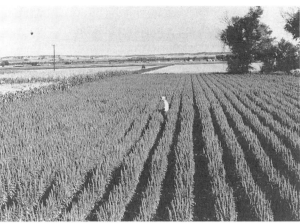

Fig. 2. 'K 432' amaranth grown under irrigation, Montana State University, Southern Agr. Res. Center, Huntley.

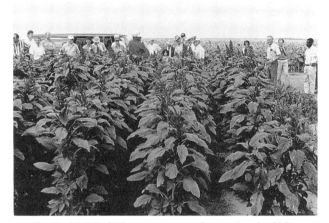

Fig. 3. Field of Pioneer amaranth growing in Sidney, Nebraska, 1991.

is grown by producers for commercial production (Fig. 2). The Nebraska Agricultural Experiment Station is presently in the process of releasing the grain amaranth cultivar, 'Plainsman' (PI 358322). 'Plainsman' is a red-flowered, golden seeded selection of *A. hypochrondriacus* (Fig. 3). 'Plainsman' was selected in part based on its early maturity. Also available as a grain amaranth line is A200D which was selected for domestic production by Nu-World Amaranth, Naperville, IL.

FUTURE PROSPECTS

It has been three years since the report on grain amaranth in the First National Symposium on New Crops (Kauffman and Webber 1990). During these past three years, United States amaranth production has risen from approximately 1,000 to 1,800 ha. Nebraska reported an estimated 1,200 ha planted in 1991, Colorado 120 ha, Minnesota 80 ha, and Montana 30 to 40 ha. Reports of production increase of 800 ha though quite small for an agronomic crop, is nearly a doubling in three years.

In a survey response sent to all 50 states, six Land Grant agronomists estimated 2 ha or less of amaranth while 26 reported that they knew of no amaranth production in their respective states. Another 10 states indicated amaranth production of 12 to 1,200 ha, with 14 states not responding to the amaranth questionnaire. Personal communication with the millers and marketers, indicated that while not all grain supplies have been sold, amaranth sales in the market place has been quite active.

Perhaps the key issue with the future of amaranth will be determined by the end-use product. If the primary amaranth product use will continue to be the niche organic health food market then we do not foresee a major expansion of production acreage. However, if amaranth can be incorporated into a major flour milling blend for large volume uses, then significant expansion could follow.

The 1988 amaranth report summarized, "grain amaranth as a new crop that is in its adolescence." In our 1991 report, we can report a small significant healthy growth in the entire industry, from basic and applied research studies, to continued grower innovations, and to a strong viable processing, milling, and marketing industry. Successful agronomic production and cultivation development will be the determining factor to both maintaining and/or expanding the amaranth industry. In Montana, the most successful method to establish amaranth stands can be achieved by fall ridging of the 76 cm rows, spring de-ridging, and planting into firm moist soil. Since the major production areas are in the semi-arid high plains area of the western United States, stand establishment will be most important along with weed control. Weed control can be successful by use of mechanical cultivation and hand weeding when necessary. Given our experiences with grain amaranth during the past nine years, we have been encouraged by the growth of the amaranth industry, particularly the positive attitude of the amaranth marketers. This in turn has encouraged us to suggest to Montana producers that they consider small trials for production considerations (Schaeffer et al. 1989, 1990, 1991).

REFERENCES

Baltensperger, D.D., D.J. Lyon, L.A. Nelson, and A. Corr. 1991. Amaranth grain production in Nebraska. NebFacts F-2, NF 91–35, Inst. Agr. and Natural Resources, Coop. Ext., Univ. Nebraska, Lincoln.

Becker, R., E.L. Wheeler, K. Lorenz, A.E. Stafford, O.K. Grosjean, A.A. Betschart, and R.M. Saunders. 1981. A composition study of amaranth grain. J. Food Sci. 46:1175–1180.

Becker, R. 1989. Preparation, composition and nutritional implications of amaranth seed oil. Cereal Foods World 34:950–953.

Breene, W.M. 1991. Food uses of grain amaranth. Cereal Foods World 36:426–430.

Brenner, D. and H. Hauptli. 1990. Seed shattering control with indehiscent utricles in grain amaranth. Legacy 3:2–3 Amer. Amaranth Inst., Bricelyn, MN.

Bressani, R. 1989. The proteins of grain amaranth. Food Rev. Int. 5:13–38.

Bressani, R. 1990. Grain amaranth. It's chemical composition and nutritive value. In: Proc. Fourth Amaranth Symp. Minnesota Ext. Serv., Minnesota Agr., Univ. Minnesota, St Paul.

Cheeke, P.R. and J. Bronson. 1980. Feeding trials with *Amaranthus* grain, forage and leaf protein concentrates. In: Proc. Second Amaranth Conf. Rodale Press. Emmaus, PA.

Elbehri, A., D. Putnam, and M. Schmitt. 1990. Evaluation of N, P, K, effects on amaranth yield using a central composite design. Proc. Fourth Amaranth Conf. Minnesota Ext. Serv., Minnesota Agr., Univ. Minnesota, St Paul.

Feine, L.B., R.R. Harwood, C.S. Kauffman, and J.P. Senft. 1979. Amaranth, gentle giant of the past and future, p. 41–63. In: G.A. Ritchie (ed.). New agricultural crops. Westview Press, Boulder, CO.

Grubben, G.J.H. and D.H. von Sloten. 1981. Genetic resources of amaranth: A global plan of action. AGP: IBPGR/80/2. Int. Board for Plant Genet. Resources. FAO, Rome, Italy.

Igbokwe, P.E., S.C. Tiwari, J.B. Collins, J.B. Tartt, and L.C. Russell. 1988. Amaranth—A potential crop for southwestern Mississippi. Res. Report 13 No. 10. Mississippi Agr. & Forestry Expt. Sta., Mississippi State Univ., Mississippi State.

Kauffman, C.S., N.N. Bailey, and B.T. Volak. 1983. Amaranth grain production guide. Rodale Press. Emmaus, PA.

Kauffman, C.S. and L.E. Webber. 1990. Grain amaranth, p. 127–139. In: J. Janick and J.E. Simon (eds.). Advances in new crops. Timber Press, Portland, OR.

Kulakaw, P.A. and S.K. Jain. 1990. Grain amaranth crop species, evolution and genetics. In: Proc. Fourth Amaranth Conf., Minnesota Ext. Serv., Minnesota Agr., University Minnesota, St Paul.

Lehman, J. 1988. Carbohydrates of amaranth. Legacy 1:4–8 Amer. Amaranth Inst. Bricelyn, MN.

Lehman, J. 1989. Proteins of grain amaranth. Legacy 2:3–6 Amer. Amaranth Inst. Bricelyn, MN.

Lehman, J. 1990. Pigments of grain and feral amaranths. Legacy 3:3–4 Amer. Amaranth Inst., Bricelyn, MN.

Lehman, J. 1991. Lipids of grain and feral amaranths. Legacy 4:2–6 Amer. Amaranth Inst., Bricelyn, MN.

Lyon, C.K. and R. Becker. 1987. Extraction and refining of oil from amaranth seed. J. Am. Oil Chem. Soc. 64:233–236.

Makus, J.D. 1984. Evaluation of amaranth as a potential greens crop in the mid-south. HortScience 19:881–883.

Makus, D.J. and D.R. Davis. 1984. A mid-summer crop for fresh greens or canning—vegetable amaranth. Ark. Farm Res. May–June.

Makus, D.J. 1989. Aluminum accumulation in vegetable amaranth grown in a soil with adjusted pH values. HortScience 24:460–463.

Makus, D.J. 1990a. Composition and nutritive value of vegetable amaranth as affected by stage of growth, environment and method of preparation. Proc. Fourth Amaranth Symp. Minnesota Ext. Serv., Minnesota Agr., Univ. Minnesota, St Paul.

Makus, D.J. 1990b. Applied nitrogen affects vegetable and grain amaranth seed yield and quality. In: Proc. Fourth Amaranth Conf., Minnesota Ext. Serv., Minnesota Agr., Univ. Minnesota, St Paul.

Meyers, R.L. and D.H. Putman. 1988. Growing grain amaranth as a specialty crop. Minnesota Ext. Serv., Ag-FS-3458. Univ. Minnesota, St Paul.

National Academy of Sciences. 1985. Amaranth: Modern prospects for an ancient crop. Natl. Acad. Sci., Washington DC.

Pedersen, B., L. Hallgren, I. Hansen, and B.O. Eggum. 1987. The nutritive value of amaranth grain (*Amaranthus caudatus*) 2. As a supplement to cereals. Plant Foods Hum. Nutr. 36:325–334.

Pedersen, B., K.E. Bach Knudsen, and B.O. Eggum. 1990. The nutritive value of amaranth grain (*Amaranthus caudatus*). 3. Energy and fiber of raw and processed grain. Plant Foods Hum. Nutr. 40:61–71.

Pond, W.G. and J.W. Lehman. 1989. Nutritive value of a vegetable amaranth cultivar for growing lambs. J. Anim. Sci. 67:3036–3039.

Pond, W.G., J.W. Lehman, R. Elmore, F. Husby, C.C. Calvert, C.W. Newman, B. Lewis, R.L. Harrold, and J. Froseth. 1991. Feeding value of raw or heated grain amaranth germplasm. Anim. Feed Sci. Technol. 33:221–236.

Putnam, D.H., E.S. Oplinger, J.D. Doll, and E.M. Schulte. 1989. Amaranth. Alternate field crops manual. Univ. Wisconsin Coop. Ext., Minnesota Ext. Serv., Univ. Minnesota, St Paul.

Putnam, D.H. 1990. Agronomic practices for grain amaranth. In: Proc. Fourth Amaranth Conf. Minnesota Ext. Serv., Minnesota Agr., Univ. Minnesota, St Paul.

Sanchez, J.M.C. 1990. Amaranth (*Amaranthus* spp.) as a forage. In: Proc. Fourth Amaranth Conf., Minnesota Ext. Serv., Minnesota Agr., Univ. Minnesota, St Paul.

Sauer, J.D. 1967. The grain amaranths and their relatives: a revised taxonomic and geographic survey. Ann. Mo. Bot. Gard. 54:103–137.

Saunders, R.M. and R. Becker. 1984. *Amaranthus*: a potential food and feed source, p. 357–396. In: Y. Pomeranz (ed.). Advances in cereal science and technology. Vol. 6. Amer. Assn. Cereal Chem., St Paul, MN.

Schaeffer, J., G. Stallknecht, H. Bowman, D. Baldridge, and C. McGuire. 1990a. A specialty crop in Montana, Part I. Montana Farmer-Stockman. Aug.

Schaeffer, J.R., C.F. McGuire, and G.F. Stallknecht. 1990b. Grain amaranth—research and potential. Proc. First Int. Conf. New Industrial Crops and Products. Oct. 8–12, Riverside, CA.

Schaeffer, J., G. Stallknecht, H. Bowman, D. Baldridge, and C. McGuire. 1991. Grain Amaranth: A specialty crop in Montana, Part II. Montana Farmer-Stockman Sept.

Schulz-Schaeffer, J., D.E. Baldridge, G.F. Stallknecht, and R.A. Larson. 1988. Grain amaranth: A way to diversify your farming enterprise. MontGuide, MT 8808. Agr. Ext. Serv. Montana State Univ., Bozeman.

Schulz-Schaeffer, J., G.F. Stallknecht, D.E. Baldridge, and R.A. Larson. 1989a. Registration of Montana-3 grain amaranth germplasm. Crop Sci. 29:244–245.

Schulz-Schaeffer, J., D.M. Webb, D.E. Baldridge, G.F. Stallknecht, and R.A. Larson. 1989b. Registration of Montana-5 grain amaranth germplasm. Crop Sci. 29:1581.

Schulz-Schaeffer, J., D.E. Baldridge, H.F. Bowman, G.F. Stallknecht, and R.A. Larson. 1991. Registration of 'Amont' grain amaranth. Crop Sci. 31:482–483.

Schulte, E.E., J.B. Peters, and K.A. Kelling. 1991. The effect of soil pH and liming on the yield and quality of crops. Ann. Rpt. to the Wisconsin Dept. Agr. Trade and Consumer Protection. Project 1813, Dept. Soil Sci., Univ. Wisconsin, Madison.

Singhal, R.S. and P.R. Kulkarni. 1990a. Some properties of *Amaranthus paniculatas* (Rajgeera) starch pastes. Starch/Starke 42:5–7.

Singhal, R.S. and P.R. Kulkarni. 1990b. Utilization of *Amaranthus paniculatas* (Rajgeera) starch in salad dressing. Starch/Starke 42:52–53.

Singhal, R.S. and P.R. Kulkarni. 1990c. Studies on applicability of *Amaranthus paniculatas* (Rajgeeraa) starch for custard preparation. Starch/Starke 42:102–103.

Stallknecht, G.F., J.E. Duffus, and J. Schaeffer. 1990. Curly Top virus in grain amaranth. Post Paper. Fourth U.S. Amaranth Conf., Minneapolis, MN Aug 23–25.

Teutonico, R.A. and D. Knorr. 1985. Amaranth: Composition, properties, and applications of a rediscovered food crop. Food Technol. 39:49–60.

Toll, J. and D.H. von Sloten. 1982. Directory of germplasm collections. Int. Board Plant Genet. Resour. Rome, Italy.

Tucker, J.B. 1986. Amaranth: the once and future crop. BioScience 36:9–13, 59–60.

Walters, R.D., D.L. Coffey, and C.E. Sams. 1988. Fiber, nitrate, and protein content of *Amaranthus* accessions as affected by soil nitrogen application and harvest date. HortScience 23:338–341.

Webb, D.M., J.R. Schaeffer, and C.W. Smith. 1984. Screening of grain amaranth for adaptation to Montana, USA. Proc. Third Amaranth Conf. Rodale Press, Emmaus, PA.

Weber, L.E., E.S. Hubbard, L.A. Nelson, D.H. Putnam, and J.W. Lehman. 1988. Amaranth grain production guide. Rodale Press, Emmaus, PA.

Weber, L.E., W.W. Applegate, D.L. Johnson, L.A. Nelson, D.H. Putnam, and J.W. Lehman. 1989. Amaranth grain production guide. Rodale Press, Emmaus, PA.

Weber, L.E., W.W. Applegate, D.D. Baltensperger, M.D. Irwin, J.W. Lehman, and D.H. Putnam. 1990. Amaranth-Grain Production Guide. Rodale Press, Emmaus, PA.

Weber, L.E. and C.S. Kauffman. 1990. Plant breeding and seed production. In: Proc. Fourth Amaranth Conf. Minnesota Ext. Serv., Minnesota Agr., Univ. Minnesota, St Paul.

Whittaker, P. and M.O. Ologunde. 1990. Study of iron bioavailability in a native Nigerian grain amaranth cereal for young children using a rat model. Cereal Chem. 67:505–508.

Wilson, R.L. 1990. Insects and disease pests of amaranth. In: Proc. Fourth Amaranth Conf. Minnesota Ext. Serv., Minnesota Agr., Univ. Minnesota, St Paul.

Row Spacing and Population Effects on Yield of Grain Amaranth in North Dakota

T.L. Henderson, A.A. Schneiter, and N. Riveland

Grain amaranth (*Amaranthus* spp.), a high protein pseudo-cereal which originated in Central and South America, was a staple crop of ancient Aztec and Inca civilizations. Since the mid-1970s, amaranth has received attention as a new crop for North America. Trials conducted in North Dakota since 1981 indicate that certain cultivars of grain amaranth are well adapted in the eastern part of this state, producing more than 2000 kg/ha (Henderson et al. 1991).

Results of research to determine optimal row spacing have been inconclusive (Robinson 1986). Grain yield response to plant density has been shown to be influenced by environments, species, and cultivars (Putnam 1990). Robinson (1986) reported a decline in yield at populations greater than 210,000 plants/ha. Yet, Haas (1983) identified a much higher range of optimal plant density, between 323,000 and 360,000 plants/ha. A positive yield response to increasing plant density was observed for lower populations (20,000 to 60,000 plants/ha) (Edwards and Volak 1980). At excessively high populations, competition for moisture and nutrients reduces grain yield (Weber 1990). The relationship between plant density and grain yield may be influenced by cultivar (Edwards and Volak 1980; Haas 1983).

This study was conducted as part of research at North Dakota State University to establish production guidelines for grain amaranth in North Dakota. Our objective was to determine the most suitable row spacing and plant population for grain amaranth production in North Dakota.

METHODOLOGY

Four grain amaranth cultivars, 'K283' and 'MT-3' (both *A. cruentus*), and 'K343' and 'K432' (both *A. hypochondriacus* x *A. hybridus*), were evaluated at Prosper and Williston, North Dakota, in 1989 and 1990. Populations of 74, 173, and 272 thousand plants/ha were established for each cultivar at narrow (30.5 cm) and wide (76.2 cm) row spacing. Stands were oversown and thinned by hand to establish the desired populations. Experimental design was a randomized complete block with a split-split plot arrangement. Row spacing, established plant population, and cultivars constituted the main, sub, and sub-sub plots, respectively. All plots were hand-harvested. Grain yield was determined for each plot. Precipitation was recorded daily at each environment.

RESULTS AND DISCUSSION

Main effects of row spacing, established population, and cultivar on grain yield for individual environments are presented in Table 1. In the combined analysis, a significant environment × cultivar interaction, which can be attributed to precipitation differences, was obtained for grain yield. All cultivars exhibited a decrease in grain yield at the driest environment, Williston 1990, which received only 9.4 cm of precipitation during the growing season, compared to 21.7 cm at Prosper 1989 and 20.0 cm at Prosper 1990. In the combined analysis, highest yields were produced by 'MT-3' and 'K283'.

In the combined analysis, established population had a significant effect on grain yield, with highest yields achieved at the lowest population. The row spacing × established population interaction was significant for grain yield as a yield advantage for wider rows at the higher populations (Fig. 1). This response occurred presumably due to increased competition within the rows which decreased plant population after establishment, resulting in more water and nutrients for surviving individual plants in the wider rows.

A similar row spacing × population interaction effect was observed at Prosper during 1990. To examine the influence of row width and established population on plant competition, final plant population at harvest was determined for each plot at the Prosper 1990 environment. A significant row spacing × established population interaction was observed for final population. Intrarow competition was greater at the 76.2 cm row width, resulting in a substantial loss of plant population by harvest time, especially at the higher established populations.

Table 1. Mean amaranth grain yield values by environment for main effects of row spacing, established population, and cultivar.

Environment	Mean grain yield (kg/ha)		
	Prosper 1989	Prosper 1990	Williston 1990
Row width (cm)	*	NS	**
30.5	867	1414	344
76.2	1228	1452	477
LSD 0.05	217	---	31
Established population (plants/ha)	NS	*	**
74000	1114	1513	479
173000	993	1450	410
272000	1035	1337	344
LSD 0.05	---	132	32
Cultivar	**	**	**
K283	1193	1467	571
K343	989	1566	291
K432	661	976	294
MT-3	1348	1724	487
LSD 0.05	180	131	47

NSIndicates not significant at the 0.05 level.
*Indicates significant at the 0.05 level.
**Indicates significant at the 0.01 level.

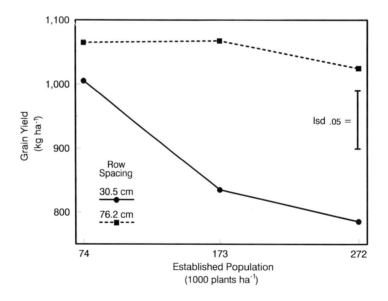

Fig. 1. Mean amaranth grain yield values for established population × row spacing interaction, based on combined analysis of three environments in North Dakota. (Least significant difference 0.05 = 93.6 kg/ha.)

Significant losses in plant population were not observed with the narrower row spacing. Grain yield increased as final population decreased (Fig. 2). Results of the combined analysis suggest that at the lowest established population, row width was not critical. At the higher established populations, a yield advantage was obtained with wider row spacing, due to lowered plant density resulting from competition within the rows.

SUMMARY

Highest amaranth grain yields were obtained at the Prosper location in eastern North Dakota, which received more precipitation during the growing season. 'MT-3' and 'K283' (*A. cruentus*) were the highest yielding cultivars in the combined experiment. The lowest established population, 74,000 plants/ha, consistently produced the highest grain yield. Row spacing had no effect at the lowest population, while at the higher populations, more grain was produced with the wider (76.2 cm) row spacing. With the wider rows, plants within each row were spaced closer together, leading to increased competition at high established populations. This intrarow competition caused substantial losses in plant numbers after establishment. Grain yield of the surviving plants was higher as a result of the lowered plant population in the wider rows.

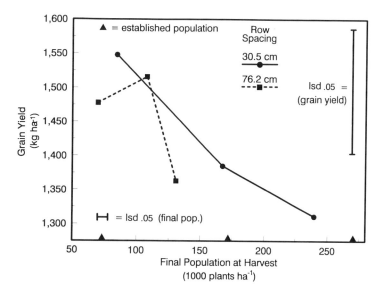

Fig. 2. Mean amaranth grain yield values as a function of row spacing and final plant population at Prosper, ND in 1990. (Least significant difference 0.05 = 185.9 kg/ha and 7781 plants/ha for grain yield and final population, respectively.)

REFERENCES

Edwards, A.D. and B. Volak. 1980. Grain amaranth: optimization of field population density, p. 91–94. In: Proc. 2nd Amaranth Conference. Rodale Press, Emmaus, PA.

Haas, P.W. 1983. Amaranth density report. Rodale Research Center Report No. RRC/NC-83-8. Rodale Press, Emmaus, PA.

Henderson, T.L., A.A. Schneiter, B.L. Johnson, N. Riveland, and B.G. Schatz. 1991. Production of amaranth in the Northern Great Plains. In: Alternative crop and alternative crop production research: a progress report. North Dakota State Univ., Fargo.

Putnam, D.H. 1990. Agronomic practices for amaranth, p. 151–162. In: Proc. 4th National Amaranth Symposium. Rodale Press, Emmaus, PA.

Robinson, R.G. 1986. Amaranth, quinoa, ragi, tef and niger: tiny seeds of ancient history and modern interest. Station Bul. AD-SB-2949. Agr. Expt. Sta., Univ. of Minn., St. Paul.

Weber, L.E. 1990. Amaranth grain production guide. Rodale Press, Emmaus, PA.

Quinoa

Duane L. Johnson and Sarah M. Ward

*On December 16, 1983, Dr. Norman Borlaugh (with others) visited the National Agrarian University in La Moina, Peru... In their talks they emphasized the development of Opaque Maize and the importance of the fact that its protein content, in the form of lysine... has been increased from 2.8 to 4%... It was pointed out (by the Andeans) that in both centers of pre-Hispanic maize cultivation, the Central Andes and Meso-America, indigenous farmers intuitively knew that maize's nutritional imbalance could be improved, not by forcing a plant to produce a balanced food, but by associating it with another crop that had a high content of the amino acids that maize was lacking... In the Andes maize was associated with quinoa... while on the Mexican plateau its relative Huazontle (*Chenopodium Nutalliae*) was cultivated.*

Editorial *of the Andean Food Crops Bulletin, March 1984*

Most of the Indian products are still under cultivation....On the plateau (Peru) the grain crops were quinoa *and* canuagua. *The* quinoa *struck me as being a crop from which a choice breakfast food could be made. It was starchy with just enough tang from its pigweed blood to produce a good flavor.*

H.V. Harlan's One Man's Life with Barley *(1953)*

TAXONOMY

Quinoa (*Chenopodium quinoa* Willd.) is generally considered to be a single species within the Chenopodiaceae. Quinoa is used much as a cereal crop, yet it is not a grass and has been classified as a pseudocereal. Wilson (1990) states that over 120 species have been found within the genus *Chenopodium*. Two species, *C. berlandieri* and *C. hircinum* contain the same chromosome number as quinoa ($2n = 36$). Wilson (1988) has obtained interspecific hybridization between these species.

Quinoa has a long and distinguished history in South America. Quinoa has been cultivated in the Andean highlands since 3,000 BC (Tapia 1982). In the Quechua language of the Incas, quinoa is the *chisiya mama* or "mother grain;" in Spanish, it is *quinoa, trigo inca,* or *arroz del Peru* (National Research Council 1989). Its adaptation to cold, dry climates, seed processing similarity to rice, and excellent nutritional qualities make quinoa a crop of considerable value to highland areas around the world which are currently limited as far as crop diversity and nutritional value. Development of other *Chenopodium* species in the United States (Wilson 1981) the Himalayas (Partap and Kapoor 1985), Mexico (Risi and Galway 1989), and Denmark (Renfrew 1973) illustrate a diverse appreciation for this genera. Even the weedy relatives, *C. alba* and *C. berlanderii*, in the United States and around the world have been utilized as a food during times of starvation.

NUTRITIONAL VALUE

In the time of the Incas, quinoa sustained armies which frequently marched for days and could eat a mixture of quinoa and fat known as "war balls" (D. Cusack pers. commun.). Nutrition, from its almost perfect amino acid composition to its high content of calcium, phosphorus, and iron to its low sodium content, still is the major contributor to quinoa's popularity.

The nutritional value of quinoa has been known for a long time to be superior to traditional cereals and is, in fact, superior to milk solids in feeding trails (White et al. 1955). Protein content ranges from 10 to 18% with a fat content of 4.1 to 8.8%. Starch, ash, and crude fiber average 60.1, 4.2, and 3.4%, respectively (DeBruin 1964; Ballon pers. commun.). The ash has been found to primarily consist of potassium and phosphorus (65% of total). Calcium and iron are significantly higher in quinoa than in rice, maize, wheat, or oats (White et al. 1955; DeBruin 1964). Variations have been observed between species and between landraces within species. Many landraces of quinoa contain saponin in the seedcoat. Saponins function as "antinutrients" and are frequently associated with plant lipids. They are not normally absorbed from the gut and have been shown to induce small intestinal damage or reduce intestinal absorption of nutrients (Jenkins 1988). Quinoa saponin is a known hemolytic when mixed with blood cells. In South America, saponin removed from quinoa is used as a detergent for clothing, washing and as an antiseptic to promote healing of skin injuries (D. Cusack pers. commun.; E. Ballon pers. commun.). Saponin can be removed either mechanically or with a water rinse (White et al. 1955; DeBruin 1964; Mahoney et al. 1975). Mechanical abrasion systems currently in use fail to remove all saponin, leaving bran with saponin attached to perisperm granules (Becker and Hanners 1991).

Mechanical abrasion of quinoa has been found to significantly increase α-amylase activity in quinoa (Lorenz and Nyanzi 1989). This appears to be due to the reduction in the pericarp content during abrasion. Quinoa has a significantly higher α-amylase content than cereals such as rice and proso millet. Amylograph analyses also show quinoa to have superior α-amylase activity to wheat (Lorenz and Nyanzi 1989). The mineral content of quinoa has been evaluated both in South America by Ballon (pers. commun.) and by the author for North American quinoa. Results indicate a mineral profile which is generally higher than comparable cereals (Table 1).

BREEDING RESEARCH

Quinoa is primarily an inbreeding species with plants bearing hermaphroditic flowers. Ward (1991) has found the hermaphroditic nature of quinoa to be variable. In a study of male sterility, male fertile plants were found to possess anthers in only 10 to 90% of the inflorescences, with fertile flowers concentrated at the distal ends of the flower cluster. Outcrossing exceeds 10% (D.L. Johnson unpublished). These outcrossing estimates are similar to those reported in South America. Wind pollination studies of fertile quinoa (CO 407) with an orange panicle by a red-panicled near-isoline (CO 407R) indicate pollen to move 36 cm. Plants samples beyond that distance show no cross pollination to the CO 407R source in any direction (S. Ward pers. commun.). No insect activity in flowers was observed, although various *Diptera* spp. have been observed to visit quinoa flowers in Colorado's San Luis Valley and may add to wind distribution of pollen.

Quinoa has received a considerable amount of attention in the Andean highlands over the past two decades (Johnson 1990). Quinoa production extends from Columbia to Chile and Argentina and a diversity of landraces have resulted. Within the major quinoa production areas of Columbia, Ecuador, Peru, and Bolivia, Gandarillas (1968) described 17 races based upon morphological characters. Galwey (1989) and Tapia (1979) proposed four main types based upon geographic location: The "Valley" type, typical from 2,000 to 4,000 m in elevation; the "Altiplano" type, typical of highland areas above 4,000 m; the "Salar" type of 4,000 m but adapted to the high pH soils typical of the Atacama region; the "Sea Level" types found in the inner valleys of Bolivia. The "Sea Level" type has been described by Wilson's electrophoretic work to be distinctly different from the other highland quinoas. Cusack (1984) proposed that quinoa within South American cultures may have arisen independently. Wilson (1990) has proposed a division of quinoa into two distinct groups: northern and southern. The northern group, being less diverse than the southern, would indicate it is derived from the southern group. In Colorado crossing trials, quinoas within Wilson's groups have shown no heterosis for yield while crosses between his groups have shown heterosis varying between 201 and 491%.

The heterosis demonstrated in quinoa initiated a search for male sterility in 1987 and 1988. Using commercial fields in Colorado, no male steriles were found in the cultivar 'CO 407'—a Southern, Sea Level type of quinoa common to Colorado. In 1989, Ward (1991) obtained two potential sources of male sterile—one from

Table 1. Mineral analysis of four selected crops (Wahli 1990).

Crop	Content (ppm)					
	Calcium	Phosphorus	Iron	Potassium	Sodium	Zinc
Quinoa	1274	3869	20	6967	115	48
Barley	880	4200	50	5600	200	15
Beans	1191	3674	86	10982	103	32
Wheat	550	4700	50	8700	115	14

the cultivar 'Amachuma' and another from the cultivar 'Apelawa'. The 'Amachuma' type appears to be a simply inherited, genetic male sterile. The 'Apelawa' type is a cytoplasmic male sterile and Ward (1991) has transferred this trait into four additional background genotypes. Other sources of male sterility in quinoa have been reported such as genic-cytoplasmic male sterility (Simmons 1971); a single gene male sterile (Gandarillas 1979); and a cytoplasmic male sterile reported by Galwey and Risi (1984). Research on male sterility in quinoa has generally not received a great deal of attention or replication and at this point, only Ward's work appears definitive.

Evaluation of germplasm can be difficult given the array of accessions available. One method to separate the diversity modern researchers have observed in quinoa is through canonical discriminate analysis. Risi and Galwey (1989) used a canonical discriminant analysis with 19 traits for accessions from sea level types, altiplano types, salar types, and valley types. Risi and Galwey found the sea level and valley types to be very homogeneous within type. Other types were difficult to discriminate. E. Ballon and D. Johnson (unpubl.) studied 15 cultivars and found altiplano, valley, and sea level types were not homogeneous within type when grown in Colorado and New Mexico.

Significant differences in agronomic value in the United States were observed between 15 cultivars for protein, seed size, and yield, with no significant location effects. There was, however, a significant cultivar by location interaction in all cases (Ballon et al. 1991). Similar yield results were observed by Galwey and Risi (1984) in England and in Finland (Carmen 1984). Ballon et al. (1991) also conducted a heritability for grain yield and grain size. Broad-sense heritabilities of 49 and 32% were estimated for yield and seed size, respectively. Heritability for protein content was not calculated.

CULTURAL PRACTICES

Nitrogen has been observed in both South America and Colorado to be very influential for yield increases. Gandarillas (1982) noted quinoa responds only to nitrogen with no measurable response being observed for either phosphorus or potassium. Under rainfed conditions, Gandarillas noted a response of 13.8 kg/ha per kg/ha of urea added. In irrigated fields, quinoa yield response was 16.6 kg/ha per kg/ha of urea applied. Currently, recommendations in South America are for 120 kg/ha of urea. Identical recommendation from field trrials in Colorado has been made by the author. Nitrogen applications have also significantly increased protein content of quinoa. The author has found protein percentage to increase by 0.1% per kg of ammonium nitrate applied. Protein in Colorado ranged from 16.2 to 18.6% in the cultivar (CO 407).

Irrigation may have a significant effect on yield. Tapia (1984) recommends an average of 550 mm of available moisture. In the loamy soils typical of the Valley quinoa types, 700 mm may be required while types which grow in the saltflats of Southern Bolivia require 350 mm. In Colorado, Flynn (1990) found maximum yields of 1439 kg/ha were obtained on sandy-loam soils with 208 mm of water (rainfall and irrigation) with available water levels of 128, 208, 307, and 375 mm being tested.

Seeding rates vary between United States recommendations and those of South America. Current United States recommendations are for seeding rates of 1 to 1.5 million plant/ha (Johnson and Croissant 1985). South American recommendations are for 8 million/ha for row cropping and 20 million/ha for broadcast cultural practices.

Weed control has had a major impact on quinoa yield. In Colorado, grassy weed control alone increased yields from 640 kg/ha to 1,822 kg/ha (Johnson 1990). Weed control via herbicides have been effective and several show promise. In England, Metamazide, Propachlor, Linuron, Propyzamide, and aloxium sodium did not significantly reduce plant stands of two quinoa cultivars (Galwey and Risi 1984). In Colorado, preliminary herbicide studies of pre-emerge herbicides with Dual, Furloe, Sutan, and Antor showed good crop safety and control of grasses and many broadleaf weeds (Westra 1988). Post-emergent control was best for Poast, Tough, and Probe, with Tough and Probe at lower rates (Westra 1988).

Salt tolerance is of concern to quinoa growers in the arid regions of the world. Preliminary work by the University of Arizona indicates that quinoa is very salt tolerant. Germination of five quinoa cultivars was unaffected by salinity levels varying from 114 to 2,169 ppm NaCl. Growth over a 6-week period shows CO 407 to be superior to other cultivars at the 2,169 ppm level with only a 40% reduction in plant height. 'Isluge' (CO 211), a salt adapted cultivar, had a 45% reduction in plant height (D. Shropshire and V. Lindley pers. commun.).

Insects are a major concern in South America and have received increasing attention in the United States. In South America, Romero (1980) has pointed out two important pests of quinoa: Kcona Kcona (*Scrobipalpula* sp.) which destroy buds, inflorescences, immature and mature grain; and "leaf miners" (*Liriomyza* sp.) which destroy leaves and occasionally stacks of quinoa. In Colorado, Cranshaw et al. (1990) found insects commonly associated with sugar beet and lambsquarters (*C. alba* L.). Seedling damage was caused by *Malanotrichus coagulatus* Ulher and *Atomoscelis modestus* Van Duzee and the seed bug, *Nysius raphanus* Howard. Foliar pests include two leaf miners, *Pegomyia hyoscyami* Panzer and *Monoxia* nr. *pallida* Blake. Also found were leaf feeding insects such as a leaf curling aphid *Hayhursita atriplicis* (L.) and various *Lepidoptera*, such as *Spodoptera exiqua* Hubner. A foot, or root feeding aphid, *Pemphgus populivenae* Fitch caused late season damage. Seed damage was due to *Lygus* spp.

PROCESSING

Saponin, a component of the pericarp of quinoa seed, is a known toxic glycoside. Saponin can be found in the pericarp of several species such as quinoa, alfalfa, hops, and soybean and is easily identified by production of a soapy lather when placed in water and by being soluble in pure alcohol. It also gives unwashed quinoa a bitter flavor and has antinutritional properties.

There are apparently two types of saponin: (1) a rarer acid and neutral saponin group (found in white quinoas) that can be used commercially in the production of pharmaceutical steroids, and (2) a more common type prevalent in the yellow quinoa cultivars which is used in soaps, detergents, beer production, fire extinguishers, photography, shampoos, cosmetics, and pharmeceuticals (synthetic hormones). Within the saponin of quinoa, two aglycones predominate: oleanolic acid and heterogenin. The ratio of oleanolic acid to heterogenin varies from 2.3 to 8.6 (Burnouf-Radosevich et al., 1983) depending upon the cultivar. Oleanolic acid and heterogenin content averaged 3.0 and 1.4 mg/g. Triterpene concentration ranged from 6.3 mg/g for 'Real de Puno' to as low as 0.06 mg/g for 'Sajama' and was found to be highly proportional to saponin content.

Once saponin is removed, protein quality was unaffected. Amino acid balance was virtually the same regardless of saponin content of the seed (Burnouf-Radossevich et al., 1983). Both soluble proteins (albumins and globulins) and the high molecular weight glutelins were measured. High saponin cultivars lacked three glutelin subunits and may be useful as protein markers for low-saponin type quinoas.

Processing quinoa to remove saponin can be done by alkaline water washing or mechanically via abrasion. Mechanical dehulling involves "pearling" the grain to remove the pericarp as bran. High saponin cultivars require more abrasion than low saponin types. Washing quinoa is probably not at the current time a viable option in developed countries due to pollution of water where potential pollution of major bodies of water may be affected. In South America, a "dry" system involving a flotation cell is used. The seed is wetted and dirt, saponin, and foreign matter are removed and the grain then subjected to forced air to dry. Foam breakdown and drying costs are serious problems in this method. The grain can also be "pre-toasted" and "polished" or abraided using a spinning stone (Gandarillas 1982). Abrasion also tends to reduce ash content in quinoa and has been demonstrated to increase α-amylase activity. Reichert et al. (1986a,b) found the saponin content of quinoa flour could be effectively reduced by minimal abrasion in a Tangential Abrasive Dehulling Device (TADD).

Becker and Hanners (1991) used three quinoas (low, medium, and high saponin content) and a Morehouse Model 350 stone mill to evaluate saponin removal. The stone mill removed 33 to 40% of the seed as bran fraction. Moisture tempering the grain from 8 to 16% did not improve milling yield or mill fraction composition. The mill fraction typically contained less than 0.3 mg/g of saponin and residual bran was left on the grain. The extremely high loss of grain via mechanical milling indicates an area of research which needs more work.

Nutritional analyses of quinoa have generally been conducted on desaponified quinoa. In one such test, Dahlin (1991) tested quinoa against high and low tannin sorghum, corn, wheat, rye, and proso millet. In the unprocessed (nonextruded) state, quinoa was found to be the most carbohydrate digestible of the seven crops. Dahlin states that this is probably due to the very high concentration of α-amylase in quinoa. Quinoa carbohydrates improved in digestibility when extruded at 25% feed moisture and a 100°/150°C initial/final food temperature, but unlike cereals, overall digestibility decreased with extrusion. Dahlin measured nitrogen solubility, a measure of biological value of protein. Nitrogen solubility was highest for quinoa and rye and ranged from 20.9 at pH 2.0 to 30.0 at pH 10.

Kleiman et al.(1972) evaluated oil from four species of the Chenopodiaceae and found most contained some unusual components. These are methyl *cis*-5-hexadecenoate (4.6 to 12%) and methyl 5-octadecenoate (1.1 to 1.2%). Kleiman et al. also observed quinoa oil to contain small amounts of $18:2^{5,9}$ and $18:3^{5,9,12}$. The majority of the oil, however was common to most seeds with oleic fatty acids composing 14 to 21% of the oil. Linoleic and linolenic fatty acids composed 53 to 57% and 3.5 to 7.8% respectively. These oil compositions are similar to those obtained from quinoa's distant relatives, spinach (*Spinacea oleracea* L.) and Russian thistle (*Salsola pestifer*).

The unusual components, methyl *cis*-5-hexadecenoate and methyl 5-octadecenoate occur in other plant species but are the highest in concentration in the Chenopodiaceae. Quinoa was unique among the four species in that it lacked methyl *cis*-5-hexadecenoate and methyl 5-octadecenoate in detectable amounts. Quinoa oil was composed of 31% oleic; 45% linoleic; and 2.7% linolenic fatty acids. The remainder of the oil was composed of 16, 20, and 22 carbon fatty acids.

REFERENCES

Ballon, E., L. Robison, D. Johnson, S. Nelson, and T. Claure. 1991. The adaptation of quinoa varieties (*Chenopodium quinoa* W.) and their implications of selection for yield and size of grain. Anales V Cogreso Internacional sobre Cultivos Andinos. (in press).

Becker, R. and G.D. Hanners. 1991. Composition and nutritional evaluation of quinoa whole grain flour and mill fractions. Lebensmittel-Wissenschaft and Technologie 23:441–444.

Burnouf-Radosevich, M., T. Burnouf, and N.E. Delfel. 1983. Saponin content and protein composition in *Chenopodium quinoa*. Abstr. Amer. Assoc. of Cereal Chem., Kansas City, MO.

Carmen, M.L. 1984. Acclimization of quinoa *Chenopodium quinoa* and *Chenopodium pallidicaule* to Finland. Ann. Agr. Fenn. 23:135–144.

Cranshaw, W.S., B.C. Kondraftieff, and T. Qian. 1990. Insects associated with quinoa, *Chenopodium quinoa*. Colorado J. Kansas Ent. Soc. 63:195–199.

Cusack, D. 1984. Quinoa: Grain of the Incas. Ecologist 14:21–31.

DeBruin, A. 1964. Investigation of the food value of quinoa and canihua seed. J. Food Sci. 29:872–876.

Flynn, R.O. 1990. Growth characteristics of quinoa and yield response to increase soil water deficit. MS Thesis, Colorado State Univ. Fort Collins.

Galwey, N.W. 1989. Exploited plants—quinoa. Biologist 36:267–274.

Galwey, N.W. and J. Risi. 1984. Development of the Andean grain crop quinoa for production in Britain. Univ. of Cambridge Annu. Rpt., Cambridge, UK.

Gandarillas, H. 1982. Quinoa production. IBTA–CIID. (Trans. by Sierra–Blanca Assoc., Denver, CO. 1985.)

Gandarillas S.C., H. 1989. Genetica y. origen, p. 45–64. In: M.E. Tapia (ed.). Quinoa y kaniwa. Cultivos Andinos. 49. Instituto Interamericano de Ciancias Agricolas, Bogata.

Gandarillas, S.C., H. 1968. Razas de quinoa. Boletin 34 Instituto Boliviano de Cultivos Andinos. La Paz. In: M.E. Tapia (ed.). Quinoa y. kaniwa. Cultivos Andinos. 49. Instituto Interamericano de Ciencias Agricolas, Bogata.

Harlan, H.V. 1953. One man's life with barley.

Jenkins, D. 1988. Carbohydrates: (B) dietary fiber, p. 52–71. In: M. Shils and V. Young (eds.). Modern nutrition in health and disease. Lea and Febiger, Philadelphia.

Johnson, D.L. 1990. Cereals and pseudocereals, p. 122–127. In: J. Janick and J.E. Simon (eds.). Advances in new crops. Timber Press, Portland, OR.

Johnson, D.L. 1992. Impact of weeds on quinoa yields. Proc. Assoc. Adv. Indust. Crops. (in press).

Johnson, D.L. and R.L. Croissant. 1985. Quinoa production in Colorado. SIA 112. Colorado State Univ. Coop. Ext., Fort Collins.

Kleiman, R., M.H. Rawls, and F.R. Earle. 1972. *cis*-5-monoenoic fatty acids in some Chenopodiaceae seed oils. Lipids 7:494–496.

Lorenz, K. and F. Nyanzi. 1989. Enzyme activities in quinoa (*Chenopodium quinoa*). Int. J. Food Sci. Tech. 24:543–551.

Mahoney, A.W., J.G. Lopez, and D.G. Hendricks. 1975. An evaluation of the protein quality of quinoa. J. Agr. Food Chem. 23:190–193.

Mather, K. 1949. Biometrical genetics. The study of continuous variation. Dover Publ., London

National Research Council. 1989. Lost crops of the Incas: Little known plants of the Andes with promise for world-wide cultivation. National Academy Press, Washington, DC. p. 149–162.

Partap and Kapoor. 1985. The Himalayan India grain chenopods II. Comparative morphology. Agr. Ecosyst. Environ. 14:201–220.

Reichert, R.D., J.T. Tatarynovich, and R.T. Tyler. 1986a. Abrasive dehulling of quinoa (*Chenopodium quinoa*): Effect on saponin content as determined by an adapted hemolytic assay. Cereal Chem. 63:471–474.

Reichert, R.D., R.T. Tyler, A.E. York, D.E. Schwab, J.E. Tataynovich, and M.A. Mwasaru. 1986b. Description of a product model of the tangential abrasive dehulling device and its application to breeder's samples. Cereal Chem. 63:201.

Renfrew, J.M. 1973. Paleoethnobotany. Meuthen, London. as cited by Ward, S. 1991. Male sterility in quinoa (*Chenopodium quinoa* Willd.) MS Thesis, Colorado State Univ., Fort Collins.

Risi, J. and N.W. Galwey. 1989. Chenpodium grains of the Andes: A crop for temperate latitudes, p. 222–234. In: G.E. Wickens, N. Haq, and P. Day (eds.). New crops for food and industry. Chapman and Hall, London.

Romero, R.O. 1980. Biological controls for grain-destroying insects and leaf-miners of quinoa (*Chenopodium quinoa* Willd.), p. 86–91. In: First meeting on genetics and improvement of quinoa. IICA–CIID/Universidad Nacional Technica del Altiplano/Instituto Boliviano de Technologia Agropecuraria.

Simmons, N.W. 1971. The breeding system of *Chenopodium quinoa*. I. Male Sterility. Heredity 27:73–82.

Tapia, M. 1982. The Environment, crops and agricultural systems in the Andes of Southern Peru. IICA.

Ward, S. 1991. Male sterility in quinoa (*Chenopodium quinoa* Willd.) MS Thesis, Colorado State Univ., Fort Collins.

Westra, P. 1988. Weed control in quinoa. Report to Sierra Blanca Assoc.

Wahli, C. 1990. Quinua hacia su cultivo comercial. Latinreco S.A. Quito.

White, P.L., E. Alvistur, C. Dias, E. Vinas, H.S. White, and C. Collazos. 1955. Nutrient content and protein quality of quinoa and canihua, edible seed products of the Andes mountains. J. Agr. Food Chem. 3:531–534.

Wilson, H.D. 1981. Domesticated *Chenopodium* of the Ozark cliff dwellers. Econ. Bot. 35:233–239.

Wilson, H.D. 1988a. Allozyme variation and morphological relationships of *Chenopodium hircinum*. Syst. Bot. 13:215–228.

Wilson, H.D. 1988b. Quinoa biosystematics. I. Domesticated populations. Econ. Bot. 42:461–477.

Wilson, H.D. 1990. Quinoa and relatives (*Chenopodium* sect. *Chenopodium* subsect. *Cellulata*. Econ. Bot. 44:92–110.

Blue Corn

Duane L. Johnson and Mitra N. Jha

Blue corn or maize (*Zea mays* L.) is an open pollinated flour corn and contains soft starch useful in the milling of specialty foods. Currently, these foods include tortillas, pancake mixes, cornbread mixes, corn chips, and cereal. Experimental extrusion of blue corn has been successful, and extruded blue corn products are now being marketed (Arrowhead Mills pers. commun.). Studies at Colorado State University indicate that the protein content of commercial blue corn is consistantly 30% higher than dent corns in adjacent fields (Johnson and Croissant 1990).

Consumption and sales of blue corn is increasing (Fig. 1). The market is in Mexican restaurants, health food stores, and some supermarkets. The term "blue corn" is a generic term with plants producing blue and mixtures of blue and white kernels. Bluecorn sales continue to show growth as shown in Fig 2.

HISTORY

Maize, has been closely associated with the culture and life of the Southwestern American Indian. This paper focuses on a maize of the Hopi Indian, one of the most adaptive of the American Indian tribes. Their culture has been predominantly agricultural throughout their long history in the arid southwest and they have established a reputation as superior dryland farmers (Carter and Anderson 1945). The conservation of their farms is reflected in their crop plants—most notably in their maize. Maize is utilized in ritual as well as a food source. The use of maize in the rituals appears to have preserved these ancient cultivars. Foreign cultures have impacted the Hopi just as they have other cultures in this region. Many of the cultivars of maize grown a century ago by the Hopi are now believed to be extinct while others show an introgression of genes from other maize populations. The number of blue corn races is unknown at this time.

MODERN EVALUATIONS OF BLUE CORN

Blue corn planted in non-irrigated conditions has yielded 1,020 to 3,360 kg/ha with market prices of approximately $0.33 to $0.35/kg paid during the last two years. Hybrid development is ongoing, but open pollinated cultivars are currently the only material available for commercial use.

These maize populations have not been utilized to a great extent in major maize improvement programs and are of value not only historically, but also as germplasm pools for future evaluation. We know that maize landraces are uniquely variable not only from region to region but also from cultivar to cultivar and from plant to plant. For geneticists, such populations provide a stockpile of genes that have rarely been sampled or studied. If these various strains are not preserved, it is inevitable that many of them will be lost to introgression. Furthermore, the germplasm of drought tolerance may reside in the southwestern Indian maizes and this material has not yet been utilized extensively in United States maize improvement programs.

Five Hopi blue flour maize populations were compared to similar populations described in the 1950s by Brown et al. (1952). Two landraces of Southwestern flour maize were obtained from the Talavaya Center (Espanola, New Mexico) and two landraces identified by Krumpacker were provided by Robin Cuany, both from Colorado State University. These maize races had been obtained from local American Indian farmers (New Mexico) and from Hispanic farmers (Colorado). A fifth population was obtained from the Talavaya Center and was identified as "Hopi blue corn." To avoid confusion, this population was referred to as "Hopi blue corn" with other populations having the designation of New Mexico and Colorado blue corn. Variances and covariances between the races of maize indicate significant differences for the traits studied and that these populations do not appear to have a common origin (Table 1). Plant height varied from 1.00 to 1.35 m for both New Mexico and Colorado populations. The Hopi blue corn population differed significantly from the other populations and reached a plant height of 1.8 to 2.4 m. Tillering was observed with eight to ten tillers per plant in the New Mexico and Colorado populations while two to three tillers were seen in the blue corn 1 population. A typical population of New Mexico blue corn is described in Table 2.

The number of rows per ear varied within each New Mexico and Colorado population from 8 to 16 and average 12.3 populations. Row number ranged from 10 to 18 in the Hopi blue corn (Fig. 2). This character is

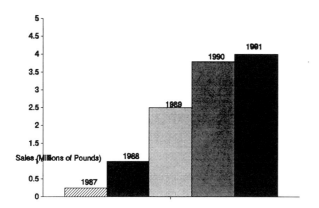

Fig. 1. Bluecorn sales by one United States company.

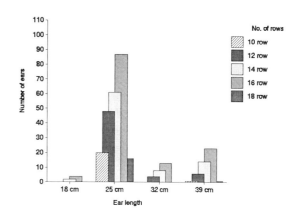

Fig. 2. Row number and ear length of Hopi blue corn populations.

Table 1. Analysis of racial variances in New Mexico and Colorado Hopi flour corns for eight traits.

Variable	MS	F	P	
Kernel yield (g)	16585	25.1	0.000	***
Shank diameter (cm)	164	0.9	0.349	NS
Ear length (cm)	15307	10.9	0.001	**
Cob diameter (cm)	168	10.1	0.002	**
Kernel width (mm)	1	3.8	3.860	NS
Kernel thickness (mm)	5.6	7.7	0.006	**
Row number	3	1.3	0.289	NS
Kernel weight (gm)	602	43.3	0.000	***

Probabilities are reported as ***($P = 0.001$)

Table 2. Description of a New Mexico Hopi corn population grown in Colorado.

Variable	Mean	SD	Min. value	Max. value
Kernel yield (g)	53.6	17.6	32.0	98.0
Shank diameter (cm)	7.4	0.3	1.0	2.6
Ear length (cm)	15.2	3.3	9.0	21.0
Cob diameter (cm)	2.9	0.4	2.2	3.8
Kernel width (mm)	6.7	0.7	5.0	8.0
Kernel thickness (mm)	4.2	2.7	3.7	4.8
Row number	12.2	1.6	8.0	16.0
Kernel weight (gm)	19.1	3.3	10.5	28.9

similar to those previously reported by Brown and Anderson (1947). The characteristic 14 row trait noted in Hopi corn was observed in all races but lacked the apparent preponderance noted by Brown et al. (1952). Ear characteristics such as yield, ear length, cob diameter, kernel thickness, and kernel weight are similar to the Hopi corns previously reported. The differences from prior research (Brown and Anderson 1947) were primarily noted to be in the greater width and reduced length of the kernels, greater ear length, reduced number of rows, greater internode length, greater tillering, and a narrowing of the leaf blades. Many of the phenotypic traits observed differed greatly from those of the Mexican dent corns and the Basketmaker corns. We anticipated that these races might have affected introgression into the Hopi corn populations.

In the Colorado and New Mexico populations, ear length and kernel yield were positively correlated in both the New Mexico ($r = 0.73$) and Colorado ($r = 0.76$) cultivars. A significant correlation between kernel thickness and cob diameter was observed in all populations. These values when compared to those reported by Brown et al. (1952) were similar to the Hopi corns of the early 1950s with one exception: Brown et al. (1952) showed that blue and white flour corn had a negative correlation between kernel width and kernel thickness. This was not been observed in the Colorado study. Positive correlations for these traits to the purple corn were, however, observed in the study. Path analysis of the five corn populations indicates kernel weight, width of kernel, and thickness of kernel are the most important components of yield in these races of blue corn and each had a positive direct influence on yield.

The Hopi corn ear possesses several characteristics not generally found in more common corn. The most conspicuous is the width of the ear at the shank end which averaged 18.5 mm in these landraces. Several traits showed significant to highly significant differences between the landraces (Table 1). These results are very similar to that of other Hopi corn races as reported by (Brown et al. 1952).

PRODUCTION PRACTICES

Production practices of blue corn will require modification of those used on conventional yellow dent corn. The seed is planted 4 to 6 mm deep in good moisture at the rate of 20 to 30 kg/ha in dryland (425 mm precipitation) environments. This will provide a final stand of 30,000 to 45,000 plants/ha. Under dryland conditions, seed must be planted into soil moisture. If high production levels are attempted using conventional high soil fertility and additional irrigation water management techniques, severe lodging may be expected. To keep plant height to a minimum, it is advantageous to stress the plants both with low soil nutrition and water until the 12 leaf stage. If irrigated prior to that time, farm experience shows burial of the culm to the last emerged leaf to be effective in reducing lodging and for weed control. All blue corn is open pollinated, therefore uniform field growth, plant size, maturity, and resistance to insect diseases that we experience with hybrid corn should not be expected.

To keep blue corn quality high and prevent cross-pollination of other types, it is recommended to maintain minimum isolation distances of 230 m from other types of corn for seed production. If minimum distances are not adhered to, F_1 seed will be blue as the blue color is dominant. Subsequent crosses may show color segregation as well as endosperm variation. Some color variation is normal in currently available cultivars.

INSECTS AND DISEASES

Western corn rootworms may be a problem on fields where corn follows corn in the rotation on hardland soils. Blue corn planted on fallow, following crops other than corn or that planted on sandy soil should escape attack by the Western corn rootworm (*Diabrotica virgifera* LeConte). Current cultivars of blue corn are very susceptible to European Corn Borer (*Ostrinia nubilalis* Hubner). In 1991, interplanting rows of amaranth with blue corn in Rocky Ford, Colorado reduced borer damage in the blue corn when compared to borer damage of surrounding dent corn. Stalk rot, (*Fusarium* spp.) a disease of the lower stalk may cause severe lodging. Lodging may be controlled to some degree by keeping plant height to a minimum or by burial.

As blue corn advances in maturity, the kernels will be white until the drydown period. At this time, the blue color appears and darkens as drydown progresses. Harvest should begin when the grain moisture reaches 18% and should progress rapidly. As kernel moisture declines, lodging increases depending on plant height, amount of stalk rot present, and the incidence of wind. Combine cylinder speeds must be reduced with special efforts to minimize seed cracking. Seedcoat cracking interferes with its removal during processing. Combined grain should be dried with aeration to less than 13% prior to shipping. Commercial operations use popcorn cleaners and baggers for their crops.

Buyers generally require delivered clean grain that is free of disease, insect, and foreign matter. Cracked and broken grain is objectionable and a 5% tolerance is allowed for total defects.

REFERENCES

Brown, W.L. and E. Anderson. 1947. The Northern flint corns. Ann. Missouri Bot. Gard. 34:1–28.

Brown, W.L., E.G. Anderson, and R. Tuchaweng, Jr. 1952. Observation on three varieties of Hopi Maize. Amer. J. Bot. 39:597–609.

Carter, G.F. and E. Anderson. 1945. A preliminary survey of maize in the southwestern United States. Ann. Mo. Bot. Gard. 32:297-322.

Johnson, D.L. and R.L. Croissant. 1990. Alternate crop production and marketing in Colorado. Colorado Expt. Sta. Coop. Ext. Serv. and Dept. of Agron. Tech. Bul. LBT 90-3.

Teff: Food Crop for Humans and Animals

G.F. Stallknecht*, Kenneth M. Gilbertson, and J.L. Eckhoff

Present day production and use of *Erogrostis tef* (Zucc.) Trotter, which means "lost" in Amharic, for grain or fodder in the United States represents re-discovery of a crop used by ancient civilizations. Teff is a C_4 plant (Kebede et al. 1989), having Kranz anatomical characteristics, and is intermediate between a tropical and temperate grass. The use of teff can be traced back to about 3359 BC (Mengesha 1965). In contrast to amaranth, which was utilized by early civilizations throughout the world, teff production and uses have been primarily restricted to the countries of Ethiopia, India and its colonies, and Australia (Anon. 1894). While teff grain still provides over two-thirds of the human nutrition in Ethiopia, it is relatively unknown as a food crop elsewhere. Teff has adaptive characteristics similar to other crops grown by early civilizations. Teff can be cultivated under a wide range of environmental conditions such as on marginal soils under water logged to drought conditions. Teff can produce a crop in a relative short growing season and will produce both grain for human food and fodder for cattle. The grain is either white or a very deep reddish brown in color. Published accounts of teff in the late 1800s report that upper class consumed the white grain, the dark grain was the food of soldiers and servants, while hay made from teff was consumed by bullocks (Anon. 1894, 1897). Late 20th century publications in the United States describes teff grain as being marketed as a health food product, or used as a late planted emergency forage for livestock (Goerge 1991, Weibye 1991).

BOTANY

Taxonomy

Eragrostis is a member of the tribe *Eragrosteae*, sub-family *Eragrostoidae*, of the Poaceae (Gramineae). There are approximately 300 species in the genus *Eragrostis* consisting of both annuals or perennials which are found over a wide geographic range. *Eragrostis* species are classified based on characteristics of culms, spikelets, lateral veins, pedicels, panicle, flowering scales, and flower scale colors. Recently, the taxonomy of teff has been clarified by numerical taxonomy techniques, cytology and biochemistry, including leaf flavanoids and seed protein electrophoretic patterns (Jones et al. 1979; Costanza et al. 1980; Bekele and Lester 1981).

Morphology

Teff is a fine stemmed, tufted annual grass (Fig. 1). The plant has the appearance of a bunch grass, having large crowns and many tillers. The inflorescence is an open panicle and produces small seeds (1,000 weigh 0.3 to 0.4 g). The roots are shallow and develop a massive fiberous rooting system. Plant height of teff varies dependent upon cultivar type and growing environments.

AGRONOMY

Agronomic production guidelines for teff cultivation were first published by westerners in the late 1800s (Anon. 1984). Teff was recommended for light moist soils using staggered planting dates. At present, a number of practical production guides are available in the United States (Goerge 1991; Twidwell et al. 1991; Weibye 1991).

Planting of teff requires a firm moist seed bed to effect good soil moisture-seed contact due to the extremely small seed size. Planting can be accomplished using a Brillion grass seeder and cultipacker combination, or by a spinner type grass seeder. Seeding rates varies from 2.3 to 9 kg/ha, with 5 to 8 kg/ha generally recommended. Teff germinates rapidly when planted an average depth of 1.2 cm, however, the initial growth is slow until a good root system has been established. Forage yields of teff in South Dakota have ranged from 4 to 11 t/ha, depending upon planting date and number of cuttings (Boe et al. 1986). In Montana, forage yields cut from dryland and

---

*The senior author acknowledges Vicki L. Bradley, Western Regional Plant Introduction Station, Washington State Univ., Pullman, and Arvid Boe, Dept. Plant Sci., South Dakota State Univ., Brookings, for assisting with the literature search.

irrigated cropping ranged from 2.2 to 15 t/ha. Teff seed yields in Montana ranged from 0.2 to 1.5 t/ha. The low seed yields were obtained at the MSU Southern Agr. Res. Center, Huntley, when planted as a non-irrigated dryland crop, due to poor stands and drought conditions. Harvesting teff for either forage or seed production is easily accomplished, as long as the combine is seed tight. Teff seed can shatter if harvest is delayed. Broad leafed weeds in teff can be easily controlled by use of broad leaf herbicides, however grass weeds if present, can outcompete the teff during the early stages of plant growth. No specific fertility studies have been conducted, but rates similar to those suggested for millets or sorghums are recommended. Green house studies on nutritional requirements of teff have been conducted at Oklahoma State University Department of Agronomy, Stillwater (pers. commun.).

Nutritive Value

The nutritive value of teff for livestock fodder is similar to other grasses utilized as hay or ensiled feeds (Boe et al. 1986; Twidwell et al. 1991). Digestability studies of cell wall contents suggests that teff has tropical grass characteristics (Morris 1980), protein and digestability as forage decreases with increased maturity. Protein content of teff forage produced in South Dakota ranged from a high of 19.5 to a low of 12% as the plant matured. In Montana, teff hay protein content ranged from 13.7 to 9.6%. Protein level (10 to 12%) of teff grain is similar to other cereal grains. Teff has a very high calcium content, and contains high levels of phosphorous, iron, copper, aluminum, barium, and thiamine (Mengesha 1965). The principal use of teff grain for human food is the Ethiopian bread (injera). Injera is a major food staple, and provides approximately two-thirds of the diet in Ethiopia (Stewart and Getachew 1962). While the reported high iron content of teff seed has been refuted, the lack of anemia in Ethiopia, is considered to be due to the available iron from injera (Mamo and Parsons 1987). Injera is described as a soft, porous, thin pancake, which has a sour taste. Teff is low in gluten and therefore, the bread remains quite flat. When eaten in Ethiopia, teff flour is often mixed with other cereal flours, but the flavor and quality of injera made from mixtures is considered less tasty. Injera made entirely from barley, wheat, maize or millet flours is said to have a bitter taste. The degree of sour taste is imparted by the length of the fermentation process. If the dough is fermented for only a short period of time, injera has a tasty sweet flavor. Research studies on the techniques used to make injera have indicated that a yeast, *Candida guilliermondii* (Cast.) Longeron & Guerra, is the microorganism primarily responsible for the fermentation process (Stewart and Getachew 1962).

Disease and Pests

Teff is relatively free of plant diseases when compared to other cereal crops. In Ethiopia, in locales where humidities are high, rusts and head smuts are important diseases. In Ethiopia, 22 fungi and 3 pathogenic nematodes have been identified on teff (Bekele 1985). Teff seedlings are also susceptable to Damping-off caused by *Drechslera poae* and *Helminthosporium poae* (Baudys) Shoemaker, when sown too early (Ketema 1987).

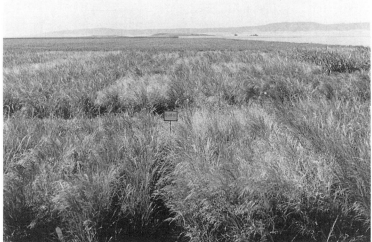

Fig. 1. Teff (*Eragrostis tef*) cultivar trial, dryland cropping, Montana State Univ., Central Research Center, Moccasin, MT, 1990.

Insect pests of teff in Ethiopia include Wello-bush cricket, *Decticoides brevipennis*, red tefworm, *Mentaxya ignicollis*, tef epilachna, and tef black beetle. Since teff has been limited to small areas in the United States few disease and insect problems have been observed. However, a serious problem was observed in South Dakota where the stem boring wasp, *Eurytomocharis eragrostidis* (Howard) reduced forage yields by over 70% (McDaniel and Boe 1990). Although the insect problem was observed in only one out of the five years in research trials, the significant losses obtained could be a deterrent to commercial expansion of teff production.

Cultivars

A detailed description of 34 named Ethiopian teff cultivars based on morphological characteristics was published in 1975 (Ebba 1975). The cultivars are described by differences in culms, panicles, panicle branches, leaves, flowers, spikelets, and grains. Studies on teff production in Montana were initiated by evaluating over 300 accessions, subsequently reduced to 12 for further study (Fig. 1). A cultivar selected from a PI accession by A. Boe, South Dakota State, has been designated SD100. In addition to SD100, a limited number of accessions have been selected by private individuals.

Attempts to develop methods to improve breeding of teff cultivars (which are self-pollinating) have met with only limited success (Mengesha et al. 1965; Berhe and Miller 1978; Berhe et al. 1989). While teff production in Ethiopia occupies large areas and is the most important staple of the country, most cultivars are selections that have been grown for thousands of years. Although cultivar development has been given a high research priority most on going studies have focused on agronomic practices.

FUTURE PROSPECTS

While teff has survived for thousands of years as a major food staple for humans and as fodder for cattle, there are some negative aspects to the nutritional value of injera. Research studies have shown that if the fermentation process is prolonged to produce the sour type of injera, essential nutrients particularly amino acids such as lysine are lost in the liquid which is removed from the dough. The nutrient loss can be reduced if the fermentation process is shortened but then the result is a sweet type of injera, which does not store as well as the sour type. Tabita is also a fermented teff flour pancake which is easily digestible and non-bitter (Anon. 1897). We do not known if the tabita bread is another name for injera.

The major advantages of teff production in Ethiopia according to Ketema (1987) are as follows:
- It can be grown under moisture-stress areas.
- It can be grown under waterlogged conditions.
- It is suitable and is used for double and relay cropping.
- Its straw is a valuable animal feed during the dry season when there is acute shortage of feed. It is highly preferred by cattle and costs higher than the straw of other cereals.
- It has acceptance in the national diet and enables farmers to earn more because of its high price.
- It is a reliable and low-risk crop.
- It is useful as rescue or catch crop in moisture-stress areas. For example, around Kobo or Zeway, farmers first plant maize around April. If the crop fails due to moisture stress, they plow it under and plant sorghum. If this one also fails, it is again plowed under and as a last resort farmers sow teff. In some areas teff is sown because farmers cannot grow wheat, maize, or sorghum due to moisture stress. However, this practice is not widespread, and farmers should be encouraged to reserve teff for use if crops of other cereals fail, especially in drought-prone areas.
- It can be stored easily under local storage conditions since it is not attacked by the weevil and other storage pests, thus reducing postharvest management costs.
- It can be stored for a relatively long period of time (a minimum of 3 years) before it loses its viability. It can be stored in moisture-stress areas where more than one sowing in one season is a common practice or where the rains can fail for more than one year. If it is required for food, it can also be stored for more than 5 years, and perhaps indefinitely.
- It has less disease and pest problems than any other cereal.

CONCLUSION

Domestic experience in teff production is limited; however, teff grain has already found a niche as grain and flour in the health food market. The future of teff forage production for livestock in the United States is unknown. Teff does have the advantage of producing a good hay or pasture crop when late season plantings are required due to a crop failure. Results of a nationwide survey indicate that this crop is virtually unknown in most states, and that production may be limited to only a few western states. Information on teff production in the United States remains scarce as most teff production is handled by private entrepreneurs.

REFERENCES

Anon. 1894. Tropical fodder grasses. Kew Bul. 95:378–380.

Anon. 1887. Teff (*Eragrostis abyssinica*). Kew Bul. 1:2–6.

Bekele, E. and R.N. Lester. 1981. Biochemical assessment of the relationship of *Eragrostis tef* (Zucc) Trotter with some wild *Eragrostis* species (Gramineae). Ann. Bot. 48:717–725.

Bekele, E. 1985. A review of research on diseases of barley, tef, and wheat in Ethiopia, p. 79–108. In: T. Abate (ed.). A review of crop protection research in Ethiopia. Proc. First Ethiopian Crop Prod. Symp. Dept. Crop Protection, Inst. Agr. Res., Addis Ababa, Ethiopia.

Berhe, T. and D.G. Miller. 1976. Sensitivity of tef [*Eragrostis tef* (Zucc.) Trotter] to removal of floral parts. Crop Sci. 16:307–308.

Berhe, T. and D.G. Miller. 1978. Studies of ethephon as a possible selective male gametocide on teff. Crop Sci. 18:35–38.

Berhe, T., L.A. Nelson, M.R. Morris, and J.W. Schmidt. 1989. Inheritance of phenotypic traits in teff: 1. Lemma color. J. Hered. 80:62–70.

Boe, A., J. Sommerfeldt, R. Wynia, and N. Thiex. 1986. A preliminary evaluation of the forage potential of teff. Proc. South Dakota Acad. Sci. 65:75–82.

Costanza, S.H., J.M.J. deWet, and J.R. Harlan. 1979. Literature review and numerical taxonomy of *Eragrostis tef* (T'ef). Econ. Bot. 33:413–424.

Ebba. T. 1975. T'ef (*Eragrostis tef*) cultivars: Morphology and classification. Part II. Expt. Sta. Bul. 66. Addis Ababa Univ. College Agr., Dire Dawa.

Goerge, D. 1991. Cattle like Love Grass. In: The Dakota farmer 109:11. Intertec Pub. Minneapolis, MN.

Jones, B.M.G., J. Ponti, A Tavassoli, and P.A. Dixon. 1978. Relationships of the Ethiopian cereal t'ef [*Eragrostis tef* (Zucc.) Trotter]: Evidence from morphology and chromosome number. Ann. Bot. 42:1369–1373.

Kebede, H., R.C. Johnson, and D.M. Ferris. 1989. Photosynthetic response of *Eragrostis tef* to temperature. Physiol. Plant. 77:262–266.

Ketema, S. 1987. Research recommendations for production and brief outline of strategy for the improvment of tef [*Eragrostis tef* (Zucc.) Trotter]. In: Proc. 19th Natl. Crop. Imp. Conf. IAR. Addis Ababa, Ethiopia.

Mamo, T. and J.W. Parsons. 1987. Iron nutrition of *Eragrostis tef* (teff). Trop. Agr. (Trinidad). 64:313–317.

Mengesha, M.H. 1965. Chemical composition of Teff (*Eragrostis tef*) compared with that of wheat, barley and grain sorghum. Econ. Bot. 19:268–273.

Mengesha, M.H., R.C. Pickett, and R.L. Davis. 1965. Genetic variability and interrelationship of characters in Teff, *Eragrostis tef* (Zucc.) Trotter. Crop Sci. 5:155–157.

McDaniel, B. and A. Boe. 1990. A new host record for *Euryto-mocharis eragrostidis* Howard (*Chalcidoidea*: *eurytomidae* infesting *Eragrostis tef* in South Dakota. Proc. Entomol. Soc. Wash. 92:465–470.

Morris, E.J. 1980. The cell walls of *Eragrostis tef*: variations in chemical composition and digestibility. J. Agr. Sci. Camb. 95:305–311.

Stewart, R.B. and S. Getachew. 1962. Investigations of the nature of Injera. Econ. Bot. 16:127–130.

Twidwell, E.K., A. Boe, and D.P. Casper. 1991. Teff: a new annual forage grass for South Dakota. ExEx 8071. Coop. Ext. Serv. South Dakota State Univ. Brookings, SD.

Weibye, C. 1990. Fast food for livestock. In: Hay & forage grower. 6:12. Intertec Pub. Minneapolis, MN.

Wild Rice: Domestication of a Native North American Genus

Ervin A. Oelke

Wild rice (*Zizania palustris* L.), Poaceae is native to North America and grows predominantly in the Great Lakes region in shallow lakes and rivers (Martin and Uhler 1939). This large-seeded species, one of four species of wild rice has been gathered, dried (Fig. 1), and eaten by people since prehistoric times (Johnson 1969). Early North American inhabitants, especially the Ojibway, Menomini, and Cree tribes in the North Central region of the continent, used the grain as a staple food and introduced European fur traders to wild rice (Jenks 1901). Manomin, the name they gave wild rice, means good berry. Early English explorers called this aquatic plant wild rice or Indian rice, while the French saw a resemblance to oats and called it *folle avoine* (Steeves 1952). Other names given to wild rice include Canadian rice, squaw rice, water oats, blackbird oats, and marsh oats. However, the name "wild rice" persisted and today it is the common name for the genus *Zizania*, even though the wild type of rice (*Oryza*) is also called wild rice.

BOTANY

Taxonomy

The genus, *Zizania*, was named by Gronovius in Leyden, Holland from a plant collected in Virginia by John Clayton in 1739 (Aiken et al. 1988). Linnaeus in 1753 provided the binomial *Zizania aquatica* from the Clayton specimen. There are four species of wild rice: *Z. palustris* L., *Z. aquatica* L., *Z. texana* Hitchcock, and *Z. latifolia* (Griseb.) Turcz. ex Stapf. The first three are native to North America and the last is native to Asia. *Z. palustris* and *Z. aquatica* are annuals, the others perennials. *Z. palustris*, the large seeded type, grows in the Great Lakes region and is the species grown as a field crop (Fig. 2). *Z. aquatica* grows in the St. Lawrence River, eastern and southeastern United States coastal areas, and in Louisiana. Its seeds are slender and are not harvested for food. *Z. texana* grows in a small area in Texas, has slender seeds, and also is not harvested for food. North American species have a chromosome number of $2n = 30$; *Z. latifolia* has $2n = 34$ (Aiken et al. 1988).

Growth Habit

Wild rice (*Z. palustris*) is an annual, cross-pollinated species that grows in flooded soils (Fig. 3). In Minnesota, it matures in about 120 days, and requires about 2,600 growing degree days (4.4°C base). Plants are 60 to 70 cm tall and can have up to 50 tillers per plant. In cultivated fields, plants usually have three to six tillers. Stems are hollow except at nodes where leaves, tillers, roots, and flowers appear. Internodes are separated by thin parchment-like partitions. The shallow root system has a spread of 20 to 30 cm. Mature roots are straight, spongy, and have very few root hairs. Ribbon-like leaf blades vary in width from 0.6 to 3.2 cm. Mature plants have five or six leaves per stem or tiller above the water.

Flowers are in a branching panicle with female (pistillate) flowers at the top and male (staminate) flowers on the lower portion. Cross pollination usually occurs since female flowers emerge first and become receptive and are pollinated before male flowers shed pollen on the same panicle. Sometimes the transition florets, which are located between the pistillate and staminate florets on the panicle, have both stigmas and anthers (pollen), and can therefore be self-pollinated. Two weeks after fertilization the wild rice seeds are visible, and after four weeks, it is ready for harvest. This seed is a caryopsis that is similar to the grain of cereals. The caryopsis has an impermeable pericarp, large endosperm, and small embryo. The grains with the palea and lemma (hulls) removed, range from 8 to 16 mm in length, and from 1.5 to 4.5 mm in diameter (Fig. 4). Immature seeds are green, but turn a purple-black color as they reach maturity. Seeds on any tiller will mature at different times, and on secondary tillers they mature later than on main tillers.

Seeds of *Z. palustris* will not germinate for at least three months after reaching maturity, even if environmental conditions are satisfactory for growth. An afterripening period is required in water at freezing or near-freezing temperatures (3°C) before the embryo breaks dormancy and develops into a new seedling. This seed

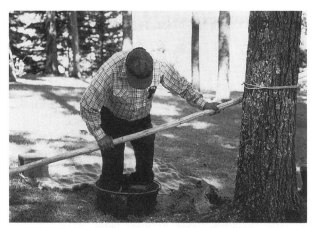

Fig. 1. The traditional hulling method "jigging" of dried hand harvested grain from lakes.

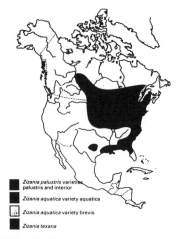

Fig. 2. Distribution of wild rice in North America. Adapted from USDA, Technical Bulletin 634.

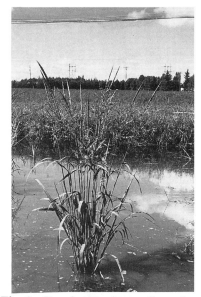

Fig. 3. *Z. palustris* plant at flowering.

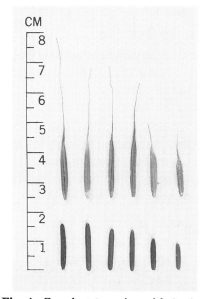

Fig. 4. *Z. palustris* grains with (top) and without lemma and palea (bottom).

dormancy is caused by the impermeable pericarp that is covered by a layer of wax, and by an imbalance of endogenous chemical growth promoters and inhibitors (Albrecht et al. 1979). In the spring, seeds will start to germinate when the water temperature reaches about 7°C. Freshly harvested seeds can be made to germinate by carefully scraping off the pericarp directly above the embryo. Nondormancy has been found in seeds from plants of *Z. aquatica* that grows in Florida.

Nutrition

This grain has a high protein and carbohydrate content, and is very low in fat (Anderson 1976). The nutritional quality of wild rice appears to equal or surpass that of other cereals. Lysine and methionine comprise a higher percentage of the amino acids in the protein than in most other cereals. The SLTM value (sum of lysine, threonine, and methionine contents) often serve as a measure of the nutritional quality of cereals, and is a little higher for wild rice than for oat groats, which is one of the better cereals for humans. Amino acid composition of processed and unprocessed wild rice is similar, which indicates little reduction in nutritional quality during processing. Wild rice contains less than 1% fat, of which linolenic and linoleic acids together comprise a larger proportion of the fatty acids (68%) than in wheat, rice, or oats. Although these two fatty acids are easily oxidized and make wild rice prone to develop rancid odors, the high levels of linolenic acid make the fat in wild rice highly nutritious. Mineral content of wild rice, which is high in potassium and phosphorus, compares favorably with wheat, oats, and corn. Processed wild rice contains no vitamin A, but serves as an excellent source of the B vitamins: thiamine, riboflavin, and niacin.

Commercialization/Domestication

Perhaps the first individuals to attempt to increase availability of wild rice for food were Native Americans (Steeves 1952). Often suitable lakes or rivers were seeded to wild rice by mixing seed into clay, rolling it into a ball and dropping the clay ball into the water. This resulted in some, but not significant, increase in natural stands.

Businessmen and botanists have thought about cultivating this plant for over 100 years (Steeves 1952). Early European explorers collected seed for planting in Europe but these failed probably because the seed was not handled properly to remain viable. In 1828, Timothy Flint in *Geography and History* wondered why so little attention has been paid to wild rice. In 1852, Joseph Bowron suggested wild rice be seeded for agricultural purposes. In 1853, Oliver Kelly, founder of the National Grange, made the same proposal. Mechanical harvesting of private lands in Canada started in 1917, by H.B. Williams and Z. Durand (Trevor 1939).

Since about 1950, wild rice has been in the process of becoming a domesticated crop in the United States and is now being grown commercially in both the United States and Canada (Oelke et al. 1982; Stevenson 1988). Prior to that time, natural stands were the only source of the grain, and supplies were limited and varied greatly from year to year. With the advent and growth of commercial production, supplies of wild rice have increased tremendously over the last 25 years. Natural stands continue to be harvested, but the proportion of total supplies derived from natural stands has steadily declined. In some areas, including the entire state of Minnesota, natural stands of wild rice, by law, must be harvested only by traditional canoe-and-flail method, whereas in some parts of Canada, mechanized harvest is permitted. Included in Table 1 are annual harvest estimates from natural stands in Minnesota since 1963. Of all the wild rice harvested by hand, Minnesota is likely to account for more than half in any given year.

In Canada, commercial production of wild rice takes place predominantly in lakes leased from the various provincial governments (Winchell and Dahl 1984). Lease provisions vary by province, but generally lease holders are permitted to seed the lakes and, in some cases, to control water levels, and are granted exclusive harvesting rights. Much of the wild rice acreage in these leased lakes is harvested with the use of airboats (Stevenson 1988). Shown in Table 1 are annual harvest estimates from lakes and rivers in four Canadian provinces since 1963.

In the United States, wild rice is being produced commercially as a "domesticated" field crop in diked, flooded fields. Minnesota and California account for most of the hectarage (8,000 and 4,000 ha, respectively, in 1992) with additional amounts in Idaho, Wisconsin, and Oregon. Table 2 shows production totals from cultivated fields in Minnesota and California since 1968.

Growing wild rice as a field crop was first attempted near Merrifield, Minnesota in 1950–1952 (Oelke et al. 1984). James and Gerald Godward diked a 0.5 ha area, planted it with seed collected from a nearby lake, and flooded the field. The field was drained before harvest and the crop was harvested by hand. An additional 16 ha were planted by them in 1953 and harvested with a small pull-type combine. They had good crops the first few years, but leaf blight (*Bipolaris oryzae* B. de Haan) caused serious losses thereafter. However, they continued their pioneering efforts, and today one of their sons has nearly 1,000 acres in wild rice production.

Initially, the only seed available for planting in fields was of shattering types found in natural stands. These early fields were harvested several times over a 2-to 3-week grain-ripening period with specially designed, multiple-pass harvesters (Fig. 5). In 1963, Dr. Paul Yagyu and Mr. Erwin Brooks with the University of Minnesota, Department of Agronomy and Plant Genetics, discovered plants in a grower's field that retained their seed longer than the rest of the plants (Oelke et al. 1984). From these few plants, they and other breeders developed cultivars with more resistance to shattering than types growing in lakes and rivers. Today, most of the wild rice being grown in fields are more shattering resistant. Yields of unprocessed grain from shattering types grown in fields typically ranged from 168 to 224 kg/ha, whereas, with shattering resistant cultivars, yields have been reported as high as 1,680 kg/ha in Minnesota and twice that amount in California.

The development of more shattering resistant cultivars of wild rice was largely responsible for a tremendous expansion in field production that occurred in the late 1960s and early 1970s. Practically all the expansion at that time was taking place in Minnesota where area increased from 354 ha in 1968 to 7,090 ha in 1973 (Oelke et al. 1982). The finding of improved shattering resistance was the development that eventually made possible the shift to more efficient harvest with grain combines (Fig. 6). The improved harvest efficiency from the use of combines, together with greater harvested yields from shattering resistant cultivars, were major contributing factors to expanded field production at that time.

Other factors that were important in the development of wild rice as a field crop were: the contracting of production by Uncle Bens, Inc., and the formation of Manomin Development Corporation for development of seed, growing, and marketing of wild rice in 1967; the formation of a Wild Rice Growers Association and the initiation of a research program on processing at the University of Wisconsin-Madison in 1970; and the initiation of a research program at the University of Minnesota on breeding, production, diseases, insects, soil fertility, machinery, and processing in 1972. In 1974, a Minnesota Paddy and Wild Rice Research and Promotion Council was formed after growers voted to contribute a specified fee for each pound of processed grain produced for promotion and research of the crop. In the early 1970s, growing wild rice as a field crop began in California and by 1987, the added production had a significant impact on supply and price. In 1982, an International Wild Rice Association was formed which now includes all producers, processors and marketers in the United States and Canada.

Marketing and processing of wild rice was significantly aided by the formation of two cooperatives in Minnesota (Winchell and Dahl 1984). In 1971, the first successful cooperative was United Wild Rice, Inc.

Table 1. Wild rice harvested from lakes and rivers in Canada and Minnesota, 1963–1987[z].

Years	Tonnes					
	Minnesota	Manitoba	Saskatchewan	Ontario	Alberta	Total
1963	583	---	---	10	---	593
1964	233	---	---	10	---	243
1965	197	---	---	5	---	202
1966	195	---	---	8	---	203
1967	477	---	---	102	---	579
1968	238	---	---	57	---	295
1969	178	---	---	28	---	206
1970	222	27	0.5	12	---	262
1971	221	91	4	55	---	371
1972	188	124	10	198	---	520
1973	184	113	2	235	---	534
1974	181	25	4	2	---	212
1975	91	26	8	17	---	142
1976	363	64	18	204	---	649
1977	198	210	15	156	---	579
1978	100	86	11	28	---	225
1979	138	109	29	54	---	330
1980	454	254	58	176	---	942
1981	181	83	91	123	---	478
1982	200	75	94	34	---	403
1983	218	61	110	34	---	423
1984	245	113	204	73	---	635
1985	73	117	53	6	2	251
1986	81	155	138	18	3	395
1987	227	300	234	261	4	1,026

[z]Estimated using 40% yield of processed from unprocessed wild rice.

Table 2. Wild rice harvested from cultivated fields in Minnesota and California, 1968–1991.

Year	Minnesota (tonnes)	California (tonnes)
1968	16	0
1969	73	0
1970	165	0
1971	276	0
1972	679	0
1973	544	0
1974	470	0
1975	559	0
1976	821	0
1977	468	0
1978	799	45
1979	978	91
1980	1,053	181
1981	1,032	227
1982	1,224	399
1983	1,452	1,134
1984	1,633	1,724
1985	1,906	3,584
1986	2,314	4,083
1987	1,906	1,905
1988	1,906	1,588
1989	1,805	1,952
1990	2,178	1,905
1991	2,405	2,495

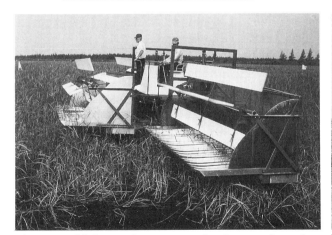

Fig. 5. Multiple pass harvester used to harvest shattering types.

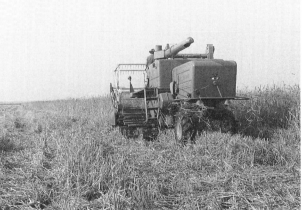

Fig. 6. Harvesting cultivars which have same shattering resistance.

(United). They constructed facilities and staffed the program with a professional manager and sales force. A second cooperative, Minnesota Wild Rice Growers (MRG) was formed in 1974. In 1983, a third cooperative was organized under the name of the Independent Wild Rice Producers Association. Later in 1987, a marketing and product development company, New Frontier Foods, Inc. was formed by some growers. In 1986, Busch Agricultural Resources purchased the processing facilities and marketing operations from United Wild Rice thus involving another large marketer in the industry. The marketing of the cultivated crop was significantly aided by the long-time harvest and marketing of the grain from natural stands. The name of the product was already established in the gourmet markets, thus the cultivated crop could exploit the gourmet nature of the grain.

Even though wild rice is grown now on hectarage in several states it is continuing to undergo domestication in that wild rice still possesses several traits of a wild species such as some seed shattering, seed dormancy, tiller asynchrony, and variable seed size (Hayes et al. 1989). However, these traits are under genetic control and given the heritability of these traits, deliberate selection should accelerate the domestication process.

AGRONOMY

Adaptation

Wild rice is well adapted to northern latitudes. It is not very productive in the southern United States since warm temperatures accelerate plant growth, and as a result, plant heights are shorter with an accompanying lower number of florets (Oelke et al. 1980). Also the high humidity may result in severe leaf diseases (brown spot, *Bipolaris* sp.). Wild rice grows well in the warmer climate of northern California, however, cultivars have been developed for that area and the humidity is very low, consequently leaf diseases are not prevalent. Presently, no resistance to brown spot exists, however variability is present in wild rice germplasm for many other characteristics so that further breeding could permit this crop to be grown in new areas in the future.

The crop is grown similarly to rice (*Oryza*), thus relatively flat areas are needed where a flood can be maintained for most of the season (Fig. 7). It will grow well on organic or inorganic soils if the proper nutrients are applied. Since the plant is relatively tall, its nitrogen requirements are lower than for rice. In addition, it will grow well in cooler and deeper water than rice, thus requiring fewer weed control chemicals compared to rice.

Wild rice seed needs to be stored for 90 days in cold (3°C) water before dormancy is released. Seed storage is an added cost in the Sacramento Valley of California compared to Minnesota. Wild rice seed loses viability, especially after dormancy release, when it is allowed to dry below 25% moisture content. Dormant seed, however, can withstand drying below 25% moisture but needs to be stored in cold (3°C) water for 90 days to release dormancy (Oelke and McClellan 1992). In contrast to rice seed, wild rice seed when planted 5 to 8 cm into the soil before flooding can still grow while rice seed cannot when covered for more than a few days by both soil and water. In Minnesota, new fields are seeded with 45 kg/ha of seed (35% moisture) while in California a seeding rate of 112 kg/ha is common. A higher seeding rate is used in California because plants don't tiller as much as in Minnesota and also a higher plant population can be utilized since no leaf diseases are prevalent.

In Minnesota and Wisconsin fields are prepared, fertilized, and seeded in the fall and flooded to a depth of about 30 cm in the spring. In California, these operations are done in the spring except in some of the higher elevations where production practices are similar to those in Minnesota.

In Minnesota, once a field is seeded to wild rice it will reseed itself due to seed shattering even when planted to cultivars with some shattering resistance. Thus, fields are generally kept in production for 3 to 4 years. It is also difficult to change a field to a new cultivar due to seed dormancy, causing volunteers the following year. Cultivars without seed dormancy are needed to allow more rapid adoption of new, improved cultivars. The plant density the second and following years is also too high making it necessary to reduce the plant population by airboats equipped with a series of V-shaped knives set 15 to 20 cm apart on a toolbar attached to the rear of the boat. The boat travels at a speed of 55 km/h with the knives riding on the soil surface, and removing about 70% of the plants. The plant density desired is 40 plants/m^2.

In Minnesota and California, fields are drained about 3 weeks before harvest with combines. Combines are often adapted with half or full tracks for ease of harvesting in moist soils. The grain is harvested at 30% moisture since seed shattering occurs if allowed to dry more on the plant. The moist grain is immediately transported to processing plants and not dried or stored on the farm like other cereals. At the processing plant the grain is cured, parched, hulled, and graded (Fig. 8).

Diseases and Pests

Diseases in natural stands of wild rice are not usually destructive, but in field-grown wild rice they can cause serious losses. In the early years of commercial production, severe epidemics of brown spot destroyed entire crops in some locations. Almost every disease pathogen of wild rice has been observed previously on rice (*Oryza*).

Brown spot (formerly called *Helminthosporium* brown spot) is the most serious disease affecting wild rice that is grown in fields in Minnesota but, is not a problem in California. This disease is caused by *Bipolaris oryzae* Luttrell (*Helminthosporium oryzae* B. de Haan) and *B. sorokiniana* Luttrell (*H. sativum* P.K. and B.). These fungi are considered to cause brown spot since both are found on infected plants and cause similar symptoms. Every cultivar of wild rice, at each stage of development, is susceptible to brown spot. This disease is most severe when day temperatures range from 25° to 35°C and nights are 20°C or warmer. High relative humidity (greater than 89%), and the continuous presence of free water on leaf surfaces for 11 to 16 h, also favor infection. All parts of the plant are susceptible to infection. The brown, oval leaf spots usually have yellow margins and are about the size of sesame seeds. These spots are uniform and evenly distributed over the leaf surface. Severe infections cause weakened and broken stems, damaged florets, and a reduced quantity and quality of grain. Yield reductions can vary from insignificant to 100%. Sanitation and a fungicide are needed for control.

Stem rot is the second most common disease in field-grown wild rice. Two fungi, a *Sclerotium* sp. and *Helminthosporium sigmoidium* Cav., may cause this disease. These fungi produce dark structures called sclerotia in culms, leaf sheaths, and stems. Small, oval, purple lesions develop initially on stems or leaves at the water surface. Extensive lodging may result after the fields are drained prior to harvest, since the infected stems become necrotic, dry, and brittle. Control of stem rot is achieved most effectively by appropriate sanitation and cultural practices. Plant residue must be removed or tilled into the soil, only clean seed should be used, and resistant crops or fallow should be in the rotation. There is no fungicide available for effective control.

Stem smut is caused by the fungus *Entyloma lineatum* (Cke.) Davis. Economic losses from this disease have not been a problem in cultivated fields.

Ergot is rarely found in cultivated fields of Minnesota, but can be a serious problem in natural stands. This disease is caused by the fungus *Claviceps zizaniae* Fyles, which is a different species than the one causing ergot in cereal grains. Wind-borne ascospores infect flowers and hard, dark sclerotia eventually develop in place of the grain. No specific control is recommended, but poisonous ergot bodies should be removed from harvested grain by flotation, or by screening.

Bacterial leaf streak and wheat-streak mosaic virus have been found in cultivated wild rice in Minnesota. Bacterial leaf streak is caused by *Pseudomonas syringae*. The wheat streak mosaic virus-wild rice is the only one known to infect wild rice. Economic losses for grain yield, if any by these diseases, have not been determined. No control measures are known.

The rice worm (*Apamea apamiformis* Guenee), which s the larval stage of the noctuid moth, is the most serious insect pest of wild rice in the Upper Midwest but not a problem in California. Significant yield losses have

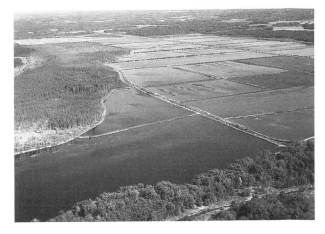

Fig. 7. Flooded wild rice fields in northern Minnesota.

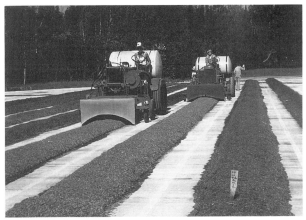

Fig. 8. Equipment used to turn and water wild rice grain daily during curing at the processing plant.

been caused by this insect. Its life cycle is coordinated closely with the growth and development of wild rice. Adult moths begin to emerge at about the same time as flowering begins in wild rice during late June or early July. Nectar from milkweed flowers serves as the primary food source for adult moths through August. Eggs are deposited in wild rice flowers over a period of 4 to 6 weeks. Larvae hatch and develop through several instars or stages, and feed as they grow. Yield potential is reduced by the initial feeding activity on the glumes of the spikelet and subsequent feeding on kernels. Rice worms bore into stems of wild rice or migrate to plants that border the production area as their growth and development nears completion. Rice worms overwinter inside the stems in the seventh instar. After a final molt and some additional feeding in the spring, the larvae usually pupate in early June, and develop into the adult moth. Research in Minnesota found that one larva per plant reduces yield by 10%. Control of the rice worm has been effective with several insecticides; yet only malathion at one pound of active ingredient per acre (1.1 kg/ha) is approved for use in Minnesota.

A number of midges use the flooded paddies for larval development. Eggs are laid in the moist soil and hatch when the fields are flooded. One of the midges, *Cricotopus* spp., has caused severe damage to first-year fields in Minnesota and California. The mosquito-like adults are so small that most growers will not see them. Algal growth is associated with paddies showing high midge numbers. A slow emergence of seedlings results in greater damage by midges since it allows more time for feeding activity. The larvae feed on leaf edges and cause frayed leaf edges with subsequent curling of leaves. The leaf curling and webbing that midges produce will interfere with seedling emergence above the water. As a result, the damaged seedlings fail to reach the floating-leaf stage and the stand is thinned severely. Midge control with malathion is often necessary in first-year fields. In the following years control is not usually necessary since there is no economic loss. This is not the result of a lack of midges, which actually increase in number, but due to higher plant numbers so the damage goes unnoticed.

Rice stalk borers (*Chilo plejadellus* Zincken), rice water weevils (*Lissorhoptrus* spp.), rice leafminer (*Hydrellia* spp.), rice stem maggot (*Eribolus longulus* Loew), and other insects will feed on wild rice plants. Research in Minnesota did not reveal any economic injury from these insects.

Crayfish (*Orconectes virilis* Hagen) are carried into paddies by flood waters where they forage and may cut back the seedlings. Once crayfish are established in a field, they persist and can increase in number. They survive in production fields by burrowing into moist soil between periods of paddy flooding. Severe stand reductions have occurred in some fields in Minnesota. No chemicals are cleared for their control.

Blackbirds are a major pest in both Minnesota and California. These birds use the paddy dikes as nesting sites and are present in large numbers in the growing areas. Birds begin feeding on wild rice when the kernels are in the milk stage. Control measures should start when blackbirds are first observed in the area.

Wild rice fields are also ideal sites for resting, foraging, nesting, and raising broods of migratory and resident water birds. Four species of ducks (mallard, pintail, blue-wing teal, and green-wing teal) and more than 35 species of shorebirds and wading birds inhabit wild rice paddies. Economic damage from waterfowl is rarely observed. Paddies are excellent areas for duck production.

Raccoon, mink, and skunk search for food on the dikes and in ditches. Deer and moose occasionally cause some damage in the fields, but it usually has no economic importance. Muskrats can cause problems by feeding on seedlings and mature plants and by burrowing holes in the sides of dikes. However, since muskrats are not permanent inhabitants due to the annual drainage of the paddies for he harvest, they do not pose a threat to the dikes.

The common broadleaf water weeds of the Upper Midwest are a more serious problem than aquatic grassy weeds. Common waterplantain (*Alisma trivale* Pursh), an aquatic perennial weed, is the most troublesome weed in wild rice fields. Early control of waterplantain is critical since competition with wild rice is greatest after 8 weeks of growth. First-year seedlings of waterplantain are usually too small and late in appearance to compete with wild rice. Water management is the major control measure.

Cultivars

Wild rice in Minnesota is produced using cultivars that have a nonshattering tendency. All the following cultivars shatter somewhat and are susceptible to lodging and diseases. The most popular is 'K2'.

'K2' has a medium height, early to medium maturity, and medium to high yield. Developed by Kosbau Brothers in 1972.

'M3' has a medium height, medium to late maturity, high yield, and variable plant and panicle type. Developed by Manomin Development Co. in 1974.

'Meter' has a shorter height, very early maturity, low to medium yield, and large seed size. Reduced foliage in the canopy compared to other varieties. Released by the Minnesota Agricultural Experiment Station in 1985.

'Netum' has a medium height, early maturity, and low to medium yield. Released by the Minnesota Agricultural Experiment Station in 1978.

'Voyager' has a short to medium height, early maturity, and medium to high yield. Should equal or exceed K2 in yield and mature a few days earlier. Released by the Minnesota Agricultural Experiment Station in 1983.

In California, cultivars developed by NorCal Seeds are the predominant ones grown.

SUMMARY AND FUTURE

Wild rice is firmly established as a new cultivated crop and should continue to expand in production and usage as yield and production efficiency are improved. Several key factors have led to its success to date: (1) the grain was recognized by consumers as a gourmet food before domestication began, thus was relatively high priced and in demand, (2) there were several champions of the crop that were willing to invest in production and marketing, (3) growers organized themselves early in the process to seek research monies, and (4) the discovery of shattering resistance trait. Continued expansion will depend on increasing the yield through breeding better cultivars which have better shattering resistance, tiller synchrony, disease resistance, grain/straw ratio, and lodging resistance. In addition, reduced seed dormancy and ability to store germplasm longer are needed. Expansion also will be dependent on increasing the market demand for this gourmet product.

REFERENCES

Aiken, S.G., P.F. Lee, D. Punter, and J.M. Stewart. 1988. Wild rice in Canada. New Canada Publication, Toronto.

Albrecht, K.A., E.A. Oelke, and M.L. Brenner. 1979. Abscisic acid levels in the grain of wild rice. Crop Sci. 19:671–676.

Anderson, R.A. 1976. Wild rice: Nutritional review. Cereal Chem. 53:949–955.

Elliott, W.A. 1980. Wild rice, p. 721–731. In: W.R. Fehr and H.H. Hadley (eds.). Hybridization of crop plants. Amer. Soc. Agron., Madison, WI.

Hayes, P.M., R.E. Stucker, and G.G. Wandrey. 1989. The domestication of American wildrice (*Zizania palustris*, Poaceae). Econ. Bot. 43:203–214.

Jenks, A.E. 1901. The wildrice gatherers of the Upper Lakes. U.S. Dept. of Interior, Bur. Amer. Ethnol., 9th Rpt. 1899:1015–1160.

Johnson, E. 1969. Archaeological evidence for utilization of wild rice. Science 163:273–277.

Martin, A.C. and F.M. Uhler. 1939. Food of game ducks of the U.S. and Canada. U.S. Dept. Agr. Tech. Bul. 634.

Oelke, E., J. Grava, D. Noetzel, D. Barron, J. Percich, C. Schertz, J. Strait, and R. Stucker. 1982. Wild rice production in Minnesota. Agr. Ext. Ser., Univ. of Minnesota, AG-BU-0546.

Oelke, E.A., J.K. Ransom, and M.J. McClellan. 1980. Wild rice production and seed research, p. 19–38. In: L. Etkin (ed.). Minnesota wild rice research—1979. Agr. Expt. Sta., Univ. of Minnesota, St. Paul.

Oelke, E.A. and M.J. McClellan. 1992. Wild rice production and seed research, p. 1–18. In: L. Etkin (ed.). Minnesota wild rice research—1991. Minnesota Agr. Expt. Sta. Misc. Pub. 74.

Steeves, T.A. 1952. Wild rice—Indian food and a modern delicacy. Econ. Bot. 26:107–142.

Stevenson, S. 1988. Wild rice report 1987—Northwestern Region of Ontario. Ont. Min. Nat. Res., Kenora, Ont.

Trevor, L. 1939. Wild rice in Canada. Can. Geographical J. 19:289–299.

Winchell, E.H. and R.P. Dahl. 1984. Wild rice: Production, processing and marketing. Agr. Expt. Sta., Univ. of Minnesota Misc. Pub. 29.

Structure and Chemical Composition of Developing Buckwheat Seed*

Ralph L. Obendorf, Marcin Horbowicz, and Douglas P. Taylor

Buckwheat (*Fagopyrum esculentum* Moench) grain is a basic food item in porridges, soups, and the preparation of "kasha" in Central and Eastern Europe. In Japan, buckwheat is used mostly for manufacturing a noodle, soba, which is prepared from a mixture of buckwheat and wheat flours (Udesky 1988). Considered a healthy food, Japan's total buckwheat consumption is about 100,000 tons/year (Komeichi et al. 1992). About 80% of Japan's consumption is imported, largely from the United States and Canada. Buckwheat produces a low grain yield because of a low incidence of seed set. Although the plants usually produce an abundant number of flowers, only 10 to 20% of the flowers develop into mature grain (Ruszkowski 1986). Yields vary from 150 to 1,200 kg/ha depending on the soil, climate, and other factors. Demand from export markets has increased the need for stabilization of yields and prompted basic research on factors regulating seed set and cessation of seed growth in buckwheat.

The structure and composition of mature buckwheat fruits has been reviewed by Pomeranz (1983), but little information is available on the changes in the fresh and dry weight and the composition of parts of the developing seeds. In this paper, we summarize our research on the reproductive biology of developing buckwheat seeds and the changes in content of sugars, organic acids, amino acids, sterols, and fatty acids in developing seeds.

REPRODUCTIVE BIOLOGY

Buckwheat flowers are perfect but incomplete. They have no petals, but the calyx has the appearance of petals. Flowers occur in compact racemes, either terminally on the main stem or on branches from the axil of leaves. Common buckwheat plants are dimorphic and heterostylous. One-half of the plants have pin-type flowers with long styles and short stamens, and one-half of the plants have thrum-type flowers with short styles and long stamens (Marshall and Pomeranz 1982). Each type is self-incompatible and cross-incompatible among plants with the same flower type. Seed set requires legitimate cross pollination, pin by thrum and thrum by pin, by insects under field conditions (Namai 1990) or by hand pollination in the greenhouse as in the present study (Horbowicz and Obendorf 1992). Temperature in the greenhouse was controlled at 24° day and 18°C night. Natural sunlight was supplemented 14 h daily with high intensity incandescent light. Buckwheat plants were watered as needed and supplemented weekly with fertilizer.

The mature buckwheat seed is an achene. The mature ovule or groat, the dehulled achene (with pericarp removed), is used for food. Seed set is defined as producing a seed that the miller can use. Seeds usually set if not aborted by 10 days after pollination (DAP). Oil, starch, and protein storage reserves in the embryo and endosperm tissues accumulate rapidly after 10 DAP, the period of seed fill. The cessation of seed growth at full development is called physiological maturity and corresponds to the time of maximum dry weight. The loss of water from the seed is desiccation and leads to harvest maturity and safe storage when sufficiently dry. A number of conditions must be met for seed set to occur.

The female parts of the buckwheat flower, an ovary with styles and stigmas receptive to pollen are illustrated in Fig. 1. Within the ovary (or developing achene), a complete and functional ovule (developing groat) must be present. The outer and inner integuments (each two cells thick) form the seed coat of the dehulled groat at maturity. At the upper end of the ovule, the integuments form an opening, the micropyle, through which the pollen tube enters. The nucellus is positioned inside the integuments. One cell of the nucellus becomes the megaspore mother cell, divides by meiosis ($2n$ to $1n$) forming four haploid ($1n$) megaspores. One of the four divides sequentially

---

*Contribution from the Department of Soil, Crop and Atmospheric Sciences, Cornell University Agricultural Experiment Station, Ithaca, NY 14853-1901. Cornell buckwheat research is supported by grants from MINN-DAK Growers Ltd., The Birkett Mills, Japan Buckwheat Millers Association, and Kasho Company Limited.

to form an egg sac with eight-nuclei (Mahony 1935). One forms the egg cell (future embryo) bordered by two synergids, two fuse to form the nucleus of the central cell (future endosperm), and three migrate to the bottom in close proximity to the hypostase, a structure analogous to the nucellar projection in wheat (Frazier and Appalanaidu 1965) and barley (Cochrane and Duffus 1980).

Viable pollen must be delivered to the stigma by legitimate cross-pollination to achieve seed set. The pollen must germinate rapidly, have vigorous growth of the pollen tube through the style and into the micropyle. The pollen tube must penetrate the nucellus and the egg sac, delivering two sperm nuclei (each $1n$) to the egg sac. One unites with the egg ($1n$) to form the zygote ($2n$) which develops into the embryo; the other unites with the fused ($2n$) nucleus of the central cell forming $3n$ nuclei which develop into endosperm cells. This double fertilization of the egg and central cells is essential for seed set.

The nucellus and embryo sac in the ovule and the tapetum and sporogenous cells of the anther are distinctly different than other tissues in the ovary and stamen. A monoclonal antibody which specifically recognizes an L-arabinose containing arabinogalactan-protein in the plasmalemma of cells reacts with all plant cells except those of the nucellus, egg sac, and embryos during early embryogenesis (Pennell and Roberts 1990). The pattern is the same in pea, maize, and *Arabidopsis*, and presumably also in buckwheat. Pennell and Roberts (1990) suggest that absence of the arabinogalactan-protein may be an essential prelude to the expression in the gametes themselves of determinants involved with fertilization. Another epitope of a plasma membrane arabinogalactan protein occurs in association with the sperm cells of pollen grains late in anther development in rapeseed flowers (Pennell et al. 1991). In ovular tissues, this epitope appears first in the nucellar epidermis near the micropylar end of the ovule and subsequently in the egg cell and both synergids. Since this epitope is not found in the central cell, Pennell et al. (1991) proposed that it is related to gamete recognition. Upon entry of the pollen tube, the sperm cells are released in a synergid before fertilization of the egg and central cell nuclei (Knox et al. 1986).

Following double fertilization, the embryo develops rapidly during the first day (Stevens 1912; Mahony, 1935), the ovary doubles in size from 1 to 2 mm in length (Fig. 2), and the ovule increases from 0.5 to 1 mm in length. Volume of the endosperm increases rapidly, remains clear and fluid, and contains multiple nuclei. By 3 DAP, the embryo forms cotyledons, the upper endosperm forms cells, and the basal endosperm remains as a thin layer of cytoplasm containing multiple nuclei and a very large vacuole (Stevens 1912). By 6 DAP, the endosperm starts to solidify along the margins (Stevens 1912), and the liquid endosperm becomes milky.

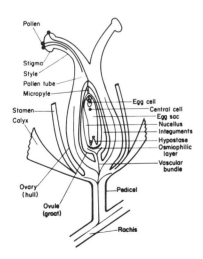

Fig. 1. Diagram of a buckwheat flower with emphasis on structures of the ovule and embryo sac.

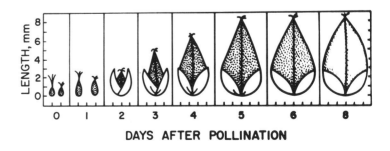

Fig. 2. Schematic development of a buckwheat seed (from M. Horbowicz, R.L. Obendorf, and W.J. Cox, unpubl.).

Vascular tissues (for transporting nutrients and water) branch from the stem into the rachis of the raceme (inflorescence), branch into the pedicel and then into the sepals and stamens (Fig. 1). Vascular tissues enter the funiculus and form a saucer-shaped "Y" at the base of the ovule (Fig. 1). Vascular tissues do not enter the integuments, nucellus, nor egg sac. Therefore, nutrients going to the developing egg sac, embryo, and endosperm must exit the symplast (cell cytoplasm), enter the apoplast ("free-space" in cell walls and between cells), and be reloaded into the symplast (cytoplasm) of the developing cells of the egg sac, embryo, and endosperm. At the basal interface between the integuments and the nucellus, and positioned across the apparent path of nutrient flow to the egg sac and developing embryo and endosperm, a group of cells accumulate an osmiophilic substance which may include polyphenols or flavonoids. This deposit may limit transport through these cells. Characterization of the basal tissues of the ovule is lacking in early reports (Mahony 1935; Stevens 1912).

Ovaries of both pin and thrum flower types are about 1 mm in length at anthesis, and the developing achene rapidly increases to maximum length at 5 or 6 DAP (Fig. 2). Width of developing achenes continues to increase until 12 to 14 DAP during the seed-filling period. The ovule undergoes characteristic changes in morphology during the development (Fig. 3). Ovules are about 0.5 mm in length at anthesis, and by 2 DAP, they are about 2 mm in length and have developed a swollen base with expanding endosperm. The vascular attachment is at the base of the bulbous structure while the embryo develops near the micropyle at the apex of the ovule and grows downward into the endosperm. Expanding pericarp tissues rapidly accumulate fresh weight between 2 and 6 DAP (Fig. 4). Ovule tissues, including the endosperm and embryo, increase rapidly in length and width between 6 and 10 DAP with a rapid increase in fresh weight after 6 DAP and a rapid increase in dry weight after 8 DAP. The embryo attains maximum fresh weight at 12 DAP, but the endosperm continues to increase in fresh and dry weights until 16 DAP (Fig. 4A,B). Cessation of achene dry matter accumulation occurs by 20 DAP. Water concentration in the endosperm decreases from 850 g/kg fresh weight at 6 DAP to 220 g/kg fresh weight at 16 DAP (Fig. 4D). Water concentration in embryo tissues declines at a slower rate. The accumulation of storage reserves in the endosperm and embryo contribute to the ovule shape conforming to the shape of the pericarp (Fig. 3). By contrast, when the endosperm does not develop, the pericarp may grow to normal length of the mature achene, but the pericarp walls are folded inward reflecting the lack of endosperm and embryo development.

SUGARS AND ORGANIC ACIDS

Whole or parts of 3 to 20 developing achenes were boiled, homogenized, and extracted in 50% ethanol/water with sedoheptulose as internal standard. Trimethylsilyl (TMS) derivatized sugars and organic acids were analyzed by capillary (DB-1701) gas chromatography (M. Horbowicz, R.L. Obendorf, and W.J. Cox, unpubl.).

Sucrose is the major sugar accumulating in buckwheat achenes. Increases in sucrose accumulation reflect periods of dry weight increases, with the embryo tissues accumulating the largest amount of sucrose (Fig. 5A). Sucrose is abundant in the seed coat and nucellus tissues from anthesis through 6 to 8 DAP and then accumulates in the developing embryo. The high concentration of sucrose in embryo tissues is typical of oilseed tissues (Duffus and Binnie 1990; Kuo et al. 1988). The starchy endosperm accumulates only low transitory levels of sucrose. The ovular maternal tissues (integuments and nucellus) accumulate sucrose before major accumulation of dry

Fig. 3. Schematic development of a buckwheat ovule (from M. Horbowicz, R.L. Obendorf, and W.J. Cox, unpubl.).

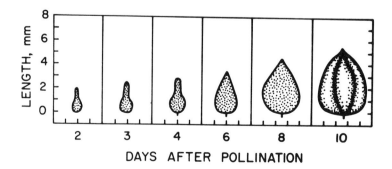

matter in the endosperm and embryo, and then, the sucrose level declines consistent with an apparent transport role to the developing endosperm and embryo.

The monosaccharides, glucose and fructose, are mostly in the pericarp and seed coat (Fig. 5B). Levels of glucose and fructose are similar (data not presented). Except in embryo tissues, increasing glucose and fructose levels precede sucrose and starch accumulation (Fig. 5B), a pattern observed in starchy endosperm of maize (Shannon 1968, 1972). Levels of inositol are low in all tissues. Inositol is detected sequentially in the pericarp, seed coat and nucellus, endosperm, and embryo during later developmental stages of each (Fig. 5C). After seed set, faster-growing achenes have higher starch levels and lower sugar levels while slower-growing achenes have lower starch levels and higher sugar levels (Dua et al. 1991), indicating that utilization of sugars may be limiting in slower-growing achenes.

Citric acid accumulates only in green pericarp tissues with peak levels at 6 to 8 DAP (M. Horbowicz, R.L. Obendorf, and W.J. Cox, unpubl.). Malic acid is detected sequentially in pericarp and maternal ovule tissues and then in endosperm and embryo tissues (Fig. 5D) with peak concentrations early in development (4 DAP in endosperm). Malic acid content is much higher than citric acid in cells and amyloplasts of starchy endosperm (Liu and Shannon 1981).

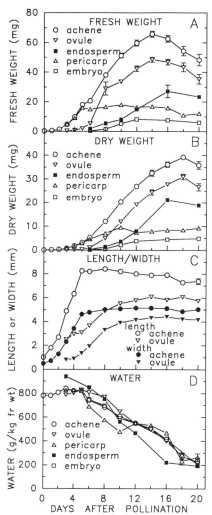

Fig. 4. Changes in fresh weight (A), dry weight (B), length and width (C), and water concentration (D) of developing achene, ovule, pericarp, endosperm, and embryo tissues in relation to days after pollination (from M. Horbowicz, R.L. Obendorf, and W.J. Cox, unpubl.).

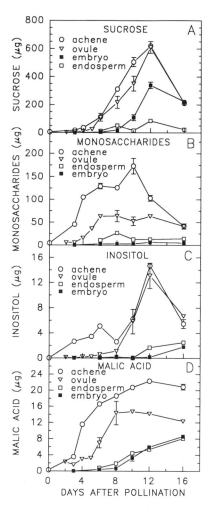

Fig. 5. Changes in sucrose (A), glucose plus fructose (B), inositol (C), and malic acid (D) in developing achene, ovule, embryo, and endosperm tissues in relation to days after pollination (from M. Horbowicz, R.L. Obendorf, and W.J. Cox, unpubl.).

CHEMICAL COMPOSITION

Free Amino Acids

Free amino acids in the ethanol/water, 1:1, extract from endosperm and embryo tissues were diluted 5 to 10 fold with water and analyzed by the ninhydrin method (Rosen 1957). Free amino acids accumulate 4 to 12 DAP primarily in the seed coat and nucellus, maternal tissues of the ovule (Fig. 6). Free amino acids in the endosperm and embryo increase to a constant level at 8 and 10 DAP. The rise in level of free amino acids in the maternal tissues of the ovule at 12 DAP and subsequent depletion by 16 DAP, when dry matter accumulation in the endosperm and embryo has nearly ceased, is indicative of the role of these tissues in transport of amino acids to the developing endosperm and embryo. The concentration of amino acids in all tissues declines during seed development with the accumulation of dry matter (M. Horbowicz, R.L. Obendorf, and W.J. Cox, unpubl.).

The protein content of mature whole grain is 13.8%, dehulled groat 16.4%, pericarp 4%, endosperm 10.1% and embryo 55.9% (Pomeranz and Robbins 1972). The amino acid content of protein in the embryo and endosperm are quite similar. Embryo proteins are enriched slightly in arginine, serine, and glutamine/glutamic acid while endosperm proteins are slightly enriched in lysine, proline, alanine, methionine, and leucine. Amino acid analysis of proteins in mature achenes has been reported (Pomeranz and Robbins 1972; Pomeranz et al. 1975; Pecavar et al. 1990). While protein concentration in the hull declines during seed development, protein concentration in the groat is more constant, and the amino acid composition of groat proteins is very similar at 7, 14, 21, and 28 DAP (Pomeranz et al. 1975). Buckwheat proteins are composed of about 18% albumins, 43% globulins, 1% prolamins, 23% glutelins, and 15% insoluble residue (Javornik et al. 1981). About 30% of the total N is non-protein N and N in molecules of <10,000 molecular mass. A 13 S globulin is 80% of the protein body proteins and 51% of the total protein in cotyledons of the embryo (Elpidina et al. 1990).

Sterols and Fatty Acids

Endosperm and embryo tissues of developing buckwheat seeds were homogenized in methanol containing methyl-heptadecanoate and dihydrocholesterol, which were added as internal standards. Fatty acids and sterols were extracted with potassium hydroxide/methanol solution at 80°C which simultaneously combined extraction and saponification steps (Horbowicz and Obendorf 1992). After addition of saturated sodium chloride solution, the non-saponified fraction containing sterols was extracted with hexane. After evaporation of hexane, extracted sterols were silylated and analyzed by capillary (DB-1701) gas chromatography (Horbowicz and Obendorf 1992). The methanol/water layer containing saponified materials was acidified and the fatty acids were extracted with hexane. After evaporation of hexane, total extracted fatty acids were converted to methyl esters (Metcalfe et al. 1966) and analyzed by capillary (DB-1701) gas chromatography (Horbowicz and Obendorf 1992).

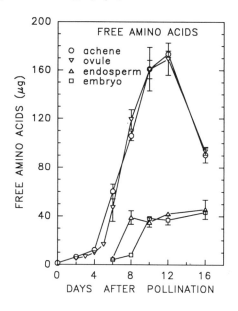

Fig. 6. Changes in free amino acids in developing achene, ovule, endosperm, and embryo tissues in relation to days after pollination (from M. Horbowicz, R.L. Obendorf, and W.J. Cox, unpubl.).

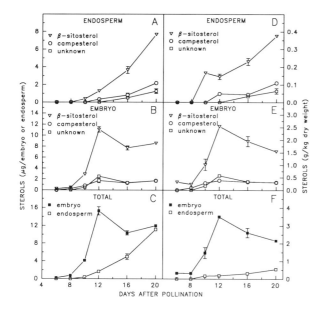

Fig. 7. Changes in total content (A, B, C) and specific content (D, E, F) of sterols in endosperm and embryo tissues in relation to days after pollination (from Horbowicz and Obendorf 1992).

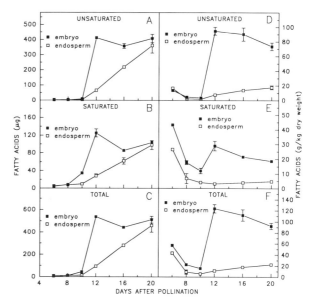

Fig. 8. Changes in total content (A, B, C) and specific content (D, E, F) of unsaturated, saturated and total fatty acids in endosperm and embryo tissues in relation to days after pollination (from Horbowicz and Obendorf 1992).

Sterols include ß-sitosterol (70% of total), campesterol, an unknown, and traces of stigmasterol (Fig. 7). Total sterol (2.1 g/kg at 20 DAP; Fig. 7F) and total fatty acid (123 g/kg; Fig. 8F) concentrations are four to five times higher in embryo tissues than in endosperm during development. The amount of each sterol increased continuously during endosperm development (Fig. 7A). In embryo tissues, however, the amount and concentration reached a maximum at 12 DAP (Fig. 7B,E).

At 6 to 10 DAP, 60 to 80% of the fatty acids are saturated (Fig. 8) with palmitic being three to five times higher in concentration than any other fatty acid at 6 DAP (Horbowicz and Obendorf 1992). By contrast, at 12 to 20 DAP, 70 to 80% of the fatty acids are unsaturated (Fig. 8) with linoleic, oleic, and palmitic representing 85% of the total (Horbowicz and Obendorf 1992). The transition at 10 to 12 DAP occurs during rapid growth of the embryo (Fig. 4) and a 10-fold increase in total fatty acids (Fig. 8); 80% of the total fatty acids in embryo tissues accumulate between 10 and 12 DAP. At 12 DAP more than 80% of the total lipids are in the embryo. As the storage lipids begin to accumulate in the achene, sterols and palmitic acid accumulate initially followed by stearic, oleic, linoleic, and linolenic acids (Horbowicz and Obendorf 1992). The long chain fatty acids, eicosenoic, arachidic, and behenic, are synthesized last at 16 DAP. The late appearance of long chain fatty acids precludes them from a role in seed set or abortion. In mature buckwheat achenes, long chain fatty acids are present in higher concentrations in neutral and free lipids but in lower concentrations in phospholipids (Mazza 1988) and milling fractions vary in concentrations of long chain fatty acids (Tauzuki et al. 1991). Lower temperatures during achene maturation result in higher concentrations of linoleic and linolenic acids, slightly lower concentrations of long chain fatty acids and no change in myristic, palmitic, or stearic acids (Taira et al. 1986).

REFERENCES

Cochrane, M.P. and C.M. Duffus. 1980. The nucellar projection and modified aleurone in the crease region of developing caryopses of barley (*Hordeum vulgare* L. var. distichum). Protoplasma 103:361–375.

Dua, I.S., U. Devi, and N. Garg. 1991. Differential distribution of different saccharides and proteins in two types of grains growing in the same ear of buckwheat (*Fagopyrum esculentum* Moench). Fagopyrum 11:19–26.

Duffus, C.M. and J. Binnie. 1990. Sucrose relationships during endosperm and embryo development in wheat. Plant Physiol. Biochem. 28:161–165.

Elpidina, E.N., Y.E. Dunaevsky, and M.A. Belozersky. 1990. Protein bodies from buckwheat seed cotyledons: Isolation and characteristics. J. Expt. Bot. 41:969–977.

Frazier, J.C. and B. Appalanaidu. 1965. The wheat grain during development with reference to nature, location and role of its translocation tissues. Amer. J. Bot. 52:193–198.

Horbowicz, M. and R.L. Obendorf. 1992. Changes in sterols and fatty acids of buckwheat endosperm and embryo during seed development. J. Agr. Food Chem. 40:745–750.

Javornik, B., B.O. Eggum, and I. Kreft. 1981. Studies on protein fractions and protein quality of buckwheat. Genetika 13:115–121.

Knox, R.B., E.G. Williams, and C. Dumas. 1986. Pollen, pistil, and reproductive function in crop plants. Plant Breed. Rev. 4:9–79.

Komeichi, M., Y. Honda, and H. Hayashi. 1992. Genetic resources of buckwheat in Japan, p. 19–31. In: buckwheat genetic resources in east Asia. Papers of an IBPGR workshop, Ibaraki, Japan, 18–20 December, 1991. Int. Crop Network Ser. No. 6, International Board for Plant Genet. Resources, Rome.

Kuo, T.M., J.F. VanMiddlesworth, and W.J. Wolf. 1988. Content of raffinose oligosaccharides and sucrose in various plant seeds. J. Agr. Food Chem. 36:32–36.

Liu, T.-T.Y. and J.C. Shannon. 1981. Measurement of metabolites associated with nonaqueously isolated granules from immature *Zea mays* L. endosperm. Plant Physiol. 67:525–529.

Mahony, K.L. 1935. Morphological and cytological studies on *Fagopyrum esculentum*. Amer. J. Bot. 22:460–475.

Marshall, H.G. and Y. Pomeranz. 1982. Buckwheat: description, breeding, production, and utilization. Adv. Cereal Sci. Tech. 5:157–210.

Mazza, G. 1988. Lipid content and fatty acid composition of buckwheat seed. Cereal Chem. 65:122–126.

Metcalfe, L.D., A.A. Schmitz, and J.R. Pelka. 1966. Rapid preparation of fatty acid esters from lipids for gas chromatographic analysis. Anal. Chem. 38:514.

Namai, H. 1990. Pollination biology and reproductive ecology for improving genetics and breeding common buckwheat, *Fagopyrum esculentum*. Fagopyrum 10:23–46.

Pecavar, A., M. Prosek, and B. Javornik. 1990. Quantitative amino acid analysis of buckwheat by reverse phase liquid chromatography. Fagopyrum 10:81–85.

Pennell, R.I., L. Janniche, P. Kjellbom, G.N. Scofield, J.M. Peart, and K. Roberts. 1991. Developmental regulation of a plasma membrane arabinogalactan protein epitope in oilseed rape flowers. Plant Cell 3:1317–1326.

Pennell, R.I. and K. Roberts. 1990. Sexual development in the pea is presaged by altered expression of arabinogalactan protein. Nature 344:547–549.

Pomeranz, Y., H.G. Marshall, G.S. Robbins, and J.T. Gilbertson. 1975. Protein content and amino acid composition of maturing buckwheat. Cereal Chem. 52:479–485.

Pomeranz, Y. 1983. Buckwheat: Structure, composition, and utilization. CRC Crit. Rev. Food Sci. Nutr. 19:213–258.

Pomeranz, Y. and G.S. Robbins. 1972. Amino acid composition of buckwheat. J. Agr. Food Chem. 20:270–274.

Rosen, H. 1957. A modified ninhydrin colorimetric analysis for amino acids. Arch. Biochem. Biophys. 67:10–15.

Ruszkowski, M. 1986. Productivity of buckwheat, p. 78–98. In: Institute of Soil Science and Plant Cultivation (ed.). Buckwheat research 1986. Proc. 3rd Int. Symp. Buckwheat, Pulawy, Poland, Part I. Laboratory of Science Publisher, Poland.

Shannon, J.C. 1968. Carbon-14 distribution in carbohydrates of immature *Zea mays* kernels following $^{14}CO_2$ treatment of intact plants. Plant Physiol. 43:1215–1220.

Shannon, J.C. 1972. Movement of ^{14}C-labelled assimilates into kernels of *Zea mays* L. I. Pattern and rate of sugar movement. Plant Physiol. 49:198–202.

Stevens, N.E. 1912. The morphology of the seed of buckwheat. Bot. Gaz. 53:59–66.

Taira, H., I. Akimoto, and T. Miyahara. 1986. Effects of seeding time on lipid content and fatty acid composition of buckwheat grains. J. Agr. Food Chem. 34:14–17.

Tauzuki, W., Y. Ogata, K. Akasaka, S. Shibata, and T. Suzuki. 1991. Fatty acid composition of selected buckwheat species by fluorometric high-performance chromatography. Cereal Chem. 68:365–369.

Udesky, J. 1988. The book of soba. Kodansha International/USA Ltd. Harper and Row, New York.

Storage, Processing, and Quality Aspects of Buckwheat Seed

G. Mazza

Buckwheat is commonly grown for its black or gray triangular seeds. It can also be grown as a green manure crop, a companion crop, a cover crop, a source of buckwheat honey, and as a pharmaceutical plant yielding rutin (Marshall and Pomeranz 1982). There are three known species of buckwheat: common buckwheat, *Fagopryum esculentum* Moench; tartary buckwheat, *F. tataricum* Gaertn; and perennial buckwheat, *F. cymosum* L. Common buckwheat, also known as *F. sagittatum* Gilib., is by far the most economically important species, accounting for over 90% of the world buckwheat production (Mazza 1992). During the past 10 years, world production of buckwheat has averaged about 2 million ha, or about 1 million tonnes, with Russia accounting for about 90% of the production. Other major producers are China, Japan, Poland, Canada, Brazil, the United States, South Africa, and Australia (Mazza 1992).

In eastern Europe, buckwheat is a basic food item in porridges and soups. In North America, it is marketed primarily in pancake mixes, which may contain buckwheat mixed with wheat, maize, rice, or oat flours, plus a leavening agent. In Japan, buckwheat is marketed primarily as flour for manufacturing a variety of noodles (soba) and as groats. Groats, that part of the grain left after the hulls are removed from the seeds, and farina, made from groats are used for breakfast food, porridge, and thickening materials in soups, gravies, and dressings. Buckwheat is also used with vegetables and spices in kasha and with wheat, maize or rice in bread and pasta products (Marshall and Pomeranz 1982; Mazza 1992).

Primary processing of buckwheat includes cleaning, dehulling, and milling. The aim of dehulling is to separate the groats from the hulls by impact or abrasion of seed against emery stones or steel followed by air or screen separation of groats and hulls. The most important quality attributes of buckwheat groats are color and flavor. The color is light green in freshly harvested seed, but gradually changes to reddish brown during storage. The color change is accompanied by loss of desirable flavor, nutrients, and formation of brown pigments.

The objectives of this investigation were to determine: (1) influence of moisture content, temperature, seed size, and shape on dehulling of buckwheat seed; (2) influence of storage, relative humidity, and temperature on color and flavor characteristics of buckwheat groats; (3) to develop recommendations for long-term storage of buckwheat seed.

METHODOLOGY

'Mancan', 'Manor', and 'Tokyo' buckwheat grown in Canada were used in this study. Processing and analytical methods were as previously described (Mazza 1985, 1986, 1988).

RESULTS AND DISCUSSION

Moisture content of seeds, dehulling recovery, percentage of whole and broken groats and Hunter color values of the groats of 'Mancan', 'Tokyo', and 'Manor' buckwheat equilibrated and dehulled at 25°C and 0.23 to 0.97 water activity are presented in Table 1. The moisture sorption isotherms of 'Mancan' buckwheat at 1°, 10°, 25°, and 40°C are shown in Fig. 1. The water concentration (X)-water activity (a_w) relationships were unaffected by temperature. However, when the data were plotted using vapor pressure instead of the corresponding activity, the higher temperature isotherms were well below those of lower temperatures, as expected, according to the physical adsorption theory (Labuza 1968).

The dehulling recovery varied between cultivar and water activity of the seed (Table 1). 'Mancan' yielded the highest amount of groats and 'Manor' the lowest. 'Mancan' had larger seeds than either 'Tokyo' or 'Manor'. The number of seeds having wings, paper-like extension of the angles of the hulls, is higher in 'Mancan', intermediate in 'Tokyo' and lower in 'Manor' buckwheat. The difference in dehulling yield between cultivars may, in part, be attributed to variations in seed characteristics as well as to differences in groat to hull ratio which is also slightly higher in 'Mancan' than in the other two cultivars.

Table 2 presents the absorbance of the extracted color and tristimulus color values of buckwheat samples stored at 25°C and 0.11 to 0.67 water activity for 19 months. The maximum concentration of browning pigments occurred at 0.45 to 0.55 water activity.

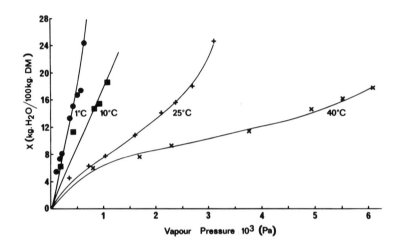

Fig. 1. Adsorption isotherms of 'Mancan' buckwheat at 1°, 10°, 25°, and 40°C.

Table 1. Influence of cultivar and moisture content on dehulling characteristics and color of buckwheat seeds stored at 25°C and water activities of 0.23 to 0.97 for 45 days.

Cultivar	Water activity	Moisture content (%)	Dehulling recovery (%)	Dehulled groat Whole (%)	Dehulled groat Broken (%)	Hunter color values[z] Whole groat L	Whole groat a	Broken groat L	Broken groat a	Mixed groat L	Mixed groat a
Mancan	0.23	5.98	69.2	30.1	69.9	52.0	+0.1	68.7	+0.3	63.5	+0.1
	0.52	9.79	67.0	33.3	66.7	53.0	−0.1	60.0	+0.4	58.7	+0.5
	0.75	13.47	65.4	44.5	55.5	52.3	+0.3	56.5	−0.4	57.4	+0.4
	0.97	19.80	65.0	68.5	31.5	51.0	+0.4	57.87	+1.3	53.2	+0.7
Manor	0.23	5.93	54.9	37.1	62.9	52.6	+1.4	60.6	+0.8	59.0	+1.0
	0.52	9.90	50.4	35.7	64.3	52.9	+1.9	58.0	+0.7	58.9	−0.7
	0.75	13.50	41.6	48.4	51.6	52.9	+1.5	56.6	+1.4	54.5	+1.2
	0.97	19.13	32.5	61.5	38.5	51.7	+2.1	61.3	+1.7	53.2	+0.4
Tokyo	0.23	5.84	66.3	28.7	71.3	51.7	+0.7	62.7	+0.5	60.6	+0.3
	0.52	9.77	60.5	33.5	66.5	51.1	+0.7	58.4	+0.1	57.6	+1.3
	0.75	13.30	58.2	45.5	54.5	51.3	+0.7	54.8	+0.3	54.6	+0.8
	0.97	18.74	51.6	75.1	24.9	50.3	+1.8	58.3	+1.1	52.1	+1.0

[z]L = lightness; a = redness when + and greenness when −.

The calculated BET monolayer for the material stored for 19 months was 7.4 g H_2O/100 g of solids. This corresponded to a water activity of 0.275. Dry foods are usually considered to be most stable to chemical reactions if their moisture content is at or near the BET monolayer (Labuza et al. 1970).

Dehulled seeds of 'Mancan', 'Tokyo', and 'Manor' were analyzed for proximate composition, selected mineral profiles and content of total, free, neutral, glyco-, and phospholipids, and each class of lipid was analyzed for fatty acid composition (Tables 3, 4). The samples contained from 2.6±0.2 to 3.2±0.1% total lipids of which 81 to 85% were neutral lipids, 8 to 11% phospholipids, and 3 to 5% glycolipids. Free lipids, extracted in petroleum ether, ranged from 2.1±0.1 to 2.6±0.1%. The major fatty acids of all cultivars and of all classes of lipids were palmitic (16:0), oleic (18:1), and linoleic (18:2) acid. Average values of these three fatty acids in the total lipids

Table 2. Absorbance of extracted color and Hunter lab tristimulus color values of 'Mancan' buckwheat samples stored at 25°C and five water activities for 19 months.

Water activity	Moisture content (% dry wt)	Absorbance index (A_{420})	Tristimulus values		
			X	Y	Z
0.11	4.1	0.257b[z]	26.3c	26.2c	15.1b
0.23	6.7	0.233c	26.7b	26.5b	15.1b
0.31	8.7	0.241c	27.1a	27.0a	15.3a
0.51	13.0	0.290a	25.3d	24.7d	13.4d
0.67	13.8	0.238c	26.4bc	25.9c	14.2c

[z] Means separated by Duncan's multiple range test, p = 0.01.

Table 3. Proximate composition and selected mineral profile of three dehulled buckwheat cultivars (dry weight basis).

Assay	Cultivar mean±SD		
	Mancan	Manor	Tokyo
Moisture (%)	16.2±0.9	10.1±0.2	10.9±0.1
Protein[z] (%)	14.2±0.6	14.6±0.3	11.9±0.4
Crude Fiber (%)	1.57±0.30	1.21±0.03	1.57±0.10
Ash (%)	1.85±0.01	1.66±0.01	1.39±0.01
Lipids[y] (%)	2.6±0.3	2.2±0.3	2.1±0.2
Carbohydrates[x] (%)	79.8±1.6	80.3±0.8	83.0±1.1
K (%)	0.44±0.01	0.42±0.01	0.41±0.01
P (%)	0.36±0.02	0.35±0.01	0.26±0.02
Mg (%)	0.21±0.01	0.20±0.01	0.20±0.01
Ca (ppm)	180.5±7.4	180.5±10.6	220.5±6.5
Fe (ppm)	24.8±1.8	21.4±0.3	21.2±0.9
Zn (ppm)	23.4±0.4	22.0±1.6	22.8±1.1
Mn (ppm)	10.2±0.2	10.0±0.5	10.2±0.4
Cu (ppm)	4.6±0.3	3.7±0.1	4.3±0.2

[z] N × 6.25.
[y] Soxhlet, petroleum ether for 8 h.
[x] By difference.

Table 4. Lipids of dehulled buckwheat seed.

Cultivar	Concentration (% dry weight)				
	Total lipids[z]	Free lipids[y]	Neutral lipids[x]	Glycolipids[w]	Phospholipids[v]
Mancan[u]	3.2a[t]	2.6a	2.6a	0.15a	0.33a
Mancan[s]	2.9b	2.4a	2.4a	0.13a	0.22a
Manor	2.6c	2.2ab	2.2b	0.09b	0.27a
Tokyo	2.9ab	2.1b	2.5a	0.13a	0.32a

[z]Chloroform-methanol determined by the Folch et al (1975) method.
[y]Soxhlet, petroleum ether for 8 h.
[x]Silicic acid column, chloroform extract.
[w]Florisil column, acetone extract.
[v]Florisil column, methanol extract.
[u]Fresh seed.
[t]Means within each column followed by the same letter are not significantly different by using Duncan's multiple range test $p = 0.05$.
[s]Seed stored for 25 months at room temperature.

of all buckwheat samples examined were 14.0±0.8, 36.3±1.9, and 37.0±1.9%, respectively. The corresponding values for the free lipids were 14.8±1.5, 36.5±2.0, and 35.5±1.9% and those for phospholipids were 9.1±0.8, 44.3±4.4, and 41.7±2.8%, respectively. Total lipid content showed significant positive correlation with free, neutral, and glycolipid contents, and there was a highly significant negative correlation between oleic and linoleic acid contents of all lipid classes. There was, however, no significant difference between new and old buckwheat in the content of free, neutral, glyco-, and phospholipids and in the fatty acid composition of total and free lipids.

The influence of water activity, temperature and cultivar on buckwheat dehulling, groat color, and lipids were examined. Of several cultivars examined, 'Mancan' yielded the most groats. Dehulled seeds contained 2.6 to 3.2% total lipids comprised of 81 to 85% neutral lipids, to 11% phospholipids and 3 to 5% glycolipids. Color and flavor characteristics of buckwheat were maximized when seed were stored at a low temperature at a relative humidity below 45%.

REFERENCES

Labuza, T.P. 1968. Sorption phenomena in foods. Food Technol. 22:263–272.

Labuza, T.P., S.R. Tannenbaum, and M. Karel. 1970. Water content and stability of low-moisture, intermediate-moisture foods. Food Technol. 24:543–550.

Marshall, H.G. and Y. Pomeranz. 1982. Buckwheat description, breeding, production and utilization, p. 157-212 In: Y. Pomeranz (ed.). Advances in cereal science and technology. Amer. Assoc. Cereal Chem., St. Paul, MN.

Mazza, G. 1992. Buckwheat (*Fagopyrum esculentum*), the crop and its importance, p. 534–539. In: R. MacRae (ed.). Encyclopedia of food science, food technology and nutrition. Academic Press Ltd., London (in press).

Mazza, G. 1988. Lipid content and fatty acid composition of buckwheat seed. Cereal Chem. 65:122–126.

Mazza, G. 1986. Buckwheat browning and color assessment. Cereal Chem. 63:261–264.

Mazza, G. and C.G. Campbell. 1985. Influence of water activity and temperature on dehulling of buckwheat. Cereal Chem. 62:31–34.

GRAIN LEGUMES

Food and Grain Legumes

F.J. Muehlbauer

COOL SEASON FOOD LEGUMES

Field pea, (*Pisum sativum* L.), lentil (*Lens culinaris* Medik.), faba bean (*Vicia faba* L.), chickpea (*Cicer arietinum* L.), and grasspea (*Lathyrus sativus* L.) are collectively known as the cool season food legumes. This group of legume crop plants grow vegetatively during the cool season and flower and produce seeds as daylengths become progressively longer. Carbonized remains indicate that peas, lentils, and chickpeas were domesticated in the Near East arc and were cultivated with the cereals as early as the seventh millennium BC (Smartt 1990). From the presumed center of origin, peas spread to the cool-temperate areas of central and northern Europe and from there were introduced into the western hemisphere soon after Columbus (Hedrick 1928; Muehlbauer 1991a). Lentils became an important crop and a dietary mainstay in the drier areas of the near east and North Africa. Lentils were successfully introduced to the Western hemisphere and are now grown extensively in the United States, Canada, Chile, and Argentina (Kay 1979). Chickpea, from their region of domestication in the Near East, quickly spread to the Indian subcontinent where it became a principal pulse crop and a dietary mainstay. Chickpea was successfully introduced to Central and South America and to the western United States (Smithson et al. 1985). Grasspea is produced throughout the arid regions of the Near East, North Africa, west Asia, and India. The grasspea crop is grown on a small scale in South America and on a very limited scale in North America (Kay 1979).

Major production areas for processing peas are the north central states of Wisconsin, Minnesota, Michigan, and the western states of Washington and Oregon. The Palouse region of eastern Washington and northern Idaho is the primary domestic production area for dry peas, lentils, and chickpeas; while the coastal region of south-central California is of equal importance for chickpeas. Faba beans are of minor importance in the United States and are most often used for livestock feeding either as grain or as green forage. Faba beans have not gained any popularity in the United States as food and overseas market outlets have not been developed. Scattered areas of faba beans can be found in western Washington, irrigated areas of Montana and Wyoming, and several northeastern states. Prospects for expanded production of the cool season food legumes depend on overseas market outlets for these crops and prospects for increased domestic usage. Large areas of the arid western states could successfully produce cool season pulses, especially chickpea, lentil, and grasspea, if uses and outlets were developed. There has been some interest in grasspea as a specialty crop for the United States; however, at the present time, low yields and neuro-toxins in the seeds are major limitations. A description of the cool season food legumes, including production methods, disease and insect pests, and their potential as alternative crops for the United States is discussed in this review.

WARM SEASON GRAIN LEGUMES

Grain legumes are a diverse group of crop plants that can be produced over a wide area, depending on the species, from the humid tropics to cool-temperate regions (Table 1). The major grain legumes such as soybean, peanut, common bean, and cowpea are warm season pulses better adapted to humid regions. The warm season pulses are characterized by epigeal germination, a period of rapid vegetative growth, followed by flowering when daylengths become progressively shorter during the growing season. In contrast, the cool season pulses have hypogeal germination, a period of rapid vegetative growth, followed by flowering when daylength becomes progressively longer.

Field Pea

Field pea, which has a wide variety of uses from dry pulses to succulent fresh peas to edible podded types, are the most widely grown of the cool season pulses (Table 2) and have the highest average grain yields (1,605 kg/ha). The production of field pea on a world basis is on the increase especially in Europe, Canada, and Oceania, where the crop is produced for expanded use in animal feeding. Domestic production of field pea (Table 3) is

Table 1. Important grain legumes and their areas of adaptation.

Scientific name	Common name	Region of adaptation
Arachis hypogaea L.	Peanut	Humid to semi-arid
Cajanus cajan (L.) Millsp.	Pigeon pea	Humid to semi-arid
Cicer arietinum L.	Chickpea	Cool season, sub-tropical semi-arid
Glycine max (L.) Merr.	Soybean	Humid to sub-humid cool season or sub-tropical
Lablab purpureus (L.) Sweet	Hyacinth bean	Sub-humid to semi-arid
Lathyrus sativus L.	Grasspea	Semi-arid
Lens culinaris Medic.	Lentil	Cool season to semi-arid
Lupinus spp.	Lupin	Humid to sub-humid
Macrotyloma uniflorum (Lam.) Verdc.	Horse gram	Sub-humid to semi-arid
Parkia spp.	Locust bean	Sub-humid to semi-arid
Phaseolus lunatus L.	Lima bean	Humid to sub-humid
Phaseolus vulgaris L.	Common bean	Humid to sub-humid
Phosphocarpus tetragonologa (L.) DC	Winged bean	Humid tropics
Pisum sativum L.	Field pea	Temperate to sub-tropical
Vica faba L.	Faba bean	Sub-tropical to temperate
Vigna aureus (Roxb.) Hepper	Green gram	Humid to semi-arid
Vigna radiata (L.) Wilczek	Mung bean	Humid to semi-arid
Vigna unguiculata (L.) Walp.	Cowpea	Humid to semi-arid

Boldface indicates international economic importance; others of regional or local importance.

Table 2. Estimated world production of cool season food legumes (FAO 1989).

Common name	Area (1000 ha)		Yield (kg/ha)		Total production (1000t)	
	1979–81	1987–89	1979–81	1987–89	1979–81	1987–89
Chickpea	9601	9593	625	713	6028	6850
Faba bean	3685	3186	1162	1309	4284	4171
Field pea	7501	9899	1140	1605	8494	15885
Lentil	2201	3217	596	795	1312	2562
World production[z] (all pulses)	61074	68886	674	815	41153	56092

[z]Excluding soybeans.

estimated at 200,000 ha and includes dry peas, processing peas, seed peas, and Austrian winter peas (Muehlbauer et al. 1983). Canadian production of field peas is currently more than three times that of the United States making that country a major competitor in world markets.

Chickpea

Chickpea is the major pulse crop in the Indian subcontinent where it is now produced on nearly 7 million ha (Smithson et al. 1985). Chickpeas are classified as either *desi* or *kabuli* types. The *desi* types are characterized by smaller, angular, and pigmented seeds; whereas the *kabuli* types are characterized by larger seeds that are more rounded and lack pigmentation. The *desi* types predominate in the Indian subcontinent while the *kabuli* types predominate elsewhere. Domestic production of chickpeas is estimated at 6,000 ha annually (Table 3) and is about

Table 3. United States production of cool season food legumes.

Common name	Area (1000 ha)		Yield (kg/ha)		Total production (1000t)	
	1979–81	1987–89	1979–81	1987–89	1979–81	1987–89
Chickpea[z]	4	6	1200	1200	4.8	7.2
Lentil[y]	78	43	1073	1314	84	60
Faba bean[z]	---	<1	---	1600	---	1.6
Field pea[y]	70	76	2310	2696	163	204

[z]Estimated by author.
[y]FAO (1989).

equally divided between California and the Palouse region of eastern Washington and northern Idaho, although there is scattered production in several other western states. *Kabuli* types predominate American production because of their high value for use as an ingredient in salad bars; however, there is a small but steadily increasing production of *desi* types. The small amount of *desi* types produced are currently marketed to ethnic communities in the large cities; however, there are prospects, yet to be explored, of developing expanded production suitable for export. Canada has not become a major competitor in chickpea production primarily because available cultivars are not particularly adapted to the short production seasons there.

Lentil

Lentil is a widely grown crop in semi-arid regions of the near east, northern Africa and the Indian subcontinent. Although mostly discontinued, lentil was a widely grown crop in southern and central Europe. The major reason lentil is not widely grown in those countries at the present time is the requirement for hand labor to harvest the crop. In these areas, the crop is planted in roughly tilled soil which are, in some cases, extremely stony. The short plant stature of lentil and the stony fields effectively preclude mechanical harvesting and consequently farmers have relied on hand pulling of the plants. With the advent of mechanical methods of harvesting crops such as wheat, barley, and oats, those crops have gradually replaced lentil. The lentil crop was effectively displaced to more marginal stony lands which are largely unsuited to mechanical harvesting methods. Poor yields and high production costs in those marginal areas eventually led to greatly reduced areas devoted to the lentil crop. Major research emphasis at the International Center for Agricultural Research in the Dry Areas (ICARDA) in Syria is toward development of tall upright lentil germplasm adaptable to mechanical harvesting. Of the southern European countries, only Spain remains as a major producer of the crop. Immigrants from central Europe brought lentils to the United States and grew the crop on a small scale for their own use. The first commercial domestic production of lentils took place in 1937 near Farmington, Washington. Production expanded until 1981 when nearly 90,000 ha were produced. Since then, production (Table 3) has stabilized at about 45,000 ha annually (Muehlbauer et al. 1985). Fluctuations in production are a response to variable export market demands as nearly 90% of the crop is exported.

Faba Bean

Faba bean production in the United States is rather limited and scattered. In the era of draft horses, the smaller seeded types were grown for feed and became known as "horse bean." In some areas of the humid northeast and in western Washington and Oregon, the crop is occasionally produced for green forage.

Grasspea

Development of grasspea into an important food legume has been hindered by the presence of a neuro-toxin in the seeds which if consumed in large quantities can cause irreversible paralysis (Smartt 1990). Grasspea could become an important feed grain crop in the semi-arid western states provided yields can be improved and low neuro-toxin cultivars can be developed.

BOTANY

Taxonomy

Peas. The genus *Pisum* contains two species, *P. sativum* and *P. fulvum*, both with $2n=14$ chromosomes (Muehlbauer 1991a). Cultivated peas are classified within *P. sativum* ssp. *sativum* which contains var. *sativum*, the horticultural types, and var. *arvense*, which are the fodder and winter types. The horticultural types are characterized by papilionaceous flowers that can be borne in singles or multiples on racemes that originate from the stem axes of viny upright plants. Flowers are usually white on horticultural types although some edible podded cultivars have violet flowers. There is a vast range in pod types from small cylindrical pods to the large and flat edible pods. Similarly, there is tremendous variation in seed sizes, shapes and colors. The wrinkled seeded types are commonly used in the immature stage for freezing and canning while the smooth seeded types are used as dry peas.

Chickpea. The genus *Cicer* contains 9 annual and 31 perennial species. Only one annual species, *C. arietinum* is cultivated. *Cicer arietinum* and *C. reticulatum* Lad., its presumed progenitor, have $2n = 16$ chromosomes as do the other annual species. Chickpea plants are usually branched and have strong woody stems that can be strongly erect or semiprostrate. Flowers are borne on racemes that originate from stem axes. Flowers of *desi* types are typically violet; whereas flowers of *kabuli* types are white. Pods are usually borne singly and contain one, two and sometimes three seeds. Seeds of *desi* types are small, sharply angular and are variously pigmented. *Kabuli* type seeds lack pigmentation and are generally larger but can vary widely in size and have a "ramshead" shape.

Lentil. The genus Lens contains two biological species *L. culinaris* and *L. nigricans* (Bieb.) Godron both with $2n = 14$ chromosomes (Muehlbauer 1991a). *Lens culinaris* contains three subspecies including ssp. *culinaris* Medic. the cultivated type, ssp. *orientalis* (Boiss.) Handel-Mazzeti, the presumed progenitor of the cultivated lentil, and ssp. *odemensis* Lad. *Lens nigricans*, the other biological species, containing ssp. *nigricans* and ssp. *ervoides* (Brign.) Grande, is not cultivated. Lentil plants, with their thin stems and small leaflets are very weakly upright. Flowers of lentil plants can range from nearly white to violet, often with blue or violet stripes on the standard, and are borne on racemes that originate from the stem axes. Pods typically have one or two and occasionally three seeds. Seeds are lens shaped and can vary in size from 2 to about 9 mm in diameter. Cotyledons can be red, yellow or green. Seeds can be variously pigmented but uniformly tan or beige seedcoats, sometimes mottled, are most common.

Faba bean. *Vicia* is a very large genus and contains over 130 species (Smartt 1990). *Vicia faba*, the cultivated species, has $2n = 12$ chromosomes. Faba beans vary greatly in seed size, seed shape, seed color, growth period, and yield. Recognized types of faba bean include two subspecies; *paucijuga* L. and *faba* L. The latter subspecies has been further divided into (i) var. *minor*, which has small rounded seeds that are about 1 cm long; (ii) var. *equina*, with medium-sized seeds that are about 1.5 cm long and are typical of the so called "horse bean" and (iii) var. *major*, the horticultural type with large, broad, flat seeds that are about 2 to 3 cm long (Kay 1979). Faba bean plants are strongly upright with stiff main stems. Flowers are borne on the stem axes and are typically white and partly deep purple. Seeds are contained in large fleshy pods that vary considerably in length from less than 5 to over 30 cm. The smaller seeded types of faba beans, vars. *minor* and *equina*, are often referred to as field beans, while the larger seeded types, var. *major*, are referred to as "broadbeans" (Bond et al. 1985). The smaller seeded minor and equina types are commonly used for animal feeding while the larger seeded major types are most often used as a green vegetable or as a dry pulse. A common food use for faba beans in the Middle East is *Foul Medanes* a common breakfast dish in Egypt. The pods are often picked green and the seeds used directly as a green vegetable. Also, in some Mediterranean countries, small amounts of faba bean flour are used in bread making (Bond et al. 1985).

Grasspea. The grasspea, *Lathyrus sativus*, is a member of a large genus which contains over 150 species (Smartt 1990). Grasspea has $2n = 14$ chromosomes. Grasspea plants are viny with flattened stems and are weakly upright. Flower morphology is similar to that of *Pisum* spp. Flowers are usually borne singly on racemes that originate from the stem axes. Pods usually contain 4 to 7 seeds that are small, usually round and heavily pigmented. Grasspea is very drought tolerant and produces some grain yield where other pulse crops are likely to fail completely. It is surprising therefore that this particular crop plant has not received much attention. Consequently, most of what is grown throughout the world are local landraces; although Kay (1979) lists several cultivars. These landraces all have a high content of ß-N-oxalyl-L-α, ß diaminopropionic acid (ODAP), the compound considered to incite the condition known as "lathyrism," an irreversible paralysis, if the seeds are consumed in excessive amounts (Smartt 1990). Progress is being made in reducing this compound in breeding lines of grasspea (A.E. Slinkard pers. commun.); a development which could lead to increased production of the crop for food in dry areas. Grasspea production, though very minor in the United States, is mostly from local landraces.

Reproductive Biology

Flowers of all the cool season food legumes have a typical papilionaceous structure. The calyx consists of five sepals and the corolla is comprised of a standard, two wings and two lower petals that lie inside the wings and are united at the lower margins to form a keel. There are 10 stamens which surround the pistil. The anthers open lengthwise and shed their pollen directly onto the stigma. After the anthers dehisce and pollination is completed, the ovary elongates. Pods of pea, lentil, faba bean, and grasspea are usually glabrous and flat and contain ovules that alternate along the margin. Pods of chickpea are round, have an inflated appearance and have glandular trichomes. Chickpea pods contain ovules that alternate along the margin.

There is minimal cross pollination in peas (Gritton 1980), lentils (Wilson and Law 1972), and chickpeas (Niknejad and Khosh-Khui 1972); however, cross-pollination can be over 50% in faba beans (Poulsen 1975; Hanna and Lawes 1967). Cross-pollination is thought to be high in grasspea, but actual data have not been reported.

AGRONOMY

Pea Cultivars

Dry pea cultivars were originally developed for use in the canning industry; however, within the past 30 years, breeding specifically for dry pea production was initiated at numerous locations including the United States, Canada, and most European countries. Cultivars of dry peas commonly grown in the United States and Canada, include 'Alaska', 'Columbian', 'Alaska 81', 'Latah', 'Umatilla', 'Trapper', 'Century ', among others. Winter pea cultivars include common 'Austrian Winter', 'Fenn', 'Melrose', and 'Glacier'. More recently, research programs have been established to develop so-called "protein peas" for which the crop is intended solely as a protein supplement for animal feeding. Protein content of protein peas is similar to other pea cultivars. For detailed information on performance and production methods see Muehlbauer (1982) and Muehlbauer et al. (1983). Brief descriptions of these cultivars follows:

'Alaska' peas are used extensively by the dry pea industry in the United States. Numerous strains are available typically with large, smooth round green seeds. 'Alaska' peas are spring sown as soon as the land can be prepared and they bloom in about the 10th node; usually about 45 days after planting. The vine type is tall and weakly upright, indeterminate, and usually nonbranching. 'Alaska' typically reaches maturity approximately 95 days after sowing. The strain locally designated as 'Columbian' in the Palouse region of Washington and Idaho is popular with producers and processors because of its consistent high yields, good seed size, and good seed color qualities. 'Alaska 81', released to producers in 1984 (Muehlbauer 1987a), has produced comparable yields and seed quality and has virus resistance.

Cultivars of the small-sieve 'Alaska' type are used less extensively and are characterized by slightly smaller seed size, earlier maturity when compared with regular Alaska types, and they tend to be slightly dimpled and more susceptible to seed bleaching. Seed bleaching is a condition in which peas that are normally green at dry seed maturity lose their color, and take on a yellow-white appearance. Bleaching is brought about by moisture imbibition following rain or heavy dews.

'Latah' is a large yellow spring sown dry pea cultivar that has a long vine habit, blooms in about the 14th node, and is relatively high yielding. The cultivar was recently replaced by 'Umatilla' (Muehlbauer 1987a).

'Umatilla' is about 16 cm shorter and 13% higher yielding when compared with 'Latah'. 'Umatilla' sets double pods compared to the single podding habit for Latah and is resistant to seed shattering. The seeds of

'Umatilla' are larger and have averaged 18.7 per 100 seeds compared to 17.1 for 'Latah'. Seeds of 'Umatilla' are bright yellow; representing a significant improvement in seed quality when compared to 'Latah' in which the seeds often have an undesirable green cast. 'Umatilla' is very well adapted to splitting, a major use for yellow peas.

Several cultivars of fall sown peas (*P. sativum* ssp. *arvense*) (referred to locally as "Austrian Winter" peas) are currently available for commercial production. Yields of common Austrian Winter peas have been extremely variable because of disease and insect problems but they tend to be tolerant of fusarium root rot (Auld et al. 1979; Murray and Slinkard 1973). In Idaho, Austrian Winter peas are seeded in the fall (late September or early October) into roughly tilled soil. Winter survival is enhanced by the rough tillage, previous crop residues and snow cover during the colder winter months. Austrian Winter peas are often used for green manure to improve organic matter and nitrogen status of soils.

'Fenn' has purple flowers, an average vine length of nearly 2 m, triple flowers per peduncle, yellow cotyledons, and speckled seedcoats (Murray and Slinkard 1973). Yield potential of 'Fenn' is slightly larger than common Austrian Winter (Auld et al. 1979).

'Melrose' is similar to 'Fenn' and has purple flowers and an indeterminate flowering habit. 'Melrose' has a vine length of about 2 m and higher yield potential than 'common Austrian Winter' or 'Fenn' (Auld et al. 1979).

'Glacier' has shorter vines and improved seed yields when compared to 'Melrose' (Auld 1982). 'Glacier', with its shorter growth habit, is not as suitable for green manuring as are other Austrian Winter cultivars.

A number of commercial dry pea cultivars are available that are representative of types grown extensively either in Canada, Europe, New Zealand, or the United Kingdom. 'Marrowfats' is a popular dry pea type grown in England and used in the canning industry. 'Marrowfats' is also used extensively in the Orient as a snack item. 'Marrowfats' tends to be late maturing and often are severely attacked by infestations of powdery mildew. The seeds of 'Marrowfats' are typically large (30 to 35 g/100 seeds), slightly flattened, dimpled, and have green cotyledons. 'Marrowfats' often bleach and are of poor quality when wet conditions coincide with crop maturity. 'Marrowfats' of acceptable color can be grown if they are swathed at about 18 to 23% seed moisture content, threshed as soon as possible, and dried artificially.

Lentil Cultivars

Lentil cultivars commonly grown in the United States and Canada include: 'Chilean 78', 'Brewer', 'Laird', 'Eston', 'Redchief', 'Indianhead', 'Emerald', and 'Crimson'. For more detailed information on cultivars and production methods, see Summerfield et al. (1982) and Muehlbauer et al. (1981). Brief descriptions follow:

'Chilean 78' is a yellow cotyledon type that requires a growth period of 95 to 110 days, depending on weather, to complete its growth cycle. 'Chilean 78' produces seeds which are about 6.5 mm in diameter and have varying degrees of seedcoat mottling.

'Brewer' (Muehlbauer 1987b) has yellow cotyledons and is earlier to flower and produces yields which average 20% greater than 'Chilean 78'. About 95 days are required for the growth period for 'Brewer'. 'Brewer' has seeds which are slightly larger and more uniform when compared to 'Chilean 78'.

'Laird' is a large yellow-seeded cultivar developed by A.E. Slinkard in Canada (Slinkard and Bhatty 1979). 'Laird' has excellent seed quality traits (large, thick seeds free of mottle and of good color); however, the major disadvantage of 'Laird' in the United States is late blooming and maturity (about 2 weeks later than 'Chilean').

'Eston' is a small-seeded yellow cotyledon cultivar developed by A.E. Slinkard in Canada (Slinkard 1981). Seeds of 'Eston' are about 40% smaller than 'Chilean 78', however, the cultivar has provided exceptionally high yields.

'Redchief' is a red cotyledon cultivar that consistently outyields 'Chilean 78'. 'Redchief' has about the same plant habit as 'Chilean 78' and requires about 95 to 105 days to mature, depending on the weather. 'Redchief' produces seeds that are about 6.0 mm in diameter, free of seedcoat mottling. Markets for large seeded red cotyledon lentils are limited; however, efforts are underway in the United States to develop suitable outlets (A.E. Slinkard pers. commun.).

'Indianhead' is a small black seeded cultivar developed in Canada also by A.E. Slinkard. 'Indianhead' is primarily used as a green manure cover crop on the Canadian prairies. The cultivar is characterized by rapid and vigorous vegetative growth.

'Emerald' is a green cotyledon cultivar recently released (Muehlbauer 1987b). The cultivar blooms several days later than 'Brewer' or 'Chilean 78'. Yields are equivalent to or slightly less than 'Brewer' in most years. The acceptability of a green cotyledon type in domestic and international markets is yet to be determined.

'Crimson' has small brown seeds with red cotyledons (Muehlbauer 1991b). The cultivar is typical of the lentils grown in the near east and northern Africa. The cultivar is well adapted to intermediate rainfall zones (350 to 400 mm annually) and therefore could become an alternative crop in rotation with wheat in those areas. Marketing of small red lentils will depend upon availability of equipment for decortication and splitting; the major process used for small red lentils.

Chickpea Cultivars

Chickpea cultivars grown in the United States and Mexico are referred to as "garbanzos" which characteristically are large seeded, usually white or cream-colored, and have rounded edges. Most of the garbanzos produced domestically are used in salad bars. For more detailed information on chickpea cultivars and production methods see Muehlbauer et al. (1982). Brief descriptions of cultivars in use in the United States are as follows:

'UC-5' is a pureline selection from 'White Spanish', a common cultivar grown in California for over 100 years. 'UC-5' is similar to both 'White Spanish' and 'Mission' but seems to have more resistance to early season root rot in California.

'Surutato 77' is a Mexican cultivar that has shown excellent resistance to fusarium wilt in California and Mexico. 'Surutato 77' blooms and matures about 7 days earlier compared to 'UC-5' and 'Mission' in California. Because of its disease resistance and excellent quality, 'Surutato 77' has become the predominant cultivar in Mexico, and appears to have replaced 'UC-5' in California. Production of 'Surutato 77' is also expanding in the Pacific Northwest.

'Tammany' is a unifoliate cultivar recently released (Muehlbauer and Kaiser 1987) for production in the Pacific Northwest. The cultivar is similar to 'Surutato 77', but is several days earlier to mature.

'Garnet' is a desi type cultivar (Muehlbauer and Kaiser 1987) with small brown angular seeds. Desi types are grown on a limited but steadily increasing area in the Pacific Northwest. *Desi* type cultivars have potential as an alternative crop to cereals in dry areas and can often replace summer fallowing.

'Sarah' originated from 'C235', an Ascochyta blight-resistant *desi* type, developed in India. 'Sarah' has shown excellent resistance to Ascochyta blight in the Palouse region of eastern Washington and northern Idaho (Muehlbauer and Kaiser 1990). Yields and quality are also very good. 'Sarah' is also adapted to dry areas and could become a significant rotational crop with the cereals if markets can be developed.

Faba Bean Cultivars

A large number of cultivars have been developed for human consumption and for animal feeding. The cultivars 'Ackerperle', and 'Diana' developed in Canada are generally used for animal feeding. In areas with mild winters, the crop can be planted in the fall and used for winter grazing.

Adaptation

The grain legumes, other than faba beans, perform well and produce acceptable yields in semi-arid regions of the world. Ranking of the grain legumes for their ability to produce under dry conditions and poor soil would place grasspea first followed by lentil, chickpea, pea, and finally faba bean. These crops are generally grown as winter annuals on soils that receive a minimum of 350 mm of annual rainfall. Of these crops, grasspea is best adapted to such dry conditions. Moisture requirements for lentil and chickpea are similar but best results are obtained where 400 to 500 mm of rainfall are received. The pea crop has a higher moisture requirement of from 450 to 500 mm annually. Faba bean has even higher water requirements and is often irrigated. The Nile valley of Egypt produces large quantities of faba beans under irrigation during the winter months. The cooler and more humid areas of Europe also produce good crops of faba beans. In all cases, the grain legumes are best adapted for production during the cool season when evapotranspiration is minimal. In many areas, these crops rely on stored soil moisture for a large part of their growth cycle.

The adaptation of lentil, chickpea, and grasspea to dry conditions make these crops suitable for production in the semi-arid regions of the western United States. In those areas, grain legumes could be ideal rotational crops with cereals or possibly can be used as fallow replacement crops in regions that receive sufficient rainfall to permit annual cropping.

Inoculation with the appropriate strain of *Rhizobia* is essential when these food legumes are seeded into fields for the first time. Fields should be reinoculated if there has been a lapse of several years between crops. *Rhizobium leguminosarum* is the appropriate inoculant for peas, lentils, grasspeas, and faba beans; whereas, chickpeas require a strain specific for *Cicer* species. Inoculants can be purchased in either the peat or the granular form. The peat form is often applied to the seeds with a sticker to improve adherence. Application of the peat inoculant over the seed in the drill hopper is not advised because it tends to settle to the bottom of the hopper and not be uniformly distributed throughout the field.

Uses and Nutritive Value

The grain legumes are major sources of dietary protein and calories for human consumption in the world but of minor importance in the United States. The cool season food legumes range in protein content from about 22% for chickpeas to 28% for lentils. These legumes are popular in the developing countries of the near east and North Africa. Also, they are a dietary mainstay on the Indian subcontinent, especially in regions where religious preferences discourage the consumption of animal protein.

The sulfur containing amino acids, methionine, and cystine, are limiting in the proteins of these grain legumes. However, a favorable amino acid profile is easily obtained with the combined use of cereal grains in the diet.

Production Methods and Weed Control

In general, the cool season food legumes perform well at high latitudes on well-drained soils on south and east facing slopes that have pH values between 6.0 and 7.5. Land that is poorly drained or excessively wet should be avoided. Land intended for these crops should be fall plowed to incorporate previous crop residues, and prepared for planting in early spring.

The cool season food legumes usually do not respond to nitrogen fertilization; but low rates, applied in bands next to but not in contact with the seeds, at planting can be beneficial to early stand establishment. There is a high requirement for phosphorous and soils should be fertilized to adequate levels. These crops seem to respond to additions of potassium and sulfur where soil tests indicate deficiencies. For additional information on mineral nutrient requirements, see Muehlbauer and Summerfield (1989).

Seed treatments. Seeds of peas, lentils, chickpeas, and faba beans should be treated with an appropriate fungicide to prevent seed decay and pre- and post-emergence damping-off. *Pythium* spp. and *Rhizoctonia* spp. can cause extensive damage to stands if not controlled. To prevent damage from wireworms and seedcorn maggots, seeds should be treated with an appropriate insecticide.

Seeding rates and depths. Optimum plant populations vary for the cool season food legumes. The optimum density is about 880,000 plants/ha for lentils and 310,000 plants/ha for chickpeas. Plant densities from 130,000 to 550,000/ha are used in faba bean production and densities of 200,000 to 250,000/ha are common for grasspea. The smaller seeded cultivars are usually seeded at slightly higher densities.

Seeding depths for peas and faba beans can be up to 7.5 cm. Deep seeding is often used to prevent phytotoxicity from shallow incorporated herbicides. Lentils and chickpeas have difficulties in emergence from deep planting and are sown no deeper than 5 cm depending on moisture conditions.

Weed problems. Weeds can compete with the food legumes and significantly lower seed yields. In addition, exudates from weeds can cause staining of the seeds and reduce crop quality. Annual grass weeds such as wild oat are a particularly serious weed problem in the food legumes. Control is most often accomplished through the use of soil incorporated herbicides. Post-emergent applications of herbicides can be effective for broadleaf weed control in peas and faba beans. Herbicides registered for use on this group of crops varies between states. In all cases, however, rates and the timing of herbicide applications are extremely important for effective weed control and to minimize crop injury.

Lentils and chickpeas are less competitive with weeds when compared to peas or faba beans. Because of their less competitive nature, careful attention must be paid to obtain optimum weed control. The best broadleaf weed control methods in these two crops have involved preemergence surface applications of herbicides.

Weed infestations can be troublesome at the time of harvest through staining of the seeds during the threshing operation. Nightshade (*Solanum* spp.) can be particularly damaging to the appearance of kabuli chickpeas and staining can be so severe as to make the crop unacceptable to processors. Seeds of the other cool season food legumes can also be badly stained by weed exudates.

Diseases and Pests

Diseases are a major factor which limit productivity of the grain legumes in the United States and worldwide. Foremost among the diseases are aphanomyces blight and fusarium root rot of pea. These root rots also affect lentil but to a lesser degree. Fusarium wilt of pea can be a serious constraint but is efficiently controlled through resistant cultivars. Likewise, fusarium wilt of chickpea is also controlled with resistant cultivars. Viruses affect all of the grain legumes and are serious constraints for peas and lentils. Foliar diseases such as sclerotinia white mold, ascochyta blight, and powdery mildew seriously affect peas but, except for ascochyta blight of chickpeas, are of lesser importance for the other grain legumes. Ascochyta blight of chickpea continues to devastate the crop in the Palouse region of eastern Washington and northern Idaho. Botrytis grey mold of faba bean can cause yield reductions in humid production areas.

Future Prospects

The grain legumes are a widely adapted group of crop plants that are generally under-utilized in cropping systems of the United States. Prospects for expanded use in rotational systems with cereals depend on development of export markets and expanded domestic use for food and feed. Pea and grasspea have potential as protein supplements for animal feeding, while lentil and chickpea will likely only be produced for food because of their relatively high value. Expansion of faba bean production does not seem likely in the United States because of its high moisture requirements and comparatively unstable yields.

Of the food legumes, chickpea, lentil, and grasspea seem to have the greatest potential for expanded production. These grain legumes are tolerant of dry conditions and can be used as fallow replacements in many areas of the arid western states. Development of grasspea as a viable drought tolerant crop will depend on the incorporation and use of low neuro-toxin germplasm.

REFERENCES

Auld, D.L. 1982. Varieties of winter hardy peas and chickpeas, p. 109–116. In: Proc. Palouse symposium on dry peas, lentils and chickpeas. Moscow, Idaho. College of Agr. Res. Ctr., Washington State Univ., Pullman.

Auld, D.L., G.A. Murray, and L.E. O'Keeffe. 1979. Melrose Austrian winter pea. Univ. of Idaho Coop. Ext. Serv. Current Information Series 497.

Bond, D.A., D.A. Lawes, G.C. Hawtin, M.C. Saxena, and J.H. Stephens. 1985. Faba bean (*Vicia faba* L.), p. 199–265. In: R.J. Summerfield and E.H. Roberts (eds.). Grain legume crops. Collins, London.

FAO. 1989. Production yearbook. FAO Statistics Series 94. p. 43:145–159.

Gritton, E.T. 1980. Field Pea. In: W.R. Fehr and H.H. Hadley (eds.). Hybridization of crop plants. Amer. Soc. Agron. Monograph. Madison, WI.

Hanna, A.S. and D.A. Lawes. 1967. Studies on pollination and fertilization in the field bean (*Vicia faba* L.). Annu. Appl. Biol. 59:289–295.

Hedrick, U.P. 1928. Vegetables of New York. Vol. 1. Peas of New York. J.B. Lyon Company, Albany, NY.

Hymowitz, T. 1990. Grain legumes, p. 154–158. In: J. Janick and J.E. Simon (eds.). Advances in new crops. Timber Press, Portland, OR.

Kay, D.E. 1979. Food legumes. Tropical Prod. Inst. Crop and Prod. Dig. No. 3. London.

Muehlbauer, F.J. 1982. Dry pea and lentil cultivars, p. 101–108. In: Proc. Palouse symposium on dry peas, lentils, and chickpeas. Moscow, Idaho, February 23–24, 1982. College of Agr. Res. Ctr., Washington State Univ., Pullman.

Muehlbauer, F.J. 1987a. Registration of 'Alaska 81' and 'Umatilla' dry pea. Crop Sci. 27:1089–1090.

Muehlbauer, F.J. 1987b. Registration of 'Brewer' and 'Emerald' lentil. Crop Sci. 27:1080–1089.

Muehlbauer, F.J. 1991a. Use of introduced germplasm in cool season food legume cultivar development. In: H.L. Shands and L.E. Wiesner (eds.). Use of plant introductions in cultivar development. Part 2. Crop Sci. Soc. Amer. Special Publ. Madison, WI. (In press).

Muehlbauer, F.J. 1991b. Registration of 'Crimson' lentil. Crop Sci. 31:1094–1095.

Muehlbauer, F.J., J.I. Cubero, and R.J. Summerfield. 1985. Lentil (*Lens culinaris* Medic.), p 266–311. In: R.J. Summerfield and E.H. Roberts (eds.). Grain legume crops. Collins, London.

Muehlbauer, F.J. and W.J. Kaiser. 1987. Registration of 'Garnet' and 'Tammany' chickpea. Crop Sci. 27:1087–1088.

Muehlbauer, F.J. and W.J. Kaiser. 1991. Registration of 'Sarah' chickpea. Crop Sci. 31:1094.

Muehlbauer, F.J., R.W. Short, W.J. Kaiser, D.F. Bezdicek, K.J. Morrison, and D.G. Swan. 1982. Description and culture of chickpeas. Coop. Ext., College of Agr., Washington State Univ., Pullman.

Muehlbauer, F.J., R.W. Short, and J.M. Kraft. 1983. Description and culture of dry peas. USDA. Agr. Rev. and Manuals, ARM-W-37.

Muehlbauer, F.J., R.W. Short, R.J. Summerfield, K.J. Morrison, and D.G. Swan. 1981. Description and culture of lentils. EB 99957, Coop. Ext. Serv., Washington State Univ., Pullman.

Muehlbauer, F.J. and R.J. Summerfield. 1989. Dry peas. In: D.L. Plucknett and H.B. Sprague (eds.). Detecting mineral nutrient deficiencies in tropical and temperate crops. Westview Trop. Agr. Ser. 7. Westview Press, Boulder, CO.

Murray, G.A. and A.E. Slinkard. 1973. Fenn Austrian winter pea. Univ. of Idaho Coop. Ext. Serv., Current Inform. Ser. 209.

Niknejad, M. and M. Khosh-Khui. 1972. Natural cross-pollination in gram (*Cicer arietinum* L.). Indian J. Agr. Sci. 42:273–274.

Poulsen, M.H. 1975. Pollination, seed setting, cross-fertilization and inbreeding in *Vicia faba* L. Z. Pflanzenzuchtg. 74:97–118.

Slinkard, A.E. 1981. 'Eston' lentil. Can. J. Plant Sci. 61:733–734.

Slinkard, A.E. and R.S. Bhatty. 1979. 'Laird' lentil. Can. J. Plant Sci. 59:503–504.

Slinkard, A.E., R.S. Bhatty, B.N. Drew, and R.A.A. Morrall. 1990. Dry pea and lentil as new crops in Saskatchewan: A case study, p. 164–168. In: J. Janick and J.E. Simon (eds.). Advances in new crops. Timber Press, Portland, OR.

Smartt, J. 1990. Pulses of the classical world, p. 190–198. In: R.J. Summerfield and E.H. Ellis (eds.). Grain legumes: evaluation and genetic resources. Cambridge Univ. Press, Cambridge.

Smithson, J.B., J.A. Thompson, and R.J. Summerfield. 1985. Chapter 8. Chickpea (*Cicer arietinum* L.). In: R.J. Summerfield and E.H. Roberts (eds.) Grain legume crops. Collins, London.

Summerfield, R.J., F.J. Muehlbauer, and R.W. Short. 1981. Description and culture of lentils. USDA, Agr. Res. Serv., Prod. Res. Rpt. 181. Washington, DC.

Wilson, V.E. and A.G. Law. 1972. Natural crossing in *Lens esculenta* Moench. J. Amer. Soc. Hort. Sci. 97:142–143.

An Interdisciplinary Approach to the Development of Lupin as an Alternative Crop

Daniel H. Putnam

From the ashen wasteland of Mount St. Helens to the barren frozen Arctic, from the heights of the Andes to the cool Mediterranean or Texas plains, over 300 *Lupinus* species have found their place in the natural world. Although its agricultural history is also thousands of years old, in many regions of the world lupin is still a "new" crop plant. Lupins are high in protein, do not contain antinutritional factors, are high N-fixers, have value in a rotation and have an upright, non-shattering habit. However, other factors such as economics and competition from established crops are important to the success of a new crop and it is not yet clear the place lupins will occupy in modern agricultural systems. This paper describes how a group of researchers approached the problem of using lupin (*Lupinus albus*) as an alternative source of protein for dairy or other livestock farmers in central Minnesota. Our experience with this crop during a collaborative project conducted between 1988 and 1991 might be of use to others who are exploring the application of lupin or similar species in different parts of the world.

CROP DESCRIPTION

Cultivated lupins are cool-season grain legumes or forage crops (Fig. 1). There are five species cultivated worldwide (*L. albus*, *L. augustifolius*, *L. luteus*, *L. mutabalis*, and *L. cosentenii*), in climates ranging from northern Europe and Russia, to the arid Australian plains and the Andean highlands. Both spring-sown and fall-sown types are grown, but only the spring types are adapted to the northern Midwest, Northeast, and Canada. Agricultural production of lupin represents a fraction of a percent of the grain legumes grown worldwide, largely because of its historically bitter seed (Williams 1986). However, lupin is one of the few grain legumes that come close to soybean in protein content of the seed (Hymowitz 1990). The large seed and lack of antinutritional factors make lupin a potential crop for many animal feed formulations, for direct feeding, and as a human food.

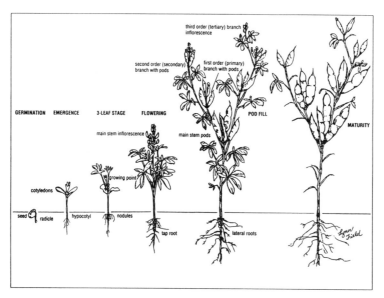

Fig. 1. Growth stages of spring-sown white lupin (*Lupinus albus*). The relatively large seed and upright habit makes lupin an attractive grain legume crop.

---

*I acknowledge the following cooperators: R.A. Meronuck, D. Otterby, K.K. Ayisi, L.A. Field, J.L. Gunsolus, L.L. Hardman, D.G. Johnson, R. Kalis-Kusnia, N. Krause, M. May, L. McCann, D. Noetzel, K. Olson, J. Orf, S.R. Simmons, E.L. Stewart, M. Wiens, and J. Wright.

HISTORY OF LUPIN

Lupin as a crop species was important to many of the Mediterranean civilizations, and was apparently independently domesticated in both the Old and New World (Gross 1986). The crop is mentioned as commonplace by the poet Virgil (70 BC), and by Greek and Persian writers (1500 AD) (Hondelmann 1984). The large seed was reportedly used as play money during Roman times. In their exploration of the New World, Spaniards noted that the Andean civilizations had lupins (Tarwi, or *Lupinus mutabilis*) "as we have in Spain" (Hondelmann 1984).

In the case of lupin, the crop introduction process seems to have occurred many times. Arab conquests spread lupin across northern Africa and into the Iberian peninsula. Frederick the Great was responsible for introducing lupin from Italy to northern Prussia. In most of these cultures, lupin was traditionally used either for grazing, or the bitter seed was soaked before use by man or animal. Shortly after WWI, the German Botanical Society held a "lupin dinner" to generate interest in the crop, featuring lupin steaks, liquor, coffee, tablecloths, napkins, and other items made from the crop (Hondelmann 1984). This sparked subsequent breeding efforts, resulting in "sweet" or low-alkaloid lupin types developed in the 1920s, essentially creating a new crop from the old, bitter types. This represents one of the first applications of Mendelian genetics to crop plants.

The process of introduction of the newer "sweet" lupins, as distinct from the older "bitter" types is still occurring. For example, Chilean researchers have introduced sweet *Lupinus albus* varieties to southern Chile, and have also developed low alkaloid *Lupinus mutabalis* varieties which may have applications in the high mountain areas where the traditional bitter *Lupinus mutabalis* (tarwi) types are grown (Von Baer 1991). Soviet, Polish, German, and South African efforts following World War II led to the development of significant, though erratic hectarage in those regions. Perhaps the largest success story for the modern development of lupin as an introduced species is in Australia, where the blue or narrow-leaf lupin (*Lupinus angustifolius* L., a more drought resistant species) was introduced in the 1960s and 1970s as a legume to rotate with wheat. In spite of early difficulties, strong cooperation between researchers (especially J. Gladstones, plant breeder), advisers, marketers, and farmers in the Geraldton area resulted in increases in planted area to currently over 900,000 ha in Western Australia. Although some of the crop is used for grazing, a large quantity of this seed is exported to the EEC or Pacific rim countries for use as a high protein animal feed.

The first experimental plantings of lupin in the United States were probably made in the 1930s by USDA researchers, primarily as a green manure or cover crop in the southern cotton belt. Area increased by 1950 to over one million hectares in the "lupin belt," the coastal plain stretching across the southeastern United States. The crop had essentially disappeared by the 1960s, largely because of availability of cheap N fertilizers and lack of government support (Reeves 1991). In the North, Fred Elliott worked for many years in Michigan developing improved white lupin lines, and later introduced several new cultivars to Minnesota and Canada in the early 1980s (Putnam 1991). Efforts by plant breeder Gene Aksland (Resource Seeds, Gilroy, CA), and experimental work in the Pacific Northwest and Canada were important in introducing the crop to those regions in the 1980s.

THE IMPETUS

The American dairy industry in the 1980s experienced increased production costs, lower milk prices, and higher debt which forced many farmers to look seriously at cutting costs, especially the possibility of reducing purchased protein inputs. In spite of the fact that Minnesota is a major soybean (*Glycine max*) producer, the purchase of soybean meal by Minnesota dairy producers is a significant expense, similar to the costs experienced by producers in protein-poor regions, such as the northeastern United States, eastern Canada, and parts of Europe. The large seed of white lupin is high in protein and oil, and has been fed directly to a wide range of livestock. Hence, it was an excellent candidate for farmers who desired to increase on-farm production of protein. In addition, there are many regions where the temperatures are too cold and the soils too sandy for soybean. There were several farmers in central Minnesota who had worked with lupin, in addition to early work at the University of Minnesota and by the Tennessee Valley Authority. A Minnesota company later developed lupin pasta and other products from white lupin (Putnam 1991). However, there was much that was not known about many aspects of production and utilization of the crop.

THE APPROACH

Several brainstorming sessions were held in 1987 with university researchers, private businesses, and others to examine the validity of lupin as a crop. These were sponsored by the Center for Alternative Plant and Animal Products, University of Minnesota. Subjects within the areas of agronomy, weed science, plant pathology, entomology, soil science, agricultural engineering, animal science, and agricultural economics were identified as important research areas, and an interdisciplinary research team was assembled from the appropriate university departments and extension. Staples Irrigation Center personnel provided technical support, and cooperating farmers in central Minnesota were identified and contacted by county extension agents.

The Central Minnesota Initiative Fund, Bremer Foundation, and the Agricultural Utilization Research Institute (all Minnesota-based foundations) provided funding. These agencies were primarily interested in developing the economy of rural Minnesota, which has been depressed for much of the 1980s despite economic growth in urban Minnesota. In addition, lupin had the potential to reduce energy and financial input costs associated with protein production, a goal in line with a more environmentally-friendly agriculture.

The objective was to focus intensive interdisciplinary efforts over a three-year period (1988–1991) to: (1) enhance probability of success by conducting research on limiting factors, (2) educate farmers and the public on the possibilities for production and utilization of lupin, and (3) assess the risk of producing lupin as an alternative protein source.

LIMITING FACTOR RESEARCH

A number of studies were undertaken in different departments to address factors which might affect the success of growing or utilizing lupin. These were conducted at the University of Minnesota Experiment Stations at Staples, Becker, Grand Rapids, Rosemount, and St. Paul. The yield potential of white lupin at some sites was relatively high (3,000 to 4,000 kg/ha), but a large yield variation from site to site and year to year was observed. The overall objectives of this research were to understand the factors which contributed to this wide yield variation, in order to enable farmers to optimize management practices for this crop.

AGRONOMY RESEARCH

Cultivars

We evaluated a number of white lupin (*Lupinus albus*) lines, as well as several *L. angustifolius* and *L. luteus* cultivars obtained from the USSR, Poland, and Australia. Both replicated yield trials and germplasm screening were conducted. White lupin was much more productive than other lupin species on the irrigated sands of central Minnesota and a number of white lupin varieties showed acceptable productivity in the north central states (Table 1). Yield differences between white lupin cultivars were highly environment-specific, and were generally non-significant when averaged over years and sites. The earlier spring-type lines were generally more productive. Factors other than cultivar selection for yield, such as seed quality, seed size, alkaloid content, or time to maturity may be more important when considering seed source for white lupin. Smaller seed size potentially allows more reliable imbibition and stand establishment in the spring, and reduces cost of seed, a major economic factor with white lupin.

Planting Date

Date of planting had a large influence on lupin performance. Mid-April planting resulted in maximum seed yield over five years of trials. Yield declined linearly about 53 kg/ha per day in plantings sown after the optimum date (11 year/location mean, Fig. 2). However, very early plantings sometimes vernalized the plants, reducing height, node number, and yield due largely to early cold effects on the seedling. Studies of yield formation on vernalized vs. non-vernalized plants indicated that pod number was dramatically altered by planting date or vernalization. Plants which had one primary branch inflorescence contributed most to yield, compared to plants which only set mainstem pods. Thermosensitivity in white lupin remains an important agronomic factor in the spring-sown crop, and the window for optimum seeding date is relatively narrow.

Table 1. Performance of lupin cultivars at Minnesota Experiment Stations.

	Seed yield (kg/ha)								
	Becker		Grand Rapids		Rosemount		Staples		Overall
Variety	1990	1987–1990	1990	1988–1990	1990	1987–1990	1990	1988–1990	avg.[z]
Blanca 101	3033	1945	4225	2547	4264	2078	2688	2576	2222
Gela x243	2509	1895	4107	2406	3960	2116	2656	2312	2157
Horizont	3223	2057	4010	2220	4240	2084	3203	2412	2176
Kiev	---	1262	---	921	---	1258	2791	2398	---
L2019 N	2766	---	4172	---	3734	---	2640	---	---
L2085 N	2862	---	4301	---	3924	---	2859	---	---
Primorski	2989	1828	4220	2330	3907	2084	2630	2160	2075
Strain 21	2791	1877	3994	2369	3917	2013	3017	2529	2160
Ultra	2848	1841	4172	2257	4316	1869	3559	2507	2081
46-10	2992	1866	4064	2311	4340	2026	3083	2421	2126
47-5	2821	2012	3661	2009	3895	1973	3320	2463	2097
LSD 5%	449	482	573	577	678	450	582	590	519

[z]Becker and Rosemount 1987–1990, Grand Rapids and Staples 1988–1990.

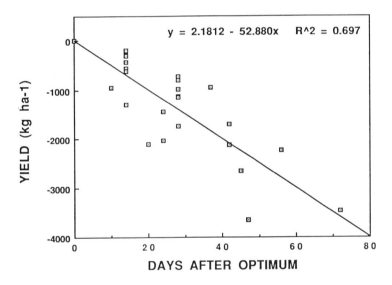

Fig. 2. Date of seeding has a strong influence on lupin performance. This graph shows the yield penalty for late planting past an optimum in central Minnesota, usually mid-April (11 year/location mean).

Inoculation

Bradyrhizobium sp. (*Lupinus*) inoculation resulted in a 1.5, 2, and 5-fold increase in yield in 1988, 1989, and 1990, respectively, compared to non-inoculated controls (Table 2). Seed protein was significantly impacted by nitrogen source, and increased 28 to 45% due to inoculation (Ayisi et al. 1992b). This was a large difference, and may explain the large variation in seed protein that is sometimes observed in lupin seed lots. White lupins were shown to fix 157 to 196 kg N/ha (1989 and 1990, respectively) from the atmosphere. *Bradyrhizobium* sp. (*Lupinus*) persisted on these soils, but populations were low with only one year of inoculation (Ayisi et al. 1992a). These results emphasized the importance of regular inoculation for white lupin yield and quality.

Table 2. Inoculation and N fertilizer effects on lupin yield and protein (Becker, MN). In our trials, N fertilizer was not required to maximize yield and inoculation significantly improved seed protein compared with non-inoculated plots, even when N fertilizer was applied.

Treatments		Seed yield (kg/ha)			Seed protein^y (%)		
N Fertilizer	Inoculum^z	1988	1989	1990	1988	1989	1990
0	+	1002	2943	2850	39.1	36.1	32.3
56	+	1187	3155	2709	40.1	32.0	31.3
112	+	1184	3260	2723	40.6	33.0	32.5
168	+	1251	3468	2161	40.7	33.8	31.4
0	−	657	1509	575	30.7	25.7	22.4
56	−	963	2180	1571	28.7	26.1	23.7
112	−	1008	2668	2483	30.5	30.2	24.8
168	−	949	2959	2346	32.5	30.7	26.5

^{z}+ = inoculated with *Bradyrhizobium* sp. (*Lupinus*); − = non-inoculated.
^{y}Dry matter basis.

Row spacing

Narrow rows (15 cm) produced 34% higher yield than wider rows (76 cm) (average of two trials). However, due to weed problems in lupin production, wider rows with cultivation should be considered in situations where chemical weed control is unavailable, unreliable, undesirable, or not economic (Putnam et al. 1991).

Weed control

Weeds are one of the biggest problems in producing lupins in this region. The lupin canopy develops and expands slowly, therefore, weeds have the opportunity to germinate and compete with the lupin crop. In Minnesota, the broadleaf weeds common lambsquarters (*Chenopodium album*) and common ragweed (*Ambrosia artemisiifolia*) were especially troublesome. The EPA-approved chemical control measures Dual (metolachlor), Prowl (pendimethalin), and Poast (sethoxydim) provide some control against some annual grassy and broadleaf weeds, but do not help in controlling these problem broadleaf weeds (especially the late-germinating weeds).

In a two-year study, the herbicide imazethapyr (Pursuit) was applied at two rates and two post-emergence dates, and provided excellent control of common lambsquarters and common ragweed. However, the lupin crop was severely injured in both years causing large yield reductions. In Wisconsin, imazethopyr-induced injury was not observed and this product is currently labeled in several states for use on heavier soils. At this point, the crop injury potential outweighs the benefits of this measure in Minnesota (Gunsolus and Wiens 1991).

Mechanical cultivation in wide rows, early seeding in narrow rows, rotary hoeing, intercropping, or other measures may improve the weed control options, but reliable weed control for production of white lupin remains a problem.

Intercropping

Lupin interplanted with peas (*Pisum sativum* L.) is an experimental practice, but has shown some promise over two years of trials. The lupins prevent lodging in the peas, and the pea provides an earlier canopy closure for weed control in the lupin. Since both crops are grown for a high protein seed, the products are compatible. Land Equivalent Ratios for this mixture have been shown to be above one for some density combinations of the two crops. In this system, peas appear to benefit more than lupins, largely because they are more competitive. Further research is needed to determine whether complementation occurs in this mixture (Putnam et al. 1991).

IRRIGATION RESEARCH

Irrigation increased lupin seed yields 553, 229, and 52% in 1988, 1989, 1990, respectively, primarily through increased pod number (Fig. 3). Optimum irrigation rates for maximizing water-use efficiency and

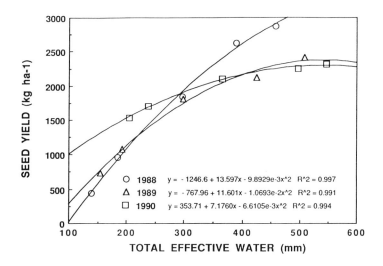

Fig. 3. Lupin response to irrigation on sandy soils has been large. White lupin is not particularly drought resistant, although narrow-leaf lupin is grown on large acreages in Australia under low moisture conditions.

economic returns were described. Seed crude protein concentration declined at high irrigation rates. Irrigation was cost-effective in most years on sandy soils (Putnam et al. 1992).

PLANT PATHOLOGY RESEARCH

Lupin pathogens common in Minnesota were identified. A number of pathogenic fungi were isolated from lupin throughout the 1989 and 1990 growing season (Table 3). *Fusarium* sp. and *Rhizoctonia* were most commonly isolated. *Fusarium* was associated with root rot and wilt symptoms and *Ascochyta* was found to cause a stem canker and pod lesions. *Ascochyta* infected seeds were found to have lower germination and emergence than healthy seed (Table 4). *Pleiocheata setosa* was found associated with a foliar and pod spot and caused plant defoliation when infections were severe. *Colletotrichum gloeosporioides* caused anthracnose on several species of *Lupinus* and appeared as a purple to pink stem lesion with resulting epinasty. This disease has the potential to cause substantial crop loss in severely infected fields and did so in the 1991 growing season.

Seed treatments of lupin were generally ineffective in improving stand establishment in our trials. Reduced stand has been a problem in many areas of the region and damping off and root rot organisms have been associated with these reduced stands. Seed treatments used on seeds of other crops (e.g., field bean) did not improve lupin stands in seed treatment trials.

Most of the diseases were found on a limited basis in production fields in Minnesota during the survey years of 1989 and 1990. The use of proper cultural control practices such as rotation and the use of clean seed must be continued to reduce the chances of crop failure due to disease.

ENTOMOLOGY RESEARCH

Results of experiments indicate that most of the commonly observed insects on lupin appear to be of little economic importance. The seedcorn maggot (*Delia platura* Meigen) has caused stand losses to the extent that yields have sometimes been decreased, but in two years of trials, insecticide treatments do not appear to be justified. The foliar insects, potato leafhopper *Empoasca fabae* (Harris), and plant bugs (*Lygus* sp. and *Adelphocoris* sp.) have been observed feeding on lupin foliage, but do not appear to be economically important. Blossom feeders, such as blister beetles and scarab beetles (*Scarabaeidae* sp.) are generally not important in Minnesota, but have been a problem in drier environments (e.g., in North Dakota trials). No insecticides are currently labeled for use on lupin, but this does not seem to be a severe limitation at this time.

Table 3. Fungi isolated from *Lupinus* spp. during the 1988 and 1990 growing seasons.

Fungus	Plant part^z	No. of isolates
Fusarium Link:Fr.	HRLS	109^y
Rhizoctonia solani Kühn AG-4^v	HR	46
Fusarium solani (Mart.) Sacc.^{v}	SR	46
Pleiochaeta setosa (Kirchn.) S.J. Hughes^v	RLP	29
Trichoderma Pers.:Fr.	R	17^y
Rhizoctonia solani Kühn	HR	17^w
Ascochyta Lib.^{v}	RSPLB	17^y
Fusarium oxysporum Schlechtend.:Fr.^{v}	RS	16
Fusarium acuminatum Ellis & Everh.^{v}	R	15
Alternaria alternata (Fr.:Fr.) Keissl.	RSLB	15
Fusarium avenaceum (Fr.:Fr.) Sacc.^{v}	SL	14
Fusarium subglutinans (Wollenweb. & Reinking) P.E. Nelson, T.A. Toussoun, & Marasas^v	R	10
Pythium Pringsh.	RH	4^y
Pythium rostratum E.J. Butler	R	3
Epicoccum purpurascens Ehrenb. ex Schlechtend.	SL	2
Colletotrichum gloeosporioides (Pens.) Pens. & Sacc. in Penz.	S	1
Curvularia protuberata R.R. Nelson & C.S. Hodges	B	1
Fusarium moniliforme J. Sheld.	R	1^x
Nigrospora sphaerica (Sacc.) E. Mason	S	1
Phoma glomerata (Corda) Wollenweb. & Hochapfel	L	1
Pythium ultimum Trow	R	1
Sclerotinia Fuckel	P	1^y

^{z}R (roots), H (hypocotyl), L (leaves), S (stem), P (pod), and B (bean or seed).
^{y}Not identified to species.
^{x}Isolated from plants in growth chamber only.
^{w}Not identified to AG group.
^{v}Pathogenticity tests were conducted on fungus.

Table 4. Effect of *Ascochyta* infection on germination and emergence of *Lupinus albus* seed.

	Distribution (%)			
	Categories^z			
Event	1	2	3	4
Germination	100.0	90.0	63.0	3.0
Emergence^y	89.0	84.0	36.0	8.0

^{z}1 = no discoloration, 2 = each seed slightly discolored, 3 = half of each seed discolored, and 4 = most of each seed discolored with ruptured seed coat.
^{y}100 seeds from each category were planted in sterilized soil and emergence counts taken after 14 days.

UTILIZATION RESEARCH

White lupins are high in protein (32 to 38%) and oil (10 to 11%) and do not contain anti-nutritional compounds, such as trypsin inhibitors. They have been fed directly to a wide variety of livestock. Lupin fed to livestock should have an alkaloid content of less than 0.02%. Palatability may still be an important factor with swine, even with seemingly "sweet" lupin types. It is possible that environment significantly impacts alkaloid level of seedlots. Several-fold variation in alkaloid content due to environment has been observed with *L. augustifolius* in Australia (J. Gladstone pers. commun.). Studies were conducted on the effect of feeding lupins to dairy cows and swine.

Conducted in Minnesota, swine trials using defatted, dehulled meal have indicated a decline in swine performance when fed this product. Results reported in the literature on swine performance with lupins have been mixed (Hill 1991). Feed intake was significantly affected in growing-finishing swine. University of Minnesota studies indicate that lupins should not be included at levels greater than 8 to 10% of dietary dry matter for swine. It appears that pigs are much more susceptible than other animals to either the alkaloid levels or the manganese content of lupins, thus it is imperative that lupins for swine be examined carefully for alkaloid level.

Dairy feeding trials indicated that cows producing less than 9,000 kg of milk per year should perform as well on lupins as on soybean meal. In addition, there was a 3.5% increase in fat-corrected milk yield when lupins supplied 75% of the supplemental protein in the diet, compared with soybean meal, possibly due to higher fat content of the lupin (Table 5). Lupins are approximately 35% protein compared with 44% for soybean meal. Because lupins are more degradable than soybean meal, they should not be the only source of supplemental protein for herds with higher production. Our trials have shown that coarse grinding of lupin seed improves protein utilization. Milk production from roasted lupins was found to be similar to that from soybean meal in trials from other regions (Singh et al. 1991). Several dairy and livestock producers in central Minnesota and Wisconsin have successfully incorporated lupin in their feeding programs.

ECONOMIC ANALYSIS

Farm enterprise budgets for lupin were developed (Table 6). Costs of production for lupin and soybean were similar with the exception of seed costs, which were higher for lupin. Since the value of lupin is currently primarily in the protein, lupin prices were determined as a percentage of soybean meal, and we calculated returns based upon several cost/price assumptions (Table 6). It is clear from this analysis that either the costs of production must decrease or the value of the product of lupin must increase to improve the economic viability of lupin as a cash crop in central Minnesota. Current cash value of lupin is about $4.00 to $4.70/bu ($147/t to $173/t) and soybean $5.50 to $5.70/bu ($202 to $209/t), and the (low) price of other protein sources (primarily soybean) is a major disincentive to lupin expansion at this time, both in Minnesota and worldwide. However, the value of lupin as an on-farm source of protein is significantly different from a cash crop, and should be assigned differently. For example, many producers place a value on the idea of self-sufficiency in producing their own feed, reducing cash requirements of such practices, and thus reduced probability of negative cash flow. Further analysis is required to estimate this value.

ON-FARM RESEARCH

On-Farm trials were conducted from 1988-1990 to understand the problems encountered in production systems and to compare lupin productivity with other crops. Non-irrigated plots were severely affected by weeds and drought in 1988 and 1989, making the data collected less useful. In 1990, a replicated on-farm comparison between lupin and soybean gave a fair comparison between the crops, and showed that lupin was similar to soybean at more southerly locations, but superior at northerly Minnesota locations (Table 7). These experiences were largely anecdotal, but were valuable in indicating where lupins would fit in Minnesota, and in describing the problems encountered by producers. A 'case-study' about the introduction of lupin as a new crop, used as a teaching tool to illustrate the problem of new crop introduction, was developed from these experiences (Simmons et al. 1992).

Table 5. Response of dairy cows fed sweet white lupins (day 22 to 140 post-partum).

Treatment[z]	No. cows	Milk yield (kg/day)		Fat yield		Protein yield		Dry matter intake (kg/day)
		uncorrected	3.5% fat corrected	(%)	(kg/day)	(%)	(kg/day)	
SSSS	11	27.3	27.5b[y]	3.7	0.97	3.0	0.82	19.9
SSSL	11	28.9	29.1ab	3.7	1.03	3.0	0.86	20.8
SSLL	10	28.4	28.6ab	3.6	1.01	2.9	0.81	20.6
SLLL	12	30.0	30.3a	3.7	1.08	2.9	0.86	21.0
LLLL	10	28.3	28.8ab	3.8	1.02	2.9	0.82	20.4
SE		0.84	0.68	0.1	0.03	0.1	0.02	0.49

All means are covariately adjusted.

[z]SSSS = 100% of supplemental protein as soybean meal. Each 'L' represents 25% of this protein being replaced by lupin protein.

[y]Treatment means with different subscripts are significantly different (P < .06).

The issue of competition from currently-used crops is important when considering any new crop alternative, and our on-farm studies indicated that there are regions in southern and central Minnesota where soybeans are more viable and regions in the north where lupin is more viable as a grain legume. There has also been a move in some quarters towards greater use of whole roasted soybean as an on-farm source of protein, a use which was also furthered by this research.

EDUCATIONAL EFFORTS AND OUTREACH

Research field days, winter meetings, and farm tours were conducted, and fact sheets were developed (Putnam et al. 1989). A Lupin Production Guide was produced which contains color photographs and a description of agronomic practices, diseases, insects, and feeding of lupin (Meronuck et al. 1991).

A symposium was held at St. Paul, MN, 21–22 March 1991 to present results of our studies with lupin and to discuss the prospects of the crop with scientists from other regions. This symposium enabled us to broaden our consideration of lupin to include those who had worked with the crop in other regions. Research results and farmers' experiences with lupins (positive and negative) were reported and published in a proceedings which serves as a record of the status of lupins in North America at the time (CAPAP 1991). This symposium and earlier contacts between researchers, resulted in the formation of the North American Lupin Association, which now publishes a newsletter (contact Dr. Paul Mask, Extension Hall, Auburn Univ., Auburn, AL 36849 for information). This has as its goal facilitation of communication between those working on this crop in either research or industry.

An interesting spin-off of the lupin project was the development of a joint US–Soviet database on lupin. In 1989, J. Orf (soybean breeder), R.A. Meronuck (plant pathologist), and D.H. Putnam (agronomist) traveled to Moscow, Kiev, and Poland to investigate the lupin work being conducted there. The contacts made during that trip resulted in the creation of a database containing over 4,500 entries from the former eastern block countries, the former USSR, and English-speaking sources. It is hoped that this database will be of use to lupin researchers and industry in years to come.

Our educational and outreach efforts with lupin underscores the importance of sharing of experiences and information networking with minor crops. There are very few individuals who have in-depth knowledge of minor crops worldwide, and still fewer who have extensive knowledge of any individual crop. In situations such as these, symposia, newsletters, and other information-sharing mechanisms become vital to the future development of that crop. This type of outreach has already yielded valuable interactions in the area of research and extension in the case of lupin.

Table 6. Simplified sample enterprise budget for irrigated lupin and soybean for Staples, MN (1991). Seed costs are a major component of production costs for lupin, but value of the product is also important. Lupin has been valued at 72 to 85% the value of soybean meal in markets in the upper Midwest. Allocated overhead costs have been estimated to be $444.53/ha for lupin and $458.25/ha for soybean (Olson and Putnam 1991).

Item	Lupin	Soybean
	Yield (kg/ha)	
Average yield (6-year mean, Staples, MN)	3158	2755
Variable costs per acre	*Budget ($/ha)*	
Seed	96.37	27.18
Fertilizer	---	30.15
Pesticides	44.50	44.48
Irrigation costs	61.16	61.16
Fuel and lubrication	27.38	30.29
Repairs and maintenance	16.38	17.79
Interest on cash expense	8.97	10.55
Total variable costs	254.74	221.60
Returns over variable costs for various lupin/soybean value/cost ratios		
($147.04/t lupin, $207.41/t soybean)	210.75	349.81
($172.54/t lupin, $207.41/t soybean)	290.14	349.81
($172.54/t lupin, $207.41/t soybean, lupin seed costs decreased by half)	338.33	349.81
($207.41/t lupin, $207.41/t soybean)	400.26	349.81
($207.41/t lupin, $207.41/t soybean, lupin seed costs decreased by half)	448.45	349.81

Table 7. Performance of lupin and soybean on six Minnesota farms, 1990, in counties ranging from south to north.

	County	Seed yield^z (kg/ha)		Crude protein (%)	
		Lupin	Soybean	Lupin	Soybean
S	Benton	1674	1769$_{NS}$^{y}	35	36$_{NS}$
↓	Stearns^x	3039	3040$_{NS}$	37	38$_{NS}$
	Stearns	2613	2508$_{NS}$	37	38$_{NS}$
	Todd	1962	839**	38	37$_{NS}$
	Wadena^x	2497	2025**	37	38$_{NS}$
N	Aitkin	151	93*	39	36**

^{z}Average of 16 observations per crop per farm.
^{y}NS, *, and ** indicate nonsignificant, significant at P=0.05, and significant at P=0.01, respectively.
^{x}Irrigated sites.

SUMMARY AND CONCLUSIONS

We analyzed the lupin crop from a production-utilization-marketing perspective, with many disciplines within the University of Minnesota, farmers and outside agencies contributing to a cooperative effort. Unlike many alternative crops, utilization pathways for lupin are broad and numerous (primarily as a dairy feed, but also for poultry and human food), and production constraints are of primary importance. Weed control, sensitivity to soil or climatic variations, diseases, and stand establishment are the primary concerns at this time. Farmers in many cases have overcome these obstacles, and some of the data we have generated may help in controlling the fluctuation in yield levels. However, further work, especially on weed control, is needed to create a reliable production management system.

It is neither likely nor necessarily desirable that lupin replace soybean or other grain legumes in areas where those crops are well adapted. However, there are many regions where lupin could make a valuable contribution to cropping systems and to farmers' economic options due to its high nutritional value and adaptation to poor sandy soils. Significant changes in the *value* of the harvested product or reduction in the *costs* of production (primarily seed costs) would give producers incentives to improve the production systems for lupin. The current use patterns for lupin have valued the crop essentially as a replacement for protein commodities traded on the world market, a comparison made in central Minnesota as well as in central Europe. Interesting ideas for the improvement in the value of lupins have been the potential for reducing saturated fats of milk or meat products from lupin-fed animals (M. McNiven pers. commun.), or the utilization of lupin alkaloids for pharmaceutical-use or plant protection (Binsack 1991). Multiple-use models have been critical to the development of other crops (e.g., soybean).

We found an interdisciplinary approach to lupin research and development to be beneficial towards a more complete understanding of the new crop development problem from a production–utilization–marketing perspective. The new-crop development process is often described as long-term, and lupin is no exception. Each piece of information and each step may move us slightly in the direction of producing a more viable new crop. It is clear, however, that cooperation between disciplines is essential to this process.

REFERENCES

Ayisi, K.K., D.H. Putnam, C.P. Vance, and P.H. Graham. 1992a. Dinitrogen fixation, nitrogen and dry matter accumulation, and nodulation in white lupin. Crop Sci. (in press).

Ayisi, K.K., D.H. Putnam, C.P. Vance, and P.H. Graham. 1992b. *Bradyrhizobum* inoculation and nitrogen effects on seed yield and protein of white lupin. Agron. J. (in press).

Binsack, R. 1991. Lupin research and development programs supported by GTZ–Germany, p. 7–12. In: Proc. Sixth Int. Lupin Conf. Nov. 25–30, 1990. Temuco–Pucon, Chile. Int. Lupin Assoc.

Center for Alternative Plant and Animal Products (CAPAP). 1991. Prospects for lupins in North America. Proc. Symp. March 21–22, 1991, St. Paul, MN.

Gross, R. 1986. Lupins in the old and new world—a biological-cultural co-evolution, p. 244–277. In: Proc. Fourth Int. Lupin Conf. Aug. 15–22, 1986. Geraldton, W. Australia. Int. Lupin Assoc.

Gunsolus, J. and M. Wiens. 1991. Postemergence weed control studies in lupin with Pursuit herbicide, p. 163–164. In: Prospects for lupins in North America. Proc. Symp. March 21–22, 1991. St. Paul, MN. Center for Alternative Plant and Animal Products, St. Paul, MN.

Harvey, R.G. 1991. Results of three years of lupin weed control research, p. 157–161. In: Prospects for lupins in North America. Proc. Symp. March 21–22, 1991. St. Paul, MN. Center for Alternative Plant and Animal Products, St. Paul, MN.

Hill, G.D. 1991. The utilization of lupins in animal nutrition, p. 68–91. In: Proc. 6th Int. Lupin Conf., Temuco–Pucon, Chile. Nov. 25–30, 1990, Int. Lupin Assoc.

Hondelmann, W. 1984. The lupin: Ancient and modern crop plant. Theor. Appl. Genet. 68:1–9.

Hymowitz, T. 1990. Grain legumes, p. 154–158. In: J. Janick and J.E. Simon (eds.). Advances in new crops. Timber Press, Portland, OR.

Meronuck, R.A., H. Meredith, and D.H. Putnam. 1991. Lupin production and utilization guide. Center for Alternative Plant and Animal Products, Univ. of Minnesota, St. Paul.

Putnam, D.H. 1991. History and prospects for lupins in the upper Midwest, p. 33–40. In: Prospects for lupins in North America. Proc. Symp. March 21–22, 1991. St. Paul, MN. Center for Alternative Plant and Animal Products.

Putnam, D.H., E.S. Oplinger, L.L. Hardman, and J.D. Doll. 1989. Lupin. In: Alternative field crops manual. Center for Alternative Plant and Animal Products, Univ. of Minnesota, St. Paul.

Putnam, D.H., L.A. Field, L.L. Hardman, and S.R. Simmons. 1991. Agronomic studies on white lupins in

Minnesota, p. 53–70. In: Prospects for lupins in North America. Proc. Symp. March 21–22, 1991. St. Paul, MN. Center for Alternative Plant and Animal Products.

Putnam, D.H., J. Wright, and L.A. Field. 1992. White lupin seed yield and water-use efficiency as influenced by irrigation, row spacing, and weeds. Agron J. (in press).

Reeves, D.W. 1991. Experiences and prospects for lupins in the south and southeast, p. 23–30. In: Prospects for lupins in North America. Proc. Symp. March 21–22, 1991. St. Paul, MN. Center for Alternative Plant and Animal Products, St. Paul.

Simmons, S.R., D.H. Putnam, and D. Otterby. 1992. Mueller Farm: Lupin as an alternative crop for on-farm protein production. J. Nat. Resour. Life Sci. Educ. 21:9–14.

Singh, C.K., P.H. Robinson, and M.A. McNiven. 1991. In: Prospects for lupins in North America. Proc. Symp. March 21–22, 1991. St. Paul, MN. Center for Alternative Plant and Animal Products, St. Paul.

Von Baer, E. 1991. New varieties of lupin, p. 376–381. In: Proc. Sixth Int. Lupin Conf. Nov. 25–30, 1990. Temuco–Pucon, Chile, Int. Lupin Assoc.

Williams, W. 1986. Current status of the crop lupins, p. 1–13. In: Proc. Fourth Int. Lupin Conf. Aug. 15–22, 1986. Geraldton, W. Australia. Int. Lupin Assoc.

White Lupin: An Alternate Crop for the Southern Coastal Plain

P.L. Mask, D.W. Reeves, E. van Santen, G.L. Mullins, and G.E. Aksland

In the 1940s, lupins (*Lupinus* spp.) were grown on over 1 million hectares in the South Atlantic and Gulf Slope Land Resource Area, i.e., the Southern Coastal Plains. At that time, lupins were mainly utilized to supply nitrogen for a subsequent crop of cotton (*Gossypium hirsutum* L.). The potential of lupins as a green manure was first reported by Warner (1939). Initial research areas (as reported in unpublished Univ. Fla. Expt. Sta. Ann. Rpts. for 1943–48), included selection for low-alkaloid blue lupin (*L. angustifolius* L.), observation and seed increases of sweet yellow lupin (*L. luteus* L.) and white lupin (*L. albus* L.), adaptation and management studies, grazing studies with cattle and hogs, seed drying and storage studies, maturity tests, and disease resistance studies. By 1952, lupins were grown to such an extent that the Coastal Plain was called the "Lupin Belt" (Weimer 1952).

Consecutive hard freezes in the winters of 1950–51 and 1951–52, severely damaged white and blue lupin, essentially eliminating lupin seed stocks (Reeves 1991; Burton et al. 1954). Loss of government price supports, low cost nitrogen fertilizer, and disease pressure also contributed to the regional decline of this crop (Reeves 1991; Burton et al. 1954). The recent interest in sustainable agriculture, and the suitability for double-cropping with winter grown lupin, however, have generated renewed interest in winter-hardy white lupin for the South.

Several characteristics of winter-hardy white lupin make it suitable as an alternative crop for the area. The species is adapted to the coarse-textured, relatively infertile, acidic soils which predominate the area. The growing season of winter-grown white lupin is similar to wheat (*Triticum aestivum* L.) and allows for double-cropping rotations with other crops grown in the area, such as sorghum [*Sorghum bicolor* (L.) Moench], late-planted tropically adapted maize (*Zea mays* L.), and soybean [*Glycine max* (L.) Merr]. Development of cropping systems with lupin as a component would: (1) provide a cover crop when erosion potential is greatest; (2) provide a rotation yield response to subsequent summer grain crops; (3) contribute to reducing or eliminating nitrogen fertilizer requirements of summer grain crops as well as replacing a winter crop requiring nitrogen fertilizer, viz., wheat; and (4) produce quantities of high protein feed grain that could be used on-farm without processing.

The main competitive crop of lupin is winter wheat. However, at current yield levels and prices, wheat is not a profitable crop for the southeastern United States. In Alabama for example, even at yield levels 20% greater than the state average, producers lose approximately $86.45/ha (Novak et al. 1991). The single largest variable production cost for wheat is nitrogen, accounting for approximately 28% of input costs. A reliable white lupin would be economically superior to wheat because it would not require nitrogen. Efficiency of nitrogen for winter wheat in the southeastern United States is low due to generally warm temperatures and excessive rainfall. This results in large nitrogen losses via leaching and denitrification. Therefore, the use of lupin also has great potential for reducing nitrogen losses to the environment, and subsequent ground and surface water contamination.

In 1987–88, a study was initiated comparing 'Tifwhite-78' white lupin, 'Tifblue-78' blue lupin, and 'Bicolor-1' lupin [*Lupinus hispanicus* ssp. bicolor (Merino)] to common cover crops used in the Southeast, i.e., crimson clover (*Trifolium incarnatum* L.) and rye (*Secale cereale* L.). The primary comparison factor was nitrogen contribution to a following crop of maize. The cover crops were planted in mid-October of 1987, 1988, and 1989. Nitrogen was applied to the maize following the cover crops at rates of 0, 56, 112, or 168 kg/ha.

A 3-day period in January of 1988, with lows of –16°C on two nights and a high during the period of only –4°C damaged all cover crops. Blue lupin was killed completely and was consequently dropped from the test. 'Bicolor-1' was dropped from the test in 1989 because even with mechanical scarification, germination was poor. 'Tifwhite-78' proved an excellent cover crop. Three year average maize grain yields indicated that 'Tifwhite-78' supplied approximately 112 kg N/ha to the subsequent maize crop.

The performance of 'Tifwhite-78' in this test prompted further research with this cultivar as an alternative feed grain. The objective was to determine the suitability of white lupin as a component in double-cropping systems for the southeastern United States, and to determine the nitrogen contribution of white lupin, harvested for grain, to summer grain crops in double-cropping systems.

This test was initiated with the planting of 'Tifwhite-78' white lupin and 'Saluda' wheat on a Lucedale sandy loam (Rhodic Paleudult) in southwestern Alabama, on 22 Nov. 1988. In 1989 and 1990, planting dates were 16 and 26 Nov. respectively. In every year, both crops were planted with a grain drill on 20-cm row drill spacing. Wheat was seeded at 100 kg/ha and lupin was seeded at 140 kg/ha. Lupin and wheat were harvested in late June of every year and tropical maize, grain sorghum, or soybean were planted following wheat and lupin harvest, approximately 10 July each year. Row spacing for all summer crops was 75 cm.

Lupin grain yields from three site-years average 1.8, 2.2, and 2.7 Mg/ha. In December 1989, 'Tifwhite-78' was subjected to a consecutive 5 day freeze with lows of –11°, –13°, –16°, –16°, and –4°C. High temperatures during the period did not exceed –2°C. Plants were killed with these freezes; in some cases severe stand loss occurred, but in elevated and well-drained sites, damage was minimal. The performance of 'Tifwhite-78' to date, suggests that white lupin is sufficiently cold hardy to become an alternative winter grain crop in the Southeast.

We are optimistic that winter-hardy white lupin can become a viable component of double-cropping systems in the southeastern United States and we are continuing studies to confirm this hypothesis. A number of problems exist, principally insufficient disease resistance, cold hardiness, and tolerance to wet soils. A strong cooperative research effort currently underway is attempting to resolve these problems in order to develop the full potential of the crop.

REFERENCES

Burton, G.W., J.L. Shepherd, and E.H. DeVane. 1954. Growing lupine on coastal bermuda sod. Univ. of Georgia College of Agr. Expt. Sta. Cir. 23.

Novak, J., P. Mask, and R. Smith. 1991. 1992 budget for wheat for grain. Ala. Coop. Ext. Ser. Pub. AECBUD Dec. 1-1, 1991. Auburn University, AL.

Reeves, D.W. 1991. Experiences and prospects for lupins in the South and Southeast, p. 23–30. In: Prospects for lupins in North America. Proc. of a Symposium Sponsored by the Center For Alternative Plant and Animal Products, Univ. of Minnesota, St. Paul. March 21–22, 1991.

Warner, J.D. 1939. Lupine, a seed-producing winter legume. Univ. of Florida, Agr. Expt. Sta. Press Bul. 541.

Weimer, J.L. 1952. Diseases of cultivated lupines in the Southeast. USDA Farmers' Bul. 2053.

The Potential of Zero Tannin Lentil

A. Matus, A.E. Slinkard, and A. Vandenberg

Lentil (*Lens culinaris* Medikus) is the fourth most important pulse crop in the world after bean (*Phaseolus vulgaris* L.), pea (*Pisum sativum* L.), and chickpea (*Cicer arietinum* L.). The four major lentil producing countries in decreasing order are Turkey, India, Canada, and the United States (FAO 1988). Turkey has been the leading lentil exporter in recent years except in 1990 when Canada temporarily became the leader. Slinkard et al. (1990) reviewed the history of lentil production in Canada.

Quality in lentil is based primarily on two factors: short cooking time and physical appearance or eye appeal. In most markets, the seed must be "big and bright." 'Laird' lentil (Slinkard and Bhatty 1979), the most widely grown cultivar in Canada and thus, in the world, is a yellow cotyledon type characterized by large seeds enclosed in a bright, light green seed coat. 'Laird' lentil is the preferred cultivar in many parts of the world, largely because of its appearance.

The seed coat of 'Laird' and all other lentil cultivars contains polyphenolic compounds (tannin precursors) which slowly oxidize and undergo a "tanning" reaction. Thus, if lentil seeds are exposed to air, the polyphenolic compounds in the seed coat oxidize and the seed coat slowly turns tan, eventually turning a dark reddish brown. These discolored seed coats are a down grading factor and the seed lot will be graded "Sample" because of damaged seed. This oxidation process proceeds slowly at room temperature and rapidly under conditions of high temperature and high humidity. Rain during the final stages of seed ripening in the field may discolor some of the seed coats, and the seed lot may be down graded. Lentil seed cannot be carried over from one year to the next because of discoloration of the seed coats; the only exception is when lentil seed is stored in large bulk bins with a small surface area. Even then, seed coats will be discolored in the surface layer, due to direct exposure to the air.

A large portion of the USDA Lentil Collection was grown at the Crop Development Centre, University of Saskatchewan in 1972. The seed was harvested and stored in a seed storage room. Germination started dropping after seven years and the entire collection was regrown to produce fully viable seed. Seed coats were dark reddish brown on all accessions except those with black seed coats and PI 345635 which still had bright white seed coats. PI 345635 was crossed with 'Laird' and 'Eston' and the mode of inheritance of this trait was studied. Vaillancourt (1984) found that this trait was due to the absence of polyphenolic compounds in the seed coat and that this was controlled by a single recessive gene, tan. Vaillancourt et al. (1986) reported that the zero tannin (ZT) gene had a pleiotropic effect on plant pigmentation (no anthocyanin pigment). In addition, the seed coat of the ZT lentil was thinner and more fragile than the normal seed coat, making the seed more susceptible to seed rot. Subsequently, over 100 F_2-derived F_4 families from the crosses PI 345635 x 'Laird' and PI 354635 x 'Eston' were selected for agronomic evaluation. The objective of this study was to determine the agronomic potential of ZT lentil, based on the performance of these 100 plus lines.

METHODOLOGY

Over 100 F_4-derived F_5 and F_6 families of ZT lentil were evaluated in 1990 at the University of Saskatchewan. 'Laird' and 'Eston' lentil were used as commercial check cultivars in all tests. Four-row plots with rows 30 cm apart and 4 m long were used in 3-replicate tests.

Fungicide Test

A paired comparison (metalaxyl fungicide at 6 g a.i./100 kg seed vs. check) was used to evaluate the need for fungicidal seed treatment in ZT lentil lines. Two check cultivars and 14 ZT lentil lines were grown in 3-replicate tests in 1990 and evaluated for emergence (plants/m of row), days to flower, plant height, 1,000-seed weight, and seed yield.

Agronomic Trials

Two check cultivars and 34 ZT lentil lines were grown in a 6 × 6 lattice with 3 replications in 1990. Three sets of 34 ZT lines were grown at two locations (Saskatoon and Sutherland). All seed was treated with metalaxyl to minimize differences in stand emergence. Data were collected on emergence (plants/m of row), days to flower, plant height, 1,000-seed weight, and seed yield.

RESULTS

Fungicide Test

Metalaxyl fungicide seed treatment had no effect on seedling emergence of the two check cultivars, indicating that fungicide is not required for these two commercial cultivars (Table 1). Seedling emergence of the untreated ZT lentil lines was only about 63% of the check cultivars. Metalaxyl fungicide treatment of the ZT lentil seeds increased seedling emergence of the ZT lentil lines to 90% of the check cultivars, indicating that metalaxyl seed treatment is beneficial to seedling emergence of ZT lentil.

The fungicide by ZT vs check cultivar interaction was significant for yield due to the effect of metalaxyl in increasing yield of the ZT lines (expected response) and decreasing yield of the check cultivars (unexpected response) (Table 1). Metalaxyl fungicide treatment had no effect on days to flower, plant height, or 1,000-seed weight (data not presented). In addition, differences among ZT lines were significant for all traits (data not presented).

Table 1. Effect of metalaxyl fungicidal seed treatment on stand establishment and seed yield of the two check cultivars and 14 zero tannin (ZT) lentil lines in 1990.

Line	Plants/m of row^z		Seed yield (kg/ha)	
	No metalaxyl	Metalaxyl^y	No metalaxyl	Metalaxyl
2 checks	38	40	2230	2021
14 ZT lines	24 (63)^x	36 (90)	1220 (55)	1324 (66)

^{z}36 plants/m of row is an excellent stand.
^{y}6 g a.i./100 kg seed.
^{x}Percent of check in parentheses.

Agronomic Trials

Results were consistent over two locations and over the three 6 × 6 lattice experiments in that in nearly every instance locations, lines and the line by location interaction were significant for every trait. The significant location effect indicated that the environmental conditions were different enough to cause markedly different responses. The significant line effects indicated large genetic differences among the ZT lentil lines for the various traits. The significant line by location interaction indicated that all lines did not respond in the same manner for all traits at the two locations. A significant line by location (genotype by environment) interaction occurs frequently among unselected lines of crops with an undeterminate growth habit such as lentil, especially in the presence of large differences in maturity.

The agronomic performance of the highest yielding 10 lines out of the 36 lines in 6 × 6 lattice test 3 averaged over two locations is presented in Table 2. Similar results occurred in 6 × 6 lattice tests 1 and 2. A general comparison of means and ranges over all three tests is presented in Table 3. Data in Tables 2 and 3 indicate that selection of some of the higher yielding ZT lentil lines would result in several lines that would approach the agronomic performance of the two check cultivars in all traits except for seed weight. The low seed weight is due to the extremely low weight of the PI 345635 parent (26 g/1,000 seeds).

Table 2. Agronomic performance of the check cultivars and the 10 highest yielding zero tannin (ZT) lentil lines out of 36 lines in 6 × 6 lattice test 3 averaged over two locations (Saskatoon and Sutherland) in 1990.

Line	Seed yield (kg/ha)	Plants/m of row	Days to flower	Height (cm)	1000-seed wt (g)
Laird	2,664	40	51	45	76
VLT-15	2,018	37	49	37	48
V2-95	1,888	36	47	43	40
V2-104	1,872	38	46	32	36
VLT-19	1,837	35	49	42	45
V6-93	1,720	35	46	37	35
Eston	1,696	38	44	32	37
VLT-20	1,668	36	48	37	43
V3-104	1,593	37	47	32	29
V8-91	1,580	35	50	32	28
V5-94	1,570	36	48	40	35
Standard error	85	1	1	1	1

Table 3. Summary of agronomic data for two check cultivars and 102 zero tannin (ZT) lentil lines (2 location average in 1990).

Line	Seed yield (kg/ha)	Plants/m of row	Days to flower	Height (cm)	1000-seed wt (g)
2 checks	2,111	36	47	37	57
102 ZT lines					
Mean	1,272	36	47	34	34
Range	(848-2,018)	(30-41)	(45-50)	(28-43)	(22-54)

DISCUSSION

Zero tannin lentil shows considerable promise as a high quality premium priced product. The seed coat does not discolor with time or weathering damage and retains its bright appearance. The first cycle of crossing produced several lines that have acceptable agronomic traits. Several of them yield 80 to 90% of the yield of the commercial cultivars and would be economically viable if they would command a price premium to compensate for the lower yield. A second cycle of crosses to adapted cultivars will result in the production of ZT lentil lines that yield competitively with standard lentil cultivars and have a wide range in seed weight as required for any market.

The ZT lentil seeds have a thinner seed coat than standard lentil seeds (Vaillancourt et al. 1984), and will imbibe water and cook more rapidly than standard lentil seeds. These ZT lentil seeds are also smaller than seeds of the commercial cultivars and thus will cook faster since speed of cooking is a function of seed size, among other factors (Bhatty 1988). The rapid cooking characteristic and the bright appealing color of the ZT lentil seeds may stimulate interest in a premium quality product for a specialty market.

The ZT lentil lines require a metalaxyl fungicide seed treatment for a normal level of seedling emergence. The seed coats of the standard lentil cultivars are thicker than the seed coats of ZT lentils and contain about 6%

polyphenolic compounds (condensed tannins) (Vaillancourt et al. 1986). These polyphenolic compounds are water soluble and exhibit fungistatic properties (Azaizeh and Pettit 1987). The thin seed coat of ZT lentil makes the seed more susceptible to mechanical damage which is further complicated by extremely rapid imbibition through the thin and/or cracked seed coat. During rapid imbibition intracellular substances, primarily starch grains and protein bodies, are extruded from the seed (Spaeth 1987). Then, soil-borne and seed-borne pathogens use these substances for nutrients, resulting in increased levels of seed rot, especially in ZT lentils which lack the fungistatic polyphenolic compounds in their seed coat. Thus, ZT lentil seeds must be treated with metalaxyl fungicide to reduce seed rot and maintain a normal level of seedling emergence.

FUTURE PROSPECTS

Zero tannin lentil seeds have a thin seed coat and will require metalaxyl fungicidal seed treatment for normal seedling emergence. Special precautions must also be taken during threshing and handling of the seed to minimize mechanical damage to the seeds. Otherwise, ZT lentil can be grown just like any other lentil.

The ZT lentil is a high quality product and will command a premium price in low volume specialty markets because of its attractive appearance. ZT lentil seeds also are excellent for producing lentil sprouts due to the absence of discolored seed coats. The first cycle of crossing produced some lines yield 80 to 90% of standard lentil cultivars. A second cycle of crossing to adapted cultivars should produce lines that yield competitively with standard cultivars.

REFERENCES

Azaizeh, A.H. and R.E. Pettit. 1987. Influence of tannin related compounds from peanut seed coats and cotyledons on *Aspergillus parasiticus* growth and aflatoxin production. Phytopathology 77:1703–1706.

Bhatty, R.S. 1988. Composition and quality of lentil (*Lens culinaris* Medik.): A review. Can. Inst. Food Sci. Technol. J. 21:144–160.

FAO. 1988. Production yearbook. Vol. 42. Rome.

Slinkard, A.E. and R.S. Bhatty. 1979. Laird lentil. Can. J. Plant Sci. 59:503–504.

Slinkard, A.E., R.S. Bhatty, B.N. Drew, and R.A.A. Morrall. 1990. Dry pea and lentil as new crops in Saskatchewan: A case study, p. 164–168. In: J. Janick and J.E. Simon (eds.). Advances in new crops. Timber Press, Portland, OR.

Spaeth, S.C. 1987. Pressure-driven extrusion of intracellular substances from bean and pea cotyledons during imbibition. Plant Physiol. 85:217–223.

Vaillancourt, R. 1984. Seed coat darkening and the inheritance of tannin content in lentil. M. Sc. thesis. Univ. of Saskatchewan, Saskatoon, Canada.

Vaillancourt, R., A.E. Slinkard, and R.D. Reichert. 1986. The inheritance of condensed tannin concentration in lentil. Can. J. Plant Sci. 66:241–245.

FORAGES

Native North American Grasses

K.P. Vogel and K.J. Moore

Two hundred years ago, grasslands occupied major portions of the North American continent. These native grasslands have been classified into seven major associations based on climax vegetation (Gould 1968). The two largest grassland associations, the true or tall grass prairie and the mixed-shortgrass prairie, covered major areas of the Midwest and Great Plains of the United States and the prairie provinces of Canada. Except for the desert plains grassland association, these grasslands have been converted into major grain crop production areas of the United States and Canada. Although much of this grassland area has been plowed for crop production, relict prairie sites exist throughout the area and can be used as a germplasm base for the native prairie grasses.

The North American grasslands contained hundreds of species of plants (Gould 1968; Weaver 1954). Sunflower (*Helianthus annuus* L.) is the only major cultivated crop that has been developed from a species native to the North American grasslands (Harlan 1975). Wild rice (*Zizania aquatica* L.) is from North America but it originates from marshy areas, not grasslands (Hitchcock 1951). The native grasslands and rangelands have and continue to provide food via meat production by native ruminants such as bison and introduced, domestic livestock for native North Americans and the subsequent European, African, and Asian immigrants who settled the continent. This report evaluates the potential of North American grasses to additionally benefit humans as new forage, grain, biomass, turf, and horticultural crops.

FORAGE CROPS

Evaluation and breeding work with native grasses prior to the 1930s was very limited. Most of the early research was botanical or ecological in nature and dealt with classifying and characterizing the grasses including their life histories. The great drought of the 1930s and the ensuing dust storms led to the establishment of grass breeding and evaluation programs in many of the Great Plains states. The mission of these breeding programs was to develop grasses that could be used to revegetate highly erodible lands that should not have been plowed.

The initial evaluation and breeding work at the various experiment stations followed a similar pattern. A large array of accessions (ecotypes or strains) of various native grasses was collected from a general geographical area. These collections were then evaluated in uniform nurseries for various agronomic traits. The better accessions of the superior grasses were increased for testing in additional environments and based on these tests released directly to the public without any additional breeding work. This procedure was used by many of the state experiment stations and the U.S. Department of Agriculture in developing the initial grass cultivars for different geographical regions of the country (Barker et al. 1985; Jacobson et al. 1985; Hassell and Barker 1985; Vogel et al. 1985a; Voigt and Oaks 1985; Heizer and Hassell 1985). Examples of grass cultivars developed by this procedure include 'Blackwell' and 'Nebraska 28' switchgrass (Hanson 1972).

Although several hundred grasses are native to the United States, after several decades of testing, only a few have proven to have value as cultivated forage grasses. Cultivated forage grasses need to be easily established, persist under grazing, have high forage yields and good forage quality, possess good disease and insect resistance or tolerance, and produce adequate seed yields. Turf grasses need to have good turf quality instead of high forage yields and quality (Vogel et al. 1989). The native grasses that meet these criteria are primarily those which were subject to heavy grazing periodically by bison (*Bison bison*). Some of these grasses, which are primarily the principal species of the tall-, mid-, and shortgrass prairie, are currently being used as cultivated species and have potential to be used to an even greater extent.

Grasses can be classified as either cool-season (C_3) or warm-season (C_4) based on their photosynthetic mechanism (Waller and Lewis 1979). Cool season grasses produce most of their growth during the cool months of spring and fall and become essentially dormant during hot, summer months. Warm-season grasses grow most efficiently during the warm months of summer and usually are relatively unproductive under cool growing conditions.

Cool-season grasses that are widely used in the United States for forage and turf include such major species as Kentucky bluegrass (*Poa pratensis* L.), tall fescue (*Festuca arundinaceae* Schreb.), smooth bromegrass

(*Bromus inermis* Leyss.), and wheatgrasses including *Agropyron* and *Thinopyrum* species (Barker and Kalton 1989; Meyer and Funk 1989). These are all introduced grasses from Europe, North Africa, and Asia where they evolved under centuries of intensive grazing by domestic livestock. The most widely utilized native cool-season grass is western wheatgrass [*Pascopyrum smithii* (Rydb.) Love]. It currently has minor use in revegetating agricultural lands in the Great Plains to which it is native. Other native cool-season grasses are utilized to a very minor extent and then usually because of legal or regulatory requirements that only native species can be used to revegetate specific sites. We believe that native cool-season grasses will have only limited use in the future as forage or turf grasses even if extensive breeding work on them is conducted. The introduced cool-season grasses can be significantly improved by breeding and the economic returns from the breeding effort would be greater than for native cool-season grasses.

The principal warm-season grasses that are being used in the southern regions of the United States are introduced grasses from Africa or Asia where they evolved under heavy grazing pressure from either wild or domestic animals. Important species are bermudagrass [*Cynodon dactylon* (L.) Pers], lovegrasses (*Eragrostis* spp.), old world bluestems (*Bothriochloa* spp.), and zoysiagrass (*Zoysia* spp.) (Burton 1989; Busey 1989). Most of these grasses cannot survive the winters in the central and northern latitudes of the United States and consequently, native warm-season grasses such as big bluestem (*Andropogon gerardii*), indiangrass (*Sorghastrum nutans*), and switchgrass (*Panicum virgatum*) have and are being increasingly utilized as cultivated grasses in these regions. These native warm-season grasses provide excellent pasture and forage during hot summer months when cool-season grasses are relatively unproductive and have poor forage quality.

Eastern gamagrass [*Tripsacum dactyloides* (L.) L.] may also have considerable potential. Its use in the past has been restricted by limited seed production. The recent discovery of a mutant that has been reported to increase seed yields by up to 20-fold (Dewald and Dayton 1985) should alleviate this problem. Eastern gamagrass is noted for high forage yields but its persistence under grazing and intensive management needs further testing. Other native grasses that are and will be utilized as cultivated grasses on a smaller scale include grama grasses (*Bouteloua* spp.) and little bluestem [*Schizachyrium scoparium* (Michx.) Nash].

There are millions of hectares in the Central Great Plains and adjacent Midwest states that need to be in permanent vegetation for erosion control. In the current Conservation Reserve Program (CRP), millions of hectares of this land was seeded to permanent vegetation. It has been predicted that over 80% of this land may be plowed when the CRP program terminates (Heimlich and Kula 1989). The production systems of the participating farmers were not adequately taken into consideration in the crash CRP program and many of the grasses and other plants used for revegetation will not be productive enough to be profitable for farmers and ranchers.

Marginal land currently in crop production often produces grain for meat production. The same land can be used to produce meat via livestock grazing in sustainable and environmentally benign integrated crop-grassland-livestock production systems if adequate plant materials are available. Research to develop sustainable *crop production* systems for erodible lands in this region have been initiated. An alternative approach would be the development of sustainable *agricultural* systems in which livestock and grasslands are integral components of the system.

Class I and II land (Klingebiel 1958) in a region can be used for grain crop production without serious erosion problems if properly managed. Land classified as having higher erosion potential should be in permanent grasslands which is the best and most cost effective method of reducing erosion to acceptable levels (Vogel et al. 1985b). Livestock are needed to utilize the forage produced by these grasslands to make the systems economically viable. Permanent grasslands could maintain livestock herds during the spring, summer, and fall months. Crop residues on the cultivated land and harvested hay would be used to maintain the livestock during the winter months. The components of this system would change from region to region. Native warm-season grasses such as big bluestem and switchgrass would provide the summer grazing component for this system in the Central and Northern Great Plains and Midwest.

One-half to one-third of the potential grasslands in Midwest and central and northern Great Plains region could be seeded to grasses such as big bluestem and switchgrass which would be approximately 5 to 10 million ha. In addition, approximately one-third of the grasslands in the fescue belt or about 5 million hectares could be converted to warm-season pastures to provide high quality grazing during the summer months by reseeding them with switchgrass and big bluestem. These grasses may also be used in the Northeastern states of the United States on marginal cropland.

Although forage yields vary with locations due to precipitation, growing season, and soil fertility, forage yields of 10 to 20 Mg/ha can be expected from switchgrass and big bluestem in the Midwest and Great Plains states. Animal gains per hectare will depend upon pasture and livestock management. Results from grazing trials indicate that the economic return from properly managed native warm-season pastures can be similar to that of grain crops grown on the same land (Table 1). The numbers of hectares of land that will be converted into grasslands seeded to native prairie grasses will be determined by economic factors including farm programs of the United States.

GRAIN CROPS

Utopian concepts for agricultural systems for the future usually include the concept of perennial grain crops. Perennial grain crops would not have to be sown annually which would eliminate the costs, labor, and soil losses that can occur with the production of annual grain crops. Recently, research on perennial grain crops has been conducted at the Rodale Research Center, Kutztown, Pennsylvania and at The Land Institute, Salina, Kansas. Two recent reviews (Jackson 1990; Wagoner 1990) summarize research at those locations and other research relevant to perennial grain crops.

The potential benefits of perennial grain crops would include reduced soil erosion due to reduced tillage, reduced production costs, and reduced energy use. Jackson (1990) has developed the concept of producing perennial grains in polycultures in grain producing "prairies" in which nitrogen fixing legumes would be part of the system.

Numerous grass species have been tested for their potential as perennial grain crops including grasses native to the North America. At the present time the seed yields of these grasses are only about a tenth to a fifth of wheat (*Triticum aestivum* L.) or maize (*Zea mays* L.) grown on similar land (Jackson 1990; Wagoner 1990). The proponents of perennial grain crops believe that the seed yields of these perennials can be improved by breeding

Table 1. Yields and economic returns from switchgrass, intermediate wheatgrass, wheat and sorghum in eastern Nebraska[1].

	Switchgrass	Intermediate wheatgrass	Wheat	Sorghum
	kg ha^{-1}			
Yields				
Forage	11,000	7,800		
Seed	450	450	4030	5040
Beef yearling gains	350	290		
	$ ha^{-1}			
Gross return ha^{-1}				
Forage[y]	605	430		
Grass Seed[x]	1980	1980		
Grain[w]	50	50	520	440
Beef gains[v]	540	445		

[z]Data are based upon USDA/ARS and Univ. of Nebrska cooperative research at the Nebraska Agricultural Research and Development Center at Mead, NE.
[y]Based on a price of $55 Mg^{-1} ($50 U.S. ton^{-1}).
[x]Based on a price of $4.40 kg^{-1} ($2.00 lb^{-1}).
[w]Based on a price of $0.128 kg^{-1} for wheat ($3.50 bu^{-1}), $0.088/kg for sorghum ($2.25 bu^{-1}), and $0.11 kg^{-1} for grasses ($0.05 lb^{-1}).
[v]Based on a price of $1.54 kg^{-1} (0.70 lb^{-1}).

to the level where they are economically competitive with grain crops. Seed yields can undoubtedly be improved but it will take a considerable sustained effort to double let alone quadruple seed yields. In the meantime, the seed yields of existing annual grain crops will not remain static. Annual genetic gains for maize from 1950 to 1980 averaged 92 kg/ha (Duvick 1984) while for wheat they increased 0.74% per year for the period 1958 to 1980 (Schmidt 1984). The increase in wheat and maize yields were due to the combined efforts of many geneticists, pathologists, entomologists, and other scientists working throughout the United States. Scientific resources of this magnitude will not be available to develop perennial grasses into grain crops, so it is doubtful if increases in seed yields of potential perennial grain crops would be equal to those that are being achieved in corn and wheat.

Breeders and production agronomists working with native North American grasses initially faced considerable seed production problems that needed to be resolved before these grasses could even be utilized as forage crops. Empirical (Schumacher 1962) and formal research (Smika and Newell 1966; Canode 1965; Kassel et al. 1985) has resulted in greatly increased seed production. By using improved seed production practices, experienced seed growers in Nebraska can produce from 250 to over 1,000 kg of seed/ha under dryland conditions and up to 2,000 kg/ha under irrigated conditions (Nebraska Crop Improvement Association pers. commun.). Since only 6 to 14 kg of pure live seed/ha are needed for grassland plantings, one seed production hectare will plant 25 to 90 hectares of grasslands which is similar to that of most cultivated crops (Vogel et al. 1989). This means that native grasses have adequate seed yields for use as *forage crops*. They do not have adequate seed yields for use as perennial grain crops.

In addition to the problem of increasing seed yields there are also problems dealing with insect and disease pests. The problems that can occur with seed pests in perennial grass production fields indicate that this problem alone may make perennial grain crops impractical. A bromegrass seed midge and a big bluestem seed midge can reduce yields of these grasses by over 50% (Neiman and Manglitz 1972; Carter et al. 1988). The biology of the bromegrass seed midge has been investigated but less is known about the biology of the bluestem seed midge (Vogel and Manglitz 1989). There are no known controls for either insect. It is very likely that similar insects exist on other prairie grasses. Based on existing knowledge of the insect, it is likely that insecticides could be used to control the insect but to date no adequate controls are available. Boe et al. (1989) recently reported evidence that there may be genetic variation for infestation by the big bluestem seed midge. The genetic differences were small and a tremendous amount of long-term breeding work would be required to produce strains that had economically improved tolerance or resistance. Because the life cycle of the seed midges matches that of the host grasses, it is apparent that they co-evolved. These insects would undoubtedly be a serious problem if a perennial grass was grown on extensive areas of land as a seed crop.

New, improved forage cultivars are already economically competitive with annual grain crops in the Great Plains (Table 1). Using these grasses in integrated crop-livestock-grassland production systems would achieve the same goals of conserving soils advocated by the proponents of perennial grain crops (Jackson 1990) and these goals can be achieved now rather than in the distant future. Additional breeding work on grasses as forage crops will only improve the economics of integrated production systems.

In addition to the production and breeding problems associated with perennial grain crops, there is also the marketing and utilization problem. This problem can be best understood by evaluating the new grain crop triticale (×*Triticosecale rimpaui* Wittm.). This new crop has not achieved its promise because no specific national markets or market channels for it have developed. It is likely that the same fate would await a perennial grain crop. If advocates of perennial grain crops want to pursue the development of a perennial grain crop in spite of these obstacles, we suggest that Canada wildrye (*Elymus canadensis* L.) and its relatives would have more potential as a perennial grain crop than other prairie grasses.

BIOMASS FUEL CROPS

Grasses could be grown on marginal land as a feedstock for ethanol fuel production from biomass (Lynd et al. 1991; Turhollow et al. 1988). Production of ethanol from perennial grass biomass has many positive attributes. Ethanol produced from biomass would be a renewable resource that would reduce America's dependence on foreign oil and it has the added environmental benefit of being a clean burning fuel. Millions of hectares of marginal cropland would be needed to produce herbage for ethanol on the scale envisioned by the planners at the U.S. Department of Energy (Lynd et al. 1991). This would take marginal land out of grain crop production and greatly reduce soil erosion problems if the herbage was produced by a perennial grass. In addition, it would alleviate the problem of crop surpluses and reduce or eliminate the need for crop subsidy payments. The U.S. Department of Energy has been funding evaluation trials of potential biomass plants and to date, switchgrass is the most promising herbaceous perennial for the midwestern states (Turhollow 1991). In our opinion, big bluestem and eastern gamagrass also have potential as biomass fuel crops because of their high yield potential.

Ethanol fuel production from biomass will be dependent upon the development of economical processes for converting the cellulose and hemicellulose in plant cell walls to extractable ethanol. Conversion technology has not reached this stage of development. We are currently evaluating switchgrass germplasm for its potential as a biomass fuel crop. This evaluation includes herbage yield, other agronomic traits, and the stability of these traits over three midwestern environments. We are unable to evaluate switchgrasses for ethanol conversion traits because development of the conversion process technology has not reached the stage at which the herbage traits most important for ethanol production can be characterized (Janet Cushman and Anthony Turhollow pers. commun. Oakridge National Laboratory). Since the important steps in the conversion process will involve biological reactions we assume that traits which improve in vitro dry matter digestibility (IVDMD) will be similar to those needed for ethanol production from biomass.

Ethanol production from herbage of perennial grasses has considerable promise and if the conversion technology can be developed, American farmers will be growing millions of acres of switchgrasses and other grasses for biomass fuel production by the year 2020. It has been estimated that ethanol could be produced from herbage using existing technology for $0.36/liter ($1.35/gallon) (Bull 1989). The use of native prairie grasses as biomass fuel crops will probably depend upon United States government energy programs and policies.

TURFGRASSES AND ORNAMENTALS

Buffalograss [*Buchloe dactyloides* (Nutt.) Engelm.] is a native prairie grass that has fine leaves, short stature, and produces a dense sod due to vigorous spreading by stolons. Although its desirable turf attributes have been known for 50 years (Frolik and Keim 1945), it is only recently that it has become increasingly important as a turfgrass for use in minimum maintenance areas (Riordan 1991; Wu et al. 1989; Pozarnsky 1983). Buffalograss can maintain a desirable turf with very limited water inputs, an important trait in the western United States. In addition, only infrequent mowings and other maintenance work are needed on buffalograss lawns. Its principal disadvantage is that it greens up later in the spring and goes dormant earlier in the fall than do cool-season turf grasses. These traits can be improved by breeding. Currently, buffalograss turf breeding programs in Nebraska and Texas are developing turf type buffalograss cultivars. Recently, the first buffalograss cultivar developed exclusively as a turf grass, 'Prairie' buffalograss, was released in Texas (Engelke and Lehman 1990). Because of its desirable attributes, buffalograss has the potential to become a major turf grass in the United States.

Many of the native grasses could be used as ornamental plants because of their striking appearance. Some landscape architects are currently using them in their planting plans and these grasses are beginning to be available in nurseries. No ornamental cultivars of these grasses have been released to date. The use of prairie grasses as ornamentals will increase because of their natural beauty and their low maintenance requirements, but the extent of use as ornamentals cannot be predicted at this time.

IMPROVING NATIVE GRASSES BY BREEDING

The improvement that can be made in a plant breeding program for a species such as switchgrass is dependent upon the genetic variability within the species for the traits being selected, the heritability of the traits, the breeder's ability to identify genetically superior plants, the intensity of selection, and the efficiency of the breeding procedure (Allard 1960; Hallauer and Miranda 1981).

The genetic variation that exists within both native and introduced cross-pollinated grasses consists of between ecotype (endemic strain) or synthesized strain variability and within strain variability. Ecotypes or endemic strains found in specific regions and sites have evolved by the genetic mechanisms of mutation, migration, selection, and random drift or chance resulting in between ecotype or endemic strain genetic variability (Falconer 1981). Eberhardt and Newell (1959) documented this between strain variability in switchgrass and we are currently conducting similar studies using germplasm of switchgrass, big bluestem, indiangrass, and Canada wildrye collected from remnant midwestern prairies in 1989. Based upon data from the first evaluation year, the between accession genetic variability is substantial.

Most of the initial breeding work with cross-pollinated grasses utilized this between strain genetic variability (Vogel et al. 1985a; Hanson 1972). Within strain genetic variability consists of the proportion of the plant-to-plant (phenotypic) variability that exists between plants of a strain that is due to genetic (genotypic) differences among plants (Falconer 1981; Hallauer and Miranda 1981). This variability is very difficult to observe or measure in a typical pasture or rangeland situation. However, if seed is harvested from the individual plants in a common native prairie site and planted in a space-planted nursery under uniform conditions, phenotypic variation among plants can be readily distinguished. By using quantitative genetics procedures, it is possible to determine the total genetic variation and the additive genetic variation in specific populations or accessions for specific traits and the heritability of those traits.

The genetics studies that have been conducted in switchgrass, big bluestem, eastern gamagrass, and indiangrass indicate that there is substantial genetic variation for important agronomic traits studied to date (Eberhardt and Newell 1959; Newell and Eberhardt 1961; Talbert et al. 1983; Vogel et al. 1981a,b; Godshalk and Timothy 1988; Godshalk et al. 1986, 1988; Gabrielsen et al. 1990; Ross et al. 1975; Glewen and Vogel 1984; Riley 1981; Boe and Ross 1988; Boe et al. 1989; Wright et al. 1983). The conclusions from these studies can be summarized as follows: (1) there is substantial genetic variability both between and within strains of these grasses for most agronomic traits including those that affect or determine forage yield and quality; (2) heritability values for most important traits range from 20 to 40% which should make it possible to improve these grasses by breeding; and (3) correlations among most desirable traits are usually positive but when negative they are usually not large indicating it should be possible to simultaneously improve several traits without adversely affecting other traits.

Almost all important native prairie grasses are cross-pollinated by wind (Hanson and Carnahan 1956). They have small florets that are difficult to emasculate, and effective mechanisms for producing hybrids such as cytoplasmic male sterility have not been developed. Thus breeders are largely limited to procedures that utilize additive genetic variability and that do not require emasculation. Fortunately, there is substantial additive genetic variability for most traits in these grasses, and breeding methods that do not require emasculation are some of the most efficient that are available. The expected gain from selection that can be made by using the breeding procedures or schemes that have been developed to date are described by Empig et al. (1972), Nguyen and Sleper (1983), and Hallauer and Miranda (1981). The two breeding methods that have the most potential of exploiting additive genetic variation are Restricted Recurrent Phenotypic Selection or RRPS (Burton 1974, 1982) and a modified form of between and within family selection (Vogel 1988; Asstveit and Asstveit 1990). Since biomass production requires traits similar to those needed for forage crops, the potential of improving these grasses as biomass fuel crops appears to be excellent.

Anderson et al.(1988) demonstrated that an increase in forage digestibility of less than two percentage units in 'Trailblazer' switchgrass resulted in about a 20% improvement in animal gains and beef production per hectare as compared to the cultivar 'Pathfinder' which had similar yields. The increase in beef production due to the small change in digestibility had a value of $89/ha ($35/acre) averaged over three years (Vogel et al. 1989). In a grazing trial completed in 1990 at Mead, Nebraska, by K.P. Vogel, K.J. Moore, B.A. Anderson, and T.J. Klopfenstein, an experimental intermediate wheatgrass produced significantly higher gains than the two leading cultivars. Averaged over a two year period, this increased gain had a value of over $50/ha. These gains were made with only initial breeding work to improve forage quality. The potential for significant economic gains by breeding for improved forage grasses appears to be the best method to improve the economic value of forage grasses. Theoretical studies evaluating the effect of increasing forage quality on animal gains indicates that exponential gains in animal performance can be achieved by breeding for improved forage quality (Fig. 1).

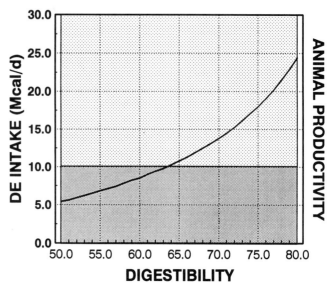

Fig. 1. Animal production increases exponentially with improvements in forage digestibility. Digestibile energy (DE) intake values are for 300 kg beef steer. The darker shaded area represents maintenance requirements.

SUMMARY

Although hundreds of grasses were native to the North American continent, only a few have the potential to become important forage, biomass, or turf crops. Switchgrass, big bluestem, and eastern gamagrass have the most potential as forage and biomass fuel crops. Indiangrass may also be important as a forage crop. Buffalograss will become an important turf grass particularly in arid regions of western states. It is doubtful if any of the native North American grasses will be developed into a perennial grain crop. Their current seed yields are currently only about a tenth of that of grain crops and even if their seed yields could be improved, substantial problems would have to be overcome in marketing the new crop.

REFERENCES

Allard, R.W. 1960. Principles of plant breeding. Wiley, New York.

Anderson, B., J.K. Ward, K.P. Vogel, M.G. Ward, H.J. Gorz, and F.A. Haskins. 1988. Forage quality and performance of yearlings grazing switchgrass strains selected for differing digestibility. J. Anim. Sci. 66:2239–2244.

Asstveit, A.H. and K. Asstveit. 1990. Theory and application of open-pollination and polycross in forage breeding. Theor. Appl. Genet. 79:618–624.

Barker, R.W., L.K. Holzworth, and K.H. Asay. 1985. Genetic resources of wheatgrasses and wildrye species native to the rangelands of western North America, p. 9–13. In: J.R. Carlson and E.D. McArthur (chair). Range plant improvement in western North America. Proc. Symp. Soc. Range Manag. Annu. Meet., 14 Feb., Salt Lake City, UT.

Barker, R.E. and R.R. Kalton. 1989. Cool-season forage grass breeding: progress, potentials, and benefits, p. 5–20. In: D.A. Sleper, K.H. Asay, and J.F. Pedersen (ed.). Contributions from breeding forage and turf grasses. Crop Sci. Special Pub. 15. Crop Sci. Soc. Amer. Madison, WI.

Boe, A., K. Robbins, and B. McDaniel. 1989. Spikelet characteristics and midge predation of hermaphroditic genotypes of big bluestem. Crop Sci. 29:1433–1435.

Boe, A. and J.G. Ross. 1988. Path coefficient analysis of seed yield in big bluestem (*Andropogon gerardii*) progenies. J. Range Manag. 36:652–653.

Bull, S.R. 1989. Advances in processes for fermentation ethanol. Paper presented at: Energy from Biomass and Wastes XIII. Feb. 13–17. New Orleans, LA.

Burton, G.W. 1974. Recurrent restricted phenotypic selection increases forage yields of Pensacola bahiagrass. Crop Sci. 14:831–835.

Burton, G.W. 1982. Improved recurrent restricted phenotypic selection increases bahiagrass forage yields. Crop Sci. 22:1058–1061.

Burton, G.W. 1989. Progress and benefits to humanity from breeding warm-season forage grasses, p. 21–29. In: D.A. Sleper, K.H. Asay, and J.F. Pedersen (eds.). Contributions from breeding forage and turf grasses. Crop Sci. Special Pub. 15. Crop Sci. Soc. Amer., Madison, WI.

Busey, P. 1989. Progress and benefits to humanity from breeding warm-season grasses for turf, p.49–70. In: D.A. Sleper, K.H. Asay, and J.F. Pedersen (eds.). Contributions from breeding forage and turf grasses. Crop Sci. Special Pub. 15. Crop Sci. Soc. Amer. Madison, WI.

Canode, C.L. 1965. Influence of cultural treatments on seed production of intermediate wheatgrass [*Agropyron intermedium* (Host) Beauv.] Agron. J. 57:207–210.

Carter, M.R., G.R. Manglitz, M.D. Rethwisch, and K.P. Vogel. 1988. A seed midge pest of big bluestem (*Andropogon gerardii*). J. Range Manag. 41:253–254.

Dewald, C.L. and R.S. Dayton. 1985. A prolific sex form variant of eastern gamagrass. Phytologia 57:156.

Duvick, D.N. 1984. Genetic contributions to yield gains of U.S. hybrid maize, 1930 to 1980, p. 15–47. In: W.R. Fehr (ed.). Genetic contributions to yield gains of five major crop plants. Crop Sci. Special Pub. 7. Crop Sci. Soc. Amer. Madison, WI.

Eberhardt, S.A. and L.C. Newell. 1959. Variation in domestic collections of switchgrass, *Panicum virgatum*. Agron. J. 15:613–616.

Empig, L.T., C.O. Gardner, and W.A. Compton. 1972. Theoretical gains for different population improvement procedures. Nebraska Agr. Expt. Stat. MP 26.

Engelke, M.C. and V.G. Lehman. 1990. Registration of 'Prairie' buffalograss. Crop Sci. 30:1360–1361.

Falconer, D.S. 1981. Introduction to quantitative genetics. 2nd ed. Longman, New York.

Frolik, E.F. and F.D. Keim. 1945. Buffalograss for lawns. Nebr. Agr. Expt. Sta. Cir. 63.

Gabrielsen, B.C., K.P. Vogel, B.E. Anderson, and J.K. Ward. 1990. Alkali-labile lignin phenolics and forage quality in three switchgrass strains selected for differing digestibility. Crop Sci. 30:1313–1320.

Glewen, G.L. and K.P. Vogel. 1984. Partitioning the genetic variability for seedling growth in sand bluestem into its seed size and seedling vigor components. Crop Sci. 24:137–141.

Godshalk, E.B., J.C. Burns, and D.H. Timothy. 1986. Selection for in vitro dry matter digestibility disappearance in switchgrass regrowth. Crop Sci. 26:943–947.

Godshalk, E.B. and D.H. Timothy. 1988. Effectiveness of index selection for switchgrass forage yield and quality. Crop Sci. 28:825–830.

Godshalk, E.B., W.F. McClure, J.C. Burns, D.H. Timothy, and D.S. Fisher. 1988. Heritability of cell wall carbohydrates in switchgrass. Crop Sci. 28:736–742.

Gould, F.W. 1968. Grass systematics. McGraw-Hill, New York.

Hallauer, A.R. and J.B. Miranda, OF. 1981. Quantitative genetics in maize breeding. Iowa St. Univ. Press, Ames.

Hanson, A.A. 1972. Grass varieties in the United States. USDA Agr. Handb. 170.

Hanson, A.A. and H.L. Carnahan. 1956. Breeding perennial forage grasses. Tech. Bul. 1145. ARS, USDA, U.S. Gov. Printing Office, Washington, DC.

Harlan, J.R. 1975. Crops and man. Amer. Soc. Agron. & Crop Sci. Soc. Amer. Madison, WI.

Hassell, W.G. and R.E. Barker. 1985. Relationships and potential development of selected needlegrasses and ricegrasses for western North American rangelands, p. 14–19. In: J.R. Carlson and E.D. McArthur (chair). Range plant improvement in western North America. Proc. Symp. Soc. Range Manag. Annu. Meet. Feb. 14. Salt Lake City, UT.

Heimlich, R.E. and O.E. Kula. 1990. Grazing lands: How much CRP land will remain in grasses? Rangelands 11:253–257.

Heizer, R.B. and W.G. Hassell. 1985. Improvement of the gramas and other shortgrass prairie species, p. 171–177. In: J.R. Carlson and E.D. McArthur (chair). Range plant improvement in western North America. Proc. Symp. Soc. Range Manag. Annu. Meet. Feb.14. Salt Lake City, UT.

Hitchcock, A.S. 1951. Manual of grasses of the United States. 2nd ed. USDA Misc. Pub. 200, U.S. Government Printing Office, Washington, DC.

Jacobson, E.T., C.M. Talilaferro, C.L. Dewald, D.A. Tober, and R.J. Haas. 1985. New and old world bluestems. p. 148–158. In: J.R. Carlson and E.D. McArthur (chair). Range plant improvement in western North America. Proc. Symp. Soc. Range Manag. Annu. Meet. Feb.14. Salt Lake City, UT.

Jackson, W. 1990. Agriculture with nature as analogy, p. 381–422. In: C.A. Francis, C.B. Flora, and L.D. King (eds.). Sustainable agriculture in temperate zones. Wiley, New York.

Kassel, P.C., R.E. Mullen, and T.B. Bailey. 1985. Seed yield response of three switchgrass cultivars for different management practices. Agron. J. 77:214–218.

Kliengebiel, A.A. 1958. Soil survey interpretation-capability groupings. Soil Sci. Soc. Proc. 22:160–163.

Lynd, L.E., J.H. Cushman, R.J. Nochols, and C.E. Wyman. 1991. Fuel ethanol from cellulosic biomass. Science 251:1318–1325.

Meyer, W.A. and C.R. Funk. 1989. Progress and benefits to humanity from breeding cool-season grasses for turf, p.31–48. In: D.A. Sleper, K.H. Asay, and J.F. Pedersen (eds.). Contributions from breeding forage and turf grasses. Crop Sci. Special Pub. 15. Crop Sci. Soc. Amer. Madison, WI.

Neiman, E.L. and G.R. Manglitz. 1972. The biology and ecology of the bromegrass seed midge in Nebraska. Nebraska Agr. Expt. Sta. Res. Bul. 252.

Newell, L.C. and S.A. Eberhardt. 1961. Clone and progeny evaluation in the improvement of switchgrass. Crop Sci. 1:370–373.

Nguyen, H.T., and D.A. Sleper. 1983. Theory and applications of half-sib matings in forage grass breeding. Theor. Appl. Genet. 64:187–196.

Pozarnsky, T. 1983. Buffalograss: Home on the range, but also a turf grass (*Buchloe dactyloides*). Rangelands 5:214–216.

Riley, R.D. 1981. Heritability of mature plant traits in sand bluestem. PhD Diss. Univ. of Nebraska, Lincoln.

Riley, R.D., and K.P. Vogel. 1982. Chromosome numbers of released cultivars of switchgrass, indiangrass, big bluestem, and sand bluestem. Crop Sci. 22:1082–1083.

Riordan, T. 1991. Buffalograss. Grounds Maint. 26:12–14.

Ross, J.G., R.T. Thaden, and W.L. Tucker. 1975. Selection criteria for yield and quality in big bluestem grass. Crop Sci. 15:303–306.

Schumacher, C.M. 1962. Grass production in Nebraska and South Dakota. USDA/SCS Technical Guide-Section IV-G.

Schmidt, J.W. 1984. Genetic contributions to yield gains in wheat, p.89–101. In: W.R. Fehr (ed.). Genetic contributions to yield gains of five major crop plants. Crop Sci. Special Pub. 7. Crop Sci. Soc. Amer. Madison, WI.

Smika, D.E. and L.C. Newell. 1966. Cultural practices for seed production from established stands of western wheatgrass. Nebraska Agr. Expt. Sta. Res. Bul. 223.

Talbert, L.E., D.H. Timothy, J.C. Burns, J.O. Rawlings, and R.H. Moll. 1983. Estimates of genetic parameters in switchgrass. Crop Sci. 23:725–728.

Turhollow, A.F. 1991. Screening herbaceous lignocellulosic energy crops in temperate regions of the United States. Biomass (in press).

Turhollow, A.F., J.W. Johnston, and J.H. Cushman. 1988. Linking energy crops to conversion: the case of herbaceous lignocellulosic crops to ethanol. RERIC Intern. Energy J. 10:41–49.

Vogel, K.P. 1988. A recurrent, multistep, between and within family breeding scheme for perennial plants. Agron. Abst. 99.

Vogel, K.P., H.J. Gorz, and F.A. Haskins. 1981a. Heritability estimates of forage yield, in vitro dry matter digestibility, crude protein, and heading date in indiangrass. Crop Sci. 21:35–38.

Vogel, K.P., F.A. Haskins, and H.J. Gorz. 1981b. Divergent selection for in vitro dry matter digestibility in switchgrass. Crop Sci. 21:39–41.

Vogel, K.P., C.L. Dewald, H.J. Gorz, and F.A. Haskins. 1985a. Improvement of switchgrass, indiangrass, and eastern gamagrass: current status and future, p.159–170. In: J.R. Carlson and E.D. McArthur (chair). Range plant improvement in western North America. Proc. Symp. Soc. Range Manag. Annu. Meet. Feb.14. Salt Lake City, UT.

Vogel, K.P., H.J. Gorz, and F.A. Haskins. 1985b. Viewpoint: Forage and range research needs in the central Great Plains. J. Range Manag. 38:477–479.

Vogel, K.P., H.J. Gorz, and F.A. Haskins. 1989. Breeding grasses for the future, p.105–122. In: D.A. Sleper, K.H. Asay, and J.F. Pedersen (eds.). Contributions from breeding forage and turf grasses. Crop Sci. Special Pub. 15. Crop Sci. Soc. Amer. Madison, WI.

Vogel, K.P. and G.R. Manglitz. 1989. Effect of the big bluestem seed midge on the sexual reproduction of big bluestem: a review, p.267–291. In: T.B. Bragg and J. Stubbendieck (eds.). Proc. Eleventh North Amer. Prairie Conf. Prairie pioneers, ecology, history, and culture. Univ. Nebraska, Lincoln.

Voigt, P.W. and W.R. Oaks. 1985. Lovegrass, dropseeds, and other desert and subtropical grasses, p. 178–187. In: J.R. Carlson and E.D. McArthur (chair). Range plant improvement in western North America. Proc. Symp. Soc. Range Manag. Annu. Meet. Feb.14. Salt Lake City, UT.

Wagoner, P. 1990. Perennial grain crop development: past efforts and potential for the future. Crit. Rev. Plant Sci. 9:381–408.

Waller, S.S. and J.K. Lewis. 1979. Occurrence of C_3 and C_4 photosynthetic pathways of North American grasses. J. Range Manag. 32:12–28.

Weaver, J.E. 1954. North American prairie. Jensen Publ. Co., Lincoln, NE.

Wright, L.S., C.M. Taliaferro, and F.P. Horn. 1983. Variability of morphological and agronomic traits in eastern gamagrass accessions. Crop Sci. 23:135–138.

Wu, L., D.R. Huff, and M.A. Harivandi. 1989. Buffalograss as a low maintenance turf. Calif. Agr. 43(2):23–25.

African Grasses

Glenn W. Burton

The grasses, Poaceae (Gramineae), are man's most useful family of plants. The cereal grasses, rice, wheat, maize, barley, oats, sorghum, and millet supply three-fourths of man's energy and over half of his protein. These, with many forage species provide the grain and forage that animals need to produce the meat, milk, and eggs that supplement the cereal diet of humans. Grasses feed the world. They also protect the soil from erosion, cover man's playing fields, and beautify his environment.

Grasses and herbivores evolved about the same time. Hyams (1971) believes that "Without the exceptional powers possessed by grasses to grow again after being eaten almost down to the roots, a large number of animal species, including nearly all farm animals could not have evolved." He says, "It is possible to argue that the astounding success of *Homo sapiens* as a species is ultimately due to the power possessed by grass to grow again after being eaten down by animals."

Grasses are cosmopolitan from the equator to the arctic circle. Wherever flowering plants will grow, grasses can be found. It is estimated that there are about 10,000 species of grasses in the world, grouped into 620 genera arranged in 25 tribes (Hubbard 1954). There are 173 genera found in South Africa, most of which are indigenous (Meredith 1955).

Grass tribes may be grouped as Panicoid grasses containing the tropical and subtropical species and Festacoid grasses containing the temperate species. The panicoid group contains most of the African grasses. The panicoid grasses (Bogdon 1977) fix carbon by the efficient C_4 pathway of photosynthesis that has optimum temperatures of 30° to 40°C and optimum light intensities of 50 to 60 klx. The festucoid grasses use the C_3 photosynthesis processes that optimizes at 15° to 20°C and 15 to 30 klx. With optimum light and temperature Panicoid grasses can fix 30 to 50 g dry matter $m^{-2}d^{-1}$ whereas Festucoid grasses can fix up to about 20 g dry matter $m^{-2}d^{-1}$. Panicoid grasses do not make use of this advantage under low temperatures and low light intensities.

IMPORTANT AFRICAN SPECIES

Annuals

Two annual grasses grown primarily for grain in Africa are pearl millet [*Pennisetum glaucum* (L.) R. Br.] and sorghum (*Sorghum bicolor* L.). Pearl millet, widely adapted, very drought tolerant and free of prussic acid glucosides, is the best annual summer grazing crop for the southeastern United States. Fifty years of genetic improvement have resulted in commercial F_1 hybrids with greater leafiness, yielding 50% more forage and animal product than the old cattail types they replaced (Burton 1983). Sudangrass and sorghum-sudangrass hybrids usually outyield pearl millet on the heavier, more fertile soils. They contain prussic acid glucosides that can kill livestock grazing them. With proper management they can be grazed with little risk of animal loss from glucoside poisoning.

Perennials

Other African grasses with sufficient forage potential to be cultivated behave as perennials. With the help of others (Bogdon 1977; Harlan 1976; Meredith 1955; Tainton et al. 1976), I have selected 16 of the most important perennial grasses for presentation in Table 1 using seven descriptors.

AFRICAN GRASSES USED IN THE UNITED STATES

Bermudagrass, *Cynodon* spp. (L.)

Cynodon dactylon (L.) Pers. is called bermudagrass in the United States because an early introduction came from the Bermuda Island. Other names include wiregrass, couchgrass, and devilgrass. *C. dactylon* is mentioned in early history. To the Hindu, it was a sacred grass because it supported their cattle. Graeco–Roman

Table 1. Selected list of the 16 most important African perennial grasses.

Scientific name	Common name	Type of growth[z]	Height (m)	Reproduction method[y]	Adaptation[x]	Planted[w]	Genetic improvement[v]	Potential future use[u] World	USA
Andropogon gayanus Kunth	Gamba	B	1–3	S?	WDtCs	SV	L	1	5
Brachiaria decumbens Stapf.	Surinam	SfS	0.3–0.6	A	WCs	VS	O	3	5
Brachiaria mutica (Forsk.) Stapf.	Para	SfS	1–2	A?	NDsCs	V	O	1	4
Cenchrus ciliaris L.	Buffel	BR	1–1.5	A	WDtCs	S	M	1	2
Chloris gayana Kunth.	Rhodes	SfS	1–2	S	WDtCt	S	M	2	4
Cynodon dactylon (L.) Pers.	Bermuda	SfSR	0.2–0.7	S	WDtCt	VS	M	1	1
Cynodon nlemfuensis Vanderyst	Star	SfS	0.3–0.9	S	WDtCs	V	S	2	2
Digitaria decumbens Stent	Pangola	SfS	0.4–0.8	V	WDtCs	V	O	1	2
Eragrostis curvula (Schrad.) Nees	Weeping love	B	0.4–1.0	A	WDtCt	S	S	1	2
Hyparrhenia rufa (Nees) Stapf	Jaragua	B	1–2	S	WDtCs	S	L	3	4
Melinis minutiflora Beauv.	Molasses	B	0.6–1.0	S	WDtCs	S	L	2	5
Panicum coloratum L.	Klein	BS	0.4–1.4	S	WDtCs	S	M	3	2
Panicum maximum Jacq.	Guinea	B	0.5–4.5	A,S	WDtCs	S	S	2	4
Pennisetum clandestinum Hochst. ex Chiov.	Kikuyu	SfSR	0.2–0.4	S	NDtCs	V	L	4	5
Pennisetum purpureum Schumach.	Napier	B	2–6	S	WDtCt	V	M	1	2
Setaria anceps Stapf ex Massey	Setaria	B	1–2	S	WDtCs	SV	L	4	5

[z]Type of growth: B = bunch, Sf = sod forming, S = stolons, R = rhizomes.
[y]Reproduction method: S = sexual, A = apomictic.
[x]Adaptation: W = wide, N = narrow, D = drought, C = cold, t = tolerant, s = susceptible.
[w]Planted: S = with seed, V = vegetatively.
[v]Genetic improvement: M = much, S = some, L = little, O = none.
[u]Potential future use: 1 = excellent, 5 = poor.

pharmacopeia described expressed juice from bermudagrass stolons as a diuretic and an astringent to stop bleeding (Harlan 1976).

Although bermudagrass originated in Africa, it is cosmopolitan today occurring in every tropical and temperate part of the world. Its seed producing ability and its woody stolons and rhizomes have made it a weed. When southern crops were grown with a man, a mule, and a plow, bermudagrass was the farmer's worst weed. Yet, it saved untold acres of soil from erosion and became the South's first and most widely grown pasture and turfgrass.

Bermudagrass is a highly variable species (Burton and Hanna 1985). One variant crossed with tall selected types from South Africa produced 5,000 hybrids, the best of which, after much testing became 'Coastal' bermudagrass, named for the Georgia Coastal Plain Experiment Station where it was bred. In numerous tests, 'Coastal' bermudagrass has yielded about twice as much as common bermudagrass. In a year with only half of the average rainfall, 'Coastal' yielded six times more than common. 'Coastal' bermudagrass crossed with a common bermudagrass from Berlin, Germany produced 'Tifton 44', the best of 3,500 F_1 hybrids (Burton 1978). Because of its greater cold tolerance, 'Tifton 44' can be grown 160 km farther north than Coastal bermuda.

'Coastcross-1' bermudagrass, an F_1 hybrid between 'Coastal' and a highly digestible bermudagrass from Kenya, yields no more dry matter but is 12% more digestible than 'Coastal' and gives 30 to 40% more average daily gains (ADGs) and liveweight gains (LWG) per unit area (Burton 1972). It is restricted to Florida and the tropics.

'Tifton 68', an F_1 hybrid between PI 255450 and PI 293606 both from Kenya, is the most digestible bermudagrass in our collection of 500 introductions (Burton and Monson 1984). It is a hexaploid, $2n = 54$.

'Callie' bermudagrass, a natural hybrid found in an old Soil Conservation Service grass nursery, yields well but lacks winterhardiness and is very susceptible to rust that reduces forage yield and digestibility.

'Tifton 78' bermudagrass, a hybrid between 'Tifton 44' and 'Callie', is immune to rust and is a little less winterhardy than 'Coastal' (Burton and Monson 1988). Compared with Coastal, it is taller, establishes easier, starts earlier in the spring and in a 3-year grazing test produced 36% more LWG/A. Fertilized with 168 kg/ha of N plus P and K, it annually produced 983 kg/ha of liveweight gain at a fertilizer cost of 11¢ per kg of gain.

'Tifton 85' is a tall, coarse, dark green F_1 hybrid between PI 290884 from South Africa and 'Tifton 68'. 'Tifton 85', $2n = 45$, is sterile but its large stolons and rhizomes make vegetative propagation easy. In a three-year replicated grazing trial, 'Tifton 85' has produced 47% more liveweight gain than 'Tifton 78'. It will be released officially in 1992. It is a little less winter hardy than 'Tifton 78', but should survive most winters in Florida and the southern half of the gulf states.

Other vegetatively propagated bermudagrass cultivars include 'Grazer', 'Midland', 'Hardie', and 'Brazos'. 'Pasto Rico' and 'Tempre Verde', commercial seed propagated mixtures of common and a tall wild type, are inferior to 'Coastal' and soon revert to low yielding common bermudagrass.

Cynodon nlemfuensis Vandeyst usually called stargrass is taller and larger than *C. dactylon* (Harland 1976). Stargrass is highly variable, spreads by seed and stolons but lacks rhizomes. It is softer, more palatable and has a higher digestibility than common bermudagrass. Stargrasses usually contains prussic acid glucosides but reports of livestock poisoning are rare. It lacks winterhardiness and is limited to South Florida and South Texas.

Buffelgrass, *Cenchrus ciliaris* L.

Buffelgrass is a drought tolerant bunchgrass that produces forage for the livestock industry in Texas. Two higher yielding more winterhardy cultivars, 'Neuces' and 'Llano' have extended the northern range of this popular grass. They are the product of plant breeding made possible by the discovery of a sexual plant that could be crossed with apomictic introductions and release their variability (Bashaw 1980).

Pangolagrass, *Digitaria decumbens* Stent

Pangolagrass is a sterile stoloniferous natural hybrid of unknown parentage. It lacks winterhardiness and is restricted to the southern two-thirds of Florida (Bennett 1973) where it has been planted on 300,000 ha. It is palatable, highly digestible and is considered an excellent pasture grass. It is less tolerant of drought and continuous close grazing than bahiagrass and bermudagrass.

Kleingrass, *Panicum coloratum* L.

Kleingrass is a leafy bunchgrass that grows well on sandy to clay soils from south Texas to Oklahoma (Voight and MacLauchlan 1985). It is drought tolerant and grows earlier in the spring and later in the fall than many warm season grasses. Two cultivars 'Selection 75' and 'Verde' give good animal gains and tolerate heavy utilization. Seed shattering is a serious problem that limits its use. It occupies about 600,000 ha, most in central Texas.

Weeping lovegrass, *Eragrostis curvula* (Schrad.) Nees

Weeping lovegrass is a bunch grass with long, narrow dropping leaves and a mature height of 0.5 to 1.5 m (Voight and MacLauchlan 1985). It grows best on sandy soils from south Texas to northern Oklahoma where is occupies some 240,000 ha. Animal performance on weeping lovegrass has been poor unless it is given intensive management. It is readily established from seeds that are easy to produce. It reproduces by obligate apomixis that has blocked genetic improvement until recently.

Napiergrass, *Pennisetum purpureum* Schumach.

Napiergrass ($2n = 28$) is a robust perennial bunchgrass that may reach a height of 6 m. It grows on a wide range of well-drained soils and is drought tolerant. Its herbage can be killed with light frosts but underground parts can remain alive if the soil is not frozen. It reproduces sexually but seed size is small, seed yields are very poor, and seedlings are weak.

Thus, napiergrass is established from stem cuttings or crown divisions. If cut only once a year, napiergrass can produce more dry matter per unit area than any other crop that can be grown in the deep south, but cutting it twice a year at Ona, Florida reduced annual yields 70% (Burton 1986). Napiergrass cut once a year will produce more dry matter per unit of N and other fertilizer nutrients removed than other biomass crops.

Blaser et al. (1955) conducted a number of management experiments from 1938 to 1944 with napiergrass in Florida. They found napiergrass inferior to maize and sorghum as a silage crop. Its coarse stems made it a very poor hay crop to cure and handle. Fertilized with 67 kg/ha of N plus adequate P and K and grazed rotationally, napiergrass maintained a stand for 3 years, provided 235 steer days, gave ADGs of 0.71 kg and produced LWG of 414 kg/ha per year. Dairy cows did well on napiergrass fertilized and managed in the same manner.

Napiergrass breeding begun in 1936 produced the eyespot immune high-yielding 'Merkeron', the best of many hybrids between outstanding tall, selection No. 1 and a very leafy dwarf No. 208 (Burton 1990). A selfed progeny of 'Merkeron' contained a number of dwarfs, the best of which has been released in Florida as 'Mott' (Sollenberger et al. 1988).

REFERENCES

Bashaw, E.C. 1980. Registration of Nueces and Llano buffelgrass. Crop Sci. 20:112.

Bennett, H.W. 1973. Pangola digitgrass, p. 339–341. In: M.E. Heath, D.S. Metcalf, and R.E. Barnes (eds.). Forages. 3rd ed. Iowa State Univ. Press, Ames.

Blaser, R.E., G.E. Ritchey, W.G. Kirk, and P.T. Dix Arnold. 1955. Experiments with napiergrass. Florida Expt. Sta. Bul. 568.

Bodgon, A.V. 1977. Tropical pasture and fodder plants. Longman, New York.

Burton, G.W. 1972. Registration of 'Coastcross-1' bermudagrass. Crop Sci. 12:125.

Burton, G.W. 1978. Registration of 'Tifton 44' bermudagrass. Crop Sci. 18:911.

Burton, G.W. 1983. Breeding pearl millet. Plant Breed. Rev. 1:162–182.

Burton, G.W. 1986. Biomass production from herbaceous plants, p. 163–171. In: W.H. Smith (ed.). Biomass energy development. Plenum Press, New York.

Burton, G.W. 1990. Grasses new and improved, p. 174–177. In: J. Janick and J.E. Simon (eds.). Advances in new crops. Timber Press, Portland, OR.

Burton, G.W. and W.W. Hanna. 1985. Bermudagrass, p. 247–254. In: M.E. Heath, D.S. Metcalf, and R.E. Barnes (eds.). Forages. 4th ed. Iowa State Univ. Press, Ames.

Burton, G.W. and W.G. Monson. 1984. Registration of 'Tifton 68' bermudagrass. Crop Sci. 24:1211.

Burton, G.W. and W.G. Monson. 1988. Registration of 'Tifton 78' bermudagrass. Crop Sci. 28:187–188.

Harlan, J.R. 1976. Tropical and subtropical grasses. In: M.W. Simmonds (ed.). Evolution of crop plants. Longman Group, London. 19:142–144.

Hubbard, C.E. 1954. Grasses: A guide to their structure, identification, uses and distribution in the British Isles. Penguin Books, London.

Hyams, E. 1971. Plants in service to man. J.B. Lippincott, Philadelphia and New York.

Meredith, D. 1955. The grasses and pastures of South Africa. Cape Times, Parow Univ. of South Africa, Johannesburg.

Sollenberger, L.E., G.M. Prine, W.R. Ocumpaugh, W.W. Hanna, C.S. Jones, Jr., S.C. Schank, and R.S. Kalmbacher. 1988. 'Mott' dwarf elephantgrass: a high quality forage for the subtropics and tropics. Univ. Florida Cir. S-356.

Tainton, N.M., D.J. Bransby, and P.de V. Booysen. 1976. Common veld and pasture grasses of Natal. Shuter and Shooten (Pty) Ltd, Pietermanitzburg, South Africa.

Voight, P.W. and M.S. MacLauchlan. 1985. Native and other western grasses, p. 177–187. In: M.E. Heath, D.S. Metcalf, and R.E. Barnes (eds.). Forages. 4th ed. Iowa State Univ. Press, Ames.

OILSEEDS

Canola Seed Yield in Relation to Harvest Methods

Casimir A. Jaworski and Sharad C. Phatak

Rapeseed/canola (*Brassica napus* L. and *B. campestris* L.) recently moved up to the world's third most important edible oil source after soybean and palm, and has the largest annual growth rate of the 10 major edible oils (Downey 1990). Canola consumption is rapidly increasing in the United States due to its lowest saturated oil (6%) of all vegetable and animal oils, the granting of GRAS (Generally Regarded As Safe) status to low erucic acid rapeseed (LEAR) oil by the Food and Drug Administration (FDA) in 1985, and allowance of the term canola on food labels by FDA in late 1988 (Neshem 1990). Most of the canola presently consumed domestically is imported.

Available area potential for double cropping with traditional summer row crops, adequate rainfall and mild winters are factors which make the southeastern United States very promising for canola production (Raymer and Thomas 1990). However, the natural dehiscent process, indeterminate growth, long period of seed maturity, and variable weather conditions such as wind and rain are some factors which can lead to large seed losses (Hall 1990; Ogilvy 1989). Seed shattering and seed loss at harvest become even more critical since late spring cultivars seeded as winter annuals in south Georgia mature earlier and produce larger yields than winter cultivars; however, these spring cultivars are more subject to seed shattering than the winter cultivars. The objective of this study was to determine if swathing canola improves seed recovery as compared to direct combining.

METHODOLOGY

Four canola harvest tests were conducted in 1990 with 'Legend' and 'Global', spring cultivars (Tables 1 and 2). Seeding for tests 1 and 2 was Oct. 12, 1989 and for tests 3 and 4 on Oct. 31, 1989. Test 1 was carried out with 'Legend' and treatments were direct harvest and swathed for 14 and 21 days. Test 2 was with 'Global' and treatments were direct harvest and swathed for 7, 14, and 21 days. Test 3 was with 'Legend' and treatments were direct harvest and swathed for 6, 12, and 19 days. Test 4 was with 'Global' and treatments were direct harvest and swathed for 7, 12, and 18 days. Swathing was done when 30% of the seeds changed from green color (Apr. 11, Apr. 25, May 2, and May 3, 1990 in tests 1, 2, 3, and 4, respectively). Clipping was carried out with a gasoline powered ornamental hedger and thrashing with a stationary harvester. The 1990 canola harvest season was unusually dry with only significant rainfall of 0.38, 0.28, and 0.61 cm on Apr. 28, May 9, and May 10, respectively.

RESULTS

'Legend' seed yields were not significantly different between harvest methods and averaged 2,173 and 1,756 kg/ha, respectively, for tests 1 and 3 (Table 1). 'Global' seed yields for direct harvest and swathed for 7 days were 2,278 and 2,778 kg/ha in test 2 and 1,650 and 2,165 kg/ha in test 4, respectively (Table 2). Harvesting after 7 days of swathed was 7 to 9 days earlier than direct harvest.

Direct harvesting of 'Global' had lower seed yields when compared to swath treatments. Seed yields from direct harvest and swathing treatments were however similar for 'Legend'. The 7 to 9 day earlier harvest for a 7 day swathing as compared to direct harvest would give more time for establishing a traditional summer row crop in a double-cropping system.

Table 1. Seed yield of 'Legend' canola as affected by harvest system (test 1 and 3).

Harvest system	Test 1		Test 3	
	Harvest date	Seed yield (kg/ha)	Harvest date	Seed yield (kg/ha)
Direct harvest	May 3	2,081[z]	May 17	1,580[z]
Swathed 6 days	---	---	May 8	1,835
Swathed 12 days	---	---	May 14	1,820
Swathed 14 days	April 25	2,285	---	---
Swathed 19 days	---	---	May 21	1,790
Swathed 21 days	May 2	2,154	---	---

[z]Each value represents mean of six and five observations in test 1 and 3, respectively. Treatment means are not significantly different.

Table 2. Seed yield of 'Global' canola as affected by harvest system (test 2 and 4).

Harvest system	Test 2		Test 4	
	Harvest date	Seed yield (kg/ha)	Harvest date	Seed yield (kg/ha)
Direct harvest	May 11	2,278b[z]	May 17	1,650b[z]
Swathed 7 days	May 2	2,778a	May 10	2,165a
Swathed 12 days	---	---	May 15	2,056a
Swathed 14 days	May 9	2,761a	---	---
Swathed 18 days	---	---	May 21	1,896a
Swathed 21 days	May 16	2,749a	---	---

[z]Mean separation within column by Duncan's multiple range test, $P \geq 0.05$. Each value represents mean of six and five observations in test 2 and 4, respectively.

REFERENCES

Downey, R.K. 1990. Canola: A quality brassica oilseed, p. 211–215. In: J. Janick and J.E. Simon (eds.). Advances in new crops. Timber Press, Portland, OR.

Hall, D. 1990. Best management practices for canola harvest. Proc. Int. Canola Conf. Foundation for Agronomy Research, Atlanta, GA. p. 201–205.

Neshem, H.E. 1990. Overview of the developing U.S. canola industry. Proc. Int. Canola Conf. Foundation for Agronomy Research, Atlanta, GA. p. 22–28.

Ogilvy, S.E. 1989. The effect of timing on the quality and yield of winter oilseed rape. Aspects of Appl. Biol. 23:101–107.

Raymer, P. and D. Thomas. 1990. Canola production systems in the southeast U.S. region. Proc. Int. Canola Conf. Foundation for Agronomy Research, Atlanta, GA. p. 271–279.

Rapeseed, a New Oilseed Crop for the United States

Matti Sovero

Rapeseed is the third most important source of vegetable oil in the world, after soybean and palm oil. During the past twenty years, it has passed peanut, cottonseed, and most recently, sunflower, in worldwide production. This is almost entirely due to the plant breeding work initiated in Canada in the 1950s and 1960s which greatly reduced the levels of two anti-nutritional compounds, erucic acid in the oil and glucosinolates in the meal, creating a new, high-value oil and protein crop known as canola in Canada and the United States. Although rapeseed has been domestically grown since World War II, it gained wider interest only after canola oil was granted GRAS status in 1985. Canola is the Canadian Canola Association trademark which refers to any rapeseed with less than 2% of erucic acid (C22:1) in the oil and less than 30 µmol of the four major aliphatic glucosinolates in a gram of air dry solids. This definition will be changed in 1995 so the limit will be 15 µmol of glucosinolates. In addition to aliphatic glucosinolates, defatted rapeseed contains usually approximately 5 µmol/g of another group of glucosinolates called indolyls.

Double low rapeseed, as defined by European Community standards, has less than 35 µmol of total glucosinolates *tel quel*. This definition will also change in 1992 with only 20 µmol of total glucosinolates being allowed after 1992. This change will bring the European and Canadian definitions of canola very close to each other.

The term "industrial rapeseed" does not have any regulatory basis but refers to any rapeseed with a high content of erucic acid in the oil. For most purposes, the limit is 45%, although higher contents are considered desirable. The term "single low" refers to high glucosinolate rapeseed with low erucic oil. High erucic cultivars with low glucosinolate content also exist.

The estimated domestic need for canola oil in 1995 is one million tons. The domestic production of this would require 1 million to 2 million hectares. Increased interest in edible rapeseed production has also resulted in renewed interest in production of high erucic rapeseed for industrial purposes.

BOTANY

Rapeseed is derived from two *Brassica* species, *B. napus* L. and *B. rapa* L. To distinguish between them *B. rapa* is often called turnip rape and *B. napus* is called Swede rape. Spring and winter types exist of both species. The rapeseed oil of world commerce comes from these two species and to a minor extent also from the mustards, especially *B. juncea* Coss. (brown mustard) and *Sinapis alba*. L. (yellow mustard).

Taxonomy

In addition to *B. napus* L. and *B. rapa* L., *Brassica* includes cultivated species *B. carinata* Braun (Abyssinian mustard), *B. nigra* Koch, and *B. oleracea* L. The four most widely cultivated species, *B. juncea*, *B. napus*, *B. oleracea*, and *B. rapa* are highly polymorphic including oilseed crops, root crops, and vegetables such as Chinese cabbage, broccoli, and Brussel sprouts.

The relationships among the cultivated species were largely clarified by cytological work of Morinaga (1934). According to his hypothesis, the high chromosome number of species *B. napus* ($2n = 38$, AACC), *B. juncea* ($2n = 36$, AABB), and *B. carinata* ($2n = 34$, BBCC) are amphidiploids combining in pairs the chromosome sets of the low chromosome number species *B. nigra* ($2n = 16$, BB), *B. oleracea* ($2n = 18$, CC), and *B. rapa* ($2n = 20$, AA). This hypothesis was verified by U (1935) with successful re-synthesis of *B. napus*. Re-synthesis of *B. juncea* and *B. carinata* was accomplished later by Frandsen (1943, 1947). The low chromosome number species may have developed from ancestral species with even lower chromosome numbers as suggested by Robbelen (1960).

Origin

Brassica crops may be among the oldest cultivated plants known to man. In India, *B. rapa* is mentioned in ancient Sanskrit literature from ca. 1500 BC and seed of *B. juncea* have been found in archaeological sites dating back to ca. 2300 BC (Prakash 1980). Rapeseed production has a long history in China. The Chinese word for rapeseed was first recorded ca. 2500 years ago, and the oldest archaeological discoveries may date back as far as to ca. 5000 BC (Yan 1990).

Historically, *B. rapa* seems to have the widest distribution of Brassica oilseeds. At least 2000 years ago, it was distributed from northern Europe to China and Korea, with primary center of diversity in the Himalayan region (Hedge 1976).

Brassica napus has probably developed in the area where the wild forms of its ancestral species are sympatric, in the Mediterranean area. Wild forms of *B. napus* are unknown, so it is possible it originated in cultivation. Production of oilseed *B. napus* probably started in Europe during the middle-ages; *B. napus* was introduced to Asia during the 19th century. The present Chinese and Japanese germplasm was developed crossing European *B. napus* with different indigenous *B. rapa* cultivars (Shiga 1970).

DISTRIBUTION

World rapeseed production exceeds 20 million hectares, making it the third most important oil plant in the world after palm oil and soybean. The leading producers in 1991 were China, India, European Community, and Canada with estimated areas of 6.13, 6.10, 2.43, and 3.14 million hectares, respectively (Oil World Statistics Update 1992). The European Community figure includes only the major producers Denmark, France, Germany, and U.K. and would be somewhat higher if smaller producers such as Italy and Spain were included. Because of its high yields, European Community was the leading producer of rapeseed oil in 1991.

Winter type *B. napus* is the main rapeseed crop in most of Europe, in parts of China and also in the eastern United States. Spring type *B. napus* is produced in Canada, northern Europe, and China. Where winters are mild enough (e.g. southeastern United States) spring type *B. napus* can be grown in the fall. In the future we should see distinct varieties developed for these areas.

Spring type *B. rapa* occupies approximately 50% of the Canadian rapeseed area and is also grown in northern Europe, China, and India. Winter type *B. rapa* has largely been replaced by more productive winter type *B. napus* and spring crops in its traditional production areas and has no significant impact on the world's rapeseed production at the present.

Only spring types exist of *B. juncea*. It is the leading *Brassica* oilseed in India and also produced in Canada and Europe but only for condiment use. Recently, low erucic, low glucosinolate types of *B. juncea* have been developed and it is possible that in the future it will be an important oilseed crop for the more arid areas of Canada and the northern United States.

The transition from high erucic to low erucic rapeseed, and the simultaneous rapid growth in the global rapeseed production began in Canada in 1968, with commercial release of single low cultivar 'Oro' followed by several other single low cultivars and the first canola Cultivar 'Tower' in 1974. In Europe, the transition started later with the release of the first single low cultivars in 1974. Almost all rapeseed produced in Canada and Europe is canola. The introduction of low erucic rapeseed is now underway in China and India.

This change in crop quality has created a need for specialized production of industrial rapeseed. Improved cultivars for this purpose have been developed in Canada, the United States and now in Europe. Because of the relatively small demand for high erucic oil and, consequently, for industrial rapeseed in comparison with edible rapeseed, most plant breeders now work exclusively on canola. This has led to a shortage of competitive new industrial rapeseed cultivars and, consequently, complicated industrial rapeseed production further.

CULTURAL AND ENVIRONMENTAL REQUIREMENTS

Heat Tolerance

Rapeseed grows best in mild maritime climates. Historically, the highest rapeseed yields have been produced in England and the Netherlands, a phenomenon which has more to do with climate and soil conditions than sophisticated crop management.

The growth of rapeseed is most vigorous in temperatures between 10° and 30°C with the optimum around 20°C. Rapeseed is very sensitive to high temperatures at the blooming time even when ample moisture is available. Long periods of over 30°C can result in severe sterility and high yield losses. During the pod-filling period rapeseed is somewhat more tolerant to high temperatures. The seed oil content, however, is highest when the seeds mature under low temperatures (10° to 15°C). Extended periods of high temperature during the seed-fill period invariably result in low oil contents and poor seed quality.

Cold Tolerance

The rapeseed plant's ability to tolerate low temperatures depends essentially on its development and the degree of hardening it has achieved. Unhardened plants can survive −4°C, while fully-hardened spring type rapeseed can survive −10° to −12°C. Hardened winter rapeseed can survive short periods of exposure to temperatures between −15° and −20°C. Dehydration during sunny and/or windy days while the soil is frozen can cause extensive winter kill in much higher temperatures even when the plants are optimally developed and fully hardened.

The hardening requirements of rapeseed have not been fully characterized. Some time in temperatures below 10°C is, however, typically required. Winter types tend to harden faster, achieve higher degree of cold tolerance and unharden slower than spring types (Paul Raymer pers. commun.), but it is likely that variable hardening requirements could also be found within both types. Some differences in cold hardiness have been observed among both winter spring types. Whether these are due to differences in ultimate achievable cold hardiness or differences in hardening requirements only is unclear.

The plants are typically best adapted to survive the winter in rosette stage with 6 to 8 leaves. Smaller plants are usually not as capable of surviving over-wintering, while plants with more leaves often start the stem elongation prematurely, exposing the meristem tissue to cold, making it more susceptible to damage.

Unhardening happens fairly fast after the plants initiate active growth. Winter type rapeseed can generally still survive temperatures down to 12°C just before the blooming begins (Cramer 1990).

Winter survival is greatly reduced by environmental factors such as occurrence of diseases and pests, grazing, inadequate, excessive or unbalanced soil fertility, and poor drainage conditions. The absence of snow cover during the coldest period of the winter decreases the plants' chances to survive. Ice formation on the soil surface can damage the crown area of the plants and reduce survival rate.

Vernalization Requirement

Most winter rapeseed cultivars will require three weeks of near-freezing temperatures in the field to get fully vernalized and start rapid generative growth. In controlled environments, eight weeks at 4°C temperature is sufficient for full vernalization. In spring planting, winter rape will typically start slow generative growth after the prolonged rosette stage, and some cultivars may start blooming towards the end of the growing season. Differences in this respect are sometimes useful in distinguishing between similar cultivars. Differences in vernalization requirements are apparent among winter rape cultivars.

Some spring type cultivars do not exhibit any vernalization response at all, but in some cases the generative development can be accelerated with brief chilling treatment. In spring planting, only a few cool nights are usually needed for this. Vernalization response in spring types also tends to disappear in a long day environment (Raymer pers. commun.). In spite of the variability in vernalization requirements within both types, the differences between the types are fairly clear with no overlap in the initiation of blooming in either spring or fall planting.

A high vernalization requirement does not necessarily result in good winter hardiness, as many of the winter type cultivars from extreme maritime environments, such as Japan, require a long vernalization period yet have little tolerance for low temperatures.

Site Selection and Cultural Practices

Good drainage is an essential. Winter rape in particular has little tolerance for heavy, wet soils and a high water table. Wet soil can significantly reduce winter survival and contribute to root disease. Establishment of uniform stands is often difficult in heavy soils. Rapeseed grows best in sandy loams, loams with high organic matter, and loamy sands. Light soils are acceptable, and even ideal when adequate moisture and nutrients are available. Boron deficiency can cause significant yield losses even if no morphological deficiency symptoms are visible.

UTILIZATION OF THE PRODUCT

Canola oil

Well-developed rapeseed seed contains 40 to 44% oil. The fatty acid composition of the oil is genetically more variable than probably the composition of any other major vegetable oil. Canola oil today contains only traces of erucic acid, 5 to 8% of saturated fat, 60 to 65% of monounsaturated fats, and 30 to 35% of polyunsaturated fats. Mutants with significantly elevated monounsaturate levels exist.

Canola oil is widely used as cooking oil, salad oil, and making margarine. Of all edible vegetable oils widely available today, it has the lowest saturated fat content, making it appealing to health-conscious consumers. Its use in continuous frying and some other industrial uses is somewhat limited by its high linolenic acid (C18:3) content (usually 8 to 12%) and, consequent, fairly high oxidation tendency. Mutant materials with only 2 to 3% of linolenic have also been developed.

The use of canola oil in non-edible uses has been studied fairly extensively and it is at the present used to some extent in lubricants and hydraulic fluids especially when there is a significant risk of oil leaking to water ways or to ground water.

High Erucic Acid Rapeseed (HEAR) Oil

High erucic rapeseed oil is used in lubricants, especially where high heat stability is required. Because of its high polarity, uniform molecule size, and long carbon chains it has greater affinity to metal surfaces and better lubricity than mineral oils. It is easily biodegradable which makes it especially appealing in environmentally sensitive uses. Although HEAR oil in many applications is superior to vegetable oils with shorter average fatty acid chain length, such as canola, it can sometimes be replaced by these. The surplus of low erucic oil in European Community countries has especially increased industry's interest in Europe to use it in place of HEAR oil. This situation has also increased public interest in promoting the production of industrial rapeseed to lower the surpluses of low erucic rapeseed.

In the oleo–chemical, industry high erucic oil is used as a source of erucic acid to produce a slipping and anti-blocking agent used in plastic foils, foaming agents used for instance in mining industry, and many other chemicals for both food and non-food industries. The long chain length of erucic acid makes it a unique raw material in oleo chemical industry. Although in some oleo chemical processes it is virtually irreplaceable, the total demand for erucic acid is fairly low and not expected to grow radically in the near future. Most likely, growth rate is approximately equal with the general growth of oleo chemical industry, which again, as typical for mature industries, is likely to be approximately equal with the overall economic growth.

Significant changes to this scenario will depend on inventions and technical breakthroughs which defy prediction. There is, however, a trend visible that is likely to work in favor of increased use of high erucic oil in future, both in oleo chemical and other uses. The development of "green technology" with increased emphasis on renewable resources and biodegradability is likely to increase interest in raw materials such as high erucic oil.

Rapeseed Meal

Rapeseed meal contains approximately 40% of protein which rates among the nutritionally best plant proteins. For monogastric diets it has better amino acid balance than soybean meal.

In traditional rapeseed cultivars the seed solids contained over 100 µmol/g of glucosinolates. The hydrolysis products of glucosinolates give cruciferous vegetables their characteristic flavor and mustard it's pungency. Some of these hydrolysis products, however, are toxic or at least anti-nutritional. Also, many of the glucosinolate derivatives decrease the palatability of the meal and, consequently, the voluntary uptake of the feed by animals. For these reasons, the use of conventional rapeseed meal was limited mainly to cattle supplementary protein formulas and had relatively low value.

With the quality of canola, significant amounts of meal can be used in virtually all animal feeds and economical disposal of the crushing residue is typically not a problem. Since some of the glucosinolates are destroyed in the crushing process, the meal of future canola cultivars will be almost glucosinolate free and can be used in feed formulas without any special limitations.

PROSPECTS

Canola

The canola industry in the United States was created after 1985 when canola oil was granted GRAS status. At present, most major food processors are using canola oil. This year the estimated imports will reach 300,000 t, while the domestic production is approximately 50,000 t.

The estimated need for canola oil in the United States by 1995 is approximately one million tonnes. The domestic production of this would require 1 million to 4 million hectares of rapeseed, depending on the production areas and cultivar types. As the by-product of the oil approximately 1.5 million tonnes of rapeseed meal would be produced. If the meal is of canola quality it should be easily absorbed by animal feed industry without burdening the crush margins for canola.

High Erucic Acid Rapeseed (HEAR)

The present consumption of HEAR oil in the United States is approximately 10,000 to 15,000 t/year. Dramatic changes in consumption are not likely to occur in the near future, although steady growth can be expected. Even if all HEAR oil will be produced domestically, and only using rapeseed, high erucic rapeseed will not develop into a major field crop in the foreseeable future, but it will remain a specialty crop for limited productions areas.

Specialty Oils

Several biotechnology companies are working to develop rapeseed with altered seed composition. Potential products could include crops which will replace foreign sources of oils and fatty acids or even produce chemicals currently for which economical plant sources are not available. The impact of these developments on the total rapeseed production is unpredictable, but it is possible that if at least some of these projects are successful, specialty rapeseed in the future will have at least as much area in the United States as canola.

Adaptation

Since little breeding work was done in the United States prior to 1985, production has mainly been based on imported cultivars, although the cultivar 'Cascade' from the University of Idaho has been grown to some extent in the Midwest and Pacific Northwest. In the summer of 1990, two cultivars 'A112' and 'A114' from Calgene/Ameri-Can's breeding program were also introduced to the market in the Southeast and have since been widely accepted to production.

Early Canadian spring types, both *B. napus* and *B. rapa,* can be produced in the northern tier states, although aridity and high summer temperatures will set limits to their adaptation. The best production areas will probably be in the western and eastern ends of the range which form the southern extensions of the "Canola Crescent" of the Canadian prairies. European winter rapeseed cultivars can also be grown successfully in the Pacific Northwest in the areas where winters are not too harsh and adequate fall moisture is available.

The Midwest, extending from central Indiana and Ohio to Central Michigan, may be the best region for the production of European type winter rapeseed cultivars, although they can be produced profitably as far south as northern Georgia. Further south, these cultivars do not reach adequate vernalization but will be extremely late if they produce any generative growth at all.

In the Great Plains area, rapeseed could possibly be grown in at least Texas, Oklahoma and parts of Kansas. Production has, to-date, suffered from multiple problems. Because of the extreme summer heat only winter rapeseed can be grown, yet the winter hardiness of present winter rape cultivars are only marginal for the region. Even if winter survival can be improved to some extent with proper cultural methods, significant genetic improvement is needed before rapeseed can be introduced to wide scale production in the Great Plains. Cultivars for this area need to be earlier than what is presently available to avoid the hot, dry summer weather which will ripen the plant prematurely and also cause extensive shattering losses.

In the Southeast, rapeseed has been very successful in the southern parts of Georgia and also in South Carolina. European spring type cultivars are well adapted to winter production in this area. Most of them have adequate winter hardiness and since they typically start blooming somewhat later than Canadian cultivars, they mostly escape the damage from spring frosts. There are regions in the Southeast where winter and spring types produce very similar yields. In those areas, however, spring cultivars typically will mature 10 to 14 days before winter cultivars and may be more appealing to producers for this reason.

Although imported cultivars have so far been fairly successful, the development of domestic, regionally-focused breeding programs is very important for the growth of rapeseed industry in the United States. In introducing rapeseed to double-cropping rotations, the lack of a high-yielding, early-maturing winter type has been a problem, and suitable cultivars need to be developed in America. It is likely that differences in cropping systems and climate will ultimately give domestic breeding programs an advantage. Imported cultivars will gradually disappear from the market once rapeseed gets established and the germplasm development in the United States starts producing results.

The development of pest and disease management strategies and availability of suitable chemicals and/or resistant cultivars is also an important factor affecting the acceptance of rapeseed to production in the United States. Diseases such as white mold, black spot, and blackleg have caused significant damage in some areas. Although the incidences have so far been isolated, the disease problem can only grow worse as production expands unless control methods become available. Cabbage seed pod weevil has established itself as a major problem in areas where rapeseed has several years of history in cultivation, and other insect pests are likely to emerge.

REFERENCES

Cramer, N. 1990. Raps Zuchtung-Anbau and Vermarktung von Kormerraps. Ulmer, Stuttgart.

Frandsen, K.J. 1943. The experimental formation of *Brassica juncea* Czern. et. Coss. Dansk Bot. Arkiv 11(4):1–17.

Frandsen, K.J. 1947. (Plant Breeding Sta., Taastrup, Denmark) The experimental formation of *Brassica napus* L. var. oleifera DC. and *Brassica carinata* Braun. Dansk Bot. Arkiv. 12(7):1–16.

Hedge, I.C. 1976. A systematic and geographical survey of the world cruciferae, p. 1–45. In: J.G. Vaughan, A.J. MacLeod and B.M.G. Jones (eds.). The biology and chemistry of Cruciferae. Academic Press, New York.

Hemmingway, J.S. 1976. Mustards: *Brassica* spp. and *Sinapis alba* (Cruciferae), p. 56–59. In: N.W. Simmons (ed.). Evolution of crop plants. Longman, London.

Morinaga, T. 1934. Interspecific hybridization in *Brassica*. The cytology of F_1 hybrids of *B. juncea* and *B. nigra*. Cytologia 6(1):62–67.

Oil World Statistics Update, 1992, 1 World p.151. ISTA, Hamburg.

Prakash, S. 1980. Cruciferous oilseeds in India, p. 151–163. In: S. Tsunoda, K. Hinata, and C. Gomez-Campo (eds.). Brassica crops and wild allies. Biology and Breeding. Japan Scient. Soc. Press, Tokyo.

Robbelen, G. 1960. Beitrage zur Analyse des Brassica-Genoms. Chromosoma 11:205–228.

Shiga, T. 1970. Rape breeding by interspecific crossing between *Brassica napus* and *Brassica campestris* in Japan. Japan Agr. Res. Quart. 5:5–10.

U, N. 1935. Genome analysis in *Brassica* with special reference to the experimental formation of *Brassica napus* and peculiar mode of fertilization. Japan. J. Bot. 7:389–452.

Yan, Z. 1990. Overview of rapeseed production and research in China. Proc. Int. Canola Conf. Potash & Phosphate Institute, Atlanta. p. 29–35.

Evaluation of Seven Species of Oilseeds as Spring Planted Crops for the Pacific Northwest

D.L. Auld, R.M. Gareau, and M.K. Heikkinen

Commercial production of oilseed crops in the Pacific Northwest region of the United States could tap both export and domestic markets for canola oil and high erucic acid industrial oils (Auld et al. 1980). Spring rapeseed and canola (*Brassica napus* L. or *B. campestris* L.) have had poor stand establishment caused by flea beetle (*Phyllotreta* spp.) feeding on young seedlings (Auld et al. 1977, 1978, 1980; Kephart et al. 1988). Even fields with good plant establishment have often yielded less than 1,000 kg/ha due to heat stress during flowering and seed fill. Damage caused by two species of aphids [cabbage aphid, *Brevicoryne brassicae* (L.) and turnip aphid, *Liaphis erysimis* (Kraft.)] have also reduced seed yields of spring rapeseed crops in this region. These factors have historically made production of spring rapeseed economically uncompetitive. The purpose of these studies was to identify exotic species of oilseed crops that produce higher seed yields in this region due to tolerance to environmental factors and plant pests.

During 1988 and 1989, seven species of *Brassica* and a single species of *Eruca* (*E. sativa* L.) were evaluated to determine if they were adapted to the Mediterranean climate of the Pacific Northwest. These species have been grown as oilseed crops in Europe, Asia, or Africa (Downey 1966; Downey and Robbelen 1989). The agronomic potential and genetic diversity of current germplasm accessions of three of the most promising species were evaluated in a series of trials during the 1989 and 1990 growing seasons.

METHODOLOGY

Species Evaluation, 1988 and 1989

Five accessions were randomly selected from the University of California–Davis (UCD) germplasm collection to represent each of the seven species: *Brassica hirta* Moench (*Sinapis alba* L.), *B. carinata* A. Braun, *B. nigra* (L.) Koch, *B. campestris* L., *B. tournefortii* (Gouan), *B. juncea* (L.) Cross, and *Eruca sativa* L. The UCD germplasm collection was made by Paul Knowles and is one of the most extensive currently available. Only five accessions were utilized in the initial screening experiments since the primary objective of the research was a more intensive evaluation of the most promising species. Individual plots consisted of two rows spaced 15 cm apart. The field plots were 2.4 m in length in 1988 and 4.2 m in 1989. The study had three replications in both years and used a split-plot design with species assigned as main plots and accessions within a species randomized as subplots. Plots were planted on 1 m centers with a planter equipped with double disc openers and packing wheels to ensure firm soil contact around the small seeds.

The 1988 study was sown on Apr. 27 at Moscow, Idaho, in a field in which spring peas (*Pisum sativum* L.) had been green manured the previous year. No additional fertilizer was applied. Flea beetle control required applications of 1.7 kg/ha of carbaryl (1-naphthyl N-methyl-carbamate) on May 14 and 1.7 kg/ha of permethrin [3-(phenoxphenyl) methyl (1RS)-cis,trans-3-(2,2-dichloroethenyl)-2,2-dimethyl cyclopropane carboxylate] on May 24 and June 13. Aphids were controlled by a single application of 1.4 kg/ha malathion (diethyl mercaptosuccinate, S-ester with 0,0-dimethyl phosphorodithioate) on July 12.

The 1989 study was sown on Apr. 26 in a field in Moscow, Idaho, which had produced a barley (*Hordeum vulgare* L.) crop the previous year. Nitrogen (76 kg/ha) was applied as ammonium nitrate (34–0–0) prior to planting. In 1989, flea beetles were controlled by applications of 2.5 kg/ha of carbaryl on May 19, May 22, June 1, and June 5. Aphids were controlled by applying 1.4 kg/ha of malathion on July 5 and July 13.

Oil yield (%) was determined using a Newport MKIIIA Nuclear Magnetic Resonance (NMR) instrument on 12 g of oven-dried, open-pollinated seed obtained from each plot. The NMR was calibrated using the cultivar 'Bridger' as a standard and all samples were analyzed with a 32 sec integration period.

Fatty acid composition was determined by the on 0.5 g of open pollinated seed. Oil was extracted from the ground seed using 4 ml of anhydrous ethyl ether. The oil solution was taken up in a syringe using a synthetic cotton

Table 1. Seed yield, seed weight, and oil content averaged over five accessions from six species of *Brassica* and a single species of *Erucal* during 1988 and 1989 at Moscow, Idaho.

Species (common name)	Seed yield (Mg/ha)			Oil content (%)			Seed weight (g/100)		
	1988	1989	Avg	1988	1989	Avg	1988	1989	Avg
B. hirta Moench. (white or yellow mustard)	2.1	3.5	2.8	22.7	27.7	25.2	0.49	0.51	0.50
B. carnita A. Braun (Abyssinian mustard)	1.1	2.5	1.8	25.6	33.6	29.5	0.49	0.38	0.39
B. nigra (L,) Koch (black mustard)	1.2	1.9	1.6	25.8	33.7	29.8	0.21	0.17	0.19
B. juncea (L.) Cross (brown, Oriental, or Indian mustard)	0.8	2.0	1.2	26.8	34.1	30.5	0.34	0.38	0.39
Eruca sativa L. (rocket salad)	0.7	1.6	1.2	26.5	30.7	28.6	0.31	0.20	0.25
B. tournefortii (Gouan) (wild mustard)	0.6	1.6	1.1	25.9	31.8	28.8	0.24	0.24	0.24
B. campestris L. (birdsrape mustard or Polish rape)	0.7	1.2	0.9	29.6	35.9	32.8	0.34	0.34	0.34
LSD (P = 0.05)	1.1	1.2		2.3	4.3		0.18	0.06	

Table 2. Flowering date, seed yield, and oil content of ten cultivars of mustard grown at Moscow Idaho in 1989 and 1990.

Cultivar	Species	Flowering date Julian		Seed yield (Mg/ha)		Oil content (%)	
		1989	1990	1989	1990	1989	1990
CJ 86/Z	*B. juncea*	172	---	4.3	---	35.2	---
Common Brown	*B. juncea*	172	180	4.1	1.5	34.0	30.8
Tilney	*B. hirta*	169	180	3.9	1.5	27.3	22.4
CW 89 TY	*B. hirta*	170	180	3.9	1.7	30.9	23.1
Blaze	*B. juncea*	172	180	3.9	0.3	33.7	29.4
Cutlass	*B. juncea*	168	178	3.8	1.7	36.2	31.7
ZEM-87-1	*B. juncea*	171	---	3.8	---	34.8	---
Lethbridge 22-A	*B. juncea*	170	177	3.7	1.4	35.5	31.1
Ochre	*B. hirta*	168	173	3.6	2.0	28.4	23.4
Gisilba	*B. hirta*	169	173	3.5	1.8	28.0	23.2
Average		171	179	3.9	1.2	34.9	30.8
LSD (P = 0.05)		1.8	1.8	0.4	0.4	2.4	0.8

ball as a filter and mixed with 200 µl of 20% tetramethylammonium hydroxide in methanol. The sample was shaken and allowed to settle for 1 min before 2 ml of distilled water was added. The sample was again shaken and allowed to settle to form an immersion layer. A 1 µl sample of the upper immersion layer was injected by a Varian model 8000 Autosampler into a Varian Model 3700 Gas Chromatograph (GC) equipped with a flame ionization detector with a Supelco 3.05 m glass column containing 3% SP-2310 and 2% SP-2300 on a 100/120 mesh chromasorb WAW support. Helium was used as the carrier gas, and the column was maintained at 220°C. Injector and detector temperatures were maintained at 250° and 300°C, respectively. A Varian Model 4290 integrator was used to determine relative concentrations of the major fatty acids by integration of total area under each curve. A rapeseed standard prepared by Supelco (Cat. No. 4-7019) was used as the control to identify the retention time of each of the seven major fatty acid found in rapeseed and run as every 20th sample.

Mustard Cultivar Trial, 1989 and 1990

Seed of several commercial several mustard cultivars was obtained from the Canadian cooperative mustard trial. The 1989 trial contained six commercial cultivars of *B. juncea* and four commercial cultivars of *B. hirta* and was planted on Apr. 26 at Moscow, Idaho using the same procedures as the *Brassica* species evaluation study with the following exceptions. Field plots contained six rows 5.2 m in length. Rows were spaced 15 cm apart and plots were planted on 1.2 m centers using a randomized complete block design with four replications.

The 1990 trial contained four commercial cultivars of *B. juncea* and four commercial cultivars of *B. hirta* and was planted on 20 Apr. in a field which had been fallowed the previous year. This study was fertilized with 90 kg/ha of nitrogen applied as urea (45-0-0) prior to planting. The six row plots were 4.7 m in length. Rows were spaced 15 cm apart and plots were planted on 1.5 m centers using a randomized complete block design with four replications. The seed was treated with carbofuran (2,3-dihydro-2,2-dimethyl-7-benzofuranyl methylcarbamate) at the rate of 2.8 kg/ha to provide flea beetle control but plots also required applications of 1.7 kg/ha of phosmet N-(mercapto-methyl)-phthalimide S-(0-0-dimethylphosphorod-ithioate) on May 17 and on June 15. Aphids were controlled by applying 1.4 kg/ha of malathion on July 17.

Germplasm Evaluation, 1989 and 1990

The 1989 germplasm evaluation of *B. hirta* contained 156 accessions and two spring rapeseed cultivars and used the procedures described for the other 1989 studies with the following exceptions. Individual plots consisted of two rows spaced 15 cm apart and 3.5 m in length. Plots were planted on 1.0 m centers using a randomized complete block design with two replications at Moscow, Idaho.

In 1990 the *B. hirta* accessions were evaluated in two trials. The two row plots contained 31 accessions and the six row plots had 28 accessions of *B. hirta* and three commercial cultivars of rapeseed. Both trials were planted on Apr. 19, 1990 using the same procedures described for the 1990 mustard cultivar trial.

The 1990, germplasm evaluation of *B. juncea* which contained trial of 383 accessions and nine commercial cultivars of *B. juncea* was planted on Apr. 18 in Moscow, Idaho. The field had produced oats (*Avena sativa* L.) the previous year. Individual plots consisted of two rows and the trial had two replications. The field was fertilized with 112 kg/ha of nitrogen and weed control was achieved with applications of 1.8 liters/ha of trifluralin (α,α,α-trifluoro-2,6-dinitro-N,N-dipropyl-p-toluidine) and 2.9 liters/hg of triallate [S-(2,3,-Trichloroallyl) diisopropylthiocarbamate].

The 1990 evaluation of *B. carinata* germplasm was unreplicated and contained 160 accessions, that were planted on Apr. 19. This study was planted and maintained using the same procedures described for the other 1990 trials.

RESULTS AND DISCUSSIONS

Species Evaluation, 1989 and 1990

The seven species produced seed yields which ranged from 1.1 to 2.8 Mg/ha averaged over both the 1988 and 1989 studies (Table 1). The *B. hirta* accessions produced the highest average seed yields in both years of the study. The average oil contents of the seven species ranged from 32.8% for *B. campestris* to only 25.2% for *B. hirta*. Largest seed were produced by *B. hirta* accessions and smallest seed by *B. nigra* (L.) Koch accessions.

The 35 individual accessions had average seed yields which ranged from 0.5 to more than 3.5 Mg/ha. In both years, the *B. hirta* accessions UCD 79 and UCD 1272 produced the highest average seed yields. These accessions also had low levels of oil and relatively large seed size. Commercial seed yields of rapeseed or canola must exceed 2.2 Mg/ha to be economically competitive with other spring planted crops currently grown in the Pacific Northwest. Both the species and individual accessions within a species showed significant variation for both oil content and seed size in this trial.

Mustard Cultivar Trial, 1989 and 1990

This trial evaluated commercial cultivars currently grown on the prairie provinces of Western Canada for their potential adaption to the Pacific Northwest. Seed yield of the mustards in 1989 ranged from 3.5 to 4.3 Mg/ha and oil contents ranged from 27.3 to 36.2% (Table 2). Generally, the commercial cultivars of *B. juncea* (brown or oriental mustard) produced higher seed yields and oil contents than the varieties of *B. hirta* (white or yellow mustard).

Seed yield of the eight cultivars included in the 1990 trial ranged from 0.3 to 2.0 Mg/ha (Table 2). The cultivar 'Blaze' had the lowest yield and very poor stand establishment, indicative of poor quality seed. Oil contents of the cultivars ranged from 22.4 to 31.7%. In the very dry conditions of 1990, *B. hirta* produced the highest seed yield, but the average oil content of the *B. juncea* was 7.7% higher.

Many of the cultivars of the two species of mustard currently grown in Canada produced excellent crops in the Mediterranean climate of the Pacific Northwest. This indicates that crops of condiment mustard could be grown commercially in this area if sufficient market could be identified. Finite markets for condiment mustard have historically limited Canadian production (Downey et al. 1975). Because of the relatively small markets for condiment mustard, larger markets could be tapped if mustard cultivars were developed that could be utilized as oilseed crops. Incorporation of high oil content, low levels of glucosinolates, and specific fatty acid composition into these two species could allow widespread commercial production of spring mustard in the Pacific Northwest.

Germplasm Evaluation, 1989 and 1990

The 1989 evaluation of 156 accessions of *B. hirta* produced seed yields which ranged from 0.5 to 4.8 Mg/ha and averaged 2.3 Mg/ha (Fig. 1). The two spring rapeseed cultivars used as controls in this trial, 'Tobin' (*B. campestris*) and 'Reston' (*B. napus*) had seed yields of only 0.9 and 0.6 mg/ha. Twenty three of the *B. hirta* accessions produced seed yields in excess of 3.0 Mg/ha indicative of the very high seed yield potential of this species of mustard. Oil contents of the accessions ranged from 21.8 to 32.6% and averaged only 28.7% (Fig. 2). Under the same conditions, oil contents for 'Tobin' was 35.2% and 39.5% for 'Reston'.

The two 1990 trials of *B. hirta* differed in relative seed yield, reflecting the inflated yield potential often observed in the smaller two row plots (Fig. 1). The two row plots had average seed yields of 3.5 Mg/ha while the six row plots grown nearby had average seed yields of only 1.0 Mg/ha. Seven accessions from the replicated six row plots produced in excess of 1.4 Mg/ha despite the extremely dry weather observed during the summer of 1990. Cultivars which produce high seed yields under the dry conditions experienced in July and August in the Pacific Northwest will need to be developed if commercial production of spring mustard is to be successful. Oil content of all the *B. hirta* accessions evaluated in 1990 were less than 33%.

As measured by the Tes-Tape procedure (Downey et al. 1975), glucosinolate levels showed a wide range of variation (Fig. 3). The two lines with the lowest Tes-Tape scores, BHLG-3553 and GHLG-3568, were obtained from Keith Downey of Agriculture Canada at Saskatoon, Saskatchewan. These lines had levels of glucosinolates that slightly exceeded the maximum level allowed in canola cultivars. Fatty acid composition of 35 select lines *B. hirta* showed a wide range of variation. Four of the lines obtained from Agriculture Canada had less than 8% erucic acid, but canola oils marketed in the United States must have less than 2% erucic acid as required by the Food and Drug Administration. This indicates that additional selection will be necessary to improve both the meal and the oil if *B. hirta* is to be developed as an economically competitive oilseed crop.

The 383 accessions and nine commercial cultivars of *B. juncea* evaluated in 1990 produced seed yields which ranged from 0.3 to 10.3 Mg/ha (Fig. 4). Four accessions, 72-525, 'Common Brown' ('ComBrown'), 77-18, and 'Juzanka', produced excellent seed yields and appeared to be well adapted to the Pacific Northwest. Oil contents of the *B. juncea* accessions and cultivars ranged from 28.6 to 41.1% (Fig. 5). Only two accessions, 'Jubileja' and 77-978, had greater than 40% oil content indicating that commercial cultivars of *B. juncea* would need to be selected for this important trait if this crop were to be grown as an oilseed crop.

Canadian researchers have recently developed *B. juncea* germplasm with low levels of glucosinolates and low levels of erucic acid (Love et al. 1990). These traits are being incorporated into commercial cultivars to allow expanded canola oil production in the drier regions of western Canada. Incorporation of these traits into the higher yielding accessions identified in this study could allow rapid development of oilseed cultivars adapted to the Pacific Northwest.

Even in small plots, only eleven accessions of *B. carinata* produced seed yields which exceeded 2.0 Mg/ha (data not presented). Oil content of these accessions ranged from 22.1 to 34.6%, indicating that additional improvement would be needed in the oil content of this species to allow commercial production. Additional

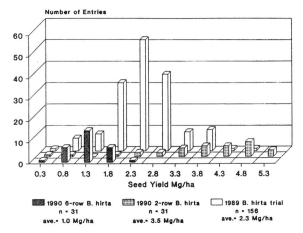

Fig. 1. Seed yield of 156 accessions of *B. hirta* evaluated in 1989 and 59 accessions evaluated in either two row or six row plots in 1990 at Moscow, ID.

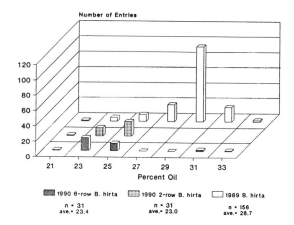

Fig. 2. Oil content of 156 accessions of *B. hirta* evaluated in 1989 and 59 accessions evaluated in two trials in 1990 at Moscow, ID.

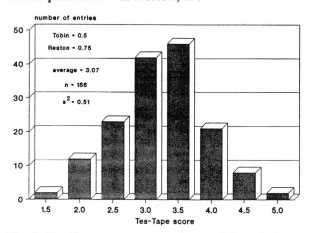

Fig. 3. Tes-Tape scores as an estimate of glucosinolate content of 156 accessions of *B. hirta* and two commercial cultivars of rapeseed evaluated in 1989 at Moscow, ID.

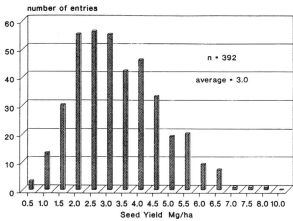

Fig. 4. Seed yield of 383 accessions and nine commercial cultivars of *B. juncea* evaluated in 1990 at Moscow, ID.

Fig. 5. Oil content of 383 accessions and nine commercial cultivars of *B. juncea* evaluated in 1990 at Moscow, ID.

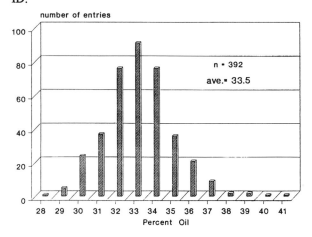

312

evaluation of *B. carinata* for the Pacific Northwest is not planned at this time since other species show more potential for this area.

SUMMARY AND CONCLUSIONS

Experiments conducted in 1988 and 1989 at Moscow, Idaho indicated that two species, *B. hirta* and *B. juncea*, have the best potential to be developed as spring planted oilseed crops in the Pacific Northwest. However, for these species to be grown as commercial crops, cultivars must be developed which combine their high seed yield potential with specific quality characteristics. Oilseed cultivars of these species would need oil contents exceeding 40% and produce either edible (canola) oils with less than 2% erucic acid or industrial oils with more than 55% erucic acid. These cultivars would also need to produce meals containing less than 30 µmol/g of defatted meal to ensure full economic value of the seed. The ability of these species to tolerate insects, diseases, heat stress, and drought would allow the commercial product of spring mustard as an oilseed crop across much of the Pacific Northwest and the Northern Plains States.

In our studies, *B. hirta* had excellent agronomic potential but currently available cultivars and accessions had low oil contents, high levels of glucosinolates, and intermediate levels of erucic acid in the oil. Selection of canola and industrial quality cultivars of *B. hirta* would allow expanded production of this drought and pest tolerant species. *Brassica hirta* (*Sinapis alba* L.) is grown as white mustard on about 57,000 ha annually in Canada for use as condiment mustard (Downey and Robbelen 1989). This species has shown tolerance to both flea beetles and selected species of aphids (Lamb 1980; Putman 1977). White mustard can tolerate drought and high temperatures during flowering and seed fill (Downey 1966; Downy et al. 1975). Selected accessions of *B. hirta* have been reported to have oil contents which exceed 42% (Persson 1986). Erucic acid levels have ranged from about 5 to 55%. All existing accessions have had relatively high levels of glucosinolates which reduces the quality of the meal residue remaining after oil extraction. Since most commercial cultivars of this species were developed for production of condiment mustard, only limited selection has been practiced on characteristics need as an oilseed crop.

Brassica juncea has been grown as brown or Oriental mustard on about 85,000 ha annually in Canada (Downey 1966; Downy and Robbelen 1989). This highly drought tolerant species originated in the Middle East but has been widely grown across Europe, Asia, and Africa (Downey 1966; Downey et al. 1975). In our studies, this species has produced good seed yields and oil contents which can approach 40%. Researchers in Canada recently reported the development of experimental lines of *B. juncea* which produce canola quality seed. Commercial cultivars of oilseed *B. juncea* should be available within three to five years (Love et al. 1990). Incorporation of these quality characteristics into adapted accessions could allow rapid development of oilseed cultivars adapted to the northern United States.

The rapeseed program at the University of Idaho will continue to evaluate accessions of both *B. hirta* and *B. juncea* for both agronomic potential and oilseed quality over the next few years. Lines with promising characteristics will be hybridized and segregating lines selected for both agronomic potential and oilseed quality. The development of improved cultivars which combine high seed yield potential with specific fatty acid composition and low levels of glucosinolates would allow expanded production of spring planted *Brassica* species as oilseed crops across the Pacific Northwest.

REFERENCES

Auld, D.L., G.A. Murray, E.F. Mink, and B.W. Studer. 1977. Alternative crops for Northern Idaho. CIS 380. Univ. of Idaho, Moscow.

Auld, D.L., G.A. Murray, J.A. Benson, E.F. Mink, C.G. Van Slyke, and B.W. Studer. 1978. Alternate crops for Northern Idaho—1977. Prog. Rpt. 203. Univ. of Idaho, Moscow.

Auld, D.L., G.A. Murray, G.G. Carnahan, J.A. Benson, and B.W. Studer. 1980. Flax, mustard, spring rape: alternative crops for Idaho's cooler regions? CIS 524. Univ. of Idaho, Moscow.

Downey, R.K. 1966. Rapeseed botany, production and utilization. In: Rapeseed meal for livestock and poultry. Can. Dept. Agr. Publ.

Downey, R.K., G.R. Stringam, D.I. McGregor, and B.R. Stefansson. 1975. Breeding rapeseed and mustard crops, p. 157–183. In: J.T. Harapials (ed.). Oilseed and pulse crops in Western Canada. Western Co-op. Fert. Limited. Calgary, Alberta.

Downey, R.K. and G. Robbelen. 1989. Brassica species. In: G. Robbelen, R.K. Downey, and A. Ashri (eds.). Oil crops of the world. McGraw-Hill, New York.

Kephart, K.D., M.E. Rice, J.P. McCaffery, and G.A. Murray. 1988. Spring rapeseed culture in Idaho. Bul. 681. Univ. of Idaho, Moscow.

Lamb, R.J. 1980. Hairs protect pods of mustard (*Brassica hirta*) 'Gisilba' from flea beetle feeding damage. Can. J. Plant Sci. 60:1439–1440.

Love, H.K., G. Rakow, J.P. Raney, and R.K. Downey. 1990. Genetic control of 2-propenyl and 3-butenyl glucosinolate synthesis in mustard. Can. J. Plant Sci. 70:425–429.

Persson, C. 1986. High erucic oil from white mustard (*Sinapis alba* L.) for technical use. Cruciferae Newsletter 11:134.

Putman, L.G. 1977. Response of four *Brassica* seed crop species to attach by the Crucifer flea beetle, *Phyllotreta cruciferae*. Can. J. Plant Sci. 57:987–989.

Camelina: A Promising Low-Input Oilseed

D.H. Putnam, J.T. Budin, L.A. Field, and W.M. Breene

The production of edible oil from crops has enjoyed unremitting growth during the latter part of the 20th century. In a six year period in the 1980s, a 26% increase in production of oils from ten oilseeds was realized. Much of this growth has been in tropical oils (oil palm, *Elaeis guinensis* L.) or high quality (low saturated fat) edible oils such as soybean [*Glycine max* (L.) Merr.], canola (*Brassica napus* L.), and sunflower (*Helianthus annuus* L.). This trend shows no signs of relenting. The demand for edible oils is increasing most in the heavily populated regions of South Asia, China, and the Far East, where vegetable oils are an important part of the diet, but demand for meal and oil is also high in the European and American markets and the Commonwealth of Independent States.

The development of soybean, sunflower, and canola, the three most significant edible oils for temperate climates, represent important new crop successes (Robinson 1973; Hymowitz 1990; Downey 1990). It is likely that these crops will continue to expand in hectarage, given increasing demand for high quality edible oils and meals, the wide adaptation of these crops, and new, improved cultivars. However, each of these major oilseeds has its limitations. For example, soybean, though ideal for most regions of the corn belt, is not well adapted to more northerly regions of North America, Europe, and Asia. Canola and sunflower are better adapted to northern climates but have high nitrogen requirements (especially canola), and are susceptible to insect or bird predation as well as diseases. These oilseed crops are not often suitable to marginal lands (low moisture, low fertility, or saline soils). In recent years, there has been increasing interest in developing agronomic systems with low requirements for fertilizer, pesticides, and energy, and which provide better soil erosion control than conventional systems (NRC 1989). This led us to examine the viability of developing camelina as an oilseed with reduced input requirements and as a crop well suited to marginal soils, or soil- and resource-conserving agronomic practices.

DESCRIPTION & ADAPTATION

Camelina sativa (L.) Crantz., Brassicaceae (falseflax, linseed dodder, or gold-of-pleasure) originated in the Mediterranean to Central Asia. It is an annual or winter annual that attains heights of 30 to 90 cm tall (Fig. 1) and has branched smooth or hairy stems that become woody at maturity. Leaves are arrow-shaped, sharp-pointed, 5 to 8 cm long with smooth edges. It produces prolific small, pale yellow or greenish-yellow flowers with 4 petals. Seed pods are 6 to 14 mm long and superficially resemble the bolls of flax. Seeds are small (0.7 mm × 1.5 mm), pale yellow-brown, oblong, rough, with a ridged surface. Morphology and distribution of camelina species has been described by Polish and Russian botanists (Mirek 1981). Camelina has been shown to be allelopathic (Grummer 1961; Lovett and Duffield 1981).

Camelina is listed as being adapted to the flax-growing regions of the northern Midwest (Minnesota, North Dakota, South Dakota) (NC-121 1981). It is primarily a minor weed in flax and not often a problem in other crops and does not have seed dormancy (Robinson 1987). However, the adaptation of camelina as a crop has not been widely explored. Similar to the other Cruciferous species, it is likely best adapted to cooler climates where excessive heat during flowering is not important. There are several winter annual biotypes available in the germplasm, and it is possible that camelina could be grown as a winter crop in areas with very mild winters. Camelina is short-seasoned (85 to 100 d) so that it could be incorporated into double cropping systems during cool periods of growth, possibly in more tropical environments.

AGRICULTURAL HISTORY

Although camelina is known in North America primarily as a weed, it was known as "gold of pleasure" to ancient European agriculturists. Cultivation probably began in Neolithic times, and by the Iron Age in Europe when the number of crop plants approximately doubled, camelina was commonly used as an oil-supplying plant (Knorzer 1978). Cultivation, as evidenced from carbonized seed, has been shown to occur in regions surrounding the North Sea during the Bronze Age. Camelina monocultures occurred in the Rhine River Valley as early as 600 BC Camelina probably spread in mixtures with flax and as monocultures, similarly to small grains, which also often spread as crop mixtures. It was cultivated in antiquity from Rome to southeastern Europe and the Southwestern Asian steppes (Knorzer 1978).

Camelina declined as a crop during medieval times due to unknown factors, but continued to coevolve as a weed with flax, which probably accounts for its introduction to the Americas. Like rapeseed oil, camelina oil has been used as an industrial oil after the industrial revolution. The seeds have been fed to caged birds, and the straw used for fiber. There have been scattered hectarages in Europe in modern times, mostly in Germany, Poland, and the USSR, and some efforts were made in the 1980s at germplasm screening and plant breeding (Enge and Olsson 1986; Seehuber and Dambroth 1983; Seehuber and Dambroth 1984: Kartamyshev 1985). Camelina has been evaluated to some extent in Canada (Downey 1971) and to a larger extent in Minnesota where R.G. Robinson conducted agronomic studies on camelina (Robinson 1987). However, there has been relatively little research conducted on this crop worldwide, and its full agronomic and breeding potential remains largely unexplored.

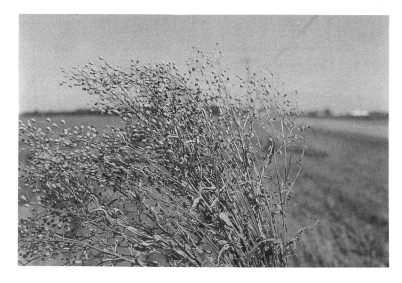

Fig. 1. Camelina plant nearing maturity. Camelina superficially resembles flax.

UNIQUE AGRONOMIC QUALITIES

Yield Potential

Field studies on camelina have been conducted at the University of Minnesota for over 30 years (Robinson 1987). In one 9-year/location yield comparison, camelina was shown to have a yield potential similar to that of many other Cruciferae (Table 1), but it differed in seed size, maturity, lodging resistance, and oil percentage. Yields of camelina cultivars (Table 2) have been in the 600 to 1,700 kg/ha range at Rosemount, Minnesota (45° N latitude), averaging about 1,100 to 1,200 kg/ha over many years of trials. It should be noted that the yield of many of these oilseeds (especially *B. napus*) has been improved significantly through plant breeding and improved agronomic practices, whereas camelina has largely not had the benefit of plant breeding. Under Minnesota conditions, yields of all spring-sown cruciferous oilseeds are much higher at more northerly locations (1,736 kg/ha long term average canola yield—Roseau, Minnesota), compared with yields at Rosemount, which is located near St. Paul. Camelina is much smaller seeded and earlier maturing than the other cruciferae tested. Lodging was comparable to or fact slightly superior to the other cruciferae oilseeds tested (Table 1), and there was significant variation for lodging among camelina varieties (Table 2).

Some variation in camelina maturity, lodging resistance, seed weight, and oil percentage was exhibited by the lines tested and by other germplasm screening not reported here, but many of these lines were similar in yield at Rosemount (Table 2). Certainly increases in yield might be generated through plant breeding. German plant breeders using the single-seed descent method, have found transgressions over parental lines in many yield traits for camelina, demonstrating both the high yield potential and capacity for yield improvement in this species (Seehuber et al. 1987). This experience indicates that camelina, unlike some wild species undergoing domestication, exhibits yield potential and oil content which are both currently agronomically acceptable and amenable to improvement through plant breeding.

Winter Seeding

The practice of broadcasting camelina seed on frozen ground in late November or early December has been tested over a number of years at Rosemount, and the practice appears to be viable (Table 3). In one four-year study, crops were sown with standard farm machinery on large plots. Camelina was sown in late fall on stubble, without seedbed preparation or herbicides, or conventionally in the spring and compared with flax sown conventionally and sprayed with herbicides (dalapon and MCPA). Performance of winter-sown camelina was equal or superior to conventionally-sown flax in these studies.

To confirm these results, a separate two-year study was conducted where camelina and flax were surface-seeded by hand in both winter and spring on tilled or stubble ground, broadcast or by machine without herbicides (Table 4). In 1990–91, surface seeding in winter was unsuccessful with flax, but was successful with camelina,

Table 1. Comparison of Camelina with other oilseeds[z].

Species	Yield[y] (kg/ha)	Oil (%)	Seed size (g/1,000 seeds)	Maturity date	Lodging (%)
Camelina sativa	1277	31	0.6–1.2	7/1–7/28	20–30
Crambe abysinica	1317	32	6–8	7/15–8/10	30–50
Brassica napus	1273	39	2.9–4.0	8/1–8/20	40–80
Brassica hirta	1319	24	4.8–5.1	7/20–8/3	20–80

[z]Data from trials conducted 1960–1985 in Rosemount and Roseau, MN; 9 year/location means (Robinson 1987).

[y]Yields of some species, especially *B. napus* have improved due to plant breeding efforts since these trials were conducted. Yields of all cruciferae were at least 50% higher at Roseau (near Canada) vs. Rosemount in these trials.

Table 2. Yield and characteristics of *Camelina sativa* lines grown in Rosemount, Minnesota, 1991.

Line (origin)	Days from planting to Full bloom	Days from planting to Maturity	Height (cm)	Lodging rating[z]	1,000 seed weight (g)	Seed yield (kg/ha)	Oil (%)
C028 (USSR)	42	77	58	7.2	1.08	1007	37.5
C037 (Germany)	45	79	67	3.4	0.98	1085	35.3
C046 (Germany)	45	78	63	1.6	1.14	1159	37.3
C053 (Germany)	46	80	64	4.2	0.72	1065	36.4
C054 (Germany)	45	81	68	1.0	1.22	1140	35.1
C082 (Germany)	45	80	67	3.1	0.94	1218	35.9
C088 (Germany)	45	79	60	2.4	0.83	1148	35.5
'Robbie' (USA)	46	78	56	1.5	0.65	1067	34.3
LSD (P≤0.05)	2	1	6	1.8	0.10	173	2.4
C.V. (%)	4	2	6	39	7	11	---

[z]1 = no lodging; 10 = severe lodging.

Table 3. Comparison of winter-sown camelina with spring-sown camelina and flax.

Crop[z]	Sowing date	Sowing rate (kg/ha)	Tillage	Weed control[y] (%)	Seed yield (kg/ha) 1970	1971	1972	1973	Ave.
Camelina	Early Dec.	12	No	77	862	840	1243	1747	1176
Camelina	Mid-April	8	Yes	69	762	840	1288	1725	1154
Flax	Mid-April	56	Yes	76	963	336	952	1848	1019
LSD (P≤0.05)				202	157	146	146	78	

[z]Camelina was grown without herbicides and flax was sprayed with dalapon and MCPA.
 Data from Robinson (1987).
[y]Percent of weeds controlled estimated by visual rating (100 = least weedy).

producing significantly earlier emergence and fewer weed problems. However, in the 1989–90 study, the winter seeding was unsuccessful for both crops, probably due to an open winter. Surface seeding of camelina seemed to work better under no-till conditions, possibly due to superior microsite protection for the small seed and seedling, and prevention of wind dispersion of the seed. Machine planting was no better than broadcasting in the spring sowings. Machine planting in December was not feasible. A winter-sown stand of camelina emerges mid-April in Minnesota, before most other spring-sown crops, and before significant weed flushes.

These trials showed that camelina sown without herbicide or tillage yielded as well or better than flax grown conventionally. These studies also showed that camelina, unlike flax, can be surface-sown on frozen ground in the late fall or winter or early spring and produce good stands and yields comparable to conventionally-sown Cruciferae crops.

Compatibility with Cover Crops

In a three-year study, winter-sown camelina yielded an average of 9% more when seeded with a fall-sown cover crop than without (Table 5). In this and in subsequent studies (Robinson 1987), camelina has produced better stands, weed control, and yields when planted in the winter with a cover crop compared with seeding after conventional tillage in the spring or surface seeding on bare ground in the fall. These data indicate that camelina is highly compatible with cover crops used for fall and early spring soil erosion control.

Table 4. Effect of tillage, seeding method, and time of seeding on camelina and flax, Rosemount, Minnesota, 1990-91.

Treatments	Stand (%)	Days from planting to		Lodging rating^z	Weeds^y (%)	Height (cm)	Seed yield (kg/ha)
		Full bloom	Maturity				
No-till stubble							
Flax winter scatter	4	6/15	7/21	1	100	52	91
Flax spring scatter	35	6/15	7/22	1	75	51	801
Flax spring machine	98	6/15	7/22	1	61	47	851
Camelina winter scatter	93	6/1	6/28	1	16	59	749
Camelina spring scatter	64	6/9	7/7	1	48	41	1008
Camelina spring machine	100	6/13	7/12	2	63	52	888
Tilled							
Flax winter scatter	3	6/14	7/21	1	100	51	142
Flax spring scatter	68	6/12	7/21	1	80	56	837
Flax spring machine	100	6/14	7/21	2	85	53	937
Camelina winter scatter	71	6/1	6/30	2	51	60	850
Camelina spring scatter	95	6/12	7/8	2	34	57	1147
Camelina spring machine	98	6/11	7/9	2	42	55	865
LSD (P_0.05)	28	4	3	n.s.	36	15	312
C.V. (%)	27	22	15	50	32	17	28

^{z}1=no lodging; 10 = severe lodging.
^{y}Weed pressure estimated by visual rating, with 100 = most weedy, 0 = least weedy.

Table 5. Influence of a cover crop on winter-sown camelina performance. Camelina was planted broadcast-sown in early December on either bare ground or on flax stubble sown in late August or early September; data from Robinson (1987).

Treatment	Stand (%)	Maturity	Weed control^z (%)	Lodging (%)	Seed yield (kg/ha)			
					1971	1972	1973	Ave.
No cover crop	77	7/11	78	37	840	1243	1747	1277
Flax cover crop	89	7/9	83	18	1120	1176	1870	1389
LSD (P_0.05)	---	---	---	---	157	146	146	90

^{z}Percent of weeds controlled estimated by visual rating (100 = least weedy).

Fertilizer and Water Needs, Insects and Diseases

The soil fertility needs of camelina are likely similar to those of other crucifers with the same yield potential. Camelina has been shown to respond to nitrogen similarly to mustard or flax (Robinson 1987).

Bramm et al. (1990) found that camelina was better able to compensate for early water deficits than flax or poppy. This drought-avoidance characteristic might make camelina better suited to drier regions than other oilseeds.

Downy mildew (*Peronospora camelinae*), a white or gray mold on the upper part of the stem is sometimes observed in camelina (Robinson 1987). Transmission of Turnip Yellow Mosaic virus by camelina seed has been reported (Hein 1984). However, camelina has been reported to be highly resistant to blackleg (*Lepotosphaeria maculans*) which is a significant disease problem with canola (Salisbury 1987). Camelina has also been found to be very resistant to *Alternaria brassicae*, compared with turnip rape or swede rape (Grontoft 1986; Conn et al. 1988).

Flea beetle [*Phyllotreta cruciferae* (Goeze)] is also sometimes observed on camelina, although it is not nearly the problem it is with canola. However, in extensive multi-year small-plot trials, damage due to insects and diseases in camelina have not been sufficient to warrant control measures (Robinson 1987).

Weed Control

The compatibility of canola with commonly used herbicides is not widely known. In one three-year trial, camelina was not injured by trifluralin incorporated either in the fall or spring, but yields were not improved over winter-seeded camelina planted without herbicide (Robinson 1987). No herbicides are currently labeled for use with camelina, and herbicides would comprise a significant cost of production should any in the future even become labeled for such use. These data however, suggest that the use of preemergence herbicides may not be necessary in camelina if it is seeded in the winter or very early spring. Winter-seeded camelina emerges earlier than conventionally seeded camelina or other cruciferous crops, and normally before any substantial weed germination in the spring. The seedlings are quite cold-tolerant, surviving several freezes in the spring. For example, in one trial, a May 12 frost (−2°C) injured mustard, rape, and flax, but did not affect camelina (Robinson 1987). Individual camelina seedlings are fairly small and non-competitive, but this early-emerging, cold-tolerant characteristic, especially when planted at high densities, provides excellent competition with many annual weeds.

Perennial or biennial weeds are likely to be more difficult to control in camelina. However, the competitiveness of camelina with annual weeds presents the possibility that camelina could be grown both without tillage and without preemergence weed control, both significant costs of production and environmental risk-factors.

UTILIZATION

Seed composition, Oil Content and Meal Quality

The oil content of camelina seed has ranged from 29 to 39% in our studies. There appears to be some variation for oil content among the cultivars tested (Table 2), but the germplasm has not been widely characterized. Studies in Germany have shown oil content to range between 37 and 41% and seed protein content 23 to 30% (Marquard and Kuhlmann 1986). Camelina appears to be similar in protein content and elemental composition to flax (*Linum usitatissimum* L.), with the exception of a higher sulfur content (Robinson 1987). Camelina meal is comparable to soybean meal, containing 45 to 47% crude protein and 10 to 11% fiber (Korsrud et al. 1978).

Zero to trace levels of volatile isothiocyanates have been found in camelina meal (Peredi 1969; Korsrud et al. 1978; Sang and Salisbury 1987) compared with crambe (*Crambe abyssinica* Hochst) or industrial rapeseed meal which contains substantially higher levels of glucosinolates. Laboratory mice fed camelina meal gained less weight than those fed casein or egg control diets, but more than those fed crambe meal (Korsrud et al. 1978). Although some essential amino acids may have been limiting in the camelina meal diets, some growth depressing factor other than glucosinolates may have been present (Korsrud et al. 1978).

Camelina has been fed to wild (Fogelfors 1984) or caged (Mabberly 1987) birds, and this is one potential use. Other potential uses include applications as an ornamental, a cover or smother crop, a border row for experimental field plots, or in dried flower arrangements (Robinson 1987).

Fatty Acid Composition and Use of the Oil

Oil was extracted from camelina and other oilseeds by the Soxhlet method using diethyl ether, and fatty acids determined using the method of Enig and Ackerman (1987). The fatty acids in camelina oil are primarily unsaturated, with only about 12% being saturated (Fig. 2). About 54% of the fatty acids are polyunsaturated, primarily linoleic (18:2) and linolenic (18:3), and 34% are monounsaturated, primarily oleic (18:1) and eicosenoic (20:1) (Table 6).

Our values for fatty acid composition of *Camelina sativa* are generally similar to those reported for *Camelina rumelica* (Umarov et al. 1972), or other reports on *Camelina sativa* (Seehuber and Dambroth 1983). With its low saturated fat content camelina oil could be considered a high quality edible oil, but it is also quite highly polyunsaturated, which makes it susceptible to autoxidation, thus giving it a shorter shelf life. With an iodine value of 144, it is classified as a drying oil (Robinson 1987). Camelina oil has been used as a replacement for petroleum oil in pesticide sprays (Robinson and Nelson 1975).

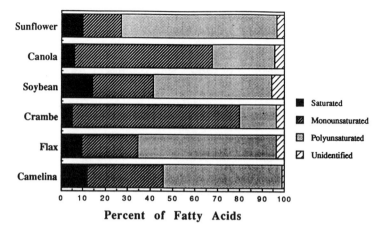

Fig. 2. Percent saturated and unsaturated fatty acids in camelina compared with other oilseeds grown at Rosemount, Minnesota, 1991. Unidentified fatty acids are those which did not match standards. Camelina is similar to soybean in balance of saturated vs. unsaturated fats, but is higher in C18:3 fatty acids.

Table 6. Fatty acid composition of camelina compared with 5 other oilseeds, grown at Rosemount, Minnesota, 1991.

Fatty acid	Fatty acid content (% of oil)					
	Canola	Soybean	Sunflower	Crambe	Flax	Camelina
Palmitic (16:0)	6.19	10.44	6.05	2.41	5.12	7.80
Stearic (18:0)	0	3.95	3.83	0.40	4.56	2.96
Oleic (18:1)	61.33	27.17	17.36	18.36	24.27	16.77
Linoleic (18:2)	21.55	45.49	69.26	10.67	16.25	23.08
Linolenic (18:3)	6.55	7.16	0	5.09	45.12	31.20
Arachidic (20:0)	0	0	0	0.50	0	0
Eicosenoic (20:1)	0	0	0	2.56	0	11.99
Erucic (22:1)	0	0	0	54.00	0.88	2.80
Other FA	4.38	5.79	3.5	6.01	3.80	3.40

Camelina oil is less unsaturated than linseed (flax) oil and more unsaturated than sunflower or canola oils (Fig. 2, Table 6). The balance of saturated vs. unsaturated fats is similar to that of soybean, but camelina contains significantly higher proportion of C18:3 fatty acids. Camelina seems to be unique among the species evaluated in having a high eicosenoic acid content in the oil, but the potential value or disadvantage of this is currently unclear.

The erucic acid content is probably too low for use in the same applications as crambe or high erucic acid rapeseed, where a high erucic acid content is desired. Most of the camelina lines evaluated contain 2 to 4% erucic acid (Table 6), which is greater than the maximum (2%) limits for canola-quality edible oil. However, in a preliminary germplasm screen, we have identified lines with zero erucic acid content (data not shown), so it is likely that this trait could readily be removed through plant breeding, as it has been with canola.

The lack of clear utilization patterns for camelina oil currently limit its use. The fatty acid composition does not currently uniquely fit any particular use. Manipulation of camelina fatty acid content, which has been achieved in other oilseeds, could greatly improve the utilization possibilities of this crop.

SUITABILITY FOR SUSTAINABLE AGRICULTURE

When analyzing the potential role of a new crop, *unique* attributes of that species must be established; it must contribute something not already provided by existing crop species. It is not sufficient, for example, for a crop simply to become "another oilseed." There must be unique and compelling properties of that crop to provide incentives for further development.

The research reported here has shown that camelina possesses unique agronomic traits which could substantially reduce and perhaps eliminate requirements for tillage and annual weed control. The compatibility of camelina with reduced tillage systems, cover crops, its low seeding rate, and competitiveness with weeds could enable this crop not only to have the lowest input cost of any oilseed, but also be compatible with the goals of reducing energy and pesticide use, and protecting soils from erosion. Camelina is a potential alternative oilseed for stubble systems, winter surface seeding, double cropping, or for marginal lands. At a seeding rate of 6 to 14 kg/ha, camelina could be inexpensively applied by air or machine-broadcast in early winter or spring on stubble ground without special equipment. Although these unimproved lines have been shown to be agronomically acceptable, modern history has indicated the Cruciferae to be highly manipulatable through plant breeding or biotechnology, and so the promise of improvement is also high. The meal does not contain glucosinolates, but the fatty acid composition of the seed needs to be modified to provide a role for the crop in the oilseeds market.

Lack of clear utilization patterns currently limit the crop, and further work on oil, meal, and seed use is required. The possibilities of using camelina in human food, as birdseed, as an edible or industrial oil, a fuel, or other applications remains largely unexplored. Further utilization and breeding research is required to more fully make use of the unique agronomic qualities that this crop possesses.

REFERENCES

Bramm, A., M. Dambroth, and S. Schulte-Korne. 1990. Analysis of yield components of linseed, false flax, and poppy. Landbauforschung Volkenrode 40:107–114.

Conn, K.L., J.P. Tewari, and J.S. Dahiya. 1988. Resistance to *Alternaria brassicae* and phytoalexin-elicitation in rapeseed and other crucifers. Plant Sci. (Irish Rep.) 55:21–25.

Downey, R.K. 1971. Agricultural and genetic potential of cruciferous oilseed crops. J. Amer. Oil Chem. Soc. 48:718–722.

Downey, R.K. 1990. Canola: A quality Brassica oilseed, p. 211–215. In: J. Janick and J.E. Simon (eds.). Advances in new crops. Timber Press, Portland, OR.

Einig, R.G. and R.G. Ackerman. 1987. Omega-3 PUFA in marine oil products. J. Amer. Oil Chem. Soc. 64:499.

Enge, G. and G. Olsson. 1986. Svavlof varieties release for cultivation in the period 1886–1986. Sveriges Utsadesforenings Tidskrift (Sweden) 96:220–235.

Fogelfors, H. 1984. Useful weeds? Part 5. Lantmannen (Sweden) 105:28.

Grontoft, M. 1986. Resistance to *Alternaria* spp. in oil crops. Sveriges–Utsadesforenings Tidskrift (Sweden) 96:293.

Grummer, G. 1961. The role of toxic substances in the interrelationships between higher plants, p. 226–227. In: Mechanisms in biological competition. Academic Press, New York.

Hein, A. 1984. Transmission of turnip yellow mosaic virus through seed of *Camelina sativa* (gold of pleasure). Zeitschrift fur Pflanzenkrankheiten und Pflanzenschutz 91:549–551.

Hymowitz, T. 1990. Soybeans: The success story, p. 159–163. In: J. Janick and J.E. Simon (eds.). Advances in new crops. Timber Press, Portland, OR.

Kartamyshev, B.G. 1985. The development of oil crop breeding on the Don. Selektsiya i Semenovodstvo (USSR) 6:9–11.

Knorzer, K.H. 1978. Evolution and spread of Gold of Pleasure (*Camelina sativa* S.L.). Bererichte der Deutschen Botanischen Gesellschaft 91:187–195.

Korsrud, G.O., M.O. Keith, and J.M. Bell. 1978. A comparison of the nutritional value of crambe and camelina seed meals with egg and casein. Can. J. Anim. Sci. 58:493–499.

Lovett, J.V. and H.F. Jackson. 1980. Allelopathic activity of *Camelina sativa* (L.) Crantz in relation to its phyllosphere bacteria. New Phytol. 86:273–277.

Lovett, J.V. and A.M. Duffield. 1981. Allelochemicals of *Camelina sativa*. J. Appl. Ecol. 18:283–290.

Mabberley, D.J. 1987. The plant book. A portable dictionary of higher plants. Camb. Univ. Press, New York.

Marquard, R. and H. Kuhlmann. 1986. Investigations of productive capacity and seed quality of linseed dodder (*Camelina sativa* Crtz.) Fette Seifen Anstrichmittel (Germany) 88:245–249.

Mirek, Z. 1981. Genus *Camelina* in Poland—Taxonomy, distribution and habitats. Fragmenta Floristica et Geobotanica. Ann. 27:445–507.

National Research Council (NRC). 1989. Alternative Agriculture/Committee on the role of Alternative Farming Methods in Modern Production Agriculture. National Academy Press, Washington, DC.

North Central Regional Technical Committee NC-121. 1981. Weeds of the North Central States. North Central Regional Res. Pub. 281. Bul. 772. Agr. Expt. Sta., Univ. Illinois, Urbana–Champaign.

Peredi, J. 1969. Fatty acid composition of the oils of Hungarian rape varieties and of other cruciferous plants, and the contents of isothiocyanates and vinyl thiooxazolidon of the their meals. Olag Szappan Kozmetika 18:67–76.

Robinson, R.G. 1973. The sunflower crop in Minnesota. Ext. Bul. 299. Agr. Ext. Serv., Univ. of Minnesota, St. Paul.

Robinson, R.G. 1987. Camelina: A useful research crop and a potential oilseed crop. Minnesota Agr. Expt. Sta. Bul. 579–1987. (AD-SB-3275).

Robinson, R.G. and W.W. Nelson. 1975. Vegetable oil replacements for petroleum oil adjuvants in herbicide sprays. Econ. Bot. 29:146–151.

Salisbury, P.A. 1987. Blackleg resistance in weedy crucifers. Cruciferae Newsl. 12:90.

Sang, J.P. and P.A. Salisbury. 1987. Wild Crucifer species and 4-hydroxyglucobrassicin. Cruciferae Newsl. 12:113.

Seehuber, R. and M. Dambroth. 1983. Studies on genotypic variability of yield components in linseed (*Linum usitatissumum* L.), poppy (*Papaver somniferum* L.) and *Camelina sativa* Crtz. Landbauforschung Volkenrode (Germany) 33:183–188.

Seehuber, R. and M. Dambroth. 1984. Potential for the production of industrial raw materials from home-grown oil plants and prospects for their exploitation. Landbauforschung Volkenrode 34:174–182.

Seehuber, R., J. Vollmann, and M. Dambroth. 1987. Application of single-seed-descent method in falseflax to increase the yield level. Lanbauforschung Voelkenrode (Germany) 37:132–136.

Umarov, A.U., T.V. Chernenko, and A.L. Markman. 1972. The oils of some plants of the family cruciferae. Khimiya Prirodnykh Soedinenii (USSR) 1:24–27.

Perilla: Botany, Uses and Genetic Resources*

David M. Brenner

Perilla [*Perilla frutescens* (L.) Britton, Lamiaceae] is a common annual weed of the eastern United States but considered a commercial crop in Asia. In the United States, perilla food products are available in Korean ethnic markets, and red-leafed cultivated plants are used in landscaping. The species has been used abroad in at least nine ways: seeds are sold as food for birds or human consumption; the seed oil is used as a fuel, a drying oil, or a cooking oil; the leaves are used as a potherb, for medicine, or for food coloring; and the foliage is distilled to produce an essential oil for flavoring (Publications and Information Directorate 1966).

BOTANY

Perilla is a member of the mint family and has the characteristic square stems and four stamens of most species in that family. Within the genus *Perilla*, the taxonomic nomenclature is controversial (Zeevaart 1969). The number of species recognized varies from one (Publications and Information Directorate 1966; Booth 1957, Koezuka et al. 1985; Misra and Husain 1987), to two (Tanaka 1976; Miller 1922), or four (Gorshkova 1954), and also includes taxonomic and horticultural varieties (Miller 1922). Historical confusion with *Ocimum* is briefly reviewed by Simon et al. (1984). The best diagnostic characteristics of *Perilla* are the net-patterned testa

---

*Journal Paper No. J.-14769 of the Iowa Agriculture and Home Economics Experiment Station, Ames, Iowa. Project No. 1018.

of the nutlets and the distinctive smell of the crushed foliage. Dry skeletons of the plants persist into the spring; their racemes retain dry papery calyces when the purple to white flowers have fallen away.

Perilla has a variable chromosome complement. Vij and Kashyap (1976) found a haploid chromosome count of fourteen, plus zero to two beta chromosomes. Yamane (1950) karyotyped four taxonomic varieties, found chromosome counts of both $n = 20$ and $2n = 38$ and distinguished three chromosome sizes.

I have seen perilla growing as a common weed of pastures and roadsides in the southeastern United States. One reason for perilla's survival in pastures, is that cattle avoid it. It stands 15 cm tall for most of the summer. In August, it blooms and its stem elongates rapidly. The plant reaches a height of approximately 1 m before being killed by frost in November.

Photoperiod

Perilla has been used by plant physiologists to investigate flower induction. The following information is modified from Zeevaart's (1969, 1985) reviews of the effect of day length on perilla. Long nights induce flowering, but different accessions have different critical night lengths. Plants become photosensitive at the fourth leaf pair stage. Flowering starts 18 to 20 days after the start of long nights. After 30 long nights, plants will bloom until they die, regardless of subsequent day length. Scions from an induced plant can induce flowering of the stock plant onto which they are grafted. Wada and Totsuka (1982) discovered another environmental influence on blooming. They forced perilla to bloom with continuous lighting by restricting nitrogen availability. I have observed plants in Ames, Iowa, that bloomed during short nights evidently because of transplanting shock.

Toxicology

Perilla is ordinarily avoided by cattle but has been implicated in cattle poisoning (Phillips and Von Tungein 1986). Plants are most toxic if cut and dried for hay late in the summer, during seed production (Kerr et al. 1986). Wilson et al. (1977) isolated the toxin "perilla ketone," which causes pulmonary edema (fluid in the lung cavity) in many animal species, although not in pigs or dogs (Garst et al. 1985). In Japan, 20 to 50% of long-term workers in the perilla industry develop dermatitis on their hands due to contact with perillaldehyde (Okazaki et al. 1982).

AGRONOMY

Perilla was never grown commercially as an oilseed in the United States, although several agronomists investigated the crop (Fox 1911; Gardener 1917, 1926; Rabak and Lowman 1945; Fuelleman and Burlison 1944; Weibel and Burlison 1948). Perilla was also experimentally grown as a crop in many parts of the British empire (Imperial Institute 1920, 1926). In contrast, production has continued in Korea (Yu and Oh 1976; Choi et al. 1980).

Fox (1911) and Gardener (1926) calculated the economic return from production of perilla as an oilseed in the United States, and found it unprofitable in comparison with linseed. Rabak and Lowman (1945) determined that although perilla is well adapted to the climate of the southeastern United States, it will be unprofitable unless seed shattering can be controlled.

Dwarf, early seed maturity types were developed in Illinois for short-season climates (Fuelleman and Burlison 1944; Weibel and Burlison 1948). Seed yields ranged from 220 to 1,400 kg/ha in Illinois research plots (Weibel and Burlison 1948), 1,020 to 1,440 kg/ha in Korean research plots (Choi et al. 1980), and 1,110 to 1,670 kg/ha in Japanese agricultural production (Imperial Institute 1920).

USES

Seed Oil

The seeds of perilla contain 31 to 51% of a drying oil similar to tung or linseed oil (Jamieson 1943). All drying oils leave a hard protective surface when dry. Perilla oil has been used as a drying oil in paints, varnishes, linoleum, printing ink, lacquers, and for protective waterproof coatings on cloth. It has also been used for cooking, and fuel (Publications and Information Directorate 1966). The spent seed meal can be fed to ruminants (Folger 1937). The oil is very unsaturated, with an iodine number of 185 to 208, and includes linolenic, linoleic, and oleic acids (Jamieson 1943; Eckey 1954; Publications and Information Directorate 1966; Park et al. 1981). One contrasting study reported a much lower iodine number, of 138 (Tsuyuki et al. 1978). Trocopherols in perilla oil reduce oxidation (Kashima et al. 1991).

The United States' importation of perilla seed oil peaked at more than two million dollars in 1939; the last report of oilseed importation was in 1943 (United States Department of Agriculture 1954). The supply was interrupted during World War II (Rabak and Lowman 1945). In Korea, the seed oil continues to be produced for cooking and industrial uses (Choi et al. 1980). Local oilseed production has also continued in Bhutan, where R.P. Croston and T. Dorji collected a seed oil accession (PI 481703) for the International Board for Plant Genetic Resources in 1981.

Ornamental

In 1922, six ornamental cultivars were listed by Miller, in whose time perilla was declining in importance: "Before the introduction of the *Coleus* this plant was much used as an ornamental flower-garden plant" he noted. Ornamental perilla is easy to grow in sun or light shade (Parke 1984) and its color is far more intense than the color of either wild or oilseed types. I have seen it grown as an attractive foliage screen behind shorter bedding plants. The purple foliage superficially resembles that of purple-leaved varieties of basil, *Ocimum basilicum* L.

Culinary

Perilla foliage "*kkaennip namul*" (Wade 1986) and seed oil (Choi et al. 1980) are used in Korean cooking. Korean markets in the United States sometimes sell perilla. An Oriental grocery in Ames, Iowa, sold bundles of fresh leaves for $6.53/kg in August, 1991. Perilla was an important vegetable in ancient China, but use in modern times has declined there (Li 1969). In Japan, the foliage of "*shiso*" serves as a garnish (Shurtleff and Aoyagi 1975). The foliage also provides a red (anthocyanin) food coloring; specialized red-leaved perilla varieties are used (Koezuka et al. 1985b) in the preparation of pickled plums (Ishikura 1981; Suyama et al. 1983; Chung et al. 1986). In addition to food coloring, perilla adds an antimicrobial substance to pickled foods (Kurita and Koike 1981). Perilla seeds are eaten in Japan (Ishikura 1981) and in parts of India (Standal et al. 1985).

Volatile Oil

In Japan, a volatile oil is distilled from the dried foliage of perilla (Guenther 1949; Nago et al. 1975). Oil of perilla is used as a flavoring agent, in which perilla aldehyde is the desirable flavoring compound (Guenther 1949; Arctander 1960). One of the aldehyde isomers is 2,000 times as sweet as sugar and four to eight times as sweet as saccharin; it is used as a tobacco sweetener (Guenther 1949). Perilla alcohol, prepared from perilla aldehyde, is used in fragrances, and has legal food status in the United States and Europe (Opdyke 1981). A perilla collection from Bangladesh is a potential commercial source of rosefuran (Misra and Husain 1987), a compound of interest in flavoring and perfumery (Ohloff and Demole 1987).

Recently, nine genotypes of perilla with different volatile oil chemistries have been crossed to allow study of the genetic control of biosynthetic pathways (Koezuka et al. 1986a; Nishizawa et al. 1989, 1990). Through this work a list of chemotypes has been developed, which show classical segregation patterns. One genotype lacks perilla aldehyde but has perilla ketone (Koezuka et al. 1986a).

Medicinal

Asian herbalists prescribe perilla for cough and lung afflictions, influenza prevention, restless fetus, seafood poisoning, incorrect energy balance, etc. (Publications and Information Directorate 1966; Hu-nan Chung i yao yen chui so. Ko wei hui 1977; Perry and Metzger 1980; Duke 1985).

Studies of perilla's volatile oil have revealed that distinct chemotypes of perilla have dramatically different biological effects (Koezuka et al. 1985a, 1986a,b,c). The perilla aldehyde chemotype is the source of Japanese "*ao-shiso*" (Arctander 1960), a medicine with an agreeable fragrance (Koezuka et al. 1986a). The perilla ketone chemotype is toxic and extremely effective as a laxative without causing diarrhea in laboratory mice (Koezuka et al. 1985a). The phenylpropanoid chemotype contains myristicin (Koezuka et al. 1986a,b), which is reported to have hallucinogenic properties (Seto and Keup 1969).

Laboratory rats had better learning ability when fed a perilla seed oil diet than with a safflower oil diet. The beneficial effect of perilla seed oil is attributable to its high α-linolenate content (Yamamoto et al. 1987).

GERMPLASM

Maintenance and Manipulation

Perilla plants are easily grown for seed. They self-pollinate without insect visits and yield well in greenhouses. The plants are most easily managed when they flower soon after planting and remain short. If planted too early, they can grow more than two meters tall in greenhouse pots. For plants 7 to 60 cm tall, seeds should be planted 30 or fewer days before the flowering date. This method allows 330 plants per square meter of greenhouse space. The minimal planting to harvest cycle is about 77 days, seeds reach maturity six weeks after the first flowering. Zeevaart (1969) used a similar schedule with controlled day length.

Koezuka et al. (1985b) emasculated perilla by removing the corolla with adhering anthers, then pollinated, and used a genetic marker (red hypocotyl) to confirm each successful cross.

The greatest difficulty in perilla germplasm maintenance is limited seed viability in storage. At room temperature, the seeds can die in less than a year, but lowered temperature or humidity improves storage life dramatically (Cho et al. 1986). At the North Central Regional Plant Introduction Station, germination percentages fell below 1% in seed lots maintained in cold dry storage for 23 years. Frequent germination monitoring and regeneration are essential for long-term maintenance.

Sources

Perilla cultivars can be purchased from at least 37 commercial suppliers (Facciola 1990). Twelve cultivars are mentioned in a recent publication from Korea (Cho et al. 1986). The many Asian cultivars are consistent with that continent's position as the center of origin of perilla.

The North Central Regional Plant Introduction Station in Ames, Iowa, maintains 17 accessions of perilla (Table 1) and distributes seeds to researchers free of charge. Plant Introduction Station holdings include long- and short-season oilseed types. Fuelleman and Burlison (1944) had success in Illinois with our short season germplasm.

Table 1. Perilla accessions and seed maturity dates in Ames, Iowa, at the North Central Regional Plant Introduction Station. The seed maturity date depends upon daylength, not planting date. These data are from plants at least four months old at maturity.

Accession	Seed maturity	Type	Source
PI 248664	Sept. 10	Oil seed	India
PI 246665	Sept. 7	Oil seed	USA
PI 248666	Sept. 7	Oil seed	USA
PI 248667	Sept. 10	Oil seed	USA
PI 248668	Sept. 4	Oil seed	USA
PI 248670	Sept. 7	Oil seed	USA
PI 248671	Sept. 27	Oil seed	USA
PI 481701	Nov. 20	Unknown	Bhutan
PI 481703	Nov. 12	Oil seed	Bhutan
PI 481704	Nov. 19	Unknown	Bhutan
PI 481705	Nov. 26	Unknown	Bhutan
PI 546459	Nov. 5	White seed	Nepal
PI 546460	Oct. 31	White seed	Nepal
PI 553074	Oct. 19	Unknown	Thailand
PI 553078	---	Red foliage	Japan
PI 557009	Nov. 26	Unknown	Thailand
Ames 18336	---	oil seed	Korea

CROP PROSPECTS IN THE UNITED STATES

Vegetable perilla has a market niche catering to people from Korea and other Asian countries. Seeds of the ornamental plants are available from United States seed companies, and use is likely to continue. Seed oil is now produced in Korea, and until new markets are found for the oil, production in the United States is unlikely. One possible new market is for use as an animal feed additive, building on the enhanced learning ability of rats on a perilla seed oil diet (Yamamoto et al. 1987). The artificial sweetener from the volatile oil (Guenther 1949) may be of value but might require an investigation of health risks before commercialization in the United States.

Perilla alcohol is a minor commercial fragrance ingredient in the United States and in Europe (Opdyke 1981). The use of perilla volatile oil as a source of rosefuran is a novel and exciting idea (Misra and Husain 1987).

REFERENCES

Arctander, S. 1960. Perfume and flavor materials of natural origin. Elizabeth, NJ.

Booth, C.O. 1957. An encyclopaedia of annual and biennial garden plants. Faber and Faber, London.

Cho, J.L., Y.W. Choi, H. Kang, S.K. Um. 1986. Studies on the germination of perilla seeds (*Perilla ocymoides* L.) I. Effects of temperature and storage method on the germinability (in Korean). Korean Soc. Hort. Sci. 27:320–330.

Choi, I.S., S.Y. Son, and O.H. Kwon. 1980. Effect of seedling age and planting density on the yield and its component of perilla (*Ocymcides* Var. *Typica* MAKINO) intercropped with tobacco or aftercropped (in Korean). Korean Soc. Hort. Sci. 25:68–75.

Chung, M.Y., L.S. Hwang, and B.H. Chiang. 1986. Concentration of perilla anthocyanins by ultrafiltration. Food Sci. 51:1494–1497, 1510.

Duke, J.A. 1985. Handbook of medicinal herbs. CRC Press, Boca Raton, FL.

Eckey, E.W. 1954. Vegetable fats and oils. Reinhold, New York.

Facciola, S. 1990. Cornucopia: a source book of edible plants. Kampong Publications, Vista, CA.

Folger, A.H. 1937. The digestibility of perilla meal, hempseed meal, and babassu meal, as determined for ruminants. Univ. of California, College of Agr., Agr. Expt. Sta., Berkeley. Bul. 604.

Fox, C.P. 1911. Ohio grown perilla. Ohio Nat. 12:427–428.

Fuelleman, R.F. and W.L. Burlison. 1944. Growing perilla in Illinois. Chemurg. Dig. 3:1, 35.

Gardener, H.A. 1917. Experimental cultivation of perilla in the United States. Paint Manufacturers Assoc. U.S. Cir. 52:1–18.

Gardener, H.A. 1926. Perilla and chia culture experiments of 1925. Paint Manufacturers Assoc. U.S. Cir. 257:216–227.

Garst, J.E., W.C. Wilson, N.C. Kristensen, P.C. Harrison, J.E. Corbin, J. Simon, R.M. Philpot, and R.R. Szabo. 1985. Species susceptibility to the pulmonary toxicity of 3-furyl isoamyl ketone (perilla ketone): in vivo support for involvement of the lung monooxygenase system. Anim. Sci. 60:248–257.

Gorshkova, S.G. 1954. Perilla, p. 452–454. In: B.K. Shishkin (ed.). Flora of the U.S.S.R. Vol. 21. Bot. Inst. Acad. Sci. USSR, Moscow. (Translated from Russian, Israel Program for Scientific Translations. 1977. Jerusalem.)

Guenther, E. 1949. The essential oils. vol 3. D. Van Nostrand, New York.

Hu-nan Chung i yao yen chui so. Ko wei hui. 1977. A barefoot doctor's manual. Running Press, Philadelphia.

Imperial Institute. 1920. The commercial utilization of perilla seed. Bul. Imp. Inst. 18:479–481.

Imperial Institute. 1926. Perilla seed. Bul. Imp. Inst. 24:205–208.

Ishikura, N. 1981. Anthocyanins and flavones in leaves and seeds of *Perilla* plant. Agr. Biol. Chem. 45:1855–1860.

Jamieson, G.S. 1943. Vegetable fats and oils. Reinhold, New York.

Kashima, M., G.-S. Cha, Yoshihiro, J. Hirano, and T. Miyazawa. 1991. The antioxidant effects of phospholipids on perilla oil. Amer. Oil Chem. Soc. 68:119–122.

Kerr, L.A., B.J. Johnson, and G.E. Burrows. 1986. Intoxication of cattle by *Perilla frutescens* (purple mint). Vet. Hum. Toxicol. 28:412–416.

Koezuka, Y., G. Honda, and M. Tabata. 1985a. An intestinal propulsion promoting substance from *Perilla frutescens* and its mechanism of action. Planta Med. 6:480–482.

Koezuka, Y., G. Honda, S. Sakamoto, and M. Tabata. 1985b. Genetic control of anthocyanin production in *Perilla frutescens*. Shoyakugaku Zasshi 39:228–231.

Koezuka, Y., G. Honda, and M. Tabata. 1986a. Genetic control of the chemical composition of volatile oils in *Perilla frutescens*. Phytochemistry 25:859–863.

Koezuka, Y., G. Honda, and M. Tabata. 1986b. Genetic control of phenylpropanoides in *Perilla frutescens*. Phytochemistry 25:2085–2087.

Koezuka, Y., G. Honda, and M. Tabata. 1986c. Genetic control of isoegomaketone formation in *Perilla frutescens*. Phytochemistry 25:2656–2657.

Kurita, N. and S. Koike. 1981. Synergistic antimicrobial effect of perilla and NaCl (in Japanese). Nippon Nogeikagaku Kaishi 55:43–46.

Li, H-L. 1969. The vegetables of ancient China. Econ. Bot. 23:253–260.

Miller, W. 1922. Perilla, p. 2553. In: L.H. Bailey. The Standard Cyclopedia of Horticulture. vol.3. Macmillan, London.

Misra, L.N., and A. Husain. 1987. The essential oil of *Perilla ocimoides*: A rich source of rosefuran. Planta Med. 53:379–390.

Nago, Y., S. Fujioka, T. Takahashi, and T. Matsuoka. 1975. Studies on the quality of the chinese drug "soyo" and the cultivation of the original plant (in Japanese). Takeda Res. Lab. 34:33–42.

Nishizawa, A., G. Honda, and M. Tabata. 1989. Determination of final steps in biosyntheses of essential oil components in *Perilla frutescens*. Planta Med. 55:251–253.

Nishizawa, A., G. Honda, and M. Tabata. 1990. Genetic control of perillene accumulation in *Perilla frutescens*. Phytochemistry 29:2873–2875.

Ohloff, G. and E. Demole. 1987. Importance of the odoriferous principle of Bulgarian rose oil in flavor and fragrance chemistry. J. Chromatogr. 406:181–183.

Okazaki, N., M. Matsunaka, M. Kondo, and K. Okamoto. 1982. Contact dermatitis due to beefsteak plant (*Perilla frutescens* Britton var *acuta* Kudo) (in Japanese). Skin Research 24:250–256.

Opdyke, D.L.J. 1981. Monographs on fragrance raw materials. Food Cosmet. Toxicol. 19:237–254.

Park, H.S., J.G. Kim, and M.J. Cho. 1981. Chemical composition of *Perilla frutescens* Britton var. *crispa* Decaisne cultivated in different areas of Korea: part 1. characteristics of lipid and fatty acid composition (in Korean). J. Korean Agr. Chem. Soc. 24:224–229.

Parke, M. 1984. The pleasures of purple mint. Horticulture 62(8):14–17.

Perry, L.M., and J. Metzger. 1980. Medicinal plants of east and southeast Asia. Massachusetts Inst. of Technol., Cambridge.

Phillips, W.A., and D. Von Tungein. 1986. Acute pulmonary edema and emphysema in steers fed old-world bluestem hay. Mod. Vet. Pract. 67:252–253.

Publications and Information Directorate. 1966. The wealth of India. vol.7. New Delhi.

Rabak, F. and M.S. Lowman. 1945. Perilla. USDA, Agriculture Research Administration, Bureau of Plant Industry, Soils, and Agricultural Engineering, Beltsville, Maryland.

Seto, T.A. and W. Keup. 1969. Effects of alkylmethoxybenzene and alkylmethylenedioxybenzene essential oils on pentobarbital and ethanol sleeping time. Arch. Int. Pharmacodyn. 180:323–240.

Shurtleff, W. and A. Aoyagi. 1975. The book of tofu. Autumn Press, Brookline, MA.

Simon, J.E., A.F. Chadwick, and L.E. Craker. 1984. Herbs: an indexed bibliography 1971–1980, the scientific literature on selected herbs, and aromatic and medicinal plants of the temperate zone. Archon Books, Hamden, CT.

Standal, B.R., H. Ako, and G.S.S. Standal. 1985. Nutrient content of tribal foods from India: *Fleminga vestita* and *Perilla frutescens*. J. Plant Foods 6:147–153.

Suyama, K., M. Tamate, and S. Adachi. 1983. Colour stability of shisonin, red pigment of a perilla (*Perilla ocimoides* L. var. *crispa* Benth.). Food Chem. 10:69–77.

Tanaka, T. 1976. Tanaka's cyclopedia of edible plants of the world. Keigaku Publishing Co., Tokyo.

Tsuyuki, H., S. Itoh, and Y. Nakatsukasa. 1978. Studies on the lipids in perilla seed (in Japanese). Bul. College Agr. Vet. Med. Nihon Univ. 35:224–230.

United States Department of Agriculture. 1954. Oilseed fats and their products 1909–1953. Sta. Bul. 147, Washington, DC.

Vij, S.P. and S.K. Kashyap. 1976. Cytological studies in some north Indian Labiatae. Cytologia 41:713–719.

Wada, K. and T. Totsuka. 1982. Long-day flowering of *Perilla* plants cultured in nitrogen-poor media. Plant Cell Physiol. 23:977–985.

Wade, L. 1986. Korean cookery. 2nd ed. Hollym International Corp., Elizabeth, NJ.

Weibel, R.O. and W.L. Burlison. 1948. Know your oilseeds: perilla. Soybean Dig. 8:14–15.

Wilson, B.J., J.E. Garst, R.D. Linnabary, and R.B. Channell. 1977. A potent lung toxin from the mint plant, *Perilla frutescens* Britton. Science 197:573–574.

Yamamoto, N., M. Saitoh, A. Moriuchi, M. Nomura, and H. Okuyama. 1987. Effect of dietary linolenate/linoleate balance on brain lipid compositions and learning ability of rats. Lipid Res. 28:144–151.

Yamane, Y. 1950. Cytogenetic studies on the genus *Perilla* and *Coleus* I. chromosome numbers (in Japanese). Jpn. Genet. 25:220.

Yu, I.S. and S.K. Oh. 1976. Effect of different defoliation periods and intensities on row leaf weight and grain yield of perilla (in Korean). Res. Rpt. Off. Rural Dev. 18:187–191.

Zeevaart, J.A.D. 1969. Perilla, p. 116–155. In: L.T. Evans (ed.). The induction of flowering: Some case histories. Cornell Univ. Press., Ithaca, NY.

Zeevaart, J.A.D. 1985. Perilla, p. 239–252. In: A.H. Halevy (ed.). CRC handbook of flowering. CRC Press, Inc., Boca Raton, FL.

Quinoa: A Potential New Oil Crop*

Michael J. Koziol

Quinoa (*Chenopodium quinoa* Willd.) is an Andean pseudocereal grain about 1.0 mm thick which ranges in diameter from 1.0 to 2.5 mm and in seed weight from 1.9 to 4.3 g/1000 seeds (Alvarez et al. 1990). From earlier investigations (White et al. 1955) to more recent reviews (Coulter and Lorenz 1990; Galwey et al. 1990), attention has focussed primarily on the content and quality of the protein in quinoa. This absorbing interest in quinoa's profile of essential amino acids has completely overshadowed another equally important nutritional characteristic of the grain when compared with cereals, namely a relatively high content of an oil which is rich in the essential fatty acids, linoleate and linolenate (Koziol 1990a). (As arachidonic acid can be synthesized from linoleic acid it will not here be considered as essential.)

The use of non-traditional oil crops, such as maize, as sources of edible vegetable oils depends partially on their oil content and composition but more importantly, on the commercialization of other major products derived from the grain; oil production is best viewed as a byproduct in such cases. Thus, as early as 1943, Jamieson stated: "Were it not for the fact that in the preparation of hominy, starch, glucose, and other corn products, the germ is almost completely separated from the rest of the kernel, corn oil would not have become an important commercial product." Production of maize oil increased proportionally with that of high-fructose corn syrup, and its consumption has been boosted by an increasing public awareness of the importance of polyunsaturated fats in the diet (Leibovitz and Ruckenstein 1983). Worldwide, the production of maize oil increased from 0.4 million t in 1965 to 1.0 million t in 1985, with a further increase to 1.5 million t predicted by 1995 (Gunstone 1989). The

---

*Gratefully acknowledged are the efforts of U. Bracco and his research group at the Nestlé Research Centre, Verschez-les-Blanc, Switzerland, for performing the fatty acid and tocopherol analyses on samples of quinoa oil.

production of maize oil as a commercially viable byproduct serves as an appropriate model with which to compare the potential of quinoa as a new oil source, with special emphasis on Ecuadorian data.

POTENTIAL OF QUINOA

Maize Oil Content and Yields

Maize cultivated in the United States contains 3 to 4% oil (Mounts and Anderson 1983). The germ, which accounts for 5 to 14% of the weight of a maize kernel (Lásztity 1984; Patterson 1989; Alexander 1989) contains about 85% of the oil (Mounts and Anderson 1983). In the starch industry, the maize germ as removed by the wet degermination (milling) process and presented for oil extraction contains about 50% oil, as opposed to the 10 to 24% oil available in germs removed by the dry process used in the production of hominy, grits, and corn flakes (Leibovitz and Ruckenstein 1983).

Breeding programs for maize with a higher oil content have successfully produced hybrids that have 6 to 8% oil with yields equivalent to those of other commercial cultivars (Weber 1983). Hybrids with higher oil contents tend to have lower yields in terms of tonnage per hectare; for example, within 22 cycles the oil content of 'Alexho Synthetic' was increased from 6.2 to 12.9%, but the yield of the maize was reduced from 8.50 to 5.69 t/ha (Alexander 1989). Given the higher oil content, oil yield per hectare actually increased from 0.53 to 0.73 t/ha. Increases in oil production, however, are accompanied by increases in germ sizes and by decreases in grain and endosperm weight and hence in starch production (Weber 1983; Alexander 1989). Despite the successes of the maize breeders, the only inducement for farmers to cultivate the higher oil content maize for milling up until the 1980s was special contracting (Weber 1983). More recently, the increased production of high-fructose sugars in the United States suggests that higher oil content maize might not be welcome by the wet millers, even though the value of maize oil is at least three times higher than that of the corn starch (Alexander 1989). Some of the dry milling processes cause excessive damage to the larger embryos of the higher oil content maize resulting not only in contamination of the endosperm by oil but also in the release of lipolytic enzymes from the embryo which can accelerate rancidity. The future of the higher oil containing hybrids of maize depends upon three factors: (1) a reassessment of the value of maize oil as a byproduct in the production of other maize products; (2) the costs of modifying existing processes and equipment to deal with the changes in the morphology of the kernels; and (3) the productivity of the new hybrids in terms of yield per hectare.

Quinoa Oil Content and Yield

On a fresh weight basis quinoa shows an oil content ranging from 1.8 to 9.5% (Table 1) with a calculated global mean of 5.8%, an oil content higher than that of normal maize. As with maize, the oil is concentrated in the germ which in quinoa represents 25 to 30% of the weight of the grain (Cardozo and Tapia 1979; Fuentes 1972). As the quinoa germ encircles the endosperm, we have found that it can easily be removed by a modified polishing procedure to give a fraction containing 19% oil.

Although special breeding programs were necessary to achieve an oil content of 6 to 8% in maize, several cultivars of quinoa already show oil contents in this range (Table 2). Unlike maize, in which an increase in oil

Table 1. Moisture and oil content of quinoa grains.

Moisture (%)			Fat (%)			
No. determinations	Mean	(Range)	No. determinations	Mean	(Range)	Reference
3	10.2	(9.8–10.5)	3	6.2	(5.5–6.7)	De Bruin (1964)
58	12.7	(6.8–20.7)	60	5.0	(1.8–9.3)	Cardozo and Tapia (1979)
58	12.9	(5.4–20.7)	54	4.6	(1.8–8.2)	Romero (1981)
127	9.6	(6.2–14.1)	92	7.2	(4.3–9.5)	Koziol (1990a)

content resulted in a decrease in starch content, increased oil content in the quinoa grain showed no significant correlation with total carbohydrate content (r = 0.348) and was negatively correlated with protein content (r = –0.910, P < 0.025) (Table 3).

Field trials were conducted with six Ecuadorian cultivars of quinoa with oil contents between 7.2 and 8.7% (fresh weight) sown at an altitude of 3,100 m and using experimental plots ranging in size from 0.2 to 0.5 ha (Burgasi et al. 1990). Converting the data from Table 4 to a dry matter basis gave no significant correlation (r = 0.648) between yield and oil content, unlike maize in which yield decreased with increasing oil content (Alexander 1989).

The potential yields of quinoa and maize oils were estimated (Table 5) for Ecuador by multiplying the ranges of average oil content by data for average crop yields as reported by the Ministerio de Agricultura y Ganadería (MAG 1985). The potential yield of quinoa oil given under the general case was calculated using the data of Nuñez and Morales (1980), who reported quinoa yields in Bolivia of 3,960 kg/ha without fertilization and of 5,420 kg/ha with fertilization. This latter value was used to calculate a maximum possible yield of quinoa. Nuñez and Morales (1980) extrapolated a yield per hectare on the basis of very small experimental plots (4 rows of 6 m spaced 0.4 m apart), and their experimental plots received eight treatments against mildew. Commercially, quinoa would likely receive one or two treatments against mildew (M. Alvarez pers. commun.). Thus, the 488 kg oil/ha reported in Table 5 is best cautiously interpreted as a maximum yield obtainable under exceedingly favorable conditions.

Conversely, the exceedingly low yield of quinoa grain of 449 kg/ha reported by MAG (1985) reflects small-scale traditional agricultural practices; hence the calculated oil yields for Ecuador based on that data from MAG

Table 2. High oil content cultivars of quinoa (data from Alvarez et al. 1990 for quinoa grown at Cumbayá, Ecuador).

Source	Accession	Moisture (%)	Oil (%)
Cambridge[z]	Chilena-B	8.9	6.7
	Chilena-T	9.6	6.8
	No. 63	8.7	7.7
	No. 63-1	6.8	6.9
INIAP[y]	Ecu Sep 17-0271	11.0	6.9
	V-8	9.4	7.5
	V-10	8.7	7.9
	V-11	9.6	8.0
	San Juan 0036	7.1	7.8
Latinreco[x]	Potoroc	7.2	7.2
	011Pn	10.1	7.6
	011Pr	9.7	7.7
	012	7.7	7.8
	012Pn	8.1	7.8
	012Pr	10.1	8.7
	013	9.4	7.5
	013Pn	9.7	8.0
	013Te	9.5	8.5

[z]Seed supplied by N.W. Galwey, Department of Genetics, University of Cambridge, England.
[y]Seed supplied by the Ecuadorian Instituto Nacional de Investigaciones Agropecuarias.
[x]Ecotypes isolated by the Department of Agronomy, Latinreco, S.A., with the exception of 'Porotoc'.

Table 3. Composition of six genotypes of quinoa on a dry matter basis (data from Alvarez et al. 1990 for quinoa grown at Cumbayá, Ecuador).

Genotype	Oil (%)	Protein (%)	Fiber (%)	Ash (%)	Carbohydrate (%)	Saponins (%)
Porotoc	7.8	19.0	3.3	2.6	67.1	0.2
V-8	8.3	18.1	3.1	3.1	66.4	1.0
012	8.5	19.0	4.2	3.4	64.7	0.2
V-10	8.7	17.6	3.7	3.6	65.7	0.7
013Te	9.4	16.7	3.5	3.1	67.1	0.2
013Pr	9.7	16.6	3.0	3.0	67.5	0.2

Table 4. Grain yield of quinoa (data from Burgasi et al. 1990; seed moisture and fat content as per Table 2).

	Grain yield (kg/ha)^z			
Accession	1986	1987	1988	Mean
Porotoc	2200	---	---	2200
V-8	1360	---	---	1360
012	---	4500	3063	3782
V-10	2200	---	---	2200
013Te	2700	4500	---	3600
012Pr	3000	4000	2956	3319

^{z}Yield data are from 0.2 to 0.5 ha experimental plots at an altitude of 3,100 m.

Table 5. Comparison of oil yields from quinoa and maize.

Source	Range of fat content (%)^z	Oil yield (kg/ha)	
		General	Ecuador
Maize	2–5^y	254^x	34–85^w
Quinoa	2–9^v	108–488^u	9–40^w
			102–306^t

^{z}At normal seed moisture content.
^{y}Duke and Atchley (1986).
^{x}Pryde and Doty (1981).
^{w}MAG (1985).
^{v}From Table 1.
^{u}Calculated on the basis of yields reported in Nuñez and Morales (1980).
^{t}Calculated on the basis of oil content from Table 2 and yield data from Table 4.

(1985) are thus also low. Better estimates of quinoa yields in Ecuador are those given by Burgasi et al. (1990) and reported in Table 4, which would then correspond to potential oil yields of 102 to 306 kg/ha (Table 5). This oil yield for quinoa compares favorably with that estimated for maize by Pryde and Doty (1981) in the United States, namely 254 kg/ha assuming an average oil content of 4.8% for maize.

Oil Composition

The fatty acid composition of quinoa oil is similar to that of maize oil (Table 6). The high concentrations of linoleic and linolenic acids normally make such oils susceptible to oxidative rancidity but both oils have relatively high concentrations of natural antioxidants, namely tocopherol isomers. The mean concentration of α-tocopherol reported for three cultivars of quinoa on a dry weight basis was 52 ppm (De Bruin 1964), which corresponds to a concentration of 754 ppm in the oil. Further analyses have shown quinoa oil to contain 690 to 740 ppm α-tocopherol and 790 to 930 ppm γ-tocopherol; upon refining these concentrations fall to 450 and 230 ppm, respectively (U. Bracco pers. commun.). In comparison, refined maize oil contains 251 ppm α-tocopherol and 558 ppm γ-tocopherol (Souci et al. 1986). As optimum antioxidant activity of the α- and γ-isomers of tocopherol has been reported at 100 to 200 ppm (Hudson and Ghavami 1984) quinoa oil would be expected to show a stability towards oxidative rancidity similar to that of maize oil.

Table 6. Comparison of the compositions of quinoa and maize oils.

Variable		Quinoa		Maize
Fatty acids (as % of lipid fraction):				
Myristic	(C14:0)	0.2^z	---	0.2^x
Palmitic	(C16:0)	9.9^z	11^y	11.2^x
Palmitoleic	(C16:1)	0.1^z	---	0.1^x
Stearic	(C18:0)	0.8^z	0.7^y	2.1^x
Oleic	(C18:1)	24.5^z	22^y	29.8^x
Linoleic	(C18:2)	50.2^z	56^y	55.0^x
Linolenic	(C18:3)	5.4^z	7^y	0.9^x
Arachidic	(C20:0)	0.7^z	---	0.4^x
Specific gravity		0.891^w		0.918-0.925^v
Refractive index		1.464^w		1.464-1.468^u
Saponification value		190^w		189-191^v
Iodine value (Wijs)		129^w		125-128^v
Unsaponifiable matter (%)		5.2^w		0.8-2.9^u
Sterols (%)		1.51^w		0.85-1.42^{t,s}
Lecithins (%)		1.8^w		1-3^r

^{z}U. Bracco (pers. commun.).
^{y}Sánchez Marroquín (1983).
^{x}Data compiled from Leibovitz and Ruckenstein (1983) and Weiss (1983).
^{w}De Bruin (1964).
^{v}Mounts and Anderson (1983).
^{u}Eckey (1954).
^{t}Souci et al. (1986).
^{s}Weber (1983).
^{r}Patterson (1989).

BY-PRODUCTS OF QUINOA OIL PRODUCTION

Saponins

Quinoa can be classified according to its saponin concentrations as either "sweet" (saponin free or having less than 0.11% saponins on a fresh weight basis) or "bitter" (containing more than 0.11% saponins) (Koziol 1990b). The saponins in quinoa are glycosidic triterpenoids (Burnouf-Radosevich et al. 1985; Mizui et al. 1988, 1990; Ma et al. 1989; Meyer et al. 1990; Ridout et al. 1991) and represent the major antinutritional factor found in the grain (Koziol 1992). Fortunately, most of these saponins are concentrated in the outer layers of the grain (perianth, pericarp, seed coat, and a cuticle-like layer) which facilitates their removal industrially by abrasive dehulling (Reichert et al. 1986) or traditionally by washing the grains with water.

The toxicity of saponins depends upon their type, method of absorption, and target organism (for a comprehensive review, see Price et al. 1987). Because of their differential toxicity to various organisms saponins have been investigated as potent natural insecticides which would have no adverse effects on higher animals and man (Basu and Rastogi 1967). Other interest in saponins is in their antibiotic, fungistatic, and pharmacological properties (Basu and Rastogi 1967; Agarwal and Rastogi 1974; Chandel and Rastogi 1980; Nonaka 1986). The pharmacological interest in saponins lies with their ability to induce changes in intestinal permeability (Gee et al. 1989; Johnson et al. 1986) which may aid the absorption of particular drugs (Basu and Rastogi 1967), and with their hypocholesterolemic effects (Oakenfull and Sidhu 1990). As the saponins in quinoa have been relatively little studied their potential commercial uses remain unknown.

Oil Press Cake as a Dietary Supplement

Both bitter and sweet quinoa are currently subjected to abrasive dehulling before export from Ecuador, resulting in one case in a material concentrated in saponins and ready for extraction and in the other a high fiber bran. A second, modified "polishing" gives the germ fraction which can be used for oil extraction. In preliminary trials, we found this germ fraction to contain 40% protein. Quinoa protein is of an exceptionally high quality. Koziol (1992) summarized the results of four different studies on the protein efficiency ratio (PER) of quinoa in feeding trials with rats, expressing the PERs as percentages of the casein control diets. Raw quinoa (both sweet and bitter) exhibited PER values from 44 to 93% and cooked quinoa PER values from 102 to 105%; in comparison, raw and cooked wheat exhibited PER values from 23 to 32% of the casein control. It is rare for a vegetable protein such as that from quinoa to approximate so closely the quality of casein.

Comparing the profile of the essential amino acids (in human nutrition) of quinoa with that of maize, rice, and wheat shows that quinoa protein is particularly rich in lysine and contains more histidine and methionine + cystine (Table 7). Of the non-essential amino acids quinoa contains more arginine and glycine but less glutamic acid and proline than the cereals. The protein in the quinoa oil press cake would be an important complementary protein for improving the nutritional quality of both human and animal foodstuffs.

Carbohydrate Cream Substitute

The endosperm remaining after degerming the quinoa grain contains a starch with rather unusual qualities. The majority of the starch grains are less than 3 μm in diameter (Wolf et al. 1950; Scarpati de Briceño and Briceño 1982; Atwell et al. 1983). Small granule starches generally exhibit gelatinization temperatures higher than those of large granule starches (Kulp 1973; Swinkels 1985) but quinoa starch initiates gelatinization at temperatures similar to those for the larger granule wheat and potato starches, i.e. 56° to 58°C (Scarpati de Briceño and Briceño 1982; Swinkels 1985). Although quinoa starch initiates gelatinization at a temperature similar to that of wheat starch, its pasting behavior is considerably different and at equal starch concentrations shows higher viscosities than wheat starch when measured with a Brabender amylograph (Atwell et al. 1983).

Table 7. Comparison of amino acid profiles (Koziol, 1992).

Amino acid	Content (g amino acid/100 g protein)			
	Quinoa	Maize	Rice	Wheat
Essential (for humans):				
Histidine	3.2	2.6	2.1	2.0
Isoleucine	4.4	4.0	4.1	4.2
Leucine	6.6	12.5	8.2	6.8
Lysine	6.1	2.9	3.8	2.6
Methionine + Cystine	4.8	4.0	3.6	3.7
Phenylalanine + Tyrosine	7.3	8.6	10.5	8.2
Threonine	3.8	3.8	3.8	2.8
Tryptophan	1.1	0.7	1.1	1.2
Valine	4.5	5.0	6.1	4.4
Non-essential:				
Alanine	4.5	7.3	6.0	3.6
Arginine	8.5	4.2	6.9	4.5
Aspartic acid	7.8	6.9	10.0	5.0
Glutamic acid	13.2	18.8	19.7	29.5
Glycine	6.1	4.0	4.7	4.0
Proline	3.3	9.1	4.9	10.2
Serine	4.1	5.1	6.3	4.8

Recently, the Nutrasweet Company exploited the properties of quinoa starch and filed a European patent for making a carbohydrate cream substitute from it (Singer et al. 1990). Although the procedure for obtaining the starch followed the method described by Atwell et al. (1983) for whole quinoa grains, there is no obvious reason why degermed quinoa could not be used instead.

CONCLUSIONS

Quinoa offers an oil rich in polyunsaturated fatty acids, a protein whose quality approaches that of casein and a starch that can be converted into a cream/fat substitute, all of which are easily marketable as products or as natural additives that should appeal to today's health conscious consumer. The saponins removed from bitter quinoa may find niches in pharmaceutical preparations or in programs of integrated pest management.

Despite being a promising "rediscovered" crop with important nutritional characteristics, the current industrial use of quinoa is limited by small-scale production which serves to keep prices for the grain too high to be commercially competitive with wheat, rice, and barley, especially in the Ecuadorian market. Fomenting further interest, research and the development of improved methods of commercial cultivation both locally and worldwide (see National Research Council 1989; Wahli 1990) will help ensure that quinoa regains the prominence it once enjoyed under the Incas.

In Ecuador, quinoa is already adapted for cultivation at altitudes from 2,300 to 3,500 m, too high for maize yields to be commercially viable (upper limits for maize for subsistence, not commercial, cultivation being 2,800 to 3,000 m; yields of wheat and barley also decline notably above 3,000 m). Quinoa should therefore be viewed as a versatile cash crop which would extend the range of commercially arable hecterage in Ecuador.

REFERENCES

Agarwal, S.K. and R.P. Rastogi. 1974. Triterpenoid saponins and their genins. Phytochemistry 13:2623–2645.

Alexander, D.E. 1989. Maize, p. 431–437. In: G. Röbbelen, R.K. Downey, and A. Ashri (eds.). Oil crops. McGraw–Hill, New York.

Alvarez, M., J. Pavón, and S. von Rütte. 1990. Caracterización, p. 5–30. In: Ch. Wahli (ed.). Quinua: hacia su cultivo comercial. Latinreco S.A., Casilla 17-110-6053, Quito, Ecuador.

Atwell, W.A., B.M. Patrick, L.A. Johnson, and R.W. Glass. 1983. Characterization of quinoa starch. Cereal Chem. 60:9–11.

Basu, N. and R.P. Rastogi. 1967. Triterpenoid saponins and sapogenins. Phytochemistry 6:1249–1270.

Burnouf-Radosevich, M., N.E. Delfel, and R.E. England. 1985. Gas chromatography-mass spectrometry of oleanane- and ursane-type triterpenes—application to *Chenopodium quinoa* triterpenes. Phytochemistry 24:2063–2066.

Burgasi, G., J. Pavón, and S. von Rütte. 1990. Cultivo comercial, p. 117–134. In: Ch. Wahli (ed.). Quinua: hacia su cultivo comercial. Latinreco S.A., Casilla 17-110-6053, Quito, Ecuador.

Cardozo, A. and M. Tapia. 1979. Valor nutritivo, p. 149–192. In: M. Tapia (ed.). Quinua y kañiwa, cultivos andinos. Centro Internacional para el Desarrollo, Bogotá, Colombia.

Chandel, R.S. and R.P. Rastogi. 1980. Triterpenoid saponins and sapogenins: 1973–1978. Phytochemistry 19:1889–1908.

Coulter, L. and K. Lorenz. 1990. Quinoa: Composition, nutritional value, food applications. Lebensm.-Wiss. u.-Technol. 23:203–207.

De Bruin, A. 1964. Investigation of the food value of quinoa and cañihua seed. J. Food Sci. 29:872–876.

Duke, J.A. and A.A. Atchley. 1986. CRC handbook of proximate analysis of higher plants. CRC Press, Boca Raton, FL.

Eckey, E.W. 1954. Vegetable fats and oils. Reinhold, New York.

Fuentes P., E.J. 1972. Importancia de la quinua (*Chenopodium quinoa* Willd.) en la solución del problema de las proteínas en la alimentación chilena. Simiente 42:15–20.

Galwey, N.W., C.L.A. Leakey, K.R. Price, and G.R. Fenwick. 1990. Chemical composition and nutritional characteristics of quinoa (*Chenopodium quinoa* Willd.). Food Sci. Nutr. 42F:245–261.

Gee, J.M., K.R. Price, C.L. Ridout, I.T. Johnson, and G.R. Fenwick. 1989. Effects of some purified saponins on transmural potential difference in mammalian small intestine. Toxicol. in Vitro 3:85–90.

George, A.J. 1965. Legal status and toxicity of saponins. Food Cosmet. Toxicol. 3:85–91.

Gunstone, F.D. 1989. Oils and fats—past, present and future, p. 1–16. In: R.C. Cambie (ed.). Fats for the future. Ellis Horwood, Chichester, UK.

Hudson, B.J. and M. Ghavami. 1984. Stabilising factors in soya-bean oil—natural components with antioxidant activity. Lebensm.-Wiss. u.-Technol. 17:82–85.

Jamieson, G.S. 1943. Vegetable fats and oils. Reinhold, New York.

Johnson, I.T., J.M. Gee, K.R. Price, C.L. Curl, and G.R. Fenwick. 1986. Influence of saponins on gut permeability and active nutrient permeability in vitro. J. Nutr. 116:2270–2277.

Koziol, M.J. 1990a. Composición química, p. 137–159. In: Ch. Wahli (ed.). Quinua, hacia su cultivo comercial. Latinreco S.A., Casilla 17-110-6053, Quito, Ecuador.

Koziol, M.J. 1990b. Afrosimetric estimation of threshold saponin concentration for bitterness in quinoa (*Chenopodium quinoa* Willd.). J. Agr. Food Sci. 54:211–219.

Koziol, M.J. 1992. Chemical composition and nutritional evaluation of quinoa (*Chenopodium quinoa* Willd.). J. Food Comp. Anal. 5:36–68.

Kulp, K. 1973. Characteristics of small granule starch of flour and wheat. Cereal Chem. 50:666–679.

Lásztity, R. 1984. The chemistry of cereal proteins. CRC Press, Boca Raton, FL.

Leibovitz, Z., and C. Ruckenstein. 1983. Our experiences in processing maize (corn) germ oil. J. Amer. Oil Chem. Soc. 60:395–399.

Ma, W.-W., P.F. Heinstein, and J.L. McLaughlin. 1989. Additional toxic, bitter saponins from the seeds of *Chenopodium quinoa*. J. Nat. Prod. 52:1132–1135.

MAG. 1985. Estimación de la superficie cosechada y de la producción agrícola del Ecuador. Ministerio de Agricultura y Ganadería, Quito, Ecuador.

Meyer, B.N., P.F. Heinstein, M. Burnouf-Radosevich, N.E. Delfel, and J.L. McLaughlin. 1990. Bioactivity-directed isolation and characterization of quinoside A: one of the toxic/bitter principles of quinoa seeds (*Chenopodium quinoa* Willd.). J. Agr. Food Chem. 38:205–208.

Mizui, F., R. Kasai, K. Ohtani, and O. Tanaka. 1988. Saponins from brans of quinoa, *Chenopodium quinoa* Willd., I. Chem. Pharm. Bul. 36:1415–1418.

Mizui, F., R. Kasai, K. Ohtani, and O. Tanaka. 1990. Saponins from brans of quinoa, *Chenopodium quinoa* Willd., II. Chem. Pharm. Bul. 38:375–377.

Mounts, T.L. and R.A. Anderson. 1983. Corn oil production, processing and use, p. 373–387. In: P.J. Barnes (ed.). Lipids in cereal technology. Academic Press, New York.

National Research Council. 1989. Quinoa, p. 148–161. In: Lost crops of the Incas: little-known plants of the Andes with promise for worldwide cultivation. Natl Acad. Press, Washington, DC.

Nonaka, M. 1986. Variable sensitivity of *Trichoderma viride* to *Medicago sativa* saponins. Phytochemistry 25:73–75.

Nuñez, Z. and D. Morales. 1980. Fertilización nitrogenada en 15 ecotipos de quinoa, p. 133–141. In: L. Corral and J.H. Cáceres (eds.). Segundo congreso internacional de cultivos andinos, 4–8 junio 1979, Riobamba. Escuela Superior Politécnica de Chimborazo, Riobamba, Ecuador.

Oakenfull, D. and G.S. Sidhu. 1990. Could saponins be a useful treatment for hypercolesterolaemia? Eur. J. Clin. Nutr. 44:79–88.

Patterson, H.B.W. 1989. Handling and storage of oilseeds, oils, fat and meal. Elsevier Applied Science, London.

Price, K.R., I.T. Johnson, and G.R. Fenwick. 1987. The chemistry and biological significance of saponins in foods and feeding-stuffs. CRC Crit. Rev. Food Sci. Nutr. 26:27–135.

Pryde, E.H. and H.O. Doty, Jr. 1981. World fats and oils situation, p. 3–14. In: E.H. Pryde, L.H. Princen, and K.D. Mukherjee (eds.). New sources of fats and oils. Amer. Oil Chem. Soc., Champaign, IL.

Reichert, R.D., J.T. Tatarynovich, and R.T. Tyler. 1986. Abrasive dehulling of quinoa (*Chenopodium quinoa*): effect on saponin content was determined by an adapted hemolytic assay. Cereal Chem. 63:471–475.

Ridout, C.L., K.R. Price, M.S. DuPont, M.L. Parker, and G.R. Fenwick. 1991. Quinoa saponins—analysis and preliminary investigations into the effects of reduction by processing. J. Sci. Food Agr. 54:165–176.

Romero, J.A. 1981. Evaluación de las características físicas, químicas y biológicas de ocho variedades de quinua (*Chenopodium quinoa* Willd.). Tesis de Maestro, Universidad de San Carlos de Guatemala, Ciudad de Guatemala, Guatemala.

Sánchez Marroquín, A. 1983. Dos cultivos olvidados, de importancia agroindustrial. Arch. Latinoam. Nutr. 23:11–32.

Scarpati de Briceño, Z. and O. Briceño. 1982. Evaluación de la composición de algunas entradas de quinua del banco de germoplasma de la Universidad Nacional Técnica del Altiplano, p. 69–77. In: Tercer congreso internacional de cultivos andinos, Feb. 8–12, 1982. Ministerio de Asuntos Campesinos y Agropecuarios, La Paz, Bolivia.

Singer, N.S., P. Tang, H.-H. Chang, and J.M. Dunn. 1990. Carbohydrate cream substitute. European Patent No. 0 403 696 A1, Office Européen des Brevets, Paris.

Souci, S.W., W. Fachmann, and H. Kraut. 1986. Food composition and nutrition tables 1986/87. Wissenschaftliche Verlagsgesellschaft, Stuttgart.

Swinkels, J.J.M. 1985. Sources of starch, its chemistry and physics, p. 15–46. In: G.M.A. Van Beynum and J.A. Roels (eds.). Starch conversion technology. Marcel Dekker, New York.

Wahli, Ch. (ed.). 1990. Quinua: hacia su cultivo comercial. Latinreco S.A., Casilla 17-110-6053, Quito, Ecuador.

Weber, E.J. 1983. Lipids in maize technology, p. 353–372. In: P.J. Barnes (ed.). Lipids in cereal technology. Academic Press, London.

Weiss, T.J. 1983. Food oils and their uses. 2nd ed. AVI, Westport, CT.

White, P.L., E. Alvistur, C. Días, E. Viñas, H.S. White, and C. Collazos. 1955. Nutrient content and protein quality of quinua and cañihua, edible seed products of the Andes mountains. Agr. Food Chem. 3:531–534.

Wolf, M.J., M.M. MacMasters, and G.E. Rist. 1950. Some characteristics of the starches of three South American seeds used for food. Cereal Chem. 27:219–222.

INDUSTRIAL CROPS

Guayule: A Source of Natural Rubber

Dennis T. Ray

Natural rubber is a commodity that accounts for an annual import deficit of nearly $1 billion for the United States. Over 2,000 rubber producing species are known, however, only two, *Hevea brasiliensis* (A. Juss.) Muell.-Arg. and guayule (*Parthenium argentatum* Gray), have been exploited as commercial sources of natural rubber. Today, *Hevea* is essentially the sole source of natural rubber, nevertheless, active research and development programs are underway to domesticate and commercialize guayule. Guayule is envisioned as a new or alternative crop for arid and semiarid areas of the southwestern United States, north central Mexico, and regions with similar climates around the world (Thompson and Ray 1989).

Although *Hevea* is the dominant rubber crop today, *Hevea* and guayule have had parallel histories of development. In both, commercialization began with the harvest of wild stands before the establishment of plantations and the initiation of cultural studies. Variability within stands and lowered yields per unit area were problems in both species. These problems continued through the early attempts at cultivation since the populations were very heterogeneous genetically due to their establishment from open-pollinated seed. Annual yields have been increased dramatically in both, from 400 to over 2,000 kg/ha for *Hevea* (Bonner 1991), and from 300 to 1,000 kg/ha for guayule (Estilai and Ray 1991). The differences in development between the two crops can be associated with the initiation of the Rubber Research Institute of Malaya, in 1925. The Rubber Research Institute has been responsible for over 60 years of continuous increases in *Hevea* yields and the production of a uniform and reliable industrial product (Bonner 1991). Guayule, on the other hand, has suffered from intermittent research efforts, which have in many cases been undermined by periods of neglect. Guayule researchers have found themselves more than once in the position of "reinventing the wheel."

Guayule is the dominant perennial xerophytic shrub found on the limestone bajadas and hillsides of the Chihuahuan desert of north central Mexico and the Big Bend region of Texas (West et al. 1991). Wild stands contain a natural polyploid series of diploids ($2n = 2x = 36$), triploids ($2n = 3x = 54$) and tetraploids ($2n = 4x = 72$); and under cultivation, individual plants have been identified with chromosome numbers up to octaploid ($2n = 8x = 144$). Diploids reproduce predominantly sexually, and polyploids reproduce by facultative apomixis. Guayule also has a sporophytic system of self-incompatibility and many plants contain B- or supernumerary chromosomes (Thompson and Ray 1989).

HISTORY

Guayule has been known as a source of rubber since the pre-Columbian times when Indians of Mexico used it to form balls for their games. In the early 1900s, guayule was first considered as an alternative source of natural rubber in the United States because of the high price of *Hevea* rubber from the Amazon region (Bonner 1991). Since this initial interest, there have been three major efforts to domesticate and commercialize guayule. The first began at the turn or the century with the harvesting of wild stands of guayule in Mexico. Several extraction methods were evaluated, and in 1904, 40 kg of guayule rubber was exported to the United States. By 1907, a total of 20 extraction plants were either operational or under construction in Mexico, and in 1910, Mexican rubber production reached a high of 10,000 t, which accounted for 24% of the total rubber imported into the United States (Bonner 1991). Production by the Continental Rubber Company continued until 1912, when the Mexican Revolution halted all commercial production. This may have been a blessing in disguise since very large areas of native shrub had been depleted, and guayule was on its way to becoming extinct in Mexico.

After the closure of the processing facilities in Mexico, commercialization efforts were moved across the border to the United States. Agronomic studies and breeding work was initiated by the newly reorganized Intercontinental Rubber Company, with efforts centered in Arizona and California. By the late 1920s, annual production of guayule rubber, from commercial plantings of over 3,200 ha, was about 1,400 t. Seventeen years (1929) after the project was moved from Mexico to the United States, production ceased because of the Great Depression (Bonner 1991).

The second major effort to domesticate and utilize guayule as a source of natural rubber came with the Emergency Rubber Project of World War II. This was an extensive effort involving over 1,000 scientists and technicians, and 9,000 laborers. Over 13,000 ha of shrub was planted at 13 sites in three states. The effort ended with the end of the war and the development of synthetic rubber (Huang 1991). During the four years of its existence, 1,400 t of guayule rubber was produced, but at the end of the war an additional 10,000 t was destroyed while still in the shrub (Bonner 1991). However, the project was very successful, and from it came the bulk of our knowledge about the basic biology of guayule and the origin of the germplasm upon which current breeding programs are based (Thompson and Ray 1991). If this work had continued, undoubtedly today guayule would have already become a commercial rubber crop.

The third effort, of which we are still a part, arose from the quadrupling of crude oil prices in the early 1970s. This led to the enactment of the Native Latex Commercialization and Economic Development Act of 1978, which has supported the current guayule research for about 12 years (Huang 1991). Although this effort is neither as concentrated, or as urgent, as the Emergency Rubber Project, a tremendous amount of work has been done, and has resulted in significant increases in yield and the refinement of cultural practices to fit today's mechanized agriculture.

CULTURAL PRACTICES

Descriptions of guayule cultivation practices have been reviewed extensively by Thompson and Ray (1989) and in *Guayule Natural Rubber*, edited by Whitworth and Whitehead (1991). The following are major points concerning cultivation gleaned from these sources and the author's experiences with guayule.

Guayule is adapted to hot desert environments, and sites with well-drained calcareous soils and relatively low concentrations of nutrients. Sandy-loam soil are most suitable since root diseases, which are exacerbated by standing water, are one of the few problems encountered in guayule cultivation (Mihail et al. 1991). Fertility treatments have been shown to have little effect on growth, and guayule is only slightly tolerant to soil salinity (Nakayama et al. 1991). The semiarid plateau region of the Chihuahuan desert (1,200 to 2,100 m in elevation) in which guayule occurs naturally has a temperature range between –18 and 49.5°C. High temperature does not appear to affect growth, but temperatures below 4°C induce semi-dormancy and extended freezing temperatures can cause plant death (Thompson and Ray 1989).

Areas with annual precipitation between 280 and 640 mm are preferable for guayule cultivation, but in order to achieve maximum yields, moderate to heavy applications of irrigation are necessary. Both dry matter production, and resin and rubber yields, have been shown to increase proportionally with increased water availability (Nakayama et al. 1991). In addition, irrigation can shorten the time until harvest. However, excess water is harmful to guayule plants of all ages, causing disease, reduced soil aeration, and increased weed competition. These problems are especially damaging to young plants (Nakayama et al. 1991).

Presently, stand establishment is accomplished by transplanting. Seeding transplants are produced in greenhouses and fields are established using typical commercial transplanting systems. Transplanting has been extremely successful, but is estimated to be more expensive than establishment by direct-seeding (Thompson and Ray 1989). Direct-seeding has been successful on an experimental scale, but no commercial scale plantings have been attempted.

Weed and pest control on a commercial scale are problematic since no compounds are presently labeled for guayule in the United States. However, pests have not proven to be a problem if sites were carefully selected, stands established by transplanting, and weeds successfully controlled (Mihail et al. 1991). If establishment via direct-seeding becomes the norm, experimental plot work has shown that damping-off of seedlings and weed control will become major areas of concern.

Mechanized techniques have been developed or adapted for all aspects of guayule cultivation. For example, the cost of transplanting may be reduced by clipping instead of digging whole plants. By clipping, the branches are cut approximately 10 cm above the soil level and regrowth occurs from the root crown. Novel equipment has been developed for this purpose and breeding programs are now selecting lines with high levels and rates of regeneration (Coates 1991).

PROCESSING

Effective processing of rubber and non-rubber coproducts is essential to a viable guayule industry. Rubber in guayule is found in the parenchyma cells, mainly in the bark, and must be released during processing. During the present effort to commercialize guayule three processing methodologies have been researched (Wagner and Schloman 1991).

The first and oldest method is flotation. This is essentially the same methodology used at the turn of the century and during the Emergency Rubber Project. In this procedure, ground shrubs are placed in a large vat of dilute sodium hydroxide until the woody tissue takes-up water and sinks to the bottom and the resinous rubber floats to the top in what are called "worms." These worms are skimmed from the top and the rubber is deresinated with acetone. Flotation was recently employed by the processing facility at Saltillo, Mexico, from which all of the guayule rubber used in test tires until 1990 was produced (W.W. Schloman, Jr. pers. commun.). The second method is sequential extraction, in which the resin is first extracted with acetone or another polar organic solvent, and then the rubber is extracted with hexane. Sequential extraction has only been used experimentally and appears not to be an economically viable method.

The third processing method is simultaneous extraction, in which a mixture of solvents, usually acetone and hexane or pentane, are used. After the initial extraction, more acetone is added to coagulate the high molecular weight rubber. This method has been used at both of the experimental processing facilities built by Texas A&M University at College Station, Texas and at Sacaton, Arizona by the Bridgestone/Firestone Corporation. Although this method has been successful in extracting rubber, engineering difficulties in handling the shrub have plagued both facilities (Wagner and Schloman 1991; N.G. Wright pers. commun.).

Economic forecasts suggest that for guayule to become a crop which can compete without subsidies, rubber yields must be increased and/or commercial utilizations of processing coproducts must be identified and developed (Wright et al. 1991). One potentially valuable coproduct is the low-molecular-weight rubber fraction, which accounts for approximately 25% of the total rubber yield. These low-molecular-weight rubber compounds have high value specialty applications as non-tire rubber (Schloman and Wagner 1991). Another processing coproduct, the resins, are only partially characterized, but are predominantly fatty-acid triglycerides and terpenoids. Resins have been used successfully as wood preservatives, a feed-stock for specialty chemicals (coatings and rubber additives), and as a high value fuel with no ash. Unfortunately, resin composition varies with shrub line, cultivation site, harvest date, and processing history (Schloman and Wagner 1991).

Guayule bagasse was used to fuel the early processing plants in Mexico and unprocessed shrub was used to fuel various processes in the Mexican mining industry. Today, bagasse is still being considered as a cogeneration fuel, as well as, a feedstock for gasification, conversion to liquid hydrocarbons, as a source of fermentable sugars, and as a fiber. These applications are not unique and are typical of other types of waste lignocellulose (Schloman and Wagner 1991).

PLANT BREEDING

Guayule breeding is the center of the present activity towards commercialization. Rubber yields must continue to increase in order for guayule to be economically competitive with other crops grown in arid and semiarid regions. The primary objective of all of the breeding programs is to improve rubber yields per unit area. Breeders are also improving rubber quality and reducing postharvest rubber degradation, improving regrowth after clipping, processing quality of the shrub, and disease and insect resistance (Thompson and Ray 1989; Estilai and Ray 1991).

Rubber yield can be expressed as a product of rubber content (% rubber) and biomass (dry weight/unit area). Thus, rubber yield may be improved by increasing either biomass and/or rubber content. An increase in rubber content is more desirable since it increases the processing efficiency of the shrub. Increased biomass involves additional costs associated with harvest, transportation, and processing (Estilai and Ray 1991). Dry weight has been found in many studies (Thompson and Ray 1989) to be the best predictor of rubber yield, with correlation coefficients between the variables typically over 0.90. Rubber content, on the other hand, has neutral to slightly positive correlation coefficients with yield, up to 0.30. There is a negative correlation observed in most studies, between biomass production and rubber content. However, gains have been made in both simultaneously by using minimum selection thresholds for both traits. In other words, a plant must have a minimum rubber content and biomass before being selected. A plant with either adequate (above the selection threshold) rubber content or biomass, but not both, would not be retained in the program.

Secondary breeding objectives are being addressed by particular breeding programs. Among these are increased resin and biomass production which have been realized in several new breeding lines. In addition, many seed characteristics have been addressed, such as size, germination rate, and yield per plant. Breeding for tolerance to environmental stresses and their interaction with rubber production have been studied, but on a very limited scale.

All breeding approaches depend upon the existing genetic variability found within available guayule germplasm. In guayule, limited genetic variability is not a problem, and has been found for every trait that has been evaluated. In fact, the facultative nature of apomixis in polyploid guayule continually releases new variability which may be exploited by plant breeders (Thompson and Ray 1989).

To date, the most extensively employed breeding approach has been single-plant selections from within apomictic polyploid populations. This has been used very successfully in increasing annual rubber yields, from approximately 300 to 1,000 kg/ha. Hybridization of polyploids is another method that has been suggested, but has been tried only sparingly. Interspecific hybridization has been discussed, but applied only on a limited scale. There is little to be gained by going to the related species to find desirable traits, since the available variability within the guayule germplasm has not yet been totally characterized and/or exploited (Estilai and Ray 1991).

Diploids have been used in guayule breeding in several ways. Because of their sexual (non-apomictic) reproduction, standard breeding methodologies may be employed, however, there are still problems in their use. Most notably, diploids yield significantly lower and are much more susceptible to root diseases than polyploids. Yields have been raised using modified recurrent selection schemes, and *Verticillium* tolerant lines have been developed through mass selection. These improved diploid lines can either be crossed to polyploids or have their chromosome numbers doubled with colchicine, producing polyploids. Diploids have also been used to release new genetic combinations from apomictic polyploids. Meiosis is normal in the pollen mother cells of apomictic polyploids, yielding potentially new and useful combinations of genes from which selections may be made. High yielding polyploids have been crossed onto diploids resulting in populations with excessive phenotypic variation (Thompson and Ray 1989; Estilai and Ray 1991).

Significant progress has been made, even though not more than 2.8 Scientific Years are presently devoted to guayule breeding each year in the United States. At the end of the Emergency Rubber Project, and through the 1950s, guayule rubber yields on an annual basis were between 220 and 560 kg/ha. This was based on the germplasm with which the current breeding programs started. By the Second Guayule Regional Variety Trials, 1985–1988, annual yields had increased to between 600 and 900 kg/ha, and in breeding plots annual yields of over 1,100 kg/ha have been estimated. These programs have been effective, but due to the limited number of researchers and resources, many aspects which might aid commercialization have been ignored. For example, coproduct production, dryland production, and screening for different environmental stresses have been addressed only indirectly.

ECONOMICS

Guayule commercialization depends upon its being economically competitive with *Hevea* rubber. But this only considers guayule as a direct substitute for *Hevea*, which means that guayule rubber must either perform the same functions at a lower cost or perform better at the same cost. Guayule researchers are not looking to replace *Hevea*, but to enhance worldwide rubber production. Demand for natural rubber continues to grow at a rate greater than new plantings of *Hevea*. Guayule should be able to fill this need, especially locally in arid and semiarid environments.

On its own, guayule is presently not economical without either greater rubber yields or identification and development of high value coproducts. Under irrigated conditions, assuming rubber at $1.21/kg, resin + low-molecular-weight rubber at $0.44/kg, and bagasse at $0.04/kg, annual rubber yields of 1,450 kg/ha (1,300 lb./acre) would have to be obtained. These are not far from our present yields. Under dryland conditions, and using the same assumptions, annual rubber yields of 640 kg/ha (600 lb./acre) must be obtained, however, this would mean an increase of 2.5 times the present dryland yields. Unfortunately, these are rough estimates at best since both the costs of production and of processing are unknown (Wright et al. 1991).

CONCLUSIONS

There currently is a group of dedicated researchers who are working to understand and improve guayule towards the goal of one day being able to supply a domestic source of natural rubber. Although not presently able to meet this goal economically, if needed in case of emergency, all of the knowledge is in place to plant, cultivate, harvest, and process guayule. With relatively few people and limited resources, yields have been improved significantly, and there is abundant genetic variability from which further progress may be made. In the past, guayule has suffered from intermittent support, and advancements often undermined by periods of indifference. It is important if guayule is to become a commercial crop to keep a sustained, even if low-level of support, since new concepts and fresh approaches result from researchers who have significant experience and familiarity with the crop.

REFERENCES

Bonner, J. 1991. The history of rubber, p. 1–6. In: J.W. Whitworth and E.E. Whitehead (eds.). Guayule natural rubber. Office of Arid Lands Studies, Univ. of Arizona, Tucson.

Coates, W. 1991. Guayule harvesting equipment, p. 241–260. In: J.W. Whitworth and E.E. Whitehead (eds.). Guayule natural rubber. Office of Arid Lands, Univ. of Arizona, Tucson.

Estilai, A. and D.T. Ray. 1991. Genetics, cytogenetics, and breeding of guayule, p. 47–92. In: J.W. Whitworth and E.E. Whitehead (eds.). Guayule natural rubber. Office of Arid Lands, Univ. of Arizona, Tucson.

Huang, H.T. 1991. Introduction, p. xv–xix. In: J.W. Whitworth and E.E. Whitehead (eds.). Guayule natural rubber. Office of Arid Lands, Univ. of Arizona, Tucson.

Mihail, J.D., S.M. Alcorn, and J.W. Whitworth. 1991. Plant health: the interactions of guayule, microorganisms, arthropods, and weeds, p. 173–216. In: J.W. Whitworth and E.E. Whitehead (eds.). Guayule natural rubber. Office of Arid Lands, Univ. of Arizona, Tucson.

Nakayama, F.S. 1991. Influences of environment and management practices on rubber quantity and quality, p. 217–240. In: J.W. Whitworth and E.E. Whitehead (eds.). Guayule natural rubber. Office of Arid Lands, Univ. of Arizona, Tucson.

Nakayama, F.S., D.A. Bucks, C.L. Gonzalez, and M.A. Foster. 1991. Water and nutrient requirements of guayule under irrigated and dryland production, p. 145–172. In: J.W. Whitworth and E.E. Whitehead (eds.). Guayule natural rubber. Office of Arid Lands, Univ. of Arizona, Tucson.

Schloman, W.W., Jr. and J.P. Wagner. 1991. Rubber and coproduct utilization, p. 287–310. In: J.W. Whitworth and E.E. Whitehead (eds.). Guayule natural rubber. Office of Arid Lands, Univ. of Arizona, Tucson.

Thompson, A.E. and D.T. Ray. 1989. Breeding guayule. Plant Breed Rev. 6:93–165.

Wagner, J.P. and W.W. Schloman, Jr. 1991. Processing, p. 261–286. In: J.W. Whitworth and E.E. Whitehead (eds.). Guayule natural rubber. Office of Arid Lands, Univ. of Arizona, Tucson.

West, J., E. Rodriguez, and H. Hashemi. 1991. Biochemical evolution and species relationships in the genus *Parthenium* (Asteraceae), p. 33–46. In: J.W. Whitworth and E.E. Whitehead (eds.). Guayule natural rubber. Office of Arid Lands, Univ. of Arizona, Tucson.

Whitworth, J.W. and E.E. Whitehead. 1991. Guayule natural rubber: a technical publication with emphasis on recent findings. Guayule Administrative Management Committee and USDA Cooperative Research Service, Office of Arid Lands Studies, Univ. of Arizona, Tucson.

Wright, N.G., S. Fansler, and R.D. Lacewell. 1991. Guayule economics, p. 351–366. In: J.W. Whitworth and E.E. Whitehead (eds.). Guayule natural rubber. Office of Arid Lands, Univ. of Arizona, Tucson.

Evaluation of Rubber and Resin Content in Lines of Guayule Collected from Nuevo Leon Province in Mexico

Sathyanarayanaiah Kuruvadi, Alfonso López Benitez, and F. Borrego

Guayule (*Parthenium argentatum*, Gray) is the most promising source of natural rubber for domestication in the semiarid regions of Mexico and the native populations are distributed in the northcentral provinces. The wild collections made from this area form the basic material for identifying high yielding rubber lines and gene reservoirs for superior agronomic characters. The purpose of this study was to evaluate 36 indigenous collections of guayule made in the province of Nuevo Leon and to identify high yielding rubber lines and localities where potential rubber genotypes existed.

METHODOLOGY

Thirty-six accessions from local germplasm of guayule were selected based on desirable plant characters such as vigor, plant height, plant spread, and stem diameter. These collections were originally made from three districts in the province of Nuevo Leon in Mexico namely: 21 collections from Dr. Arroyo; 2 from Arramberi; and 12 from Galeana. The seeds of these accessions along with a control selection (G.11605) were soaked in running water for 8 h and treated and germinated according to the procedure of Naqvi and Hanson (1980) for breaking seed dormancy. Twelve day old seedlings were transplanted individually into polyethylene bags containing about 300 g of sieved and fumigated soil. Seedlings were irrigated twice a week. After 65 days of growth in the greenhouse, the seedlings were transplanted into the field at the Dryland Experimental Station, Ocampo, Coahuila, using a spacing of 80 cm between rows and 100 cm within the row. Each accession was transplanted into a single row 10 m long, using a randomized block design with two replications. Plants were irrigated immediately after transplanting; further growth depended on natural precipitation.

The data were obtained from five plants at random when the plants were approximately 32 month old. The lowest branch from each plant was sampled for rubber and resin analysis using standard extraction procedure (Spence and Caldwell 1933).

RESULTS AND DISCUSSION

Significant genetic differences were obtained in percent rubber, percent resin, plant height, and top diameter, indicating that a selection and breeding program could improve these traits. These results are in agreement with Tipton (1982), Kuruvadi (1985), Benitez and Kuruvadi (1987), and Kuruvadi (1991) who evaluated 158, 346, 45, and 38 guayule collections and reported significant differences between lines for these traits.

The percentage of rubber varied from 3.9 to 11.3 with a mean of 7.2 (Table 1). Accession 4142, yielded the highest rubber concentration (11.3%), followed by accessions 4144 (11.2%), 4437 (11.2%), 4592 (10.9%), and 4288 (10.6%). These accessions yielded higher rubber content than the control line G.11605 (9.1%). Variation in rubber concentration has been observed previously within and among populations (Tipton 1982; Naqvi 1985; Kuruvadi 1985). The collections from the district of Dr. Arroyo demonstrated highest rubber content when compared to other districts in the province of Nuevo Leon. Drought and cold stress stimulate rubber biosynthesis (Tipton 1982) while interspecific hybridization with mariola (*Parthenium incanum* H.B.K.) reduces rubber producing potential in the progeny. Resin, another major byproduct of guayule, ranged from 7.1 to 10.5 with a mean of 8.6%. Accessions 4599, 4093, 4409, 4175, and 4240 produced the most resin.

Many of the collections made from Trinidad and Tanquecillo of the district of Dr. Arroyo and El Salero and Boca del Refugio belonging to the district of Galeana yielded higher rubber content when compared to the other populations. Plant height was greatest in accessions 4448, 4380, 4338, 4597, and 4596 while, the largest top diameters were observed in accessions 4167, 4596, 4093, 4288, and 4488. The combination of desirable traits are not present in a single genotype, but are distributed in several genotypes. Hence, hybridization between

Table 1. Mean values for different agronomic characters in guayule.

District name	Accession no.	Rubber (%)	Resin (%)	Plant height (cm)	Top spread (cm)
Dr. Arroyo	4175	4.8	10.1	44.5	75.6
	4288	10.6	8.3	49.0	83.4
	4488	4.7	7.4	51.0	81.1
	4491	9.5	8.9	41.8	67.7
	4492	9.3	8.7	43.5	69.0
	4409	5.1	10.2	49.0	79.1
	4437	11.2	9.1	39.0	70.4
	4439	6.5	7.8	45.5	66.1
	4442	7.3	7.8	37.5	65.7
	4123	8.4	7.8	44.0	74.0
	4142	11.3	8.5	38.0	63.1
	4144	11.2	8.3	44.0	67.1
	4161	5.6	7.8	42.5	80.3
	4163	5.7	9.1	39.5	80.2
	4167	4.9	7.2	49.5	86.9
	4590	8.2	8.5	43.0	71.6
	4592	10.9	7.4	38.0	61.9
	4593	8.0	8.3	34.4	62.4
	4596	4.1	8.5	49.8	84.2
	4597	7.8	7.1	50.5	77.3
	4599	7.1	10.5	35.5	67.1
Arramberri	4087	5.2	7.8	48.0	74.5
	4093	3.9	10.3	41.0	84.1
Galeana	4240	5.3	9.9	47.0	79.5
	4232	7.3	9.2	46.5	68.5
	4233	7.6	7.6	40.5	63.3
	4380	5.3	9.7	50.5	74.9
	4384	4.9	9.3	45.5	70.5
	4489	9.1	7.8	45.0	72.9
	4338	5.7	9.3	50.5	68.2
	4350	7.4	8.1	43.3	55.7
	4354	4.5	8.2	40.5	70.1
	4357	7.7	8.1	48.5	80.7
	4308	4.9	7.3	47.0	79.6
	4265	9.1	9.5	46.0	69.5
Check	G11605	9.1	9.9	44.0	72.2
Mean		7.2	8.6	44.3	72.7

accessions with the highest rubber concentration and those with greatest plant height and largest top diameter are recommended in order to obtain superior recombinants. Guayule rubber yields should be improved as well through single plant selection from highly vigorous plants in the native population.

REFERENCES

Benitez, A.L. and S. Kuruvadi. 1987. Variability in rubber content of three guayule populations in Durango, Mexico. El Guayulero 9(1, 2):3–7.

Kuruvadi, S. 1985. Evaluation of genetic resources of guayule in Mexico. El guayulero 7 (1, 2):24–26.

Kuruvadi, S. 1991. Estimation of rubber and resin content in guayule from a diverse breeding population in Mexico. Bioresource Tech. 35:167–171.

Naqvi, H.H. 1985. Variability in rubber content among USDA guayule lines. Bul. Torr. Bot. Club 112:196–198.

Naqvi, H.H. and G.P. Hanson. 1980. Recent advances in guayule seed germination procedures. Crop Sci. 20:501–504.

Spence, D. and M.L. Caldwell. 1933. Determination of rubber in rubber bearing plants. Ind. Eng. Chem. Anal. 5:371–375.

Tipton, J.L. 1982. Variation in rubber concentration of native Texas guayule. HortScience 17:742–743.

Rubber and Resin Content in the Bark and Wood Portions of the Root Stem and Branches in Guayule

Sathyanarayanaiah Kuruvadi and Diana Jasso de Rodriguez

Guayule (*Parthenium argentatum* Gray), a perennial shrub, is a potential source of natural rubber for the arid zones of Mexico and other countries. Natural rubber is superior to synthetic rubber derived from petrochemicals and is preferred where low heat buildup, elasticity and resilience are necessary (Fangmeir et al. 1984).

Rubber in guayule occurs as a colloidal suspension in the individual cells in the tissues of cortex and vascular rays of phloem and xylem (Foster et al. 1980). The bark portions of the roots, stems, and branches contain the majority of the rubber (Estilai 1987) and branches contain a higher percentage of rubber and resin than the main stem and roots (Jasso and Kuruvadi 1991). The objective of this investigation was to determine the variability of rubber and resin content in the bark and wood portions of root, stem, and branches and to identify higher rubber yielding lines associated with the production of thick bark.

MATERIALS AND METHODS

Ten accessions were selected from the local germplasm collection of guayule and were seeded in the greenhouse. Fifteen day old seedlings were transplanted individually in polyethylene bags containing approximately 500 g of sieved and fumigated soil and irrigated when necessary. After 65 days of growth in the greenhouse, the seedlings of each accession was transplanted individually at the Dryland Experimental Station, Ocampo, Coahuila, Mexico, using a spacing of 80 cm between rows and 100 cm between plants within a row. When the plants were approximately 32 month old, three entire plants were sampled per treatment. The leaves, peduncles, dried inflorescences, and small branches were pruned and the root system was cleaned. Then each plant was sectioned into three parts: root system, main stem, and branches. The bark and wood tissue were separated from each part by hammering lightly; 5 g of ground sample of each tissue was utilized for quantitative estimation of rubber and resin content using standard soxhlet extraction procedure. The means of rubber and resin in the three plant parts and two tissues were analyzed statistically using completely randomized block of three factor $10 \times 2 \times 3$ (10 entries, 2 tissues, and 3 plant parts) factorial design.

RESULTS AND DISCUSSION

The analysis of variance (not presented) indicated significant differences for percent rubber, percent resin, and diameter of bark and wood tissues between genotypes, between three plant parts, and two tissues indicating that the ten accessions of this investigation differed greatly with respect to the diameter of bark, wood, and their rubber and resin concentration (Table 1). Selection and breeding could further improve these traits.

Rubber percent varied from 3.94 to 11.42% (root), 4.80 to 12.23% (stem), and 4.92 to 11.01% (branches) in the bark, and ranged from 0.38 to 1.55% (root), 0.46 to 4.44% (stem), and 0.72 to 5.00% (branches) in the wood. The mean percent rubber was 7.3% for the bark and 1.4% for wood tissue in the three plant parts; the bark contained 421% more rubber than wood tissue. The total bark and wood portions of these genotypes contain approximately 83.8 and 16.2% of the rubber in the plant. Estilai (1987) estimated that the bark of the plant of guayule contains about 70 to 85% of the rubber in the plant depending on the genotype. Maximum percent rubber was observed in accession 4599 (7.6%), followed by accessions 4580 (5.7%), 4144 (4.8%), 4358 (4.7%), and 4443 (4.3%).

Table 1. Mean of rubber and resin content in the bark and wood portions of the root, stem, and branches in ten guayule accessions.

Accession	Root Bark	Root Wood	Stem Bark	Stem Wood	Branch Bark	Branch Wood
Rubber (%)						
4123	4.91	0.56	6.79	0.91	8.13	0.72
4130	5.79	0.95	7.97	0.46	5.75	0.94
4144	6.62	1.09	8.28	1.44	7.76	3.64
4161	3.94	0.62	4.80	1.03	4.92	1.55
4338	5.48	0.56	5.35	0.84	6.64	0.86
4358	9.53	0.38	8.92	0.70	7.35	1.05
4443	5.86	0.73	7.37	1.12	7.91	2.99
4580	8.60	0.70	10.57	3.19	9.98	1.12
4597	3.94	0.62	4.80	1.03	4.92	1.55
4599	11.42	1.55	12.23	4.44	11.01	5.00
Mean	6.61	0.78	7.71	1.51	7.44	1.94
Resin (%)						
4123	11.78	2.68	11.79	3.59	11.09	3.64
4130	13.49	4.58	11.91	4.38	12.17	5.23
4144	11.68	5.81	12.82	6.46	13.47	7.23
4161	14.92	2.84	13.46	3.19	9.84	3.44
4338	11.59	4.55	12.36	4.66	10.29	5.89
4358	12.54	2.05	10.60	3.45	10.35	2.79
4443	15.03	4.19	13.37	5.20	12.25	6.57
4580	12.21	4.67	12.22	5.64	11.34	5.09
4597	11.77	3.13	11.81	3.59	11.08	3.62
4599	9.05	3.09	10.04	3.51	11.50	5.49
Mean	12.41	3.76	12.16	4.37	11.34	4.90

Resin is another important byproduct of guayule; average resin percentage was 11.9 for the bark and 4.3 for wood. The total bark and wood tissue of these accessions contains nearly 73.4 and 26.6% resin in the plant. Superior genotypes identified were 4144, 4443, 4130, 4580, and 4338 which ranged from 8.2 to 9.6% resin.

The thickness of the bark is one of the important characters influencing the total production of rubber and resin in the plant. The mean thickness of the bark was 0.13 cm (root), 0.42 cm (stem), and 0.23 cm (branches). Superior genotypes for bark diameter were 4144, 4161, 4338, and 4597 (root); 4123, 4144, and 4599 (stem); and 4597, 4144, and 4161 (branches). Accession 4144 contained thicker bark in the three parts of the plant studied.

The majority of the rubber and resin accumulation occurs in the bark of the plant. Hence in breeding, high priority should be given to combining bark thickness, higher rubber percent and high biomass yield.

REFERENCES

Estilai, A. 1987. Molecular weight of rubber contained in guayule bark, wood and whole stem. Rubber Chem. Tech. 60:245–251.

Fangmeir, D.D., D.D. Rubis, B.B. Tylor, and K.E. Foster. 1984. Guayule for rubber production in Arizona. Univ. of Arizona, Tucson.

Foster, K.E., W.G. McGinnies, J.G. Taylor, J. Maloney, and R.C. Wyatt. 1980. A technology assessment of guayule rubber commercialization. Office of air land studies, Univ. of Arizona, Tucson and Midwest Research Institute, Kansas City, MO, p. 22.

Jasso. R.D. and S. Kuruvadi. 1991. Comparison of soxhlet and homogenizer extraction methods to determine rubber and resin content of Mexican guayule plants. Bioresource Tech. 35:179–183.

Interspecific Hybridization Between *Parthenium argentatum* Gray and *Parthenium lozanianum* Bartlett

A. López Benitez, F. Ramirez, S. Kuruvadi, and F. Borrego

The genus *Parthenium* has been classified into 16 different species (Rollins 1950) from which only guayule (*P. argentatum*) contains substantial amounts of good quality rubber. Interspecific hybridization in guayule as a means of introducing desirable traits, requires basic information on the breeding behavior of the interspecific hybrids with regard to fertility and type of inheritance of the traits studied. In F_1 hybrids between *P. argentatum* and *P. hispidum* var. *auriculatum*, Hashemi et al. (1987), reported that meiotic behavior was irregular as indicated by a low pollen stainability and the limited number of viable BC_1 seeds. In contrast, Estilai et al. (1985), showed that guayule and *P. schottii* are readily crossed and the F_1 hybrids produced showed a partial fertility and high degree of chromosome pairing. The inheritance of rubber content and morphological characters in interspecific hybrids have been described by Naqvi et al. (1984), as due to multiple gene action. A similar type of gene action has also been described by Naqvi et al. (1987) for growth habit, morphological traits, rubber, and resin contents of hybrids between guayule and *P. fruticosum*. In this paper, we report the morphological characters, rubber content and molecular weight, and resin content for hybrids between guayule and *P. lozanianum*, and compare the hybrids to their progenitors.

METHODOLOGY

Seed of diploid guayule and *P. lozanianum* were grown in the greenhouse. Chromosome counts on *P. lozanianum* at meiosis indicated $2n = 108$. Diploid guayule proved to be self-incompatible, and was utilized as the female without emasculation. Crosses were made in one direction transferring pollen from *P. lozanianum* directly to the stigmas of guayule. Seed of parental species and hybrids were collected when ripe, seeded separately in the greenhouse and allowed to grow for 20 months. Plants were then sampled for plant growth characteristics; and for rubber and resin analysis. Plant height, plant spread, leaf length, leaf width, and peduncle length were determined from 10 individual plants of each parent and F_1 hybrids. Rubber and resin analysis were performed on the same 10 plants according to Holmes and Robbin (1974). Rubber quality as estimated by molecular weight was determined for both parents and F_1 hybrids according to Campos Lopez and Angulo Sanchez (1975).

RESULTS AND DISCUSSION

Table 1 presents morphological data, rubber content, rubber molecular weight, and resin content of *P. argentatum*, *P. lozanianum*, and their interspecific F_1 hybrids. Plant height and spread, and leaf shape, length and width were the most conspicuous morphological differences between *P. argentatum* and *P. lozanianum*. Average leaf length of *P. argentatum* and F_1 hybrids was about 30% lower than *P. lozanianum*. Leaf widths of *P. lozanianum* were 30% of guayule and hybrids. Peduncle length of the hybrids was larger than either parent. Hybrids were easy to recognize because of the intermediate nature of many morphological and agronomic traits as compared to the two parental species. The intermediate nature of the morphological characteristics of interspecific F_1 hybrids in the genus *Parthenium* has been pointed out by Naqvi et al. (1984, 1987) who suggested a polygenic type of gene action for these traits. Rubber content in guayule (6.82%) was about 12 times greater than *P. lozanianum* (0.56%) but F_1 hybrids had an average of 4.6% which is about 67% of that in guayule. Although *P. lozanianum* did not improve the rubber percentage of the hybrids, the total rubber production could be improved if biomass increased as indicated by Tysdale (1950).

The small traces of rubber found in *P. lozanianum* showed higher molecular weight than guayule. This trait was found in the hybrids indicating a dominant type of gene action. Campos Lopez and Angulo Sanchez (1975) indicated that the rubber from either *Hevea* or guayule should have a molecular weight of at least 2 million to be considered of good quality. Our results suggest that *P. lozanianum* could be utilized to improve rubber quality of guayule.

Table 1. Morphological traits and rubber content of *P. argentatum*, *P. lozanianum* and their F_1 hybrids grown in the greenhouse for 20 months.

	Mean±SD		
Variable	*P. argentatum*	*P. lozanianum*	F_1 hybrid
Plant			
Height (cm)	46.7±3.0	110.6±6.9	64.7±9.2
Width (cm)	42.0±3.1	84.5±5.2	47.0±10.7
Leaf			
Length (cm)	6.0±0.8	8.3±3.0	5.6±0.4
Width (cm)	1.7±0.3	5.4±2.9	1.7±0.2
Inflorescence			
Peduncle length (cm)	12.2±1.7	10.6±2.2	17.6±4.5
Head width (cm)	5.3±0.3	5.1±0.3	5.3±0.4
Rubber			
Content (%)	6.8±0.7	0.6±0.1	4.6±0.7
M.W.	1.95×10^6	2.27×10^6	2.21×10^6
Resin (%)	8.3±0.9	5.3±0.9	7.8±1.2

REFERENCES

Campos Lopez, E. and J.L. Angulo Sanchez. 1975. Molecular weight characterization of natural guayule rubber by gel-permeation chromotography. Polymers Letters Edition 14:649–652.

Estilai, A., A. Hashemi, and, V.B. Yougner. 1985. Genomic relationship of guayule with *Parthenium schottii*. Amer. J. Bot. 72:1522–1529.

Hashemi, A., E. Estilai, and J.E. West. 1987. Relationship of woody *Parthenium argentatum* and herbaceous *P. hispidum* var. *auriculatum* (Asteraceae). Amer. J. Bot. 74:1350–1358.

Holmes, R.L. and H.W. Robbins. 1947. Rubber determination in young guayule. Studies on the Spence and Caldwell method. Anal. Chem. 19:313–317.

Naqvi, H.H., A. Hashemi, J.R. Davey, and J.B. Waines. 1987. Morphological and cytogenetic characters of F_1 hybrids between *P. argentatum* and *P. fruticosum* var *fruticosum* and their potential rubber improvement. Econ. Bot. 41:66–67.

Naqvi, H.H., V.B. Yougner, and E. Rodriguez. 1984. Inheritance of rubber content and morphological traits in F_1 hybrids between *Parthenium argentatum* and *P. schottii*. Bul. Torrey Bot. Club. 3:337–382.

Rollins, R.C. 1950. The guayule rubber plant and its relatives. The Gray Herbarium of Harvard University, Cambridge, MA.

Tysdale, H.M. 1950. Apomictic interspecific hybrids are promising for rubber production from guayule. Agron. J. 42:351–355.

Salt Tolerance in Relation to Ploidy Level in Guayule

Ali Estilai and Michael C. Shannon

Guayule (*Parthenium argentatum* Gray) is a promising alternative to rubber tree (*Hevea brasiliensis* Muel. Arg.) for production of natural rubber in semiarid regions of the world. For the United States, which is totally dependent on foreign sources of natural rubber, developing guayule as a commercial crop should be a high priority. A domestic source of natural rubber is vital to our national defense and helps balance the budget by reducing the one billion dollars spent annually for the imports of *Hevea* rubber from southeast Asia.

Guayule grows naturally in the semiarid Chihuahuan Desert region of north central Mexico and the Big Bend area of Texas in the southwestern United States. The native stands are restricted to outwash fans and rocky slopes of calcareous soils. In general, guayule is considered to be only slightly tolerant to soil salinity (Hammond and Polhamus 1965). Although guayule seeds germinate successfully in highly saline solutions of up to 22 dS/m, seedling emergence is reduced severely when saline waters are used for irrigation (Miyamoto et al. 1984). Salinity of irrigation water has been reported to decrease rubber yield and water use efficiency (Miyamoto and Bucks 1985). Experiments conducted in the 1940s at Texas indicated that salinity greater than 3.3 dS/m would be unsuitable for guayule culture (McGinnies and Mills 1980). In a more recent study, conducted at Brawley, California, guayule appeared more salt tolerant than many crops that were considered tolerant at the 6 dS/m level (Maas et al. 1986). The apparent disagreement between the findings of the two studies is due to the high sodium content found in the Texas water versus the high calcium content in the California water (Nakayama et al. 1991). Greenhouse sand culture experiments have shown the detrimental effects of high sodium concentration as compared to calcium on guayule growth (Wadleigh and Gauch 1944). No statistically significant interaction effects were found between plant population and salinity (Hoffman et al. 1988).

Salt-tolerant guayule cultivars are needed for economic production of rubber on marginal lands and in areas with low quality saline water. The available guayule germplasm which is being used to develop new guayule cultivars are $2n = 36$, 54, or 72 (Bergner 1944, 1946; Stebbins and Kodani 1944). Plants with $2n = 36$ are considered to be diploid (Bergner 1944; Estilai et al. 1985; Hashemi et al. 1989). Diploids reproduce sexually and, because of a sporophytic system of self-incompatibility, they produce seed by cross-pollination (Gerstel 1950; Estilai 1984). Plants with $2n = 54$ and 72 are polyploid (triploid and tetraploid, respectively), and their mode of reproduction is by facultative apomixis, the simultaneous occurrence of sexual and apomictic modes of reproduction (Esau 1944; Gardner 1947; Powers and Rollins 1945). Information on salt tolerance of guayule plants with different chromosome number is unavailable. The primary objectives of this study were to compare diploid, triploid, and tetraploid guayule germplasm, irrigated with saline water, for important agronomic traits and to identify salt tolerant individuals for development of improved cultivars.

METHODOLOGY

Open-pollinated seeds from diploid, triploid, and tetraploid guayule germplasm were planted in a greenhouse at the University of California, Riverside in January 1989 following procedures described previously (Estilai and Waines 1987; Estilai 1991). Seedlings were hand-transplanted into experimental plots at Brawley, California on May 24, 1989. The experimental design was a randomized complete block with four replications. Each entry in a replicate was planted in a plot consisting of two rows, each 16 m long, with the interrow and interplant spacing of 1 m and 0.45 m, respectively. Approximate population density was 22,200 plants/ha. Experiments were surrounded by a row of border plants.

Seedlings were irrigated with normal water until Nov. 6, 1989 when the first measurements were obtained for plant height and width. Plots were then irrigated with saline water of electrical conductivity of 7.5 dS/m. Prior to harvest on Feb. 26, 1991 (when plants were 21 months old), height and width were measured for 10 plants per plot. The 10 plants were cut at 0.05 m above ground, leaves and peduncles removed, and plants weighed and chipped. Immediately after chipping, two samples were taken to determine percent dry weight and rubber and resin contents. Samples used to determine the percent dry weight were dried in a forced air oven at 75°C and reweighed.

Samples used for rubber and resin analyses were stored in a freezer and later were ground in the presence of liquid nitrogen. Resin and rubber were extracted from the finely ground plant materials using acetone and cyclohexane, respectively. Detailed procedures for determination of rubber and resin contents have already been reported (Black et al. 1983; Estilai and Mayhew 1990).

RESULTS AND DISCUSSION

Table 1 compares the three germplasm lines for nine agronomic traits. The polyploid germplasm was significantly superior to the diploids for all traits. The triploid and tetraploid germplasm were similar in performance except for resin content and resin yield. The triploid germplasm had the highest annual resin content of 10.7% and the highest resin yield of 420 kg/ha. Diploid, triploid, and tetraploid germplasm, respectively, produced 60, 64, and 40% more resin than rubber (Table 1). Resin is an important co-product, and may provide an additional revenue for guayule commercialization. Possible applications of resin include use as an adhesion modifier for strippable coatings and as wood preservative.

Annual rubber yield, the most important trait for guayule commercialization, varied from a minimum of 125 kg/ha for the diploid germplasm to a maximum of 256 kg/ha for the triploid germplasm. These levels of productivity are far below the annual rubber yield of 1,000 to 1,500 kg/ha needed to make guayule a successful irrigated crop in prime agricultural lands. However, considering the reduced value of lands in semiarid regions and lower costs for the low quality saline water, annual rubber yield of 500 kg/ha may be acceptable for low input agriculture.

The guayule germplasm showed variation for all traits studied. More than 20 plants with annual rubber yield of 40 g (potential rubber yield of 500 kg/ha) were identified and will be used to develop cultivars with increased rubber production under irrigation with saline water.

FUTURE PROSPECTS

The variation observed for salt tolerance among the germplasm with different chromosome number suggests the possibility of selecting ecotypes for arid, semiarid, and marginal lands. This variability also provides suitable material to study the genetic basis and the physiological nature of salt tolerance in guayule.

Table 1. Comparison of diploid, triploid, and tetraploid guayule entries for nine agronomic traits.

	Guayule entries					
	Diploid		Triploid		Tetraploid	
Plant traits	Range	Mean	Range	Mean	Range	Mean
Height (cm)	47–66	56.5a[z]	52–64	59.5a	48–67	60.5a
Width (cm)	54–69	61.8a	65–75	69.5b	62–76	70.5 b
Dry weight (kg ha^{-1} yr^{-1})	2,029–2,689	2,334a	3,590–4,351	3,856b	3,513–4,338	3,758b
Rubber content (%)	4.9–5.7	5.3a	6.3–7.2	6.6b	6.3–6.8	6.5b
Resin content (%)	7.9–9.4	8.6a	9.2–12.2	10.7b	7.9–10.3	9.2c
Rubber+resin (%)	12.9–14.6	14.0a	15.9–18.5	17.5b	14.4–16.9	15.7c
Rubber yield (kg ha^{-1} yr^{-1})	105–147	125 a	224–279	256b	228–272	245b
Resin yield (kg ha^{-1} yr^{-1})	178–241	200 a	332–503	420b	277–380	345c
Rubber + resin yield (kg ha^{-1} yr^{-1})	296–388	325a	574–781	677b	506–654	590c

[z]Row means followed by the same letter are not significantly different at the p = 0.05 level as determined by Duncan's new multiple range test.

REFERENCES

Bergner, A.D. 1944. Guayule plants with low chromosome numbers. Science 99:224–225.

Bergner, A.D. 1946. Polyploidy and aneuploidy in guayule. USDA Tech. Bul. 918. U.S. Government Printing Office, Washington, DC.

Black, L.T., G.E. Hamerstrand, F.S. Nakayama, and B.A. Rasnik. 1983. Gravimetric analyses for determining resin and rubber content of guayule. Rubber Chem. Technol. 56:367–371.

Esau, K. 1944. Apomixis in guayule. Proc. Natl. Acad. Sci. (USA) 30:352–355.

Estilai, A. 1991. Biomass, rubber, and resin yield potentials of new guayule germplasm. Bioresource Tech. 35:119–125.

Estilai, A., and R.C. Mayhew. 1990. Automated gravimetric analyses of guayule rubber and resin contents. El Guayulero 12:5–11.

Estilai, A. and J.G. Waines. 1987. Variation in regrowth and its implications for multiple harvest of guayule. Crop Sci. 27:100–103.

Estilai, A., A. Hashemi, and V.B. Youngner. 1985. Genomic relationship of guayule with *Parthenium schottii*. Amer. J. Bot. 72:1522–1529.

Estilai, A. 1984. Inheritance of flower color in guayule. Crop Sci. 24:760–762.

Gardner, E.J. 1947. Studies on the inheritance of apomixis and sterility in the progeny of two hybrid plants in the genus *Parthenium*. Genetics 32:262–267.

Gerstel, D.U. 1950. Self-incompatibility studies in guayule. II. Inheritance. Genetics 35:482–506.

Hammond, B.L. and L.G. Polhamus. 1965. Research on guayule (*Parthenium argentatum*): 1942–1959. USDA Tech. Bul. 1327. U.S. Government Printing Office, Washington, DC.

Hashemi, A., A. Estilai, and J.G. Waines. 1989. Cytogenetics and reproductive behavior of induced and natural tetraploid guayule (*Parthenium argentatum* Gray). Genome 32:1100–1104.

Hoffman, G.J., M.C. Shannon, E.V. Maas, and L. Grass. 1988. Rubber production of salt-stressed guayule at various populations. Irrigation Science 9:213–226.

Maas, E.V., T.J. Donovan, L.E. Francois, and G.E. Hamerstrand. 1986. Salt tolerance of guayule, p. 101–107. In: D.D. Fangmeier and S.M. Alcorn (eds.). Guayule a natural rubber source. Guayule Rubber Society.

McGinnies, W.G. and J.L. Mills. 1980. Guayule rubber production. The world war II emergency rubber project: A guide to future development. Office of Arid Lands Studies, Tucson, AZ.

Miyamoto, S. and D.A. Bucks. 1985. Water quantity and quality requirements of guayule: Current assessment. Agr. Water Manag. 10:205–219.

Miyamoto, S., K. Piela, J. Davis, and L.G. Fenn. 1984. Salt effects on emergence and seedling mortality of guayule. Agron. J. 76:295–300.

Nakayama, F., D.A. Bucks, C.L. Gonzalez, and M.A. Foster. 1991. Water and nutrient requirements of guayule under irrigated and dryland production, p. 145–172. In: J.W. Whitworth and E.E. Whitehead (eds.). Guayule natural rubber. Office of Arid Lands Studies, Tucson, AZ.

Powers, L., and R.C. Rollins. 1945. Reproduction and pollination studies on guayule, *Parthenium argentatum* Gray and *P. incanum* H.B.K. Amer. Soc. Agron. J. 37:96–112.

Stebbins, G.L. and M. Kodani. 1944. Chromosomal variation in guayule and mariola. J. Hered. 35:162–172.

Wadleigh, C.H. and H.G. Gauch. 1944. The influence of high concentrations of sodium sulfate, sodium chloride, calcium chloride, and magnesium chloride on the growth of guayule in sand cultures. Soil Sci. 58:399–403.

Growth of Direct Seeded and Transplanted Guayule Seedlings

James L. Fowler and Robert Tinguely

Guayule (*Parthenium argentatum* Gray), a semi-desert shrub native to the Trans-Pecos Region of southwest Texas and northcentral Mexico, is a potential domestic source of rubber for the United States (National Academy of Sciences 1977). The feasibility of domestic rubber production from guayule is dependent on improved rubber yield, increased rubber prices, and the reduction of production costs (Foster and Moore 1987). One of the major production costs of guayule is stand establishment by transplanting nursery seedlings into the field which can cost $900 to $1,200/ha (Bucks et al. 1986). Recent advances in direct seeding techniques have resulted in a less costly option of stand establishment of guayule than transplanting (Bucks et al. 1986). Seedlings for transplanting are grown in a greenhouse or nursery in small, root restricting containers and generally have a two to four month growth advantage over direct seeded guayule. The objective of this study was to determine if transplants maintain this initial growth advantage over direct seeded guayule and whether the restricted root of the transplant limits shoot and root development.

METHODOLOGY

Seeds of guayule cultivar Cal-6 were planted in a greenhouse in a soil mixture in 5 × 5 cm peat pots on Feb. 8, 1989. Seedlings were thinned to one seedling per pot and maintained in the greenhouse until transplanted to containers (polyvinylchloride pipe, 15 cm in diameter × 76 cm high, filled with very fine sandy loam soil) in a shade house (30% shade) on June 30. Seeds were also planted in similar containers in the shade house on June 30. Transplant containers and direct seeded containers were arranged in a randomized complete block design with five replications. The direct seeded containers were thinned to one plant per container. Sufficient containers of transplanted and direct seeded plants were planted for four harvests [57, 87, 117, and 146 days after planting (DAP)] over a 146 day growth period. Two containers per treatment per replication per harvest were fractionated into leaves, stems, and roots. Leaf area, leaf dry weight, shoot dry weight, root length, root volume, and root dry weight were measured. Roots were removed from the containers by cutting the containers in two, lengthwise, and gently washing the roots from the soil. Fine roots were collected by straining the soil-water mixture through a fine mesh screen several times. Nonroot plant debris and other foreign particles were removed from the roots by hand. Roots were stored in glass jars in FAA solution (Sass 1958) until processed for root length, root volume, and dry weight. Root volume was determined by displacement and root length was measured using a Delta-T Area Meter (Delta-T Devices Ltd., Cambridge, England). The shoot was separated into leaves and stem. Leaf area was measured with a LiCor, Inc. Model 3000 Leaf Area Meter with Transparent Conveyor Belt Accessory (LiCor, Inc., Lincoln, Nebraska). Dry weights of leaves, stems, and roots were determined by drying in a forced draft oven for 48 h at 70°C and reported on a dry weight per plant basis. All data were subjected to analysis of variance (SAS 1985).

RESULTS AND DISCUSSION

The increase in leaf area of guayule transplants exceeded that of the direct seeded plants for the first two harvest dates (57 and 87 DAP), but leaf area of the transplants and the direct seeded plants tended to level out between 117 and 146 DAP (Fig. 1). Leaf weight of both the transplants and direct seeded plants increased throughout the experimental period but at a greater rate in the transplants (Fig. 2). The shoot dry weight advantage of the transplants increased over the direct seeded plants throughout the experimental period (Fig. 3). Leaves from transplants had higher specific leaf weights (leaf weight/leaf area) than leaves from direct seeded plants except for the second harvest (no significant difference) which may account for the high rate of dry matter accumulation of the transplants over the last growth period (between 117 and 146 DAP) when leaf area was leveling off. Root growth as measured by root length (Fig. 4), root volume (Fig. 5), and root dry weight (Fig. 6) followed a similar growth pattern as that of the shoot with the rate of transplant root development exceeding that of the direct seeded plants throughout the measurement period.

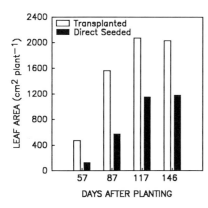

Fig. 1. Leaf area of direct seeded and transplanted guayule.

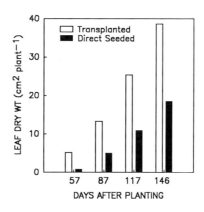

Fig. 2. Leaf dry weight of direct seeded and transplanted guayule.

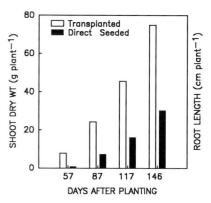

Fig. 3. Shoot dry weight of direct seeded and transplanted guayule.

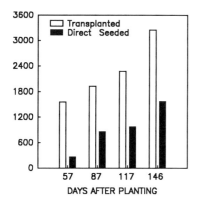

Fig. 4. Root length of direct seeded and transplanted guayule.

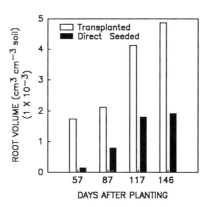

Fig. 5. Root volume of direct seeded and transplanted guayule.

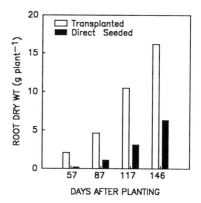

Fig. 6. Root dry weight of direct seeded and transplanted guayule.

CONCLUSIONS

The initial growth advantage of the transplants over the direct seeded plants increased with time over the 146 day growth period for both shoots and roots. There was no indication that the initial restricted root growth of the transplants had any adverse effects on subsequent root or shoot development. If the growth advantage of the transplants over the direct seeded plants is maintained through the second year of growth, the initial cost advantage of direct seeding would be decreased. A field study comparing the growth of transplanted and direct seeded guayule plants is needed to determine if the initial growth advantage of the transplants is maintained through harvest and this would permit a detailed economic comparison.

REFERENCES

Bucks, D.A., R.L. Roth, D.E. Powers, and G.R. Chandra. 1986. Direct seeding for economical guayule field establishment, p. 71–87. In: D.D. Fangmeier and S.M. Alcorn (eds.). Guayule, a natural rubber source. Proc. Fourth Intl. Guayule Res. and Dev. Conf., Tucson, AZ. 16–19 Oct. 1985. Guayule Rubber Soc., Inc.

Foster M.A. and J. Moore. 1987. Guayule: a rangeland source of natural rubber. Rangelands 9:97–102.

National Academy of Sciences. 1977. Guayule: an alternate source of natural rubber. National Academy of Science, Washington, DC.

SAS Institute. 1985. SAS user's guide: Statistics. Version 5. SAS Institute, Cary, NC.

Sass, J.E. 1958. Botanical microtechniques. The Iowa State College Press, Ames.

Impact of Seeding Rate and Planting Date on Guayule Stand Establishment by Direct Seeding in West Texas

Michael Foster, Greg Kleine, and Jaroy Moore

Transplanting of greenhouse-grown seedlings has been the only reliable method of guayule stand establishment. Bucks et al. (1986) estimated that development of direct seeding methods could reduce the cost of establishment to below $400/ha versus $900 to $1,200/ha for transplanting. Recently, Foster et al. (1991) calculated that the cost of establishment could be reduced to $250/ha or less.

Foster and Moore (1991) demonstrated that guayule stand establishment was possible with conditioned seed and precision planting. Seeding rate and the optimum date of planting still must be defined throughout the potential guayule production region. The objectives of this study were to examine the effects of seeding rate and planting date on guayule stand establishment by direct seeding in west Texas.

METHODOLOGY

The study was conducted during 1991 at the Texas Agricultural Experiment Station Guayule Research Site near Fort Stockton. A split plot design arranged in a randomized complete block with four replications was used with date of planting (31 May, 28 June, 15 Aug., and 1 Oct.) and seeding rate (30, 40, 50, 60, 80, 100 seeds/m) as main and subplots, respectively. Main plots were 6 m wide (six 1 m wide rows) and 9 m long. Subplots consisted of single rows 9 m long seeded with a Gaspardo SV 255 pneumatic planter. Mexican bulk guayule seed was conditioned by the process outlined by Chandra and Bucks (1986). Seed germination was 80%. Seedling density (Fig. 1) was not adjusted for percentage germination. The plots were sprinkler irrigated and kept moist during germination and emergence.

RESULTS AND DISCUSSION

Initial germination and emergence was greatest in August (Fig. 1). Seedling density was consistently greater in the 80 and 100 seeds/m treatments as compared to the lower seeding rates. Based on plant spacing recommendations for transplants, 2 to 3 established seedlings/m would be required for an acceptable stand (27,500/ha or 11,500/acre). Even the lower seeding rates (30 to 60 seeds/m) satisfied these requirements. Seeding rate may need to be adjusted for seed quality (% germination), weather factors (heavy rain and hail), insect damage to young seedlings, and reduced germination by preemergence herbicides. Therefore, rates of 40 or 50 seeds/m

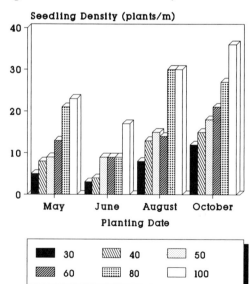

Fig. 1. Average number of guayule seedlings/m row in plots planted at 100, 80, 60, 50, 40, and 30 seeds/m.

may be more realistic, and would require 0.22 to 0.30 kg of seed/ha (0.20 to 0.22 lb./A). Initial seed quality can affect the germination rate of conditioned seed.

Just after plant emergence, the May seeding was damaged by heavy rain and hail, which can occur throughout the growing season. Seedlings in the cotyledon stage were damaged by fall armyworms (*Spodoptera frugiperda*) in the July study.

CONCLUSIONS

Direct seeding guayule during 1991 in west Texas was successful in May, June, and August. Seedling density was greatest in the 100 and 80 seeds/m treatments. Based on plant population recommendations for guayule transplants, even lower seeding rates (30 to 60 seeds/m) were acceptable for stand establishment. Seeding rates of 40 to 50 seeds/m may be more realistic and should be adjusted for seed quality, weather factors, insect damage to young seedlings, and possible reduced germination by preemergence herbicides.

REFERENCES

Bucks, D.A., R.L. Roth, D.E. Powers, and G.R. Chandra. 1986. Direct seeding for economical guayule field establishment, p. 77–87. In: D.D. Fangmeier and S.M. Alcorn, (eds.). Proc. Fourth Int. Guayule Res. Dev. Conf., Tucson, AZ, 16–19 Oct. 1985. Guayule Rubber Soc., Inc., College Station, TX.

Chandra, G.R. and D.A. Bucks. 1986. Improved quality of chemically treated guayule (*Parthenium argentatum* Gray) seeds, p. 59–68. In: D.D. Fangmeier and S.M. Alcorn, (eds.). Proc. Fourth Int. Guayule Res. Dev. Conf., Tucson, AZ, 16–19 Oct. 1985. Guayule Rubber Soc., Inc., College Station, TX.

Foster, K.E., N.G. Wright, and S.F. Fansler. 1991. Guayule natural rubber commercialization: a scale-up feasibility study. Univ. Ariz., Office of Arid Lands Studies, Tucson, AZ.

Foster, M.A. and J. Moore. 1992. Direct seeding techniques for guayule stand establishment in West Texas. J. Prod. Agr. (in press).

Chrysothamnus: A Rubber-producing Semi-arid Shrub

D.J. Weber, W.M. Hess, R.B. Bhat, and J. Huang

Chrysothamnus, a multi-use desert shrub which can grown in a wide range of environmental conditions, has potential uses for revegetation (Sankhla et al. 1987), as a forage for wildlife and livestock (Bhat et al. 1989), for production of natural rubber (Hall and Goodspeed 1919), for production of hydrocarbons from its biomass (Buchannon et al. 1978), for resin for polymer plastics (Thames 1988), as a landscape shrub (Weber et al. 1986), and as a potential source of natural chemical compounds (Hegerhorst et al. 1987a,c). Production of natural rubber can be obtained from *Chrysothamnus* grown on semi-arid lands where cold temperatures would exclude guayule and it could provide resin for polymer plastics and specific chemical compounds for the chemical industry.

BOTANY AND HORTICULTURE

The genera, *Chrysothamnus* (Asteraceae), is endemic to the western United States with 5 sections, 16 species, and 41 subspecies (Anderson 1986). Plants in this genera can grow from Mexico to Canada and from sea level to 3,000 m.

The species, *Chrysothamnus nauseosus* (Pallas) Britt. (rubber rabbitbrush) is a vigorous pioneer plant in disturbed sites. Plants can reach heights of 30 to 180 cm with a few reaching heights of 366 cm. Rubber rabbitbrush has a high rate of photosynthesis and does not become light saturated at full sun (Davis et al. 1985). The average dry weight biomass per plant is 29 kg and the average number of plants per ha in a normal population is 2,632 (McKell and Van Epps 1980). *Chrysothamnus nauseosus* blooms in the fall and the flowers are born in heads that in turn are raised into cymes, racemes, or panicles. The heads contain five yellow disc flowers and are subtended by involucral bracts. Each flower contains a pappus of abundant white slender capillary bristles. The plant is self-fertile and entirely diploid, although polyploidy does occur in one species.

Chrysothamnus nauseosus is a prolific producer of easily harvestable seeds. Seeds germinate on most soils including saline sites in a few days under cool nights (5°C) and warm days (15°C) (Khan et al. 1987). Propagation by cuttings is difficult though possible, and in vitro propagation techniques have been developed (Upadhyaya et al. 1985). The plants grow well under arid conditions but produce more biomass with increased moisture. *Chrysothamnus nauseosus* can tolerate both low freezing and hot arid temperatures.

A number of the species of *Chrysothamnus* particularly *nauseosus* contain rubber up to 7% dry weight. The average molecular weight of the rubber varies in the species, but some species contain rubber with an average molecular weight of 585,000 (Weber and Fernandes 1991). Rubber content was found to be highest under stress conditions (Hegerhorst et al. 1987b).

The resin content of *Chrysothamnus* may be as high as 35% in some species (Bhat et al. 1989) and the resin has potential use as a plastic extender (Thames 1988). The resin, located in the leaves and in the glandular trichomes, contain a range of terpenoid compounds including monoterpenes and pregnanes (Weber and Fernandes 1991). The resin chemicals can be extracted and have potential as a source of natural terpenes and insect inhibitors. The pregnanes are chemically related to animal hormones (Deepak et al. 1989).

LEAF TRICHOMES

Plants and seeds of species and subspecies of *Chrysothamnus* were collected from the western United States from a range of environmental conditions and planted in a uniform garden. Leaf samples were collected from the uniform garden when the leaves were fully mature. The leaf samples were fixed, dehydrated, gold coated, and then observed with a scanning electron microscope. There were two major types of trichomes observed, filiform and glandular. A total of six variants of the filiform or glandular trichomes could be distinguished (Fig. 1). In

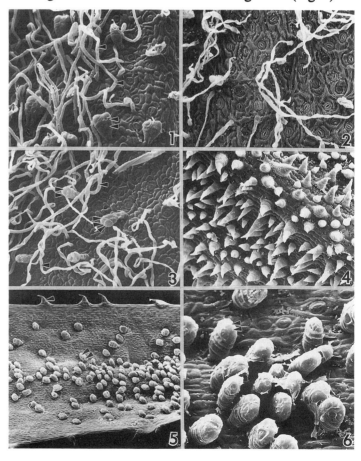

Fig. 1. Leaf surfaces of *Chrysothamnus* showing trichome types. (1) *C. nauseosus* ssp. *consimilis* (Greene) Hall & Clem. showing filiform tubular (arrow) and glandular biseriate (double arrows) types ×225. (2) *C. nauseosus* ssp. *viridulus* (Hall) Hall & Clements showing ribbon types ×225. (3) *C. nauseosus* ssp. *salicifolius* (Rydb.) Hall & Clem showing filiform ribbon (arrow), glandular uniseriate (double arrows), and glandular biseriate (triple arrows) types ×225. (4) *C. viscidiflorus* ssp. *lanceolatus* (Nutt.) Hall & Clem showing prickle types ×225. (5, 6) *C. viscidiflorus* ssp. *viscidiflorus* (Hook.) Nutt. showing prickle multicellular (arrow) and glandular (double arrows) types. ×90; ×450.

some cases, two or three types of trichomes were present on the same leaf. In other cases, only one type of trichome was present. The ratio of filiform to glandular trichomes on a single leaf ranged from 1 in *C. nauseous* ssp. *iridis* L.C. Anderson to 11.9 in *C. nauseous* ssp. *salicifolius* (Rydb.) Hall & Clem. The density varied greatly on the leaves of the different species. The number of total trichomes per mm^2 ranged from 1 in *C. nauseous* ssp. *graveolens* (Nutt.) Piper to 301 in *C. nauseous* ssp. *viridulus* (Hall) Hall & Clements. The number of trichomes per mm^2 did not correlate with resin content, amount of precipitation, or summer temperatures.

REFERENCES

Anderson, L.C. 1986. An overview of the genus *Chrysothamnus* (Asteraceae). In: E.D. McArthur and B.L. Welch (eds.). Proc. symposium on the biology of *Artemisia* and *Chrysothamnus*. USDA Report INT 200. Ogden, UT.

Bhat, R.B., B.L. Welch, D.J. Weber, and E.D. McArthur. 1989. Winter nutritive value of *Chrysothamnus nauseous* ssp. J. Range Manag. 43:177–179.

Buchannon, R.A., I.M. Cull, F.H. Otey, and C.R. Russell. 1978. Hydrocarbon and rubber producing crops. Econ. Bot. 32:131–145.

Davis, T.D., N. Sankhla, W.R. Anderson, D.J. Weber, and B.N. Smith. 1985. High rate of photosynthesis in the desert shrub *Chrysothamnus nauseous* ssp. *albicaulis*. Great Basin Natur. 45:520–526.

Deepak, D., A. Khare, and P.K. Maheshwari. 1989. Plant pregnanes. Phytochemistry 28:3255–3263.

Hall, H.M. and T.H. Goodspeed. 1919. Rubber-plant survey of western North America. Univ. Calif. Pub. Bot. 7:159–278.

Hegerhorst, D.F., D.J. Weber, and E.D. McArthur. 1987a. Resin and rubber content in *Chrysothamnus*. Southwestern Natur. 32:475–482.

Hegerhorst, D.F., D.J. Weber, R.B. Bhat, T.D. Davis, S. Sanderson, and E.D. McArthur. 1987b. Seasonal changes in rubber and resin in *Chrysothamnus nauseous* ssp. *hololeucus* and ssp. *turbinatus*. Biomass 15:133–142.

Hegerhorst, D.F., R.B. Bhat, D.J. Weber, and E.D. McArthur. 1987c. Seasonal changes of selected secondary plant products in *Chrysothamnus nauseous* ssp. *turbinatus*. Great Basin Natur. 48:1–8.

Khan, M.A, N. Sankhla, D.J. Weber, and E.D. McArthur. 1987. Seed germination characteristics of *Chrysothamnus nauseous* ssp. *viridulus* (Astereae, Asteraceae). Great Basin Natur. 47:220–226.

McKell, C.M. and G. Van Epps. 1980. Biomass energy production from large growing rangeland shrubs. Utah State Univ, Logan.

Sankhla, N., T.D. Davis, D.J. Weber, and D. McArthur. 1987. Biology and economic botany of *Chrysothamnus* (rabbitbrush): a potentially useful shrub for arid regions. J. Econ. Tax. Bot. 10:481–496.

Thames, S.F. 1988. Agriculture products-their value to the polymer industry. Guayule Rubber Society, 8th Annual Conference, Mesa, AZ.

Upadhyaya, A., N. Sankhla, T.D. Davis, and D.J. Weber. 1985. In vitro propagation of a rubber-producing desert shrub, *Chrysothamnus nauseous* ssp. *albicaulis*. HortScience 20:864–865.

Weber, D.J., T.D. Davis, D. McArthur, and N. Sankhla. 1986. *Chrysothamnus nauseous* (rabbitbrush) multi-use shrub of the desert. Desert Plants 7:172–202.

Weber, D.J. and G.W. Fernandes. 1991. Insect galls and chemical composition of leaves of *Chrysothamnus nauseous* ssp. *hololeucus* in riparian and dry sites. In: Proc. Symposium on riparian sites. USDA Report INT 200. Ogden, UT.

Variation and Broad Sense Heritability of Branching Frequency of Jojoba

Damian A. Ravetta and David A. Palzkill

Flower buds (and later fruit) are typically produced at every other node on new growth near branch tips of jojoba, *Simmondsia chinensis* (Link) Schneid, Buxaceae (Gentry 1958). Because of this, the number of nodes produced puts an upper limit on the number of flowers, fruit, and seed that a plant can produce. Casual observation of many plants and clones suggested that, in general, highly branched plants have more flowers and are more productive, and indicated that this could be a useful trait to select for in a breeding program. To begin to test this, variability of this trait must be quanified to obtain an estimate of its heritability.

Since the variance of a non-segregating population (i.e. cloned plants) must be environmental, such populations have been used to estimate the environmental component of the total observed variance (Falconer 1990). Once the environmental component is known, the genetic variation can be calculated by subtracting environmental variance from the total phenotypic variance observed. The genetic variance calculated this way includes not only additive variance, but also dominance, interaction, and epistatic components. The relationship between genetic variance and total phenotypic variance is, then broad sense heritability. The objectives of this work were to document the natural variation in branching frequency within 58 jojoba clones and to calculate broad sense heritability using the observed variability for branching frequency.

METHODOLOGY

To evaluate the effects of branching frequency on flower bud production, a survey of 58 jojoba clones growing in a production field near Hyder, Arizona was conducted during the summer 1989. The number of nodes, number of branches (tips) and the number of flowers were measured on three branches per plant and three plants per clone. The length of each branch was fixed by marking on each major branch the tenth node from the tip. All the tips, nodes, and flowers above that mark were counted. In a sampling done on a wide range of jojoba clones with different branching habits, ten nodes was found to be the minimum length of a branch needed to give an accurate portrayal of branching frequency of a complete plant.

The same population of jojoba clones was used to calculate broad sense heritability (H) for branching related traits. Genetic variance for the number of tips per branch, the number of nodes per branch and the relationship tips to nodes was derived from the mean squares of clones (MSc) and error (MS_E) in a regular analysis of variance by separating out the variance components (σ_2) according to the following formula

$$H = \frac{\sigma^2_c}{(\sigma^2_c + \sigma^2_E + \sigma^2_{cr})} \quad \text{where} \quad \sigma^2_{cr} = \frac{(MS_{cr} - MS_E)}{n_r} \quad \text{and} \quad \sigma^2_c = \frac{(MS_c - MS_{cr})}{n_r \, n_{obs}}$$

(MS_{cr} = mean square of clone by replicate; MS_E = mean square of the error term; MS_c = mean square of clones; n_r = number of replicates; n_{obs} = number of observations.)

RESULTS AND DISCUSSION

The results of the survey of 58 jojoba clones illustrate the relationship between branching frequency and flower bud production (Fig. 1). The number of flower buds along the main stem of 10 nodes was not only correlated with the number of nodes per branch but also with the amount of branching along the stem. The relationship between the number of nodes and flowers is illustrated in Fig. 1a, where line A illustrates the regression for all 58 clones (three plants of each clone and three branches/plant). As the number of nodes in a branch segment increases, there is a linear increase in the number of flowers. The slope of 0.49 reflects that on average there is one flower at every other node. Line B shows the regression for three selected clones that have an average of about one flower per node (a slope of 0.93). Thus, the number of flowers increases as the number of nodes increases.

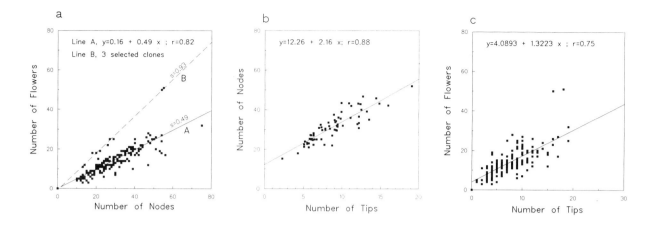

Fig. 1. Relationship between number of nodes, number of tips, and number of flowers for 58 jojoba clones growing at Hyder, AZ. Counts were done on three branches of equal length per plant, and three plants per clone. Each branch had 10 nodes along the main stem axis. (a) Regression for number of nodes and number of flowers, line A for the 58 clones, line B for three selected clones with an average of 0.93 flowers/node; s = slope of regression line. (b) Regression for number of tips and number of nodes. (c) Regression for number of tips and number of flowers.

A positive relationship also exists between the amount of branching (number of tips) along the stem segment and the number of nodes (Fig. 1b). Clones with more branching showed an increase in nodes. As a consequence of the relationship illustrated in Fig. 1a and 1b, the amount of branching (number of tips) was also correlated with the number of flowers per branch (Fig. 1c). We conclude that an increase in branching frequency (number of branch tips/number of nodes) would likely increase node production (everything else remaining constant), and if the ratio of flower buds to nodes remains constant, then the number of flower buds would be increased.

Calculated broad sense heritability was estimated to be 0.36 for the number of tips per branch, 0.19 for the number of nodes per branch, and 0.84 for the tip to node ratio.

The low heritability estimates for number of nodes produced by a particular branch indicates high influence of many conditions which affect growth. The number of tips per branch is less influenced by the environment, although it has been shown that the dormancy observed in lateral buds can be overcome with the external application of plant growth regulators (Ravetta and Palzkill 1990; Ravetta 1990). Increases in the number of tips per plant 17 months after treatment application of up to 120% have been observed with applications of 6-benzyladenine and Promalin (a combination of 6-benzyladenine and gibberellic acid$_{4+7}$). The use of gibberellic acid produced an increase of more than 150% probably as a consequence of a change in the plant's architecture. The ratio of tips to number of nodes is little influenced by environmental factors and this is borne out by results of plant growth regulators experiments. In conclusion, selection for branching frequency, which is related to flower bud production and presumably yield, should be effective.

REFERENCES

Falconer, D.S. 1990. Introduction to quantitative genetics. 3rd ed. Longman Scientific and Technical. p. 125–141.

Gentry, H.S. 1958. The natural history of jojoba (*Simmondsia chinensis*) and its cultural aspects. Econ. Bot. 12:261–295.

Ravetta, D.A. and D.A. Palzkill. 1990. Effect of growth regulators and pinching on branching frequency and flower bud production of jojoba. Proc. 8th Int. Conf. Jojoba. Asuncion, Paraguay, June 17–22 1990

Ravetta, D.A. 1990. Branching in jojoba (*Simmondsia chinensis*): natural variation and effects of plant growth regulators and pruning. MS Thesis, Univ. of Arizona, Tucson.

Irrigation Effects on Growth, Cold Tolerance of Flower Buds, and Seed Yield of Jojoba

J.M. Nelson and D.A. Palzkill

Jojoba [*Simmondsia chinensis* (Link) Schneid., Buxaceae] is being grown commercially in the very hot arid areas of the southwestern United States for the production of seed containing a high quality liquid wax. One factor limiting jojoba production has been damage to flower buds caused by freezing temperatures. Most of the regions where jojoba is being grown are subject to episodes of freezing temperatures in the winter. Flower buds are present on the plants during the winter months and can be damaged or killed by temperatures of $-2°$ to $-5.5°C$.

The possibility of using water stress to increase frost resistance of jojoba, although recognized (Yermanos 1983), has not been properly studied. The objective of this research was to determine the effect of early irrigation termination dates on growth and seed production following a cold winter.

METHODOLOGY

This study was conducted in the 1990-91 seasons in a planting established from cuttings in 1984 at the University of Arizona Maricopa Agricultural Center, Maricopa. The planting contained six pistillate clones in groups of five with a plant spacing of 1.2 by 4.1 m. Each sixth plant in the row was staminate. The planting was flood irrigated until March 1988. At that time three irrigation treatments were established (Table 1).

The wet treatment was irrigated using a drip system to provide water based on estimated seasonal evapotranspiration. Medium and dry treatments were flood irrigated with 115 mm of water per irrigation. Data presented in this paper are from the 1990 growing season and include 1991 seed production. In the 1990–91 winter there were several frost episodes in which the air temperature dropped below $-5°C$ in the planting. The lowest temperature recorded was $-8°C$.

RESULTS

Growth

In the third year after irrigation, treatments were established. In 1990, the wet treatment produced 43 and 75% more growth in height than the medium and dry treatments, respectively (Table 2). Plants in the dry treatment produced only an average of 7 cm of growth which greatly reduced flower bud production. A factor that may have contributed to reduced growth in the drier treatments was differential seed yields. In 1990, plants in the medium and dry treatments produced over 400 g of seed per plant compared to 120 g per plant in the wet treatment.

Flower Bud Survival

Flower bud survival was very low in the wet treatment, in which plants were well-watered going into and during the early winter (Table 3). The medium and dry treatments had significantly greater bud survival than the

Table 1. Irrigation treatments applied 1988–1990 at Maricopa, Arizona.

Irrigation treatment	Date irrigated	Total irrigation (mm)			Total water (mm)		
		1988	1989	1990	1988	1989	1990
Wet	Biweekly Mar.–Nov.	386	548	832	529	647	1064
Medium	Mar., May July, Sept.	460	460	460	621	559	692
Dry	Mar., May	230	230	230	391	329	462

Table 2. Irrigation effects on plant height of six jojoba clones, 1990.

Irrigation treatment[z]	Plant height (cm)						
	Clone						
	01	03	04	06	15	21	Avg
Wet	33	31	30	21	27	28	28
Medium	13	19	25	12	14	11	16
Dry	5	11	13	3	5	5	7

[z]LSD (P = 0.05) for irrigation treatments = 4.

Table 3. Irrigation effects on flower bud survival of six jojoba clones following the winter of 1990–91.

Irrigation treatment[z]	Flower bud survival (%)						
	Clone						
	01	03	04	06	15	21	Avg
Wet	2	0	0	0	0	6	1
Medium	61	59	65	15	29	85	52
Dry	20	29	43	9	15	65	30
Avg	28	29	36	8	15	52	

[z]LSD (P = 0.05) for irrigation treatments = 5; for clones = 10.

Table 4. Irrigation effects on seed yield of six jojoba clones, 1991.

Irrigation treatment[z]	Seed yield (g/plant)						
	Clone						
	01	03	04	06	15	21	Avg
Wet	177	163	10	62	9	407	138
Medium	493	457	400	149	476	727	450
Dry	25	175	164	16	186	224	132
Avg	232	265	191	76	224	453	

[z]LSD (P = 0.05) for irrigation treatments = 164; for clones = 155.

wet treatment. Plants in the medium and dry treatments were water-stressed before and during frost episodes. Large differences among clones in bud survival were observed.

Seed Yield

The highest seed yield came from plants grown under the medium irrigation treatment (Table 4). Yields in the wet and dry treatments were not different even though bud survival was greater in the dry treatment. The lower than expected seed yield in the dry treatment was apparently caused by a combination of factors—reduced shoot growth in 1990, and heavy pruning in the winter of 1990–91, which limited the number of flower buds for 1991 seed production.

CONCLUSIONS

Jojoba plants maintained in a water-stressed condition going into the winter greatly improved the chances of their flower buds surviving frost. Plants which received their final irrigation in September produced significantly more seed than plants which received water until late November. Plants which received their final irrigation in May produced less growth than well-watered plants.

Clones differed in their response to frost in the irrigation treatments and between years. Several clones averaged over 454 g of seed per plant over a two year period in which winter temperatures were low (–8°C). These results indicate that frost resistant jojoba cultivars can increase seed yield and performance under conditions of low temperatures.

REFERENCES

Yermanos, D.M. 1983. Performance of jojoba under cultivation between 1973–1982: Information developed at the University of California, Riverside, p 197–211. In: A. Elias-Cesnik (ed.) Proc. 5th Int. Conf. Jojoba and Its Uses through 1982. Univ. of Arizona, Tucson.

Vernonia and *Lesquerella* Potential for Commercialization

David A. Dierig and Anson E. Thompson

Potential exists for the diversification of agricultural products in the United States by developing alternative plants suitable for commercialization. Such products could have a positive, significant effect on the American trade balance. Vernonia and lesquerella are two promising oilseed crops with potential to provide a domestic source for currently imported oils and the development of new applications.

Vernonia galamensis (Cass.) Less. produces high quantities of epoxy fatty acids useful in the reformulation of oil based (alkyd-resin) paints to reduce emission of volatile organic compounds that contribute to production of smog (Perdue et al. 1986). Other potential markets for the fatty acids include plasticizers, additives in polyvinyl chloride (PVC), polymer blends and coatings, cosmetic, and pharmaceutical applications (Carlson and Chang 1985). About 38% of the seed is oil, with about 72% vernolic acid. No other available germplasm containing naturally occurring epoxy oils, with good potential for commercialization, exists in the United States. Present needs are met with petrochemicals or by chemical epoxidation of fats and vegetable oils such as soybeans and linseed (Carlson et al. 1981). The unique structure of the vernolic acid, if left unmodified, may have a much wider use than epoxidized oils, and further epoxidation of this oil would require only about half the cost of soybean and linseed oils (Carlson and Chang, 1985).

Lesquerella fendleri (Gray) Wats. contains a seed oil high in a hydroxy fatty acid that is similar to imported castor oil, which is on the Department of Defense Critical Materials list. The United States presently spends about $40 million a year on castor imports from China, India, Thailand, and Brazil (Roetheli et al. 1991). Supply reliability and price stability are major concerns of castor oil importers and users (Roetheli et al. 1991). About 25% of the lesquerella seed is oil, of which about 55% is a hydroxy fatty acid. Castor oil is used in numerous products including adhesives, lubricants, plasticizers, pharmaceutical and medical products, waxes and polishes, soaps, inks, caulks and sealants, primers and appliance finishes, detergents, inks, and cosmetics (Roetheli et al. 1991). Lesquerella may be able to directly substitute for castor in many of these applications. Additionally, the longer fatty acid carbon chain of lesquerolic acid, compared to ricinoleic oil of castor (C_{20} vs. C_{18}), could permit development of new products that would not be possible with castor. A task force of the USDA Office of Agricultural Materials has recently completed a thorough evaluation of the feasibility of commercialization of lesquerella as a new industrial oilseed crop and their conclusions were favorable (Roetheli et al. 1991).

VERNONIA

Germplasm and Origin

Vernonia galamensis is an herbaceous annual member of the Asteraceae and is widely distributed in regions of Africa. The *V. galamensis* species complex is now recognized according to Gilbert (1986), to include six subspecies, with one subdivided into four varieties:

1. ssp. *galamensis*
   a. var. *galamensis* M. Gilbert
   b. var. *petitiana* (A. Rich.) M. Gilbert
   c. var. *australis* M. Gilbert
   d. var. *ethiopica* M. Gilbert
2. ssp. *mutomoensis* M. Gilbert
3. ssp. *nairobensis* M. Gilbert
4. ssp. *gibbosa* M. Gilbert
5. ssp. *afromontana* (R.E. Fries) M. Gilbert
6. ssp. *lushotoensis* M. Gilbert

The ssp. *galamensis* and *mutomoensis* in general are found in areas of low rainfall, some as little as 200 mm per year, with no well defined dry season. The ssp. *nairobensis* and *gibbosa* occur in dry evergreen forests, while ssp. *afromontana* and *lushotoensis* are generally found at higher elevations and areas of highest rainfall (Perdue et al. 1986; Perdue 1988). Similar qualities and quantities of vernolic acid are found in the seed oil of all the subspecies of *galamensis*.

MORPHOLOGY

The capitula of *V. galamensis* contain hermaphroditic florets that are protandrous. The pistil emerges through an anther sheath as pollen is shed. As the stigma emerges and fully opens, pollen has reached its surface. This would appear to be an important opportunity for auto-fertility. Controlled crosses of ten capitulum on each of five plants were made on a number of different subspecies accessions (Table 1). Only one accession (V013) uniformly set viable seed on all five self-pollinated plants. Five of ten accessions tested appear to be completely autosterile, and produce essentially no seed following self pollinations (V003, V004, V021, V022, V018). Four accessions appear to segregating for this trait and contain both autofertile and autosterile plants. Variability of this characteristic allows selection and breeding for the desired type of mating system. Even though there appears to be a high amount of variation among plants within a given accession, there was little variation in response among

Table 1. Average number of filled seeds per head from ten controlled self-pollinations within five plants of ten accessions of *Vernonia galamensis* (Cass) Less.

Accession	Ssp./Variety		Avg. no. filled seeds/head for 5 plants				
			1	2	3	4	5
V001	*galamensis*	*ethiopica*	0	0	2.6	17.5	36
V008	"	*australis*	0	0.4	5.3	10	16.2
V009	"	*australis*	0	0	0	1.4	7.4
V004	"	*galamensis*	0	0	0.8	1.3	2
V003	"	*galamensis*	0	0	0	0	0
V013	"	*petitiana*	3.1	6.3	8.8	9.3	10.4
V020	*afromontana*		0	0	0	0.8	8.8
V021	*gibbosa*		0	0	0	0	0.2
V022	*gibbosa*		0	0	0	1.5	2.2
V018	*mutomoensis*		0	0	0	0	0.1

flowers within a single plant. In most cases, the amount of selfed seed was a low percentage of the total possible seed produced in a given capitulum. An average number of total possible seeds per head is about 80, with a range between 60 and 155. In contrast to greenhouse grown plants, most open-pollinated plants in the field have percentages of 95 to 100% viable seed. Under favorable environmental conditions, high activity of bees and other pollinating insects are readily observed in field plantings.

We have concluded that low seed set following controlled self-pollinations of certain accessions, and among certain plants within other accessions is due to self incompatibility. This is most likely a genetic trait that may have a selective advantage. Even though high pollinating insect activity is observed in the field, we believe that autofertility would be most desirable for maximization of seed set in field plantings.

Culture and Breeding

The short day photoperiodic response to flowering is a problem in all the subspecies that needs to be overcome before *Vernonia galamensis* can be successfully grown in the United States. Under normal cultural practices of spring planting, the plants remain vegetative and do not flower until the fall season. Seeds fail to mature before frost. An accession of the variety *petitiana* (V029), is presently the only one available that will flower any time of year in Arizona, regardless of planting date. In Tifton, Georgia, it was classified as a quantitative short day plant (Phatak et al. 1989). However, in Arizona, it behaves as a day neutral plant, indicating that an interaction with temperature may occur. Others accessions of var. *petitiana* (V014, V015, V027, V032, and V035) require short day induction for flowering. The collection from Ethiopia (var. *ethiopica*, V001) required ten photocycles for induction, the Nigerian collection (var. *galamensis*, V004) flowered after five photocycles (Phatak et al. 1989). In Arizona, when days are short enough to induce flowering of these photosensitive subspecies, temperatures are still too cold to bring the plants to maturity for harvest before frost. The photoperiod problem may be overcome by searching for natural genetic variation within the desirable subspecies and selecting for this trait.

Another approach we are taking at the USDA/ARS, U.S. Water Conservation Laboratory, is hybridizing among subspecies and looking for favorable recombinations. The accessions we are focusing on are selections of V029 (var. *petitiana*), since it flowers readily under long day conditions and the seed oil content is around 40%. However, V029 is generally self-incompatible, indeterminate in flowering, and does not have good seed retention. V029 is being hybridized with V001 (var. *ethiopica*), which has good plant vigor, and has large seed in large seed heads (capitula) with the best seed retention of any of the germplasm in our collection. We have also identified plants of V001 that are highly autofertile. We are also interested in V013, which has not been taxonomically classified, but is from Tanzania and looks like a vigorous *petitiana* with a larger seed size. V013 appears to have at least partial auto-fertility, which we believe is a desirable trait. The F_1 generation is now being grown in a greenhouse for evaluation along with the parents. Segregating F_2 and backcross generations are being developed for selection and determination of heritability of autofertility, photoperiodic response, and possibly seed retention.

In 1989, observational plots of the different subspecies were planted at two locations, Phoenix and Yuma, Arizona. These were established by transplanting month-old seedlings into the field in mid-February. By mid-April, 100% of the plants of all varieties of the *galamensis* subspecies were flowering. All subspecies had 100% of the plants flowering by June 8, except for accessions of subspecies *nairobensis*, where the range was between 30 and 100%. Since these plants were started in the greenhouse in January, flowering was induced in most cases before field planting. These plantings gave an indication of the potential for vernonia production in temperate climates and variability in flowering habits. It also allowed for seed increase of many of the accessions.

During the 1991 growing season in Arizona, a date of planting study was conducted with accession V029 var. *petitiana* to determine the earliest time when vernonia can be direct seeded in the field. The earlier it can be planted without the danger of a frost, the shorter the days are for flower induction. Good stands were obtained at each planting date. Seeding rates were also tested in this experiment at 1.4, 2.8, 5.6, and 11.2 kg/ha. All except the lowest seeding rate had acceptable stands. The practice of "topping" plants was experimented with by removing the terminal buds when plants were about 0.15 m tall. This practice did not seem to enhance yields in the petitiana variety since this germplasm is shorter in stature than that of V001, where the treatment significantly enhanced yields in Zimbabwe. Some of the other subspecies may grow up to 2.8 m tall and may respond positively to topping (Anon. 1989).

The most important plant characteristics inherent to the success of vernonia domestication and production in temperate climates are day neutral flowering response, autofertility, non-dormant seed germination, good seed retention, high oil and vernolic acid content, and increased uniformity of seed maturity. In the evaluation of germplasm thus far, these characteristics appears to be present. It is matter of taking advantage of the natural genetic diversity, manipulating and recombining these traits to produce fully adapted, high yielding selections.

LESQUERELLA

Germplasm and Origin

Lesquerella, (*Lesquerella* spp.) a member of the Brassicaceae, consists primarily of herbaceous annuals, biennial, and perennial plants that occupy dry open spaces (Rollins and Shaw 1973). Most current interest for agronomic purposes is in the species *L. fendleri*, which occurs over the southwestern United States and northern Mexico. The plant is naturally found at elevations between 600 and 1,800 m in areas of annual average rainfall ranging from 250 to 400 mm (Gentry and Barclay 1962).

Other species are found throughout North America and may be grouped according to the major hydroxy fatty acid content in the seed oil. These three groups are: lesquerolic acid species, $C_{20:1\text{-}OH}$ (western United States), densipolic acid species, $C_{18:2\text{-}OH}$ (east of the Mississippi), and auricolic acid species, $C_{20:2\text{-}OH}$ (Texas and Oklahoma) (Roetheli et al. 1991). If production and commercialization are successful for *L. fendleri*, domestication of other species for production of densipolic and auricolic acid is likely to be feasible in adapted areas.

Morphology

Lesquerella fendleri is grown as a winter annual. Plants have an indeterminate growth habit, reaching a height up to 45 cm in a cultivated field and is said to be the most polymorphic species of the genus. In Arizona, plants begin flowering in February, in response to warming temperatures, and continue until May. It can be distinguished from other species by the combination of the yellow flowers with glabrous siliques and trichomes that are fused not more than half their length (Rollins and Shaw 1973). Lesquerella has hermaphroditic flowers and appears to be mainly allogamous. Male sterility has been observed in populations.

Culture and Breeding

Cultural studies on lesquerella production have been carried out by USDA/ARS, U.S. Water Conservation Laboratory, Phoenix, Arizona over the past six years (Thompson and Dierig 1988; Thompson et al. 1989). In central Arizona, lesquerella is planted in October and harvested in early June, similar to a winter wheat cropping system. Seedling growth is slow in the first few months after planting due to cool temperatures. By mid-February more rapid growth takes place when temperatures warm and supplemental irrigations begin. A full plant canopy is reached by mid-March. The fruits (seeds) are usually mature by early May and plant biomass begins to dry. Upon drying, plants can be harvested using a conventional combine equipped with small sized sieves to accommodate the small seed size. This growing season time frame has also been successful in small research plots in central Texas (Fort Stockton). In southern Oregon (Medford), lesquerella may be better adapted as a summer annual; planted in late March and harvested in September. Optimum planting dates still need to be ascertained within specific growing locales.

The most successful method of planting has been with a broadcast Brillon seeder. This type of seeder is readily available to farmers that grow such crops as alfalfa and clovers, and thus, would not involve additional expenses. We compared this method with row type vegetable planters and found it superior due to the even seed distribution and the easy adjustment of rate setting for desired plant populations. Although the row plantings had more plants per square meter area, the broadcast plantings had higher yields. Plants were better distributed throughout the field when broadcast planted and were able to develop better. Yields were higher as a consequence when compared to being planted in a crowded row.

We found no significant differences in yields between planting on raised beds and level fields. The advantage of raised beds is in weed and insect control, and, if water quality is a problem, salts are easier to manage. The disadvantage of the raised bed method is the difficulty of harvesting. Dried plants tend to lodge down into the furrow at harvest, making them difficult to recover with the combine. Slight modification to the combine could solve this problem. We are currently experimenting with 0.5, 0.75, and 1 m (20, 30, and 40 inch) bed widths. The shallower furrow of narrow beds may minimize combine difficulty. Higher plant populations were obtained on a raised bed compared to the level basin method. Seeding rates of 4.5, 6.75, and 9.0 kg/ha were compared for both treatments. The yields from the 6.75 kg/ha rate were the highest, but this was not statistically significant in the one year test. Once a desirable plant population is reached, a higher population may not significantly contribute to yield. Planting rate also depends on the seed quality and germination. *L. fendleri* does not have a seed dormancy problem as is the case with many of the other lesquerella species.

Breeding improvements are focused on developing lines with higher oil content. Another trait of interest includes earlier flowering so the growing season takes place before the onset of high temperatures when consumptive use of water is the highest, so water is conserved. We have selected and produced yellow seeded lines. Lesquerella seedcoats are normally orange-brown in color. Since pigmentation of the seed oil is a slight problem, it may be overcome if the seed coat did not contain this darker pigment. Oil content may also be higher in these lines as was found in rapeseed and flax because of the thinner seed coat (Knowles 1983). This remains to be tested.

Pollination mechanisms are being investigated. We have observed that our large acreage plantings were not as productive as smaller research plots. This could be attributed to a lack of adequate number of bees and insect pollinators for optimum seed set in large populations. We believe that for lesquerella to be fully successful, autofertility must be incorporated. We are presently attempting to select for this trait. We have identified a number of male-sterile lines, and are currently studying the mode of inheritance. These may be useful for hybrid seed production in the future.

In the 1990-91 season, the initiation of a cooperative venture took place between two private industrial companies, Agrigenetics Company and the Jojoba Growers and Processors, Inc., USDA/ARS, and the University of Arizona. Eight hectares of lesquerella were planted on the University of Arizona, Maricopa Agricultural Center in central Arizona. The seed oil harvested from this planting is being used to formulate products for testing. Research on processing methodology and utilization is being conducted at the USDA/ARS National Center for Agricultural Utilization Research (NCAUR) Peoria, IL. The meal is being evaluated in mice and chick feeding trials at Kansas State University and in cattle feeding trials at the University of Arizona. Approximately 30 ha have been planted by farmers in California, Arizona, Texas, and Oklahoma in 1991-92 for increased pilot scale production and utilization. These fields will be in addition to the agronomic and breeding research plots that have been planted in Arizona, Texas, and Oregon.

REFERENCES

Anon. 1989. Vernonia-bursting with potential. Agr. Engin. 70:11-13.

Carlson, K.D., W.M. Schneider, S.P. Chang, and L.H. Princen. 1981. *Vernonia galamensis* seed oil: A new source for epoxy coatings. Amer. Oil Chem. Soc. Monogr. 9:297-318.

Carlson, K.D. and S.P. Chang. 1985. Chemical epoxidation of a natural unsaturated epoxy seed oil from *Vernonia galamensis* and a look at epoxy oil markets. J. Amer. Oil Chem. Soc. 62:934-939.

Gentry, H.S. and A.S. Barclay. 1962. The search for new industrial crops III: prospectus of *Lesquerella fendleri*. Econ. Bot. 16:206-211.

Gilbert, M.G. 1986. Notes on East African Vernonieae (Compositae). A revision of the *Vernonia galamensis* complex. Kew Bul. 41:19-35.

Knowles, P.F. 1983. Genetics and breeding of oilseed crops. Econ. Bot. 37:423-433.

Perdue, R.E., K.D. Carlson, and M.G. Gilbert. 1986. *Vernonia galamensis*, potential new crop source of epoxy acid. Econ. Bot. 40:54-68.

Perdue, R.E. 1988. Systematic botany in the development of *Vernonia galamensis* as a new industrial oilseed crop for the semi-arid tropics. Symb. Bot. Ups. 28:125-135.

Phatak, S.C., A.E. Thompson, C.A. Jaworski, and D.A. Dierig 1989. Response of *Vernonia galamensis* to photoperiod. First Annual Conference of the Association for the Advancement of Industrial Crops. Peoria, IL (Abstr.).

Roetheli, J.C., K.D. Carlson, R. Kleiman, A.E. Thompson, D.A. Dierig, L.K. Glaser, M.G. Blase, and J. Goodell. 1991. Lesquerella as a source of hydroxy fatty acids for industrial products. An assessment. USDA/CSRS Office of Agricultural Materials, Washington, DC.

Rollins, R.C. and E.A. Shaw. 1973. The genus *lesquerella* (Crucifererae) in North America. Harvard University Press, Cambridge, MA.

Thompson, A.E. and D.A. Dierig. 1988. Lesquerella—a new arid land industrial oil seed crop. Al Guayulero 10:(1&2)16–18.

Thompson, A.E., D.A. Dierig, and E.R. Johnson. 1989. Yield potential of *Lesquerella fendleri* (Gray) Wats., a new desert plant resource for hydroxy fatty acids. J. Arid Envir. 16:331–336.

Development of a Cosmetic Grade Oil from *Lesquerella fendleri* Seed

James G. Arquette and James H. Brown

Lesquerella fendleri L., Brassicaceae, is an annual native to the arid southwestern United States and has been under study by the USDA Agricultural Research Service since the 1960s. The fatty acid composition of the oil is a blend of lesquerolic acid, a C-20 monounsaturated hydroxy acid, and highly unsaturated C-18 fatty acids. As such, lesquerella oil represents an alternative to castor oil as a source of hydroxy fatty acids. Both the similarities and differences with castor provide a stimulus for application trials involving lesquerella. Initial testing of lesquerella oil indicate extremely low levels of toxicity or irritation (oral, dermal, and ocular). The lesquerella meal resulting from oil extraction is rich in protein and is being evaluated as a source of natural antioxidants, gums, colorants as well as animal feed. A low volume specialty oil market, such as cosmetics, has been identified for product development and is the subject of this paper.

AGRICULTURE

Lesquerella is a New World genus of over 70 species (Gentry and Barclay 1962). Producing abundant nonshattering seed, the species, *L. fendleri*, has been found to have superior agronomic potential. The species is native to the states of Arizona, New Mexico, Oklahoma, and Texas and found in regions of poor soil and low rainfall (25 cm/yr). Its low water demand may make it an attractive potential substitute for certain heavily irrigated crops in these regions. Current seed yields of 950 to 1,120 kg/ha and the 21% seed oil content must still be improved through breeding and agricultural practices.

OIL EXTRACTION

The cosmetics industry desires a solvent free product and often stipulates that the processing be solvent free. For this reason, the lesquerella seed is being cold press extracted. The seed is preconditioned in a steam tube drier modified to allow contact with live steam. The oil is then mechanically extracted from the seed. This system of crushing lesquerella seed produced favorable results with a crude yield of 85% of available oil. The crude oil contained an excessive amount of gums that were unfilterable and did not decant upon washing. Centrifugal degumming is required. Gum contamination of the oil can be minimized by controlled conditioning of the seed prior to extraction. As more seed becomes available, cold press extraction followed by solvent extraction of the meal will provide maximum yields and deliver both a solvent free oil for cosmetic applications and a solvent extracted oil for other industrial applications.

LABORATORY REFINING PROCEDURE

Crude lesquerella oil is the color of molasses, often too dark to measure with a Lovibond Tintometer 1" cell. The oil also posses a distinct odor. Both the color and odor must be reduced for cosmetic applications.

Refining of lesquerella has been limited to laboratory studies until now. Crude oil decanted from the gums was filtered. Free fatty acid content was reduced by spraying 0.7% excess 16° Bé sodium hydroxide over the top of the oil at room temperature. After 1 h the temperature was raised to 65°C for 5 min. Heat was then turned off, allowing the soap stock to break and settle. The oil was decanted, water washed, and dried under vacuum. Bleaching consisted of addition of 10% Filtrol 160 at 90°C for 20 to 30 min with good agitation and under vacuum. Activated carbon and Trisyl have been used as bleaching agents without significant improvements. Laboratory deodorization consisted of steam sparging at 220° to 230°C for 2 h at 5 mm Hg pressure.

The procedure described above followed conventional oil refining procedures and did not result in any significant reduction in hydroxyl content. As more oil becomes available, investigations will continue to determine the effects of using neutral bleaching clays and physical refining to remove free fatty acids and odor simultaneously.

This process produced a superior quality oil of good color but with a slight residual odor. Large scale continuous deodorization equipment must be examined in an effort to further reduce odor levels.

LESQUERELLA MEAL

The meal resulting from oil extraction has an excellent distribution of amino acids being particularly high in lysine (Carlson et al. 1990). Preconditioning the seed is necessary for deactivation of the thioglucosidase enzyme system so that the meal can be used for animal feed. Meal feeding studies are in progress for a variety of livestock. Unlike castor, lesquerella does not contain toxic moieties like the very lethal protein, ricin; the poisonous alkaloid, ricinine; or the very potent allergen, CB-1A. There is significant interest in the lesquerella meal as a source of natural antioxidants, pigments, gums, and protein extracts as well as for animal feed.

PHYSICAL PROPERTIES

The *L. fendleri* seed contains approximately 21% triglyceride oil with nine fatty acids (Table 1). Moisture content at harvest was 5 to 6%.

Current breeding programs need to increase both the oil content of the seed and the lesquerolic acid content of the oil. The highly unsaturated fatty acid portion resembles linseed oil and contributes significantly to the characteristics of the oil and unique derivative potential. The structure of lesquerolic acid, 14-hydroxy, *cis*-11-eicosenoic acid bears a close relationship to ricinoleic acid found in castor oil (Fig. 1). Table 2 presents physical properties of the cold pressed and refined oils currently being produced.

Table 1. Fatty acid composition of *Lesquerella fendleri* seed oil.

Fatty acid		Concentration (%)
Palmitic	C 16:0	1.3
Palmitoleic	C 16:1	0.7
Stearic	C 18:0	2.1
Oleic	C 18:1	18.1
Linoleic	C 18:2	9.3
Linolenic	C 18:3	14.0
Arachidic	C 20:0	0.2
Gadoleic	C 20:1	1.2
Lesquerolic	C 20:1(OH)	51.4

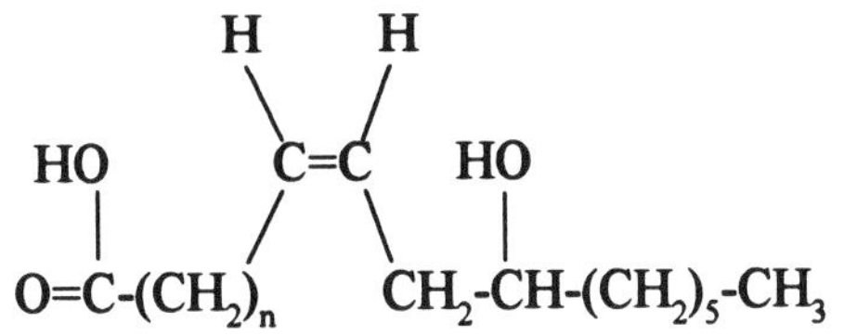

$$\text{HO} - \overset{H}{\underset{O=C-(CH_2)_n}{C}} = \overset{H}{\underset{CH_2-CH-(CH_2)_5-CH_3}{C}} - \text{OH}$$

Fig. 1. Structure of ricinoleic and lesquerolic acid (n = 7, ricinoleic acid; n = 9, lesquerolic acid).

Table 2. Physical properties of crude and refined lesquerella oil.

Property	AOCS Method	Crude	Refined
Iodine value	Cd 1-25	107	104
Hydroxyl value	Cd 4-40	102	
Free fatty acid	Ae 4-52	1.5	0.7
Color (5.25" Lovibond	Cc 136-45	too dark	4.1R; 37Y
Gardner)		14	5
Saponification number	Cd 3-25	168	
Peroxide values	Cd 8-53	1.6	0.40
Refractive index 40°C		1.4719	1.4710
Phosphorous (ppm)	Ca 12b-87	0.41	
Metals (ppm):	Ca 15-75		
Fe		0.1	
Mg		0.16	
Cu		1.1	
Ni		0.08	
Ca		1.9	

Table 3. Relative stability of triglyceride oils with added antioxidants.

Oil	Iodine value	Tocopherols (ppm)	AOM[z] (h)	Increased stability (%)
Cashew	87	0	13	---
		365	20	54
		1050	27	108
Brazil Nut	101	0	10	---
		360	13	30
		930	16	60
Lesquerella	106	0	35	---
		375	40	14
		915	46	31

[z]Active oxygen method, AOCS Method Cd 12-57.

STABILITY

Lesquerella oil contains an almost equal blend of highly unsaturated fatty acids and hydroxy unsaturated fatty acids. As oxidative stability of an oil tends to be inversely proportional to the degree of unsaturation, tests were conducted to determine the relative stability of lesquerella oil (Table 3). The AOCS Method Cd 12-57 was used to determine the stability of the oil under prescribed conditions. In this case, active oxygen method (AOM) hours to an endpoint of 100 meq/kg are reported. The oils selected for examination were provided by Jojoba Growers and Processors Inc. The tests were conducted by Henkel Corp., supplier of the mixed tocopherol antioxidant, Covi-Ox. Covi-Ox is a registered trademark of the Henkel Corp.

Cashew and Brazil nut oil were included in the study as they have comparable Iodine Values. The results indicate that Lesquerella oil is stable beyond what might be expected given the Iodine Value of 106. Whether lesquerella might be a source for new potent natural antioxidants warrants further study.

TOXICOLOGY

Acute Oral Toxicity (Single Dose)

The acute single dose oral toxicity was determined on Sprague-Dawley rats. Lesquerella oil was found to have an apparent LD_{50} Single Oral Dose of greater than 15 g/kg of body weight. No larger dosages are administered in this test. Lesquerella, according to this test, achieved the lowest rating of "Practically Non-Toxic" (Gleason et al. 1969). Of the ten animals tested, three females exhibited a slight weight loss during the first week, but all animals went on to show positive weight gain by the end of the test period with no other signs of toxicity. The observation criteria is extensive. Noteworthy was the lack of diarrhea at these high dosages indicating that lesquerella is no substitute for castor oil in the purgative market.

Eye Irritation Test (Draize)

The extent of eye irritation was determined in New Zealand rabbits. The highest mean score was 0.0. No positive reactions were exhibited in any of the six animals. Lesquerella oil was rated as Non-Irritating and passed the eye irritation test. For all seven potential ocular reactions monitored, the results were consistently zero (lowest possible) for the entire 72 h test period.

Primary Dermal Irritants

The degree of irritation (erythema-eschar and edema) elicited by the lesquerella oil was determined on the abraded and non-abraded skin of six New Zealand white rabbits over a 72 h observation period. The Primary Dermal Irritation Score was 1.67 (mild irritant) and is not considered to be a Primary Dermal Irritant. At the 24 h observation, three animals exhibited well defined erythema and three animals exhibited very slight erythema. At the 48 h observation, five animals exhibited well defined erythema and one very slight erythema. All six animals exhibited no edema.

Comedogenicity

This test (Morris and Kwan 1983) is designed as a screen for any material which may be a potential acnegen. The test is conducted on the ear canals of four New Zealand white rabbits which are inspected for comedomes (acne) whose size is proportional to the potency of the test substance. Lesquerella oil's Comedogenic Grade is 0.0, noncomedogenic. This test is critical for cosmetic ingredients. Since the 1980s formulators have carefully selected ingredients to reduce the possibility of "acne cosmetics," the technical name for acne attributed to makeup, skin, and hair care products. The unequivocal low result will promote applications' studies within the cosmetics industry.

Allergenicity

This test (Magnusson and Kligman 1969) is designed to determine if a given material causes allergenic responses. Albino guinea pigs are used with positive and negative controls. Intradermal injections and topical applications were used. No allergenic responses were observed in the ten test animals (or in the two unsensitized

Table 4. Toxicological test results for cold pressed lesquerella oil.

Test	Results
Acute oral toxicity	LD_{50} Single Dose > 15 g/kg body wt.
Eye irritation (Draize)	0.0, Non-Irritating
Primary dermal irritation	1.67, Mild irritant, not considered a primary irritant
Comedogenicity	0.0, Non-comedogenic
Allergenicity	Grade I, Non-sensitizing

and two negative controls, the two positive controls exhibited positive allergenic response). The test showed 0% sensitization. A 0 to 8% sensitization is considered Grade I, Non-sensitizing or at most a weak agent. The summary of toxicological testing conducted to date is presented in Table 4.

These toxicological test results indicate an extremely low potential for irritation. For use as a cosmetic material, this is extremely important. Lesquerella has potential for broad based application (e.g. stick deodorant, lip and eye care products, soaps, etc.) including pharmaceutical applications.

FUTURE PROSPECTS

While optimum genetic material and agronomic practices are still a few years from realization, the immediate potential for lesquerella oil and its derivatives as raw materials for the cosmetic industry appears very promising. Studies are underway to improve oil processing technology for optimum quality and yields. Initial examinations of partially and selective hydrogenated lesquerella oil have produced derivatives with very distinct properties. Formulation work has begun incorporating lesquerella oil into lip care products. Lipstick, which may contain as much as 80% castor oil, provides an initial focus for lesquerella. Lipstick has been successfully manufactured using lesquerella oil instead of castor oil. Product evaluation will begin in early 1992.

REFERENCES

Carlson, K.D., M. Bagby, and A. Chaudry. 1990. Analysis of oil and meal from *Lesquerella fendleri* seed. J. Amer. Oil Chem. Soc. 67:438–442.

Gentry, H.S. and A. Barclay. 1962. The search for new industrial crops II: Lesquerella (Cruciferae) as a source of new oilseeds. Econ. Bot. 16:95–100.

Gleason, M.N., R.E. Gosselin, H.C. Hodge, and R.P. Smith. 1969. Clinical toxicology of commercial products. 3rd ed. Williams and Wilkens, Baltimore, MD.

Morris, W.E. and S.C. Kwan. 1983. Use of the rabbit ear model in evaluating the comedogenic potential of cosmetic ingredients. J. Soc. Cosmet. Chem. 34:215–225.

Magnusson, B. and A. Kligman. 1969. The identification of contact allergens by animal assay. The guinea pig maximization test. J. Invest. Dermatol. 52:268–276.

Breakthroughs Towards the Domestication of *Cuphea**

Steven J. Knapp

Over three decades ago, several species of *Cuphea* of the Lythraceae (Graham 1988) were found to be rich sources of medium-chain fatty acids (MCFAS) (Earle et al. 1960; Miller et al. 1964). These fatty acids and medium-chain triglycerides (MCTS) are used worldwide as industrial feedstocks and foods. They are commercially supplied by the tropical oil crops coconut (*Cocos nucifera* L.) and oil palm (*Elaeis guineensis* Jacq.); no temperate oilseed crops supply these lipids (Ignacio 1985; Arkcoll 1988). Many of the MCT-rich species of *Cuphea* are summer annuals which, if domesticated, could become domestic sources of MCTs for the United States and other importing countries, thereby breaking the tropical oilseed monopoly. Toward this end, a project was undertaken by G. Roebbelen and his colleagues at Georg August University in Goettingen, Germany to evaluate different species and to determine the feasibility of domesticating *Cuphea* (Hirsinger 1980; Hirsinger and Roebbelen 1980; Hirsinger and Knowles 1984; Hirsinger 1985; Roebbelen and von Witzke 1989). A project to domesticate Cuphea is currently underway at Oregon State University (OSU) (Knapp 1990).

Several species native to Mexico are adapted to the United States and Europe (Hirsinger and Roebbelen 1980; Hirsinger and Knowles 1984; Hirsinger 1985; Knapp 1990). At OSU, we work extensively with *C. viscosissima*, the only species native to the United States, and *C. lanceolata*, a species native to the Sierra Madre of Mexico (Graham 1988). These species are grown as summer annuals in the United States. The seed and oil yields of these species seem to be sufficient for them to compete as oilseed crops (Knapp 1990b); however, this must be substantiated using non-shattering cultivars, which are presently being developed. Seed shattering and seed dormancy are the major domestication barriers within the genus (Knapp 1990a,b); the seed dispersal mechanism is a characteristic which unifies the genus (Graham 1988). Only a fraction of the total seed yield of *Cuphea* is recovered by combine harvesting, the remainder being lost to seed shattering. This trait must be eliminated to domesticate and commercialize *Cuphea*.

Seed shattering has frustrated the endeavor to domesticate Cuphea. This problem has persisted because no natural diversity has been found for seed shattering (Graham 1988, 1989; Roebbelen and von Witzke 1989; Knapp 1990b); however, over the last three years, important breakthroughs have been made at OSU towards eliminating seed shattering and seed dormancy by exploiting interspecific diversity. These breakthroughs have significantly brightened the commercial outlook for *Cuphea*. In this paper, I report the discovery of non-shattering phenotypes within the *C. viscosissima* x *C. lanceolata* f. *silenoides* population VL-119, the only non-shattering phenotypes known within the genus, and review the development of autofertile non-dormant and non-shattering *C. viscosissima* x *C. lanceolata* f. *silenoides* germplasm and cultivars at OSU. The development of autofertile non-dormant germplasm has been enormously important to the development of *Cuphea* as a crop (Knapp 1990a,b), but this has been overshadowed by the genesis of interspecific diversity for seed retention. This has greatly increased the commercial promise of *Cuphea* by creating the basis for eliminating the most serious barrier to the domestication of this crop.

SEED SHATTERING AND SEED DORMANCY

Throughout the history of agriculture, non-shattering and non-dormant populations have arisen within numerous species, thereby leading to their domestication (Renfrew 1969; Ladizinsky 1985; Kadkol et al. 1984a,b, 1989). The discovery of non-shattering populations of seed crops was critical to the shift from hunting and gathering to agrarian cultures (Renfrew 1969). The non-shattering phenotypes of many diploid seed crops have been shown to be caused by single gene mutations—events which have overwhelmingly affected human history and culture (Renfrew 1969; Ladizinsky 1985; Kadkol et al. 1984a,b, 1989). Natural selection has maximized

---

*This work was funded by grants from the USDA (58-5114-9-1002 and 91-37300-6569), Soap and Detergent Association, and Procter and Gamble Company. Oregon Agricultural Experiment Station Technical Paper 9994.

seed dispersal within *Cuphea*, thus optimizing its survival in the wild. *Cuphea* has not been subjected to selection against seed shattering over the last several millennium because it has been of no use to humans as a seed crop. The economic value of this genus as an oilseed only became known late in this century. Domesticating *Cuphea* means reversing 12 to 14 million years of evolution to perfect seed dispersal, yet, as history teaches us, this reversal might be achieved by a simple mutation.

Until 1987, *Cuphea* was a completely undomesticated genus. When we initiated domestication work in 1986, the entire germplasm base was comprised of wild populations, and no species had been selected for intense breeding and domestication work. Seed of most species was very scarce, and no species had been extensively collected from the wild for germplasm preservation and plant breeding work. Despite this, our initial goal was to rapidly narrow the field of species down to the one or two with the greatest promise as oilseed crops.

Between 1986 and 1988, we tested many of the more promising species evaluated by Hirsinger and Knowles (1984), Hirsinger (1985), and Roebbelen and von Witzke (1989). From this group, which was entirely made up of Section Heterodon species, we selected *C. lanceolata* and *C. viscosissima* for intense domestication work (Table 1). Their selection was partly motivated by the discovery of fertile interspecific hybrids between them (Table 1).

In 1987, Anson Thompson (USDA/ARS, Phoenix, Arizona) reported fertile F_1 progeny from *C. viscosissima* × *C. lanceolata* matings (Ronis et al. 1990). We subsequently discovered thousands of *C. viscosissima* × *C. lanceolata* seedlimgs within a *C. lanceolata* population. That arose from natural outcrossing between these species. We began using *C. viscosissima* × *C. lanceolata* matings for breeding work because *C. lanceolata* is an extremely useful source of diversity for many important traits, e.g., seed dormancy. We had been selecting, for example, for increased oil percentage within each species separately, but shifted to selecting for increased oil percentage within the *C. viscosissima* × *C. lanceolata* population VL-119. This population was created by intermating *C. viscosissima* and *C. lanceolata* progeny selected for increased oil percentage (Fig. 2).

Because chiasma frequencies within *C. viscosissima* × *C. lanceolata* populations are less than those within either species (Brandt and Knapp 1992), we intermated VL-119 for an additional generation without selection as *C. viscosissima* × *C. lanceolata* populations are allogamous. The additional intermating proved to greatly increase recombination between the genomes of these species and led to phenotypes transgressing the range of these species (Fig. 2). Non-shattering phenotypes (Fig. 1) were among the transgressive segregates which sprang from this population (Fig. 2). At least 15 out of 500 spaced plants of VL-119 had some seed retention. Many of the 15 show great promise and are the focus of intense breeding work.

Wildtype *Cuphea* disperses seed through a dorsal abscission layer along the corona tube. The placenta of the wildtype rotates upward 100 to 120° from its origin within the corolla tube. The fully exposed seeds mature and dehisce after the placenta separates from the corolla tube, the parchment thin fruit carpels remain within the corolla tube. The non-shattering phenotypes we discovered disrupt this process. Placentas of 100% of the fruits of non-shattering individuals fail to rotate, so the seeds mature and dehisce within the corolla tube (Fig. 1). The dorsal abscission layer arises within these phenotypes, but most of the seed is retained within the corolla tube. The placenta dries over the developing seed, further decreasing shattering (Fig. 1). The carpels are torn irregularly by the expanding and maturing seed.

Since the selection of non-shattering progeny within VL-119, we have developed progeny from these selections with fruits which fail to split open. Numerous S_1 individuals have been tested from a promising selection. The corolla tubes of certain individuals within this S_1 family did not split open; the corolla tube encased the fruit carpels, placenta, and mature seed, thereby conferring complete seed retention. Naturally, these progeny are exactly what we have been striving to develop and what everyone has been hoping to find. Their development has been pivotal for *Cuphea*.

The precise biological and genetic underpinnings of the non-shattering trait are unknown. The non-shattering phenotypes came from wildtype genetic backgrounds of the progenitor species. They are not the consequence of induced mutations, rather they are the consequence of wide hybridization which led to genotypes which cannot arise and phenotypes which seemingly do not arise within either species alone. At the very least, the natural diversity within a given species of *Cuphea* is probably not sufficient to lead to non-shattering progeny purely by hybridization and selection alone. We have not observed phenotypic differences within any species

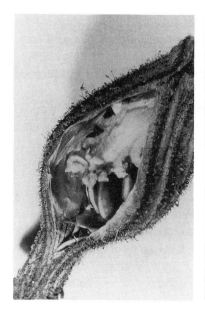
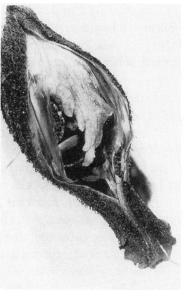

Fig. 1. Non-shattering phenotypes from the *C. viscosissima* x *C. lanceolata* f. *silenoides* population VL-119.

Fig. 2. History and pedigree of the *C. viscosissima* x *C. lanceolata* f. *silenoides* population VL-119.

Table 1. History of *Cuphea* domestication and breeding work at Oregon State University marking the major events which led to domesticated germplasm of *C. viscosissima* x *C. lanceolata* f. *silenoides*.

Date	Event
August of 1987	Fertile *C. viscosissima* x *C. lanceolata* progeny are discovered.
January of 1988	*C. viscosissima* and *C. lanceolata* are selected as targets for domestication. Breeding work within these species is significantly increased, while work with other species ceases.
March of 1990	Autofertile non-dormant phenotypes are discovered among *C. viscosissima* x *C. lanceolata* BC_1S_1 progeny.
September of 1991	Non-shattering phenotypes are discovered within the *C. viscosissima* x *C. lanceolata* population VL-119.
December of 1991	Fully non-dormant autofertile *C. viscosissima* x *C. lanceolata* lines are developed.
May of 1992	Non-splitting phenotypes are observed within S_1 families from non-shattering individuals selected from VL-119.

sufficient for developing non-shattering germplasm. The phenotypic diversity within VL-119 significantly increased with repeated intermating. Ongoing recurrent selection work should perpetuate this trend for many years since we have kept the 'effective population size' very great for certain selection projects. Because *C. viscosissima* x *C. lanceolata* hybrids are fertile, breeding them is no different from breeding intraspecific populations, save for understanding and compensating for reduced recombination (Brandt and Knapp 1992). Many additional nonshattering phenotypes should arise from VL-119 and other extensively intermated interspecific populations. Naturally, we are aggressively developing non-shattering populations, lines, and cultivars for the eventual commercialization of *Cuphea*.

As a whole, seed dormancy is less severe of a problem than seed shattering for *Cuphea*; however, seed dormancy is severe within wild populations of *C. viscosissima*. Seed dormancy has been observed within *C. lanceolata*, but it is not severe within many populations, and non-dormant populations and lines of this species have been developed (Knapp 1990; Knapp and Tagliani 1990). We have developed a fully non-dormant inbred line, $(LN-61ND)S_5$, of *C. lanceolata*; freshly harvested seed of this line germinates. It is the only fully non-dormant line which has been reported within the genus.

Until the spring of 1990, breeding work with *C. viscosissima* was impeded by severe seed dormancy. The initial aim of our interspecific breeding work was to introgress genes for non-dormancy from *C. lanceolata* to *C. viscosissima*, while retaining the autofertility of *C. viscosissima* (Table 1). In retrospect, this was not especially difficult to achieve. We originally selected within BC_1S_1 populations using *C. viscosissima*, an autogamous species, as the recurrent parent. We have not recovered autofertile progeny within F_2 populations; however, they arise with great frequency within BC_1S_1 populations. Using *C. viscosissima* as the recurrent parent circumvents the negative consequences of the genetic load of the *C. lanceolata* genome. As most allogamous species, *C. lanceolata* manifests inbreeding depression and heterosis (Ali 1991; Knapp et al. 1991). Breeding work is underway to develop autofertile *C. viscosissima* x *C. lanceolata* inbred lines for F_1 hybrids which retain a significant percentage of the *C. lanceolata* genome and exploit the heterosis between *C. viscosissima* and *C. lanceolata* and within *C. lanceolata*.

The development of autofertile non-dormant lines has significantly affected our work to induce seed retention mutants within these species. We are advancing our mutation breeding work, despite the discovery of non-shattering phenotypes, because of the merits and utility of having induced mutations affecting fruit morphology and dehiscence, e.g., mutations which eliminate the dorsal suture of the mature fruits could be very useful. Our original objective was to mutagenize *C. viscosissima*, but severe seed dormancy has prevented us from developing and screening large mutagenized populations of this species. The only consistent way to overcome the seed dormancy problem within this species is to excise embryos from whole seeds after-ripened for two to three months. This was done to develop ~2,000 M_2 lines of *C. viscosissima*. Seventy-two mutations affecting seed oil fatty acid percentages have been isolated from these lines (Knapp and Tagliani 1990; Knapp 1992). Non-shattering mutants were not observed among this limited sample of lines. Many more M_2 progeny must be screened to recover mutations affecting fruit morphology or dehiscence. The seed dormancy problem was solved by the development of autofertile non-dormant *C. viscosissima* x *C. lanceolata* lines (Table 1). We have since used these lines to develop M_2 populations originating from at least a quarter of a million mutagenized M_1 individuals. The screening of these populations for mutations affecting fruit morphology and dehiscence and other traits should be completed within the next two years.

Mutation breeding of *Cuphea* has been underway for several years (Hirsinger 1980; Hirsinger and Roebbelen 1980; Campbell 1987; Roebbelen and von Witzke 1989; Roebbelen 1991). This was motivated by the lack of natural diversity for seed shattering, but non-shattering mutants have not yet been isolated. Roebbelen and von Witzke (1989) reported a 'radial' flower mutant of *C. calophylla*, but this phenotype was not shown to affect fruit dehiscence or to decrease seed shattering (Roebbelen and von Witzke 1989). Seed shattering seems to be as great for the radial flower phenotype as for the wildtype of *C. calophylla*. A shift from zygomorphic to actinomorphic flowers should not be presumed to lead to seed retention.

Roebbelen and von Witzke (1989) screened M_2 progeny from 9,312 M_1 progeny of *C. tolucana* and M_2 progeny from 3,693 M_1 progeny of *C. wrightii*. These progeny were developed by EMS mutagenesis. Mutations affecting fruit dehiscence were not observed within either species; however, mutations affecting several morphological traits were observed within *C. tolucana* (Roebbelen and von Witzke 1989). Mutation rates for *C. tolucana* and *C. wrightii* were 1.4 and 0.0% (Roebbelen and von Witzke 1989). The lack of mutations within *C. wrightii* is not surprising. This species is undoubtedly an allotetraploid ($2n = 4x = 44$) and, as such, the phenotypes of most induced mutations are masked by duplicate genes. Additional evidence for this comes from the mutagenesis experiments of Campbell (1987) who observed no mutant phenotypes within *C. wrightii* using mutagen dose rates several fold greater than those used to induce mutations within the diploid species *C. tolucana* ($2n=2x=20$).

The question of inducing non-shattering mutants is still very much open. Extensive breeding work with an autogamous diploid species, e.g., *C. viscosissima* x *C. lanceolata* or *C. viscosissima*, is essential to maximize the probability of isolating non-shattering mutants, and this has not been done.

INSECT POLLINATION AND AUTOFERTILITY

Many productive *Cuphea* species are allogamous, e.g., *C. lanceolata* (Knapp et al. 1991), *C. laminuligera* (Krueger and Knapp 1991), and *C. leptopoda*. Most allogamous species of *Cuphea* are pollinated by bumblebees and other Hymenopteran and Lepidopteran insects. The long length of the floral tubes of most allogamous species prevents honeybees from foraging for nectar. Ironically, *C. viscosissima*, an autofertile species with a fairly short floral tube (Graham 1988), is regularly pollinated by honeybees. Honeybees do forage within *C. lanceolata*, *C. leptopoda*, and many other large flowered allogamous species, but not effectively.

Insect-pollinated allogamous species of *Cuphea* probably cannot be produced commercially. Even if honeybees or some other domesticated pollinator effectively pollinated these species, their commercial use is impractical and prohibitively expensive. This was a major factor which led us to select *C. viscosissima* for intense domestication and breeding work.

Because it is feasible to transfer genes between *C. viscosissima* and *C. lanceolata* (Table 1), we initiated breeding work to exploit the hybrid vigor of *C. lanceolata* (Ali 1991) by developing autofertile inbred lines for F_1 hybrids. Naturally, by introgressing genes for autofertility from *C. viscosissima* to *C. lanceolata*, the subsequent inbreeding within autofertile lines leads to inbreeding depression within those lines or populations where a significant percentage of the *C. lanceolata* genome is retained. These lines can be effectively exploited by using F_1 hybrids; however, mechanisms have not yet been developed for producing F_1 hybrid seed of *Cuphea*.

STICKY HAIRS, INDETERMINATE FLOWERING, AND CROP ARCHITECTURE

Most *Cuphea* species are characterized by sticky or glandular hairs covering their stems, leaves, and flowers (Graham 1988; Amarasinghe et al. 1991). These hairs have been repeatedly cited as a negative trait which must be eliminated to advance *Cuphea* (Hirsinger 1980; Hirsinger and Roebbelen 1980; Thompson 1984). The stickiness of *Cuphea* is unpleasant, but it is not a barrier to the commercialization of *Cuphea*. Although some of the sticky residue *from* Cuphea chaff accumulates in harvesting equipment, it does not seem to hinder harvesting; however, commercial scale tests have not yet been done. Sticky non-shattering *Cuphea* cultivars can be handled and harvested like other summer annuals, such as sunflower or soybean, by direct combining the crop after killing frosts destroy the foliage. Whether or not glabrous or non-sticky cultivars should be used is a subject for debate. Sticky hairs may be an effective defense against many insect pests. Aphids and many other insects are immobilized by the sticky hairs of *C. viscosissima* and *C. lanceolata*. At the very least, many insects cannot navigate wildtypes of many *Cuphea* species, among them *C. viscosissima* and *C. lanceolata*, and eliminating the sticky hairs might increase their vulnerability to many insect pests. Non-sticky mutants have been reported for *C. lanceolata* (Hirsinger 1980; Hirsinger and Roebbelen 1980), and the non-sticky trait might prove useful, but additional work is needed to determine the role of sticky hairs as a defense mechanism against insect pests before non-sticky cultivars are used. Regardless, stickiness should be repeatedly branded as a negative trait. It might ultimately be vindicated by serving as a defense against an otherwise serious insect pest. Indeed, it might be useful to breed for increased hairiness and stickiness, which is an unpleasant thought for anyone who has worked with this genus.

In addition to sticky hairs, indeterminate flowering has been cited as a negative trait of *Cuphea* (Hirsinger 1980; Hirsinger and Roebbelen 1980; Thompson 1984). It might be useful to develop determinate flowering *Cuphea*, but indeterminate flowering poses no problem for the production or harvest of *Cuphea*. Indeterminate flowering has not been shown to positively or negatively affect the seed yields of *Cuphea*. This cannot be determined until determinate flowering phenotypes are discovered or developed. Determinate flowering phenotypes might well be lower yielding than indeterminate flowering phenotypes.

Crop architecture has been cited as another problem trait (Roebbelen and von Witzke 1989); however, the wildtype crop architectures of *C. viscosissima* and *C. lanceolata* pose no problem for the production or harvest of *Cuphea*, nor do they negatively affect seed yield. These species grow upright, and very strong upright growth can be achieved by planting densely. It might be useful to modify the architecture of these species, e.g., to develop monoculm cultivars, but the merits of a 'monoculm' architecture (Roebbelen and von Witzke 1989) are uncertain. Furthermore, useful monoculm phenotypes have not yet been developed. Hirsinger (1980) and Roebbelen and von Witzke (1989) reported a monoculm mutant of *C. lanceolata*, but this mutant is unproductive and inferior to the wildtype. The negative characteristics of this phenotype seem to be a consequence of pleiotropy. Additional work to modify architecture might be useful, but a monoculm architecture is not necessarily going to lead to seed yield increases.

THE MARKET FOR MCT OILS

Estimates of coconut and palm kernel oil imports for North American and Europe from 1986 to 1988 (Mackie and Calhoun 1991) can be used to estimate the demand for MCT-rich oils (Table 2). North America and Europe imported 1.72 billion kg of coconut and palm kernel oil per year from 1986 to 1988. Assuming a seed yield of 2,500 kg/ha and an extracted oil percentage of 25% for *Cuphea*, 100% of the North American and European demand for MCT-rich oil could be met by producing 2.75 million ha of *Cuphea*. With a price of $0.65/kg for the seed, the projected revenue from the seed alone is 1.12 billion dollars. *Cuphea* cannot be expected to capture all of the market, but it should capture some of it. Furthermore, it might significantly restructure the market because of the many new kinds of oils it can supply (Knapp 1992). Although these demand estimates are rather crude, they demonstrate the underlying economics of MCTS.

The demand for MCT-rich oils is expected to steadily increase over the next several decades as the world population increases. As documented by Mackie and Calhoun (1991), world trade in oils from plants and oilseed meals "tripled from 1962 to 1988, while the number of countries participating in world trade increased by 85%." Mackie and Calhoun (1991) further stated, "Oilseed, oil, and meal consumption in most countries outpaced production during this period. Consequently, more countries have turned to world markets for a growing part of their oilseed product needs. These developments not only increased the volume of world trade in oil products between a larger group of countries, but also changed the pattern and direction of trade flows for these products." *Cuphea* could become a significant factor in oilseed trade over the next several years since virtually 100% of the MCT needs of many countries are being met by imports.

These demand estimates for MCT-rich oils do not account for new food and industrial uses of caprylic, capric, lauric, and myristic acid-rich oils from *Cuphea*. The great diversity of fatty acid phenotypes of *Cuphea* could greatly impact the demand for different oils (Knapp 1992). MCTs are presently used for infant feeding and hyperalimentation, especially for the critically ill, and they have been shown to decrease heart disease, breast cancer, colon cancer, and other diseases when used as the primary dietary lipid source (Babayan 1981; Bach and Babayan 1982; Babayan 1987). As a consequence, the use of MCTs in the human diet might increase if an inexpensive source such as *Cuphea* oil is developed. Present use of MCTs is severely restricted by the cost of synthesizing them from 8:0 and 10:0 fractions of coconut and palm kernel oils.

SUMMARY AND PROSPECTUS

The development of autofertile non-dormant and non-shattering germplasm has created the basis for developing profitable cultivars of *Cuphea*. Although much effort remains in order to commercialize *Cuphea*, the

Table 2. Mean coconut (copra) and palm kernel oil imports by North America and Europe from 1986 to 1988. Import estimates were compiled from USDA/ERS statistics (Mackie and Calhoun 1991).

		Imports (1,000 Tonnes)			
Importer[z]	Commodity	1986	1987	1988	Mean
North America	Palm Kernel Oil	181	196	233	203
Europe	Palm Kernel Oil	351	354	395	367
North America	Copra Oil	558	533	470	520
Europe	Copra Oil	645	639	601	628
Total		1,735	1,722	1,699	1,718

[z]Statistics for North America are sums for the United States, the U.S. Virgin Islands, Canada, Puerto Rico, St. Pierre, and Miquelon. Statistics for Europe are sums for the EC10 (Belgium–Luxemborg, Denmark, France, the Federal Republic of Germany, Greece, Ireland, Italy, the Netherlands, and the United Kingdom), other western European countries (Andorra, Austria, the Faeroe Islands, Finland, Gibraltar, Greenland, Iceland, Malta, Norway, Portugal, Spain, Sweden, and Switzerland), and eastern European countries (Albania, Bulgaria, Czechoslovakia, the German Democratic Republic, Hungary, Poland, Romania, USSR, and Yugoslavia) (Mackie and Calhoun 1991).

development of non-shattering germplasm eliminates the risk which has heretofore made investments by agribusiness and state agricultural experiment stations risky and impractical. As the risk further diminishes over the next several years, cultivar testing and agronomic extension must be developed to give farmers the information needed to maximize seed yields and profitability, while processing and distribution networks must be developed. Beyond this, more plant breeders must endeavor to advance this crop. Decreased risk should catalyze an increase in the scale of breeding, genetic, and biotechnology efforts within this important and useful genus. Significant expansion cannot take place, however, until the commercial promise of autofertile non-shattering cultivars is demonstrated.

REFERENCES

Ali, S. 1991. Cytology, inbreeding depression, and heterosis of *Cuphea lanceolata*. PhD Thesis, Oregon State Univ., Corvallis.

Amarasinghe, V., S.A. Graham, and A. Graham. 1991. Trichome morphology in the genus *Cuphea* (Lythraceae). Bot. Gaz. 152:77–90.

Arkcoll, D.B. 1988. Lauric oil resources. Econ. Bot. 42:195–205.

Babayan, V.K. 1981. Medium chain length fatty acid esters and their medical and nutritional applications. J. Amer. Oil Chem. Soc. 58: 49–51.

Bach, A.C. and V.K. Babayan. 1983. Medium-chain triglycerides: an update. Amer. J. Clinical Nutr. 36:950–962.

Babayan, V. 1987. Medium chain triglycerides and structured lipids. Lipids 22:417–420.

Brandt, T. and S.J. Knapp. Genetics and cytogenetics of *Cuphea lanceolata* x *Cuphea viscosissima* populations. Crop Sci. (in press).

Campbell, A. 1987. Chemical mutagenesis of two *Cuphea* species. Can. J. Plant Sci. 67:909–917.

Earle, F.R., C.A. Glass, C. Geisinger, I.A. Wolff, and Q. Jones. 1960. Search for new industrial oils. IV. J. Amer. Oil Chem. Soc. 37:440–447.

Graham, S.A., F. Hirsinger, and G. Roebbelen. 1981. Fatty acids of *Cuphea* (Lythraceae) seed lipids and their systematic significance. Amer. J. Bot. 68:908–917.

Graham, S.A. 1988. Revision of *Cuphea* section Heterodon (Lythraceae). Sys. Bot. Mono. 20:1–168.

Graham, S.A. 1989. *Cuphea*: A new plant source of medium-chain fatty acids. CRC Crit. Rev. 28:139–173.

Hirsinger, F. 1980. Untersuchungen zur beurteilung der anbauwurdigkeit einer neuen MCT olpflanze *Cuphea* (Lythraceae). 2. Chemische mutaggenese bei *Cuphea* aperta Koehne. Z. Pflanzenzuchtg. 85:157–169.

Hirsinger, F. and G. Roebbelen. 1980. Studies on the agronomical value of a new MCT oil crop, *Cuphea* (Lythraceae). 3. Chemical mutagenesis of *C. lanceolata* and *C. procumbens*, and general evaluation. Z. Pflanzenzuchtg. 85:275–286.

Hirsinger, F. and P.F. Knowles. 1984. Morphological and agronomic description of selected *Cuphea* germplasm. Econ. Bot. 38:439–451.

Hirsinger, F. 1985. Agronomic potential and seed composition of *Cuphea*, an annual crop for lauric and capric seed oils. J. Amer. Oil Chem. Soc. 62:76–80.

Ignacio, L.F. 1985. Present and future position of coconut in world supply and trade. J. Amer. Oil Chem. Soc. 62:192–204.

Kadkol, G.P., G.M. Halloran, and R.H. MacMillan. 1989. Shatter resistance in crop plants. CRC Crit. Rev. 8:169–188.

Kadkol, G.P., R.H. MacMillan, R.P. Burrow, and G.M. Halloran. 1984. Evaluation of *Brassica* genotypes for resistance to shatter. I. Development of a laboratory test. Euphytica 33:63–73.

Kadkol, G.P., R.H. MacMillan, R.P. Burrow, and G.M. Halloran. 1984. Evaluation of *Brassica* genotypes for resistance to shatter. II. Variation in siliqua strength within and between accessions. Euphytica 33:915–924.

Knapp, S.J. 1990. Recurrent mass selection for reduced seed dormancy in *Cuphea laminuligera* and *Cuphea lanceolata*. Plant Breed. 104:46–52.

Knapp, S.J. 1990. New temperate oilseed crops, p. 203–210. In: J. Janick and J.E. Simon (eds.). Advances in new crops. Timber Press, Portland, OR.

Knapp, S.J. 1992. Modifying the seed oils of *Cuphea*—a new commercial source of caprylic, capric, lauric, and myristic acid. Amer. Oil Chem. Soc. Monograph. Amer. Oil Chem. Soc., Champaign, IL.

Knapp, S.J. and L.A. Tagliani. 1990. Genetic variation for seed dormancy in *Cuphea laminuligera* and *Cuphea lanceolata*. Euphytica 47:65–70.

Knapp, S.J. and L.A. Tagliani. 1991. Two medium-chain fatty acid mutants of *Cuphea viscosissima*. Plant Breed. 106:338–341.

Knapp, S.J., L.A. Tagliani, and W.W. Roath. 1991. Fatty acid and oil diversity of *Cuphea viscosissima*: A source of medium-chain fatty acids. J. Amer. Oil Chem. Soc. 68:515–517.

Knapp, S.J., L.A. Tagliani, and B.H. Liu. 1991. Outcrossing rates of experimental populations of *Cuphea lanceolata*. Plant Breed. 106:334–337.

Krueger, S.K. and S.J. Knapp. 1991. Mating systems of *Cuphea laminuligera* and *Cuphea lutea*. Theor. Appl. Genet. 82:221–226.

Ladizinsky, G. 1985. Founder effect in crop-plant evolution. Econ. Bot. 39:191–199.

Mackie, A.B. and S.D. Calhoun. 1991. World oilseed and products trade, 1962–1988. Agriculture and Trade Division, Economic Research Service, U.S. Department of Agriculture. Statistical Bul. 819.

Miller, R.W., F.R. Earle, I.A. Wolff, and Q. Jones. 1964. Search for new industrial oils. IX. *Cuphea*, a versatile source of fatty acids. J. Amer. Oil Chem. Soc. 41:279–280.

Renfrew, J.M. 1969. The archaeological evidence for the domestication of plants: methods and problems. In: P.J. Ucko and G.N. Dimbleby (eds.) The domestication and exploitation of plants and animals. G. Duckworth, London.

Roebbelen, G. 1991. Mutation breeding for quality improvement: a case study for oilseed crops. Proc. IAEA Symp. Vol. 2:3–30. Vienna, Austria.

Roebbelen, G and S. von Witzke. 1989. Mutagenesis for the domestication of *Cuphea*. Plant domestication by induced mutations. IAEA, Vienna, Austria.

Ronis, D.H., A.E. Thompson, D.A. Dierig, and E.R. Johnson. 1990. Isozyme verification of interspecific hybrids of *Cuphea*. HortScience 25:1431–1434.

Thompson, A.E. 1984. Cuphea a potential new crop. HortScience 19:352–354.

Wolf, R.B., S.A. Graham, and R. Kleiman. 1983. Fatty acid composition of *Cuphea* seed oils. J. Amer. Oil Chem. Soc. 60:27–28.

Castor: Return of an Old Crop

Raymond D. Brigham

Production of castor (*Ricinus communis* L., Euphorbiaceae) is needed in the United States to supply castor oil for the hundreds of products using this versatile chemurgic raw material. Forty to 45 thousand tonnes of castor oil and derivatives are imported each year (Roetheli et al. 1991) to supply the entire needs of our domestic industries. The United States is the largest importer and consumer of castor oil in the world. Castor oil is classed as a strategic material critical to our national defense by the Agricultural Materials Act P.L. 98-284 passed by Congress in 1984. Other "strategic" materials include natural rubber and sperm whale oil substitutes. Public Law 81-774 requires that sufficient supplies of these materials be acquired and stored in the United States to meet national defense needs in case of war (Roetheli et al. 1991).

HISTORY OF PRODUCTION IN THE UNITED STATES

Castor was in production as early as the mid-1850s in the central part of the United States, and over 23 crushing mills reportedly were operational at that time (Zimmerman 1958). Sporadic production caused mills to eventually locate on the east and west coasts to crush imported seed. In the mid-1930s, Baker Castor Oil Company began a program to develop domestic production to supply their processing plant in California. Contracts were offered to growers, and limited production developed in the Imperial and San Joaquin Valleys (Zimmerman 1958). During World Wars I and II, domestic production was encouraged because of castor oil's strategic value. Derivatives of castor oil are key ingredients in hydraulic fluids, greases, and lubricants for military equipment. During the Korean conflict, castor production was stimulated by a government sponsored procurement program. The production area reached over 20,000 ha in 1951, mainly in Texas, Oklahoma, California, and Arizona. Improved cultivars and harvesting equipment allowed the crop to compete favorably with other field crops. By 1959, Texas became the leading producer of castor, and production was centered near Plainview (Brigham and Spears 1961). In the late 1960s, over 30,000 ha were grown in Texas. The seed was shipped to the crushing facility of Baker Castor Oil Company, Bayonne, New Jersey. A small crushing facility with solvent extraction was built in Plainview in the early 1960s by the Plains Cooperative Oil Mill of Lubbock. This plant operated until castor production ceased in the early 1970s. Castor production and processing was discontinued due to: (1) low world prices for castor oil; (2) higher prices being paid for competing crops grown in the High Plains area; (3) the cooperative oil mill and castor oil buyers not agreeing on a contract price for the oil in 1972, and (4) elimination of the government price support for castor in 1972. Since that time, only limited plantings for seed production have been made. Some planting seed of the cultivar 'Hale' was exported to other countries during the 1980s.

THE PLANT

Although commonly referred to as a "bean," castor is not a legume. The plant has also been called the "castor oil plant." Castor oil, one of the oldest commercial products, was used in lamps by the Egyptians more than 4,000 years ago, and seeds have been found in their ancient tombs (Weiss 1971). Castor is considered by most authorities to be native to tropical Africa, and may have originated in Abyssinia (Weiss 1971).

Although grown as annual plants, they act as perennials in the tropics and subtropics and the plants reach heights of 9 to 12 m. The dwarf-internode cultivars 'Hale' and 'Lynn', and hybrids using them as the pollen parent, vary in height from 0.9 to 1.5 m, compared to 1.8 to 3.7 m for the normal-internode types formerly grown (Brigham 1970a,b). Soil conditions, availability of moisture, and levels of nutrients can cause considerable variation in height of plants. Plants have a tap root, plus prominent lateral roots below the soil surface.

The large leaves are palmately lobed, (hence the name Palma Christi used for castor) and are borne more or less alternately on the stems, except for the two opposite leaves at the node just above the two cotyledonary leaves. The petioles are usually several times as long as the long axis of the leaves. The main stem is terminated by the first or primary raceme, which often is the largest on the plant. The primary raceme of early dwarf-internode cultivars usually occurs after the 6th to 10th node. On later cultivars, the primary raceme may occur after the 8th to 16th node. In introductions from other countries, dwarf-internode types flowering after 40 or more nodes are known.

After the first raceme appears, branches originate at the nodes below it. The number of branches depends on plant spacing and in some cases the cultivar. Under field conditions, two or three branches occur at almost the same time, but generally in the following order: the first branch at the node immediately beneath the primary raceme, the second at the second node, and the third at the third node below the primary raceme. The first racemes formed on the branches are commonly called the "second set" of racemes. Subsequent branches arise from the nodes just beneath the racemes of the second set. This sequence of development continues as long as the plant remains alive and growing actively. Thus, the development of racemes along any one axis is sequential, making it possible for a plant to have racemes in all stages of development from bud stage to complete maturity.

Typically, the racemes usually bear pistillate flowers on the upper 30 to 50% and staminate flowers on the lower 70 to 50% of the raceme. Number of staminate and pistillate flowers can vary greatly, depending upon raceme size. The flowers are without petals. After the pollen is shed, the staminate flowers dry up and usually drop. The pollen, which is discharged forcibly from the anthers, is carried to stigmas mainly by wind (Brigham 1967). After fertilization, the pistillate flowers develop into spiny capsules, though spineless types are known. At maturity, the hull (pericarp) of the capsule may split along the outside seam (dorsal suture) of each of the three capsule segments (carpels). If splitting is violent, as in wild types, the seed will be ejected and scattered on the ground around the plant. This type of splitting (dehiscence) is not present in cultivars grown for mechanized production. Seeds of present cultivars are held within the capsule for several weeks after frost with no appreciable loss.

Seeds of current cultivars weigh from 3.0 to 3.5 g. Seed color ranges from light to dark brown, with various mottling patterns. The seed coat makes up about 25% of the weight of the seed. Oil content averages 50% on a dry weight basis.

Chromosome number of castor is $2n = 20$. Autotetraploids have been produced using colchicine, and haploids have been reported, but in nature, castor is found mainly in the diploid form. There is little or no loss of vigor when castor plants are inbred (Moshkin 1980).

AGRONOMY

Adaptation

Highest yields of castor are produced under irrigation on fine or medium textured soils, and where low relative humidity prevails. Areas where soils are infested with the cotton root-rot fungus should not be considered for growing castor, because the plants are highly susceptible to this disease (Brigham and Spears 1961). At least a 140-day growing season is required (from planting until first killing frost) to produce satisfactory yields of castor seed, and a 150 to 160-day season is more desirable.

Cultural Practices

Seedbed preparation is similar to cotton, maize, sorghum, soybean, and other row crops. Deep tillage, such as chiseling 20 to 30 cm deep, encourages development and deeper penetration of the tap root. Castor is usually planted in a shallow furrow by opening a bed with a lister-type planter, or planting can be on low beds. Beds usually are irrigated before planting by running water down the furrows. Land should be prepared for 0.96 to 1.01 m rows to fit the available harvesters.

Castor should be planted when the soil is warm—a 10 day average of 15.6°C at 20 cm depth at 8 a.m. In the Plainview, Texas, area, May 5 to 25 is usually satisfactory. Castor should not be planted after June 10 in that area. Only seed of high germination and of good quality should be planted to assure timely emergence and adequate plant populations. Seed treatment materials may be applied if needed to control damping-off in cold soils.

Castor seeds are large and slow to germinate; emergence of the seedlings may take 7 to 14 days. Castor seeds require moist soil over a longer period than maize or cotton. Seeds should be planted 6.3 to 7.6 cm deep, depending on texture and condition of the soil. If press wheels are used in contact with the seed, care should be taken that they do not crush the seed. Castor is planted in 0.96 to 1.01 m rows, with a seeding rate of 11.2 to 15.7 kg/ha and plant spacing of 20 to 25 cm within the row. Special care must be taken to prevent crushing the fragile seed in the planter box. Air planters are ideal, and can space seeds precisely. Use of an inclined-plate planter is also a preferred method, but a cotton planter box can be used if properly modified (Brigham and Spears 1961).

Adequate amounts of nitrogen, phosphorus, and potassium must be available to produce high yields of castor seed. Levels of these nutrients should be determined by soil test. If the soil is deficient in nitrogen, 90 to 135 kg/ha of nitrogen usually are needed for maximum yields. A split application of nitrogen is often used, with the second half sidedressed between the rows at last cultivation. If phosphorus is needed, application should be made before planting time. Potassium can be applied at planting time. A minimum of 37 to 56 kg/ha of P is needed for production of castor, and 15 to 19 kg/ha of K.

Where preplant furrow irrigation is applied, castor plants should not require irrigation until the first racemes appear on the plant. Under normal conditions, 12 to 14 days between irrigations should keep plants from stressing for moisture, but high temperatures and high winds during the peak growing and fruiting periods may cause the plants to need more frequent irrigation. Castor requires 20.6 to 24.7 cm/ha of water annually to produce high yields. The time of last irrigation is usually from 1 to 10 Sept.

Cultivation is much the same as for controlling weeds in cotton or soybeans. Rotary hoes are often used before or after the plants emerge to control small annual weeds and grasses. Cultivation with sweeps should be as shallow as possible to prevent damage to the fibrous root system of the plants. Trifluralin is labelled as a preplant incorporated herbicide for control of certain broadleaf weeds and grasses.

INSECTS AND DISEASES

The castor plant is not toxic to most insects, even though small amounts of the toxic protein, ricin, and the alkaloid tricinine, occur in vegetative parts of the plant (Weiss 1971). However, only infestations of false chinch bugs have become serious enough to warrant control measures in the Texas High Plains, and those occur only in a few fields every few years. Thrips, corn earworms, armyworms, spider mites, leaf miners, lygus bugs, and green stink bugs have been observed in castor fields with minimal damage.

Castor plants are attacked by numerous diseases under high relative humidity conditions, but only a few occur in the High Plains area. Alternaria leaf spot, caused by *Alternaria ricini* (Yoshii) Hansf., caused defoliation to varying degrees of earlier susceptible cultivars, but later released cultivars such as 'Hale' and 'Lynn' (Brigham 1970a,b) show resistance to this fungus. Bacterial leaf spot, caused by *Xanthomonas ricinicola* (Elliott) Dowson, also caused serious damage to susceptible cultivars, but the above dwarf-internode cultivars have moderate resistance to bacterial leaf spot. Gray mold, caused by *Botryotinia ricini* (Godfrey) Whetzel, has been observed a few times in the Plainview area, but has never been considered a problem. The organism causing cotton root rot, *Phymatotrichopsis omnivara* (Duggar) Hennebert, attacks castor, and plants should not be grown on infested soils. Charcoal rot, caused by *Macrophomina phaseolina* (Tassi) Goidanich, has been observed on plants that were stressed for soil moisture. Capsule mold, incited by a complex of fungi, causes capsules to stop development and turn bluish-purple or brown to black. This only occurs after high rainfall periods, so is usually not a problem on the High Plains. The dwarf-internode castor cultivars are resistant to Verticillium wilt caused by *Verticillium* species (Brigham and Minton 1969).

HARVESTING

Dwarf-internode castor plants are usually ready to harvest about 10 days after a killing frost, if normal drying weather prevails. Capsules should be dry enough for the seed to hull when rubbed between the hands (Schoenleber 1961). The newest harvester has a 4-row header that uses rotating brushes to remove the capsules from the plants. This harvester, adapted to a grain combine, uses rubber-covered cylinders to hull the seed. Ground speed under favorable conditions can be 8 km/hr. Relative humidity must be below 40% when harvesting castor seed, and moisture content of the seed should be 6% or lower. Castor seed stores well, and does not deteriorate significantly in storage for at least 2 years.

Yields of irrigated castor range from 2,242 to 3,363 kg/ha, and some fields have produced 3,811 to 4,035 kg/ha. The seed is usually bought at a price directly related to the world market. There are no government acreage controls or price support programs.

NEEDS AND FUTURE PROSPECTS

To restart domestic production, industries in the United States which are large users of castor oil will need to make contractual agreements on the price to be paid for oil which will attract both grower and processor. To encourage sufficient production of castor seed to supply the castor oil needs of our domestic industries the following factors need to be addressed:

- Grower contracts at a price which will attract hecterage now devoted to other crops.
- Adequate supplies of high-quality planting seed of dwarf-internode, open-pollinated cultivars or F_1 hybrids.
- A sufficient number of special built harvesters to harvest the seed from plants after a killing frost.
- A crushing/processing facility, dedicated to crushing castor seed, located in the production area.
- A contractual agreement by the processor to market castor oil over a period of years.
- Bridge financing for seed inventory from the time seed is received at the plant until oil is sold.
- Acceptance of the crop by growers and the agricultural community.
- Detoxification and deallergenation of castor meal to allow use in livestock feeds.
- Government programs with incentives to produce alternative crops not in surplus.

If castor production can be stimulated and production can again be realized, research priorities include:

- Development of improved hybrids to increase yield and oil percentage of castor seed.
- Development of breeding lines with improved disease and insect resistance, drought tolerance, and shatter resistance.
- Mutagenesis and genetic research to eliminate ricin, the toxic seed protein.
- Acquisition and preservation of germplasm useful to a breeding program.
- Improvement of harvesters to more efficiently harvest and hull the seed.
- Investigation of more economical and efficient methods of oil extraction, such as use of extruders.

REFERENCES

Brigham, R.D. 1967. Natural outcrossing in dwarf-internode castor, *Ricinus communis* L. Crop Sci. 7:353–355.

Brigham, R.D. 1970a. Registration of castor variety Hale. Crop Sci. 10:457.

Brigham, R.D. 1970b. Registration of castor variety Lynn. Crop Sci. 10:457.

Brigham, R.D. and E.B. Minton. 1969. Resistance of dwarf-internode castor (*Ricinus communis* L.) to Verticillium wilt. Plant Dis. Rptr. 53:262–266.

Brigham, R.D. and B.R. Spears. 1961. Castorbeans in Texas. Texas Agr. Expt. Sta. Bul. 954.

Moshkin, V.A. 1980. Castor. Kolos Publishers, Moscow. (English translation by American Publishing Co. Pvt. Ltd., New Delhi, 1986).

Roetheli, J.C., L.K. Glaser, and R.D. Brigham. 1991. Castor: Assessing the feasibility of U.S. production. Workshop summary, Plainview, TX, Sept. 18–19, 1990. USDA/CSRS Office of Agr. Materials. Growing Ind. Material Ser.

Schoenleber, L.G. 1961. Mechanization of castorbean harvesting. Oklahoma Agr. Expt. Sta. Bul. 591.

Weiss, E.A. 1971. Castor, sesame, and safflower. Leonard Hill, London.

Zimmerman, L.H. 1958. Castorbeans: a new crop for mechanized production. Adv. Agron. X:257–288.

Potential of Fanweed and Other Weeds as Novel Industrial Oilseed Crops*

Patrick M. Carr

Diversification has been suggested as a possible strategy for improving the financial condition of United States crop producers (Jolliff and Snapp 1988; Jolliff 1989). Agricultural production of industrial feedstocks, for example, would open additional markets to farmers who typically grow only food and feed crops. In some instances, farm production of industrial feedstocks could be quite profitable since high-value specialty chemicals are contained in the seeds of some plants (Hinman 1986).

While crambe, (*Crambe abyssinica* Hochst.), ironweed [*Vernonia galamensis* (Cass.) Less.], and several other plant species have been identified as promising industrial crops (Princen 1983), few studies have evaluated the potential of present weed species as sources of high-value specialty chemicals and industrial feedstocks (Clopton and Triebold 1944; Shultz et al. 1983). There are several weeds that are well adapted to growing conditions in different regions of the United States and could be grown as sources of industrial chemicals if domesticated. While a plant may contain desirable chemicals or have valuable properties, it is unknown if these plant species could be developed for field production. The objective of this research was to evaluate the agronomic potential of four weeds occurring in the Northern Great Plains: fanweed [*Thlaspi arvense* (L.)], black mustard [*Brassica nigra* (L.) Koch], wild mustard [*Brassica kaber* (DC.) Wheeler], and hare's ear mustard [*Conringia orientalis* (L.) Dumort]. These four weeds were studied since previous work indicated that each contained valuable specialty chemicals (Appelqvist 1971), or were related to other plant species which were sources of valuable chemicals. The potential of *Euphorbia lagascae* Spreng., as a field crop was also considered since past research indicates it may have potential as an industrial crop (Krewson and Scott 1966), even though this plant species is neither native to, nor naturalized in, the United States.

METHODOLOGY

1990

A field evaluation was conducted under dryland management at the Carrington Research/Extension Center (47°30' N, 99°7' W) in central North Dakota. Seed samples of a single accession of black mustard, hare's ear mustard, and *Euphorbia lagascae* were obtained from the USDA/ARS National Center for Agricultural Utilization Research in Peoria, Illinois, while seed of wild mustard and fanweed were collected from wild stands. Seed of each species along with crambe, an industrial crop which is grown in North Dakota, was planted in nonreplicated 1.4 m² plots on May 17. The agronomic potential of each species was rated on the basis of its ease of establishment, rate of growth, initiation and duration of flowering, susceptibility to lodging and pests, seed development (determinate or indeterminate), susceptibility of seeds to shatter, and other factors. Height of 10 plants of each species was measured prior to harvest. A 0.7 m² area was harvested by hand for determination of dry matter, grain yield, and seed weight.

1991

The six plant species included in the 1990 field experiment were each planted in 8.2 m² plots in a randomized complete block design with four replicates. The agronomic potential of each plant species was evaluated as

---

*Sincere appreciation is extended to R. Kleiman, research leader for new crops and K. Carlson, a research chemist, both at the USDA/ARS National Center for Agricultural Utilization Research, for providing seed, seed oil composition data, and helpful advice, and to N. Hettiarachchy, Associate Professor of Cereal Science and Food Technology at North Dakota State University, for determining the seed oil content and composition of the plant species included in this investigation.

described. A sunfleck ceptometer (Decagon Devices, Inc., Pullman, WA) was used to quantify the amount of photosynthetically active radiation (PAR) that was intercepted by the plant canopy in plots of two replicates on selected dates during the growing season. Plants in a 1.9 m² area from the central portion of each plot were harvested for determination of dry matter, grain yield, and seed weight. Seed oil content and fatty acid distribution of the oil were determined for a representative sample of each species by mass spectroscopy at the Food and Cereal Science Laboratory at North Dakota State University, in a manner previously described (Riveland 1991).

RESULTS AND DISCUSSION

Fanweed

Fanweed (*syn.* stinkweed, field pennycress, pennycress) was rated as having excellent potential as a new crop if established in the fall (Table 1). Poor germination of spring-sown fanweed seed was a problem. As a result, yield of fanweed was low when planted in the spring. Metzger (1990) reported that exposure to temperatures of 0° to 10°C for 3 to 6 weeks can break the dormancy of fanweed seed. Dormancy can be broken if seed is scarified by scratching the seedcoat (Best and McIntyre 1975), although this was not true for spring-sown seed in this study. Broadcast planting rather than seed drilling is desirable, since exposure to light seems to enhance seed germination. Overwintering fanweed plants were in full-flower by mid-May, while other plant species were still seedlings. Hence, seed production by most fanweed plants was completed prior to the relatively hot, dry conditions which developed by mid-July during 1990 and 1991.

Seeds, contained in pods, tended to shatter as plant moisture levels declined; however, plants could be swathed to minimize harvest loss from shattering and to promote uniform seed maturation. If swathed, fanweed could be harvested in mid-June in the Northern Great Plains, possibly enabling a second crop to be planted in the field during the same growing season. Double cropping would likely be possible in more southern portions of its range in North America.

Individual fanweed plants established in the fall produced an average of 1,600 seeds, translating into an estimated yield of about 1,500 kg/ha for both years. This yield is similar to that reported in Montana during the 1940s when fanweed was experimentally grown under irrigated management (Clopton and Triebold 1944), and to seed production estimates of wild stands in Canada (Best and McIntyre 1975). Seed yields in excess of 1,300 kg/ha are not unusual when seed from wild fanweed stands is grown in the northern United States.

Fanweed demonstrated potential as an industrial crop on the basis of seed oil content and composition (Table 2). Fanweed seed contained about 26% oil by weight; the oil, in turn, was close to 40% erucic acid (22:1). Erucic acid is an unusual fatty acid with several industrial applications (Van Dyne et al. 1990). While the level of erucic acid in the seed produced by crambe was greater than that produced by fanweed, consideration of pests, crop rotations, and other factors could make fanweed a promising candidate for new crop development.

Black Mustard

Black mustard was rated as having very good to excellent agronomic potential. Plants were easy to mechanically sow and manage. Growth was vigorous and large plants developed (Table 1). Seed production was underway by early July; the seeds which developed were contained in pods from 1.3 to 1.9 cm long which tended to shatter as plant moisture levels declined. Plants would probably need to be swathed prior to harvesting. Black mustard may fit as a short season crop in some crop rotations in the Northern Great Plains.

Black mustard produced relatively large amounts of seed (>1,200 kg/ha) during 1990 and 1991 (Table 1). In 1991, close to 1,900 kg/ha of seed was produced, making black mustard the highest yielding species evaluated. By comparison, yield of crambe averaged 1,820 kg/ha in 1991. Unlike fanweed, seed dormancy was not a serious problem with black mustard, so relatively good plant stands were fairly easy to establish in the spring.

Black mustard produced seed that was 32% oil (Table 2). Of this, roughly 40% was erucic acid. As with fanweed, black mustard demonstrated potential as an industrial crop, even though crambe seed contained greater amounts of erucic acid.

Table 1. Selected agronomic characteristics of weed species evaluated during 1990 and 1991 in central North Dakota.

Plant	Date established		Duration of flowering		Lodging[z]		Plant ht (cm)		Seed yield (kg/ha)		Seed weight (g/100 seed)	
	1990	1991	1990	1991	1990	1991	1990	1991	1990	1991	1990	1991
Fanweed	June 19	May 13	July 15–Aug 13	June 7–July 1	0.5	0.5	43	27	200	119	0.09	0.07
	Sept 1	Aug 25	May 20–June 15	May 13–June 15	0.5	0.5	28	67	1628	1414	0.08	0.08
Black mustard	May 27	May 10	June 29–Aug 8	June 13–Aug 20	1.0	1.0	176	126	1243	1875	0.17	0.16
Wild mustard	May 27	Apr 29	June 8–July 26	June 5–Aug 14	1.0	1.0	67	83	2005	1849	0.24	0.25
Hare's ear mustard	June 11	May 26	July 9–July 29	June 3–July 21	1.0	1.0	37	27	901	549	0.16	0.19
Euphorbia lagascae	May 29	May 15	July 6–Sept 20	June 12–Sept 28	1.0	1.0	72	42	201	147	0.91	1.18
Crambe	May 24	Apr 26	June 26–July 31	June 1–July 29	1.0	1.0	89	61	1997	1820	0.64	0.62

[z]0 = none, 1 = severe.

Table 2. Fatty acid acid composition of the seed oil.

Plant	Fatty acid composition (% of total seed oil)					
	16:0	18:0	18:1	18:2	20:0	22:1
Black mustard	4.8	0.0	14.3	17.9	14.0	37.6
Wild mustard	3.9	2.2	35.7	22.7	17.6	6.4
Crambe	1.4	0.8	14.0	6.2	1.0	62.9
Fanweed	2.7	0.0	13.8	20.2	9.0	37.8
Hare's ear mustard	2.5	0.0	5.8	27.5	2.2	26.9

Wild Mustard

Wild mustard (charlock, kaber mustard) was considered to have very good to excellent agronomic potential. Plants were easy to mechanically sow and manage, and seeds appeared to lend themselves to mechanical harvesting methods. As with fanweed and black mustard, seeds of wild mustard were susceptible to shattering so plants would probably be swathed prior to harvesting the seed if grown on a field-scale.

Wild mustard produced roughly 2,000 kg/ha of seed during 1990 and 1991 (Table 1). Individual plants produced an average of 2,076 seeds which were contained in pods approximately 2.5 cm in length. The seed contained about 26% oil but failed to be comprised of a high percentage of highly valued fatty acids (Table 2). For this reason, wild mustard was considered to have low potential as an industrial crop.

Hare's Ear Mustard

Hare's ear mustard (*syn.* hare's mustard) was considered to have moderate agronomic potential. Plants were generally easy to mechanically sow and manage. However, about 15% of the stand was destroyed by an unknown pathogen in 1991. Plants were short (<40 cm) and some seed pods were less than 10 cm above the soil surface (Table 1). This could present difficulties in the mechanical harvesting process. Seed could be harvested without first swathing the plants since seed pods were not susceptible to shattering.

Hare's ear mustard produced relatively low quantities of seed in 1990 and 1991 field evaluations; yields averaged 901 kg/ha in 1990 and only 549 kg/ha in 1991 (Table 1). Individual plants produced an average of 590 seeds which were contained in seed pods about 5 cm in length.

Hare's ear mustard produced seed containing about 30% oil, with close to 30% of the oil being comprised of erucic acid (Table 2). Other research indicates that the oil contains additional fatty acids with industrial applications (Appelqvist, 1971). It seems that further consideration of hare's ear mustard as an industrial crop is warranted.

Euphorbia lagascae

Euphorbia lagascae was considered to have the lowest agronomic potential of all plant species. Seed development was indeterminate and fruits containing the seed burst violently as the seed approached maturity. Still, this plant species was agronomically attractive in several respects. The seed was large and easy to mechanically sow. Seedlings grew rapidly and were easy to manage. Grasshoppers and other insect pests did not appear to feed on *Euphorbia lagascae*. Improvements in seed retention are needed.

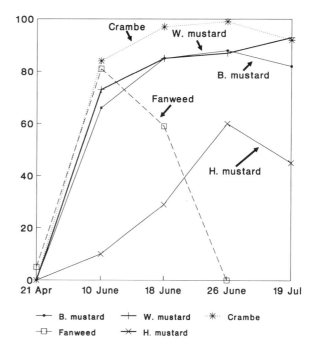

Fig. 1. Percent of photosynthetically active radiation intercepted by the plant canopy.

Euphorbia lagascae produced an abundance of seed in 1990 and 1991 field evaluations, but much of the seed could not be collected due to seed shattering. Hence, harvested seed only amounted to about 200 kg/ha during 1990 and 150 kg/ha during 1991 (Table 1). Further studies are needed to assess seed yields when plants are swathed prior to harvesting.

Euphorbia lagascae produced seed which contained over 50% oil by weight. Past research determined that the oil contained over 50% vernolic acid (K. Carlson 1991 pers. commun.), making it a promising candidate for new crop development if genetic improvements and/or management practices could enhance the mechanical harvestability of seed.

Weed Control

Weeds were a problem and had to be removed by hand throughout the growing season. Effective weed control strategies must be developed for each plant species. The plant canopy produced by crambe intercepted more than 90% of the incident PAR after June 13 in the 1991 field evaluation (Fig. 1). Only small amounts of PAR could penetrate the canopy after this date and reach weed seedlings which were developing underneath. This may explain why weed pressure was much greater in hare's ear mustard than in crambe plots, since more than 50% of the incident PAR reached weed seedlings developing under a canopy of hare's ear mustard through most of the growing season.

SUMMARY

Fanweed, black mustard, hare's ear mustard, and *Euphorbia lagascae* contain fatty acids with important industrial applications. These plants have varying degrees of potential as novel industrial crops. Fanweed is adapted to growing conditions in the Great Plains and seems suited to field production methods. Approximately 1,500 kg/ha of seed was produced in 1990–91 field evaluations in North Dakota. This seed contained about 180 kg/ha of erucic acid, an unusual fatty acid with several industrial uses. Black mustard and hare's ear mustard also produced seed containing erucic acid, but these weed species appeared to have less potential than fanweed as industrial crops when agronomic factors were considered. Seed harvesting difficulties with *Euphorbia lagascae* and failure of wild mustard seed oil to contain high-value fatty acids presently limit their potential as industrial crops.

REFERENCES

Appelqvist, R.K. 1971. Lipids in cruciferae VIII. The fatty acid composition of some wild and partially domesticated species. J. Amer. Oil Chem. Soc. 47:740–744.

Best, K.F. and G.I. McIntyre. 1975. The biology of Canadian weeds. 9. *Thlaspi arvense* L. Can. J. Plant Sci. 55:279–292.

Clopton, J.R. and H.O. Triebold. 1944. Fanweed seed oil: potential substitute for rapeseed oil. Ind. Eng. Chem. 36:218–219.

Hinman, C.M. 1986. Potential new crops. Sci. Amer. 255:33–37.

Jolliff, G.D. 1989. Strategic planning for new-crop development. J. Prod. Agr. 2:6–13.

Jolliff, G.D. and S.S. Snapp. 1988. New crop development: opportunity and challenges. J. Prod. Agr. 1:83–89.

Krewson, C.F. and W.E. Scott. 1966. *Euphorbia lagascae* Spreng., an abundant source of epoxyoleic acid: seed extraction and oil composition. J. Amer. Oil Chem. Soc. 43:171–174.

Metzger, J. 1990. Stories on the control of flowering in field pennycress (*Thlaspi arvense* L.), p. 3. In: Proc. North Dakota Acad. Sci. 44:3. 82nd Annual Meeting. April 19–20, Fargo, ND.

Princen, L.H. 1983. New oilseed crops on the horizon. Econ. Bot. 36:478–491.

Riveland, N. 1991. Oil quality and quantity of alternative oil seeds, p. 8–15. In: Alternative crop and alternative crop production research: a progress report. North Dakota State Univ., Fargo, ND.

Shultz, E.B., Jr., W.P. Darby, H.M. Draper III, and R.P. Morgan. 1984. Novel marginal-land oilseeds: potential benefits and risks, p. 13–42. In: E.B Shultz, Jr. and R.P. Morgan (eds.). Fuels and chemicals from oilseeds: technology and policy options. AAAS Selected Symposia Ser. 91. Westview Press, Boulder, CO.

Van Dyne, D.L., M.G. Blase, and K.D. Carlson. 1990. Industrial feedstocks and products from high erucic acid oil: crambe and industrial rapeseed. Univ. Missouri–Columbia, Columbia., MO.

Marigold Flower Meal as a Source of an Emulsifying Gum

Ana L. Medina and James N. BeMiller

Marigold (*Tagetes erecta* L., Asteraceae) is not only grown as an ornamental, cut flower, and landscape plant, but also as a source of pigment for poultry feed. The pigment is added to intensify the yellow color of egg yolks and broiler skin. It is composed of esters of xanthophyll (lutein). Finely ground blossom meal, often enriched with an extract, or the extract itself, usually saponified for better absorption, is added to the feed. Marigolds are grown for this purpose in various locations in the western hemisphere, primarily in Mexico and Peru, by and for various companies who produce feed additives.

One interest of the Whistler Center for Carbohydrate Research is to search for ways to meet the need for an alternative to gum arabic, the supply of which has been variable and uncertain. Unique properties of gum arabic are its ability to emulsify and its ability to form high-solids, low-viscosity solutions. The marigold flower meal that remains after removal of the xanthophyll esters by extraction was chosen as a potential source of such a gum because it was believed to contain a polysaccharide component that had the ability to protect hydrophobic substances from oxidation. To remove pigment, blossoms, either fresh or after having been stored in silos, are pressed to remove water. The resulting cake is dried, pelletized, and extracted with hexane. The remaining meal was used as a source of MFP in this work (Fig. 1).

CULTIVATION

Field production of marigolds is well established, especially for the Americas, and has been studied elsewhere, particularly in South Asia (C.G. Fohner pers. commun.). Marigolds are sown directly into a finely prepared seed bed. The crop requires supplemental irrigation. Both overhead and furrow irrigation should be available. The soil surface must be kept moist for uniform germination and emergence; irrigation by sprinkler is advised to enhance seedling establishment and minimize soil crusting. After the stand is established, water is best applied by furrow irrigation.

Marigolds are usually grown in double rows on 75- or 100-cm beds. The crop is sown as early as possible, for an early start promotes flowering. Final stands in the row should be 15 to 25 cm. Under optimal germination rates, the seeding level should be 0.37 kg/ha.

Phosphorus is required to promote flowering. Nitrogen should be applied two or three times during the growing season. The effects of nutrients, growth regulators, planting time, and plant density on plant growth, flower yield and quality, and seed yield have been reported elsewhere (Parmar and Singh 1983; Arora and Khanna 1986; Gowda and Jayanthi 1986; Ravindran et al. 1986; Shedeed et al. 1986; Anuradha et al. 1988a, 1988b, 1990; Yadav and Bose 1988; Arulmozhiyan and Pappaiah 1989; Girwani et al. 1990; Tolman et al. 1990).

Marigold is often intercropped with other plants. Rotation with marigolds reduces diseases of other crops (Medhane et al. 1985; Ijani and Mmbaga 1988; Perwez et al. 1988; Abid and Maqbool 1990), and reduces nematode populations (Prasad and Haque 1982; Baghel and Gupta 1986; Reddy et al. 1986; Alam et al. 1988). No pesticides are registered in the United States for use on marigolds grown for xanthophyll production, so proper site selection to minimize pest problems is important. Marigolds are susceptible to root diseases, but risk can be minimized by not planting marigolds in fields previously planted to peppers and by avoiding fields that are prone to standing water. Mites can be a severe problem on marigolds, but miticides are not registered for use on marigolds grown for xanthophyll production or feed use.

Cultivation to control weeds is advised until the crop canopy has closed because as no herbicides are registered for use on marigolds grown for direct use in poultry feed or for xanthophyll production. Flowers are harvested by hand when plants have, on the average, two or three fully developed flowers (about 90 days after planting). Subsequent harvests (up to two) can be made at intervals of 3 to 5 weeks, depending on plant vigor. Mechanical harvesters are also used; they generally limit the number of harvests to one because of plant damage.

METHODOLOGY

Marigold Flower Polysaccharide (MFP)

MFP can be extracted from the meal with warm (50° to 55°C) water (BeMiller et al. 1989). MFP was determined to be a protein-polysaccharide. One purified fraction of the polysaccharide portion was found to contain 3.75% galacturonic acid and neutral sugars in the molar ratio: galactose (15): glucose (7): arabinose (3). Methylation analysis indicates a highly branched, acidic arabinoglucogalactan. Partial characterization of the protein part indicated the presence of at least two very hydrophobic polypeptide constituents (Wickramasingha 1990).

The crude extract was dark, and a procedure involving an oxidative pretreatment of the meal prior to extraction of the gum was worked out to give preparations of minimal color (BeMiller et al. 1989). Both the crude-extract and the bleached MFP had emulsifying and emulsion stabilization powers for limonene equivalent to those of gum arabic at equal concentrations (1 and 2.5%) and slightly less than those of gum arabic for olive and castor oils (BeMiller et al. 1989). It was not, however, possible to prepare high-solids, low-viscosity solutions of MFP and, hence, not possible to prepare concentrated emulsions. It was hypothesized that the difference in negative charge on the two molecules (ca. 16% uronic acid in gum arabic vs. 3.75% uronic acid in MFP) might be the reason for their different rheological behaviors. A project was undertaken to increase the negative charge on MFP by sulfation. The net negative charge was increased to 14.3 mole% without decreasing its emulsion-stabilizing properties. The reduction in viscosity was, however, only slight and remained much higher than that of gum arabic (Medina Fuentes 1991).

MFP was characterized from material subjected to two different treatments before pigment extraction, as well as from fresh petals after removal of pigments. Storage of blossoms in silos before pigment extraction resulted in a MFP preparation of slightly less viscosity and protein content as compared to MFP obtained from nonensiled blossoms. The former MFP also required a slightly higher concentration to achieve equivalent emulsion stability. MFP obtained from fresh petals had poorer performance as an emulsifier and higher solution viscosity (Medina Fuentes 1991). Covalently attached phenolic compounds were present in all three sources of MFP.

Sources

The source of the meal obtained from Prodomex S.A. de C.V. (Prodomex meal) was marigolds grown near Los Mochis, Sinaloa, México, that had been picked both by hand and by machine. Fresh blossoms were heated, then pressed. The resulting cake was dried, extruded into pellets, and extracted with hexane. The source of the meal obtained from Kemin Industries, Inc. (Kemin meal) was marigolds grown in Peru. Blossoms were stored in a silo before being pressed, dried, and hexane extracted. The source of the fresh marigold flowers was Alternative Agriculture Cooperative, Sedalia, Missouri; they were kept frozen until used.

Preparation of MFP

Removal of pigments from fresh flowers. Petals were separated from the rest of the flower and extracted in a Soxhlet apparatus with methanol. The methanol was removed, and the petals were soaked in a mixture (2:1 v/v) of benzene and ethanol at room temperature for 1 h and then extracted again in a Soxhlet apparatus with the same solvent. The petals were extracted twice with hexane in a Soxhlet apparatus. The remaining colorless petals were dried at room temperature.

Extraction of MFP. Dry meal (300 g) or extracted petals (55 g) were soaked in water (1,500 ml) for 3 h at room temperature. The suspension of swollen material was then heated for 3 h with constant stirring in a water bath at 55°C. The suspension was centrifuged at 3,000 rpm (Beckman model J-6B) for 25 min at 22°C, and the supernatant was filtered. The filtrate was acidified with acetic acid to pH 4.5, and 95% ethanol (3 volumes) was added in a thin stream to the rapidly stirred solution. The precipitate was collected by centrifugation (3,000 rpm, 25 min, 22°C) and dissolved in 0.5 liters of water. The resulting solution was filtered through a layer of diatomite filter-aid (Celite, Manville Products Corp.) in a Buchner funnel (Wickramasingha 1990).

The aqueous solution was passed through a column of Amberlite IR-120(H^+) cation-exchange resin to remove proteinaceous material. All effluent with an acidic pH (pH 3) was collected and dialyzed against distilled water. The retentate was concentrated and lyophilized (Wickramasingha 1990).

Sulfation (Medina Fuentes 1991)

Sulfation with methyl sulfoxide-sulfur trioxide complex. MFP was dissolved in DMSO (1 g/10 ml). After solution was complete, the reaction mixture was cooled to 15° to 17°C. The complex (Whistler and Spencer 1961) was added, and the mixture was stirred at 15° to 17°C for 15 min. Ice (10 g) and water (25 ml) were added, and the solution was neutralized to pH 7 with 10% ammonium hydroxide solution. A 5% excess of alkali was added, and the mixture was stirred for 15 min. The Prodomex MFP derivative was precipitated with ethanol (3 volumes), redissolved, and dialyzed 24 h against a pH 8 solution of ammonium hydroxide and 48 h against distilled water. The final product was obtained by freeze-drying.

Sulfation with triethylamine-sulfur trioxide complex. A mixture of triethylamine-sulfur trioxide complex (Aldrich Chemical Co.) and 250 ml of dimethylformamide was cooled to 0°C. Prodomex MFP (1 g) was added, and the reaction was allowed to proceed 24 h at 0°C with stirring. The material was then dialyzed 24 h against a solution of 10% ammonium hydrogen carbonate, and 48 h against distilled water. The sulfated product was precipitated with ethanol (3 volumes), collected by centrifugation (3,000 rpm, 25 min, 22°C), and freeze-dried.

Samples (0.05 g) were analyzed for sulfur content using the method described by Ma and Crattner (1970). Removal of cationic interferences prior to analysis was necessary. This was done by adding 0.15 g of cation-exchange resin (Amberlite IR-120 [H⁺]) to solutions of samples, stirring for 20 min, and removal of an aliquot after settling (Hoffer et al. 1979).

Emulsion Stability

Emulsions were prepared with a Vibra Cell Sonifier (Sonics & Materials, Inc.). A mixture of either limonene or olive oil (0.25 ml), and gum solution (2.25 ml of a 1% w/v solution) was sonicated for two 90-s periods, first placing the tip of the instrument's tapered probe into the surface of the mixture, and then lowering the probe into the middle of the sample. The instrument was used in a continuous mode at a power setting of 3 (75 watts) (Dea and Madden 1986). In the case of diluted emulsions, 1 ml of emulsion was diluted with 9 ml of distilled water (1:10 dilution). After 2 min, another 1:10 dilution was made (1:100 dilution) (Prakash et al. 1990).

Emulsion stability was determined by diluting the emulsion and monitoring turbidity as a function of time at a wavelength of 500 nm with a Varian Model DMS80 double-beam spectrophotometer (Pearce and Kinsella 1978). Gum arabic was used as a standard. All three emulsions were diluted appropriately to give a final 1:1000 dilution.

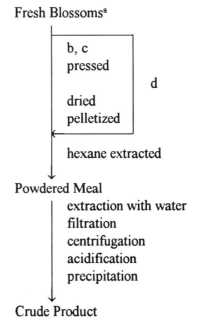

Fig. 1. Preparation of MFP. [a]Hand or machine picked. [b]Prodomex MFP (not ensiled). [c]Kemin Industries MFP (ensiled). [d]Pigment was removed from fresh petal MFP by extraction with methanol and benzene-ethanol, in that order, then hexane.

CONCLUSION

Marigold flower petal meal contains a water-soluble gum (MFP) that has been characterized as a protein-polysaccharide. MFP has emulsifying and emulsion-stabilizing properties equivalent to those of gum arabic towards limonene and slightly less than those of gum arabic towards olive and castor oils. It is, however, not possible to prepare concentrated emulsions with MFP because of the high viscosity of its solutions at concentrations above about 5%. A test of the hypothesis that the reason for the difference in rheological behavior between MFP and gum arabic, also a protein-polysaccharide, was the much lower charge density of MFP did not support it for increasing the anionic charge on MFP to a value close to that of gum arabic reduced its viscosity only slightly.

REFERENCES

Abid, M. and M.A. Maqbool. 1990. Effects of inter-cropping of *Tagetes erecta* on root-knot disease and growth of tomato. Int. Nematol. Network Newsl. 7:41–42.

Alam, M.M., A.M. Khan, and S.K. Saxena. 1988. Management of plant parasitic nematodes by different cropping sequences. Indian J. Plant Pathol. 6:102–109.

Anuradha, K., K. Pampapathy, and N. Narayana. 1988a. Effect of N and P_2O_5 on the nutrient composition and uptake by marigold (*Tagetes erecta* L.). S. Indian Hort. 36:209–211.

Anuradha, K., K. Pampapathy, and R. Sreenivasalu. 1988b. Effect of N and P_2O_5 on flowering and yield of marigold (*Tagetes erecta* L.). S. Indian Hort. 36:321–323.

Anuradha, K., K. Pampapathy, and N. Narayana. 1990. Effect of nitrogen and phosphorus on flowering, yield and quality of marigold. Indian J. Hort. 47:353–357.

Arora, J.S. and K. Khanna. 1986. Effect of nitrogen and pinching on growth and flower production of marigold (*Tagetes erecta*). Indian J. Hort. 43:291–294.

Arulmozhiyan, R. and C.M. Pappaiah. 1989. Studies on the effect of nitrogen, phosphorus and ascorbic acid on the growth and yield of marigold (*Tagetes erecta* L.) cv. MDU 1. S. Indian Hort. 37:169–172.

Baghel, P.P.S. and D.C. Gupta. 1986. Effect of intercropping on root-knot nematode (*Meloidogyne javanica*) infesting grapevine (var. Perlette). Indian J. Nematol. 16:283–284.

BeMiller, J.N., A.K. Gupta, and D.S. Wickramasingha. 1989. Structure and properties of the water-extractable polysaccharide of marigold (*Tagetes erecta*) petals, p. 1–14. In: R.P. Millane, J.N. BeMiller, and R. Chandrasekaran (eds.). Frontiers in carbohydrate research-1. Elsevier Applied Science, London.

Dea, I.C.M. and J.K. Madden. 1986. Acetylated pectic polysaccharides of sugar beet. Food Hydrocolloids 1:71–88.

Girwani, A., R.S. Babu, and R. Chandrasekhar. 1990. Response of marigold *Tagetes-erecta* to growth-regulators and zinc. Indian J. Agr. Sci. 60:220–222.

Gowda, J.V.N. and R. Jayanthi. 1986. Studies on the effect of spacing and season of planting on growth and yield of marigold *Tagetes erecta* Linn. S. Indian Hort. 34:198–203.

Hoffer, E.M., E.L. Kothny, and B.R. Appel. 1979. Simple method for microgram amounts of sulfate in atmospheric particulates. Atmos. Environ. 13:303–306.

Ijani, A.S.M. and M.T. Mmbaga. 1988. Studies on the control of root knot nematodes (*Meloidogyne* species) on tomato in Tanzania using marigold plants (*Tagetes* species), ethylene dibromide and aldicarb. Trop. Pest Management 34:147–149.

Ma, T.S. and R.C. Crattner. 1979. Modern elemental analysis. Marcel Dekker, New York.

Medhane, N.S., G.B. Jagdale, A.B. Pawar, and K.S. Darekar. 1985. Effect of *Tagetes erecta* on root-knot nematodes infecting betelvine. Intl. Nematol. Network Newslett. 2:11–12.

Medina Fuentes, A.L. 1991. Marigold (*Tagetes erecta*) flower polysaccharide: (1) comparison of preparations from different sources; (2) viscosity and emulsion stabilizing properties of sulfated gum. MS Thesis, Purdue University, West Lafayette, IN.

Parmar, A.S. and S.N. Singh. 1983. Effect of plant growth regulators on growth and flowering of marigold (*Tagetes erecta*). S. Indian Hort. 31:53–54.

Pearce, K.N. and J.E. Kinsella. 1978. Emulsifying properties of proteins: evaluation of a turbidimetric technique. J. Agr. Food Chem. 26:716–723.

Perwez, M.S., M.F. Rahman, and S.R. Haider. 1988. Effect of *Tagetes erecta* on *Meloidogyne javanica* infecting lettuce. Int. Nematol. Network Newslett. 5:18–19.

Prakash, A., M. Joseph, and M.E. Mangino. 1990. The effects of added proteins on the functionality of gum arabic in soft drink emulsion systems. Food Hydrocolloids 4:1177–184.

Prasad, D. and M.M. Haque. 1982. Reaction on varieties of marigold against root-knot nematode, *Meloidogyne incognita*. Indian J. Nematol. 12:418–419.

Ravindran, D.V.L., R.R. Rao, and E.N. Reddy. 1986. Effect of spacing and nitrogen levels on growth, flowering and yield of African marigold (*Tagetes erecta* L.). S. Indian Hort. 34:320–323.

Reddy, K.C., A.R. Soffes, G.M. Prine, and R.A. Dunn. 1986. Tropical legumes for green manure II. Nematode populations and their effects on succeeding crop yields. Agron. J. 78:5–10.

Shedeed, M.R., K.M. El-Gamassy, M.E. Hashim, and A.M.N. Almulla. 1986. Effect of some growth regulators on the growth, flowering and seed production of some summer annuals. Ann. Agr. Sci., Ain Shams Univ. 31:677–689.

Tolman, D.A., A.X. Niemiera, and R.D. Wright. 1990. Influence of plant age on nutrient absorption for marigold seedlings. HortScience 25:1612–1613.

Whistler, R.L. and W.W. Spencer. 1961. Preparation and properties of several polysaccharide sulfates. Arch. Biochem. Biophys. 95:36–41.

Wickramasingha, D.S. 1990. Partial characterization of the structure and properties of the water-extracted polysaccharide of marigold (*Tagetes erecta*) flowers. MS Thesis, Purdue University, West Lafayette, IN.

Yadav, L.P. and T.K. Bose. 1988. Influence of planting time and plant density on growth, flowering and seed yield in marigold. Bangladesh Hort. 16:17–21.

Sweet Sorghum for a Piedmont Ethanol Industry

Glen C. Rains, John S. Cundiff, and Gregory E. Welbaum

One method to reduce air pollution in EPA non-attainment areas is to mandate oxygenated fuel for vehicles operating in those areas. Currently 8% of the United States gasoline supply is an ethanol blend (USDA 1990), and the importance of ethanol use is expected to increase as more health issues are related to air quality. The current budget bill approved by the Congress included an extension of the partial excise tax exemption and the blenders income tax credit for ethanol blended gasoline to the year 2000. With the tax incentive in place for another 10 years, ethanol production capacity is expected to double by 1995 and triple by the year 2000 (Dinneen 1991).

Both herbaceous and woody crops represent possible sources of fiber for conversion to ethanol. Herbaceous crops harvested as hay are generally field-dried and stored outside in round bales. Woody crops have the advantage of a relatively long harvest season (40 weeks annually) which reduces storage requirements. They too are dried naturally and stored in open-air storage facilities.

Sweet sorghum can produce large quantities of both readily fermentable carbohydrate, and fiber for conversion via enzymatic hydrolysis, per unit land area. In fact, on the average, sweet sorghum produces more carbohydrate per unit land area than maize in the drought-prone southeastern Piedmont of the United States (Parrish et al. 1985). Unlike maize, sweet sorghum does not concentrate carbohydrates in grain, but stores them in the stalk. Many tons of high moisture content material must be handled to collect the fermentable constituent, and equipment and transportation costs are directly related to tonnage handled. Also, the harvest season is short, only 4 to 6 weeks. The challenge is to harvest the crop, separate it into juice and fiber, and utilize each constituent for year-round production of ethanol.

This study determines the cost, expressed in $/liter of ethanol, to deliver sweet sorghum to an ethanol production facility in the Piedmont. Options exist for each step of the process—harvesting and field processing, use of rind-leaf fraction, and final processing to ethanol—and costs vary according to option.

OVERVIEW

The southeastern Piedmont, a physiographic region extending from the southeastern corner of Pennsylvania to the middle of Alabama, has relatively small, irregularly-shaped fields on rolling terrain. The Piedmont was chosen for sweet sorghum production because much effort has been expended to develop drought-tolerant crops for this region, and sweet sorghum has emerged as a leading candidate for carbohydrate production with minimum inputs.

In developing a concept for a sweet sorghum-for-ethanol industry in the Piedmont, an attempt was made to encourage the involvement of a large number of growers with varying production units, perhaps as small as 10 hectares. It is hypothesized that a centralized ethanol production plant will buy whole-stalk sorghum standing in the field and will be responsible for harvesting, processing, and transporting the crop. The grower will provide bunk silo space to store the fiber constituent. The central plant could own the necessary harvesting equipment, or perhaps will contract with a harvesting company. In either case, farmers will not be required to own harvesting equipment, used only a small fraction of the year, to harvest their crop.

COST OF ETHANOL FEEDSTOCK

Field Production

Based on data reported by Maxey et al. (1989) and Worley and Cundiff (1991), the calculated cost to produce sweet sorghum, up to harvest, is $365/ha. If a sweet sorghum-for-ethanol industry is organized in the Piedmont, and a central plant is responsible for harvesting, it is probable that Piedmont farmers would grow sweet sorghum for a net return of $125/ha. Gross return to the farmer is then $365 + 125 = $490/ha. Assuming an average yield of 40 Mg/ha, achievable with modest inputs, the cost to the central ethanol production facility is $12.25/Mg whole stalks standing in the field.

Harvesting/Field Processing of Sweet Sorghum

Presently, there are no commercially available sweet sorghum harvesters designed specifically for conditions found in the Piedmont. However, with possible modifications, equipment for silage-making appears to be a reasonable harvesting option. For this study, three sweet sorghum harvesters were considered: (1) conventional forage chopper, (2) "pith combine" consisting of a conventional forage chopper, modified to collect the pith fraction and to drop the rind-leaf fraction back on the field, and (3) pull-type harvester that will cut whole stalks and place them in a windrow in the field.

The following is envisioned for the forage chopper option: whole-stalk sorghum is chopped with a conventional forage chopper, blown into forage wagons or trucks, and transported to a truck-mounted screw press parked inside a bunk silo. Chopped sorghum is passed through the press to express the juice, and the residue is conveyed immediately into the silo. Juice is collected in a storage tank which is emptied periodically (twice daily, or more if indicated) by a tanker truck. At the ethanol production plant, juice is fermented directly. This system, hereafter referred to as the "forage chopper" system, could be implemented today with existing technology. Performance parameters for the various pieces of equipment in the forage chopper system are known, except for the screw press.

Research conducted by Cundiff and Worley (1991) and Crandell et al. (1989) indicates that a forage chopper could be modified to collect sweet sorghum pith and drop rind-leaf back on the field. This machine, referred to as a "pith combine", is envisioned as an assembly of the following subsystems: a forage chopper pickup mechanism, slightly modified forage chopper feed rolls and chopper assembly, a set of straw walkers mounted behind the chopper, and a conveyor to load pith into a forage wagon. For this study, a "pith combine" system is defined by replacing the forage chopper in the forage chopper system with a pith combine. All features of the forage chopper and pith combine systems are identical except the pith combine leaves a rind-leaf fraction equal to 10% of the whole-stalk mass on the field.

A whole-stalk harvester is being developed for the Piedmont (Rains et al. 1990). A system, hereafter referred to as the Piedmont system (Fig. 1), is expected to operate as follows: The whole-stalk harvester cuts stalks and deposits them in windrows. A field loader dumps stalks onto trailers for transporting and stockpiling at a processing site adjacent to a bunk silo. At some later time, perhaps after 30 to 60 days storage, stalks are loaded into a processor consisting of feeder, chopper, and pith separator. The processor is mounted on a flat-bed trailer for transport from farm to farm. Stalks are fed into the chopper/separator, which operates like the pith combine, except that it separates out a rind-leaf fraction equal to 30% of the whole-stalk mass. After passage through the

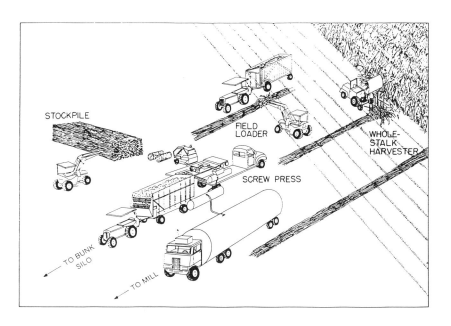

Fig. 1. The Piedmont harvest system. A whole-stalk harvester cuts sorghum and deposits it in windrows, and a field loader dumps the stalks onto a trailer for transport to the field processing site.

screw press to capture juice, pith presscake is recombined with the rind-leaf fraction and conveyed into the bunk silo. Resulting silage is identified as "combination" silage to differentiate it from silage produced with the pith combine system, which does not include the rind-leaf fraction. Juice produced by the Piedmont system is handled in the same manner as the other two systems.

The forage chopper system has one key disadvantage compared to the pith combine or Piedmont system. Passing chopped whole stalk through the press reduces press capacity and juice yield. Little sugar is contained in the fibrous leaf and rind, but it absorbs juice, thus reducing the total juice that can be expressed. Because juice expression is a relatively expensive processing step, it is important to investigate options which maximize juice yield per hour of press operating time.

Using the assumption that sugar content of juice remaining in the presscake (fiber that exits the screw press), is equal to sugar content of the expressed juice, Cundiff (1991) presents a procedure to calculate the sugar collected in the juice for several whole-stalk fractionation options. Using the expression ratio (defined as juice mass divided by input mass to press) and the juice Brix, quantity of sugar collected in the juice can be calculated for each system. Crandell et al. (1989) conducted a single experiment for a 65 to 75% pith fraction and found that the expression ratio was 0.625 and 0.60, respectively. Cundiff and Rains (1991) later completed a replicated experiment and found that the expression ratio for chopped whole stalks was 0.36, and for a 90% pith fraction it was 0.46. Based on these limited data, the following expression ratios were assumed for the material produced by the three systems: forage chopper (0.35), pith combine (0.45), and Piedmont (0.55).

Stripping away rind-leaf mass equal to 10% of the whole stalks mass (pith combine system) increases the sugar yield per Mg of input to the press by 29%. When a 30% rind-leaf fraction is eliminated (Piedmont system), sugar yield per Mg input is increased by 57%. The increase in whole-stalk sugar captured in the juice is 16% for the pith combine system and 10% for the Piedmont system. If the press has the same capacity (Mg/h) for the pith fractions as the chopped whole stalk, then press operating cost per unit of sugar captured in the juice is minimized for the 70% pith fraction. The 90% pith fraction represents a compromise choice which maximizes whole stalks sugar yield in the juice, and still achieves a 29% increase in screw press performance.

The forage chopper system requires the lowest equipment investment and the Piedmont system requires the greatest. A key question is, does increased yield of juice fermentables pay for the additional equipment investment?

The Piedmont system has one key advantage over the forage chopper and pith combine systems—it allows for whole-stalk storage. Without whole-stalk storage, sorghum must be processed (juice expressed and residue ensiled) as it is harvested. Therefore, harvest and juice expression operations are tied together—if one machine breaks down, the entire system is delayed. Whole-stalk storage allows the harvest season to be extended at least 30 days, and perhaps up to 60 days, without significant degradation of sugars. Extension of harvest season results in cost savings at an ethanol production plant by reducing peak capacity requirement. If the harvest season can be extended from 8 to 12 weeks, processing equipment capacity can be reduced by one-third.

Worley and Cundiff (1991) developed a systems model of sweet sorghum harvesting, and estimated costs for harvesting and juice expression via forage chopper, pith combine, and Piedmont systems. Costs were $13.25/Mg whole stalk (forage chopper), $9.05 (pith combine), and $16.20 (Piedmont). Assuming a 40 Mg whole stalk/ha yield, costs were $530/ha (forage chopper), $362 (pith combine), and $648 (Piedmont).

Options for Fiber Fractions

The by-products of sweet sorghum processing (whole-stalk presscake or rind-leaf fraction and pith presscake), represent a significant percentage of a sweet sorghum crop, and their use (and associated value) significantly impacts the economics of ethanol production. Possible uses for sweet sorghum by-products include burning to provide heat energy, pulp for paper or fiber board manufacture, hay, silage for animal feed, and silage for use as a feedstock in fiber conversion to ethanol. Worley et al. (1991) considered possible uses and determined monetary values for by-products. Harvest system selection determines in part which uses are feasible and the relative yields of juice and ensiled fiber residue. Total value on a per hectare basis ranged from $318 for combination silage (pith presscake and rind-leaf fractions recombined after juice expression) fed to cattle on the grower's farm, to $155 for combination silage delivered to a central plant for fiber conversion at $44/dry Mg.

Conversion Efficiencies

The juice sugar is assumed to be converted at 85% theoretical, or 54.4 liter ethanol per 100 kg. Costs in this paper are calculated based on an average juice sugar concentration of 15 kg/kg solution (approximately 17° Brix), which is attainable in the Piedmont. Juice Brix of 18° have been reported in Louisiana (Ricaud and Arcemeaux 1989), and some higher sugar varieties tested in Georgia have produced 22° Brix juice (Bryan and Monroe 1985).

Potential ethanol yield from the fiber is more difficult to predict. Emerging enzymatic hydrolysis technology has not been proven on a commercial scale. Since sweet sorghum is not currently a commercial crop, and is not expected to compete with maize as an ethanol feedstock until fiber conversion is a commercial option, it is appropriate to use the projected conversion efficiency for the mid-1990s, i.e., 420 liter/dry Mg (Norman Hinman, Manger, Biofuels Program, Solar Energy Research Institute, 1617 Cole Boulevard, Golden, CO 80401-3393), which equates to 147 liter/Mg silage at 35% dry matter. Based on an average yield of 40 Mg whole stalks/ha, the total potential ethanol yield per hectare from both juice and fiber is 5,025 (forage chopper), 4385 (pith combine), and 4790 (Piedmont). These results were based on expected silage yields of 0.617 Mg silage/Mg whole stalks (forage chopper), 0.47 (pith combine), and 0.553 (Piedmont). Juice yields were 332 liter/Mg whole stalks (forage chopper), 385 (pith combine), and 365 (Piedmont).

Cost to Transport Feedstock

Based on the potential ethanol yields, the maximum production area required for a 3.8 million liter per year (LPY) (1 million GPY) production facility ranges from 860 ha (pith combine) to 750 ha (forage chopper), or about 1% of the total land area in a 15 km radius. Many locations with sufficient surrounding row cropland for a 3.8 million liter plant are available, and it is probable that locations can be found for 10 million LPY facilities.

Road networks in the Piedmont are such that, within a 15-km radius, estimated average trucking distance to bring feedstock to a central facility is about 15 km. Energy in the diesel fuel to truck juice 15 km is equivalent to 1.5% of the energy in the ethanol produced. With silage, the transport energy is 1% of the energy in the ethanol. For comparison, the average energy to move petroleum from the wellhead to a retail outlet is 4% of the energy in the petroleum.

Trucking cost was determined by contacting companies engaged in trucking operations similar to the needed operations. A molasses hauler reported a cost of $0.93/km for short deliveries. (All trucking costs are presented as a per-km charge for travel out empty and return loaded). A logging contractor reported a trucking cost of $0.78/km, and a feed mill reported $0.75/km. Cost to haul silage was taken to be $0.78/km and cost to haul juice was taken to be $0.93/km.

Cost to Transport Expressed Juice and Silage

Assuming a tanker truckload carries 21 Mg (20,000 liter of juice) and each load requires a 30-km round trip at $0.93/km, transportation cost is $0.0014/liter juice. Assuming an average load of 21 Mg, round trip travel of 30 km, and a cost of $0.78/km, transportation cost is $1.11/Mg silage.

Storage Costs

It is anticipated that juice will be fermented directly as it is produced during the harvest season. Cost of storing 65% moisture content material in a bunk silo was estimated to be $5.38/Mg (Worley et al. 1991). It is probable that the central plant will rent silo space on the grower's farm. This option will allow the silage to be trucked in as needed, and permits the use of a small fleet of trucks operating year-round rather than a large fleet operating only during the short harvest season. Assuming the grower must receive at least 5% profit on his storage lease, total cost to the central plant is $1.05 \times 5.38 = \$5.65$/Mg silage, which is equivalent to $0.038/liter expected ethanol yield.

Total Feedstock Cost

Costs to deliver sweet sorghum fermentables for year-round ethanol production at a 3.8 million LPY facility are presented in Table 1. For comparison purposes, it is instructive to consider sweet sorghum as a fiber crop

Table 1. Total cost of feedstock ($/liter expected ethanol yield) when the juice is fermented as harvested and the fiber is ensiled and converted year-round.

	Cost ($/liter expected ethanol yield)			
	Forage chopper			
Operation	Fiber only	Juice+fiber	Pith combine	Piedmont system
Field production	0.099	0.073	0.083	0.076
Harvest/field processing	0.066	0.105	0.083	0.135
Storage	0.038	0.028	0.024	0.026
Transportation	0.008	0.009	0.010	0.009
Total	0.211	0.215	0.200	0.246

only (no juice expression). Total cost ($/ha) to harvest with conventional silage equipment, ensile in a bunk silo, and transport to a fiber conversion plant is: Production ($365) + Harvesting ($246) + Storage ($152) + Transportation ($133) = Total ($896).

Potential return at $44/dry Mg is $499/ha. A fiber conversion plant would have to pay $79/dry Mg for a grower to break even on sweet sorghum. These costs are shown in Table 1 on a per-liter-of-expected-ethanol-yield basis for comparison with the other systems.

DISCUSSION

The forage chopper system uses existing commercial equipment, consequently it is appropriate to discuss this option in detail. The total cost (Table 1), $0.215/liter expected ethanol yield, is equivalent to $31.60/Mg silage, assuming the silage yields 147 liter/Mg. At 65% moisture content, $31.60/Mg silage is equivalent to $90/dry Mg, or approximately twice the feedstock cost assumed for some fiber conversion studies. What opportunities exist to reduce cost? By eliminating juice expression, the total cost was reduced 12% to $79/dry Mg. Ethanol yield was 3,700 liter/ha for the forage chopper system (fiber conversion only) as compared to 5,025 liter/ha, or 36% more, when the juice is also collected and fermented.

The pith combine and Piedmont system options were developed in an attempt to reduce the cost of fermentables collected in the juice. Using the assumption of 420 liter/dry Mg for fiber conversion of the silage, the yield from the juice is a minor part of the total yield per ton of whole stalks, 28% (forage chopper), 37% (pith combine), and 32% (Piedmont). Differences between these systems and the forage chopper system are obscured by the silage yield. The analysis does show a slightly lower cost for the pith combine, suggesting that return of a 10% rind-leaf fraction to the field as a contribution to sustainable agriculture may be a viable option. The Piedmont system offers the advantage of whole-stalk storage, and subsequent extension of the harvest season from 8 to 12 weeks. Since this system only has a cost 14.4% higher than the forage chopper system, it also merits further study.

CONCLUSIONS

Three harvesting/handling systems were analyzed to determine the cost for delivery of sweet sorghum fermentables for year-round operation of an ethanol plant. Predicted feedstock cost ranged from $0.200 to $0.246/liter expected ethanol yield. (No conversion costs are included.) For comparison, maize at $2.50/bu represents a feedstock cost of $0.264/liter expected ethanol yield. Wet milling of maize spins off an array of co-products including ethanol, high fructose corn syrup, gluten feed, oil, and carbon dioxide. Just as high-value chemicals help pay the distillation cost of gasoline, these co-products help pay the cost of producing the ethanol. It is probable that a fiber conversion plant will have to produce a range of higher-value co-products along with ethanol, if it is going to compete with the wet milling of maize.

Net feedstock cost in a maize wet milling plant typically ranges 20 to 25% of the total ethanol production cost (Fuel Ethanol Cost-Effectiveness Study 1987). Remaining costs (all other than feedstock) range from $0.159 to $0.359/liter, and if costs at a fiber conversion plant are similar, total cost of producing fuel ethanol from sweet sorghum will range from $0.200 (feedstock) + $0.159 (conversion) = $0.359 (total) to $0.246 (feedstock) + $0.359 (conversion) = $0.605 (total). Current selling price of ethanol as a fuel additive is $0.30 to $0.35 per liter (Oxyfuel News 1992); consequently, the market must change before sweet sorghum can be competitive.

There is so little difference in the projected cost for the three harvest systems, none should be excluded from further study at this time. Should the market change, and a central plant be built to operate on sweet sorghum, it is probable that a mix of all three harvesting systems would be used.

Two forage chopper options were considered, harvesting the crop for silage only, and harvesting for juice expression and silage. Feedstock cost, computed up to the point conversion begins, ranged from $79 to $90/dry Mg. If the objective is simply the delivery of a Mg of fiber for a conversion process, it does not appear that a high moisture crop like sweet sorghum, which must be stored by ensiling, can be delivered at a cost competitive with high-yielding perennial grasses which are harvested and stored like hay. Ensiling does provide an opportunity for biochemical modification of the fiber during storage, and this advantage may increase the competitiveness of an ensiled crop.

REFERENCES

Audubon Sugar Institute. 1983. Sweet sorghum studies. Louisiana State University, Baton Rouge, 1984; Unpublished Report.

Bryan, W.L. and G.E. Monroe. 1985. Sweet sorghum cultivation comparison. Proc. 5th Annual Solar and Biomass Workshop. Atlanta, GA. p. 125–128.

Crandell, J.H., J.S. Cundiff, and J.W. Worley. 1989. Methods of separating pith from chopped sweet sorghum stalks. Amer. Soc. Agr. Engr. Paper 89-6572. St. Joseph, MI.

Cundiff, J.S. and G.C. Rains. 1991. 1990 Annual report, Sweet sorghum for a Piedmont ethanol industry. Va. Poly. Inst. & State Univ., Blacksburg. Unpublished report.

Cundiff, J.S. and J.W. Worley. 1991. Chopping parameters for separation of sweet sorghum pith and rind-leaf. Bioresources Tech. (in press).

Dinneen, R. 1991. Congress acts to increase the production of ethanol. Biologue 8(1):11–14.

Fuel Ethanol Cost-Effectiveness Study. 1987. USDA Office of Energy, 14th and Independence Avenue, Room 438A, Administration Building, Washington, DC.

Maxey, H.T., T. Covey, B. McKinnon, and A. Allen. 1989. West central district crop budgets. Virginia Cooperative Extension Service Periodic Extension Memorandum. Va. Poly. Tech. Inst. & State Univ., Blacksburg.

Oxyfuel News. 1992. Information Resources, 499 S. Capitol Street SW, Suite 406, Washington, DC.

Parrish, D.J., T.C. Gammon, and B. Graves. 1985. Production of fermentables and biomass by six temperate fuel crops. Energy in Agr. 4:319–330.

Rains, G.C., J.S. Cundiff, and D.H. Vaughan. 1990. Development of a whole-stalk sweet sorghum harvester. Trans. Amer. Soc. Agr. Engr. 33(1):56–62.

Ricaud, R. and A. Arcemeaux. 1989. Sweet sorghum for biomass and sugar production in Louisiana. Agronomy Department. Louisiana State Univ., Baton Rouge. Unpublished report.

USDA. 1990. USDA backgrounder. News Division, Office of Public Affairs Room 404-A, Washington, DC.

Worley, J.W., J.S. Cundiff, and D.H. Vaughan. 1991. Potential economic return from fiber residues produced as by-products of juice expression from sweet sorghum. Bioresource Technology (In press).

Worley, J.W. and J.S. Cundiff. 1991. System analysis of sweet sorghum harvest for ethanol production in the Piedmont. Trans. Amer. Soc. Agr. Eng. 34(2):539–547.

FIBER CROPS

Kenaf: an Emerging New Crop Industry

Charles S. Taylor

This report describes an on-going adventure with a new crop called kenaf, *Hibiscus cannabinus* L, a new annual fiber crop with a wide range of exciting product applications. This report will identify the numerous individuals and institutions that have been instrumental in bringing kenaf up to and across the threshold of commercialization. A brief review of the major events that have brought kenaf to this juncture will also be made. Finally, the emergence of commercial scale activities by both Kenaf International and Natural Fibers of Louisiana, Inc. will be discussed.

THE KENAF HALL OF FAME

Kenaf is now crossing the commercial threshold, and it is no longer necessary to recite the physical and chemical attributes that make kenaf an interesting source of natural fibers for a wide range of industrial applications. The attributes of kenaf have been extensively reviewed by Dempsey (1975). While a solid reservoir of technical information is critical to the successful introduction of a new crop industry such as kenaf, the best way to view such information is as a prerequisite. In other words, before initiating new crop development activities, research activities should have already determined the basic set of information necessary for decision makers to consider. Then, once the development of the new crop industry warrants a serious consideration of commercial potentials and options, much of the key information on product/process developments and market strategies will no longer be freely circulated in the public sector. So it is now with kenaf.

This will cause some concern in the future as it will become increasingly more difficult for those of us in the private sector to find much that can be discussed in public regarding kenaf. One aspect that remains is the human factor, the men and women and institutions that have searched for potential and nurtured it into being. Citing a list of contributors to the development and commercialization of a new crop industry like kenaf is risky business, as some will be overlooked and under recognized. Regardless, new crop developers should be well known for their risk-taking propensity.

Before 1977

The watershed event for kenaf in the United States was the successful conclusion of the USDA Search for New Pulp Fibers that culminated in the pressroom of the *Peoria Journal Star* on August 8, 1977. This work effort was initiated on a limited scale in the 1940s when government agencies became concerned about the need to replace imported jute supplies from the Far East due to market disruptions caused by the Japanese. Some of this early work took place in the lower Rio Grande Valley of South Texas under the supervision of W.R. Cowley of Texas A&M University.

The literature is fairly complete on those who contributed to the exploratory research activities of the 1940s and 1950s and the more applied research efforts that began in the late 1950s and continued through 1977. Dempsey's 1975 classic, Fiber Crops, offers a comprehensive narrative of the work that went on prior to the printing of the *Peoria Journal Star* on kenaf newsprint. Most of the key individuals were USDA staff members at both the National Program level and at the regional research centers, particularly the laboratory at Peoria, Illinois. Leadership was provided by Tom Clark and later by Marvin Bagby. Many others on the USDA utilization research team contributed significantly to this effort. Credit should be given here to the chemurgic movement, which gave rise to interest in industrial applications of agricultural based materials such as kenaf.

Agronomic studies were also conducted by both the USDA and land grant university personnel. During the 1960s and 1970s, work coordinated by USDA's George White involved yield trials ranging from the Pacific Northwest to Texas and Florida (White et al. 1971). Much of this work was based on research that had taken place in the Caribbean (primarily Cuba before Castro) and Central America. In addition to the late Jack Dempsey, individuals like Joseph Atchison and Edwin Sholton served as consultants on the new fiber crop's potential for the world's pulp and paper industry. These two were responsible for some of the early feasibility work that eventually led to the world's first kenaf pulp mill in Khon Kaen, Thailand. They, along with USDA personnel, were instrumental in getting the Technical Association of the Pulp and Paper Industry (TAPPI) to form a Non-Wood Pulp Fiber Committee. This committee then became the principal source of information about kenaf as a potential fiber source for the pulp and paper industry.

On the private side, most of the work focussed on harvesting and processing kenaf bast fibers for the twine and burlap industries. Various small companies were formed in Florida, Mexico, El Salvador, and Guatemala to compete with jute/kenaf fibers from the Far East. A company called North American Kenaf International, Inc. developed seed supplies and field decortication equipment in the early 1960s. However, by the early 1980s only a small bag operation in Guatemala called Productos de Kenaf, S.A. was still operating. These initial efforts caused the technology to be field tested in the western hemisphere and kenaf became well exposed to the United States agricultural research community. As documented in a TAPPI report (Atchison and Collins 1976), numerous pulp and paper companies around the world conducted their own investigations into kenaf during this time period.

Although key questions remained regarding the dependability of an industrial raw material supply based on an annual crop (primarily logistics, economics of scale, and need to develop and structure a harvesting—handling—storage—delivery system), kenaf benefitted greatly from the two-pronged approach used by USDA during the last decade of their early work on kenaf, i.e., the focus on both agronomic and industrial aspects. Of special note here is the remarkable breeding accomplishments of the USDA Kenaf Breeders led by F. Douglas Wilson, Charles Adamson, and Austin Campbell. Their work resulted in the release of the two Everglades varieties as well as several other promising lines.

After 1977

The 1977 printing of the *Peoria Journal Star* ironically represented the end of the USDA/land grant university work on kenaf. The basic technical feasibility of using kenaf in the manufacture of newsprint had been demonstrated, and national program priorities shifted, primarily to focus on "energy" crops. Except for the extra-curricular efforts of key individuals such as Bagby, Adamson, and the late Eli Whiteley (Texas A&M University), the USDA kenaf program would be dormant until late 1985.

However, to USDA's credit, sufficient work of significant quality had been done to encourage a more serious private sector look at kenaf by the North American Pulp and Paper Industry. Most businessmen appreciate that it is important to be prepared when "opportunity knocks." Whereas low wood and paper prices in the 1960–75 period had discouraged spending much time and funds, looking for alternatives, the economy had changed somewhat by the late 1970s. Donald N. Soldwedel, the publisher of the *Yuma Daily Sun* in Arizona, convinced his colleagues in the American Newspaper Publishers Association (ANPA) to support a series of studies, which followed up on the USDA work.

Industry support of the ANPA initiative came from the Newsprint Division of the International Paper Company, where Charles A. Thompson succeeded in getting CIP's Research Lab to refine the Thermo-mechanical pulping process (TMP) defined in the earlier USDA work. The late Walt Kammann of Yuma, Arizona grew about 100 acres (40 ha) of kenaf in 1978 and some of this fiber was used by International Paper (IP) in cooperation with what is now Andritz Sprout-Bauer, Inc. to conduct the first commercial machine trial with kenaf-based newsprint. The pulp was made at the Bauer pilot plant in Springfield, Ohio and made into newsprint at IP's mill in Pine Bluff, Arkansas. Six newspapers tested the kenaf newsprint with encouraging results. In 1981 a follow up trial took place at the IP mill in Mobile, Alabama. This time, eight newspapers tested the product successfully.

Meanwhile, two unrelated events were taking place. In Thailand, a financial consortium made the decision to proceed with the Phoenix Pulp & Paper Company's 200 ton/day kraft pulp mill that was initially based on whole-stalk kenaf. The mill initiated operations in late 1981, under the technical leadership of P.K. Paul. Back in the United States, Melvin G. Blase and Fred L. Mann committed the University of Missouri to a National Science Foundation-supported research effort looking for more efficient approaches to the introduction of new crops for American farmers. In 1979, this author became committed to the study of kenaf as a possible model for testing a "systems" approach for new crop introductions.

Sometimes the methodology of a dissertation takes on more lasting significance than the research itself. To gather the information necessary to assess the status of the embryonic kenaf system, the Soil and Land Use Technology, Inc./University of Missouri team adapted the Delphi Technique (Taylor and Whiteley 1981). This enabled them to rather quickly develop direct contacts with everyone from plant breeders to newsprint experts. The research effort after several months became essentially self-fulfilling as key members of the research team were contracted by the ANPA to study the general feasibility of using kenaf as a fiber source for the manufacture of newsprint in the United States. The study was the focus of the First International Kenaf Conference held 29 April 1982 in San Francisco, where more than 100 participants reviewed its conclusions (Taylor et al. 1982).

While the above study was still in progress, the research team was approached by *The Bakersfield Californian* (newspaper) and Agri-Future, Inc. (an agri-management company also from Bakersfield). The discussions resulted in the formation of Kenaf International, which next month will celebrate its first decade. This new kenaf champion immediately proceeded to attack some of the gaps remaining in the kenaf to newsprint system.

The first action preceded the formation of the joint venture company by a few months as the partners-to-be agreed that it was urgent to commence increasing the available kenaf seed supply. Contact was made with Eli Whiteley who had participated in the earlier studies and he, after consulting with his former professor, W.R. Cowley, recommended that Kenaf International contract with Andrew W. Scott, Jr. at the private research farm known as Rio Farms, Inc. in the Rio Grande Valley of Texas. Thus, began a relationship that has survived 10 long years and enabled Kenaf International to (1) develop over the next nine years an American based commercial seed inventory capable of meeting the needs of large scale kenaf projects and (2) eventually recognize that the lower Rio Grande Valley offered an ideal location for industries based on kenaf.

During the next four years, Kenaf International was disappointed when political forces caused International Paper to divest its newsprint division and interrupt its interest in developing kenaf. Other companies seemed only casually interested in kenaf, asking questions that called for extensive growing experience. Little funding could be found in the United States for the work required, and Kenaf International spent time in Thailand, Zimbabwe, Belize, the Dominican Republic, Pakistan, Italy, Trinidad, and Puerto Rico, developing the field based technologies necessary to support a kenaf-based pulp and paper project.

After conducting a third feasibility study in the Caribbean only to listen to the bankers complain about the small country's fiscal irresponsibility, Kenaf International was invited home in late 1985 to meet with then Deputy Secretary of Agriculture, John Norton, and discuss how the USDA could re-establish its work with kenaf. After a series of meetings and visits to American newsprint mills, Kenaf International and the USDA signed, in early 1986, a Cooperative Agreement that soon led to the Kenaf Demonstration Project, which has been well chronicled by Daniel E. Kugler (1988). Incidentally, these decisions also rescued young Daniel from the den of the Economic Research Service and gave us a tireless spokesperson for industrial crops who understands that cooperation between public agencies and private companies is a two-way street. Kenaf also recaptured some of Marvin Bagby's time. A couple years later, Frank X. Werber of the Agricultural Research Service added invaluable insight and experience to product development efforts with kenaf.

Our five years of seed production with Rio Farms led us to look at that area as a potential site for a kenaf based project. Rio Farms' Andy Scott suggested that we introduce ourselves to their Congressman Kika de la Garza who chairs the House Agriculture Committee. He and his excellent staff have been a source of constant support and encouragement. The USDA was particularly responsive in adding the services of Charles G. Cook to their experiment station in Weslaco, Texas.

The Kenaf Demonstration Project over the next five years proved to be an excellent example as to how a system-wide group of companies, agencies, and individuals could cooperate to develop and demonstrate the technologies necessary to launch a new crop industry. Not only did we succeed in demonstrating our ability to produce high quality newsprint from kenaf, covering each step from field to pressroom runs, but the initial work on separating kenaf fibers for a variety of other products was also initiated. Simply put, we grew kenaf in Texas, pulped it in Ohio, made it into newsprint in Quebec, and printed on it in California, Texas, and Florida. This made for some well traveled fiber. Special acknowledgements are due Andritz Sprout Bauer, Canadian Pacific Forest Products Limited, the Beloit Corporation, and Daniel Engineering. Key leadership was provided by Bauer's

Joseph A. Kurdin and William Bohn.

It is sometimes too easy to focus on the results as being the major accomplishments. To be sure, Kenaf International and the USDA as well as all of the other parties involved are justifiably proud of the kenaf newsprint that was made in July 1987. We're equally pleased with the auto parts and other natural fiber products that were made earlier this year. However, the principal successes were in the field. During the past four years, 12 farmers grew approximately 300 acres (125 ha) of kenaf. Surviving both hurricanes and drought, average harvestable yields were in the 6 to 8 dry tons/acre (13 to 17.5 t/ha) range. The leadership of Rio Farms was invaluable during this period.

When it came to harvesting the kenaf, we confronted a long learning curve. The literature suggested that we could use forage choppers and so we did. The program would have ended there in a field near Monte Alto, Texas had we not captured the interest (and sympathy) of Harold A. Willett, who had retired from several careers in the sugar industry and was looking for new challenges. Upon review, he reminded the team that we needed a harvesting system not harvesting equipment. We agreed and H. Willett & Associates, Inc. began work on developing the system and equipment necessary to harvest the 1988 crop. That August found key team members in the hospital and Hurricane Gilberto visited in September. In October, we ran our field tests. The unanimous opinion of the observers was that we had a proven harvesting system for kenaf. Since 1988, Kenaf International and Natural Fibers of Louisiana have harvested approximately 1,000 acres (400 ha) of kenaf in Texas and Louisiana.

As far as the newsprint project was concerned, the technology was ready. It now became the responsibility of engineers, bankers, and corporate attorneys. The Kenaf Paper Company was formed in 1989 and has essentially completed its project development phase. Meanwhile the focus of the USDA/Kenaf International cooperation shifted to an investigation of the possibility of achieving an acceptable mechanical separation of the kenaf bast and core fibers.

The kenaf stalk contains two distinct fibers, i.e., long, jute-like bast fibers in its bark and the short, balsawood-like core fibers. The bast fibers have been used traditionally in the manufacture and trade of cordage products such as burlap cloth, twine, and ropes. General Felt Industries, a major importer of jute/kenaf fibers, had followed the kenaf work since the late 1970s, and Kenaf International was aware of their interest and requirements. The pulp trials at Andritz Sprout Bauer required milling the whole-stalk fibers in order to get the material into the pulping system. The milling itself caused some natural separation and caused us to consider that it might be possible to claim specialized markets for natural fibers for United States farmers.

Follow up work over the next two years, led to a decision by the USDA and Kenaf International, that a pilot plant separation trial was warranted. Believing that it was logical to go to the cotton gin industry for the necessary technology, the Lummus Development Corporation was asked to conduct some lab tests with kenaf. The initial results were quite promising and plans were made to proceed with a pilot plant trial in the Rio Grande Valley. This approach proved to be too expensive in terms of capital and operating requirements, but more importantly it failed to produce a saleable product. We also learned the importance of fire prevention as we lost about 200 tons of stalks in less than 15 minutes one hot May afternoon in 1989.

The pilot trial's disappointing results led Kenaf International to explore other equipment options, and lab scale trials with European machinery kept hope alive that our objectives were possible, however, feasibility was a more elusive issue. Small scale and high horsepower were the major concerns. Meanwhile the worldwide search for processing equipment was helping us to identify a wider range of potential applications and markets for natural fiber products.

Chief among the latter was a call from Hunter Brooks who at that time headed up a task force at Cadillac Motor Car Company. He wanted some kenaf to use in the manufacture of car interior parts like headliners. This particular technology holds the potential of opening up very wide horizons for a natural fiber substitute for fiberglass in certain applications. This work has continued with Kirk Cunningham of the PresGlas Corporation. Similar possibilities began to develop for the core material, primarily as a poultry litter medium thanks to initial work by George Malone in Delaware with additional trials by Dale Hyatt at Texas A&M University. These and other opportunities were investigated and evaluated. However, without an effective and cost efficient process, such markets could not be accessed.

The scene shifts to Cajun Country in South Louisiana where Harold Willett has his headquarters. He and his crew had been directly involved in the 1989 separation trial and understood the limitations of the Lummus approach. Willett began tinkering with a much simpler process and has applied for a patent after running a pilot plant operation since January 1991. Kenaf has been grown in Louisiana since 1988 to assist in the testing of the harvesting equipment. Charles Lanie and other local farmers in New Iberia parish became interested in kenaf as a crop for their seed fallow cane acreage. They joined with Willett to form Natural Fibers of Louisiana, Inc. on August 28, 1990 to finance the further work necessary to establish a commercial fiber separation business.

Since the formation of Kenaf International, we have cooperated closely with others working on kenaf around the globe, particularly in Thailand with P.K. Paul of Phoenix Pulp and Paper Company and in Australia with I.M. Wood of CSIRO. These contacts have helped us assess the viability of various technologies that have been advanced from those areas and stay abreast of new developments. Kenaf International maintains close contacts with a growing number of American and overseas entities, particularly within the pulp and paper industry's research community. This helps us to stay abreast of new developments around the world. In cooperation with the USDA and local governments, Kenaf International introduced kenaf to Oklahoma in 1986 where it is presently being studied as a possible niche forage crop by Bill Phillips at USDA/ARS in El Reno, Oklahoma and Mike Dicks of Oklahoma State University.

Kenaf International was also the first to explore kenaf's potential in other states like Delaware, Mississippi, and California. While kenaf can be considered a prospective crop in those areas under certain conditions and some efforts are purportedly underway in each of those states, Kenaf International's initial doubts have not been adequately overcome.

KENAF COMMERCIALIZATION ACTIVITIES

Although Kenaf International initiated its seed increase operations in 1981, only in 1990 did its management decide that it was appropriate to commence commercial seed sales. Sales in 1991 are expected to show an increase over 1990 and projections call for steady but not spectacular growth in seed sales through the next few years or until a commercial project begins using kenaf on a significant scale. Sales to date are primarily domestic, but a significant portion is entering the international market. Kenaf International is dedicated to maintaining a commercial scale inventory of viable seed for the principal kenaf cultivars in a manner that will keep the cost of seed reasonable for farmers.

Reference has already been made to the successful efforts of Natural Fibers of Louisiana, Inc. to start up the first commercial kenaf fiber separation facility in the United States. Their pilot operation has enabled them to began supplying various users with small volumes for test marketing for the past 10 months, and the new commercial facility is scheduled to initiate operations in December 1991 with the harvest of approximately 650 acres (265 ha) of kenaf in South Louisiana. Their plans call for planting about 1,500 acres (612 ha) in 1992. It should be emphasized that these efforts in Louisiana, as well as those in Texas, have been *solely* supported by the private sector without any direct assistance from public institutions. Their capital costs are slightly under $1 million.

Similarly, Kenaf International is finalizing plans to proceed with its own fibers project in South Texas. The first phase will be initiated with the planting of approximately 200 acres (82 ha) in February 1992 with expansion scheduled later next fall. Local markets have been identified and most of the equipment is already in place. Once the expansion planned for late 1992 is complete and full capacity is attained (projected for 1995), the annual acreage requirements are projected to be 5,000 acres (2,040 ha) with a total capital investment will be about $2 million for harvesting and processing equipment, site, engineering, permits, and initial working capital.

Kenaf International's primary goal since its inception has been to develop kenaf as a commercially viable fiber for the pulp and paper industry. While good progress has been made, we have not yet realized this objective. Plans to build and operate a 85 t/day newsprint mill based on a combination of kenaf and recycled fibers in the Rio Grande Valley are on hold pending a restructuring of financing arrangements. About $4 million of the anticipated $50 million capital requirements has already been invested in acquiring site, permits, and key equipment as well as basic engineering. Farmers and engineers are ready to roll should the project be restructured and attain sufficient financing.

The proposed "K-Chico" Project's combination of annually renewable and recycled fibers has some unique economic and environmental implications. A "tree-free" paper that requires relatively minimal chemical inputs in either field or mill operations reduces both costs and environmental concerns. Energy consumption is 15 to 25% lower for kenaf than what is required to pulp southern pine using the TMP process and the treated wastewater can be used to irrigate nearby fiber crops. The USDA's Forest Products Lab and the ANPA deserve much of the credit for testing the concept of combining the two fibers. The future implications could become quite important as the use of kenaf and old newspapers in relatively tiny but profitable mill operations could eventually have a dramatic impact on the world's pulp and paper industry, which is what we've believed all along.

REFERENCES

Atchison, J.E. and T.T. Collins. 1976. Worldwide developments in kenaf. TAPPI Non-wood Pulp Fiber Committee Progress Report 7, p. 15–17. Atlanta, GA.

Dempsey, J.M. 1975. Fiber crops. Univ. of Florida Press, Gainesville, FL.

Kugler, D.E. 1988. Kenaf newsprint: realizing commercialization of a new crop after four decades of research and development. USDA Cooperative State Research Service, Washington, DC.

Taylor, C.S. and E.L. Whiteley. 1981. Kenaf, p. 22–72. In: E.G. Knox and A.A. Theisen (eds.). Feasibility of introducing new crops: production—marketing—consumption (PMC) systems. Rodale Press, Emmaus, PA.

Taylor, C.S., G.L. Laidig, R.S. Puls, and J.G. Udell. 1982. Kenaf newsprint system. American Newspaper Publishers Association, Reston, VA.

White, G.A., D.G. Cummins, E.L. Whiteley, W.T. Fike, J.K. Greig, J.A. Martin, G.B. Killinger, J.J. Higgins, and T.F. Clark. 1970. Cultural and harvesting methods for kenaf. USDA Production Research Report 113. Washington, DC.

Response of Kenaf to Multiple Cutting

Frank E. Robinson

Kenaf thrives in the desert area of El Centro, California (Robinson 1988). The high protein content of the leaves may offer promise as a forage crop, if the plant can survive multiple harvest as it does in Oklahoma (Phillips 1989). A project was initiated to examine the response of 11 kenaf cultivars to multiple cutting. Treatments consisted of: (1) a single cut in the fall on Oct. 24, 1990; (2) two cuts on July 2 and Nov. 9, 1990; and (3) three cuts July 2, Sept. 10, and Nov. 7, 1990.

METHODOLOGY

The plot area was 56 rows wide by 12 m long. The kenaf was field sown on Apr. 3, 1990 with two rows per 1 m bed and furrow irrigated. Soil was an Imperial clay; fertilization was 110 kg N/ha applied as urea preplant, and two sidedress applications of 55 kg N/ha. Superphosphate was applied preplant at 110 kg P/ha. Colorado river irrigation water contained 5 ppm K, so the 20 irrigation applications made during the 30 week crop period supplied approximately 101 kg K/ha. We left 3 m of each row uncut until final harvest. The remaining 9 m of each 4 row plot was cut two nodes above the soil surface (Phillips 1989) on July 2; of these 3 m were allowed to regrow until harvest. On Sept. 10, 6 m of the original 9 m of the plot were cut again and allowed to regrow until harvest. This produced 3 m cut once at the final harvest, 3 m cut twice i.e. on July 2 and at final harvest, and 6 m cut three times July 2, Sept. 10, and at final harvest. At each cutting, the diameter of the stems in the center 3 m of two rows in each cultivar were measured either at the ground surface or next to the main stem where side shoots originated. Stem heights and weight, leaf weight, and plant density were determined. Sub-samples were taken and oven dried at 65°C to calculate percent dry weight. A single 6 m strip of two rows on the border was cut at the soil surface to observe regeneration.

Table 1. Total kenaf dry matter yields with either one harvest on Oct. 24, total of two harvests on July 2 and Nov. 9, or total of three harvests on July 2, Sept. 10, and Nov. 7.

Cultivar	Stalk (t/ha) Harvests 1	2	3	Leaf (t/ha) Harvests 1	2	3	Leaf (%) Harvests 1	2	3	Total yield (t/ha) Harvests 1	2	3
CV-34Sp	22.1	18.3	12.4	2.6	4.3	5.0	13.7	19.2	28.9	25.0	22.6	17.4
Xiang	21.6	20.1	13.0	2.7	4.4	5.1	12.9	17.9	28.1	24.7	24.5	18.1
E-41	20.4	18.4	8.9	3.2	5.2	5.3	10.4	21.9	37.0	23.9	23.6	14.2
Tainung 1	19.7	16.7	8.8	3.0	5.2	4.5	13.0	23.6	33.8	23.1	21.9	13.3
45-9X	19.3	13.0	10.2	3.0	3.4	4.5	11.9	20.9	30.8	22.8	16.4	14.7
RS-10	18.9	16.4	10.2	2.8	4.8	5.0	13.3	22.5	33.0	21.9	21.2	15.1
CV-34	18.8	17.0	11.4	2.2	4.0	4.8	10.2	19.2	29.8	21.5	21.0	16.2
G-45	18.8	16.4	8.9	3.0	4.0	4.4	10.9	19.8	32.8	22.1	20.4	13.3
E-71	18.2	17.7	11.7	3.0	3.1	4.5	12.4	14.8	27.7	21.6	20.8	16.1
C-108	17.8	15.9	8.7	2.5	3.9	4.3	13.4	19.6	32.8	20.7	19.8	13.0
C-2032	17.0	16.1	9.2	2.7	4.9	5.3	13.2	23.3	36.5	20.2	21.0	14.6
Mean	19.3	16.9	10.3	2.9	4.3	4.8	12.3	20.3	31.9	22.5	21.2	15.1
SD	1.5	1.7	1.5	0.3	0.7	0.4	1.2	2.5	3.0	1.5	2.0	1.6

RESULTS

The stems cut for the first time had no side shoots and only 30% of the stalks cut at the soil surface regenerated. Those that grew after being cut two nodes above ground developed multiple side shoots. Cultivar means were 2.6±1.1 shoots for second cutting (10 Sept.) 2.3±0.9 shoots (Nov. 9), and 2.6±1.3 for a third harvest on Nov. 7.

The multiple cuts produced thinner stems. Shoot diameters were 9.9±4.2 mm and 8.4±6.8 mm for second cuts, 7.6±3.8 mm for the third cut as compared to 17.5±1.0 mm for the single cut at final harvest.

The height of the stalks was greatly reduced by multi-cutting. The treatment with the tallest stalks (3.1±0.2 m) was uncut until final harvest. The stalks cut on 2 July were 1.4±0.2 m with regrowth reaching 1.5±0.7 m by Nov. 9. The treatment with three cuts was 1.1±0.3 m on first regrowth and 0.4±0.2 m at the second regrowth at final harvest.

The cumulative result of the shorter, thinner, multiple stems on the cut treatments was a leafier harvest which should provide a more palatable forage. Total yield comparisons are shown in Table 1.

DISCUSSION

Our results indicate that kenaf grown for forage should be cut two nodes above ground, rather than at the soil surface as is alfalfa. The treatment with one intermediate cut before the final harvest produced the best forage with highest leaf percentage and thinnest stems. A 2.5 t loss in total stalk yield was accompanied by a 1.4 t increase in total leaf production increasing the percent leaf dry matter in the total harvest from 12 to 20%. A second intermediate cut in September caused a large 6 t reduction in total stalk yield while increasing the total leaf yield only 0.5 t as compared to the single intermediate cut. Moving the first and second cuts up to earlier dates may produce a higher total yield and should be explored.

REFERENCES

Phillips, W.A., S.C. Rao, and T.H. Dao. 1989. The nutritive value of immature whole plant kenaf and tops of mature kenaf for growing ruminants. First Annu. Conf. Assoc. Adv. Ind. Crops. Pub. 63.

Robinson, F.E. 1988. Kenaf: a new fiber crop for paper production. Calif. Agr. 42(5):31–32.

Kenaf in Irrigated Central Washington

David W. Evans and An H. Hang

Kenaf (*Hibiscus cannabinus* L., Malvaceae) is an annual crop with uses for fiber, forage and paper pulp (White et al. 1970; Husingi 1989). In the continental United States, kenaf has been most productive in the southern states, but it may also have potential in northern regions. We are investigating the plant development and yield of irrigated kenaf in central Washington State where an annual pulp crop could further broaden our agricultural diversity and reduce pressure on forest resources.

MATERIALS AND METHODS

Three cultivars of kenaf were tested on a preliminary basis in 1987 and four were tested in 1990 at WSU-Prosser. This site is 46° 15' N, 119° 45' W and 275 m above sea level. It averages 160 frost-free days and 0.19 m annual precipitation, mostly in the winter months. Kenaf was raised both years on a silt loam (coarse-silty, mixed, mesic, Xerollic Camborthids) fertilized and furrow irrigated as for maize (*Zea mays* L.) grain production. The crop was seeded in rows spaced 0.76 m apart at a target population of 25 thousand/ha. Both plantings were surrounded by maize. Stands were hand weeded.

In 1987, single, 6 m long, unreplicated plot rows of 'Everglades 41' ('EV41'), 'Everglades 71' ('EV71'), and 'Tainung 1' ('T1') were planted on 7 May. In 1990, 'EV41', 'EV71', 'T1', and 'Cuba 2032' ('C2032') were seeded on 11 May, in plots 6 rows wide by 20 m long using a randomized complete block design with 5 replications. Plant height was measured monthly in 1987; both height and leaf and stem weight (10 plant samples) were determined weekly from 23 July to 8 Oct. on 'EV41', 'EV71', and 'C2032' in 1990. Defoliated stem yield was determined on all entries from 3 m of each single row in 1987 and from 4.6 m of an interior row of each plot in 1990.

RESULTS

Monthly degree days (10°C base) as determined from air temperatures recorded 600 m from the plot area were warmer than average in May and June 1987, and in July–September 1990 (Table 1). Kenaf grew taller early in the season and reached a greater final height in 1987 than in 1990 (Fig. 1). Flowering began in mid-September both years which was too late to result in viable seed production.

Leaves made up a constantly decreasing fraction of total top weight over the period July 23–Oct. 8 in 1990 (Fig. 2). The leaf fraction in 1990 was described by the relationship $y = 35 - 3.67 + 0.014 x^2$ ($r^2 = 0.898$), where y = fraction of leaf in total top growth (g leaf/kg total top, dry matter basis) and x = days with July 23 = day 1. Prior to the final yield harvest both years, frost killed the leaves which dried and dropped from the plants, leaving bare stalks.

Yields of 'EV41' and 'T1' exceeded 22 Mg/ha in 1987 (Table 2). 'EV71' did not establish well and consequently yields were very low. In 1990, yields ranged between 11 and 14 Mg/ha with 'T1' yielding most, but differences were only significant at the 10% level. The upper ends of kenaf stems may be discarded when kenaf is harvested for fiber (Hays 1989). This stem tip material has potential as animal feed. At yield harvest in 1990, kenaf tops were separated by hand into the basal 6 m and all material above 6 m, and weighed separately. The basal 6 m ranged from 9.3 to 10.4 Mg/ha with no significant cultivar differences. The stem tips ranged between 2.0 ('C2032') and 2.6 ('T1') Mg/ha which was significant only at the 10% level.

DISCUSSION

A yield of 11 to 23 Mg/ha compares favorably with an average hybrid poplar yield of 23.6 Mg/ha per year over a four year period in Washington (Heilman and Stettler 1985). This kenaf yield, however, was obtained on single unreplicated rows and is likely to represent an upper extreme. Average yields of 11 to 14 Mg/ha, as found in 1990, appear more realistic and still approach those reported from some of the more southern growing areas [e.g. 13 to 21 Mg/ha for 1988 in Oklahoma as reported by Dag et al. (1989); 13.6 to 20.1 Mg/ha for 1986 in

Table 1. Monthly mean degree days (°C; 10°C base) at Prosser, Washington.

Month	Degree days		
	52-yr.	1987	1990
May	147	216	128
June	247	332	281
July	351	332	414
Aug.	328	352	366
Sept.	203	261	299
Oct.	28	74	33

Table 2. Kenaf stand and dry matter yield at Prosser, Washington.

Year	Cultivar	No. plant/ha (000)	Total top dry yield (Mg/ha)
1987	Everglades 41	254	23.1
	Everglades 71	56	6.3
	Tainung 1	185	22.3
1990	Everglades 41	144	11.4
	Everglades 71	198	12.4
	Tainung 1	205	14.0
	Cuba 2032	196	11.4
	LSD (5%)	28	---
	CV (%)	11.1	13.8

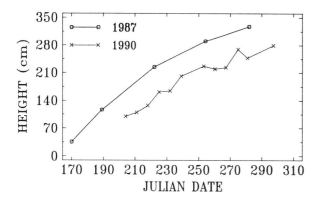

Fig. 1. Kenaf heights at Prosser, Washington; averages of 'EV41' and 'EV71'.

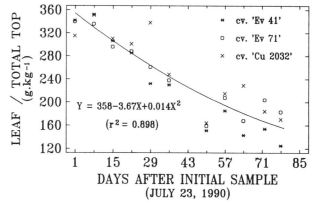

Fig. 2. Leaf fraction of Kenaf at Prosser, Washington in 1990; g dry leaf/kg total dry top.

California as reported by Robinson (1988)]. Based on the height and yield comparisons of 1987 and 1990, it appears that warm temperatures early in the growing season may have an important influence in establishing early growth and maximum performance. The economic prospect of kenaf as a viable central Washington crop, however, will require a stable production area, consistent high yields and the availability of a processing facility set up to handle the pulping requirements.

REFERENCES

Dao, T.H., W. Lonkerd, S. Rao, R. Meyer, and L. Pellack. 1989. Kenaf in a semi-arid environment? Its water requirement and forage quality in Oklahoma. Agron. Abstr. p. 130.

Hays, S.M. 1989. Kenaf tops equal high-quality hay. Agr. Res. 37(6):19.

Heilman, P.E. and R.F. Stettler. 1985. Genetic variation and productivity of *Populus trichocarpa* and its hybrids. II. Biomass production in a 4-year plantations. Can. J. For. Res. 15:384–388.

Husingi, G. 1989. Agricultural fibres for paper pulp. Outlook on Agr. 18(3):96–103.

Robinson, F.E. 1988. Kenaf: a new fiber crop for paper production. Calif. Agr. 42(5):31–32.

White, G.A., D.G. Cummins, E.L. Whitely, W.T. Fike, J.K. Greig, J.A. Martin, G.B. Killinger, J.J. Higgins, and T.F. Clark. 1970. Cultural and harvesting methods for Kenaf . . . an annual crop source of pulp in the southeast. Production Res. Rpt. 113, USDA/ARS. Washington, DC.

Utilization of Methanol Stress for Evaluating Kenaf Quality

Charles G. Cook and Andrew W. Scott, Jr.

Problems encountered in the establishment of uniform, vigorously growing kenaf (*Hibiscus cannabinus* L.) may result from poor seed quality. Although germination may remain relatively high, poor quality seeds often lack seedling vigor and are more susceptible to diseases and environmental stresses. Studies with soybeans (Mugnisjah and Nakamura 1986) and cottonseed (Hernandez 1987) show that methanol stress mimics the effects of weathering and accelerated aging, and may be a useful screening tool for evaluating seed quality and seedling performance. The objective of this study was to determine whether methanol stress could be used in the evaluation of kenaf seed to rapidly ascertain seed quality.

METHODOLOGY

Seed of five kenaf genotypes with similar seed production and weather exposure history were immersed in 20% methanol-water solutions for four selected durations (0, 1, 3, 5 h), and sown in the field. Genotypes included: 'Everglades 71' (E71), 'Tainung 1' (T1), 'Cuba 108' (C108), '15-2' (X15), and '19-117-2' (X117). The study was conducted at two Texas locations, Weslaco and Monte Alto. Experimental design was a randomized complete block, with four replications. Single row plots were 6.7 m in length and spaced 1.0 m apart. One hundred seed were planted with a cone planter in each plot and the number of emerged seedlings were counted on weekly basis for six weeks. Initial emergence and final stand establishment were determined at seven and 42 days after planting respectively. Post-emergence damping off was determined throughout the six week period and expressed as the percentage of dead emerged seedlings.

RESULTS

No significant genotype × location or treatment × location interaction was observed for initial emergence, final stand establishment, or post-emergence damping-off. Therefore, results presented here were combined over the two locations. Genotypes differed for initial emergence under the methanol treatments (Table 1). Emergence of E71 and T1 was greater than X117 under the control treatment. Differences also occurred among genotypes in the methanol treatments, with E71 consistently having the highest emergence. In the 3 and 5 h treatments, lower seedling emergence occurred for T1, X15, and X117, with X15 having the least emergence in the 5 h treatment.

Final stand establishment differed among genotypes across treatment durations. In the control treatment, final stand of E71 was significantly greater than X15 and X117. All genotypes produced greater stands than X117

Table 1. Effect of simulated aging by 20% methanol-water seed treatment on initial plant emergence and final stand of five kenaf genotypes[z].

Methanol treatment (h)	Emergence (%)[y]					Final stand (%)[y]				
	Genotype					Genotype				
	E71	T1	C108	X15	X117	E71	T1	C108	X15	X117
0	60.3a[x]	55.8a	52.3ab	49.5b	42.5b	53.3a	50.7ab	46.2abc	43.2bc	36.8c
1	57.5a	55.6ab	55.5ab	48.8b	39.0b	51.1a	48.9a	48.7a	45.5a	36.7b
3	52.0a	39.8b	47.8ab	41.2b	39.8b	45.1a	35.3b	42.0ab	36.1b	36.3b
5	44.2a	33.6b	35.4b	26.7c	34.3b	40.4a	30.5b	31.3b	24.8c	30.3b

[z]Initial plant emergence and final stand establishment were recorded at 7 and 42 days after planting, respectively, and expressed as % of total seed planted.
[y]Combined over the Weslaco and Monte Alto, TX locations.
[x]Means in a row followed by the same letter are not significantly different according to Duncan's multiple range test (P = 0.05). Data were arc sin transformed for statistical analysis, actual means presented.

Table 2. Initial plant emergence, final stand, and post-emergence damping-off of kenaf seed across five genotypes under 20% methanol-water treatments to simulate artificial aging.

Methanol treatment (h)	Emergence (%)	Final stand (%)	Damping-off (%)
0	52.1a[z]	46.0a	21.5a
1	51.3a	46.2a	22.2a
3	44.7b	39.0b	25.4b
5	34.8c	31.6c	23.9ab

[z]Means in a column followed by the same letter are not significantly different according to Duncan's multiple range test. (P = 0.05). Data were arc sin transformed for statistical analysis, actual means presented.

in the 1 h treatment. For the 5 h treatment, E71 had significantly greater stands than the other genotypes. In the 5 h treatment X15 produced the lowest final plant stands.

Initial emergence and final stand establishment differed significantly between treatments (Table 2). Compared to the control, seed and seedling performance were adversely affected in the 3 and 5 h treatments. Post-emergence damping-off in the 3 h treatment was observed to be significantly greater than in the untreated control and 1 h methanol treatments.

DISCUSSION

Genotypes differed significantly in seed quality. When the control and 5 h treatments were compared, stand reductions due to artificial aging were greatest for X15 (43.2 vs 24.8%) and T1 (50.7 vs 30.5%). Except for T1, emergence and final stand were not severely reduced until seeds were soaked with methanol for 3 h. Although X117 exhibited poorest seed quality in the untreated treatment, T1 and X15 showed the greatest deterioration when exposed to the longer methanol treatments. These results suggest that methanol stress may be used to artificially deteriorate kenaf seed for the evaluation of seed quality. Such a methanol stress test may possibly be utilized as a selection tool for genetically improving or for screening kenaf seed quality.

REFERENCES

Hernandez, V.H. 1987. Effects of cultivar, seed quality, pathogen virulence, inoculum density, and seed depth on host resistance to the seed-seedling disease complex of cotton. PhD diss. Texas A&M University, College Station.

Mugnisjah, W.Q. and S. Nakamura. 1986. Methanol and ethanol stress for seed vigour evaluation in soybean. Seed Sci. Technol. 14:95–103.

The Effects of Metolachlor and Trifluralin on Kenaf Yield Components

Charles L. Webber III*

While kenaf (*Hibiscus cannabinus* L.) shows great promise as a new source of fiber, commercialization depends on successful development of production systems. Researchers have reported that kenaf is a good competitor with weeds once the plants are of sufficient size to shade the ground (Burnside and Williams 1968; Orsenigo 1964), yet weeds can significantly reduce kenaf yields. Weed control therefore becomes an important consideration in obtaining optimum kenaf yields.

Williams (1966) reported that weed competition, with moderate weed pressure, reduced stalk yields during one season by an average of 1.0 t/ha. Weed competition in a three year Nebraska study significantly reduced yields by an average of 9.0 t/ha (69%) and reduced plant height and stalk diameter (Burnside and Williams 1968).

Presently, no herbicides are registered for kenaf in the United States. Literature examining the effects of preemergence herbicides on kenaf development and stalk yields is limited. Many herbicides originally evaluated for use in kenaf production are either no longer available, phytotoxic to kenaf, or reduce kenaf populations (Orsenigo 1964; Williams 1966; Burnside and Williams 1968). Two efficacious herbicides that have registration potential are trifluralin and metolachlor; trifluralin has been the standard herbicide used by kenaf researchers (White et al. 1970).

Burnside and Williams (1968) tested seven herbicides and found that kenaf was most tolerant to trifluralin, which also provided excellent weed control. However trifluralin, at 2.2 kg/ha, significantly reduced kenaf yields by 3.9 t/ha (25%) during the first year; although stalk heights and diameters were unaffected by the application of trifluralin. Orsenigo (1964) reported a 50% phytotoxicity and a 50% stand reduction when trifluralin was applied to kenaf at 6.7 kg/ha, but 100% tolerance and no stand reductions when applied at 2.2, 3.4, and 4.5 kg/ha. In south Texas, trifluralin, at 0.9 and 1.7 kg/ha, and metolachlor at 3.4 kg/ha provided excellent (90%) grass control while acceptable (80%) total weed control was obtained with metolachlor at 3.4 kg/ha (Hickman and Scott 1989). Trifluralin did reduced stalk yields at the rates tested. In Mississippi, metolachlor (3.0 kg/ha) gave no visual injury to the kenaf, although stalk yields may have been reduced (Kurtz and Neill 1990).

As the commercial production of kenaf in the United States grows closer, weed control strategies must be developed and the best herbicides identified and registered. The objective of this research was to determine the effects of metolachlor and trifluralin on kenaf plant development and stalk yields.

MATERIALS AND METHODS

A two-year field plot study was conducted at Lane, Oklahoma on a Bernow fine sandy loam, 0 to 3% slope, (fine-loamy, siliceous, thermic Glossic Paleudalf). Fertilizer was applied and incorporated prior to herbicide application at a rate of 168-72-139 kg/ha (N–P–K). Trifluralin [2,6-dinitro-N,N-dipropyl-4-(trifluoromethyl) benzenamine] and metolachlor [2-choro-N-(2-ethyl-6-methylphenyl)-N-(2-methoxy-1-methylethyl) acetamide] were applied at 0.56, 1.12, and 2.24 kg ai/ha using fan nozzles at 187 liters/ha. The trifluralin treatments were incorporated twice to a depth of 5 to 7.5 cm, with the second incorporation at 90° to the first. A combination secondary tillage tool with cultivator shovels, cutting blades, spike tooth harrow, and rolling baskets was used for the trifluralin incorporation and to prepare the seedbed for all treatments prior to planting. Metolachlor was applied after seedbed preparation and prior to planting. The experiments also included a weed-free (kept as such via handweeding) and weedy check treatments.

Plots were 3 m wide (four 76-cm rows), 6 m long, and were oriented in a east-west direction. Kenaf cultivar 'Tainung #1' was planted on June 22, 1989 and June 12, 1990. All plots were planting the same day as herbicide application.

---

*I am indebted to David A. Iverson, Research Technician, Agricultural Research Service, South Central Agricultural Research Laboratory, Lane, Oklahoma for field plot work, data entry and data analysis.

Crop injury ratings were collected at two and four weeks after planting using a 0 to 5 rating system; 0 represents no visual injury, 5 represents crop death. Grass and broadleaf weed control ratings were collected at four weeks after planting, using a 0 to 10 rating system; 0 represents no weed control, 10 represents 100% weed control. Kenaf plant populations, plant heights, and stalk data were collected at harvest. Kenaf plots were hand-harvested 18 weeks after planting on Oct. 23, 1989 and Oct. 17, 1990. A 2.25 m² (1.5 by 1.5 m) quadrant was harvested from the center of the second and third row of each plot. Plant counts from the harvest quadrant were used to determine plant populations. The harvested plants were cut at ground level and fresh weights determined. Three plants were randomly selected from the harvested material for plant height. Leaves, flowers and flower buds were removed from the stalks and weighed separately before and after samples were oven dried at 66°C for 48 h. The fresh and oven dry weights of the three plants were used to determine the percent moisture of the plants and the percent stalks by weight. The percent plant moisture and percent stalks were used to convert the fresh weight of the 2.25 m² quadrant sample to dry weight of stalks. Stalk yields are based on oven dry weights.

In both years, the experiments were randomized complete block designs with four replications. Crop injury and weed control data were converted to percentages and transformed using an arcsin transformation before analysis (Snedecor and Cochran 1967).

Rainfall during the growing season, from planting to harvest, was 6.1 cm below and 9.2 cm above the 20-year average rainfall for 1989 and 1990 respectively.

RESULTS

Plant Injury and Weed Control

No visual crop injury was observed during 1989 or 1990 as a result of the herbicides applied at the given rates (data not shown). The only year by treatment interaction detected was reflected in the degree of grass weed control, which was less in 1990 by metolachlor (Table 1). Metolachlor at 0.56 kg/ha, in 1990, was the only herbicide treatment in either year that had less grass weed control than any other herbicide treatment (Table 1). Broadleaf weed control data showed no differences in weed control (Table 1).

The primary weeds present during both years were large crabgrass [*Digitaria sanguinalis* (L.) Scop.] and tumble pigweed (*Amaranthus albus* L.). Both these weed species were present at moderate populations.

Table 1. Influence of herbicide application on the percentage of grass and broadleaf weed control in 1989 and 1990.

Herbicide treatment	Rate (kg/ha)	Weed control (%)			
		Grass		Broadleaf	
		1989	1990	1989	1990
Trifluralin	0.56	98a[z]	93b	99a	99a
	1.12	99a	95b	98a	99a
	2.24	100a	96b	100a	100a
Metolachlor	0.56	99a	70c	99a	98a
	1.12	99a	91b	100a	97a
	2.24	100a	96b	100a	100a
Weedy Check	---	0b	0d	0b	0b
Weed-Free	---	100a	100a	100a	100a

[z]Means within each column followed by the same letters are not significantly different at the 0.05 level using LSD.

Plant Populations

Except for metolachlor at 0.56 kg/ha and trifluralin at 1.12 kg/ha all herbicide treatments reduced plant populations compared to the weed-free plots (Table 2). No kenaf population differences were detected between the herbicide treatments or between the herbicide treatments and the weedy check plots (Table 2). No weed control by year interactions were detected for plant populations, plant heights, or stalk yields as a result of the combined analysis of the eight weed control treatments and the two years. Populations, when combined over weed control treatments, were greater in 1990 than those in 1989 (Table 2). The differences in populations were attributed to less than ideal planting conditions and less rainfall in 1989 compared to 1990.

Plant Heights

Plant heights were greater in 1990 (311 cm) than in 1989 (176 cm) when combined over all weed control treatments (Table 2). Increased height in 1990 may in part be from an earlier planting date (10 days) and 15.3 cm greater seasonal rainfall. No differences in plant height were detected between herbicide rates within either trifluralin or metolachlor (Table 2).

Stalk Yields

Stalk yields were greater in 1990 (21.3 t/ha) than 1989 (5.2 t/ha) (Table 2). An earlier planting date in 1990 (10 days) and greater seasonal rainfall contributed to greater stalk yields. No differences in stalk yields were detected between any of the weed control treatments indicating that rates of trifluralin and metolachlor which decrease plant populations and plant height did not significantly reduce stalk yields (Table 2).

CONCLUSIONS

Trifluralin and metolachlor provided excellent (>90%) weed control of moderate weed populations. The herbicides did not induce visual injury or reductions in stalk yields, though plant populations were adversely affected. The moderate weed populations did not reduce stalk yields, but weed interference did reduce kenaf heights and populations. Trifluralin and metolachlor are promising for use in kenaf production. The probability of expanding the registration label of these herbicides to include use in kenaf remains a serious problem to overcome.

Table 2. Influence of trifluralin and metolachlor on kenaf stand establishment, heights, and stalk yields for 1989 and 1990.

Herbicide treatment	Rate (kg/ha)	Plant pop. ($\times 10^3$/ha)	Plant heights (cm)	Stalk yields (t/ha)
Trifluralin	0.56	116	245	13.6
	1.12	137	240	13.7
	2.24	115	235	13.2
Metolachlor	0.56	134	251	13.6
	1.12	117	248	13.1
	2.24	117	253	13.5
Weedy Check	---	124	232	12.2
Weed-Free	---	154	247	13.3
LSD (0.05)		26	12	NS
Across all herbicide treatments				
1989		107	176	5.2
1990		147	311	21.3
LSD (0.05)		13	6	1.0

REFERENCES

Burnside, O.C. and J.H. Williams. 1968. Weed control methods for kinkaoil, kenaf, and sunn crotalaria. Agron. J. 60:162–164.

Hickman, M.V. and A.W. Scott. 1989. Preemergence herbicides for kenaf production. Proc. Assoc. Adv. Indust. Crops. (Abstr.)

Kurtz, M.E. and S.W. Neill. 1990. Possible herbicides for use in kenaf. Proc. Second Annu. Int. Kenaf Assoc. Conf. (Abstr.)

Orsenigo, J.R. 1964. Weed Control in kenaf. Proc. Int. Kenaf Conf. 2:177–187.

Snedecor, G.W. and W.G. Cochran. 1967. Statistical methods. 6th ed. Iowa State University Press, Ames.

White, G.A., D.G. Cummins, E.L. Whiteley, W.T. Fike, J.K. Greig, J.A. Martin, G.B. Killinger, J.J. Higgins, and T.F. Clark. 1970. Cultural and harvesting methods for kenaf. USDA Prod. Res. Rpt. 113.

Williams, J.H. 1966. Influence of row spacing and nitrogen levels on dry matter yields of kenaf (*Hibiscus cannabinus* L.). Agron. J. 58:166–168.

Kenaf: Production, Harvesting, Processing, and Products

Charles L. Webber III and Robert E. Bledsoe*

Kenaf (*Hibiscus cannabinus* L., Malvaceae) is a warm season annual closely related to cotton (*Gossypium hirsutum* L.) and okra (*Abelmoschus esculentus* L.). Initial interest in kenaf in the United States was as a domestic supply of cordage fiber as a jute substitute in the manufacture of rope, twine, carpet backing, and burlap (Wilson et al. 1965). Later, kenaf was identified as a very promising fiber source for production of paper pulp (Nieschlag et al. 1960; White et al. 1970). Researchers have processed kenaf fibers into both newsprint and bond paper (Bagby et al. 1979; Clark et al. 1971). Agricultural research starting in the early 1940s focused on the development of harvesting machinery, high yielding anthracnose resistant cultivars, and cultural practices for kenaf as a cordage crop (Nieschlag et al. 1960; White et al. 1970; Wilson et al. 1965).

In addition to the use of kenaf for paper pulp and cordage, researchers have investigated its use as an animal feed (Killinger 1967; Phillips et al. 1989, 1990; Webber 1990b), a poultry litter (Tilmon et al. 1988), and as a bulking agent for sewage sludge (Webber 1990a). Additional products that could possible use kenaf as a raw material include automobile dashboards, carpet padding, corrugated medium (Kugler 1988) and as a "substitute for fiberglass and other synthetic fibers" (Scott and Taylor 1988).

The United States acceptance of kenaf as a commercial crop would be strengthened if additional uses for kenaf can be established in the United States. These and other possible kenaf uses need to be further investigated to increase the potential use of kenaf plant products in the United States and therefore encourage the commercial establishment of the kenaf industry.

LADONIA MARKET CENTER

Demonstration Projects

Starting in 1988, the Ladonia Market Center, Ladonia, Texas, has conducted kenaf research, development, and demonstration work. In addition to expanding the list of possible uses of kenaf fibers, the Ladonia Market Center is a primary proponent of kenaf as a livestock feed. Kenaf demonstration projects have included kenaf production, harvesting, processing, and product evaluations.

---

*We acknowledge David A. Iverson, Research Technician, Agricultural Research Service, South Central Agricultural Research Laboratory, Lane, Oklahoma for field plot work, data entry, and data analysis; Vee Hiltbrunner-Bledsoe, Leon Hurse, and Foy Burns for their constant encouragement and support.

Production

Fiber and Forage. In addition to cooperative research with the USDA evaluating kenaf cultivars and their protein content, the Ladonia Market Center was involved in a demonstration project evaluating the effect of row spacings on kenaf dry matter yields. Production size (10 ha) kenaf plantings produced 10.3 t/ha on 25-cm row spacings and 14.0 t/ha on 76-cm row spacings when harvested at 97 days after planting as a forage crop.

Seed. Ladonia Market Center has also demonstrated the feasibility of producing seed from photo-insensitive kenaf cultivars in northern Texas. Typically, photosensitive kenaf cultivars are preferred for use in the production of kenaf fiber in the United States. Two of these cultivars, 'Everglades 41' and 'Everglades 71', were developed by USDA researchers (Wilson et al. 1965) to extend the growing season of kenaf plant before the plants initiate flowering. These photosensitive cultivars initiate flowering when daylengths decrease to approximately 12.5 h, mid-September in southern states (Scott 1982). In photosensitive cultivars, the initiation of flowering results in plant growth reductions (Dryer 1967). Because of late floral initiation and inability to produce mature seed prior to a killing frost, seed production in the United States for these cultivars is limited to southern Florida, the Lower Rio Grande Valley of Texas, and southernmost Arizona and California (Scott 1982).

Unlike photosensitive cultivars, photo-insensitve cultivars (i.e. Guatemala series) can initiate flowering and produce mature seed before a killing frost (Dempsey 1975). Photo-insensitive cultivars such as 'Guatemala 4', 'Guatemala 45', 'Guatemala 48', 'Guatemala 51', 'Cuba 2032' can initiate flowering after 100 days and prior to a decrease daylength of 12.5 h (Dryer 1967; Dempsey 1975). Photo-insensitive plants can, therefore, be planted during May or early June and still have ample time to produce mature seed. The earlier production of mature seed for photo-insensitive cultivars greatly expands the potential seed production areas. After floral initiation, photo-insensitive cultivars continue to grow without as much reduction in growth rate as with photosensitive cultivars (Dryer 1967; Webber 1990b). As a livestock feed, kenaf is often harvested at an earlier stage of growth than as a fiber crop, 60 to 90 days after planting (DAP) compared with 120 to 150 DAP (Webber 1990b). A shorter growing season for kenaf as a livestock feed enables a producer to use kenaf cultivars of the photo-insensitive group to produce equivalent dry matter productions as with photosensitive cultivars while using seed that can be produced further north and in a larger geographic area (Webber 1990b). Seed production of photo-insensitive cultivars in more northern areas is often overlooked as a result of the demand for and production of photosensitive cultivar seed which cannot be typically produce outside a few selected southern locations (Scott 1982).

Harvesting

The evaluation of field equipment for use with kenaf continues to be an important aspect in commercializing kenaf. Standard cutting, chopping, and baling equipment can be used for harvesting kenaf as a forage and fiber crop. Kenaf was baled into both small square and large round bales. It is an economic advantage to use presently available commercial harvesting equipment if possible rather than investing in the development and production of kenaf specific equipment. Appropriate harvesting equipment is readily available throughout the United States, and the on-farm cost can be distributed over that of other crops produced on the farm.

Processing and Product Development

Research demonstrated the feasibility of pelletizing kenaf as a fiber and forage crop. Pelletizing kenaf increases the density of the kenaf plant material, reducing both transportation and storage costs. Kenaf stalks and whole plants (stalks and leaves) were pelletized with standard commercial equipment in widespread use for existing livestock feeds. Kenaf stalks with an initial density of 0.31 g/cm^3 were transformed into pellets with a 13.2 mm diameter and a density of 1.21 g/cm^3, a 390% increase in density. Whole plant kenaf, produced as a livestock feed, was pelletized into pellets with a 10.4 mm diameter and a density of 1.22 g/cm^3, a 395% increase in density. The pelletizing research is an important element in moving the harvested kenaf crop from the field to a packaged kenaf product.

In addition to processing and product development work with kenaf as a livestock feed, Ladonia Market Center developed kenaf particle boards (K-Board) of various densities, thicknesses, and fire and insect resistances. Kenaf fibers were also successfully used in product development evaluations with extraction molded plastics.

FORAGE EVALUATION

Kenaf was recognized as having high protein levels and therefore might be a potential livestock feed (Killinger 1964). Crude leaf protein levels in kenaf range from 18 to 30% (Cahilly 1967; Killinger 1967; Killinger 1969; Suriyajantratong et al. 1973; Swingle et al. 1978) stalk crude protein levels from 5.8 to 12.1% (Phillips et al. 1989; Swingle et al. 1978) and whole plant crude protein levels from 11 to 25% (Clark and Wolff 1969; Killinger 1965; Phillips et al. 1989; Powell and Wing 1967; Swingle et al. 1978).

Cahilly (1967) reported that the amino acid composition of kenaf was similar to that of alfalfa (*Medicago sativa* L.). Kenaf can be ensilaged effectively, and as such has satisfactory digestibility, and an outstanding amount of digestible protein (Wing 1967). Digestibility of dry matter and crude proteins for kenaf feeds have ranged from 53.5 to 82.4%, and 59 to 70.6% respectively (Phillips et al. 1989; Powell and Wing 1967; Suriyajantratong et al. 1973; Swingle et al. 1978; Wing 1967). Kenaf meal, used as a supplement in a rice ration for sheep, compared favorably with a ration containing alfalfa meal (Suriyajantratong et al. 1973). Clark and Wolff (1969) determined that crude protein content of kenaf decreased from 90 to 244 DAP. Powell and Wing (1967) and Hurse and Bledsoe (1989) have reported whole plant kenaf yields of 13.4 and 13.9 t/ha respectively at approximately 98 DAP. The objective of the forage evaluation research was to determine the effect of cultivars and harvest date on plant growth, protein content, and kenaf dry matter yields.

Materials and Methods

In 1989, and 1990, a research study was conducted at Ladonia, Texas (Lat. 33°, Long. 96°) which included six kenaf cultivars and three harvest dates. The six kenaf cultivars evaluated were 'Guatemala 4', 'Guatemala 45', 'Guatemala 48', 'Guatemala 51', 'Cuba 2032', and 'Everglades 41'. Each cultivar was harvested at 76, and 99 DAP to evaluate kenaf as a livestock feed. A full season harvest sample was also collected at 184 DAP (27 Oct. 1989) and 154 DAP (25 Oct. 1990) to comparatively evaluate the cultivars as a source of fiber. The experiments were planted on 26 Apr. 1989 and 24 May 1990. Plots were 3 by 6 m with 50 cm row spacing. A 2.25 m^2 (1.5 by 1.5 m) quadrant was harvested from the center three rows of each plot. The plants in the entire quadrant were harvested at ground level and weighed to determine the fresh weight of plants per hectare. Three plants from this area were measured for plant height, and vegetative growth stage (V-Stage). The kenaf vegetative growth stage was determined by adapting the soybean [*Glycine max* (L.) Merrill] index system developed by Fehr et al. (1971) to kenaf. The index system counts the number on vegetative nodules on the primary plant stalk. Leaves and reproductive parts (flowers and flower buds) were removed and stalks cut into 20 cm lengths. Leaves, reproductive parts, and stalks were weighed before and after being oven dried at 66°C for 48 h. Total dry matter, stalk yields, percent leaves, and percent stalks were based on oven dry weights. Leaf, and stalk samples from harvest dates 76, and 99 DAP were ground using a Wiley mill with a #10 mesh screen and then reground using a #20 mesh screen. The Texas A&M analytical laboratory at College Station, Texas analyzed the ground kenaf leaf and stalk samples for crude protein (Techcon Method 334-74-W/B).

The studies were randomized complete block designs with four replications and mean differences were determined using a least significant difference (LSD) test level of 0.05 as described by Snedecor and Cochran (1967).

Results and Discussion

'Guatemala 4' was shorter than all other cultivars except 'Everglades 41' (Table 1). Vegetative development was greater for 'Guatemala 45' than either 'Guatemala 4' and 'Cuba 2032' (Table 1). Cultivars and harvest dates affected the percentage of kenaf leaves (Table 1). 'Guatemala 45' with 31% leaves was significantly greater than either Guatemala 48 or Everglades 41 (Table 1). Other researchers have also reported significantly less leaf percentages for 'Everglades 41' compare to other cultivars (Wilson et al. 1965; Webber 1990b). Percent leaves decreased 36% for the first harvest to 20% for the third harvest (Table 1). As kenaf plants increase in height and maturity, the lower leaves senesce, resulting in a decreased percentage of leaves (Webber 1990b; Clark and Wolff 1969).

Kenaf cultivars did not affect the percent crude protein in the leaves or stalks (Table 2). Percent whole plant crude protein was the only crude protein percentage which resulted in differences between cultivars (Table 2).

Table 1. Two year means of yield components of kenaf as influenced by cultivars and harvest dates.

Variable	Height (cm)	V-Stage (no.)	Leaves (%)	Total dry matter (kg/ha)
Cultivar[z]				
Everglades 41	180	54.4	27	9160
Cuba 2032	185	50.8	28	9195
Guatemala 4	171	50.7	29	7883
Guatemala 45	183	56.1	31	7713
Guatemala 48	187	54.9	28	9345
Guatemala 51	185	52.8	30	8831
LSD[y] (0.05)	10	4	3	1269
Harvest date[x]				
76 DAP	123	32.7	36	4764
99 DAP	171	48.7	30	7512
169 DAP	252	78.4	20	13788
LSD[w] (0.05)	7	3	2	898

[z]Cultivar means averaged over three harvest dates.
[y]LSD for comparison between cultivars.
[x]Harvest means averaged over six cultivars.
[w]LSD for comparison between harvest dates.

Table 2. Two year means of crude protein percentages and whole plant protein yields as influenced by cultivars and harvest dates.

	Crude protein			
Variable	Leaves (%)	Stalks (%)	Whole plant (%)	Whole plant (kg/ha)
Cultivar[z]				
Everglades 41	15.2	3.0	6.9	436
Cuba 2032	14.5	2.6	6.2	435
Guatemala 4	14.4	2.6	6.6	325
Guatemala 45	14.9	2.9	7.2	369
Guatemala 48	15.5	2.8	7.2	558
Guatemala 51	14.9	2.8	6.7	395
LSD[y] (0.05)	NS	NS	0.9	116
Harvest date[x]				
76 DAP	15.6	3.2	7.7	390
99 DAP	14.2	2.4	5.9	449
LSD[w] (0.05)	0.7	0.3	0.5	NS

[z]Cultivar means averaged over two harvest dates (76 and 99 DAP).
[y]LSD for comparison between cultivars.
[x]Harvest means averaged over six cultivars.
[w]LSD for comparison between harvest dates.

'Guatemala 48' had significantly greater percent whole plant crude protein than 'Cuba 2032' (Table 2). Crude protein for leaves, stalks, and whole plants were adversely affected by harvest date and decreased from 76 DAP to 99 DAP (Table 2).

'Guatemala 48', 'Everglades 41', and 'Cuba 2032' had significantly greater whole plant yields than either 'Guatemala 4' or 'Guatemala 45' (Table 2). The combination of high whole plant protein and whole plant yields for Guatemala 48 resulted in this cultivar yielding the greatest total crude protein produced per ha (Table 2).

The selection of a harvest date and kenaf cultivar are important variables in producing maximum protein and dry matter yields. 'Guatemala 48' percent whole plant protein was greater than 'Cuba 2032' and greater than all other cultivars in its production of crude protein production per ha (Table 2). An early harvest date (76 DAP) produced the greatest percentage leaf, stalk, and whole plant protein (Table 2). Kenaf can produce a large amount of dry matter, 7,512 kg/ha, within 90 DAP (Table 1). Results suggest that kenaf should continue to be studied, not only as a fiber crop for the production of paper pulp, but as a viable source for livestock feed. Future research should focus on differences in percent crude protein between cultivars, and maximizing total protein production per ha.

SUMMARY

The possible acceptance of kenaf as a commercial crop within the United States is increased as additional production, harvesting, processing, and product development evaluations are conducted. The establishment of small diversified uses for kenaf may offer certain advantages over the large capital investment in a single large kenaf paper or newsprint mill. The increased production, processing, and product development work being conducted within private industry is encouraging and suggests a bright future for the establishment of kenaf as a commercial crop within the United States.

REFERENCES

Bayby, M.O., R.L. Cunningham, F.G. Touzinsky, G.E. Hamerstrand, E.L. Curtis, and B.T. Hofreiter. 1979. Kenaf thermomechanical pulp in newsprint. TAPPI/NPFP Committee Progr. Rpt 10. Atlanta, GA.

Cahilly, G.M. 1967. Potential value of kenaf tops as a livestock feedstuff. Proc. First Conf. Kenaf For Pulp. Gainesville, FL. p. 48. (abstr.)

Clark, T.F., R.L. Cunningham, and I.A. Wolff. 1971. A search for new fiber crops. TAPPI 54:63–65.

Clark, T.F. and I.A. Wolff. 1969. A search for new fiber crops, XI. Compositional characteristics of Illinois kenaf at several population densities and maturities. TAPPI 52:2606–2116.

Dempsey, J.M. 1975. Fiber crops. The Univ. Presses of Florida, Gainesville.

Dryer, J.F. 1967. Kenaf seed varieties, p. 44–46. Proc. First Conf. Kenaf for Pulp. Gainesville, FL.

Fehr, W.R., C.E. Caviness, D.T. Burmood, and J.S. Pennington. 1971. Stage of development descriptions for soybeans (*Glycine max* L. Merrill). Crop Sci. 11:929–931.

Hurse, L. and R.E. Bledsoe. 1989. Kenaf grown as a forage crop in Northeast Texas. Proc. Assoc. Advancement of Industrial Crops. Peoria, IL. p. 13. (Abstr.)

Killinger, G.B. 1964. Kenaf, a potential paper-pulp crop for Florida. Second Int. Kenaf Conf. Palm Beach, FL. p. 54–57.

Killinger, G.B. 1965. Kenaf, *Hibiscus cannabinus* L. and *Erucastrum abyssinica* as potential industrial crops for the south. Proc. Assoc. Agr. So. Workers. Dallas, TX. p. 54–55.

Killinger, G.B. 1967. Potential uses of kenaf (*Hibiscus cannabinus* L.). Fla. Soil Crop Sci. Soc. Proc. 27:4–11.

Killinger, G.B. 1969. Kenaf (*Hibiscus cannabinus* L.), a multi-use crop. Agron. J. 61:734–736.

Kugler, D.E. 1988. Non-wood fiber crops: Commercialization of kenaf for newsprint, p. 289–292. In: J. Janick and J.E. Simon (eds.). Advances in new crops. Timber Press, Portland, OR.

Nieschlag, H.J., G.H. Nelson, I.A. Wolff, and R.E. Perdue, Jr. 1960. A search for new fiber crops. TAPPI 43:193–201.

Phillips, W.A., S. Rao, and T. Dao. 1989. Nutritive value of immature whole plant kenaf and mature kenaf tops for growing ruminants. Proc. Assoc. Advancement of Industrial Crops. Peoria, IL. p. 17–22.

Phillips, W.A., S.C. Rao, and T.H. Dao. 1990. Kenaf production with sewage sludge and fertilizer. Proc. Sec.

Annu. Int. Kenaf Assoc. Conf. Tulsa, OK. p. 9. (Abstr.)

Powell, G.W. and J.M. Wing. 1967. Kenaf as silage. Proc. First Conf. Kenaf for Pulp. Gainesville, FL. p. 49. (abstr.)

Scott, A. 1982. Kenaf seed production: 1981–82. Rio Farms, Inc. Biennial Rpt. 1980–1981. Monte Alto, TX. p. 60–63.

Scott, A.W. Jr. and C.S. Taylor. 1988. Economics of kenaf production in the lower Rio Grande Valley of Texas, p. 292–297. In: J. Janick and J.E. Simon (eds.). Advances in new crops. Timber Press, Portland, OR.

Snedecor, G.W. and W.G. Cochran. 1967. Statistical methods. 6th ed. Iowa State Univ. Press, Ames.

Suriyajantratong, W., R.E. Tucker, R.E. Sigafus, and G.E. Mitchell, Jr. 1973. Kenaf and rice straw for sheep. J. Anim. Sci. 37:1251–1254.

Swingle, R.S., A.R. Urias, J.C. Doyle, and R.L. Voigt. 1978. Chemical composition of kenaf forage and its digestibility by lambs and in vitro. J. Anim. Sci. 46:1346–1350.

Tilmon, H.D., R. Taylor, and G. Malone. 1988. Kenaf: an alternative crop for Delaware, p. 301–302. In: J. Janick and J.E. Simon (eds.). Advances in new crops. Timber Press, Portland, OR.

Webber, C.L. III. 1990. Kenaf production with sewage sludge and fertilizer. Proc. Second Annu. Int. Kenaf Assoc. Conf. Tulsa, OK. p. 15. (abstr.)

Webber, C.L. III. 1990. Kenaf protein and harvest dates. Proc. First Annu. Int. Conf. New Industrial Crops and Products. Riverside, CA. p. 19. (abstr.)

White, G.A., D.G. Cummins, E.L. Whiteley, W.T. Fike, J.K. Greig, J.A. Martin, G.B. Killinger, J.J. Higgins, and T.F. Clark. 1970. Cultural and harvesting methods for kenaf. USDA Prod. Res. Rpt 113. Washington, DC.

Wilson, F.D., T.E. Summers, J.F. Joyner, D.W. Fishler, and C.C. Seale. 1965. 'Everglades 41' and 'Everglades 71', two new varieties of kenaf (*Hibiscus cannabinus* L.) for the fiber and seed. Florida Agr. Expt. Sta. Cir. S-168.

Wing, J.M. 1967. Ensilability, acceptability and digestibility of kenaf. Feedstuffs 39:26.

The Milkweed Business

Herbert D. Knudsen and Richard D. Zeller

John Conrad from the staff of the House Agriculture Committee provided an important guideline for the development of new crops (Conrad 1992): "Congress is looking for tangible useful results from the funds expended to develop new opportunities." Natural Fibers Corporation of Ogallala, Nebraska is working diligently to achieve "tangible useful results" through its efforts to commercialize milkweed. Our goal is to create a major new agricultural industry based on milkweed.

Choosing milkweed to develop causes problems right from the start. Almost every farmer in our area has a ditch with a wonderful stand of healthy milkweed, whereas many of our cultivated fields look sick and full of disease. People wonder why we cannot grow it as well as it grows in the wild, and I envy those of you working on crops without the disadvantage of this close comparison.

Trials and tribulations abound for companies in new crops. The most recent setback for our Company occurred when a major loan application to finance our business was rejected. Nonetheless, you have to move forward. Like Satchael Paige said, "you can glance back, but you shouldn't stare." We feel you must move on rather than concentrate on the past. In this paper, I present an overview of how we analyzed and organized the milkweed opportunity as a start-up, and what we did to achieve the early tangible useful results with our Ogallala Down comforters and pillows.

BACKGROUND

From a historical perspective, milkweed pods were gathered from the wild, and the floss was extracted and used as fill for life jackets during World War II. After the War, these efforts were abandoned. Standard Oil of Ohio became involved with milkweed in the late 1970s. Nobel Laureate, Melvin Calvin, and others projected that billions of barrels of synthetic crude oil could be recovered from the biomass of milkweed. A research program in cooperation with Native Plants, Inc. was started to produce a synthetic crude oil from milkweed biomass. Milkweed was grown like hay—it was cut, dried, and baled. The dried biomass was then subjected to a hexane extraction and a few chemical processes to produce a crude oil substitute. The unfortunate conclusion from these studies was that the price was too high and the yield was too low. Economically, it was totally unfeasible.

This is where I entered the milkweed picture in the mid-1980s. As Manager of Corporate Ventures for Standard Oil, I was in charge of starting up new businesses and was asked to take a look at the milkweed opportunity. During the process, I made contact with William G. Wilson of Kimberly-Clark in Neenah, Wisconsin, who was looking for someone who knew how to grow milkweed. At that time, we had about five years' experience growing milkweed in research plots and there seemed to be a good fit between our interests. Arrangements were made for Kimberly-Clark to handle product development and for Standard Oil to handle growing milkweed.

When British Petroleum took over Standard Oil, they were not interested in promoting diversification efforts. In 1987, I acquired the milkweed venture and founded Natural Fibers Corporation with the dream of creating a new agricultural industry based on milkweed.

ANALYZING THE MILKWEED OPPORTUNITY

Starting up a business on your own is much different than producing new businesses with the extensive financial and people resources of Standard Oil. In the beginning, we wanted to continue the thrust of Kimberly-Clark and Standard Oil into the nonwovens market.

In milkweed or any alternative crop, the market in terms of volume and price needs to be matched with what you can do. With all the resources of Standard Oil, it was a reasonable dream to go into the nonwovens market. To compete in the $2 billion nonwovens market you needed at least a quarter of a million kilograms of fiber and a price less than $20 per kilogram.

We took a hard look at the opportunity from the perspective of small Natural Fibers without Standard Oil's financial resources. How much was this start-up really going to cost? We produced financial projections, a critical part of any alternative crop's planning process, and determined that penetrating the nonwovens market would require at least $6 million of investment in our Company.

To Standard Oil, $6 million is a modest investment. For Natural Fibers, six million is a lot of money. When we counted the potential sources of financing, there was no chance of raising that kind of capital. Thus, penetrating the nonwovens market in the short term was out of the question. Rather than targeting this high volume, low value nonwovens market, we had to back up to target a lower volume, higher value market.

Milkweed floss showed properties similar to goose down. The United States waterfowl down market has an annual volume of less than 5 million annual kilograms at a price in the range of $20 to $70 per kilogram. We chose to target our commercialization efforts on the waterfowl down market where milkweed floss could be substituted for goose down.

Based on this strategy choice, we made our projections and came up with a projected investment of $1.5 million to enter the down market—a challenging but more realistic number. So far, we have raised and spent about $900,000 of that amount. According to our original projections, we have about $600,000 more to raise. Recent projected numbers indicate that we might be able to achieve breakeven with as little as an additional $250,000 in investment, but $600,000 will probably be more accurate.

From its founding in 1987, Natural Fibers Corporation has made considerable progress toward achieving its ambitious goal of creating a new milkweed industry. The progress achieved is the result of efforts not only by me, but also the result of major contributions from our Board of Directors and the extended entrepreneurial team. Each person brings their unique skills to bear on the problems faced.

A vigorous Board of Directors is a necessary component of a successful business. I recruited internal Boards for all of my ventures in Standard Oil and have an active Board at Natural Fibers. Our Board consists of six people: Robert L. Raun and Ralph Holzfaster, who are growers in our milkweed program; William G. Wilson, a former Vice President at Kimberly-Clark; J. David Hopkins, a former Vice President at Springs Industries; the President of the Enterprise Fund, a State of Nebraska sponsored venture capital fund; and me. This Board functions to see the forest rather than the trees. We have plenty of brush fires and need a Board to help us see the overview of our activities.

In the very beginning of the start-up of this business, we decided to do only two things—grow milkweed and process milkweed pods to recover salable floss. With this focus in mind, we set out to recruit the people needed to accomplish these two broad tasks.

First, we needed people who want to grow milkweed. I was extremely fortunate to find Richard D. Zeller, an agribusiness professional. What he really wanted to do has to learn how to grow milkweed. He has been a real blessing for us and has worked hard to learn as much as possible about this plant. He is our expert and works closely with our research plots and with farmers to raise experimental production fields of milkweed.

Of course, one also needs farmers who are willing to grow milkweed. Robert L. Raun, former Director of Agriculture for Nebraska, is doing a great job of raising this new crop. Ralph Holzfaster and Edward D. Perlinger, farmers in the Ogallala area, also have acreage in milkweed.

Second, we needed people who would take up the challenge to make a beautiful clean floss from milkweed pods. George Ragsdale headed these operations and was provided very able assistance from Jerry L. Quick and my son, Peter D. Knudsen. These three worked diligently on equipment that we could beg or burrow to develop our milkweed pod processing system.

Our main processing unit is a 1940 John Deere combine that had been the home of raccoons for 40 years. George Ragsdale cleaned and modified it with a cutting torch so that floss could be separated from seed and pod hulls. Two of our other separating units are cracked fertilizer tanks converted for use in our process. The end result is a minimum investment processing facility that works very nicely to produce the developmental quantity and quality of milkweed floss that we needed for our operations.

Finally, we needed someone that could hold things together. LaVae H. Fattig is absolutely expert in taking care of the many administrative tasks from ordering to reports. She has expanded her role into sales as products were developed and sales effort was required. My wife, Karen M. Knudsen, also has important responsibility in comforter sales.

Soon after our start-up, we found other tasks needed to be addressed. Product development activities were needed because people in the goose down market wanted to see the practical results that could be achieved with milkweed floss. General scientific data was not enough. Down users were not inclined to conduct research on this new product, but wanted to see what we could do. Patricia C. Crews, at the University of Nebraska and Elizabeth McCullough, at Kansas State University, took on the responsibility for product research work and Natural Fibers staff did most of the production development.

Because our nuts and bolts people were fully occupied with the processing end of the milkweed floss production, we separated out the agricultural equipment issues. Kenneth Von Bargen and David D. Jones, of the University of Nebraska were recruited to develop harvesting, drying, and transfer systems. They, along with a number of their graduate students, accepted the challenge and have done an outstanding job of providing what we need when we needed it.

Historically, our efforts are based on research developed at Standard Oil of Ohio by Steven Price, Melvin Keener, and Janis Farmer. Jess Martineau at Native Plants Incorporated in Salt Lake was also responsible for developing a good share of this agricultural technology.

Currently, a number of researchers help us with the agronomic issues. Merle D. Witt, Paul Nordquist, and Lenis Nelson help us with our field research and production problems. Anne K. Vitivar and Michael G. Boosalis assist us with research related to milkweed plant pathology. We have also recognized the need for a milkweed breeding program, and efforts to organize and fund these activities are underway. These efforts are critical to our long term success in dealing with the many issues of growing milkweed.

Natural Fibers Corporation is aggressively pushing its way into the commercial market, but it is important to have timely and skilled research input to overcome the many obstacles faced. We have certainly had plenty of problems. The research component helps you analyze the situation encountered and helps you develop possible solutions that can be implemented.

"Partnership" is the word used to describe our relationship with the university research component available to us. In my past experience, there is cause for skepticism as to the practical utility of what university people are willing to do, what time frame they respect, and what drives their efforts. The people we are working with provided the data, equipment, samples, and advice on time and within budget. It is a model for public/private cooperation.

GROWING MILKWEED

Milkweed grows in about the same regions as maize. For the farmer, milkweed is planted and cared for with traditional row crop equipment. The milkweed plant is a deep rooted perennial that produces beautiful flowers in early summer. Pollinated flowers form pods which contain seed and silky white seed hairs.

Our general theory of economics for farmers is to provide them a crop that will produce the same revenue as maize with only half of the input costs. Milkweed requires less fertilizer, chemicals, and water than maize. The major agricultural problems the farmers face are weeds and disease. Weeds stress the plant reducing the yield and disease kills the plant—prematurely opening the pods before they can be harvested. Solutions for these problems in a milkweed monoculture still need to be found.

With specialized equipment operated by Natural Fibers, milkweed pods are harvested, dried, and processed. We harvest with a modified ear corn picker at about 70% moisture while the pod is still closed. The pods are opened in a modified rolling mill and dried to about 30% moisture on the farm.

Partially dried pods are then transported to our processing facility where they are dried to 10% moisture. At 10% moisture, the dried pods can be stored or processed. Processing ten units of pods yields two parts of floss, three parts of seed, and five parts pod hulls and other biomass.

Floss is collected in a hopper and then bagged for future use. We have an inventory of 3,000 kg of floss. Translated into comforters, this inventory is about 6,000 comforters which have an average retail price of about $200. Thus we have enough floss to support about $1.2 million in retail sales for comforters.

MILKWEED PRODUCT DEVELOPMENT

To us, product development is an interactive process considering fiber properties, markets, and prototype products. These topics will be discussed in separate sections, but, in the real world, product experience, data and observations are made in each area simultaneously over an extended period of time.

Floss Economics and Potential Floss Markets

I am a strong believer in prototype products. Make a prototype product as best you can and find a potential customer. Put the product in their hands and tell them the price. Then keep lowering the price until you cannot get the product back. This process develops prices and questions that need to be answered for the customer.

With this information you look at the floss fiber economics. Can we make any money at the price the customer is willing to pay? You have to generate revenue from customers in the business of alternative crops, or it does not make any difference.

Considering the commercialization of milkweed floss, we looked at the value of milkweed floss products in a number of markets. Four of these markets are analyzed in Table 1.

Our experience is that we can produce floss for $17/kg. To develop a start-up business strategy, the estimated cost of producing floss fiber was evaluated against the projected milkweed floss market price information (Table 1), the market volume, and the amount of money available. Our inability to raise larger sums of money to finance extended losses while penetrating the large, lower price nonwovens, yarn and paper markets, led us to adopt a strategy of focusing on the down market to begin our business.

The down market is a high value use of milkweed floss. Down prices of $20 to 70/kg were expected to support floss prices of $15 to 30/kg. These economics are approximations, but close enough to establish a commercial direction. At this point, product development issues and market penetration factors have a much greater impact on the viability of the business than refined economic numbers.

Moreover, fiber economics are not stagnant in a developing business and factors that will drive costs down would be aggressively pursued. About 90% of our fiber cost is growing the crop. To push floss fiber costs down, the yields need to be dramatically increased, more experience in growing the crop is required and uses of the seed by-product could be developed.

Our goal is milkweed floss prices of less than a $2/kg. Confirmation that this goal is realistic comes from cotton, a similar crop in many respects, where the cost of cotton fiber is less than $2/kg.

The prospect of lower cost floss fiber drives our dream that milkweed could become a major new crop. With slightly improved fiber prices, initial penetration of the $2 billion nonwovens market may be possible. With greatly improved economics and much lower fiber prices, penetration of the enormous yarn and paper markets with milkweed floss fiber may be feasible.

Table 1. Value of floss products in different markets.

Market	Floss value ($/kg)
Down	15–30
Nonwovens	1–20
Cotton/milkweed yarn	1–5
Pulp and paper	0.5–1.5

Floss Properties and Image

Analyzing product properties gives you something to discuss when you put a prototype product in the customer's hands. Floss properties are not only physical and chemical properties, but include the image of the product.

Focusing on milkweed floss properties important in the down market, we found that floss is: a non-allergenic cellulose fiber; with a fill-power of about 350 cm^3/g which is comparable to high quality goose down; white in color; 50% more breathable than down; 20% more durable than down; and 10% warmer per unit of weight than down.

Milkweed has a positive image, but the name "weed" detracts from peoples' positive reaction to the product. Floss is a natural vegetable fiber and not an animal byproduct. Environmentally, milkweed is attractive because it is grown in low impact agriculture or collected from native stands. Milkweed is a plant known to consumers. In a national survey, 59% of those surveyed in the United States were familiar with the plant. Milkweed provides habitat for Monarch butterflies; it is the subject of extensive native American lore, foods and medicines; and milkweed is the subject of many artists renditions of Autumn.

To our surprise, publicity about our efforts identified many people who are in love with the milkweed plant. Nellie Skipper of Oklahoma sent us a beautiful floral arrangement using milkweed floss, a woman from New York photographs milkweed as her avocation and presented us with photographs for our office. Artists from all over North America have provided us paintings, paper weights, Christmas decorations, and needlepoint art depicting milkweed. Fourth grade students in Iowa Falls are conducting milkweed floss mitten experiments on the playground this winter. It is a special treat for us to find such great interest and fascination with our product.

Prototype Products

The importance of prototype products cannot be overstressed. What can we sell? Unfortunately, the answer is not often clear and can be the subject of much debate.

When we were just beginning our milkweed processing operations, initial tests of our modified 1940 John Deere combine spewed out a cloud of milkweed floss into a gunny sack. To us that was our product, but to anyone else, such a small bag of milkweed floss certainly is not an attractive product. Real products are needed for real people.

We develop prototype products for all the potential markets we can envision. We also encourage others to develop new prototype products with our milkweed fiber. You cannot, however, dilute your commercial thrust spreading limited resources over a broad range of products—you need to focus on a product that makes the most sense. Our general strategy was to focus on products for the down market.

Our initial down prototype product was jackets. Jackets with milkweed floss alone, milkweed floss and down, and down alone were prepared and tested. Thermal insulation and other properties were good, but milkweed floss alone matted upon washing. The mixture of milkweed floss and down, however, worked well. The volume and economics of using milkweed floss in jackets were a good fit with our capability so we began promoting a mixture of down and milkweed floss for jackets and showing off our prototype product.

Presentation of our milkweed jacket prototype to customers evoked the reaction that the jacket market would be very difficult to penetrate. It is better to switch than fight—you need the easiest target you can find.

We then switched down products and made prototype comforters first hand stuffing milkweed floss and down into comforter shells (this is not fun), and then by borrowing some time on another company's down filling equipment. Experiencing acceptance, we built a small developmental comforter filling facility so that more prototype comforters were supplied to potential customers.

In the comforter development process, we found that the mixture of milkweed floss and down needed to be changed from our initial blend to assure excellent washability. None of our technical data showed this, but experimentation by our customers with our prototype comforter products demonstrated this need.

Down Market Segments

Down is used in the home furnishings, clothing and sleeping bag market segments. We studied these opportunities by reading current articles surveying the trends in these market segments and by talking to participants and trade reporters who were active in the markets.

Our initial prototype products were jackets, but our market analysis led us to focus on the down comforter segment of the home furnishings market. The market is growing at a rate of 10% per year, 2.3 million units were sold in 1989 for $250 million and comforters were competitively produced in the United States. There are no strong brand names. Milkweed floss has fiber property advantages primarily in allergenic properties and breathability; it was as good as or better than down in thermal insulation and durability; and, washability problems could be solved by mixing floss with down.

Our choice to initially focus on the down comforter market was also guided by the unattractive features of the sleeping bag and jacket markets. Down sleeping bags are a small segment with little or no growth, and we felt milkweed fiber resilience properties were not as good as we would like to assure successful market entry. About 90% of all down jackets are manufactured offshore, jackets involve strong brand names and use small quantities of down per unit. Style trends in jackets were away from the very full look of down.

To us, the high quality down pillow segment of the home furnishings market was hidden by the dominance of very low price feather pillows. We also had concerns about the resilience of floss. Even though milkweed floss had good resilience, it was not superior to down. We, therefore, focused on the down comforter market where thermal insulation and comfort were important. This focus on comforters continued for two years with only occasional customer requests for pillows. After the CBS Sunday Morning television program with Charles Kuralt aired a segment about our Company in June of this year, we had orders for 10 high quality pillows with milkweed floss, and we entered the pillow business. Customers judge allergenic properties and quality important in their buying decision.

Product Promotion

You have to make the product attractive and to inform potential customers of the benefits and features of your product to gain their acceptance. No product sells itself, promotion is essential.

Our original promotions in 1989 were rather crude. We provided potential customers a detailed message of milkweed development and promoted sales with an Indian maiden named Flame, an Ogallala Sioux legend, and Monarch butterflies. About $20,000 in sales were achieved, but it was tough.

From experience, we found out that touting comforters containing milkweed floss did not result in significant customer acceptance. We needed an attractive product name. Natural Fibers logo was and still is a milkweed pod opening. I like it, but it is not a strong logo for promoting a consumer product. We had no positioning statement.

These three deficiencies were corrected about a year ago. We adopted the name "Ogallala Down" for our blend of milkweed floss and down. We adopted a strong simple logo of a rounded lower case "d" that could be interpreted to be an "o" and a "d" for Ogallala Down. We invented the positioning statement "Nothing Warms You Up Like Ogallala Down" and made everyone swear allegiance to use this statement in all our promotions.

With these three decisions made, we developed and produced sales materials including an attractive high quality brochure on our products, labels and product inserts for the comforter and package. Product information sheets were also written.

Quality, price, and value of the product need to be designed to attract target customers. Who buys? When do they buy? Why do they buy? Retail sales are a fourth quarter business, but wholesale sales are made in the second quarter. To our retail customers, we stress the benefits of the product: exceptional comfort and warmth, non-allergenic floss, a good night's rest, light weight, and easy care. Continued experimentation with different messages and sensitivity to customer feedback develops the best message.

Our experience allows us to further segment our market. For example, environmental consumers show special interest in Ogallala Down comforters. We target these customers and gear our message to meet their needs. Environmental customers want a clean environmental history of the product and environmental benefits of using the product. In response, we stress that milkweed floss is a vegetable fiber produced in low impact agriculture and that our warm comforters allow users to turn back their thermostat in the winter saving energy and money.

Distribution is a key issue. We adopted the strategy of demonstrating acceptance of Ogallala Down products by retail customers so that wholesale customers would be willing to carry our product. Retail sales require a solid promotional program to convince ultimate consumers to buy your product. Successful wholesale sales require contacts with innovative retailers who like your story and are willing to take a risk.

In 1990, our second year of comforter sales, we achieved almost a five fold increase in sales to a little over $100,000. About two-thirds of our comforter business in 1990 was wholesale sales, and the remainder was direct retail sales throughout the United States and Canada.

In retrospect, it seems more planned than it actually was at the time. We used the trial and error approach, mainly error. We started by promoting jackets, but that was not the right market fit. We got sidetracked on nonwoven batting. The few hundreds of yards of experimental batting we have, make wonderful jackets and blankets. When that inventory is gone, however, we would be out of business. That thrust was stopped.

We also developed a new rugged comforter product, the Bunk Buddy. The comforter has a durable cover, and we tried to promote it to over-the-road truck drivers, owners of recreational vehicles, and couch potatoes. We love the product, but it was a lethal combination—a new company, new product, and new market with too many hurdles to overcome. We cut back and now focus on being a new company producing traditional comforters and pillows containing a new fill in the existing home furnishings market.

Through all of the trials and tribulations, however, we achieved "tangible useful results" with milkweed. Many formidable challenges remain to be conquered, but these successes lay a strong foundation for future development of this new crop.

REFERENCES

Conrad, J. 1992. National new crops policy. In: J. Janick and J.E. Simon (eds.). Progress in new crops. Wiley, New York.

Milkweed Cultivation for Floss Production

Merle D. Witt and Herbert D. Knudsen

Field plot studies of milkweed, *Asclepias speciosa* and *A. syriaca*, as a row crop, were initiated in 1985 at Garden City, Kansas. Potential cultivars and interspecies hybrids were evaluated for their floss production potential. Milkweed floss is usable as a hollow, cellulose, insulative, batting fiber and competes readily with the more traditionally used white goose down, which costs $66.00/kg. Fifteen lines of these two species yielded a 4-year annual average of 212 kg floss/ha from dried pods that averaged 21.8% floss. Thirty-five interspecies hybrids yielded a 4-year annual average of 350 kg/ha from dried pods that averaged 22.7% floss. Approximately 227 pods were required to produce a kilogram of floss. In view of the high-value application of floss and a projected market use of 1.27 million kg/year, *Asclepias* species appear to be worthy of further crop development.

The genus *Asclepias* is composed of approximately 140 species worldwide (Woodson 1954, 1962) with 108 species identified in North America, where this dicotyledonous plant is a native. *Asclepias* species are generally considered as being persistent, perennial, hardy weeds containing cardiac glycosides that are toxic when ingested by livestock (Muenscher 1975). Because of the negative aspects of milkweed as a pest, research efforts have most often dealt with techniques associated with control of these resilient plants (Timmons 1946; Wyrill and Burnside 1976). At the same time, milkweed has been of interest to agriculturalists for many years because of its potential economic value as a new crop (Stevens 1945; Moore 1946; Berkman 1949).

Various plant components have been identified as having potential uses, including insulative and absorptive materials made from the floss (Adams et al. 1984), and liquid fuel and rubber (Buchanon et al. 1978), as well as oil and polymeric hydrocarbons (Adams et al. 1987), from the latex sap. The only plant component used in quantity to date is floss, which emerged as the most feasible alternative to replace kapok when imported supplies during World War II were halted. The suggestion of such a potential use (Groh and Dore 1945) was followed quickly by a report of floss being collected and used as a kapok substitute (Gladfelter 1946). Eventually 11 million kg of pods were consumed to fill 1.2 million "Mae West" life jackets.

The currently preferred batting product of high insulative quality is goose down, but it costs $66.00/kg to import from China. At present, milkweed floss is being utilized to blend with white goose down or synthesized polypropylene in insulative batting for such products as comforters, sleeping bags, and arctic apparel.

Inadequate information exists on the production potential of milkweed as a cultivated crop. Initial interest suggested that if milkweed is to be considered as a crop plant, attention should be given first to selection of superior strains (Stevens 1945). Naturally occurring interspecies hybrids with variable characteristics were soon reported (Moore 1946; Nicholsen and Russel 1955). However, we found no evidence that replicated production evaluations of milkweed germplasm strains were ever conducted. This research effort was designed to evaluate the agronomic potential and variability of 50 collected milkweed ecotype strains and hybrids of *Asclepias speciosa* (showy milkweed) and *Asclepias syriaca* (common milkweed) when grown in monoculture as a new fiber-producing row crop. By providing an alternative cash crop, milkweed farming could strengthen the agricultural diversity and economy of the western Great Plains.

METHODOLOGY

Two field studies were established in a small, leveled flood irrigation basin and treated similarly. Plots were established from seed collected through efforts funded previously by the Standard Oil Company of Cleveland, Ohio. Seeds that had been repeatedly water soaked and dried to break dormancy were planted in 76.2 cm rows in a Keith Silt Loam type soil on May 30, 1985. A John Deere 71 flex-planter with cone seeding units and disk openers with depth bands was used to plant all plots with seed placed 1.27 cm deep. A seeding rate of 5.6 kg/ha placed approximately 1,111,500 seeds/ha into the seedbed. Stands were thinned to 10 cm between plants, when they had reached 8 cm in height on July 10, 1985. Two adjacent field studies were established.

Study I—Line Ecotypes

Fifteen randomly collected entries from 10 states (Colorado, Idaho, Kansas, Maine, Montana, New Mexico, North Dakota, Oregon, Utah, and Washington) included 12 showy milkweeds, two common milkweeds, and a single interspecies hybrid from two parent entries. The accessions were seeded in a randomized complete block design using three replications with three row plots and 3.04 m row length.

Study II—Hybrid Ecotypes

Thirty-five entries originating in Kansas and eastern Colorado and identified taxonomically by Kansas State University herbarium personnel as naturally occurring showy milkweed × common milkweed crosses were included. Because of limited seed quantity, these were seeded in a randomized complete block design using two replications with single-row 3.04-m-long plots.

All plots were overhead irrigated for 3 weeks after sowing to aid seedling emergence. Thereafter, irrigation was applied to plots 2 or 3 times each summer. Ammonium nitrate fertilizer granules were broadcast each season at 67.2 kg N/ha. Milkweed beetle (*Tetraopes tetraphthalmus* Forst.) control was initiated in 1989, using Malathion 25% WP at 0.56 kg/ha. Trifuralin applications were incorporated between rows each year in early May for weed control.

Summer harvest of pods began each season when approximately 10% of the pods had burst open. Ten representative pods from each entry were separated into floss, seed, and empty shell and weighed. The resulting dry weight proportions were used to partition total harvested pod weights per plot into calculated components from 4.18 m^2 harvest areas for the line ecotypes and from 1.39 m^2 harvest areas for the hybrid ecotypes. Harvest dates over the years ranged from July 24 to Aug. 15.

RESULTS AND DISCUSSION

Crop Establishment

Establishment was excellent, with seed germination as high as 80% resulting in uniform stands. Initial year stands were totally vegetative and reached average heights of 20 to 48 cm by the first killing freeze. Starting in 1986 and thereafter, the crop began to grow each spring from underground buds in late April, flowers appeared in early June, and pods were harvested 6 to 8 weeks later.

Plants were vigorous and developed extensive root systems with numerous viable root buds. Roots spread outward as much as 2 m from the unbordered perimeter rows by the end of 1986. Root spreading within and between plots was much more restricted, apparently due to plant competition and between-row cultivation that excised unwanted shoots so that the 76.2 cm row spacing could be maintained.

Pod Components

Harvested plant pods had a similar ratio of component parts for both species and for the interspecies hybrids (Fig. 1.). About 24% of the dried weight of pods was floss. The seed comprised the largest portion of the pod mass (about 40%). The shell component of 36% included the outer wall (34%) and the central placenta (2%). The exterior shell surface generally displayed more roughness with the showy milkweed species than did the shell of the common milkweed pods. However, shell wall thickness was similar between species.

Floss Production

Average annual productions of floss by the hybrid ecotypes and by the line ecotypes during the 4 years are indicated in Fig. 2. The hybrid ecotypes as a group averaged 349 kg floss/ha annually over the 4 years. The hybrid ecotypes consistently outproduced the line ecotypes. A direct statistical comparison between the two studies cannot be made. However, in comparison to line ecotypes, the hybrid ecotypes bloomed an average of 4 days later, stood 5 cm taller, and produced 58% more pods per area with 71% more pods per stem and 65% more floss per unit area.

Of the line ecotypes, the 12 showy milkweed ecotypes averaged 207 kg floss/ha, and the two common milkweed ecotypes yielded a similar level of 187 kg floss/ha over the 4-year period. Floss yields of the line ecotypes varied with differing state origins but did not appear to be highest from any particular state or region.

Yields of harvested floss were high in 1986 and 1988. Yields were hampered in 1987 and 1989. On June 16, 1987, during flowering, hail destroyed approximately 80% of the potential fruiting sites. In 1989, stands were reduced approximately 50% due to larvae of the milkweed beetle which had fed and tunnelled into the plant's root system following the 1988 harvest. Diseases were not a serious problem, although black bacterial leaf spot, leaf rust, and pod blight infections were observed late in the season in 1985 and 1986.

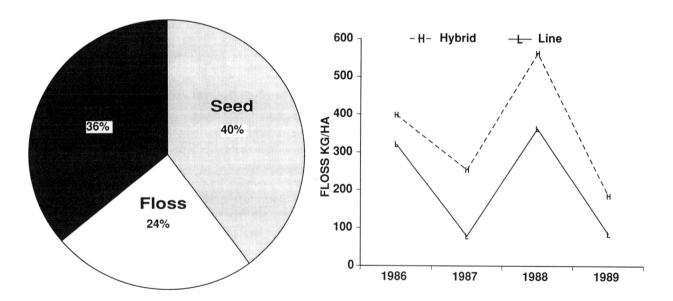

Fig. 1. Components of a typical dried milkweed pod. Proportions did not differ significantly between *A. speciosa*, *A. syriaca*, and interspecies hybrids between them.

Fig. 2. Average floss yield of 35 hybrid ecotypes and 15 line ecotypes.

Flowering

Milkweed is an obligate outbreeder, so that cross pollination is essential. Isolated colonies of wild plants were observed to bear few fruits in comparison with plantings of several colonies close together (Stevens 1945). We had hoped to provide adequate cross pollination in this study by rearing 50 different milkweed acquisitions within a 600 square meter area. The close proximity of these variable strains should have provided adequate pollen for maximum pod production.

Each single plant stem usually had about four flower clusters with about 40 flowers/cluster. Thus, there were about 160 flowers with two ovaries each, for a potential of about 320 pod sites/stem. However, this theoretical number was never approached. The best year (1988) allowed an overall average of 1.56 pods/stem for the variety ecotypes and an overall average of 2.3 pods/stem for the hybrid ecotypes.

FUTURE PROSPECTS

As with all new crops, development of milkweed is a high risk, long-term venture. At the same time, the need for alternative crops to overproduced crops has never been greater. A market for a product is a crucial ingredient in the successful development of a new crop. Fortunately, the thermal impedance level of milkweed floss equals that of the well known goose down. This helps provide an already developed market and a major incentive for addressing remaining considerations in production and processing. Additionally, the production, harvesting, and floss extraction procedures and equipment needed by a new milkweed industry closely parallel the procedures and equipment already in use by the well established cotton industry. In this study, we have produced floss yields considerably beyond the 56 kg/ha minimum that we felt would be adequate to compete with goose down. The transition to greater usage of domestically grown milkweed floss in place of imported goose down would be a positive step, with substantial benefits for both consumers and producers.

REFERENCES

Adams, R.P., M.F. Baladrin, and J.R. Martineau. 1984. The showy milkweed, *Asclepias speciosa*, a potential new semi-arid land crop for energy and chemicals. Biomass 4:81–104.

Adams, R.P., A.S. Tomb, and S.C. Price. 1987. Investigation of hybridization between *Asclepias speciosa* and *A. syriaca* using alkanes, fatty acids and triterpenoids. Biochem. Syst. Ecol. 15:395–399.

Berkman, B. 1949. Milkweed—a war strategic material and a potential industrial crop for submarginal lands in the United States. Econ. Bot. 3:223–239.

Buchanon, R.A., I.M. Cull, F.H. Otey, and C.R. Russell. 1978. Hydrocarbon- and rubber-producing crops. Econ. Bot. 32:131–145.

Evetts, L.L. and O.C. Burnside. 1973. Competition of common milkweed with sorghum. Agron. J. 65:931–932.

Gladfelter, C.F. 1946. Milkweed floss collections in Kansas. Kansas Acad. Sci. Trans. 49:217–218.

Groh, H. and W.G. Dore. 1945. A milkweed survey near Ontario in adjacent Quebec. Sci. Agr. 25:463–481.

Moore, R.J. 1946. Investigations on rubber bearing plants. IV. Cytogenetic studies in *Asclepias* Torr. L. Can. J. Res. (Sect. C) 24:66–73.

Muenscher, W.C. 1975. Poisonous plants of the United States (Rev. ed.). Collier MacMillan, New York. p. 195–199.

Nicholsen, D. and N.H. Russell. 1955. The genus *Asclepias* in Iowa. Proc. Iowa Acad. Sci. 62:211–215.

Schwartz, D.M. 1987. Underachiever of the plant world. Audubon Sept:46–61.

Stevens, O.A. 1945. Cultivation of milkweed. North Dakota Agr. Expt. Sta. Bul. 333.

Timmons, F.L. 1946. Studies of the distribution and floss yield of common milkweed (*Asclepias syriaca* L.) in northern Michigan. Ecology 27:212–225.

Woodson, R.E., Jr. 1954. The North American species of *Asclepias*. Ann. Mo. Bot. Gand. 41:1–211.

Woodson, R.E., Jr. 1962. Butterflyweed revisited. Evolution 16:168–185.

Wyrill, J.B., III and O.C. Burnside. 1976. Absorption, translocation, and metabolism of 2,4-D and glyphosate in common milkweed and hemp dogbane. Weed Sci. 24:557–566.

Black Locust: An Excellent Fiber Crop*

James W. Hanover

Black locust, (*Robinia pseudoacacia* L., Fagaceae), is a remarkable yet relatively neglected tree species with untapped potential which much of the rest of the world already appreciates. The native range is east- and west-central United States (Hanover 1992), but the species now grows wild in all of the contiguous states. It is ironic that one of our common native species may now be considered as a new crop for fiber. An intensive research and development effort for black locust has the goal of exploiting one of our most valuable plant resources with a multitude of uses including fiber production.

ATTRIBUTES OF BLACK LOCUST

Black locust is a nitrogen-fixing legume (Hanover and Mebrahtu 1991). When mature, it can reach 35 m in height and 1.0 m in diameter and such trees are usually found on upland sites in hardwood forests with black oak, red oak, chestnut oak, pignut hickory, yellow poplar, maple, and ashes. It tolerates a wide range of soil pH (4.6 to 8.2), but grows best in calcareous, well-drained loams. The species is intolerant of water logged soils and shading. Black locust reproduces prolifically from root sprouts and dominates early forest regeneration in native forest stands and areas disturbed by man. Black locust possesses virtually all of the characteristics that define a typical weed (Hanover 1992; Keeler 1989).

Other important attributes of black locust are its extremely rapid early growth rate, very high density wood, high resistance to wood decay fungi, tolerance to low fertility sites, drought resistance, abundance of natural product chemicals in its wood, bark and leaves, and large amount of genetic variation in most attributes (Barrett et al. 1988). On the negative side, black locust has been plagued by the locust borer, *Megacyllene robiniae* Forster, which attacks the stem and causes deformation or breakage. This single factor has been primarily responsible for the lack of attention to the species for lumber production. In other areas of the world where black locust has been introduced and the borer does not exist, the species is attracting wide interest and utilization (Keresztesi 1988). The tree also tends to have a crooked stem but this defect has been remedied by selection and breeding (Keresztesi 1983; Hanover et al. 1989). For the fiber production systems proposed here both borer attack and crooked stems would be of little consequence due to the short rotations used.

BLACK LOCUST FOR FIBER AND BIOMASS

There are at least six ways in which black locust can be used as a fiber crop or to generate large amounts of biomass at relatively low energy inputs. These include pulp for paper, leaves and young stems for fodder, leaves and young stems for solid, liquid or gaseous fuels, and extraction of specialty chemicals such as natural wood preservatives. There now exists a substantial natural resource of black locust timber and poles of fence post size growing throughout its natural range and now appearing in colonized areas outside that range. The species is prized for making fencing and post products and paper companies harvest it for pulp. Due to its dispersion or lack of concentration in pure stands and usually poor stem form, there is virtually no black locust lumber used in commerce. This situation could change when new, improved genetic materials become widely planted and commercially available because the wood is of very high quality; in many respects superior to species like teakwood or black walnut.

What are the specific characteristics of black locust which make it a desirable fiber source? Black locust wood has a large portion of uniformly distributed libriform fibers which confers great strength to wood. It has an average specific gravity of 0.68 compared to other North American hardwoods which average 0.51. Its average fiber length is 1.05 mm, slightly shorter than other hardwoods which average 1.13 mm. The central stem or pith of young black locust has a fiber length of 0.75 mm and specific gravity of 0.57, still well above the average mature hardwood values.

---

*This research was supported by the Michigan State University/USDA/CSRS Eastern Hardwood Utilization Research Special Grant Program (Grant No. 91-34158-5895).

Some other important characteristics of the wood of black locust are listed in Tables 1 and 2. Of particular interest are: (1) very young plant material contains no heartwood with all of its associated extractive chemicals; (2) the caloric content of young material is high and unchanged with age; and (3) the moisture content is very low relative to other species.

Less information is available regarding the chemical and physical characteristics of black locust leaves compared with the wood. Leaves are very high in nitrogen and have been used in animal feeding trials with mixed success (Baertsche et al. 1986; Cheeke et al. 1983). Baertsche et al. (1986) compared leave-stem mixtures of ten woody plants and alfalfa for chemical compositions and found black locust to be superior to all species in crude protein content (22.3% of dry matter).

Black locust also has potential to serve as a source of energy. According to Abelson (1991) there is great potential for energy crops in the United States in the future, and this species should be considered along with a wide array of other species. The wood is also a veritable chemical storehouse with extractives comprising 11% of dry weight (Table 1). Thus, black locust should be considered as a potential source of natural products just as other crops are being developed for their unique extractable natural products (Hanover 1990; Simon et al. 1990; Turick et al. 1991).

Table 1. Main-stem wood properties of ten- to twelve-year-old black locust trees[z].

Property	Average	Range
Stem volume (m^3)	0.043	0.03–0.05
Wood (%)	84.7	80.0–86.3
Heartwood (%)	54.1	34.8–60.2
Specific gravity	0.68	0.65–0.71
Ash content (% dry mass)	0.62	0.47–0.74
Fiber length (mm)	1.05	0.94–1.11
Extractives (% dry mass)		
Benzene–EtOH	3.5	2.7–3.9
EtOH	1.1	0.7–1.6
H_2O (hot)	2.8	2.4–3.1
Total	7.4	6.2–8.3

[z]Modified from Stringer and Olson (1987). Main-stem defined from groundline to 80% total tree height. Mean dbh (diameter at breast height) and height of the 10 trees sampled was 12.5 cm and 10.5 m, respectively.

Table 2. Stem diameter variation in wood properties[z].

| Diameter class (cm) | Mean±SE | | | |
	Specific[y] gravity	Caloric content[x] (cal/g)	Moisture content[x,w] (%)	Heartwood content[y] (%)
0.1–2.5	0.549	4641±52	41.1±16.5	absent
2.6–5.0	0.588	4644±58	38.0±16.1	3.4
5.1–7.5	0.644	4637±34	33.2±9.7	28.2
7.6–10.0	0.658	4665±42	26.7±6.4	38.0
Mean	0.609		33.1	

[z]Includes mainstem and branch material from 2- to 10-year-old black locust trees.
[y]From Stringer (1981).
[x]From Stringer and Carpenter (1986).
[w]% wet-weight basis.

A critical consideration in evaluating the potential of a new crop for fiber production and commercial utilization of its components is the efficiency and economy of producing the new crop usually under quite different or non-conventional cultural conditions. It is in this context that we are focusing on black locust, i.e., development of very efficient, large scale cultural systems for furnishing the raw material to be used for any of the purposes stated above.

CULTURAL SYSTEMS

Black locust lends itself admirably to direct seeding much as is now done conventionally with agricultural row crops. The seed must be pretreated with acid (H_2SO_4 for 50 min.) to allow it to germinate and germination rates are very high. We have successfully drill-sown several plantations and achieved good stands rather rapidly. Because black locust is one of the fastest growing species in North America, it literally appears to outcompete weed competition early in development. Individual trees can reach 3 m in height in one year, but the average is closer to 1 to 2 m, depending on soils and other conditions. Genetic selection and breeding efforts now underway should further enhance yields (Hanover et al. 1989).

Because black locust sprouts readily from the roots and regrows from cut stems, we have several options for regenerating another crop either in one growing season or over several seasons. Thus, the need to reestablish by seed is eliminated at considerable reduction in energy inputs for many years. A drill-sown, vigorous stand of closely spaced (30 cm) black locust can be harvested in July, in Michigan, and by early September another crop will have regrown. Alternatively, the initial crop can be allowed to grow the entire season and be harvested before or after leaf fall in October, depending upon the product to be extracted. Each of the six potential uses of the material generated now need to be closely examined to determine the best methods for harvesting and overall economic feasibility.

SUMMARY

Black locust has physical and biological characteristics that make it a prime candidate for fiber production. These include: very rapid early growth; the ability to fix N_2; reproduction from root sprouts and coppice; wide climatic and edaphic adaptation; good fiber quality; high density wood; high caloric content; low moisture content; high protein content; high genetic variation; potentially useful chemical extractives; amenable to intensive culture management. Research should now focus on the genetic improvement and cloning, the utilization of leaves and stems, and the development of high yield production systems.

REFERENCES

Abelson, P.H. 1991. Improved yields of biomass. Science 252:1469.

Baertsche, S., M.T. Yokoyama, and J.W. Hanover. 1986. Short rotation, hardwood tree biomass as potential ruminant feed-chemical composition, nylon bag ruminal degradation and ensilement of selected species. J. Anim. Sci. 63:3028–2043.

Barrett, R.P., T. Mebrahtu, and J.W. Hanover. 1988. Black locust: a multi-purpose tree species for temperate climates, p. 278–283. In: J. Janick and J.E. Simon (eds.). Advances in new crops. Timber Press, Portland, OR.

Cheeke, P.R., M.P. Geoeger, and G.H. Arscott. 1983. Utilization of black locust (*Robinia pseudoacacia*) leaf meal by chicks. Nitrogen Fixing Tree Res. Rpt. 1:41.

Hanover, J.W. 1990. Chemical basis for resistance of black locust to decay. In: K. Miller (ed.). Advanced technology applications to eastern hardwood utilization. Prog. Rpt. No. 3, Michigan State Univ. Agr. Expt. Sta., East Lansing.

Hanover, J.W. 1992. *Robinia pseudoacacia*: A versatile legume tree for temperate/subtropical regions. Proc. Int. Conf. Black Locust: Biology, Culture and Utilization. June 17–21, 1991, Michigan State Univ., East Lansing.

Hanover, J.W., and T. Mebrahtu. 1991. *Robinia pseudoacacia*: temperate legume tree with worldwide potential. Nitrogen Fixing Tree Highlights 91:03.

Hanover, J.W., T. Mebrahtu, and P. Bloese. 1989. Genetic improvement of black locust: a prime agroforestry species. In: P. Williams (ed.). Proc. First Conf. on Agroforestry in North America. August 1989, Guelph, Ontario, Canada.

Keeler, K.H. 1989. Can genetically engineered crops become weeds? Bio/Technology 7:1134–1139.

Keresztesi, B. 1983. Breeding and cultivation of black locust, *Robinia pseudoacacia*, in Hungary. Forest Ecol. Mgt. 6:217–244.

Keresztesi, B.. 1988. Black locust: the tree of agriculture. Outlook on Agr. 17:77–85.

Simon, J.E., D. Charles, E. Cebert, L. Grant, J. Janick, and A. Whipkey. 1990. *Artemisia annua* L.: A promising aromatic and medicinal, p. 522–526. In: J. Janick and J.E. Simon (eds.). Advances in new crops. Timber Press, Portland, OR.

Stringer, J.W. 1981. Factors affecting the variation in heat content of black locust biomass. MSc. Thesis, Univ. of Kentucky, Lexington.

Stringer, J.W. and S.B. Carpenter. 1986. Energy yield of black locust fuel. Forest Sci. 32:1049–1057.

Stringer, J.W. and J.R. Olson. 1987. Radial and vertical variation in stem properties of juvenile black locust (*Robinia pseudoacacia*). Wood Fiber Sci. 19:59–67.

Turick, C.E., M.W. Peck, D.P. Chynoweth, and D.E. Jerger. 1991. Methane fermentation of woody biomass. Bioresource Technol. 37:141–147.

Development of *Hesperaloe* Species (Agavaceae) as New Fiber Crops

Steven P. McLaughlin

"Hard fibers" are the bundles of fiber cells obtained by decorticating the leaves of abaca (*Musa textilis* Née), sisal (*Agave sisalana* Perrine), henequen (*A. fourcroydes* Lem.), and other monocots. These fiber bundles are used mostly in cordage products (rope, twine, canvas, burlap), but can be pulped for use in specialty papers (Clark 1965; Corradini 1979; da Silva and Pereira 1985), which include such products as tissue papers, filter papers, tea bags, currency papers, and security papers. The very long and thin fiber cells of these plants produce papers that are strong yet fine-textured. The crop plants that produce the hard fibers of commerce are all frost-sensitive tropical species. The objective of my research program is to develop domestic production of a cold-tolerant source of hard fibers for use in specialty papers.

SCREENING STUDIES

Abaca and sisal pulps command premium prices in the paper industry (Clark 1965; Baker 1985). Tensile strength, tearing resistance, and bursting strength, are largely determined by fiber morphology (Horn and Setterholm 1990). The fiber cells of abaca and sisal are as long or longer yet much thinner than those of softwoods. Abaca fibers may average 6.0 mm in length and 24 µm in width, for a length-to-width ratio (L/W) of 250. Sisal fibers are closer to 3.0 mm in length with a L/W of 150.

We examined several species of Agavaceae native to the southwestern United States and northern Mexico to determine if any of these plants possessed fibers similar to those of abaca and sisal (McLaughlin and Schuck in press). An updated summary of our results is presented in Table 1. Native species of *Agave*, *Nolina*, and *Dasylirion* have relatively short fiber cells. Species of *Yucca* and *Hesperaloe* have much longer and narrower cells. Those of *Hesperaloe* species are comparable to abaca in their L/W. From this screen, we selected *Hesperaloe* for further study.

BOTANY OF *HESPERALOE*

Taxonomy

The genus Hesperaloe consists of three described and two or more as yet undescribed species; all are native to northern Mexico. *Hesperaloe* is probably most closely related to the larger genus *Yucca* (Smith and Smith 1970). *Hesperaloe funifera* (Koch) Trel. (Fig. 1A) is found at lower elevations in the east-central part of the Chihuahuan Desert in Coahuilla and Nuevo Leon. Its Spanish common name is samandoque or zamandoque. *H. parviflora* Torr. is the most widespread species, occurring at higher elevations in the northern Chihuahuan Desert of Texas, Chihuahua, and Coahuilla. It is widely cultivated as an ornamental plant in the southwestern United States where it is called "red yucca." *H. nocturna* Gentry (Fig. 1B) is a recently described species from the Sierra Madre Occidental area of northeastern Sonora; it has no Spanish or English common name. There are two recently discovered *Hesperaloe* forms that probably represent new species, one from the southeastern Chihuahuan Desert of San Luis Potosi and the other from southern Sonora.

Morphology

Hesperaloe species are long-lived, evergreen, acaulescent plants. As in all Agavaceae, the basic module of growth is the rosette, a cluster of leaves produced from a single meristem. This meristem produces several leaves before switching from vegetative to reproductive mode. Once the flower stalk is produced, the rosette ceases to grow. In *Hesperaloe* (as in most *Yucca*) lateral or secondary rosettes are produced from the crown after the primary rosette becomes reproductive. Although an older *Hesperaloe* plant has the appearance of a closely packed, often grass-like clump of leaves with several flower stalks, the plant actually consists of a cluster of separate but closely-spaced rosettes. The older flowering rosettes are found at the center of the clump; younger vegetative rosettes are on the periphery of the clump.

The species of *Hesperaloe* differ in their leaf morphology. The leaves of *H. funifera* (Fig. 1A) and the undescribed species from San Luis Potosi are 1 to 2 m long, 3 to 6 cm wide toward the base, and stiffly erect. Those of *H. funifera* are cresent-shaped in cross section while those of the undescribed species are more strongly folded into a V-shape. Leaves of *H. parviflora* are less rigid, arching away from the crown, shorter (mostly <1 m), narrower (1 to 2 cm), and cresent-shaped in cross section. Leaves of *H. nocturna* (Fig. 1B) and the undescribed species from southern Sonora are long (1 to 2 m), very narrow (mostly <1.5 cm wide), and hemispherical in cross section. Leaves of all species bear marginal fibers. Older plants of *H. funifera* typically consist of 10 or fewer rosettes while those of *H. nocturna* and *H. parviflora* often have many more than 10 rosettes.

All *Hesperaloe* species produce relatively large flower stalks—those of *H. funifera* may be 3 to 4 m tall. The flowers of *H. parviflora* and the undescribed species from Sonora are pink to red; those of the other species are white to green.

AGRONOMIC STUDIES

There are no published studies on the agronomy of *Hesperaloe* species. Our initial trials therefore, concentrated on determining the potential biomass production of *Hesperaloe funifera*. This species was selected

Table 1. Average fiber lengths, widths, and cell-wall thicknesses for five genera of Agavaceae from the southwestern United States and northern Mexico.

Genus	No. species examined	Fiber length (mm)	Fiber width (μm)	Cell-wall thickness (μm)	Lumen diameter (μm)	L/W ratio
Agave	7	1.14	27.0	5.4	16.3	42
Dasylirion	2	0.89	16.9	6.4	4.1	53
Nolina	3	0.94	19.1	4.9	9.2	49
Hesperaloe	5	3.55	14.7	3.6	7.5	241
Yucca	9	2.38	14.3	5.8	2.7	166

because its fibers are very long and thin and small amounts of seed were available from landscape plants growing in Tucson. While seed of *H. parviflora* are more readily available, its fibers are consistently shorter than those in *H. funifera* (McLaughlin and Schuck in press).

In the following text, standing crops and yields will be reported as fresh weights. Standing crop refers to the amount of biomass present at any particular time; yield refers to the amount of biomass obtained when the stand is harvested. Because whole, cut leaves do not readily lose moisture, it is most convenient to measure biomass as fresh weights. In addition, it is likely that leaves would be transported and pulped as fresh material. Dry matter and dry fiber contents of fresh leaves are approximately 32.5 and 10%, respectively.

Size-Biomass Relationships

H. funifera would be grown as a perennial crop (Fig. 2). Several years would be required from the time of stand establishment to first harvest. Plants harvested near ground level can regrow by (1) elongation of cut leaves (monocot leaves grow from a basal meristem), (2) production of new leaves from cut rosettes, and (3) production of new rosettes. It seems likely, therefore that cut plants will regrow to produce several subsequent harvests.

Replicated production plots for *H. funifera* were established at three densities: 6,800, 13,500, and 27,000/ ha. Plots measured 9.75 by 30.5 m with two plots at each density level. The low-density plots consist of 8 rows of 25 plants; medium-density plots have 8 rows of 50 plants, and high-density plots have 16 rows of 50 plants. Plant spacings within the plots are: low density, 1.22 m between and within rows; medium density, 1.22 m between rows by 0.61 m within rows; and high density, 0.61 m between and within rows. Plots were established from transplants (3- to 5-month old seedlings) in March 1988; they receive irrigation and fertilization through a below-ground drip irrigation system. Soil moisture was monitored with gypsum blocks.

The key problem in monitoring growth and yield in such a perennial crop is developing nondestructive methods of biomass estimation. We have measured standing crops each year by randomly sampling 5 plants per row. On each plant, basal circumference and average length of the five longest leaves were measured. Two of the five plants in each row were harvested for fresh-weight determinations. The number of plants harvested from the production plots each year varied between 4 and 8% of the stand, depending on the density. Sampling was done February 1989 (stand age 11 months), November 1989 (20 months), and November 1990 (32 months).

The data on basal circumferences (cm), leaf length (cm), and fresh weights (g) have been used to develop size-biomass relationships. Scatter diagrams show that there is not a particularly good fit between either basal circumference (Fig. 3A) or leaf length (Fig. 3B). However, basal area (BA, in cm^2) can be calculated from basal circumference (BC) as: $BA = BC^2/(4\pi)$. I then defined a new variable, SIZE2, as: SIZE2 = (BA)(Leaf Length)/ 1000. SIZE2 is proportional to the volume of the plant; it is linearly related to fresh weight (Fig. 3C). Plotted on log-log scale the relationship is linear with a very high R^2 (Fig. 3D). We used the equation for the relationship shown in Fig. 3D to estimate fresh weights on a large sample of plants in the Production Study in August 1991;

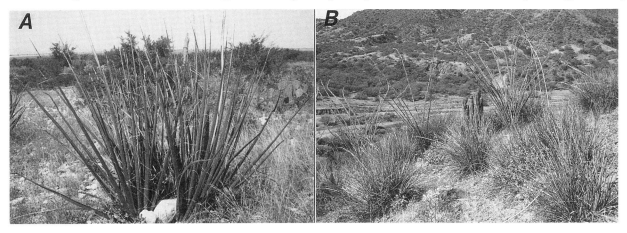

Fig. 1. *Hesperaloe funifera* in the Chihuahuan Desert of central Coahuilla (Fig. 1A) and *H. nocturna* in desert-woodland transitional vegetation in northeastern Sonora (Fig. IB).

we also have used it to estimate fresh weights nondestructively in other studies. This equation works well for plants with a single rosette; a different size-biomass equation probably will have to be developed for plants regrowing with two or more rosettes.

Biomass Production

The development of the standing crops of *Hesperaloe funifera* at three densities is shown in Fig. 4. During the first growing season, accumulation of aboveground biomass is very slow as plants establish a large crown and an extensive root system. Growth in subsequent years is rapid. Estimated standing crops (leaves only) at the end of the third growing season were 22.1 46.7, and 77.4 Mg fresh weight/ha for the low-, medium-, and high-density plots, respectively.

Standing crop to date is nearly directly proportional to density. Individual plant size is inversely proportional to density but the effect so far is small. Average plant size in the high-density plots at the end of 1990 (year 3) was 2632 g/plant compared to 3535 g/plant in the low-density plots.

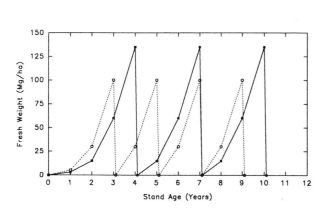

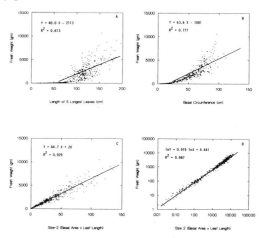

Fig. 2. Projected stand dynamics for *Hesperaloe funifera* grown as perennial crop. We originally estimated that the plant would require 4 years to reach a first harvest with subsequent harvests every 3 years thereafter (solid line): it now appears that a harvestable stand can be produced in 3 years with reharvests every 2 years thereafter (dashed line).

Fig. 3. Size-biomass relationships in *Hesperaloe funifera*: scatter diagrams showing the relationships between fresh weight and leaf length (Fig. 3A), basal circumference (Fig. 3B), and the product of leaf length and basal circumference on a linear plot (Fig. 3C) and a log-log plot (Fig. 3D).

Fig. 4. Growth in standing crops of *Hesperaloe funifera* at three stand densities (6,800, 13,500, and 27,000/ha): March 1988 to August 1991. Bars show ± 1 standard error (SE); for data points without error bars, SE <1 Mg fresh weight.

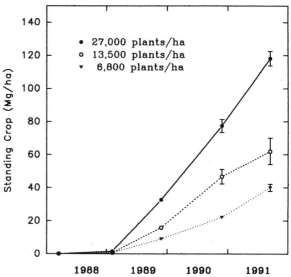

Regrowth

Half of each of the 6 plots in the production study were harvested in November 1990. Plants are vigorously regrowing from the 5- to 8-cm stubble left from the harvest, as expected (Fig. 5). Regrowth is occurring both from the harvested rosettes and from new lateral rosettes. The average number of rosettes per plant in these harvested plots is now 2.39, 1.88, and 1.56 in the low-, medium-, and high-density plots, respectively. Since the basic unit of growth is the individual rosette, the effective densities of these plots have increased to 16,000, 25,000, and 42,000/ha, respectively.

Water Requirements

To get a first approximation of this potential crop's water requirement, we examined biomass production as a function of the amount of water applied. While we have tried to balance water applications to rates of soil moisture depletion, our system for monitoring soil moisture is not sophisticated and irrigation schedules are far from optimized. Nevertheless, *Hesperaloe* appears to have a rather low water requirement for an arid-land crop (Table 2). In the high density plots, a total of 38.5 Mg dry weight has been produced with a total application of 238 cm of irrigation, equivalent to a water requirement of 6.2 cm/Mg dry weight of leaves. In comparison, alfalfa grown in Final Co., Arizona, requires 11.6 cm/Mg dry weight and kenaf grown in Imperial Co., California, requires 13.0 cm/Mg dry weight.

Fertilizer Requirements

Leaf nitrogen levels were measured on leaves from 6 plants at the end of the 1990 growing season. Average N content was 1.42% (dry-weight basis) and did not vary with density level or leaf age. Harvest of 77 Mg fresh

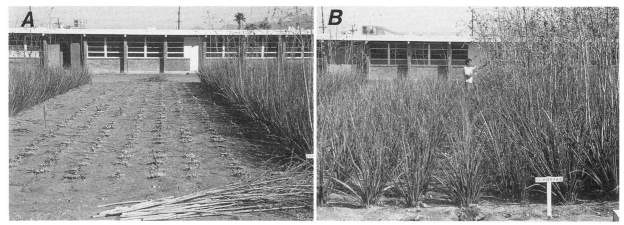

Fig. 5. High-density plot of *Hesperaloe funifera* immediately after harvest in November 1990 (Fig. 5A) and in September 1991 (Fig. 5B), showing the rapid regrowth of the harvested stand.

Table 2. Water requirement and productivity of *Hesperaloe funifera* in the high-density treatment (27,000/ha).

Year	Water applied (cm)	Estimated aboveground annual productivity (Mg dry weight/ha)	Water requirement (cm/Mg dry weight)
1988	42	0.5	---
1989	46	10.1	4.6
1990	74	14.6	5.1
1991[z]	76	13.3	5.7
4-year total	238	38.5	6.2

[z]Through August, 1991.

weight/ha from the high-density treatment at the end of the third growing season represents a withdrawal of 358 kg N/ha; additional N is removed in the flower stalks, flower parts, capsules, and seeds. The high-density plots were fertilized with only 120 kg N/ha over the first three years. Plants clearly used considerable residual N in our plots and it is likely that growth has been limited by low N to some unknown degree in our study.

Phosphorus contents averaged 0.13% of leaf dry weights, corresponding to a removal rate of 32 kg P/ha over the first three years in the high-density plots.

Flowering

Hesperaloe produces a fairly large flower stalk. In the 43 randomly selected plants that flowered in 1990, the flower stalk (excluding dehisced flowers and dispersed capsules and seeds) constituted 27% of the aboveground fresh weight. At the end of the 1990 growing season (after the third growing season), percentage of plants in flower ranged from 31% in the low-density plots to 18% in the high-density plots. At the end of August 1991 (in the fourth growing season) percentage of plants in flower in the unharvested portions of our production plots averaged 57% and did not vary among density treatments.

Monthly Growth Rates

We have been monitoring growth rates in a population of 20 *Hesperaloe funifera* plants on a monthly basis since February 1990. These plants are approaching the end of their second growing season. Number of leaves increases most rapidly between June and October; rates of leaf elongation are greatest during the same period. Basal circumference, however, continues to increase through December. Thus, our estimates for fresh weight, which are based on basal area and leaf length, continue to rise through December of the first year. Estimated fresh weight begins increasing rapidly by May of the second growing season (Fig. 6), consistent with our findings from the production study.

Other *Hesperaloe* Species

Hesperaloe nocturna has been grown in a small observation plot and several plants of this species have been harvested on a yearly basis. Fibers of this species are nearly as long as those of *H. funifera*; if *H. nocturna* can be harvested at yearly intervals rather than the projected 2-year interval for *H. funifera*, the former species might be a superior crop plant. In October 1989, sufficient seed of *H. nocturna* was collected from the wild for establishing a series of production plots. We transplanted replicated plots of this species at densities of 6,800, 10,000, 13,500, and 20,000/ha in October 1990. Initial growth appears to be good; these plots will be monitored for biomass production as they mature.

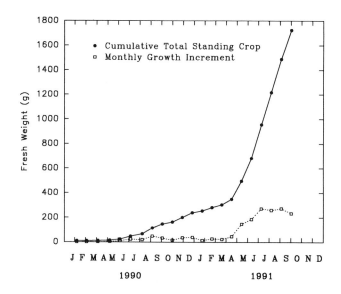

Fig. 6. Estimated standing crops (Mg fresh weight/ha) and growth rates (Mg fresh weight ha^{-1} month^{-1}) at 4-week intervals in a sample of 20 plants of *Hesperaloe funifera*.

DISCUSSION

It is difficult at this initial stage of research and development on *Hesperaloe funifera* to evaluate this plant's potential as a new crop. We estimate that stands of *Hesperaloe* will need to produce annual yields of 30 to 45 Mg fresh weight/ha (ca. 10 to 15 Mg dry weight) to produce biomass at $40 to $60/Mg fresh weight (N.G. Wright and S.P. McLaughlin unpublished analyses). This would correspond to a feedstock cost of $400 to $600/Mg dry fiber. Leaf standing crop at the end of the third year was approximately 78 Mg fresh weight/ha in the high-density plots, corresponding to an annual productivity of 26 Mg fresh weight/ha. First-year aboveground growth rates, however, were low. We estimate that the standing crop at the end of the fourth year will be between 120 and 140 Mg fresh weight/ha, corresponding to an annual productivity of 30 to 35 Mg fresh weight/ha. The rate of regrowth during the first year after harvest appears to be much higher than the initial growth rate during the first year after stand establishment.

The literature on cultivated *Agave* species indicates the magnitude of yields that might be possible from perennial rosette plants in the Agavaceae. *Agave* species are more succulent than *Hesperaloe* species (12% dry matter vs. 32.5% dry matter, respectively, in the leaves) so that direct comparisons of fresh weights are not meaningful. Nobel (1988) reported the following dry-weight standing crops for 7-year-old stands of cultivated *Agave* species: *A. sisalana*, 70 Mg/ha; *A. fourcroydes*, 80 Mg/ha; and *A. tequilana*, 90 Mg/ha. These would correspond to annual yields of 10 to 13 Mg dry weight/ha similar to the targets I have set for *Hesperaloe*. Nobel (1991) reported annual yields of 38 to 42 Mg/ha in special plantings of *A. mapisaga* and *A. salmiana* at Tequexquinahuac, Mexico. These yields are comparable to the maximum yields observed in experiment station plants of C_3 and C_4 crops.

Initial predictions that 4 years would be required to reach a first harvest and that subsequent harvests might be made every three years thereafter were proved wrong. Stands should reach a harvestable standing crop after three years and the amount of regrowth may be enough that subsequent harvests could be obtained every two years.

Hesperaloe funifera, like *Agave*, is a CAM (crassulacean acid metabolism) plant (Damian Ravetta unpublished data). The photosynthetic pathways of other *Hesperaloe* species have not yet been determined, but it is of interest to note that in *Yucca*, *Hesperaloe*'s closest relative, there are both CAM and C_3 species (Kemp and Gardetto 1982). The very low water requirement of *H. funifera* is consistent with CAM photosynthesis (Nobel 1991). High water-use efficiency, and hence low water requirement, is an important criterion for potential new crops for arid regions (McLaughlin 1985).

There appears to be a trade-off between flower-stalk production and leaf production in *H. funifera*, i.e., investment of photosynthetically-fixed carbon into flower stalks may decrease the amount of leaf production. Selection for plants with delayed flowering might result in greater leaf production at the first harvest. However, all rosettes must eventually terminate in a flower stalk. Delayed flowering will only result in improved leaf yields if it is accompanied by formation of an increased number of leaf primordia. Also, flowering is correlated with the production of lateral rosettes and an increased number of rosettes probably will result in larger subsequent harvests. Determining what controls the number of leaves produced by a rosette and what triggers production of flower stalks and lateral rosettes will be critical to improving yields in this species.

REFERENCES

Baker, D.M. 1985. Alternative uses for sisal fiber, p. 177–186. In: C. Cruz, L. del Castillo, M. Robert, and R.N. Ondara (eds.). Biologia y aprovechamiento integral del henequen y otros Agaves. Centro de Investigacion Cientifica de Yucatan, A. C.

Clark, T.F. 1965. Plant fibers in the paper industry. Econ. Bot. 19:394–405.

Corradini, F.T. 1979. Companhia de Celulose da Bahia, p. 70–74. In: L.E. Hass (ed.). New pulps for the paper industry. Proceedings of the Symposium on New Pulps for the Paper Industry. Brussels, Belgium. May 1979. Miller Freeman Publ., Inc., San Francisco.

da Silva, N.M. and A.D. Pereira. 1985. Experience of a pioneer—sisal—simultaneous resource for pulp and energy, p. 63–69. In: A.J. Seaquist and E.C. Cobb (compilers). Nonwood plant fiber pulping: progress report no. 15. TAPPI Press, Atlanta.

Horn, R.A. and V.C. Setterholm. 1990. Fiber morphology and new crops, p. 270–275. In: J. Janick and J.E. Simon (eds.). Advances in new crops. Timber Press, Portland, OR.

Kemp, P.R. and P.E. Gardetto. 1982. Photosynthetic pathway types of evergreen rosette plants (Liliaceae) of the Chihuahuan Desert. Oecologia 55:149–156.

McLaughlin, S.P. 1985. Economic prospects for new crops in the southwestern United States. Econ. Bot. 39:473–481.

McLaughlin, S.P. and S.M. Schuck. 1992. Fiber properties of several Agavaceae from the Southwestern United States and Northern Mexico. Econ. Bot. (in press).

Nobel, P.S. 1988. Environmental biology of agaves and cacti. Cambridge University Press, Cambridge.

Nobel, P.S. 1991. Achievable productivities of certain CAM plants: basis for high values compared with C_3 and C_4 plants. New Phytol. 119: 183–205

Smith, C.M. and G.A. Smith. 1970. An electrophoretic comparison of species of *Yucca* and of *Hesperaloe*. Bot. Gaz. 131:201–205.

Sweetgrass: History, Basketry, and Constraints to Industry Growth

Robert J. Dufault, Mary Jackson, and Stephen K. Salvo

Sweetgrass is a native, perennial, warm-season grass found growing sparsely in the coastal dunes extending from North Carolina to Texas. The "treads" or long, narrow leaf blades of this grass have been harvested by direct descendents of enslaved Africans of antebellum South Carolina and used as the principle foundation material for constructing African coiled basketry in the Southeast, especially near Charleston (McKissick Museum 1988). Originally, these graceful products provided useful, practical objects or "work baskets" for agricultural and household use on the plantations; today, they have evolved as souvenirs treasured by tourists, and elegant objets d'art (Fig. 1).

Basketmakers are faced with changes and challenges that threaten the existence of their craft. The supply of sweetgrass is becoming more difficult to acquire because the natural habitats of sweetgrass have significantly diminished. Two primary factors have led to this situation. First, the urbanization of the area around Mt. Pleasant has led to the destruction of much of the natural sweetgrass plant communities. Second, the traditional gathering areas on the Barrier Islands off the coast of Charleston, have been developed as beach resorts or private communities with restricted access. Basketmakers now have to travel to Georgia and Florida to find adequate supplies.

Natural habitats of sweetgrass need to be preserved, protected, or relocated if this industry is to continue. The basketmaking community will need help from local governments to continue to sell baskets along the old Ocean Highway (Hwy 17) or relocate the stands to equally visible, safe locations. Alternatively, the ability to cultivate sweetgrass on inland soils in the Mt. Pleasant area would enable the production of readily available raw material. These practices would help to insure that the heritage of basketmaking will continue to flourish into the 21st century.

SWEETGRASS INDUSTRY

Mt. Pleasant, South Carolina, is located four miles north of Charleston on U.S. Hwy 17. Baskets are sold in a variety of places in the Charleston area. About 75 basket stands dot the old Ocean Highway in Mt. Pleasant.

Baskets are also sold by the "basket ladies" in Charleston's Market area and even on major intersections within the historic areas of the city.

About 300 families are involved in sweetgrass basketry of which approximately 75% are full-time basketmakers and 25% are part-time (Mary Jackson pers. commun.). Twenty-five years ago, approximately 1,200 families were involved in basketmaking and this represents a 75% decline in the basketmaking community.

HISTORY

The variability of African baskets is as diverse as the 800 different ethnic groups that comprise the African people (Vlach 1978). Only certain African people however, especially those from Senegal, were brought to South Carolina as early as 1505 with the advent of the slave trade in the New World. By the end of slavery around 1808, Africans were abducted from areas down to Central Africa and Mozambique.

Rice was the main cash crop of South Carolina during the colonial period and the base of the State's economy until the 19th century. Slavers were paid premium prices for Africans from the West African Rice Kingdoms of the Windward Coast (Senegal to the Ivory Coast) and the mouth of the Congo River (Gabon, Zaire, and Angola) (Littlefield 1981). A man or women who made baskets was worth more than one who did not, age, strength, and other skills being equal (Chas. Gaz. Adv. 1791). Since colonial South Carolinians knew little of rice culture, the success of the American Rice Kingdom is credited to enslaved Africans (Joyner 1984).

The technique of basketmaking crossed the Atlantic in slave ships and took root in the new land. The art of making sweetgrass baskets is a three-century old African-American tradition that has been "passed-down" over the centuries from parent to offspring. Sweetgrass basketmaking is one of the earliest traditional rafts with a rich documented history from "carryover" from African enslavement and plantation days to the present (McKissick Museum 1988). Although the materials used are different in the United States, the form and function of the African counterparts of sweetgrass baskets are unchanged to this day (Mary Jackson pers. commun.).

Folk history recounts that enslaved men and women weaved African coiled baskets to fan rice in order to separate the grains from the chaff. After the Emancipation Proclamation in 1863, former slaves were dedicated to preserve the African traditions of their ancestors. A reaffirmation of this goal has been made by each generation of the descendants of enslaved Africans and sweetgrass basketry is a symbol of this devotion.

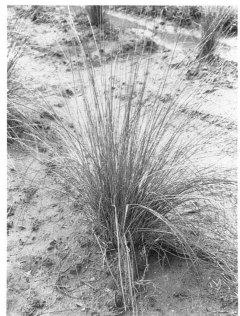
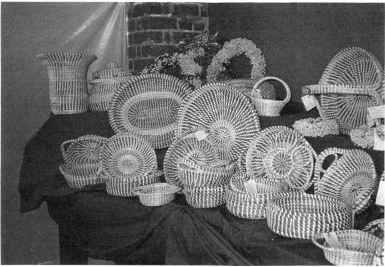

Fig. 1. Sweetgrass plant and baskets.

SWEETGRASS IDENTITY AND HABITAT

Sweetgrass (*Muhlenbergia filipes* Curtis, Poaceae) was first identified and described botanically by Moses Ashley Curtis in 1843 and later by Pinson (1971). There is still a dispute as to whether sweetgrass should be identified as a variety of *Muhlenbergia capillaris* or remain a distinct genus and species (Rosengarten 1987). There is a lack of concise, comprehensive descriptive information on this species (Pinson and Batson 1971.)

Sweetgrass grows in bands about 50 to 75 m from the mean high tide line in undulating sand dunes usually behind the first dune along the ocean from North Carolina to Texas. Occasionally, plants are found growing on well-drained, sandy uplands bordering brackish marshes and in open maritime forests (Pinson and Batson 1971). Sweetgrass grows on many of the barrier islands along South Carolina's coast, such as, Kiawah, Seabrook, Dewees, Bulls, Fripp, and Hilton Head.

BASKET CONSTRUCTION

Rosengarten (1987) has provided an excellent review of basketry technique. Coiled basketry involves sewing or stitching unlike other types of baskets that are woven. Each basket begins with a small knot of long-leaf pine needles (*Pinus palustris* Mill.) or the fine-threaded sweetgrass. Pine needles may be used throughout the basket to provide a russet color that contrasts well with the more yellow sweetgrass. Coarse, thicker gauge black rush (*Juncus roemerianus* L.), also known locally as "bulrush, rushel, or needlegrass", may be added to the inside of the baskets for strength. Black rush turns a rich tawny color when dried. Strips of palm leaf (*Sabal palmetto* Lodd.) are used to sew the rows of coils to each other. A hole for the palm strips is made with a bone (a spoon with the bowl removed and the end smoothed and polished), nail, or bagging needle. Shape of the baskets is created by building upon the foundation, one row at a time and then row upon row. The coils of material must constantly be fed with new grasses to maintain a constant foundation of uniform thickness. The strength of the basket depends on how firmly the stitches are pulled. Today, baskets of great variability are constructed by modifying the amounts of these materials to create subtle changes of tone and radical change of texture.

CONSTRAINTS TO INDUSTRY GROWTH

The development of South Carolina's barrier islands and beach fronts has increased the areas economic prosperity and tourism which has been helpful to the basketmakers. However, changes in land ownership, land use and lifestyles have destroyed many plant communities or restricted access to remaining local sweetgrass habitats. Expensive and long journeys to Georgia or Florida are now necessary to gather raw materials. Political help is needed to preserve and protect natural sweetgrass habitats from destruction. Research is needed to learn how to domesticate this wild plant and cultivate sweetgrass as a row crop.

JUSTIFICATION FOR PRESERVING SWEETGRASS BASKETRY

The traditional basket stands along the Ocean Highway are being unintentionally forced out of the community by construction of shopping malls and business parks with road frontage along the highway. These stands have been located on this highway for over 60 years. The display of African baskets has been a major source of income for many basketmakers as well as providing tourists an appreciation of the beauty, significance, and value of this ancient art form. The danger in displacement from traditional marketing areas is that basketmakers would have very few alternatives to sell their baskets in highly visible locations. This frustration may require them to seek other sources of income and cause a loss of basketmakers from the community.

The Mt. Pleasant basketmaking community has become known throughout the United States and abroad for their art. Today, the baskets have become a symbol of coastal South Carolina. The downtown area of Charleston has over 2,000 buildings registered with the Historic Society, yet basketmaking is truly the only "live" viable symbol or relic of the extinct plantation days of colonial times. After 300 years, this tradition, as well as historic buildings, are the trademarks of Charleston. Postcards and photographic illustrations commonly depict basketmakers and their art. African coiled basketry are objects of scholarly research and commonly are featured in newspaper and magazine articles in the United States and abroad. Sweetgrass baskets are displayed in art galleries, traveling exhibits, and have been displayed in the Smithsonian, Vatican, and Gibes Art Museum in Charleston and other museums.

In 1988, the Mt. Pleasant Basketmakers' Association was formed. The function of the Association is to organize the basketmakers into a cohesive group and to form a common voice to influence the management of their resources. The Association's purpose is to promote, preserve, and protect the tradition of sweetgrass basketmaking.

The first Sweetgrass Basket Conference was held on March 26, 1988 to discuss the basketmaking tradition, biological assessment and ecology of sweetgrass resources, impact of coastal development and public and private concerns in relation to the basket industry (McKissick Museum 1988). Through the activities of the Conference, many immediate pledges of public and private aid were offered.

In October, 1988, the Town Council of Mt. Pleasant resolved to make preservation of the basket stands a goal of the zoning process. In December, 1991, the Sweetgrass Preservation Society was formed by the Mayor of Charleston to help the basketmakers work on strategies to help protect and preserve their craft and tradition.

The art of sweetgrass basketmaking has evolved from a practical craft, to a curio, to a genuinely valuable artform. The sweetgrass basketmaking tradition is a crucial element of the African cultural tradition. The descendents of enslaved Africans possess an intimate, loyal, and loving bond of their ancestry and heritage in colonial South Carolina and Africa. Sweetgrass basketmaking is the "living" symbol of this passion.

REFERENCES

Charleston Gazette and Advertiser. 1791. Feb. 15 ed. South Caroliniana Library, Columbia.

Joyner, C. 1984. Down by the riverside: A South Carolina slave community. Univ. of Illinois Press, Urbana.

Littlefield, D. 1981. Rice and slaves: Ethnicity and the slave trade in colonial South Carolina. Baton Rouge.

McKissick Museum, Univ. of South Carolina. 1988. Proc. Sweetgrass Basket Conf. Charleston, 26 Mar. 1988.

Pinson, J. and W. Batson. 1971. The status of *Muhlenbergia filipes* Curtis (Poaceae). J. Elisha Mitchell Sci. Soc. 87(4):188–191.

Rosengarten, D. 1987. Row upon row: Sea grass baskets of the South Carolina lowcountry. McKissick Museum, Univ. of South Carolina.

Vlach, J. 1978. The Afro-american tradition in decorative arts. Cleveland Museum of Art, Cleveland, OH.

FRUITS AND NUTS

Commercialization of Carambola, Atemoya, and Other Tropical Fruits in South Florida

Jonathan H. Crane

Introduction and commercialization of tropical fruit crops into south Florida has been occurring for over 100 years. Two of these crops, carambola and atemoya have begun to be grown commercially in the past 10 to 20 years. This paper will discuss the introduction and culture of tropical fruit crop production in southern Florida with emphasis on carambola and atemoya. Factors which enhance and inhibit commercialization of new tropical fruit crops will also be highlighted.

CARAMBOLA

Carambola or star fruit (*Averrhoa carambola* L., Oxalidaceae) was introduced into Florida over 100 years ago (Knight 1969; Knight 1987; Wolfe 1937) from Southeast Asia (Martin et al. 1987). However, until the early 1970s (Table 1), carambola had been grown only as specimen trees in botanical gardens and experiment stations and as a curiosity in home landscapes.

Carambola was thought to have commercial potential as early as 1941 (Anon. 1941). During the 1960s, there was a resurgence of interest in this fruit which was sold to local restaurants and specialty shops (Vines and Grierson 1966; Knight 1969). Interest was based mostly on its attractive star shape when cut in cross-section and yellow to golden color. Fruit from early introductions were however, sour and sometimes considered unpalatable. This limited market and public acceptance, inhibiting development and expansion of carambola as a commercial fresh fruit.

During the past 56 years introduction, evaluation, and selection of carambola fruit has been actively pursued in South Florida (Table 2) (Campbell 1970; Knight 1982; Wagner et al. 1975). Seeds and/or budwood have been introduced from Hawaii, Malaysia, Taiwan, and Thailand and numerous seedlings have been evaluated by the USDA Subtropical Horticultural Research Station and Germplasm Repository in Miami, Florida. Organizations such as the Rare Fruit Council International, nursery tradesman, and fruit growers have also planted, evaluated, and selected many new cultivars.

During the mid to late 1970s, Morris Arkin, a local nurseryman in Miami, selected a sweet carambola with good handling characteristics from a seedling population which was subsequently named 'Arkin'. Soon afterward, the limited commercial area of carambola under cultivation in south Florida (4 to 12 ha) was top-worked to 'Arkin' and this new cultivar lead to a rapid increase in consumer demand for the fruit which further stimulated interest in establishing new commercial plantings (Table 1).

Table 1. Estimated hectares of commercial carambola in Florida from 1971 to 1991.

Year	Hectares	Reference
1971	4	Campbell 1971
1983	12	Campbell 1983
1984	16	Knight et al. 1984
1985	24	Campbell et al. 1985
1986	61	Campbell 1986
1987	81	Campbell 1988
1988	137	Crane 1991
1989	176	Crane 1989
1990	192	Crane 1991
1991	243	Crane 1991

Table 2. Carambola cultivars introduced or developed and selected in South Florida[z].

Cultivar	Origin of introduction	Flavor	Selected in Florida	Commercial potential	Comments
Arkin	Thailand	Sweet	yes	Excellent	Major cultivar at present
B-2	Malaysia	Sweet	no	Unknown	Under evaluation
B-10	Malaysia	Sweet	no	Unknown	Under evaluation
B-16	Malaysia	Sweet	no	Unknown	Under evaluation
B-17	Malaysia	Sweet	no	Unknown	Under evaluation
Dah Pon	Florida	Sweet	yes	Poor	Poor color, insipid
Demak	Indonesia	Sweet	no	Poor	Bitter after-taste
Fwang Tung	Thailand	Sweet	no	Fair	Poor color, thin ribs
Golden Star	Hawaii	Tart	yes	Poor	Sweet when fully mature
Hew-1	Thailand	Sweet	no	Poor	Whitish spots on fruit
Kary	Hawaii	Sweet	no	Unknown	Under evaluation
Maha	Malaysia	Sweet	no	Poor	Poor color, thin ribs insipid
Mih Tao	Taiwan	Sweet	no	Poor	Insipid
Newcomb	Florida	Tart	yes	Poor	Too tart
Sri Kembangan	Malaysia	Sweet	no	Unknown	Under evaluation
Star King	Florida	Tart	yes	Poor	Too tart
Tean Ma	Taiwan	Sweet	no	Poor	Insipid
Thayer	Florida	Tart	yes	Fair	Too tart, poor flavor

[z]Only named cultivars have been included. Numbered selections from open and hand pollinations have been evaluated but not listed here.

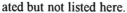

Fig. 1. 'Arkin' carambola.

Today, there is about 243 ha of commercial carambola in south Florida (Table 1). Production for the 1989–90 season was estimated at 1.1 million kg (packed) and production for the 1990–91 season is estimated at 1.6 million kg. The value of the crop is now estimated to be between $1.5 to $2 million annually (Tropical Fruit Advisory Council 1990).

Botany

The carambola is a small tree (7 to 10 m high). Mature seedling trees having a symmetrical canopy (Campbell and Malo 1981); grafted trees a range of shapes (e.g., upright or spreading) and growth habits. Leaves are compound with five to eleven leaflets (Ruehle 1967). Flowers are borne in panicles on twigs and small diameter branches in the leaf axils of present or fallen leaves (Ochse et al. 1961), along larger diameter branches including scaffolding limbs, and occasionally on the main trunk. Flowers are small (1 cm diam.) and perfect with five sepals and petals and pink to lavender in color (Campbell and Malo 1981). The fruit (Fig. 1) is a four to five celled fleshy berry, 5.0 to 12.5 cm long and 3 to 6 cm in diameter with five (sometimes 4 to 6 or more) longitudinal ribs (Ochse et al. 1961). Fruit weight ranges from 100 to 110 g or more (Campbell and Koch 1989) and the waxy exocarp is thin, smooth, and light yellow to dark orange-yellow (Campbell and Malo 1981; Ochse et al. 1961). Fruit flesh is yellow, crisp, and juicy with a mild to strong sour or sweet taste.

Horticulture

Adaptation. Carambola trees are best adapted to hot, humid, wet tropical or subtropical lowland areas (Campbell and Malo 1981; Martin et al. 1987). Air temperatures at or below –1.7° to –2.8°C may kill young trees and damage leaves and twigs on mature trees (Campbell et al. 1985). Mature trees may be severely damaged or killed at temperatures of –4.4° to –6.7°C (Campbell et al. 1985). Overhead, high volume sprinkler irrigation has been observed to be effective in protecting trees and fruit from prolonged freezing temperature.

Carambola cultivars grown and tested in Florida vary in wind tolerance. For instance, 'Golden Star' appears more tolerant to planting in areas exposed to high winds (e.g., >40 km/h) and constant buffeting, whereas newly planted 'Arkin' trees may be stunted and unhealthy in the same location. Constant and strong winds during early to mid-spring can cause desiccation, defoliation, twig and stem dieback, and fruit scarring. Observations indicate planting carambola trees adjacent to natural wind-breaks such as pinelands, hammocks, and Australian pines, within manmade wind-breaks, or interplanting with other crops (e.g., papaya, avocado) enhances the growth, development, and production.

Carambola trees are tolerant of a variety of soil types as long as they are well drained (Campbell and Malo 1981). Joyner and Schaffer (1990) report that carambola trees are moderately flood tolerant. Young 'Golden Star' trees survived continuous or intermittent flooding over an 18 week period. However, flooding decreased carbon assimilation, transpiration, and biomass accumulation compared to non-flooded controls.

Carambolas grow best in neutral to mildly acid pH soils (Campbell et al. 1985) while trees growing in the calcareous high pH soils (pH 7.5 to 8.5) of south Florida often show symptoms of iron, manganese, and magnesium deficiency. These deficiencies may be prevented by periodic foliar applications of micronutrients and soil drenching with iron chelated materials.

Propagation, rootstocks, and cultivars. Trees can be propagated by seed, grafting, budding, and air layering (Campbell et al. 1985). Recently, gibberellic acid applied in a lanolin paste to the basal stem of young seedlings increased stem diameter growth rate, thus reducing the time for plants to reach graftable stem diameter from an average of 93 days to 47 days (Marler and Mickelbart 1991). Currently, a plant is ready for field planting 16 to 24 months after grafting. Propagation by tissue culture has been only partly successful, as shoots but not roots have been regenerated (Litz and Griffis 1989).

Generally, seedlings derived from open pollinated 'Golden Star' and 'Dah Pon' (M-18690) are used as rootstocks in south Florida. This is based on limited rootstock development and selection which compared seedling survival and deficiency symptoms of several crosses over a two-year period (Knight 1982).

Many cultivars have been introduced and evaluated in south Florida during the past 50 odd years (Table 2). Of these, two cultivars stand out: 'Arkin' the primary sweet cultivar grown in south Florida, comprising at least 98% of the current hectarage (Crane 1989); and 'Golden Star' the primary tart cultivar (Campbell 1965). Many of the cultivars introduced into south Florida have proved unsatisfactory for one reason or another. For example, although 'Fwang Tung' is a sweet cultivar, but its large, thin ribs are easily damaged during handling and 'Demak', also sweet, has a bitter after-taste.

Plant spacing, fertilization, and irrigation. There is a broad range of plant spacings and densities (173 to 701 trees/ha) used in carambola production (Crane 1989). However, most (about 60%) of the groves currently employ a 4.6 to 6.1 m spacing within rows and 6.1 to 7.6 m spacing between rows resulting in between 286 to 356 trees/ha. Optimum plant spacing and densities have not been investigated.

Little work has been done concerning fertilizer and irrigation practices for carambola. Current recommendations are based on observation. General fertilizer recommendations include 4 to 6 or more applications of a 6–2.6–5.0 or 11–1.7–10 (NPK) or similar material applied at a rate of 560 kg/ha per application, 1 to 3 foliar applications of micronutrients (manganese, zinc), and 2 to 3 soil drench applications of chelated iron (Campbell et al. 1985; Campbell and Malo 1981). Ferguson et al. (1988) found no difference in trunk calipers and tree heights between young carambola trees fertilized with slow release and standard materials suggesting application frequency could be reduced without reducing tree growth.

The water requirements of carambola have not been determined. Currently 2.54 to 5.1 cm of water are applied after 7 to 10 days of little or no rainfall.

Pruning and tree size control. Little research has been conducted in south Florida on carambola pruning. Generally, young trees are not trained and because the industry is only about 10 years old, tree size control is only now becoming critical in commercial groves. Preliminary results from current field trials on selectively pruned six year old carambola trees has shown the lower and mid-tree canopy remain productive despite pruning of the upper canopy. Furthermore, because only fruit from the ground to about 3.7 m is easily picked, annual pruning at a 3.7 to 4.3 m height may be feasible and result in commercially acceptable yields.

Diseases and insect pests. Several insects may cause damage to carambola fruit including stink bugs, *Acanthocephala* sp., fruit blotch miner (Pena 1986), red-banded thrips [*Selenothrips rubrocinctus* (Giard)], and soft brown scales [*Coccus hesperidum* (L.)] (J.E. Pena pers. commun.). Other pests such as Plumose scale [*Morganella longispina* (Morgan)] and Philephedra scale [*Philephedra tuberculosa* (Nakahara & Gill)] attack twigs and small stems causing defoliation and stem die-back (Pena 1986). Reniform nematodes [*Rotylenchulus reniformis* (Linford & Oliveira)] have been associated with tree decline (Campbell et al. 1985). Birds may attack fruit especially early in the harvest season.

Several leaf spot diseases caused by *Cercopsora averrhoae* Petch., *Corynespora cassiicola* Berk. & Curt. (McMillan 1986), *Phomopsis* sp. and *Phyllosticta* sp. (Campbell et al. 1985), may cause premature leaf drop. Ripe and injured carambola fruit may be attacked by anthracnose (*Colletrotrichum gloeosporioides* Penz.) (McMillan 1986) while a *Leptothyrium* sp. has been identified with "sooty-mold" symptoms on fruit (Simone and Kuchareck 1988). *Pythium splendens* Braun has been recently identified as the cause of a general tree decline syndrome which includes defoliation, twig and root die-back, and reduced fruit production (Ploetz 1991).

Harvest, handling, and utilization. Carambola trees are precocious and generally begin fruit production within the first 12 to 18 months of planting. Five year old trees may produce 45 kg per tree per year while more mature trees (8 to 13 years old) may produce between 90 to 181 kg per tree per year (Campbell et al. 1985). In Florida, some carambolas are available all year, but the commercial season generally ranges from July to February/March. Fruit development takes about 61 to 70 days depending upon cultivar and weather conditions (Campbell and Koch 1989).

Proper harvesting is critical to successful storage and marketing of the fruit. Fruit are carefully harvested by hand at "color break," placed in field boxes, and transported to packinghouses for grading, packing, and storing. Carambolas are non-climacteric (Osland and Davenport 1983) but will develop normal color if picked at color break (Campbell et al. 1987). Fruit can be stored for up to 44 days at 5°C and 85 to 95% relative humidity without suffering chilling damage and develop normal color when transferred to 23°C (Campbell et al. 1987).

Carambola is primarily sold as a fresh fruit although small quantities are sold pickled, in sauces, and jellies. Fresh fruit is incorporated into a wide variety of dishes, salads, desserts, and drinks. Carambola can also be cut in cross-section and dried (Campbell and Campbell 1983).

ATEMOYA

Atemoya trees are hybrids of *Annona squamosa* L. (sugar apple) x *A. cherimola* Mill. (cherimoya) which either result from natural crosses (Morton 1987) or result from a breeding program (Fairchild 1974; Fairchild 1990; Morton 1987). The first recorded manmade crosses occurred in Miami in 1908 (Fairchild 1990; Morton 1987). Natural hybrids have been found in Venezuela (Popenoe 1974) and chance hybrids were noted in adjacent sugar apple and cherimoya groves in Israel during the 1930s and 1940s (Morton 1987). The name atemoya was proposed by P.J. Wester for these sugar apple, cherimoya hybrids and combines "ate," an original name for sugar apple, with "moya" taken from the last two syllables of cherimoya (Fairchild 1990).

The purpose of the initial crosses among sugar apples and cherimoyas was to incorporate the excellent fruit quality and cold tolerance of the subtropically adapted cherimoyas (which did not grow or fruit well in humid lowland areas like south Florida) with the sugar apple which is well adapted to warm, humid, subtropical, and tropical climates (Fairchild 1990). Some seedlings of these early crosses appeared to produce fruit with excellent quality (Fairchild 1990) and possessed sufficient cold hardiness to have survived freezing weather (−3.1°C) in 1917 (Morton 1987).

Despite these early breeding successes and introduction of numerous cultivars (Table 3) from countries such as Israel and Venezuela (Popenoe 1974), atemoyas remained a home garden and specimen tree in botanical gardens and germplasm repositories until the early (Campbell 1983) to mid-1980s (Anon. 1986) (Table 4). This was due to poor fruit set and yields, alternate bearing, splitting of mature fruit, and uneven ripening of these early selections (Popenoe 1974).

Commercial development of the crop was greatly facilitated by the introduction 'Gefner' atemoya from Israel which is a fairly reliable bearer of good quality fruits. Even so, the search and development for superior atemoya cultivars continues in south Florida, both by private individuals (Mahdeem 1989; Mahdeem 1990) and at the USDA Subtropical Research Unit and Germplasm Repository in Miami.

Today, south Florida has about 49 ha of commercial atemoyas (Table 4). Production is estimated to be about 68 to 91 kg annually and the crop worth $250,000 to $400,000.

Botany

The atemoya is a member of the Annonaceae and is a small tree (up to 10 m) with a symmetrical, globose, dense canopy. Leaves are lanceolate, ovate, or elliptic, and deciduous (Campbell and Phillips 1980). Flowers possess 3 fleshy petals, are yellowish-green, and are borne singly or in clusters of 2 to 3 in leaf axils on new shoots or 1 to 2 year old wood (Campbell and Phillips 1980). Fruit type is aggregate, formed by the coherence of many pistils (Fig. 2). Fruit is green to greenish-yellow, conical to ovate shaped, with slight to pronounced surface protuberances (Campbell and Malo 1980). Pulp is white, smooth textured, containing 10 to 40 dark brown to black seeds per fruit. Fruit weigh between 225 to 450 g (Campbell and Malo 1980).

Table 3. Atemoya cultivars introduced or developed and selected in South Florida[z].

Cultivar	Origin of introduction[y]	Selected in Florida	Commercial potential	Comments[x]
African Pride[w]	South Africa	no	Poor	Requires hand pollination, uneven fruit ripening
Bernitski	Israel	no	Poor	Poor fruit set, may require hand pollination
Bradley	Florida	yes	Poor	Requires hand pollination, fruit splits
Caves	Florida	yes	Poor	
Cherimata	Egypt	no	Poor	
Chirimorinon A	Venezuela	no	Poor	
Chirimorinon B	Venezuela	no	Poor	
Chirimorinon C	Venezuela	no	Poor	
Finny	Egypt	no	Poor	
Gefner	Israel	no	Excellent	Major cultivar in south Florida
Island Beauty	Australia	no		
Island Gem	Australia	no	Poor	Small fruit, poor fruit set
Lindstrom	Australia	no	Poor	
Malali#1	Israel	no	Poor	Poor fruit set
Malamud	Israel	no	Poor	
Page	Florida	yes	Poor	Fruit splitting
Pinks's Mammoth	Australia	no	Poor	Poor fruit set
Priestly	Australia	no	Poor	Requires hand pollination
Stermer	Hawaii	no	Poor	

[z]Only named cultivars are included in the table.
[y]Florida cultivars were selected from seedling populations.
[x]Blank space indicates insufficient data to comment.
[w]Synonymous with 'Kaller' which originated in Israel.

Table 4. Estimated hectares of commercial atemoya in Florida from 1985 to 1991.

Year	Hectares	Reference
1985	8	Anonymous 1986
1986	12	Campbell 1986
1988	18	Anonymous 1989
1989	19	Crane 1989
1990	28	J.H. Crane unpublished
1991	49	J.H. Crane unpublished

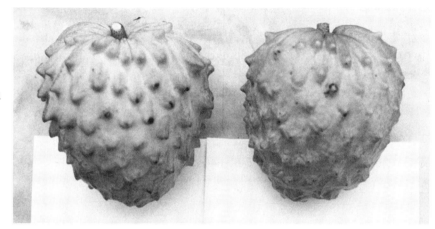

Fig. 2. 'Gefner' (left) and 'African Pride' (right) atemoya.

Horticulture

Adaptation. Atemoyas are adapted to a wide range of temperatures, from lowland tropical to cool subtropical climates. In south Florida during January 1977, young trees were killed or severely injured by prolonged temperatures between $-6.7°$ to $-3.9°C$ whereas mature trees withstood those temperatures with slight to moderate damage (Campbell et al. 1977). High volume overhead and under tree irrigation were observed to protect young and mature trees during the 1989 freeze in South Florida.

Observation by the author suggests strong, constant winds during late winter and spring may cause young atemoya trees to either lean in the leeward direction and/or to develop canopy and limbs only on the leeward side giving trees an unbalanced canopy.

Atemoyas are adapted to a range of soil types as long as the soils are well drained (Campbell and Phillips 1980; Morton 1987). Micronutrient deficiencies appear to be less of a problem in soils with a neutral to moderately acid pH (5 to 7). In the high pH calcareous soils of South Florida, micronutrient deficiencies can be prevented with the use of micronutrient foliar sprays of manganese and zinc and chelated iron soil drenches.

Propagation, rootstocks, and cultivars. Atemoyas may be propagated by seed, grafting, and budding. However, fruit quality and production of seedlings is extremely variable. Trees may be veneer, cleft or whip grafted (Campbell and Phillips 1980; Morton 1987) and pre-graft preparation of budwood increases success (Ogden et al. 1981). Grafted trees begin to produce fruit in 3 to 4 years.

Several rootstocks have been recommended for atemoya, including pond apple (*Annona glabra* L.), custard apple (*A. reticulata* L.), sugar apple (*A. squamosa* L.), and atemoya (Campbell and Phillips 1980). However, delayed incompatibility problems occur with pond apple (Campbell and Phillips 1980) and custard apple (Cockshutt 1990). At present, sugar apple and atemoya seedlings are the most commonly used rootstocks. Seeds of atemoya and sugar apple appear to have an after ripening requirement of 3 to 6 months which delays planting for seedling rootstocks.

A number of cultivars have been selected in south Florida or introduced from other countries (Table 3). However, problems such as poor natural fruit set, fruit splitting, and uneven ripening have precluded their use commercially. Only the 'Gefner', introduced from Israel has proven commercially viable. However, local nursery people (Hahdeem 1990) and researchers at the USDA Subtropical Research Station, Miami, continue to develop and evaluate new germplasm in search of improved cultivars.

Plant spacing, fertilization, and irrigation. Moderate plant spacings (6 to 7 × 6 to 9 m) and plant densities (158 to 277 trees per ha) are suggested for atemoya groves. An industry survey found 42% of the current south Florida hectarage at low plant densities (143 to 215 trees per ha) and wide spacings (6.1 to 8.2 × 7.6 to 8.5 m), 34% at moderate plant densities (268 to 431 trees per ha) and spacings (3.8 to 6.1 × 6.1 to 7.0 m), and 24% at high plant densities (528 trees per ha) and close spacings (3.1 × 6.1 m) (Crane 1989). Most low density plantings are interplanted with another fruit crop such as sugar apple or carambola. Optimum plant spacings and densities have not yet been determined.

Little research has been conducted to determine the optimum fertilizer recommendations for atemoya. Current recommendations for young trees include bimonthly applications of 6–2.6–5.0 (NPK) or similar material at 100 g per tree (Campbell and Phillips 1980). As trees mature an 8–1.3–7.5 (NPK) or similar material should be applied 3 to 4 times per year at the rate of 450 g per tree per 2.5 cm of trunk diameter per application. To prevent micronutrient deficiencies, foliar application of magnesium, manganese, and zinc and soil drenches of chelated iron are typically made 2 to 4 times per year.

Irrigation is recommended during dry periods and has been observed to be important during bloom, fruit set, and fruit development (Campbell and Phillips 1980). Excessive irrigation or rainfall during fruit maturation may increase fruit splitting.

Pruning and tree size control. To date, little work has been done on the training and pruning of atemoya trees. Early recommendations (Campbell and Phillips 1980) suggested training young trees to an open center form to increase scaffold strength. Periodically thereafter, shoots should be headed back to keep trees manageable and easy to harvest.

Pollination. Atemoya flowers are protogynous with the flowers first functionally female; flowers begin to open in the late afternoon and by the following morning are fully open and receptive (Nagel et al. 1989). The flowers begin functioning as males by the late afternoon and early evening following the female stage. Usually, by this time however, the stigmas are dry and unreceptive, precluding self-pollination.

Atemoyas are successfully pollinated by a complex of beetles in the family Nitidulidae (commonly called sap beetles) (Nagel et al. 1989). These sap beetles are most abundant from 8:00 am to 4:00 pm and remain at the base of the flower for many hours. Hand-pollination is also practiced by some growers to insure adequate fruit set, increase early fruit set, and enhance fruit uniformity (Cockshutt 1990). Attempts to induce parthenocarpic fruit with gibberellic acid have not been successful (Campbell 1979).

Disease and insect pests. Atemoya fruit are attacked by the annona seed borer [*Bephratelloides cubensis* (Ashmead)], mealy bugs (*Pseudococcus* sp.), and Philephedra scale [*Philephedra truberculosa* (Nakahara & Gill)] (Pena 1986). Leaves and stems are attacked by Cyanophyllum scale [*Abgrallafpif cyanophylli* (Signoret)], Philephedra scale (Pena 1986), and ambrosia beetles (stems only) (*Xylosandrus* sp.) (Campbell and Phillips 1980).

Several diseases affect the fruit including anthracnose (*Colletotrichum gloeosporioides* Penz.) and *Botryodiplodia theobromae* Pat. (McMillan 1986). A rust fungus (*Phokospora cherimoliae* Cumm.) attacks leaves causing early defoliation (McMillan 1986). Recently, *Pythium splendens* Bruan has been shown to be the cause of a tree decline in commercial groves (Ploetz 1991). This decline is more prevalent in poorly drained or excessively wet groves.

Harvest, handling, and utilization. The atemoya season is generally from August to January with the peak during August through October. About 100 to 120 days are required from flowering to horticultural maturity and this depends upon the weather and cultural conditions. Mature trees may produce from 23 to 34 kg per tree, possibly more with good management.

Atemoya fruit are carefully clipped from the branches, leaving a small portion of the peduncle. Fruit are harvested when they have turned from green to greenish-yellow and the area between protuberances has filled out. Fruit have limited storage life (5 to 10 days) but can be held for several days at 13°C to slow ripening. The atemoya is primarily consumed as a fresh fruit but the pulp is used in desserts, salads, ice creams, and milk shakes.

MISCELLANEOUS COMMERCIAL TROPICAL FRUITS

In 1991, there were approximately 9,308 ha of commercial tropical fruit crops in south Florida (Table 5). Dade County had about 96% (8,903 ha), Lee County had about 353 ha, Collier and Broward Counties had 20 ha each, and Palm Beach County about 12 ha. A recent study (Mosely 1990) found gross sales of tropical fruits from Dade County, Florida, to be about $74 million annually (Table 6).

Avocados, limes, and mangos make up about 83% of the hectarage (Table 5). Smaller but significant commercial hectarage of atemoya, banana, carambola, mamey sapote, longan, lychee, papaya, passion fruit, and sugar apple also exist. There is also minor but increasing commercial hectarage of Barbados cherry, guava, kumquat, and sapodilla. A number of entrepreneurs have establish small plantings of canistel, black sapote, jaboticaba, jackfruit, pummelo, wampee, wax jambu, and white sapote.

Although many tropical fruit crops were introduced into Florida during the past 70 to 490 years (Table 7) (Knight 1987; Krome and Goldweber 1987; Wolfe 1937), only limes, grapefruit, avocados, mangos, and papayas have been successfully grown commercially (Krome and Goldweber 1987; Wolfe 1937). For the past 20 to 30 years, Barbados cherry, sapodilla, guava, banana, mamey sapote, and lychee have been grown on a limited commercial scale (Campbell 1970; Campbell 1971), and only during the last 5 to 10 years has commercial hectarage of carambola, atemoya, sugar apple, longan, kumquat, and passion fruit been established (Campbell 1983; Campbell 1986).

The potential for continued or expanded commercial development of various tropical fruit crops in south Florida varies by plant species (Table 5). For example, the outlook for increased avocado and mango hectarage is poor due to foreign competition from Central and South America; the outlook for increased lychee, pummelo, jackfruit, and sugar apple appears promising because of increasing demand by Asian and Hispanic Americans; the outlook for increased longan and canistel hectarage is limited by lack of improved cultivars or selections.

In South Florida, horticultural practices for crops such as avocados, limes, and mangos has been well researched and are well known (see references cited by Lamberts and Crane 1990). However, horticultural information on crops such as atemoya, Barbados cherry, passion fruit, and carambola is limited. For some crops, such as canistel, jaboticaba, wax jambu, and wampee information is almost nonexistent.

References to available literature concerning horticultural practices for the tropical fruit crops listed in Table 5, were compiled and discussed previously (Lamberts and Crane 1990). The following section will highlight some of the issues and problems facing new fruit crop development.

TROPICAL FRUIT INDUSTRY DEVELOPMENT

Limitations

There are numerous factors which impede the commercial development of new tropical fruit crops in South Florida. These include unfamiliarity with the crop by the general public, lack of funds for marketing and promotion by producers, limited production volume and season of availability, financial risk for the entrepreneur, marginally acceptable cultivars or selections from the producers standpoint, lack of pesticides and the recalcitrance of regulators to assist in registering pesticides for "minor" crops, and reluctance by county tax assessors to grant agricultural exemptions for land with new crops.

Unfamiliarity by the general population is one of the most limiting factors encountered when marketing any new tropical fruit crop. People unfamiliar with the crop usually do not know how to tell when the fruit is mature enough to eat, how to prepare it, and perhaps not even what part is edible. In addition, if the price per fruit is too high they may not want to risk buying something they may not like. Basically, exposure to the fruit and education of people in the wholesale and retail trade as well as the consumer must occur to create consumer demand for these new crops.

Funding for market development and promotion is a limiting factor for increasing the demand for tropical fruit crops. Generally, new tropical fruit crops are grown by entrepreneurs who have spotted a potential niche, such as an ethnic or novelty market. Local marketing and promotion of the crop is by word-of-mouth. This was the case with carambola and was probably the case for most of Florida's tropical fruit crops at one time or another.

Table 5. Current estimated hectarage of tropical fruit crops in south Florida.

Common name	Scientific name	Estimated area of production (ha)	Potential for commercial expansion
Atemoya	*Annona cherimola* L. x *A. squamosa* L.	49	Excellent
Avocado	*Persea americana* Mill.	3,642	Poor
Banana	*Musa* sp. hybrids	162	Good
Barbados cherry	*Malpighia glabra* L.	11	Excellent
Black sapote	*Diospyros ebenaster* Retz.	<1	Fair
Canistel	*Pouteria campechiana* Baehni	<1	Fair
Carambola	*Averrhoa carambola* L.	243	Good
Guava	*Psidium guajava* L.	31	Excellent
Jaboticaba	*Myrciaria cauliflora* Berg.	<1	Fair
Jackfruit	*Artocarpus heterophyllus* Lam.	<1	Good
Kumquat	*Fortunella* sp.	10	Good
Tahiti lime	*Citrus* x 'Tahiti'	2,865	Excellent
Longan	*Euphoria longana* Steud.	30	Fair
Lychee	*Litichi chinensis* Sonn.	81	Excellent
Mamey sapote	*Calocarpum sapota* Merr.	108	Fair
Mango	*Mangifera indica* L.	1,172	Fair
Papaya	*Carica papaya* L.	142	Good
Passion fruit	*Passiflora edulis* Sims	41	Excellent
Plantain	*Musa* sp.	81	Good
Pummelo	*Citrus grandis* (L.) Osbeck	8	Good
Sapodilla	*Manilkara zapota* Van Royen	8	Fair
Sugar apple	*Annona squamosa* L.	41	Good
Wampee	*Clausena lansium* (Lour.) Skeels	<1	Fair
Wax jambu	*Syzygium samarangense* Merr. et Perry	<1	Good
White sapote	*Casimiroa edulis* Llav. et Lex.	<1	Excellent

This seems to be adequate only initially, prior to increased competition among producers. Marketing and promotion on a larger scale is then necessary, but the funds are usually not available.

The volume and availability of fruit may also impede or limit commercial development. Production volume of new crops is almost always limited. This is because expansion of production may pose large financial risk by the entrepreneur and the area of production is limited. Early entrepreneurs may for various reasons wish for the volume of production to remain limited so prices remain high and/or they cannot afford to expand. In addition, a limited season of availability may in some cases limit demand for the tropical fruit crop because it must essentially be reintroduced each season.

The lack of suitable cultivars has had a pronounced negative effect on the commercial development of some tropical fruit crops such as longan, white sapote, and canistel. Sometimes, current cultivars may be adequate to meet local demand for quality and storage life but not withstand handling and storage requirements for longer distance distribution. Cultivars may also be unsuitable because of low yields (e.g., 'Brewster' lychee), unreliable bearing (e.g., 'Kohala' longan), short storage and shelf life (e.g., sugar apple, atemoya), poor taste, and insect and disease susceptibility.

Another impediment to the commercial development of tropical fruit crops in south Florida is the lack of registered pesticides for even basic cultural practices like weed control. The lack of chemicals increase the financial risk to growers who may loose their crop to insect and/or diseases and must use more costly and less efficient pest control methods. The lack of understanding and unwillingness on the part of the pesticide regulatory community to facilitate new crop development by streamlining the pesticide registration process slows new crop development at best and prevents it at worst. Programs such as the Interregional Project-4, designed to assist

Table 6. Current estimated gross crop value of tropical fruit crops produced in Dade County, Florida[z].

Commodity	Total crop value (millions $)
Limes	28.4
Avocados	17.8
Mangos	14.9
Mamey sapote	2.5
Banana/plantain	1.2
Papayas	0.9
Others[y]	8.3
Total	74.0

[z]Data modified from Mosely (1990).
[y]Includes carambola, passion fruit, lychee, atemoya, sugar apple, guava, kumquat, longan, and Barbados cherries.

Table 7. Year selected tropical fruit crops were introduced into Florida.

Tropical fruit	Year introduced	Reference
Atemoya[z]	1908	Fairchild 1990; Morton 1987
Avocado	1833	Morton 1987
Banana[y]	1887	Knight 1987; Wolfe 1937
Barbados cherry[y]	1887	Knight 1987; Wolfe 1937
Black sapote	1919	Morton 1987
Canistel[y]	1887	Knight 1987
Carambola[y]	1887	Knight 1987; Wolfe 1937
Guava[x]	1500s(1912)	Ledin 1957; Morton 1987; Wolfe 1937
Jaboticaba	1913	Morton 1987
Jackfruit	1887	Morton 1987
Kumquat	1885	Ziegler and Wolfe 1981
Tahiti lime	1883	Morton 1987: Ziegler and Wolfe 1981
Longan	1903	Morton 1987
Lychee[y]	1883	Morton 1987: Wolfe 1937
Mamey sapote[y]	1887	Morton 1987; Wolfe 1937
Mango[w]	1833/1862	Crane and Campbell 1991; Morton 1987
Papaya	1500s	Ledin 1957
Passion fruit[y]	1887	Knight 1987; Wolfe 1937
Plantain	1500s	Ledin 1957
Pummelo[y]	1887	Knight 1987
Sapodilla[y]	1889	Knight 1987
Sugar apple[y]	1887	Knight 1987; Wolfe 1937
Wampee	1908	Morton 1987
Wax jambu	1953	Whitman and Wirkus 1957
White sapote[y]	1887	Wolfe 1937

[z]Hybrid of sugar apple and cherimoya developed in Florida.
[y]Introduced sometime before 1887.
[x]First formal commercial planting established in 1912 (Morton 1987).
[w]Introduced in 1833 but not successfully established until 1862 or 1863 (Morton 1987).

minor crop producers register pesticides, is of great assistance. However, the time frame from requesting the use of a particular pesticide to actual registration may take 2 to 5 years.

Finally, due to the unfamiliarity of local tax assessors with new crops, some entrepreneurs are denied agricultural exemptions for their groves. This increases the financial risk of the enterprise and may forestal or prevent the entry of potential producers.

Facilitation

There are several factors which may facilitate the commercial development of new tropical fruit crops in Florida, including large ethnic populations familiar with tropical fruit crops, potential for some tropical fruit crops to appeal to the general population, entrepreneurial producers and packinghouses, marketing and promotion, development and selection of improved cultivars, applied and basic research at federal and state institutions, and federal-state programs to facilitate pesticide registration, and tax breaks.

The development of local demand and markets for many of the tropical fruit crops grown in south Florida stems from Florida's large Hispanic (about 49%) (Israel and Stephenson 1990; Anon. 1991) and substantial Caribbean and Asian populations. Many people from Hispanic, Asian, and Caribbean countries are familiar with the tropical fruit crops which can be grown in south Florida and will pay good prices for the locally available fresh fruit.

The capacity for a new crop to be accepted by the general population is a primary factor in its potential demand and expanded commercial production. Tropical fruit crops currently seen to have appeal to the general public include carambola, lychee, guava, and passion fruit. Others such as jackfruit, pummelo, wax jambu, and white sapote have a good chance for increased production and commercialization to meet increasing ethnic demand.

Critical to the introduction and development of new tropical fruit crops are those individuals and companies willing to facilitate commercial development of tropical fruit crops by their efforts at producing and promoting them. These entrepreneurs base their efforts on early experiences with the crop on a small scale, investigation of potential markets, and a vision that the crop can succeed commercially. Local marketing and promotion of the crop by word-of-mouth or local advertising can help establish a consumer base from which to build. This is true of atemoyas, sugar apples, lychees, sapodilla, and guava, to name a few. Later, as the industry develops, professional literature and advertising by individuals and packinghouses becomes necessary to continue and expand consumer demand.

Institutions such as the USDA Subtropical Research Station and Germplasm Repository, the University of Florida's Tropical Research and Education Center, and Fairchild Tropical Garden Tropical Fruit Program assist in the development and commercialization of new tropical fruit crops by introducing, evaluating, and disseminating new plant material. Some horticultural research is being conducted on underdeveloped tropical fruit crops by researchers at these institutions during the early stages of commercialization. Of great importance also, are individuals in the nursery business involved in their own breeding and/or selection of new cultivars and the propagation and dissemination of this new material.

Registration of pesticides for use on "minor" crops is greatly facilitated by the Interregional Research Project-4 which is a joint effort by the USDA, State Agricultural Experiment Stations, Environmental Protection Agency, Food and Drug Agency, pesticide manufacturers, and growers (Anon. 1988). This program has enabled the generation of scientific data and information required by EPA and the States for registering a number of pesticides for use in tropical fruit production in south Florida.

Finally, agricultural tax exemptions, which lower the tax rates on property used for commercial agriculture can help to lower the financial risk many entrepreneurs have when beginning to produce a new crop on a commercial scale.

REFERENCES

Anon. 1941. Tropical fruit in Florida with commercial possibilities. State of Fla. Dept. Agr., Tallahassee.

Anon. 1986. Dade County Florida minor tropical fruit crops, p. 39. In: Marketing Florida tropical fruits and vegetables—summary 1985–86. Federal-State Market News, Winter Park, FL.

Anon. 1988. Project statement: A national agricultural program to clear pest control agents and animal drugs for minor uses. Communications Services, New York State Agr. Expt. Sta., Geneva.

Anon. 1989. Dade County Florida minor tropical fruit crops, p. 41. In: Marketing Florida tropical fruits and vegetables—summary 1988–89. Federal-State Market News, Winter Park, FL.

Anon. 1991. Census: S. Florida grows to a Latin beat. The Miami Herald, Sect. 22A.

Campbell, B.A. and C.W. Campbell. 1983. Preservation of tropical fruits by drying. Proc. Fla. State Hort. Soc. 96:229–231.

Campbell, C.A. and K.E. Koch. 1989. Sugar/acid composition and development of sweet and tart carambola fruit. J. Amer. Soc. Hort. Sci. 114:455–457.

Campbell, C.A., K.E. Koch, and D.H. Huber. 1987. Postharvest response of carambolas to storage at low temperatures. Proc. Fla. State Hort. Soc. 100:272–275.

Campbell, C.W. 1965. The golden star carambola. Cir. S-173. Univ. of Florida, IFAS, Coop. Extn. Serv., Gainesville.

Campbell, C.W. 1970. Minor tropical fruit cultivars in Florida. Proc. Fla. State Hort. Soc. 83:353–356.

Campbell, C.W. 1971. Commercial production of minor tropical fruit crops in Florida. Proc. Fla. State Hort. Soc. 84:320–323.

Campbell, C.W. 1979. Effect of gibberellin treatment and hand pollination on fruit-set of atemoya (Annona hybrid). Proc. Trop. Reg., J. Amer. Soc. Hort. Sci. 23:122–124.

Campbell, C.W. 1983. Tropical fruit produced commercially in Florida. Proc. Amer. Soc. Hort. Sci. Trop. Reg. 27(A):101–110.

Campbell, C.W. 1986. Tropical fruit crops—A rapidly changing situation. Proc. Fla. State Hort. Soc. 99:217–219.

Campbell, C.W. 1988. Tropical fruits produced and marketed in Florida. HortScience 23:247.

Campbell, C.W. and S.E. Malo. 1981. The carambola. Fruit Crops Fact Sheet FC-12. Univ. of Florida, IFAS, Coop. Extn. Serv., Gainesville.

Campbell, C.W. and R.L. Phillips. 1980. The atemoya. Fruit Crops Fact Sheet FC-64. Univ. of Florida, IFAS, Coop. Extn. Serv., Gainesville.

Campbell, C.W., R.J. Knight, Jr., and R. Olszack. 1985. Carambola production in Florida. Proc. Fla. State Hort. Soc. 98:145–149.

Campbell, C.W., R.J. Knight, Jr., and N.L. Zareski. 1977. Freeze damage to tropical fruits in southern Florida in 1977. Proc. Fla. State Hort. Soc. 90:254–257.

Cockshutt, N. 1990. Annona problems and prospects in south Florida. Fairchild Tropical Garden—Tropical Fruit World. 1:123–125.

Crane, J.H. 1989. Acreage and plant densities of commercial carambola, mamey sapote, lychee, longan, sugar apple, atemoya, and passion fruit plantings in south Florida. Proc. Fla. State Hort. Soc. 102:239–242.

Crane, J.H. and C.W. Campbell. 1991. The mango. Fruit Crops Fact Sheet FC-2. Univ. of Florida, IFAS, Coop. Extn. Serv., Gainesville.

Crane, J.H., C.W. Campbell, and R. Olszack. 1989. Current statistics for commercial carambola groves in south Florida. Proc. Interamer. Soc. Trop. Hort. 33:94–99.

Fairchild, W. 1974. The annonaceous fruits, p. 161–195. In: Manual of tropical and subtropical fruits. Hafner Press, New York.

Fairchild, D. 1990. Who knows the annonas? Fairchild Tropical Garden—Tropical Fruit World. 1:99–108.

Ferguson, J.J., J.H. Crane, and R. Olszack. 1988. Growth of young carambola trees using standard and controlled-release fertilizers. Proc. Interamer. Soc. Trop. Hort. 32:20–24.

Hadeem, H. 1989. Reaching for perfection—future focus on annonas. Tropical Fruit News 23:12,16–19.

Hadeem, H. 1990. Zill's annona project. Fairchild Tropical Garden—Tropical Fruit World 1:109.

Israel, G.D. and W.C. Stephenson. 1990. Population and agriculture in Florida: A new look at trends and characteristics—Challenge '95, excellence in Florida extension programs (PE-13). Univ. of Florida, IFAS, Coop. Extn. Serv., Gainesville.

Joyner, M.E.B. and B. Schaffer. 1989. Flooding tolerance of 'Golden Star' carambola trees. Proc. Fla. State Hort. Soc. 102:236–239.

Knight, Jr., R.J. 1969. The carambola: A fruit for south Florida. Muse News 1:60–61, 75.

Knight, Jr., R.J. 1982. Response of carambola seedling populations to Dade County's oolitic limestone soil. Proc. Fla. State Hort. Soc. 95:121–122.

Knight, Jr., R.J. 1987. New tropical fruit crops of 1887—A blueprint for today, and a sweepstakes. Proc. Fla. State Hort. Soc. 100:265–268.

Knight, Jr., R.J. 1988. Miscellaneous tropical fruits grown and marketed in Florida. Proc. Interamer. Soc. Trop. Hort. 32:34–41.

Knight, R.J., M. Lamberts, and J. Bunch. 1984. World and local importance of some tropical fruits grown in Florida. Proc. Fla. State Hort. Soc. 97:351–354.

Krome, W.H. and S. Goldweber. 1987. Commercial fruit production in Dade County 1990–1987. Proc. Fla. State Hort. Soc. 100:268–272.

Lamberts, M.L. and J.H. Crane. 1990. Tropical fruits, p. 337–355. In: J. Janick and J.E. Simon (eds.). Advances in new crops. Timber Press, Portland, OR.

Litz, R.E. and J.L. Griffis, Jr. 1989. Carambola, p. 59–67. In: Y.P.S. Bajaj (ed.). Biotechnology in agriculture and forestry. vol. 5. Trees II. Springer-Verlag, Berlin.

Ledin, R.B. 1957. Tropical and subtropical fruits in Florida (other than citrus). Econ. Bot. 11:349–376.

Marler, T.E. and M.V. Mickelbart. 1991. Basal GA_{4+7} application enhances carambola seedling growth. Subtrop. Trop. Hort. (in press).

Martin, F.W., C.W. Campbell, and R.M. Ruberte. 1987. Perennial edible fruit of the tropics. USDA/ARS Agr. Handbk. 642.

McMillan, Jr., R.T. 1986. Serious diseases of tropical fruits in Florida. Proc. Fla. State Hort. Soc. 99:224–227.

Morton, J.F. 1987. Annonaceae, p. 65–90. In: Fruits of warm climates. J.F. Morton Publisher, Miami, FL.

Moseley, A.E. 1990. Economic impact of agriculture and agribusiness in Dade County, Florida. Industry Report 90–94. Food and Resource Economics Dept., Univ. of Florida, IFAS, Gainesville, FL.

Nagel, J., J.E. Pena, and D. Habeck. 1989. Insect pollination of atemoya in Florida. The Fla. Entom. 72:207–211.

Ochse, J.J., M.J. Soule, Jr., M.J. Dijkman, and C. Wehlburg. 1961. Tropical and subtropical agriculture. Macmillan, New York.

Ogden, M.H., C.W. Campbell, and S.P. Lara. 1981. Grafting annonas in southern Florida. Proc. Fla. State Hort. Soc. 94:355–358.

Oslund, C.R. and T.L. Davenport. 1983. Ethylene and carbon dioxide in ripening fruit of *Averrhoa carambola* L. HortScience 18: 229–230.

Pena, J.E. 1986. Status of pests of minor tropical fruit crops in south Florida. Proc. Fla. State Hort. Soc. 99:227–230.

Ploetz, R.C. 1991. Species of Pythium as pathogens of perennial, woody fruit crops in south Florida. Phytopathology 81:699 (Abstr.).

Popenoe, J. 1974. Status of annona culture in south Florida. Proc. Fla. State Hort. Soc. 87:342–344.

Ruehle, G.D. 1967. Miscellaneous tropical and subtropical Florida fruits. Agr. Ext. Serv., Univ. of Florida, IFAS, Bul. 156A.

Simone, G. and T. Kucharek. 1988. Extension plant pathology report. Coop. Ext. Serv., Univ. of Florida, IFAS, Gainesville.

Tropical Fruit Advisory Council. 1990. The south Florida tropical fruit plan. Fla. Dept. Agr. and Consumer Services, Tallahassee.

Vines, H.M. and W. Grierson. 1966. Handling and physiological studies with the carambola. Proc. Fla. State Hort. Soc. 79:350–355.

Whitman, W.F. and L.V. Wirkus. 1957. Rare fruit council activities, 1956–57. Proc. Fla. State Hort. Soc. 70:307–314.

Wolfe, H.S. 1937. Fifty years of tropical fruit culture. Proc. Fla. State Hort. Soc. 50:72–78.

Ziegler, L.W. and H.S. Wolfe. 1981. The kinds of citrus fruits, p. 12–62. In: Citrus growing in Florida. 3rd ed. The Univ. Presses of Fla., Gainesville.

Rambutan and Pili Nuts: Potential Crops for Hawaii

Francis T. Zee

Rambutan and pili nuts are important crops of commerce in Southeast Asia but are relatively unknown in the United States. The lack of a postharvest quarantine treatment for fruit fly infestation in rambutan, and the inconsistent production and lack of quality control in pili nuts are some of the causes hindering the expansion of these crops. With the decline of the sugar industry and the diversification of its agricultural industries, Hawaii could become a potential production and launching site for these crops into the mainland United States.

RAMBUTAN

Rambutan fruits are consumed fresh, canned, or preserved. The colorful fruits of rambutan are frequently used in displays with flower and fruit arrangements.

Origin

Nephelium lappaceum Linn., Sapindaceae, is native to Malaysia and Indonesia. Rambutan, a tropical relative of the lychee (*Litchi chinensis* Sonn.), is grown in Southeast Asia, Australia, South America, and Africa, but only exported from Malaysia and Thailand (Laksmi et al. 1987).

Morphology

The word *rambutan* is derived from the Malay word "hair," which describes the numerous, characterizing, long, soft, red or red and green colored spine-like protuberances (spinterns) on the surface of the fruit. The pericarp of this attractive oval-shaped fruit can be red, orange, pink, or yellow in color and is removable by a twist of the hands. The edible, pearlish white, juicy, crispy, sweet and subacid flavored flesh (sarcotesta) conceals a single seed with a thin, fibrous seed coat (testa).

Rambutan is an evergreen tree about 10 to 12 m tall, has pinnately compound leaves without the presence of an end-leaflet. On the lower surface of each leaflet are the domatia, small crater-like hills located in the axils between the mid and secondary veins. The function of the domatia is unknown (Van Welzen et al. 1988).

Rambutan has perfect flowers, however, they are functionally pistillate or staminate. Most commercial cultivars behave hermaphroditically and are self fertile, with 0.05 to 0.9% of the functional females possessing functional stamens. Insect pollination is needed. Flowers are produced on matured terminal or sub-branches in panicles; they are small, greenish white in color and in large numbers (1,200 to 1,700 flowers per panicle). Depending on the cultivar, flowering may spread over a period of 23 to 38 days, with an average of 3.4% setting fruit. Fruits may be produced in large bunches, with 40 to 60 fruits per panicle, but most often only 12 to 13 per panicle are retained to maturity. Final fruit set is usually between 0.7 to 1.45%. Time required from fruit set to harvest is about 107 to 111 days (Van Welzen et al. 1988).

Fruit size ranges from 27 to 80 g. Edible flesh weight, depending on season and cultivar, may range from 28 to 54% of the fruit weight. Total soluble solids can reach 24% (Lye et al. 1987). Economic life of a tree is about 15 to 20 years and may be up to 30 years. Depending on the location, rambutan can produce up to two crops a year (Laksmi et al. 1987).

Culture

Rambutan trees prefer deep, loamy, well drained soil with a high organic content. Optimum temperature range is above 22°C. An absolute temperature of 5° to 6°C will cause defoliation and poor cropping. Trees need to have well distributed rainfall and wind protection.

At the National Clonal Germplasm Repository, USDA/ARS, in Hilo, Hawaii, rambutan seedlings grew best in full sun, protected from wind, in a 1:1:1 medium of soil, macadamia compost, and volcanic cinder, and fertilized with a high potassium (10–2–33 NPK) fertilizer. Young seedlings given a lower potash formulation (16–7–13 NPK) produced severe marginal necrosis of leaves, stunted growth, and die-back of apical growth.

Well grown rootstocks are bud grafted at 8 to 12 months. Dormant buds with well-healed petiole scars from one to two year old branches averaged 80% success between May and October. Rootstocks should be cut back 25 cm above the bud union and all foliage removed at two weeks after budding. This cutback and defoliation promoted bud break of the new graft 14 to 17 days later (Zee and Kaneshiro unpub.).

Rambutan trees exhibit strong apical dominance and have a tendency to produce long, upright growth if not properly managed. Early pruning and training in the field is needed to develop proper branch scaffolds.

Over 187 clones of rambutan are registered in Malaysia and over 25 additional cultivars are known in Indonesia, the Philippines, Thailand, and Singapore (Lye et al. 1987). Some of the most popular and recommended rambutan cultivars are 'Lebakbulus', 'Benjai' and 'Rapiah' (Indonesia); 'Seematjan', 'Seejonja', and 'Maharlika' (Philippines); 'Deli Cheng' and 'Jitlee' (Singapore); 'Gula Batu' (R3), 'Muar Gading' (R156), 'Khaw Tow Bak' (R160), 'Lee Long' (R161), 'Dann Hijau' (R162), R134, and R167 (Malaysia); 'Rongrien', 'Seechompoo', 'Seetong', and 'Namtangruad' (Thailand).

Postharvest Diseases

Most postharvest problems are related to latent infection, injuries incurred during harvesting, and high humidity and temperature during packaging and transport. The major postharvest diseases are caused by *Botryodiplodia theobromae*, *Gliocephalotrichum bulbilium*, and *Colletotrichum* spp. A survey conducted in Bangkok markets identified about 30% of the postharvest diseases caused by *Colletotrichum* spp., 10% by *Gliocephalotrichum bulbilium*, and 5% by *Botryodiplodia theobromae*. Postharvest storage of fruit in the dark, with low temperatures, may discourage fruit rot (Visarathanonth and Ilag 1987).

Insects

Rambutan is host to 118 different species of insects, but only 17 were identified as attacking rambutan fruits. The following pests are listed in the order of importance: *Acrocercops cramerella* Snell., *Phenacaspis* sp., *Planacoccus citri* Risso., *Dichocrocis punctiferalis* Guen., *Dacus dorsalis* Hend., *Carpophilus dimidatus* L., *Carpophilus marginelius* Mot. (Osman and Chettanachitara 1987). Rambutan infested with *Acrocercops cramerella*, cacao pod moth, showed no external symptoms, with up to 40% infestation observed in some cultivars and damage generally between 10 to 15%.

Wild *Nephelium* species

Some native *Nephelium* species in Malaysia and Indonesia are *N. aculeatum*, *N. maingayi*, *N. reticulatum*, *N. compressum* Radlk., *N. uncinatum* Leenh., *N. muduseum* Leenh., *N. laurinum* Blume., *N. daedaleum* Radlk., *N. juglandifolium* Blume, *N. hypoleucum* Kurz. (also in Thailand), *N. cuspidatum* var. *eriopetalum*, *N. cuspidatum* var. *robustum*, *N. lappaceum* var. *lappaceum*, *N. lappaceum* var. *pallen*, *N. lappaceum* var. *xanthioides*, and *N. ramboutan ake* (Van Welzen et al. 198?). Species in other Southeast Asian countries include *N. obovatum* L. (Thailand); *N. bassacense* Pierre (Malaysia and Vietnam); *N. chryseum* Blume, *N. philippinense*, and *N. xerospermoides* R.D.K. (Philippines) (Martin et al. 1987).

Future Prospects

Thailand is the leading producer of rambutan in the Asian region with about 60,000 ha and 430,000 t (1983/84). Production is concentrated in the provinces of Chanthaburi, Rayong, Trad, and Prajineburi in the east and Surattani, Choomporn, Naratiwart, and Nakornsritummarart in the south. Peak harvest season is between May and August (Laksmi et al. 1987). In recent years, many rambutan plantings in the Chanthaburi area have been replaced by durian, *Durio zibethinus* L., due to overproduction, high postharvest costs (Hiranpradit pers. commun. 1991) and low return—U.S. $0.10/kg for rambutan vs. U.S. $2.00/kg for durian.

In the northern territory of Australia, rambutan plantings have increased to about 20,000 trees. Production is geared for November and December, when the value of the fruit is the highest at between $7 to $16/kg (Lim 1991).

In Hawaii, small plantings of rambutan are coming into production on the islands of Kauai and Hawaii. Average price is between $9 to $13/kg. The current nursery price for a grafted plant is about $45.

Rambutan can become a potential industry in Hawaii. The population of 1.1 million residents and approximately the same number of visitors each year are potential customers of this exotic fruit. Moreover, the west coast of the United States is only six hours away by air for a potentially feasible export market.

A market analysis conducted by the University of Hawaii for exotic tropical fruit in 1990 identified the lack of a postharvest fruit fly disinfestation treatment and the lack of a cultivar testing program as the major obstacles to rambutan production (unpublished); additionally, the high cost of production and the presence of large competitors in Southeast Asia contributes to the risk. To avoid direct competition with large producers in Southeast Asia and poor market price, the production of rambutan in Hawaii should be geared towards the winter months of November to January, which can be achieved through the use of selected cultivars and better understanding of the environmental, cultural, and cultivar interactions.

PILI NUTS

Origin

Canarium ovatum Engl., one of 600 species in the Burseraceae (Neal 1965), is native to the Philippines and is abundant and wild in the southern Luzon part of Visayas and Mindanao. The Philippines is the only country that produces and processes pili nuts commercially. Production centers are located in the Bicol region, provinces of Sorsogon, Albay, and Camarines Sur, southern Tagalog, and eastern Visaya. There is no commercial planting of this crop, fruits are collected from natural stands in the mountains near these provinces. In 1977, the Philippines exported approximately 3.8 t of pili preparation to Guam and Australia (Coronel et al. 1983).

Morphology

Trees of *Canarium ovatum* are attractive symmetrically shaped evergreens, averaging 20 m tall with resinous wood and resistance to strong wind. *C. ovatum* is dioecious, with flowers borne on cymose inflorescence at the leaf axils of young shoots. As in papaya and rambutan, functional hermaphrodites exist in pili. Pollination is by insects. Flowering of pili is frequent and fruits ripen through a prolonged period of time. The ovary contains three locules, each with two ovules, most of the time only one ovule develops (Chandler 1958).

Pili fruit is a drupe, 4 to 7 cm long, 2.3 to 3.8 cm in diameter, and weighs 15.7 to 45.7 g. The skin (exocarp) is smooth, thin, shiny, and turns purplish black when the fruit ripens; the pulp (mesocarp) is fibrous, fleshy, and greenish yellow in color, and the hard shell (endocarp) within protects a normally dicotyledonous embryo. The basal end of the shell (endocarp) is pointed and the apical end is more or less blunt; between the seed and the hard shell (endocarp) is a thin, brownish, fibrous seed coat developed from the inner layer of the endocarp. This thin coat usually adheres tightly to the shell and/or the seed. Much of the kernel weight is made up of the cotyledons, which are about 4.1 to 16.6% of the whole fruit; it is composed of approximately 8% carbohydrate, 11.5 to 13.9% protein, and 70% fat (Coronel and Zuno 1980a,b). Kernels from some trees may be bitter, fibrous or have a turpentine odor.

Culture

Pili is a tropical tree preferring deep, fertile, well drained soil, warm temperatures, and well distributed rainfall. It can not tolerate the slightest frost or low temperature (Chandler 1958). Refrigeration of seeds at 4° to 13°C resulted in loss of viability after 5 days. Seed germination is highly recalcitrant, reduced from 98 to 19% after 12 weeks of storage at room temperature; seeds stored for more than 137 days did not germinate (Coronel et al. 1983).

Asexual propagations using marcotting, budding, and grafting were too inconsistent to be used in commercial production. Young shoots of pili were believed to have functional internal phloems, which rendered bark ringing ineffective as a way of building up carbohydrate levels in the wood. Success in marcottage may be cultivar dependent. Production standards for a mature pili tree is between 100 to 150 kg of in-shell nut with the harvest season from May to October and peaking between June and August. There are high variations in kernel qualities and production between seedling trees.

Most pili kernels tend to stick to the shell when fresh, but come off easily after being dried to 3 to 5% moisture (30°C for 27 to 28 h). Shell nuts, with a moisture content of 2.5 to 4.6%, can be stored in the shade for one year without deterioration of quality (Coronel et al. 1983).

The most important product from pili is the kernel. When raw, it resembles the flavor of roasted pumpkin seed, and when roasted, its mild, nutty flavor and tender-crispy texture is superior to that of the almond. Pili kernel is also used in chocolate, ice cream, and baked goods (Rosengarten 1984). The largest buyers of pili nuts are in Hong Kong and Taiwan, the kernel is one of the major ingredients in one type of the famous Chinese festive desserts known as the "moon cake."

Nutritionally, the kernel is high in calcium, phosphorous, and potassium, and rich in fats and protein. It yields a light yellowish oil, mainly of glycerides of oleic (44.4 to 59.6%) and palmitic acids (32.6 to 38.2%) (Mohr and Wichmann 1987; Coronel et al. 1983).

The young shoots and the fruit pulp are edible. The shoots are used in salads, and the pulp is eaten after it is boiled and seasoned. Boiled pili pulp resembles the sweet potato in texture, it is oily (about 12%) and is considered to have food value similar to the avocado. Pulp oil can be extracted and used for cooking or as a substitute for cotton seed oil in the manufacture of soap and edible products. The stony shells are excellent as fuel or as porous, inert growth medium for orchids and antherium.

Future Prospects

According to Richard A. Hamilton, University of Hawaii at Manoa (macadamia breeder), the current status of the pili is equivalent to that of the macadamia some 30 years ago. It has great potential to develop into a major industry. The immediate concern in pili production is the difficulty of propagation. The lack of an effective clonal propagation method not only hampers the collection of superior germplasm but also makes it almost impossible to conduct feasibility trials of this crop. Few elite pili trees, such as 'Red', 'Albay', and 'Katutubo' were selected in the Philippines (Coronel et al. 1983). The National Clonal Germplasm Repository at Hilo, USDA/ARS, has initiated studies in in vitro and vegetative propagation for the multiplication and long-term preservation of pili.

A recently released pili cultivar in Hawaii may further stimulate the interest in this crop. This new selection, known as 'Poamoho', was released by R.A. Hamilton. Besides the desirable production and quality attributes, its kernels separate easily from the hard shell without the need of prior drying (30°C for 27 to 28 h). This is an important cost saving feature for processing.

REFERENCES

Rambutan

Laksmi, L.D.S., P.F. Lam, D.B. Mondoza Jr., S. Kosiyachinda, and P.C. Leong. 1987. Status of the rambutan industry in ASEAN, p. 1–8. In: P.F. Lam and S. Kosiyachinda (eds.). Rambutan: fruit development, postharvest physiology and marketing in ASEAN. ASEAN Food Handling Bureau, Kuala Lumpur, Malaysia.

Lim, T.K. 1991. Rambutan industry in the Northern Territory current status, research and development emphasis, p. 119. In: International symposium on tropical fruit, working abstracts. May 20–24, 1991. Pattaya, Thailand.

Lye, T.T., L.D.S. Laksmi, P. Maspol, and S.K. Yong. 1987. Commercial rambutan cultivars in ASEAN, p. 9–15. In: P.F. Lam and S. Kosiyachinda (eds.). Rambutan: fruit development, postharvest physiology and marketing in ASEAN. ASEAN Food Handling Bureau, Kuala Lumpur, Malaysia.

Martin, F.L., C.W. Campbell, and R.M. Ruberte. 1987. Perennial edible fruits of the tropics: An inventory. USDA/ARS. Agr. Handb. 642.

Morton, J.F. 1987. Fruits of warm climates. Julia F. Morton, 20534 SW 92 Ct. Miami FL. p. 262–265.

Osman Mohd, S.B. and C. Chettanachitara. 1987. Postharvest insects and other pests of rambutan, p. 57–60. In: P.F. Lam and S. Kosiyachinda (eds.). Rambutan: fruit development, postharvest physiology and marketing in ASEAN. ASEAN Food Handling Bureau, Kuala Lumpur, Malaysia.

Van Welzen, P.C., A. Lamb, and W.W.W. Wong. 1988. Edible Sapindaceae in Sabah. Nature Malaysiana. 13:10–25.

Visarathanonth N. and L.L. Ilag. 1987. Postharvest diseases of rambutan, p. 51–57. In: P.F. Lam and S. Kosiyachinda (eds.). Rambutan: fruit development, postharvest physiology and marketing in ASEAN. ASEAN Food Handling Bureau, Kuala Lumpur, Malaysia.

Pili

Chandler, W.H. 1958. Evergreen orchards. Lea & Febiger, Philadelphia.

Coronel, R.E. and J.C. Zuno. 1980a. Note: The correlation between some fruit characters of pili. Philippine Agriculturist 63:163–165.

Coronel, R.E. and J.C. Zuno. 1980b. Note: Evaluation of fruit characters of some pili seedling trees in Calauan and Los Banos, Laguna. Philippine Agriculturist 63:166–173.

Coronel, R.E., J.C. Zuno, and R.C. Sotto. 1983. Promising fruits of the Philippines, p. 325–350. Univ. Philippines at Los Banos, College of Agr., Laguna.

Mohr, E. and G. Wichmann. 1987. Cultivation of pili nut *Canarium ovatum* and the composition of fatty acids and triglycerides of the oil. Fett Wissenschaft Technologie 89(3):128–129.

Neal, M.C. 1965. In gardens of Hawaii. Bernice P. Bishop Museum. Special Pub. Bishop Museum Press.

Rosengarten, F. Jr. 1984. The book of edible nuts. Walker and Company, New York.

Introduction and Evaluation of Pejibaye (*Bactris gasipaes*) for Palm Heart Production in Hawaii

Charles R. Clement, Richard M. Manshardt, Joseph DeFrank, Francis Zee, and Philip Ito*

Hawaiian agriculture has always been based upon "new crop" introductions. The first Hawaiians brought their Pacific crop complex with them, which included coconut (*Cocos nucifera* L.), breadfruit [*Artocarpus altilis* (Sol. ex Park) Fosb.], banana and plantains (*Musa* spp), sugarcane (*Saccharum officinarum* L.), taro [*Colocasia esculenta* (L.) Schott] and other minor crops (Lebot in press). With the arrival of European colonists in 1778, a new period of crop introductions began. Among the most important were pineapple [*Ananas comosus* (L.) Merril], papaya (*Carica papaya* L.), macadamia nuts (*Macadamia integrifolia* Maiden & Betche), guava (*Psidium guajava* L.), coffee (*Coffea arabica* L.), ginger root (*Zingiber oficinale* Roscoe), plus numerous other fruits, vegetables, flowers, and livestock (HASS 1990). The continued viability of Hawaiian agriculture depends fundamentally upon research directed at raising yields through improved agronomy and genetics, lowering production costs, and introducing new specialty crops with which Hawaii can develop a production and marketing edge.

Among the options is pejibaye (*Bactris gasipaes* Kunth), also known as the peach palm (Hamilton 1987; Roecklein and Leung 1987; Clement 1990). The pejibaye is the Neotropic's only domesticated palm and is well suited to modern agriculture. Its palm heart has potential as a gourmet fresh vegetable. The palm heart is composed of the tender leaves that originate in and grow from the palm meristem and are consumed before they expand and green. Palm heart can supply both the tourist's desire for exotic foods and west coast markets for exotic vegetables. Its multiple potentials in modern agriculture have been examined by Mora Urpí (1984) and Clement and Mora Urpí (1987).

The pejibaye fruit has four uses: cooked fruit for human consumption, flour for bread and confectionaries,

---

*The authors thank Dr. Marilene L.A. Bovi, Instituto Agronômico de Campinas, for information about *E. oleracea*.

vegetable oil, and animal ration. Its unique flavor and texture, however, is unknown to the public outside of tropical America and would require a concerted marketing effort to promote acceptance.

The palm heart, in contrast, is well known and its consumption is expanding rapidly worldwide (Mora Urpí et al. 1991). Palm heart production and canning is already a rapidly growing industry in Latin America. The pejibaye palm heart has been on international markets since 1978 and is expanding in market share in both Europe and the United States (Mora Urpí et al. 1991). The United States currently (1989) imports 2000 t of canned palm heart (up from 900 t in 1980), valued at $4.5 million, of which 700 t is from pejibaye (U.S. Dept. Commerce 1990).

The palm heart market is based upon a processed product, which, although popular, has limited culinary potential because it is pre-cooked in a slightly salty, strongly acidic solution (Quast and Bernhardt 1978). Nonetheless, the value of current world trade in canned palm hearts is estimated to be close to $50 million. World consumption is much greater, because humid tropic populations consume the bulk of locally available fresh palm heart. Brazil, for example, is both the largest producer and largest exporter (70% of world trade): in 1988, 100,000 t of fresh palm heart were produced, but only 9,500 t were exported (Coradin and Clement 1989). Brazil's production is based upon the palm *Euterpe oleracea*, which occurs in large natural populations in the Amazon River estuary. *E. oleracea* has several characteristics that limit its potential for the fresh market. The most important of these is the presence of enzymes that discolor the palm heart upon contact with air.

The popularity of fresh palm heart in Latin America suggests that a strong demand can be created for this product in countries that currently know only the canned product. The pejibaye is ideally suited for the fresh market, because its palm heart does not discolor upon cutting and has good shelf life. Production of pejibaye for the fresh market could permit higher returns to growers. This includes the Hawaiian farmer, who has excellent growing conditions, an efficient agro-industrial infrastructure, and a large tourist market in search of novel foods.

In this paper we will discuss the commercial potential of pejibaye, the current American palm heart market, and the role that Hawaii can play in the crop's further expansion and commercialization.

SELECTION OF PEJIBAYE FOR PALM HEART PRODUCTION

There are several thousand palm species distributed around the tropical world. All have edible hearts. Perhaps 100 species have hearts that are large enough to be commercialized and most are used in local cuisines. Within this group of large palms, there are some with hearts that are slightly sweet, others that are bland, and a few that are bitter. The pejibaye is a member of the sweet group, as are many other well known species of the Cocosoide sub-family, including the coconut (*Cocos nucifera* L.) and the African oil palm (*Elaeis guineensis* Jacq.). As a domesticate, it is adapted to agroecosystems and grows rapidly. These traits, combined with its caespitose (multistemmed) growth habit and non-discoloring palm heart, are its major advantages over other palm heart species.

In spite of these advantages, international trade in palm hearts is based upon the genus *Euterpe*, of South and Central America. Brazil started exporting *E. edulis* in the 1950s (Renesto and Vieira 1977). This agro-industry was based upon extraction of wild palms from the Atlantic forests of southern Brazil and soon decimated the wild populations, since it is a single-stemmed species with very slow growth rates. The industry then shifted to the estuary of the Amazon River to exploit *E. oleracea*, a smaller statured, caespitose species (Calzavara 1972). The majority of Brazil's exports (>90%) are now derived from this species, although Brazilians still consider *E. edulis* to be the premier palm heart (Coradin and Clement 1989).

Quality Distinctions

Ferreira et al. (1982a,b) compared *E. edulis* and pejibaye palm hearts, and M.L.A. Bovi (Instituto Agronomico de Campinas pers. commun.) and her colleagues provided information on *E. oleracea*. Fig. 1 presents four important compositional characteristics that differ amongst the three species. Tannins in the *Euterpe* are double those in pejibaye, which explains the slight bitterness of the *Euterpe* (Ferreira et al. 1982b). Total sugars in pejibaye are triple those in the *Euterpe*, which explains the sweetness of the pejibaye (Ferreira et al. 1982b). Most important, the levels of the polyphenoloxidase and peroxidase enzymes, which cause the rapid tissue discoloration in *Euterpe* spp., are nearly absent in pejibaye (Ferreira et al. 1982a).

Fig. 1. Four important quality characteristics of palm heart species. Note that *B. gasipaes* has no oxidases to discolor the fresh palm heart.

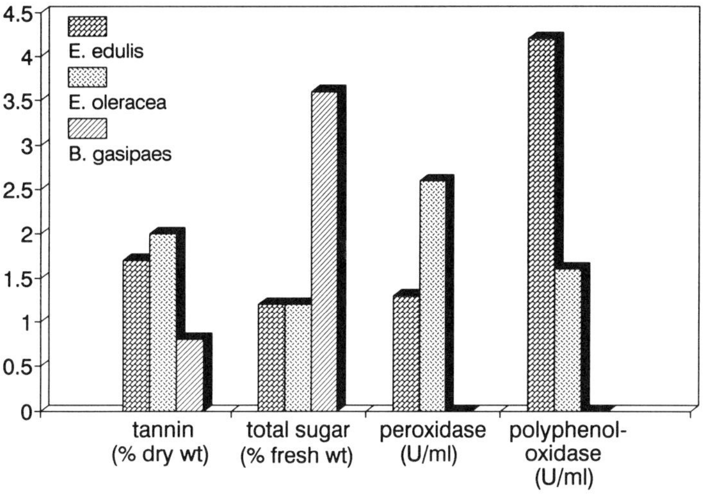

The pejibaye palm heart is yellower than that of *E. edulis* (Ferreira et al. 1982a), a slight disadvantage in a market accustomed to a bone-white product. The texture of pejibaye is somewhat firmer than that of *E. edulis*, due to slightly lower water and higher fiber contents.

A Brazilian test panel accustomed to *E. edulis* found the pejibaye acceptable (7.0 vs 8.5 for *E. edulis*, on a 1 to 9 scale) (Ferreira et al. 1982a). Several restaurant chefs in Ubatuba, Sao Paulo, Brazil (in the heart of *E. edulis*' distribution), were extremely enthusiastic about pejibaye's culinary potential after evaluating this new product in direct comparison with *E. edulis*.

Precocity and Yield Distinctions

Of the three palm heart species discussed here, only the pejibaye is a full domesticate. *E. edulis* is a native of the nearly extinct Atlantic forest of coastal Brazil and requires moderate shade during its early development (Bovi et al. 1988). *E. oleracea* is a native of the floodplain swamps of the eastern Amazon River basin, where it occurs in large, nearly monospecific stands (Peters et al. 1989). The pejibaye is native to the plateaus of western Amazonia and was domesticated in Native American agroecosystems (Clement 1988).

E. edulis must be planted with light to moderate shade during the first 3 to 5 years, and suffers high plant mortality during establishment (Bovi et al. 1988). At very high plant densities (6,666 and 10,000 plants/ha), yields are excellent (2.9 and 2.5 t/ha, respectively), but the palm hearts are small (200 to 250 g). At lower densities, yields are lower (1 to 2 t/ha), but palm hearts are larger (to 600 g) (Bovi et al. 1988). Harvest size is only attained at 6 to 8 years and, since the plants have only one stem, the plantation must be replanted (Bovi et al. 1988). Annual yields, in uneven aged natural stands, are therefore estimated at 0.5 t/ha (2.9 t/ha after 6 years).

E. oleracea grows faster than *E. edulis*, attaining harvest size in 4 to 6 years, both in its natural, nutrient rich ecosystem and in plantation (Bovi et al. 1988). This species should be planted in light shade, which can be removed within a year. Compared to *E. edulis*, plant mortality during establishment is low in humid soils (Calzavara 1972), but high on plateau soils in Amazonia (Gomes 1983). Yields are similar to those of *E. edulis* and show similar size to density trends. Because it is a caespitose palm, management for continuous cropping is possible (Calzavara 1972). Each clump yields another palm heart after 18 to 24 months (Bovi et al. 1988). Annual yields of *E. oleracea* are estimated at 1.4 t/ha after the first harvest.

Pejibaye can be planted in full sun, after light shade in the nursery. If correctly handled, it does not suffer plant mortality during establishment. In agroecosystems, it grows rapidly and responds readily to applications of fertilizers and other inputs, and attains harvest size in 18 to 30 months (Mora Urpí 1984). Yields and size to density trends are similar to the *Euterpe* species. Like *E. oleracea*, it is caespitose and is managed for continuous cropping and each clump yields another palm heart after 9 to 15 months (Clement et al. 1988). Annual yields are 2 t/ha after the first harvest in Costa Rica (Mora Urpí et al. 1991).

Although Brazil has a strong *Euterpe* tradition, there is currently strong interest in planting pejibaye in high density monocultures, because of the above mentioned advantages. In Acre state, 300+ ha are in production (A. Vieira, BONAL SA pers. commun.). Numerous agribusinessmen from Sao Paulo, Espirito Santo, and Bahia are starting to plant and have created an over-heated market for seeds of spineless pejibaye. The only national producer of these seeds, located in Manaus, received requests for 3+ million seed in 1989, but could only supply 0.5 million. Recent (1991) Brazilian government environmental regulations require management plans for extraction of *Euterpe* species from natural stands. This new factor will probably encourage palm heart agribusinesses to plant more pejibaye.

THE UNITED STATES IMPORT MARKET

Compared to the French import market, the United States palm heart market is still very small, consuming 2,000 t in 1989. This is equivalent to an annual consumption of only 8 g/person, versus about 100 g/person in France.

In the United States market, imports of *E. oleracea* have been extremely erratic over the last two decades. In 1977, the Organization of American States reported poor quality control as the major factor limiting imports of *Euterpe* palm hearts. As Mora Urpí et al. (1991) explain, exploitation of wild populations of *E. oleracea* by poorly trained harvesters results in an extremely variable product, frequently too fibrous or discolored for canning (Quast and Bernhardt 1978). These defects are not always handled adequately in the canning plants, and fibrous or discolored palm hearts are occasionally marketed. This lack of rigorous quality control in the canning plant has not been addressed by most Brazilian exporters to date, so that considerable volatility can continue to be expected.

Pejibaye palm heart entered the American market in 1978. Since then it has continued to expand its market share, except in 1988, when it contracted as a result of Brazil's introduction of a minimum price for its palm heart, which increased prices for all tropical American palm hearts and lowered demand. The current Brazilian government eliminated this price support in 1990. In 1989, Costa Rican pejibaye accounted for 22.5% of the domestic US market, versus only 3% in 1982. During this period, the American palm heart import market more than doubled in size

Fig. 2 presents the palm heart imports observed during the 1980s in the American market. *Euterpe* imports are extremely volatile, but did not previously have competition from another high quality palm heart. This new factor may be fatal for the Brazilian *Euterpes*, unless the Brazilian exporters start practicing good quality control. The pejibaye trend, based only upon Costa Rican exports, is strongly upward. If the Brazilian *Euterpe* exporters do not institute quality control and Costa Rican exports continue to expand, Fig. 2 suggests that pejibaye could become the major palm heart in the American market by the late 1990s.

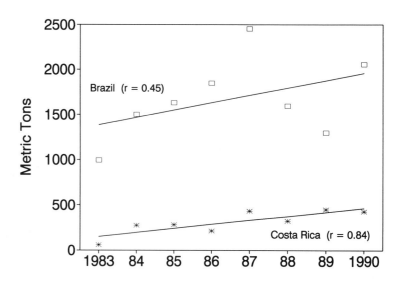

Fig. 2. Imports of canned palm hearts from Brazil and Costa Rica during the period 1983–1990. Small amounts are also imported from 10 to 15 other countries but rarely amount to more than 10% of the total. Note the extreme volatility of the Brazilian product.

SUITABILITY OF HAWAII

Hawaii is the only state in the United States with a tropical climate to grow this tropical crop commercially. There are three other reasons for being optimistic that Hawaii can develop a successful market for its pejibaye palm heart.

A Large Tourist Market for Exotics

Hawaii's annual tourist population is 2 to 3 times larger than its permanent population of 1 million. This transient population, obviously wealthy enough to make the trip, is searching for, or at least receptive to exotic experiences, especially exotic foods. For the Asians, who make up a large fraction of the tourist population, western style foods are in demand, while for the Americans and Europeans, the Asian foods are an attraction. The pejibaye palm heart can provide an exotic touch to any meal and will be perfectly acceptable in the cuisine of both hemispheres.

An ideal way to penetrate this market is through the chef's clubs in Honolulu and on the Island of Hawaii. The imagination of these master chefs in developing new culinary uses for fresh palm heart could be essential. Through their restaurants, an initial test of the tourist and local markets can be made.

Excellent Environmental Conditions

The Hawaiian islands contain a wide array of soil and climatic conditions, some of which are ideal for pejibaye. Many areas have been in sugarcane, and these farmers are seeking new crop options. Preliminary observations suggest that yields close to those currently attained in Latin America will be possible.

An Active Diversified Agriculture Sector

In 1989, 17% of Hawaii's agricultural hectarage (excluding pastures) was occupied by diversified agriculture, defined in Hawaii as excluding sugarcane and pineapple. The diversified sector produced 37% of Hawaii's nearly $500 million dollar agricultural income (excluding livestock) (HASS 1990). Both the agricultural community and the state realize that Hawaiian agriculture must diversify to survive in the face of rapidly rising land prices (driven by tourism and urbanization) and competition from abroad.

The state of Hawaii recently initiated a crop diversification program, coordinated by the Council for Agricultural Product Expansion (CAPE), an advisory group to the Governor's Agricultural Coordinating Committee. The University of Hawaii and an active agribusiness sector are also involved. Continued diversification will depend upon the imagination, energy and cooperation of these three groups.

THE INTRODUCTION PROGRAM

The University of Hawaii and private individuals have introduced pejibaye into the islands occasionally during the last several decades. The most notable introductions were carried out from the late 1960s to the late 1970s by Richard A. Hamilton, Department of Horticulture, who introduced pejibaye as a fruit crop. The pejibaye's rather starchy texture and uniquely nutty sweet flavor limited its acceptance. Furthermore, the initial introductions were of spiny stemmed plants and did not attract much attention from the diversified agricultural community in Hawaii.

In the early 1980s, the United States Agency for International Development sponsored a series of pan-Amazonian germplasm explorations that collected and mapped a considerable portion of the genetic diversity inherited from the Native Americans in the Neotropics (Clement and Coradin 1988). In the final report of that project, Mora Urpí and Clement (1988) classified and mapped 8 landraces of pejibaye and numerous hybrid populations. Clement and Mora Urpí (1987) and Clement (1988) proposed improvement programs for pejibaye's five major potential uses based upon different landraces and hybrid populations.

The spineless hybrid population found at Yurimaguas and the associated Pampa Hermosa landrace were suggested for use in the palm heart improvement program, combined with spineless germplasm available from the Benjamin Constant population of the Putumayo landrace and the San Carlos population of the Central American complex (Clement et al. 1988). With this germplasm identified and available from several Latin American germplasm collections, a new introduction of pejibaye into Hawaii was organized.

The USDA Project

A project designed to introduce pejibaye for palm heart is now financed by a USDA Special Research Grant for Tropical Agriculture and carried out by the Department of Horticulture, University of Hawaii, on the island of Oahu, in collaboration with the USDA National Clonal Germplasm Repository and the University of Hawaii Beaumont Research Center, both on the island of Hawaii.

Open-pollinated progenies from each of the two major Amazonian spineless populations identified above have been introduced. Seed from Benjamin Constant and Yurimaguas included both selected and non-selected spineless genotypes from the collections of the National Research Institute for Amazonia—INPA, of Brazil's National Research Council. Additional germplasm from San Carlos, Costa Rica, is expected in 1992. This germplasm will provide a wide genetic base from which to identify promising accessions for the diverse Hawaiian agroecosystems.

This germplasm will be maintained at two sites, the National Clonal Germplasm Repository's Waiakea station, at Hilo, on the island of Hawaii, and the University of Hawaii's Waimanalo Experiment Station, on the island of Oahu. The environmental conditions at Hilo are characterized by thin soils of recent volcanic origin. The climate provides abundant rainfall and lacks a pronounced dry season, although any dry spell on these shallow soils can become serious, if prolonged for more than a week or two. Environmental conditions at Waimanalo are unique in Hawaii, with a rich loamy soil, abundant rainfall (October–March) with a pronounced dry season and strong trade winds. Nonetheless, pejibaye does well there, if sheltered from the wind.

Progeny × density trials are being planted with germplasm from each base population. The densities used are 3,333, 5,000, and 6,666 plants/ha. Current commercial density in Costa Rica is 5,000 plants/ha, but larger or smaller palm hearts may be required for the fresh market. After the first harvest, the plants will be managed to have two stems each, thus doubling densities.

The progeny trials are located in environments representative of major Hawaiian agricultural zones. The choice of sites provides information that can be extrapolated to almost any likely plantation site for pejibaye in Hawaii, Latin America, or elsewhere in the Pacific basin.

Growth and yield data will be collected at 6 month intervals. This will permit timely evaluation of pejibaye populational adaptation to the conditions chosen and will permit early modification of cultural practices to enhance growth, should this prove necessary. Several physiological parameters of interest in plant improvement and agronomy will be estimated from the growth and yield data (Corley 1983). Genotype–environment interactions will be examined to improve the extrapolation of results from this experiment to other areas.

The CAPE Project

The costs of installing and maintaining a hectare of pejibaye plantation for palm heart in Hawaii were estimated as part of a feasibility study. In general, this crop option looks promising, but the study identified the high maintenance cost of weed control as a problem. In Latin America, most pejibaye is hand-weeded, since the herbicides used there have suppressed growth and reduced palm heart quality (Mora Urpí, Univ. Costa Rica pers. commun.).

Yet, Hawaiian agriculture depends upon herbicides for weed control, as labor is both scarce and expensive (DeFrank 1990). The Environmental Protection Agency regulations are constantly narrowing the number of herbicides that can be used in the United States and registration for new crops is becoming increasingly difficult and expensive. Consumers are also demanding less pesticide residues in their foods and are willing to pay more for products produced in herbicide-free environments (DeFrank 1990). To evaluate the effect of herbicides on pejibaye in Hawaii and look at "organic" alternatives, a second project was designed and approved by the CAPE. The major points to be evaluated include:

Three herbicides (Gramoxone, Goal, and Surflan) will be tested with pejibaye at commercial density (5,000 plants/ha). A non-bearing EPA approval will be requested for the most efficient.

Ground covers, including *Desmodium ovalifolium*, *D. heterophyllum*, *Arachis pintoi*, and *Cassia rotundifolia*, will be tested with pejibaye at the same commercial density. These species are prostrate non-climbers and relatively shade-tolerant. *D. ovalifolium* has given good results at pejibaye fruiting densities (400 plants/ha) in Brazil and Peru, but has not been tested at palm heart densities. If one or more of these species forms a good cover and does not compete with the crop, it will help control weeds, as well as offer the other agroecological advantages expected from cover crops (DeFrank 1990).

Black plastic mulch sheets have a long tradition in Hawaii as a crop establishment aid for controlling early weed growth. Recent advances in plastic technology allow mulch to remain in the field for up to five years for efficient weed control (DeFrank and Easton-Smith 1990). This mulch will be combined with both the herbicides and the ground covers and evaluated as an aid in further reducing costs.

REFERENCES

Bovi, M.L.A., G. Godoy Jr., and L.A. Saes. 1988. Pesquisas com os generos *Euterpe* e *Bactris* no Instituto Agronômico de Campinas. Anais 1º Encontro Nacional de Pesquisadores em Palmito, Centro Nacional de Pesquisas de Florestas, Curitiba, Parana.

Calzavara, B.B.G. 1972. As possibilidades do açaizeiro no estuário Amazônico. Boletin 5, Faculdade de Ciências Agrárias do Pará, Belém.

Clement, C.R. 1988. Domestication of the pejibaye palm (*Bactris gasipaes*): past and present. Adv. Econ. Bot. 6:155–174.

Clement, C.R. 1990. Pejibaye, p. 302–321. In: S. Nagy, P.E. Shaw, and W. Wardowski (eds.). Fruits of tropical and subtropical origin: Composition, properties, uses. Florida Science Source, Lake Alfred.

Clement, C.R. and J. Mora Urpí. 1987. The pejibaye (*Bactris gasipaes* H.B.K., Arecaceae): multi-use potential for the lowland humid tropics. J. Econ. Bot. 41:302–311.

Clement, C.R. and L. Coradin (eds.) 1988. Final report (revised): Peach palm (*Bactris gasipaes*) germplasm bank. US-AID project report, Manaus.

Clement, C.R., W.B. Chavez F., and J.B.M. Gomes. 1988. Considerações sobre a pupunha (*Bactris gasipaes* H.B.K.) como produtora de palmito. Anais 1º Encontro Nacional de Pesquisadores em Palmito, Centro Nacional de Pesquisas de Florestas, Curitiba, Parana. p. 225–248.

Coradin, L. and C.R. Clement. 1989. Brazilian palm hearts: present status and future prospects. Consultation Meeting on Palm Hearts. FHIA/US-AID, San Pedro Sula, Honduras.

Corley, R.H.V. 1983. Potential productivity of tropical perennial crops. Expt. Agr. 19:217–37.

DeFrank, J. 1990. Ground cover management in reduced tillage cropping systems in Hawaii. Proc. Int. Conf. Agr. 21st Century. Maui, HI. October 12–14, 1990. p. 51–52.

DeFrank, J. and V.A. Easton-Smith. 1990. Evaluation of preemergence herbicides on four proteaceous species. Trop. Agr. (Trinidad) 67:360–362.

Ferreira, V.L.P., M. Graner, M.L.A. Bovi, I.S. Draetta, J.E. Paschoalino, and I. Shirose. 1982a. Comparição entre os palmitos das palmeiras *Guilielma gasipaes* Bailey (pupunha) e *Euterpe edulis* Mart. (juçara). I. Avaliações físicas, organolépticas e bioquímicas. Coletânea Inst. Tecnologia de Alimentos, Campinas 12:255–272.

Ferreira, V.L.P., M. Graner, M.L.A. Bovi, I.B. Figueiredo, E. Angelucci, and Y. Yokomizo. 1982b. Comparição entre os palmitos das palmeiras *Guilielma gasipaes* Bailey (pupunha) e *Euterpe edulis* Mart. (juçara). II. Avaliações físicas e químicas. Coletânea Inst. Tecnologia de Alimentos, Campinas 12:273–282.

Hamilton, R.A. 1987. Ten tropical fruits of potential value for crop diversification in Hawaii. Univ. Hawaii, Res. Ext. Ser. 85, Honolulu.

HASS. 1990. Statistics of Hawaiian agriculture, 1989. Hawaii Agr. Statistics Serv., Dept. Agr., Honolulu.

Lebot, V. Genetic vulnerability of Oceania's traditional crops. Expt. Agr. (in press).

Mora Urpí, J. 1984. El pejibaye (*Bactris gasipaes* H.B.K.): origen, biologia floral y manejo agronómico, p. 118–160. In: Palmeras poco utilizadas de América tropical. Turrialba (Costa Rica): FAO/Centro Agronomico Tropical de Investigación y Enseñanza.

Mora Urpí, J. and C.R. Clement. 1988. Races and populations of peach palm found in the Amazon basin, p. 79–94. In: C.R. Clement and L. Coradin (eds.). Final report (revised): Peach palm (*Bactris gasipaes*) germplasm bank. US-AID project report, Manaus.

Mora Urpí, J., A. Bonilla, C.R. Clement, and D.V. Johnson. 1991. Mercado Internacional de Palmito y Futuro de la Explotación Salvaje vs. Cultivado. Série Técnica Pejibaye 3:6–27.

OAS. 1977. Market profile: Palm hearts. CECON-Organization of American States, Washington, DC.

Peters, C.M., M.J. Balick, F. Kahn, and A.B. Anderson. 1989. Oligarchic forests of economic plants in Amazonia: Utilization and conservation of an important tropical resource. Conserv. Biol. 3:341–349.

Quast, D.G. and L.W. Bernhardt. 1978. Progress in palmito (heart-of-palm) processing research. J. Food Protection 41:667–674.

Renesto, O.V. and L.F. Vieira. 1977. Análise econômica da produção e processamento do palmito em conserva nas regiões sudeste e sul do Brasil. Estudos Econômicos—Alimentos Processados 6. Instituto de Tecnologia de Alimentos—ITAL, Campinas.

Roecklein, J.C. and P.S. Leung. 1987. A profile of economic plants. Transaction Inc., New Brunswick, NJ.

Garcinia hombrioniana: A Potential Fruit and an Industrial Crop

Hj. Serudin D.S. Hj. Tinggal*

Southeast Asia is regarded as a major center of origin and evolution of many cultivated crops particularly tropical fruits. A great variety of fruits, some wild, others cultivated are located in Brunei. Species of *Artocarpus*, *Durio*, *Garcinia*, *Mangifera*, *Musa*, and *Nephelium*, to mention only a few, occur as scattered species amidst forest trees or growing alongside homes, in backyards or mixed orchards. These indigenous species together with introduced cultivars represent invaluable genetic resources waiting to be collected, identified, and tested for commercial development.

One of these potential new fruit crops is *Garcinia hombrioniana* Pierre, locally called Assam Aur Aur, a close relative of the mangosteen, *G. mangostana* L. The attractive fruit contains white segmented luscious pulp, sweet with a pleasing fragrance similar to apricot (Fig. 1). The pulp has many uses. The dried crimson rind of the fruit for example, is commercially important and used extensively as sour relish in curries and culinary dishes requiring an acidulous base. Demand for this condiment is seemingly unsatisfiable and at every fruit season, housewives gather the fruits, remove the pulp, and sun-dry the rind (Fig. 2). The market price is attractive and keeping quality for properly dried pulp is good.

BOTANY

Origin

Assam Aur Aur is native to the Brunei Bay region of the states of Sabah and Sarawak of Malaysia and Brunei. The tree probably originated in the rainforests and was cultivated in the coastal and riverine regions to serve the culinary uses of the early settlers. Currently, the distribution is still restricted to the riverine and coastal alluvial regions. Some trees are found in the interior settlements, probably introduced, as coastal and riverine dwellers moved to settle inland. The fruit has never achieved the importance of mangosteen and early explorers and naturalists have largely neglected the small fruit for the larger, sweeter mangosteen.

---

*There is no known published data on Assam Aur Aur. The information presented has been collected by the author during various field trips to the countryside and discussion with farmers and their families. Officers of the Department of Agriculture provided valuable information on its culture and food processing.

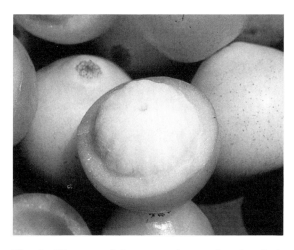

Fig. 1. Close up of the savory Assam Aur Aur fruit.

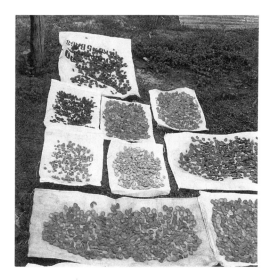

Fig. 2. Sun-drying of Assam Aur Aur rind with the pulp removed.

Morphology

Assam Aur Aur is a handsome evergreen closely resembling the mangosteen in shape and canopy structure, except that Assam Aur Aur has smaller, more elliptical leaves. Mature trees can reach 10 m in height with numerous radially arranged spreading branches. Much of the leaves are held by tertiary branches. Inflorescence are borne on these branchlets in clusters of not more than five small flowers. Very little is known about the morphology of the flowers and owing to the smallness and almost fused structures, the flowers have received very little attention. It is likely that the flowers are hermaphroditic and the few seeds produced apomictic. Seedlings derived from seeds are always identical to the mother plant; there is no known genetic variation. Subtle differences in size (3 to 5 cm in diameter) and shape of fruits could be attributed to environmental influence. The population is generally homogeneous making selection for superior types difficult. However, this homogeneous attribute can be advantageous as fruit and fruit products derived from the fruits are fairly uniform.

HORTICULTURE

Culture

Assam Aur Aur is a tropical species requiring humid conditions of uniform annual rainfall exceeding 2,000 mm and mean temperature of 27°C. The tree shows a wide range of soil adaptability and will grow on damp alluvial soil as well as free draining upland soils. However, the preference is for well-drained fertile alluvial soil where water is not limiting.

Seeds, with the pulp removed, germinate within one week and can be shown direct into plastic bags. Early growth requires protection from full sunlight; 50% shading is recommended and progressively removed to harden the seedlings for field planing when 6 to 8 months old.

There is no commercial planting of Assam Aur Aur to provide cultural recommendations. However, based on observations and experiences, trees grow best at 5 m spacing. Nurse shade between 50 to 60% is essential at planting. Growth is rapid. Prunning of lower branches, weeding, and fertilization will bring the trees to bear after four years. Recommended fertilizers consist of NPK (12–5–14) to enhance fruiting. Mulching with dry litter will help to retain soil moisture and prevent erosion which appears to be essential for healthy growth of the plant.

As long as the trees are healthy, problems of diseases appear minimal. However, ripe fruits are susceptible to infection by fruit flies (*Dacus* spp) causing damage to the pulp. The rind is unaffected and can still be processed into condiments. Fruit fly damage is more prevalent when few fruits are in season. Spraying with insecticides may reduce the damage, but, generally control of fruit fly is difficult in the tropics.

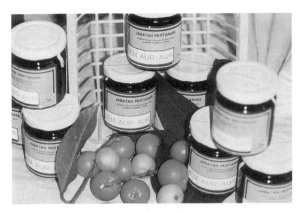
Fig. 3. Assam Aur Aur conserve produced by the Department of Agriculture, Brunei.

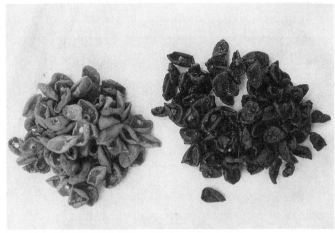
Fig. 4. Dried rind of Assam Aur Aur used as sour relish (left: freshly dried; right: after six months storage).

UTILIZATION

Bruneians, for centuries, have found many uses for the fruits. The young fruits that drop to the ground are collected and sliced into thin pieces or chunks and sun-dried. The final product is a fig brown condiment ready to give the needed tang to Brunei dishes. Currently, there is a limited amount in the market. The mature fruit has multiple uses with a fragrance reminiscent of apricot. Early Bruneians fermented the pulp into organic vinegar. The flavor is distinct, fruity, and strong. In recent years, efforts of the Department of Agriculture have produced suitable cordials and jams from the pulp (Fig. 3). The quality of the cordial is still questionable but the jams have penetrated a limited market. Research is still in progress.

The greatest commercial value of the fruit is the crimson rind. Dried in the sun, the shiny rind turns dull mauve in the process. Packed into small plastic bags, the rind is ready for sale as an essential ingredient for many Brunei dishes. The best condiment exudes some oil when pressed between fingers and quality rind, properly dried, will eventually turn black without being moldy (Fig. 4). Dark colored rind does not affect the culinary quality.

FUTURE PROSPECTS

Assam Aur Aur has tremendous opportunity as a specialty fruit. Strong promotional support will strengthen marketing. The research programs of the Department of Agriculture can explore postharvest and handling technology to establish quality and standards. However, it is the inherent quality of fruit that will attract connoisseurs. The strategy is to introduce this fruit into specialty markets.

Another area of interest is the acidulous quality of the rind. It is already in great demand. Opportunity exists for more systematic and scientific approach to rind processing, packaging, and marketing. Greater efforts will be required to evaluate value-added products such as jams, juices, and food colors.

New Products from Theobroma cacao: Seed Pulp and Pod Gum

Antonio Figueira, Jules Janick, and James N. BeMiller

Theobroma cacao L. (Sterculiaceae), an important tropical rain forest species, is grown for its oil-rich seed, to produce cocoa and cocoa butter. Cocoa seeds are a major cash crop of the tropical world, but prices fluctuate widely and economic hardships occur when prices are low. Despite this, only about 10% by fresh weight of the fruit is commercialized, although several promising commercial products could be obtained from the fruit (Greenwood-Barton 1965).

One strategy to increase income for cocoa growers is to identify and commercialize new products that will not interfere with the main seed crop. In this paper, we review a number of new products that have potential for increasing returns to cocoa growers. These include seed pulp and products from pod husk waste; byproducts from the chocolate processing industry, such as cocoa shell, cocoa cake, and cocoa dust (Abiola and Tewe 1991) are not included.

COCOA PULP

Cocoa seeds are surrounded by an aromatic pulp which arises from the seed teguments (technically an aril). The mucilaginous pulp is composed of spongy parenchymatous cells containing cell sap rich in sugars (10 to 13%), pentosans (2 to 3%), citric acid (1 to 2%), and salts (8 to 10%) (Lopez 1986).

During on-farm processing of cocoa seed (the exportable products), the pulp is removed by fermentation and is hydrolyzed by microorganisms. Hydrolyzed pulp is known in the industry as "sweatings." During fermentation, the pulp provides the substrate for various microorganisms which are essential to the development of chocolate flavor precursors, which are fully expressed later, during the roasting process. Fermentation was once thought to be simply an easy way to remove the pulp to facilitate drying, but its importance to cocoa quality has been well established (Lopez 1986).

The schedules for fermentation vary according to location and season, chamber size, depth of seed layer, and physical turning of the seed. Although pulp is necessary for fermentation, often more pulp occurs than is needed. Excess pulp, which has a delightful tropical flavor has been used to produce the following products: cocoa jelly, alcohol and vinegar, nata, and processed pulp.

Approximately 40 liters of pulp can be obtained from 800 kg of wet seeds. Cocoa jelly is produced by cooking fresh pulp mixed with sugar at the rate of 300 to 600 g to one liter pulp. The pulp contains about 1% pectin (Wood and Lass 1985). The jelly has a fruit-acid flavor and is a popular delicacy in Bahia, Brazil.

By controlled fermentation and distillation, sweatings can be made into an alcoholic spirit with 43% ethanol. Alcohol produced can be further fermented by *Acetobacter* sp. to produce acetic acid, but vinegar is not yet a commercial product (Samsiah et al. 1991).

Cocoa sweatings have been shown to be a suitable substrate for fermentation to produce nata (Samsiah et al. 1991), a product usually obtained from fermentation of coconut water by *Acetobacter aceti* subspecies *xylinum*. Nata is processed to an agar-like product, packed in syrup, and is consumed as a dessert in Asia.

Recently, a small industry utilizing fresh pulp has been established in Bahia for a number of tasty products. The pulp can be consumed fresh in the form of juices and "shakes." In small stalls, seeds with pulp are extracted from individual pods and placed, as ordered, in a modified food blender in which a metal disc with holes instead of blades. Milk or water is added, and after a few seconds of blending, the contents are poured through a strainer, producing a frothy, delicious, refreshing beverage. Enough pulp is usually left on the seed for normal fermentation, but pulpless seeds can also be added to intact seed to complete fermentation. Pulp can be preserved by freezing and used for ice-cream, yogurt flavoring, and juice concentrates. Because of the expense of the freezing process, cocoa pulp has not been marketed outside Bahia. It is our belief that this product could have large scale accep-tance, and we recommend market studies in temperate countries.

Extraction of pulp does not interfere with subsequent seed fermentation, and reduction of pulp before fermentation may be beneficial to cocoa quality (Schwan and Lopez 1988). In Brazil, seed quality is improved by the removal of pulp in order to reduce acidity. Commercial depulping machines of various sizes have been developed based on a revolving cylinder, which removes about 60% of the pulp and does not injure the seeds. Bahia alone produces about 300,000 tonnes of dry cocoa seeds. Each ton of dry seeds represents 300,000 t of pulp, of which 60% will be needed for fermentation, leaving an excess of 120,000 t. If only 10% of this quantity would be utilized in Bahia alone, there would be sufficient raw product available to produce 12,000 tons of pulp.

CACAO POD HUSK

Each ton of dry seeds represent about 10 tons of husk (fresh weight). At the present time, pod husks are a waste product of the cocoa industry, and present a serious disposal problem. They become a significant source of disease inoculum when used as a mulch inside the plantation. Fresh or dried husks may be used as livestock feed, but theobromine content (ca. 0.4%) restricts the proportion that can be consumed, and its use has been limited. Although acceptability by animals is satisfactory, digestibility is considered poor and dependent on processing cocoa pod husk (Adomako and Tuah 1988). Reports indicate that pod meal can constitute 20% of ration for poultry, 30 to 50% for pigs, and 50% for sheep, goats, and dairy cattle, but these values may be too high (Wood and Lass 1985). The toxic dose of theobromine for rats (LD_{50}) is 1254 mg kg^{-1} (Abiola and Tewe 1991).

Low digestibility of polysaccharides restrict the use of pod husks for methane production in biodigestor (Lopez et al. 1985).

Potassium Salts for Soap

Cocoa pod husks contain 3 to 4% potassium on a dry basis (Wood and Lass 1985). Pod husk ash has been used to make soap in Ghana and Nigeria (Oduwole and Arueya 1990; Arueya 1991).

Cacao Pigment

A cocoa husk extract called cacao pigment, which is a mixture of condensed or polymerized flavonoids (such as anthocyanidins, catechins, leukoanthycyanidin), sometimes linked with glucose, has been utilized in Japanese food industries (Kimura et al. 1979). Recently this extract has been shown to inhibit cytopathic effects of HIV in cell culture (Unten et al. 1991). The anti-HIV activity was attributable to interference with the virus adsorption, rather than inhibition of the virus replication after adsorption.

Pod Gums

In cacao, lysigenous cavities filled with mucilaginous substances occur in roots, stems, flowers, and leaves (Brook and Guard 1952) as well as fruit husks (Figueira et al. 1992). Krishna Moorthy and Subba Rhao (1976, 1978, 1980) also isolated gums from the seed pulp. Polysaccharides of cacao were first characterized by Whistler et al. (1956), who found differences in hot-water-soluble polysaccharides between seed and pod husks. Blakemore et al. (1966) examined the hot-water-soluble fraction of husk polysaccharide and concluded that the major part of this fraction was a pectic material. Cocoa pod husks were examined as a source of pectin by mild acid extraction by Adomako (1972) and Berbert (1972), but yields were low and the pectin was inferior to apple or citrus pectin in gel-forming ability. Krishna Moorthy and Subba Rhao (1978, 1980) found that gums from seed pulp were effective in low concentrations as a binder for pharmaceutical pills, and reported that suspending properties were superior to tragacanth, sodium alginate, sodium carboxy-methyl cellulose, and methyl cellulose.

Gum karaya produced from various *Sterculia* species, Sterculiaceae, mainly *S. urens* Roxb., has been used in the food and medical industry (Glickman 1982), but its use has diminished because its supply is variable and unreliable. We have recently characterized cocoa gums from pod husks and stems to evaluate their potential as a replacement for gum karaya or as a new commercial product (Figueira et al. 1992).

Yield averaged 1.5% of fresh weight and 8.4% dry weight for stem gum, and 0.7% of fresh weight and 8.7% dry weight for pod gum. Cacao pod gum was closer in composition to gum karaya than was stem gum (Table 1). Both cocoa gums contained the same monosaccharides as gum karaya but with the addition of arabinose and

Table 1. Sugar comparison of cacao gum and gum karaya.

Gum source	Sugar composition (molar ratio)[z]							
	Rhamnose	Arabinose	Galactose	Glucose	Xylose	Mannose	Galacturonic acid	Glucuronic acid
Gum karaya	1.6	0.0	1.0	0.1	0.0	0.0	1.3	0.6
Cacao stem gum	2.0	1.7	1.0	2.8	0.0	0.0	1.1	1.4
Cacao pod gum[y]	2.4	2.1	1.0	0.1	0.1	0.0	1.1	0.6
Cacao pod gum[x]	1.0	0.3	1.0	0.0	0.0	0.3	0.0	0.0
Cacao pod gum[w]	0.4	0.2	1.0	0.4	trace	0.3	1.3	0.0
Cacao pod gum[v]	0.6	0.4	1.0	trace	0.3	0.0	13.4	0.0

[z]All monosaccharides were standardized for galactose molar concentration.
[y]Figueira et al. (1992)
[x]Whistler et al. (1956)
[w]Blakemore et al. (1966)
[v]Adomako (1972)

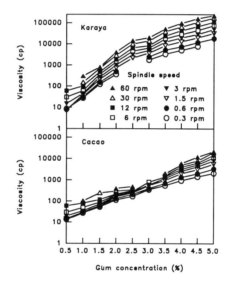

Fig. 1. Viscosity changes with concentration of cacao pod gum and gum karaya at different spindle speeds.

with higher proportions of rhamnose. The major component of stem gum was glucose, not found in the other two gums and also contained more glucuronic acid. Cacao stem gum has a higher viscosity at concentrations below 1% than gum karaya (Fig. 1).

SUMMARY

Unutilized portions of cocoa pods contain many potential new products that could provide extra income for cocoa growers. The most promising products appear to be cocoa pulp and the gums from pod husks. Although cocoa pulp is now essentially a waste product, exploitation will require a considerable investment in freezer processing equipment. Potential uses for pod gums include binders for such products as pet food, emulsifiers, and fixatives. More research is needed to discover economic uses of this product. For maximum efficiency, we foresee a combination of seed fermentation, pulp and gum extraction in a single operation. This may be carried out by medium to large growers in an on-farm operation, or by a cooperative facility that will service small growers.

REFERENCES

Adomako, D. 1972. Cocoa pod husk. Phytochemistry 11:1145–1148.

Arueya, G.L. 1991. Utilisation of cocoa pod husk in the production of washing powders. In: Abst. Int. Cocoa Conf.: Challenges in the 90s, Kuala Lumpur, Malaysia, 25–28 Sept. 1991.

Abiola, S.S. and O.O. Tewe. 1991. Chemical evaluation of cocoa by-products. Trop. Agr. 68:335–336.

Berbert, P.R. 1972. Estudo da pectina do mel e da casca do fruto do cacau. Rev. Theobroma 2(2):49–51.

Blakemore, W.S., E.T. Dewar, and R.A. Hodge. 1966. Polysaccharides of the cocoa pod husk. J. Sci. Food Agr. 17:558–560.

Brooks, E.R. and A.T. Guard. 1952. Vegetative anatomy of *Theobroma cacao*. Bot. Gaz. 13:444–454.

Figueira, A., J. Janick, M. Yadav, and J.N. BeMiller. 1992. Cacao gum: a potential new economic product. In: Proc. Int. Cocoa Conf. Challenges in the 90s (in press).

Greenwood-Barton, L.H. 1965. Utilisation of cocoa by-products. Food Manufacture 40(5):52–56.

Kimura, K. 1979. Manufacturing procedure of natural pigment from cacao bean. Japanese Patent no. Showa 54-10567.

Krishna Moorthy, N. and B. Subba Rhao. 1976. Study of the gum from cocoa (*Theobroma cacao*) seed husk. Eastern Pharmacist XIX, 224:121–123.

Krishna Moorthy, N. and B. Subba Rhao. 1978. Binding properties of the mucilage of cocoa gum (*Theobroma cacao*) for tablets. Indian J. Pharm. Sci. 40:175–177.

Krishna Moorthy, N. and B. Subba Rhao. 1980. Suspending properties of the mucilage of cocoa gum. Indian J. Pharm. Sci. 42:46–48.

Lopez, A.S. 1986. Chemical changes occurring during the processing of cacao. In: P.S. Dimick (ed.). Proc. Symp. Cacao Biotechnology. The Pennsylvania State Univ., University Park.

Lopez, A.S., H.I.S. Ferreira, A. Llamosas, and A.P. Romeu. 1985. Situaçao atual da utilizaçao de subprodutos de cacau no Brasil. Boletim Tecnico 133. CEPLAC, Bahai, Brazil.

Odwole, O.O. and G.L. Aruyea. 1990. An economic analysis of soap production from cocoa pod husk. Café, Cacao, Thé 34:231–234.

Samsiah, S., Y.Q. Lan, and C.E. Chong. 1991. Development of food products from cocoa pulp and sweatings. In: Abstracts Int. Cocoa Conf.: Challenges in the 90s, Kuala Lumpur, Malaysia, 25–28 Sept. 1991.

Schwan, R.F. and A.S. Lopez. 1988. Mudanca no perfil da fermentacao de cacau ocasionada pela retirada parcial da polpa da semente. Rev. Theobroma 18:247–257.

Unten, S., H. Ushijima, H. Shimizu, H. Tsuchie, T. Kitamura, N. Moritome, and H. Sakagami. 1991. Effect of cacao husk extract on human immunodefficiency virus infection. Letters Appl. Microbiol. 14:251–254.

Whistler, R.L., E. Masak, and R.A. Plunkett. 1956. Cacao polysaccharides. J. Amer. Chem. Soc. 78:2851–2853.

Wood, G.A.R. and R.A. Lass. 1985. Cocoa. 4th ed. Longman, Essex, England.

Goldenberry, Passionfruit, & White Sapote: Potential Fruits for Cool Subtropical Areas

Richard McCain

In the West, as in other agricultural regions of the United States, many farmers, especially small growers, have recently been looking at new and unusual crops to diversify their operations. Factors leading to diversification include water limitations, pressures from the development sector, overproduction of many traditional local crops, competition (i.e., lower prices) from out-of-state or foreign growers, and increasing labor costs.

The central coast region of California has a variety of soils and climates conducive to the growing of a large assortment of crops. While this region is well known for its production of strawberries, lettuce, and artichokes, its unique conditions have encouraged farmers to experiment with many unusual crops as well.

For example, since it was founded in 1979, the author, a partner in Quail Mountain Herbs, has grown herbs, salad crops, edible flowers, subtropical fruits, and other specialty produce in the Monterey Bay region of the central coast. Since its inception, Quail Mountain has successfully marketed over 100 different crops nationwide. Quail Mountain's growing grounds are located in several different microclimates. Due to this region's unique geography, at least 25 different microclimates have been reported.

The author has conducted research on a wide variety of herbs, flowers, vegetables, and fruits over the years. Most of the research has focused on finding or creating plants with superior taste, appearance or cultural requirements. This is done through selection and hybridizing to achieve desirable traits. The following fruits are among those crops that show the most potential.

GOLDENBERRY

Botany

First described by Linnaeus in 1753, the cape gooseberry or goldenberry, *Physalis peruviana* L., Solanaceae, has been cultivated for many decades along the Andes Mountains of South America. Goldenberry, the proposed name (Legge 1974) now being used to avoid any confusion with the common gooseberry (*Ribes* ssp.), has been spread by explorers and travelers worldwide, but is still considered a backyard fruit in most areas. Small industries are developing around the goldenberry in countries in central and south Africa, Australia, New Zealand, and India but nowhere has it really achieved large commercial success (Morton 1987). The plant's productivity in poor soils, its ease of cultivation, and low requirement for water and fertilizer has made it an attractive potential crop.

The goldenberry is an herbaceous, erect, alternate-branched shrub with pubescent slightly toothed heart-shaped leaves that appear irregularly along the stems (Moriconi et al. 1990). Yellow, pendulous flowers have campanulate corollas with purple to purplish brown spots. The genus, *Physalis*, with 100 or so species of annual and perennial herbs, is characterized by the fruit being enclosed in a papery husk or calyx. The goldenberry has a particularly delicious fruit with a tangy pineapple-like flavor. Several members of the genus are exploited for their berries. Among them are the ground cherry, *P. pruinosa* L. and the tomatillo of Mexico, *P. ixocarpa* Brat.

Horticulture

Dried ripe fruits from selected clones of the previous seasons are fermented in water for up to 5 days. After the seeds are separated from the pulp, they are planted in flats of sterile peat-lite mix. The flats are kept continually moist. Seeds germinate in 8 to 14 days in an unheated greenhouse. The seedlings are field planted when they are 15 to 20 cm tall with at least 1.0 m between each plant. The plants are watered by either drip irrigation or overhead sprinklers, although drip irrigation provides more control of water consumption and weeds. The plants appear to need little or no fertilizer. Fruit production decreased significantly when fertilizer was applied. When fish emulsion or 12-5-10 (NPK) fertilizer were applied at rates approximately 45 lb. N/acre (50 kg/ha), the plants exhibited a great deal of vegetative growth but produced few flowers or fruit. Plants planted in sandy soil without any amendment or fertilizer produced 150 to 300 flowers per plant with a corresponding number of fruit. Plants typically have a sprawling habit similar in size and growth pattern to their relative, the tomato. The plants should be trellised or staked.

The first yellow, bell-shaped flowers appear 4 to 5 weeks after transplanting during the onset of warm spring days in April and continue flowering through November unless damaged by an early frost. The plants are pollinated by wind and local insects including bees. While pollination is not a problem, inconsistency in fruit size is a problem.

Goldenberry plants typically are heavy fruit producers. Fruit production begins in August and continues until the plants are killed by frost (usually early December in this area). Yields of 150 to 300 fruits per plant are not unusual. The fruits are ripe when they turn yellow-gold. Unripe fruits are green. The fruits are 1.25 to 2.5 cm in diameter and are encased in a papery, tan husk. When fully ripe, the fruits and husk will naturally dehisce or fall when given a good shake. Harvesting can be accomplished by allowing the fruit to fall on fabric or plastic placed under the plants. Collection is either done by hand picking, or by gathering up the plastic and pouring the fruit into containers. Vacuum harvesting the fruit should be explored. Hand collection is preferable if the fruit is to be sold on the fresh market, to avoid bruising. The fruit is quite durable when left in the husk. Goldenberries are generally sold with the husk left on as many chefs use the husk for decorative purposes. After harvest, the ripe fruit may last several months without refrigeration, if kept dry. They also may be picked partially green and allowed to ripen, but these fruit never become as sweet as vine-ripened fruit.

Fruits seen on the market vary in taste and size. The fruits grown at Quail Mountain have a sweet, tangy taste while some cultivars are mealy and tasteless. There is great genetic variability. The fruit is eaten fresh or cooked. The fruit makes excellent pies and jellies and is very high in pectin. The fresh fruit may be served with husk pulled back for fondue. Goldenberry sauce is a nice accompaniment to a meat dish. While not well known by the retail consumer, the fruit has a strong following among chefs and the market is likely to grow for good quality, vine-ripened fruit.

The plant has been primarily pest and disease free at Quail Mountain. Botyritis mold has been found on ripe fruit. This may be caused by the frequent fog in this area.

PASSIONFRUIT

Botany

The Passifloraceae contains nearly 600 species in 12 genera, four of which are found in the New World. Of the 500 species of the genus *Passiflora*, only 10 to 12 have been exploited for their fruits (Menzel 1990; Howell 1989). Most commercial production around the world is based on cultivars of *P. edulis* Sims, its yellow form *P.e.f. flavicarpa* or their hybrids, which are species of the subgenus *Granadilla*. There are more than 60 other *Passiflora* species with edible fruits, many that should excite consumer interest.

The subgenus *Tacsonia* contains over 40 species with edible fruit (Escobar 1980). Originating from the cool, middle to high altitude regions of the Andes, most of the *Tacsonia* are suited to the ocean-influenced microclimates of Western North America. The arid inter-Andean valleys are veritable biogeographic islands, each with many endemic species that are isolated from other such valleys by wet tropical forests below and cold Andean tundras above, a situation favoring speciation (Iltis 1988). Although there is much genetic variation in the *Tacsonias*, a few natural hybridizations do occur (Killip 1938; Escobar 1980), and members of *Tacsonia* hybridize readily under cultivation. The feasibility of cross-breeding *Passifloras* to improve their fruits has been demonstrated by Rupert-Torres and Martin (1974) and Escobar (1980).

At Quail Mountain, the author started collecting *Passifloras* in 1979 and began hybridizing them in 1984. Hybridizing for fruit production has focused primarily on the subgenus *Tacsonia*. At the present time there are over 100 species of *Passifloras* in this collection, 15 of which are *Tacsonias*. Through numerous generations of hybrids and a continuous process of selecting superior plants from hundreds of hybrids, several very promising cultivars have been developed.

The very diverse genus *Passifloras* is characterized by woody or herbaceous vines furnished with tendrils in the leaf axils. The polymorphic, alternate leaves can be extremely variable in size and shape. Some species produce egg mimics to avoid predation by members of the *Lepidoptera* family or other pests (Gilbert 1975; K.W. Williams and L.E. Gilbert unpub.). The angular leaf stalks usually contain excrescences called glands along the petioles. The flowers located in the leaf axils are extremely colorful and elaborate in most species. The floral parts consist of a calyx with 5 lobes or sepals and 5 petals. Inside the petals are one to several series or rings of filaments forming the corona, the center of which is filled with nectar. The outer rings compose a perfect target for hummingbirds, bats, bees, moths, and other pollinators.

The main characteristics that set the *Tacsonia* apart from other subgenera in the family are that the filaments are reduced to nubs or tubercles in the corona and the calyx tube is much longer than the sepals. The male and female parts are raised aloft by the narrow columnar gynophore. At the top of the gynophore is the ovary with 5 stamens below and 3 stigmas above.

Many species of *Passifloras* are self-infertile, but if pollinated, the ovary swells into a fruit that is botanically classed as a berry. Hand pollination greatly increases fruit size. In over 60 species, fruits, that vary in size from that of a marble to a small melon, are filled with a deliciously sweet or tangy acidic pulp. The juice is widely used in many countries as a flavoring for juices, confections, ice cream, and other products. Demand in the United States has been growing steadily in the last few years for fruit which can be sold fresh or juiced for use in other products.

Horticulture

While the cultivation of the many *Passifloras* may be similar, the following is derived from the author's experimentation with selected *Tacsonia* species. Each year, passionfruit vines are selected from a growing area of about 1 ha based on overall vigor, consistent flowering and fruiting, fruit size and flavor, time of ripening, and disease resistance. Cuttings from these selected clones are rooted in a propagation house in the fall and over-wintered. Selections are propagated by dipping cuttings with 5 to 10 nodes from vigorous growing shoots in rooting hormone (IBA/IAA combination at a concentration of 1,500 ppm) and placed into flats containing a fast draining mix of perlite and sand on a bench with bottom heat and intermittent mist. Rooting takes three to five weeks. During the winter, well-rooted cuttings are transplanted into containers with a peat-lite mix and receive organic fertilizer once in late January.

The vines are set out in fields at the beginning of February (3×1.8 m spacing) and are drip irrigated weekly. The soil is amended with bone meal, blood meal, and seaweed meal prior to planting. The vines are trellised as they perform poorly when sprawling along the ground. The vines commence flowering in May and continue nearly year-round unless killed by a hard freeze. At Quail Mountain, nearly every flower sets a fruit. Pollination is by bees, hummingbirds, and wind. Hand pollination can increase fruit size. Vines produce 50 to 120 fruits each. With 740 vines/ha, estimates of harvest yield are 16,800 to 22,400 kg/ha.

Passifloras

The following *Passifloras* have commercial possibilities but require further breeding efforts. Most of the author's selections are *Tacsonia* or other cool growing *Passifloras* which have not had widespread commercial use in the United States.

Passiflora ampullacea is one of the only white flowered *Tacsonias*. This *Passiflora* has not flowered yet in Northern California, but flowered in San Diego, in 1988. Fruits are reported to be larger and with a thicker rind than *P. mollissima* (NRC 1989). Hardiness is unknown. It is found in the mountains of Southern Ecuador at elevations of 2,600 to 2,800 m.

P. antioquiensis thrives in shade, and must have large amounts of water. Flowers are brick-red, 15 cm across and hang down on peduncles up to 32 cm long. It has flowered and fruited at Quail Mountain and as far north as San Francisco. The fruit (to 12 cm) is similar in taste to the sweet *granadilla*, (*P. ligularis*), which is one of the sweetest passionfruits. Originally from the mountains of Colombia up to 3,000 m, it cannot survive more than a light frost.

P. cumbalensis fruits have long been used in South America for flavoring. Escobar (1987) reports at least seven distinct varieties of *P. cumbalensis* with variety *goudatiana* the best tasting. Flowers are rose to purple and fruits are red and banana shaped. It has flowered in San Francisco but not at Quail Mountain. *P. cumbalensis* can be found in the Andes from western Venezuela to northern Peru at elevations of 1,800 to 4,100 m.

P. manicata flowers and fruits nearly year round at Quail Mountain. The flowers are bright reddish-orange and attract hummingbirds. The fruits are small, (2.5 × 5 cm) with good flavor. Widely distributed in the Andes from 1,500 to 2,500 m in elevation.

P. mollissima is a widespread and variable species found from Venezuela down the central cordillera of Columbia to southeastern Peru and western Bolivia at 2,000 to 3,200 m in altitude. It is grown commercially in many areas and is reputed to be one of the best for juice. *P. mollissima* flowers from May to the first freeze (December-January). The yellow oblong fruits are approximately 10 to 15 cm long and have overtones of citrus. Some clones can be sweet. The species grows vigorously and shoots develop from the roots after frost injury.

P. mixta is a very diverse species found at higher elevations than *P. mollissima* (2,500 to 3,600 m) but with a similar range in the Andes. *P. mixta* has survived –7°C. Flowers are light pink to rosy-peach and bloom in successive flushes throughout the year in a cool coastal climate. The fruits are 2 to 3 cm wide and 8 to 12 cm long and are usually yellow-green when ripe. Fruits have a hint of raspberry flavor.

P. trisecta is found from southern Peru to Bolivia within a very limited range of elevation (2,400 to 2,800 m). It has broad white flowers with a short calyx tube. The anthers and stigmas are all located on one side of the flower. *P. trisecta* has flowered and fruited at Quail Mountain. The fruits are green and egg-shaped, 3 to 4 × 7 to 8 cm. Plant hardiness is unknown.

P. trifoliata is found in the Andes of central and southeastern Peru at 3500 to over 4000 m. The plant is very pubescent, appears to be hardy, but is susceptible to spider mites. Flowers are pink and similar to *P. mixta* although miniature in size (2 to 3 × 7 to 8 cm). Fruit is egg-shaped (3 to 4 × 5 cm) with three indentations longitudinally.

P. tripartita may be a variant of *P. mollissima*, but is limited to Columbia. The flowers are similar in color to *P. mollissima* but the petals and sepals flare open more. Fruit is similar in size, shape, and color to *P. mollissima* but tastes tarter.

Hybrids

P. antioquiensis (*P. mollissima* x*P. exoniensis*) is an extremely vigorous plant. The flowers are larger than *P. antioquiensis* and darker pink than *P. mollissima*. The fruit reported to be delicious (Vanderplank 1991).

P. manicata x*P. mollissima* flowers all year round on the coast of California. It must be hand pollinated to produce fruit. Fruit is larger than *P. manicata*, but smaller than *P. mollissima*.

P. mixta x*P. mollissima* is a vigorous grower but not as floriferous as *P. mixta*, nor as self-fertile as *P. mollissima*.

P. mollissima x*P. mixta* is fast growing and hardier than either parent with showier, vibrant pink flowers. Fruit is much larger and juicier than either parent with a different, but delicious flavor.

P. tripartita x*P. mollissima* is a weak grower with bright green leaves. The flowers are similar to the *P. tripartita* parent. The fruit retains the sour flavor of *P. tripartita*.

P. trisecta x*P. mixta* is fast growing, but has not flowered or fruited yet.

(*P. manicata* x*P. mollissima*) x*P. mollissima* is vigorous and hardier than either original parent. The fruit is delicious and as large as *P. mollissima* but pointed at the end.

Conclusions

Passionfruit vines are easy to bring to fruit if their basic cultural needs are met. Mixed-cropping or perennial cropping systems hold the most promise. At Quail Mountain, vines grow between rows of white sapotes in an orchard-like fashion. Between these rows, are rows of goldenberry and Yacon (*Polymnia sonchifolia*). At the ground level, a variety of herbs flourish. All of these crops seem to be very compatible with minimal disease or pest problems. Herbs in the Lamiaceae and *Apiaceae* are advantageous as they attract bees and other pollinating insects when they flower. Many *Passifloras* are self-infertile, so a sister seedling or closely related species must be in the vicinity to benefit pollination. Hand pollination is very labor intensive and expensive. Combinations of compatible species or clones need to be examined further to improve pollination in larger plantings. Fruits of many *Tacsonias* are soft and may bruise with mechanical harvesting, so clones must be selected for thicker skins. Selection of superior clones with larger sizes and improved fruit flavor will be continued. Processing and storage of fruit pulp needs to be investigated further. *Passiflora* fruits produce ethylene gas and need to be packed, stored, and shipped in such a way that this is not a hindrance to fruit quality. There is every reason to believe that with more research a greater variety of passionfruit flavors could be made available to the American consumer.

WHITE SAPOTE

Botany

The white sapote, *Casimiroa edulis* Llave & Lex, *Rutaceae*, has attracted interest among rare fruit growers and orchardists in California. The genus *Casimiroa* contains 5 or 6 species (Thompson 1972; Morton 1987). Among these are three little-known shrubs or small trees from Mexico, *C. pubescens* Ramirez, *C. pringlei* Engl., and *C. watsonii* Engl. Another species, *C. emarginata* Standley & Steyerin, was described in 1944 from a single specimen found in Guatemala (Morton 1987). The *C. sapota* Oerst, *matasano*, is very similar to and often confused with *C. edulis*, along with *C. tetrameria* Millsp., the wooly-leaved white sapote. Although these last two species sometimes hybridize with *C. edulis*, their flavor is considered inferior (Thompson 1972). *C. edulis*, *C. sapota*, and *C. tetrameria* are found in central Mexico. Their range is broad, extending down into Central America as far as Costa Rica. The white sapote, *C. edulis*, remains the preferred fruit of the genus due to its delicious flavor and wide appeal.

In its native habitat, trees are found at altitudes of 750 to 2,700 m. They do not flourish in the hot, tropical lowlands (Morton 1987), but are cultivated around the world in subtropical areas and regions with a mild Mediterranean climate. The trees have been planted in the northern part of South America, the Caribbean region, Spain, Portugal, Southern France, and Italy. They are grown commercially on a small scale in New Zealand, Australia, and South Africa. White sapote have not been successfully grown in the Philippines, but have been cultivated in other islands of the East Indies (Morton 1987). There are small plantings in Florida, Hawaii, and experimental plantings in three different regions in Israel (Nerd et al. 1990). The white sapote has grown well in California since the early 1800s (Schneider 1986). It is thought to be first introduced by Franciscan monks along with figs, olives, and grapes (Thompson 1972). Some cultivars have fruited well as far north as San Francisco (Thompson 1972).

White sapotes are medium to large-sized, fast growing trees with aggressive spreading roots that help them withstand periods of drought. Mature trees can reach 15 to 18 m in height and produce 900 kg (2,000 lb.) of fruit per year. Thompson, (1972) reported a tree of 'Chestnut' produced nearly 2,700 kg (6,000 lb.) of fruit in 1971 in Vista, California. Grafted trees remain smaller and develop a better canopy than seedlings.

Horticulture

The author first planted a few white sapote trees at Quail Mountain in 1983. In 1986, 190 two-year-old grafted trees, representing 18 cultivars, were planted approximately 6 m apart (346/ha). The trees were drip fertigated weekly, for the first two years, and bi-monthly thereafter. After the trees were two years old, yearly top dressings of goat manure were added to the base of each tree and the trees were foliar fed with seaweed solution in the summer and fall. Very light skirt pruning is practiced annually.

The first cultivars to fruit were 'Suebelle' in 1988 followed by 'Lemon Gold' in 1989. The first frost of the decade occurred in the winter of 1988 (29° to 30°F; –1.7° to –1.1°C), followed by another series of frosts in 1989 (lows to 28°F; –2.2°C). These frosts injured the young growing shoots and caused fruit to drop, but there was otherwise no severe damage and the trees recovered rapidly in the spring. In December of 1990, a devastating "freeze of the century" struck California. Low temperatures in the sapote orchard were 20°F (–6.7°C) followed by 21°F (–6.1°C) and then two weeks of 25 to 28°F (–3.9° to –2.2°C) nights. The cultivars most susceptible to

Table 1. Performance of white sapote cultivars planted as 2-year-old trees in 1986 in central California (Monterey Bay region).

Cultivar	Tree response to 1990 freeze[z]			Fruit	Comments	Tree type
	No. survive above graft	No. survive below graft	No. dead			
Chestnut	6	2	2	Large, round, good flavor	Commercial cv. in California	Vigorous, upright
Denzler		2	4		Hawaiian cv.	
Fred	9		1		Hardy	Vigorous
Guinn	3	5	2		Performs poorly	
Lemon Gold	1	5		Medium, round, good flavor	Good producer in Southern California	Small to medium
Malibu	1	2	3		Not vigorous	
Miller	5	1			Flowers early	Strong grower
McDill	7	2	1	Lg., round, yellowish		Vigorous
Ortega	1	2	3		Weak grower	
Pike	4	2		Lg., pointed, execellent flavor	Prolific	Small tree
Rainbow	2	7	1		Fast grower	Bushy growth
Suebelle	10			Small, green	Attracts pests	Very bushy
T.S. Suebelle	3	3		Small, yellow	Medium vigor	Bushy growth
Sunrise		6		Small, green		Mostly dead
White		3	3		Poor	Mostly dead
Wilson	5	1		Execellent flavor, green	Vigorous	Bears year-round
Vernon	6			Medium to large	Fast grower	Rounded
Vista	6			Small, oval, good flavor	Alternate bearing	

[z]December 1990 freeze; low temperatures of –6.7°C followed by –6.1°C and 2 weeks of –3.9° to –2.2°C nights.

freeze damage were killed below the graft, although most survived to come back from the roots (Table 1).

In California, the trees do well on well drained sandy loam or clay soils. They grow and fruit well on the deep sands of Florida, but may become chlorotic on oolitic limestone (Morton 1987). The young branches are bright green but turn gray and become very strong with age. Trunks of older trees can become buttressed. Leaves are shiny above, glabrous below, and palmately compound with 3 to 5 pointed leaflets.

The small flowers are 5-petaled, creamy white with a greenish tinge, and occur in panicles of 5 to 100 in number. In California, many cultivars bloom in spring, summer, and fall. Blooming time varies among the cultivars which prolongs fruit harvest. Most trees have two successive blooming flushes, separated by several months. The panicles are usually held terminally or in bases of the branch shoots or axils of mature leaves. The flowers sometimes are cauliflorous (Batten 1984). If bees are in the area, pollination is no problem, but many flowers and immature fruits abort naturally. For maximum fruit size, the fruit should be thinned. Fruits ripen gradually about 4 to 5 months after pollination occurs. On most cultivars, the fruit remains green when ripe. The fruit is ripe when the skin yields to slight pressure. Fruits are spherical to slightly oval in shape and are 6 to 11 × 6 to 12 cm in size. Fruits have a cream to yellowish custard-like pulp with a melting flavor of banana, peach, and pear. Each fruit has one to four seeds which resemble those of a large orange or grapefruit and are reportedly fatally toxic if eaten (Morton 1987). The fruit quality is quite good in coastal areas of California (Chandler 1950).

Fruit should be hand harvested as many varieties bruise easily. The fruit may be harvested early, which may be an advantage if the fruit is to be shipped for the fresh market. The fruit is high in ethylene so postharvest handling procedures should avoid prolonged storage. Separation of fruit or wrapping individually may retard ripening. The fruit lasts up to two weeks when ripe, under refrigeration. Fruit should be packaged in a manner that avoids bruising. Many new packaging methods are being used for other crops, such as Asian pears, that may be easily adapted to the sapote. Cultivars with thicker skin are needed. The fruit is liked by most all who try it, so it may "market itself" once it becomes more readily available to the general public.

REFERENCES

Goldenberry

Chia, C.L., M.S. Nishina, and D.O. Evans. 1987. Poha. Commodity Fact Sheet-Poha-3(A). Hawaii Cooperative Extension Service Univ. of Hawaii at Manoa, Honolulu.

Heiser, C.B., Jr. 1969. Nightshades the paradoxical plants. W.H. Freeman Co., San Francisco.

Miller, C.D., K. Bazore, and M. Bartow. 1981. Fruits of Hawaii. Reprint Univ. Press of Hawaii, Honolulu.

Moriconi, D.N., M.C. Rush, and H. Flores. 1990. Tomatillo: A potential vegetable crops for Louisiana, p. 407–413. In: J. Janick and J.E. Simon (eds.). Advances in new crops. Timber Press, Portland, OR.

Morton, J.F. 1987. Fruits of warm climates. Julia F. Morton, 20534 S.W. 92nd Ct., Miami, FL.

Quiros, C.F. 1984. Overview of the genetics and breeding of husk-tomato. HortScience 19:872–874.

Yamaguchi, M. 1983. World vegetables. AVI, Westport, CT.

Passionfruit

Erlich, P.R. and P.H. Raven. 1964. Butterflies and plants: A study in co-evolution. Evolution 18:568–608.

Escobar, L.K. 1980. Interrelationships of the edible species of *Passifloras* centering around *P. mollissima* (H.B.K.) Bailey, subgenus *Tacsonia*. Doctoral Thesis, Univ. of Texas, Austin.

Escobar, L.K. 1987. A taxonomic revision of the varieties of *Passifloras cumbalensis* (Passiflorasceae). Syst. Bot. 12:238–250.

Gilbert, L.E. 1975. Ecological consequences of a co-evolved mutualism between butterflies and plants, p. 210–240. In: L.E. Gilbert and P.H. Raven (eds.). Co-evolution of animals and plants. Univ. of Texas Press, Austin.

Holm-Nielsen, L. 1974. Notes on Central Andean Passiflorasceae. Bot. Notiser 127:338–351.

Howell, C.W. 1989. Tropical fruit news. (July) 23:67–76.

Iltis, H.H. 1988. Serendipity in the exploration of bio-diversity. (What Good Are Weedy Tomatoes?). In: E.O. Wilson (ed.). Bio-diversity. National Academy Press, Washington, DC.

Janzen, D.H. 1968. Reproductive behavior in the Passifloraceae and some of its pollinators in Central America. Behavior 32:33–48.

Killip, E.P. 1938. The American species of Passiflorasceae. Publ. Field Mus. Nat. Hist. (Bot. Ser.) 19:1–613.

Martin, F.W. and H., Nakasone. 1970. The edible species of *Passifloras*. Econ. Bot. 24:333–343.

Menzel, C. 1990. Looking for a better passionfruit. California Grower May p. 32–33.

Morton, J.F. 1987. Fruits of warm climates. Julia F. Morton, 20534 S.W. 92nd Ct., Miami, FL.

National Research Council. 1989. Lost crops of the Incas. National Academy Press, Washington, DC.

Nishida, T. 1958. Pollination of the passionfruit in Hawaii. Econ. Ent. 51:146–149.

Popenoe, W. 1920. Manual of tropical and subtropical fruits. Hafner Press/Macmillan, New York. p. 241–249.

Rupert-Torres, R. and F.W. Martin. 1974. First-generation hybrids of edible Passionfruit species. Euphytica 23:61–70

Smiley, J.T. 1978. Plant chemistry and the evolution of host specificity: New evidence from *Heliconius* and *Passiflora*. Science 201:745–747.

Snow, D.W. and B.K. Snow. 1980. Relationships between hummingbirds and flowers in the Andes of Columbia. Bul. Brit. Museum (Zool.) 38:105–139.

Vanderplank, J. 1991. Passionflowers and passionfruit. MIT Press, Cambridge, MA.

White Sapote

Batten, D.J. 1979. White sapote, p. 171–174. In: Tropical tree fruits for Australia. Queensland Dept. of Primary Industries Information Series, Australia.

Martin, F.W., C.W. Campbell, and R.M. Ruberte. 1987. Perennial edible fruits of the tropics: An inventory USDA Agr. Handb. 642, Washington, DC.

Morton, J.F. 1987. Fruits of warm climates. Julia F. Morton, 20534 S.W. 92nd. Ct., Miami, FL.

Neal, M.C. 1965. In gardens of Hawaii. Bishop Museum Press, Honolulu, HI.

Nerd, A., J. Aronson, and Y. Mizrahi. 1990. Introduction and domestication of rare and wild fruit and nut trees for desert areas, p. 355–363. In: J. Janick and J.E. Simon (eds.). Advances in new crops. Timber Press, Portland, OR.

Roecklein, J.C. and P.S. Leung. 1987. A profile of economic plants. Transaction Books, New Brunswick, NJ.

Schneider, E. 1986. Uncommon fruits and vegetables. A common sense guide. Harper & Row, New York.

Development of *Cereus peruvianus* (Apple Cactus) as a new crop for the Negev desert of Israel

Julia Weiss, Avinoam Nerd, and Yosef Mizrahi*

Cereus peruvianus (L.) Mill., Cactaceae (apple cactus) is a large erect, thorny columnar cactus found in South America (Fig. 1). It is an unexplored, underutilized cactus, grown only as an ornamental plant, even though it produces attractive, edible fruits, which are known as pitaya in Latin America (Morton 1987). The nocturnal flowers remain open for one night. The fruits are thornless and vary in skin color from violet-red to yellow. The flesh, which is the edible part of the fruit, is white and contains small, edible, and crunchy seeds. Fruits of a number of other columnar cacti, also belonging to the subfamily Cactoideae, tribe Cereeae, are known to be of economic significance for native use in South America (Felger and Moser 1974).

The aims of this study were to investigate growth and fruiting of *C. peruvianus* under different climatic, soil,

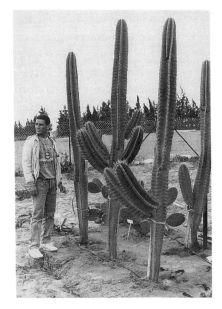

Fig. 1. *Cereus peruvianus* tree (5-year-old) at Besor (October 1991).

---

*The authors thank the following agencies: US-AID-CDR; Rich Foundation; and P.E.F. Moriah Foundation.

and water conditions in the Negev desert of Israel and to study the biology of pollination and fruit maturation.

METHODOLOGY

Seeds were obtained from (private and public botanical gardens in California). The seeds germinated easily and after two years in the nursery reached 25 cm height. The plants were then transplanted into four orchards in the Negev desert, varying in climatic, soil, and water conditions as described (Nerd et al. 1990). Besor is characterized by moderate temperatures and fresh water irrigation, whereas high temperatures and saline irrigation prevail at Qetura and Neot-Hakikar. Ramat Negev is characterized by low winter temperatures and fresh water irrigation. A smaller orchard was also established on the grounds of our institute (Beer–Sheva). The compatibility system was tested by experimental pollinations.

Fruits were picked at weekly intervals from first color change until 29 days after full color change and the fruit quality parameters [total soluble solids (TSS), reducing sugars, titratable acidity and pH] were analyzed in the pulp. Changes in fruit length and diameter were determined during fruit development for attached fruits.

RESULTS AND DISCUSSION

Plant performance

Annual growth occurred in the warm months, but plants started to grow at Qetura earlier (March) than at the other orchards (April, May). Growth occurred at a relatively constant rate at Qetura and Ramat Negev, but at Besor the onset of the summer was associated with faster growth (Fig. 2).

The total shoot length and the biomass were higher at Besor than at Ramat Negev and Qetura, while at Neot Hakikar growth was almost arrested (Table 1). Plants at Ramat Negev showed visible cold injury such as brown spots or yellowing after temperatures dropped to –7°C for several hours. Since the plant material and the agrotechniques used were similar (plants were propagated from the same batch of seeds) in all the plots, variations in growth can be attributed to the diverse environmental conditions prevailing at the different locations. The fresh water and moderate temperatures favored growth at Besor, while water salinity at Qetura and Neot Hakikar, and low temperatures at Ramat Negev inhibited growth. Sensitivity to low salinity was also shown for other cacti species such as *Opuntia ficus-indica* (Nobel 1988; Nerd et al. 1990). The salinity at Neot Hakikar caused greater stress to the plants than that at Qetura, probably because the main salt ions, sodium and chloride, in the water at Neot Hakikar, are more toxic than the ions, calcium, magnesium, and sulfates, in the water at Qetura.

Flower production was negligible at Neot-Hakikar and Ramat Negev, but abundant at Besor and Qetura. The low winter temperatures at Ramat Negev and the water salinity at Neot–Hakikar may have inhibited flowering.

Table 1. Plant biomass, plant size and flowering of 3.5-year-old *Cereus peruvianus* plants at four sites in the Negev desert of Israel[z].

Site	No. of plants	Biomass (kg dw)	Total stem length (m)	No. of flowers per plant
Besor (Western Negev)	15	7.2	15.8±1.0[y]	75±5
Ramat Negev (Negev Heights)	12	4.5	8.5±0.6	2
Qetura (Arava Valley)	10	3.2	8.1±0.2	68±7
Neot Hakikar (Arava Valley)	12	1.0	3.9±0.6	1

[z]Segments, 30 to 40 cm in length, were sampled from three plants at each site. Plants were oven dried at 70°C, and the total stem length used to calculate plant dry weight.
[y]±SE

The natural fruit set of 15 individual plants at Besor varied in the summer, 1990, between 0 and 95%, and pollination studies were conducted to evaluate the origin of this variation.

Pollination

The compatibility system of various individual plants was tested by comparing fruit set with cross, self, and open pollinations in summer 1991 at the Besor orchard and at Beer-Sheva. Flowers that were covered with bags before anthesis and were hand-self-pollinated did not set fruit (Table 2). This suggests that *C. peruvianus* is self-incompatible. Hand-cross-pollination led to 100% fruit set. Open-pollinated flowers set fruit at Besor but not at Beer-Sheva (Table 2). Fruits from hand-cross-pollinations were heavier and had a higher pulp to peel ratio than fruits which derived from open-pollinated flowers. They also had more seeds/g pulp tissue and the seed number was positively correlated to the pulp weight. Open-pollination did not lead to optimal fruit development compared to experimental cross-pollination. These results indicate that it is necessary to plant two or more different clones

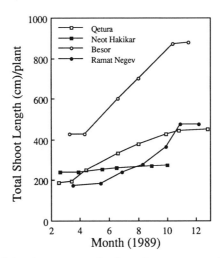

Fig. 2. Growth of *Cereus peruvianus* plants at four sites in the Negev desert of Israel during 1989. Values are means of ten plants.

Table 2. Effect of pollination on fruit set, seed development, and selected parameters of fruit quality for four individual plants[z].

Site	Seedling no.	Pollination[y] treatment	Fruit set (%)	No. seeds/ fruit	Seeds/g pulp tissue	Fruit weight	Pulp/Peel ratio
Besor	1	Cross	100	3222a	13a	401a	1.56a
		Self	0	---	---	---	---
		Open	20	399b	6b	124b	1.13b
Besor	5	Cross	100	1993a	13a	194a	3.00a
		Self	0	---	---	---	---
		Open	37.5	384b	7b	78b	1.93b
Beer–Sheva	7	Cross	100	1289	16	149	1.79
		Self	0	---	---	---	---
		Open	0	---	---	---	---
Beer–Sheva	16	Cross	100	2879	17	239	2.31
		Self	0	---	---	---	---
		Open	0	---	---	---	---

[z]Values are means of 7 to 10 fruits. Values followed by different letters for each seedling were significantly different at $p \geq 0.05$.

[y]Flower buds or the stigmata were covered with cloth bags before anthesis to prevent cross- or self-pollination. Flowers were then hand-cross- or self-pollinated at anthesis. Flowers remained unbagged for open-pollination.

in close proximity and which flower over the same time period. One reason for the low fruit set of some seedlings in open pollination might be a lack of other flowering plants in the vicinity.

The main insects visiting the flowers were bees, although small flies were also observed. The insects visited the flowers when the flowers are opening before sunset, and after sunrise, when the flowers are closing. The placing of beehives in an plantation would increase fruit set and improve fruit production.

Differences Among Seedlings of *C. peruvianus*

Seedlings varied in thorn development on the shoots, in onset and duration of the flowering period, and in fruit appearance and quality (Table 3). The ribbed stems of *C. peruvianus* bear thorns (Morton 1987). Nevertheless, some of our seedlings exhibited a reduction in thorn length with increasing age, leading to thornless upper stem parts. Cuttings taken from such thornless stem parts produced thornless plants, which indicates that this is a growth phase phenomenon and genetically controlled. Thornlessness would obviously be an important advantage for cultivating this plant.

Flowering of *C. peruvianus* occured in two waves. The first wave starts in spring (May) and the second in mid-summer (July). Detailed observations made on the first wave in 1991 showed that there are considerable variations between the various seedlings in both the onset and the duration of flowering period, which may last from two weeks to one month.

The color of the fruits varies from violet-red through orange to yellow and the fruit length ranges from 7 to 10 cm. The taste of the fruits also varies markedly, some fruits are juicy and aromatic, whereas others are mucilagenous and inferior in taste. Furthermore, the fruits differ in their tendency to burst upon ripening. A reduction of irrigation during the critical stage of fruit development might prevent this phenomenon.

Fruit quality parameters (TSS, reducing sugars, and titratable acidity of the pulp), fruit weight, pulp to peel ratio, and percentage of peel and pulp dry weight of different individual plants from Besor and Beer–Sheva are shown in Table 2 and 4. Significant differences were found in titratable acidity of the pulp and dry weight of the peel as well as in fruit weight and pulp to peel ratio. Preliminary taste-tests showed, that fruits with a higher content of titratable acids were less tasty than the fruits with a lower acidity. Fruits of the various individual plants were all harvested in the stage of full color change, but since they were not tagged at the beginning of color change, they might have reached different stages of ripeness at harvest and this fact might partially be responsible for the differences in the quality parameters.

Maturation and Harvest

CO_2 and ethylene evolution were measured in ripening fruits. No increase in gas evolution was observed indicating that the fruits of *C. peruvianus* are nonclimacteric. The TSS and reducing sugars increased and the

Table 3. Variation in thorn development, flowering period, and fruit appearance for four exemplary individual plants growing in Beer–Sheva.

Seedling no.	Thorn development	First flowering period (1991)	Fruit appearance[z] Peel color	Fruit length (cm)	Comments
7	Thorny	May 24–June 12	Orange	8.2	Fruits burst on ripening Ripe fruits are mucilagenous
8	Thornless	June 28–July 1	Dark-red	7.1	Fruits burst upon ripening Ripe fruits are mucilagenous
10	Thorny	June 14–June 29	Violet-red	7.5	Fruits do not burst on ripening Fruits are juicy and aromatic
16	Thorny	May 20–June 21	Violet-red	10.3	Fruits do not burst on ripening Fruits are juicy and aromatic

[z]Descriptions of the fruits refer to fruits at full color change.

Table 4. Fruit quality parameters for five exemplary individual plants growing at Besor[z].

Seedling no.	Pulp (% dry wt)	Peel (% dry wt)	Pulp		Titratable acidity (meq/g fw)
			TSS (%)	Reducing sugars (mg/g fw)	
1	14.6±0.7	6.40±0.20	9.3±0.2	101±3	61.7±5.6
5	12.8±0.5	10.90±1.27	8.2±0.6	83±9	17.4±1.9
7	13.7±0.9	13.73±1.14	11.6±0.5	91±10	26.8±1.6
12	15.4±0.9	6.64±0.83	9.3±0.3	106±4	65.4±3.5
16	15.3±1.1	12.39±1.09	10.8±0.2	107±8	17.6±1.6

[z]Values are means of 7 to 10 fruits ±SE.

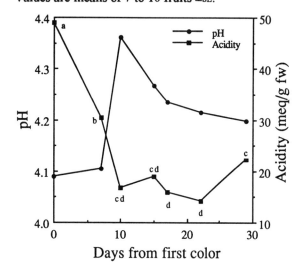

Fig. 3. Acidity and pH in fruits of *Cereus peruvianus* during color change. Values are means of 4 to 12 fruits from 15 plants, growing at Besor. Values followed by different letters were significantly different (p≥0.001)

Fig. 4. TSS and reducing sugars in fruits of *Cereus peruvianus* during color change. Values are means of 4 to 12 fruits from 15 plants, growing at Besor. Values followed by different letters were significantly different (p≥0.01)

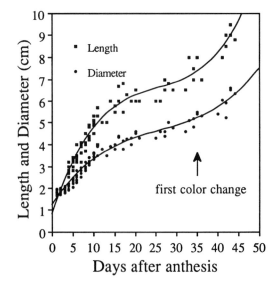

Fig. 5. Changes in length and diameter of *Cereus peruvianus* fruits. Values are separate readings of 10 fruits of one individual plant growing in Beer–Sheva.

titratable acidity decreased significantly within 10 days after first color change (Fig. 3, 4). No distinct changes in the amount of reducing sugars and the titratable acidity occurred until ripeness, whereas the TSS increased significantly upon ripeness. Fruit growth followed a sigmoidal growth pattern (Fig. 5). These results indicate that the time of full color change is the most favorable harvest time in terms of fruit size, but the optimal harvest time in terms of taste and postharvest behavior is still unclear.

CONCLUSION

Optimal conditions for growth and flower production of *C. peruvianus* were moderate temperatures and fresh water irrigation; low winter temperatures and saline irrigation inhibited growth.

Plants propagated by seeds were self-sterile. Open pollination led to a fruit set of between 0 and 95%, depending on the individual plant, but experimental cross-pollination resulted in 100% fruit set and heavier fruits with more seeds. The pulp weight was positively correlated to the seed number. Bees were the main insects visiting the flowers. The placement in the orchard of beehives may be desirable to maximize fruit yield. Selection for plant appearance, flowering time, and fruit appearance and quality is now needed for the commercialization of *C. peruvianus*.

REFERENCES

Felger, R.S. and M.B. Moser. 1974. Columnar cacti in Seri Indian culture. Kiva 39:257–275.

Morton, J.F. 1987. Cactaceae, strawberry pear, p. 347–348. In: Fruits of warm climates. J.F. Morton, Miami, FL.

Nerd, A, J.A. Aronson, and Y. Mizrahi. 1990. Introduction and domestication of rare and wild fruit and nut trees for desert areas, p. 353–363. In: J. Janick and J.E. Simon (eds.). Advances in new crops. Timber Press, Portland, OR.

Nobel, P.S. 1988. Environmental biology of agaves and cacti. Cambridge Univ. Press, Cambridge.

Pitayas (Genus *Hylocereus*): A New Fruit Crop for the Negev Desert of Israel*

Eran Raveh, Julia Weiss, Avinoam Nerd, and Yosef Mizrahi

Members of the genus *Hylocereus* (Pitaya) (Fig. 1), Cactaceae are epiphytes which produce high-quality fruits that resemble those of the prickly pear (*Opuntia ficus-indica* Mill.) in appearance but differ from the prickly pear in that they contain very small seeds. Unlike the prickly pear, the peel of pitaya fruits is thornless or becomes thornless during ripening. Attempts are currently being made to domesticate species of the shrub in Central America and in Israel (Barbeau 1990; Nerd et al. 1990). Some agrotechniques methods have been developed (Barbeau 1990; Arcadio 1986), but there remains a lack of detailed information about conditions required for growth and fruit production.

Twenty three genotypes of various *Hylocereus* species were first introduced and propagated in our institutes nursery in 1986. The plants characteristics were studied in our greenhouse, and some genotypes were planted in four experimental orchards at various sites in the Negev Desert (Nerd et al. 1990). When the shrubs were planted in the open sun, they developed bleaching symptoms and growth was inhibited. Plants recovered only after they were shaded.

In this paper, we describe fruiting in several selected clones and the effect of shading on photosynthesis and growth in two of these clones.

---

*The authors would like to thank the following agencies: US-AID-CDR and the Rich Foundation for partial support of this research.

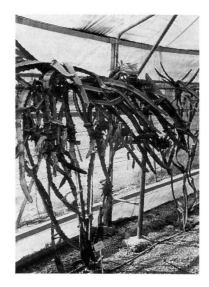

Fig. 1. *Hylocereus paolyrhi*, 3-years-old, growing on trellis system under netting, at Beer-Sheva (October 1991).

Table 1. Fruit appearance of pitayas under shade in the greenhouse in the third year.

Hylocereus species	Peel color	Pulp color	Peel morphology
H. sp. type Alon	Light red	White	Large scales with light green tips, fruit oblong
H. costaricensis	Dark red	Violet	Small scales, fruit round
H. sp. type Katom	Yellow	White	Spines, easy to remove, peel bearing warts, fruit oblong
H. paolyrhi	Dark red	Violet red	Large scales with dark green tips, fruit oblong
H. sp. type Equador	Yellow	White	Spines, easy to remove, peel bearing warts, fruit oblong

METHODOLOGY

Seeds and cuttings of various *Hylocereus* species obtained from individuals, and botanical gardens in California, Columbia, Equador, and Israel were propagated in our nursery. In greenhouse studies, three plants of each clone were planted, and plant development, flowering and fruit set, and quality were evaluated. A shading experiment was carried out with cuttings of *H. polyrhizus* and *Hylocereus* sp. type Equador (species not yet defined) planted in 15-liter buckets filled with a nursery mixture were placed in a nethouse. Three levels of shading, 30, 60, and 90%, were provided by means of nets of different densities. Each treatment contained 16 plants of each species. Growth parameters (length and weight) were measured during the winter-spring (November–April) of 1990–1991.

RESULTS AND DISCUSSION

The species can be divided into two groups according to fruit characteristics and fruit development: those having large red fruits and short fruit development time (group Alon), and those having smaller yellow fruits and longer time of fruit development (group Katom) (Table 1, Fig. 2). Katom fruits were judged to be superior (by our team of tasters), probably because they had the highest total soluble solids content (Table 2). In general, fruits of all the species were very juicy, with a pleasant sweet-sour taste.

Pollination

Hylocereus species are described as being self-compatible, but cross-pollination by insect occurs frequently (Cacioppo 1990). We found that some species set fruit after hand-self pollination, whereas others did not (Table 3). Thus, within the genus *Hylocereus*, there are both self-compatible and self-incompatible species. In one species, *H.* sp. type Katom, we found that self-pollination occurred without a pollen vector. Hand-cross

Table 2. Fruit quality if pitayas under shade in the greenhouse in the third year[z].

Hylocereus species	Fruit weight (g)	Pulp/peel fresh weight basis	Pulp				
			DW (%)	TSS (%)	Reducing sugars (mg/g fw)	Titratable acidity (meq/g fw)	pH
H. sp. type Alon	595±32	3.7±0.4	16.4±0.8	10.9±0.5	107.2±7.8	32.3±6.9	4.9±0.02
H. costaricensis	308±15	3.1±0.4	16.2±0.8	12.2±0.8	84.6±7.3	50.6±8.9	4.7±0.02
H. sp. type Katom	96±8	1.1±0.1	20.9±0.3	16.6±2.5	93.7±13.3	23.1±3.5	4.6±0.00
H. paolyrhi	327±24	2.0±0.1	17.2±1.2	10.5±0.5	68.8±6.4	63.8±2.0	5.2±0.50
H. sp. type Equador	115±8	---	---	---	---	---	---

[z]Values ±SE

Table 3. Compatibility systems of various *Hylocereus* species[z].

Plant species	Hand-cross pollination (% fruit set)	Hand-self pollination (% fruit set)	Covered, no hand pollination (% fruit set)
H. sp. type Alon	100	47	0
H. costaricensis	100	0	0
H. sp. type Katom	100	100	100
H. paolyrhi	100	0	0
H. sp. type 10487	100	67	0

[z]Six to ten flowers were used for each treatment.

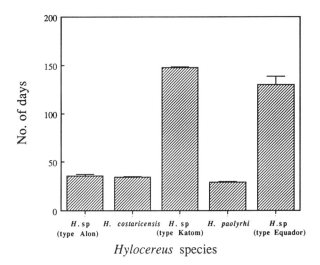

Fig. 2. Length of fruit development stage in fruits of various species of the genus *Hylocereus*. Bars represent ±SE.

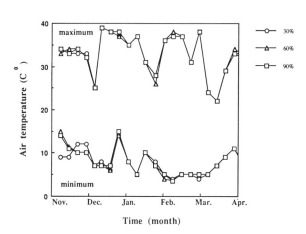

Fig. 3 Maximum and minimum air temperatures at three levels of shading.

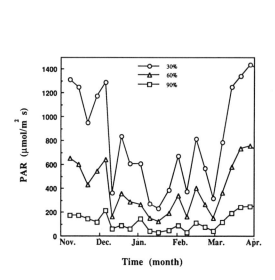

Fig. 4. Noon PAR at three levels of shading.

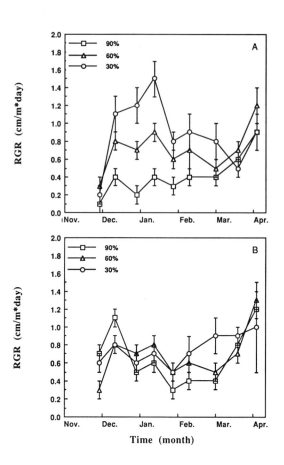

Fig. 5. Relative growth rate (RGR) of *H. polyrhizus* (A) and *Hylocereus* sp. type Equador (B).

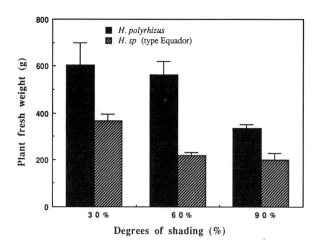

Fig. 6. Fresh weight of *H. polyrhizus* and *Hylocereus* sp. type Equador after five months in the shadehouse. Mean fresh weight of plant at planting was 148±13 g for *H. polyrhizus* and 60±4 g for *Hylocereus* sp. type Equador. Bars represent ±SE.

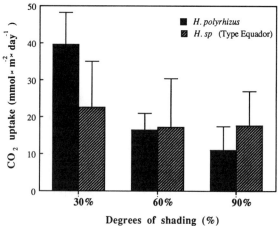

Fig. 7. Daily CO_2 uptake of *H. polyrhizus* and *Hylocereus* sp. type Equador. Measured mid March 1991. Values are means for five plants. Bars represent ±SE.

pollination between the various species led to 100% fruit set indicating no incompatibilities among these species. The flowering period of *Hylocereus* genus starts in mid-May and the last flowers appear in November. Flowering occurs in two or three waves. For the cultivation of self-sterile plants, we recommend that several species be planted together to guarantee the availability of cross-pollination partners. Flowers of all species were opened for only one night between two hours before dusk and three hours after dawn. Other reports claim that *Hylocereus* flowers are open during several nights (Cacioppo 1990; Barbeau 1990).

Shading

Maximum and minimum air temperatures fluctuated around 30° and 8°C, respectively, during the 150 days of the experiment (mid-October to mid-March), and the three parts of the nethouse exhibited similar maximum and minimum temperatures (Fig. 3). Maximum levels of photosynthetic active radiation (PAR) increased with decreasing shading (Fig. 4), i.e., the main difference among the three sections of the nethouse lay in the radiation intensity.

Growth was expressed as the relative growth rate (RGR) which is defined as: $(Lt_2-Lt_1)/Lt_1 \Delta$ day, where Lt_1 is total stem length at time t_1 and Lt_2 is total stem length at time t_2.

Growth of *H. polyrhizus* increased significantly in the winter time (November–February) with decreasing shading. This tendency was also found less significantly for *Hylocereus* sp. type Equador (Fig. 5).

The fresh weight of the plants on the 150th day is shown in Fig. 6. The weight increase in *H. polyrhizus* was greater than that in *Hylocereus* sp. type Equador (fresh weight at zero time was 148±13 g SE and 60±4 g, respectively), particularly at the lowest and medium levels of shading. These findings are compatible with those for the RGR measurements, indicating that *H. polyrhizus* exhibits a higher tolerance to high radiation than the Equador type. The two species differed in CO_2 uptake rate (Fig. 7), the rate being correlated to growth. Values of CO_2 uptake at the lowest shading level were in the range found by Nobel and Hartsock (1990) for other epiphytic cacti.

CONCLUSIONS

Cultivation of *Hylocereus* plants in the Negev will have to be restricted to shadehouses, with the shading level being adapted to the specific species. To ensure maximum pollination, compatible clones or species will have to be planted in close proximity and pollinating insects will need to be made available in the shadehouse, perhaps by placing beehives in the shadehouse. Crossing between various species of the genus *Hylocereus* is feasible and could lead to improved types.

REFERENCES

Arcadio Luis, B. 1986. Cultivo de la Pitaya. Federacion Nacional de Cafeteros. Bogota, D.E. p. 1–18.

Barbeau, G. 1990. La pitahaya rouge, an nouveau fruit exotique. Fruits 45:141–147.

Cacioppo, O.G. 1990. Pitaya: una de las mejores frutus producida por Colombia. Inforamtive Agro Economico. Feb. p. 15–19.

Nerd, A., J.A. Aronson, and Y. Mizrahi. 1990. Introduction and domestication of rare and wild fruit and nut trees for desert areas, p. 353–363. In: J. Janick and J.E. Simon (eds.). Advances in new crops. Timber Press, Portland, OR.

Nobel, P.S. and L. Hartsock. 1990. Diel patterns of CO_2 exchange for epiphytic cacti differing in succulence. Physiologia Plant. 78:628–634.

Domestication and Introduction of Marula (*Sclerocarya birrea* subsp. *Caffra*) as a New Crop for the Negev Desert of Israel

Avinoam Nerd and Yosef Mizrahi*

Marula (*Sclerocarya birrea* subsp. *caffra*, Anacardiaceae) is a large dioecious deciduous tree found in southern Africa, mostly south of the Zambesi river (Palgrave 1984). The tree is highly prized by local people for its fruits. Female trees bear plum-sized stone fruits with a thick yellow peel and a translucent, white, highly aromatic, sweet-sour flesh which is eaten fresh, or used to prepare juices and alcoholic beverages. The seeds inside the stone are also eaten they have a delicate nutty taste and a high nutritive value and high (up to 56%) oil content (Shone 1979).

Recently, an effort has been made to domesticate the tree in southern Africa and Israel in order to establish orchards that will supply both fresh fruit and fruit for the canning and beverage industry (Fig. 1) (Weinert et al. 1990; Nerd et al. 1990). This paper describes plant performance in four introduction orchards established at different locations in the Negev Desert of Israel and postharvest physiology of the fruits.

METHODOLOGY

Seeds collected from trees growing in central and northern Botswana were used for propagation. One-year-old plants were planted in 1985–87 in introduction orchards established at the following four sites in the Negev Desert: Besor—moderate temperatures, fresh water (EC about 1 dS·m^{-1}); Ramat Negev—subfreezing temperatures, fresh and brackish (EC 3.5 dS·m^{-1}) water; Qetura and Neot Hakikar high summer temperatures and warm winters, brackish water (EC fluctuating between 3.5 and 4.5 dS·m^{-1}). Additional details on the climate and soil and water properties of the four sites have been published previously described (Nerd et al. 1990).

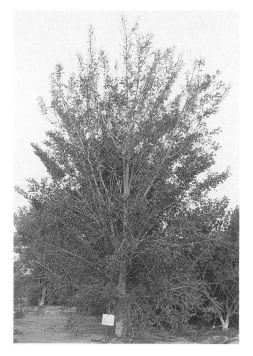
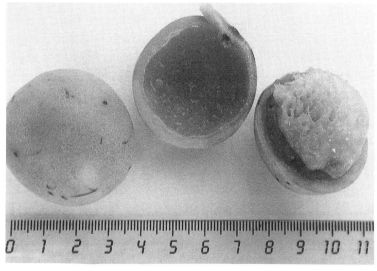

Fig. 1. Five-year-old marula tree at Qetura (December 1992) (A), marula fruit showing thick peel and soft fibrous flesh containing nut (B).

*The authors express their thanks and appreciation to Ehud Tzeeri from Neot-Hakikar, Elaine Soloway from Kibbutz Qetura, Rafi Rotem from the Besor Experimental Station, David Itzhak from the Ramat-Negev Experimental Station, Eyal Naim of the Institutes for Applied Research for their skillful help in this research. This research was partially supported by the following agencies: US–AID CDR; GIARA–Germany–Israel Agriculture Research Agreement; Moriah fund and the Israeli Minitry of Agriculture.

About thirty plants were planted in each orchard, in six blocks at Ramat Negev and in three blocks at the other plots. The plants were drip fertigated every one or two days in the summer and every three to five days in the winter. In the fourth year, the amount of water supplied was determined according to the evaporation rate (pan class A), and the plant cover, was 17 m³ per tree per year at Besor and Ramat Negev and 25 m³ per tree per year at Neot Hakikar and Qetura. At Ramat Negev, brackish water was applied to three of the blocks after two years of establishment with fresh water and the other three were irrigated only with fresh water. Growth and phenological data were recorded periodically for each orchard. Fruits collected at Qetura were used for postharvest physiology studies.

PLANT PERFORMANCE AND PHENOLOGY

The height of four-year-old plants was much greater at Qetura and Besor than at Neot Hakikar and Ramat Negev. Trunk circumference (30 cm above trunk base) usually correlated with tree height, except for the plants at Ramat Negev whose circumference was larger than the value predicted from the height (Table 1). The small size of the plants at Ramat Negev may have been related to frost damage. After one night in February 1989, when temperatures fell to −7°C, all the branches died almost to the base of the trunk. However, all plants resumed growth the following summer (dead portions of branches were cut back in the spring), and the trees tended to develop more than one main stem (Table 1). The recovered plants also produced sprouts from roots close to the base of the tree. This phenomenon coincides with that manifested in another of our studies, which showed that marula root cuttings prepared in the summer easily developed new shoots. Although climatic conditions are similar at Qetura and Neot Hakikar and both sites were irrigated with brackish water, growth at Qetura was more rapid than that at Neot Hakikar. This finding can be related to the higher Ca^{2+}/Na^+ ratio in the water at Qetura (1.2 at Qetura versus 0.8 at Neot Hakikar), which probably moderated the retarding effect of salinity on growth. Brackish water irrigation of two year-old-trees at Ramat Negev did not inhibit their growth. These results together with those obtained at Neot Hakikar and Qetura indicate that marula has tolerance to salinity of ~4 dS·m⁻¹.

Breaking of winter dormancy (late spring, April–May), occurred earlier at the warmer sites, Qetura and Neot Hakikar, than at the cooler sites, Besor and Ramat Negev (Fig. 2). It is of interest that the initiation of seasonal growth in common deciduous fruit trees such as peaches and apples in the Besor area took place 1 to 2 months earlier than that in marula.

Leaf abscission started in December in all the orchards. Plants at the cooler sites lost all their leaves within a few weeks, but those at the warmer sites maintained up to 50% of the leaves until the next summer. Although the breaking of dormancy can be retarded in deciduous trees that have not shed all their leaves in the winter (Saure 1985), we did not find any inhibition of breaking of bud dormancy in trees at the warm sites.

Yields were obtained only from the trees at Qetura. Eight of 20 trees planted in 1985–86 produced fruits, five giving reasonable yields in 1990, with an average yield of 26.8±10.4 kg and an average fruit weight of 28.3±2.5 g. These fruits are relatively small in comparison with those obtained from some selected trees in Botswana and South Africa, where average fruit weight may reach 80 g (F.W. Taylor and L.C. Holtzausen pers. commun.).

Table 1. Plant performance of four-year-old marula trees[z].

Site	Height (cm)	Trunk circ. (cm)	No. main stems/tree
Besor	533±60	50±2	1
Ramat Negev[y]	290±25	54±3	2–3
Qetura	620±30	58±2	1
Neot Hakikar	413±38	40±4	1

[z]Values for height and trunk circumference are means ±SE for 30 plants.
[y]Data for plants irrigated with fresh water and those irrigated with brackish water were combined, since plants of the two treatments did not differ significantly in size.

FRUIT RIPENING

Marula fruits abscise before ripening; at this stage the skin color is green and the fruit is firm. Time of fruit abscission varied among trees at Qetura. Of the eight yielding trees, fruits abscised mainly in August in six trees and in late October in the other two. This can be attributed to genetic variation, which can be exploited for expanding the harvest period by planting clones that ripen at different times. The pattern of fruit abscission differed among trees, but in all the examined trees, 80% of the fruits abscised within two weeks (Fig. 3).

Production of CO_2 and ethylene was studied in marula fruits collected immediately after abscission. The fruits were enclosed in an air flow system kept at 20°C, and samples of exiting air were analyzed for CO_2 and ethylene concentrations by gas chromatography (Mizrahi 1982).

The respiration rate (CO_2 production) increased to a temporary peak on day 9, and ethylene production rose concomitantly with the rise in respiration (Fig. 4). Skin color started to change on day 3, and a completely yellow color was obtained by day 12. These results indicate that climacteric processes start after abscission.

Our results contradict those of Redelinghuys (cited by Weinert et al. 1990), who showed that abscised fruits had high respiration rates which dropped markedly over 7 days at 23°C. However, the pattern of respiration we observed for abscised fruits was the same as that demonstrated by Redelinghuys for picked fruits.

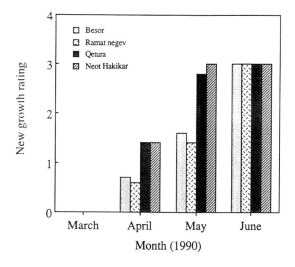

Fig. 2. Development of new growth at various orchards. The percentage of the tree canopy covered with new leaves was estimated visually at the middle of each month on a scale of 0 to 3; 0 = no new growth, 1 = less than 20%, 2 = 20 to 60%, 3 = 60 to 100%.

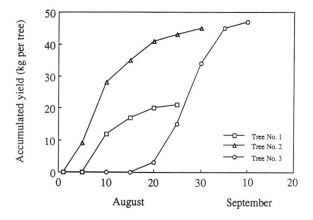

Fig. 3. Abscission of fruits during the ripening period in three high-yielding trees at Qetura.

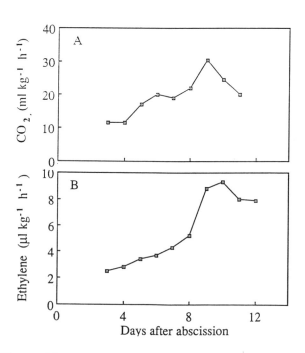

Fig. 4. CO_2 evolution rate (A) and ethylene evolution rate (B) in abscissed marula fruits stored at 20°C. Each value is mean of 10 individuals fruits.

Table 2. Characteristics of fruits stored at various temperatures for 14 days[z].

Storage temp. (°C)	Skin color rating[y]	Juice content (% of fw)	Juice acidity (meq/ml)	Total soluble solids (%)	Reducing sugars (%)
4	1	---[x]	---	---	---
12	2.8±0.3	33.7±2.1	0.21±0.05	14.0±1.4	0.97±0.04
20	4	47.4±3.2	0.15±0.05	13.8±1.9	1.11±0.03

[z]Values are means ±SE for 10 fruits. Fruit fresh weight ranged between 20 and 38 g.
[y]Color was estimated visually using a scale of 1 to 4, where 1 = pale green, 2= green-yellow, 3 = pale-yellow, 4 = deep yellow.
[x]Fruits remained firm and juice could not be squeezed out.

Ripening of abscised fruits was affected by storage temperatures. After 14 days of storage, fruits kept at 4°C remained green and firm, while those kept at 12° and 20°C developed a yellow color and could be squeezed for juice (Table 2). Fruits stored at 20°C were riper than those kept at 12°C: they had a deeper yellow color, a higher juice content, and lower acidity. The fruits stored at 4°C for 14 days were damaged by low temperatures: brown spots developed on the green skin within five days when they were transferred to 20°C and off-flavor taste developed.

CONCLUSIONS

Marula was established well at various sites in the Negev Desert, differing in environmental conditions. Brackish water (EC ~4 dS·m^{-1}) can be used to irrigate the crop, and warm winters (mean temperature of the coldest month is 15°C) do not limit the breaking of winter dormancy. Cultivation at sites with subfreezing temperatures may not be feasible since branches may be damaged by frost events (−7°C). However, it is possible that hardening the trees before winter by withholding irrigation may increase their tolerance to cold and thus enable cultivation at such sites.

Trees started to bear fruits in the fourth year, and reasonable yields (above 20 kg per tree) were obtained one year later. Full ripening (climacteric type) occurs after abscission, and fruits can be stored for two weeks at 20°C and longer at 12°C, while low temperatures (4°C) damage the fruits.

REFERENCES

Mizrahi, Y. 1982. Effect of salinity on tomato fruit ripening. Plant Physiol. 69:966–970.
Nerd, A., J.A. Aronson, and Y. Mizrahi. 1990. Introduction and domestication of rare and wild fruit and nut trees for desert areas, p. 355–363. In: J. Janick and J.E. Simon (eds.). Advances in new crops. Timber Press, Portland, OR.
Palgrave, K.C. 1984. Trees of Southern Africa. C. Struik, Cape Town, Republic of South Africa.
Saure, M.C. 1985. Dormancy release in deciduous fruit trees. Hort. Rev. 7:239–300.
Shone, A.K. 1979. Notes on the marula. Bul. 58, Dept. of Forestry, Pretoria, Republic of South Africa.
Weinert, I., A.G., P.J. van Wyk, and L.C. Holtzhausen. 1990. Marula, p. 88–115. In: S. Nagy, P.E. Show, and W.F. Nardowsky (eds.). Fruits of tropical and subtropical origin. Florida Science Source, Lake Alfred, FL.

Chinkapin: Potential New Crop for the South

Jerry A. Payne, George P. Johnson, and Gregory Miller*

Chinkapins, also spelled chinquapins and sometimes called dwarf or bush chestnuts, are shrubs and small trees commonly found throughout the East, South, and Southeast. They are characterized by usually bearing one nut per bur and having burs that open into two halves like a clam shell. Some taxonomists and geneticists have separated the chinkapins into eight or more poorly defined taxa based on growth form, leaf morphology, bur characteristics, habitat, and blight susceptibility (Jaynes 1975; Graves 1950, 1961; Ashe 1923, 1924). These include: *Castanea pumila* (L.) Mill., *C. ozarkensis* Ashe, *C. ashei* (Sudw.) Ashe, *C. alnifolia* Nutt., *C. floridana* (Sarg.) Ashe, *C. paucispina* Ashe, *C. arkansana* Ashe, and *C. alabamensis* Ashe. Other taxonomists (Tucker 1975; Johnson 1987, 1988) have reduced most of these taxa to synonymy within *C. pumila* var. *pumila* and indicate that the chinkapin is but a single species, *C. pumila*, comprising two botanical varieties: vars. *ozarkensis* (Ashe) Tucker and *pumila*. Only the Allegheny chinkapin, *C. pumila* var. *pumila* (Terrell 1977) is discussed in this report.

The Allegheny chinkapin, also called the American, common, or tree chinkapin, may well be our most ignored and undervalued native North American nut tree. It has been widely hailed as a sweet and edible nut; a wood source for fuel, charcoal, fence post and railroad ties; and a coffee and chocolate substitute (Porcher 1970; Gillespie 1959). In addition, the tree's root has folkloric history as an astringent, a tonic, and a febrifuge (Krochmal and Krochmal 1982). However, chinkapin's great potential lies in its value to commercial chestnut breeding programs and as a source of food and cover for wildlife (Halls 1977; Jaynes 1979; Bailey 1960).

DESCRIPTION AND DISTRIBUTION

Castanea pumila var. *pumila* can be characterized as a large, spreading, smooth barked multistemmed shrub, 2 to 4 m tall, occasionally single stemmed and 5 to 8 m tall. Large trees are sometimes found, especially under human intervention when some of the competing trees have been removed. According to Bailey (1960), *C. pumila* attains a height of 15.2 m; however, the National Register of Big Trees (Pardo 1978) lists its two *C. pumila* record specimens at 12.5 and 12.8 m in height. Johnson (1988) reports an individual tree from Liberty County, Florida that was 15 m tall with a 1.1 m diameter at breast height.

The Allegheny chinkapin is found in dry sandy woods and thickets from southern New Jersey and Pennsylvania to Kentucky and Missouri, south to Florida and Texas (Fig. 1). According to Hooker (1967), *C. pumila* is rare and widely scattered in the extreme eastern counties of Oklahoma on dry, rocky or gravelly ridges, or silicious uplands.

BOTANY AND HORTICULTURE

In Georgia, bud break normally occurs during the last week of March or the first week of April. The leaves are borne alternately along the slender pubescent to glabrescent reddish brown twigs. The simple leaves are acute, elliptic to obovate, 4.1 to 21.7 cm long, 1.5 to 8.3 cm wide, bright yellowish-green to light green and glabrous above, whitish and densely tomentose beneath. The leaf margins are coarsely serrate and bristle tipped and the petiole is stout and glabrous but can be pubescent. There is much variation among leaves in shape, size, color, and pubescence even when growing on the same tree (shrub).

Flowering occurs after the first leaves have expanded. Two or three types of flowers and inflorescences are borne in the leaf axils of current season's growth (Fig. 2). Unisexual male catkins appear near the bases of the shoots and bisexual catkins containing both male and female flowers are found nearer the terminal ends of the

---

*We gratefully acknowledge the following for freely sharing their knowledge, experience and unpublished data on chinkapin acreage, blight, culture, pesticides, yields, products, breeding and cultivars: Connecticut (Sandra Anagnostakis; Richard Jaynes); Georgia (Rose Payne, Mike Moore); Kansas (Bill Reid); Kentucky (Laura Ray); Missouri (Dan Millikan); New Jersey (Jerry Baron); New York (Alfred Szego, Brian Caldwell); Ohio (Diane Miller); Ontario (Doug Campbell, Ernie Grimo); Pennsylvania (Tucker Hill); Tennessee (Spencer Chase).

shoots. The female or pistillate flowers occur near the bases of these bisexual catkins and the male or staminate flowers near the tips. Occasionally, bisexual catkins are replaced by female catkins (catkins bearing only pistillate flowers).

In Middle Georgia, pollen shed of the unisexual male catkins normally occurs during the first week of May. The pistillate flowers of the bisexual catkins are normally receptive during the second week of May, several days before the staminate flowers of these bisexual catkins shed pollen. This type of blooming sequence or maturation of flowers has been called duodichogamy and hetero-duodichogamy (Stout 1928; Vilkomerson 1940). Chinkapins are rarely self-fruitful and cross pollination is necessary to ensure a good nut crop. However, Morris (1914) reported that plants of *C. pumila* may set viable seeds without pollination. This apomictic behavior has been reported in Chinese chestnuts by McKay (1942).

The Allegheny chinkapin is normally ready for harvesting in early September. Harvest must be prompt in order to gather nuts before wildlife (birds and small mammals) remove the entire crop (Fig. 3). One single brown, lustrous, rounded nut is contained in each spiny green involucre (bur) (Fig. 4). The burs of chinkapin are normally

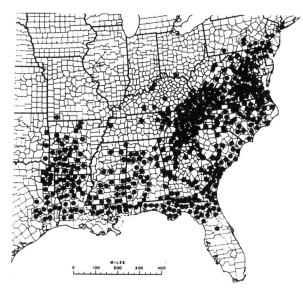

Fig. 1. Distribution of *Castanea pumila* var. *pumila*, based on herbarium specimens (Johnson 1988).

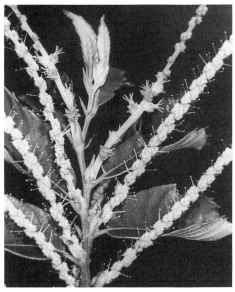

Fig. 2. The flowers are borne on erect, horizontal, or pendant axillary spikes on branches of the current season's growth. There is one inflorescence per leaf axil.

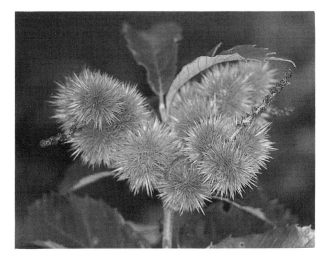

Fig. 3. Chinkapins normally bear 1 to 5 spiny burs per spike; however, 5 to 8 burs or more are encountered.

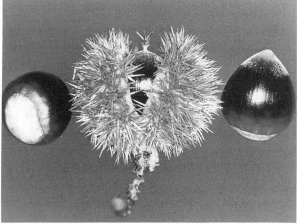

Fig. 4. Chinkapin nuts are 7 to 19 mm in diameter, chocolate to blackish brown, ovate, pointed at one end, and are enclosed in a spiny bur 1.4 to 4.6 cm in diameter.

no more than 1.4 to 4.6 cm in diameter and split into 2 valves at nut maturity. In contrast to other chestnut species, chinkapins normally remain attached to the bur at the hilum for several days after the bur has opened. Also, the burs and catkins do not abscise at harvest time, but remain attached until later in the fall or even until the following season. On each catkin, the more basal burs usually ripen before the more distal ones. These characteristics make chinkapins very difficult to harvest. The burs cannot be shaken or easily picked from the trees. After the burs open, but before the nuts fall, the exposed nuts are tempting morsels for birds or climbing mammals. Even at the peak of harvest, shaking a chinkapin branch will bring down only a small percentage of its crop, since half of the nuts are already gone, and the other half have not opened yet. If the unopened burs are cut or torn from the branches, very few of them will subsequently open, with most requiring a tedious threshing. Complicating the harvest and subsequent use is the fact that chinkapins are fall germinating. Often the radicle emerges while the nuts are still on the tree. Some of the chinkapin clones from isolated sites in Georgia bear nuts averaging 480/kg (fresh weight); however, the normal range is 800 to 1,320/kg (Fig. 5). According to Bailey (1960), *C. pumila* has been marketed in considerable quantities and for more than two centuries (Woodroof 1979); however, we seldom see mention of chinkapins for sale in any recent state market bulletins.

Chinkapins contain 5% fat, 5% protein, 40% starch, and 50% water (Woodroof 1979). Caloric content is 4,736±98 cal/g ash-free dry weight; ash content is 4.0±4% (Payne et al. 1982). Caloric and ash content were determined by standard methods (Paine 1971) with a Parr Model 1341 oxygen bomb calorimeter from four 1 g samples of *C. pumila* kernels.

YIELDS

Yield estimates are difficult to ascertain, as commercial plantings are practically nonexistent. However, nurseries have established this species for seeds and breeding research. Yield extrapolations from a 6 row planting

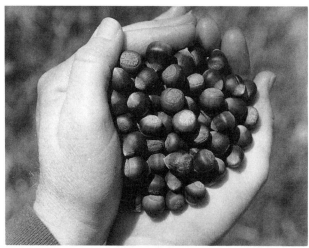

Fig. 5. Chinkapins are precocious and prolific with yields of 2 kg per plant in 6 to 8 years.

Table 1. Advantages and problems associated with development of Allegheny chinkapin as a crop.

Advantages	Problems
Precocious, produces nuts in 2 to 3 years	Excessive bird and mammal feeding
Prolific; large number of female flowers per catkin, large number of female catkins per shoot	Difficult to harvest
	Fall germination
Distinct flavor and aroma (sweet and edible)	Small nut size
Attractive foliage, flowers and burs	Adherence of nuts in the bur and germination in the bur
Wildlife food and cover crop	
Dry site plant and reclamation plant	Susceptible to blight
Dwarfing rootstock possibility	Multistemmed-suckering
	Lack of pesticide registrations

of 30 trees of *C. pumila* in southeastern Kentucky with a spacing of 3 m between trees and 6 m between rows would give 1,230 kg/ha in the 12th year and 3,100 kg/ha in the 14th year. These yields are lower than expected due to fall germination and adherence of nuts in the bur. Yield was also measured from a 7-year-old, closely-spaced (1 × 2 m) planting of seedlings in east central Ohio. The planting had reached crown closure, but had not yet suffered much branch loss due to shading. Individual tree yields varied considerably from nothing up to 1 kg or more. Average yield from trees in the middle of the planting was 5,000±1,500 kg/ha. This yield equals or exceeds the level expected for other chestnuts. In other words, the prolific production of chinkapins compensates for their small size.

PEST PROBLEMS

While there is limited information on the pest management of chinkapins, it is known they are susceptible to many of the insects, mites, and diseases that attack other native and introduced *Castanea* species (Crops Res. Div. 1960; Forest Service 1985; Payne and Johnson 1979). Several insects including two chestnut weevils, *Curculio caryatrypes* (Boheman) and *C. sayi* (Gyllenhal); a nut curculio, *Conotrachelus carinifer* Casey; Asiatic oak weevil, *Cyrtepistomus castaneus* (Roelofs); Japanese beetle, *Popillia japonica* Newman; yellownecked caterpillar, *Datana ministra* (Drury); and pinkstriped oakworm, *Anisota virginiensis* (Drury) feed on the flowers, fruit and foliage of chinkapin. The Oriental chestnut gall wasp, *Dryocosmus kuriphilus* Yasumatsu, has recently been found on chinkapins near Americus, Georgia. It is also a serious pest of Chinese chestnut, *Castanea mollissima* Blume, and Japanese chestnut, *Castanea crenata* Sieb. & Zucc., in Georgia, Japan, China and Korea; no control is presently known (Payne et al. 1983).

Chinkapins are susceptible to *Phytophthora cinnamomi* root rot (Crandall et al. 1945). The Allegheny chinkapin is reported to be rather resistant to the chestnut blight fungus caused by *Cryphonectria (Endothia) parasitica* (Murr.) Barr (Chandler 1957); however, diseased and heavily cankered trees have been found in Georgia and Louisiana (Wallace and Peacher 1970). Chinkapins blight to some degree, but they continue to sucker and send up shoots from the root collar and, despite cankering, produce fruit. *Castanea pumila* has been widely used in the breeding programs for blight resistance (Graves 1950; Jaynes 1975). 'Alamoore', a *C. crenata* × *C. pumila*, was introduced in 1952 by the Alabama Agr. Expt. Sta. because it was blight resistant, prolific, and early bearing (Brooks and Olmo 1972). According to a blight researcher (S. Anagnostakis pers. commun.) the chinkapin hybrids are as susceptible to chestnut blight as American chestnuts, *C. dentata* (Marsh.) Borkh., based on inoculation tests with two strains of *Cryphonectria parasitica*.

PROSPECTS

According to Bailey (1960), two cultivars of *C. pumila*, 'Fuller' and 'Rush', have been named, but neither is listed in *Register of New Fruit and Nut Varieties* (Brooks and Olmo 1952, 1972). In 1983, the Soil Conservation Service and the University of Kentucky Agricultural Experiment Station and Kentucky Department of Fish and Wildlife jointly released 'Golden' for commercial production.

Our native Allegheny chinkapins are prolific producers of sweet, nutty flavored, small chestnuts (Table 1). They have attractive foliage and flowers, although the odor at blossoming time is considered unpleasant by some. If the sweetness, texture, and flavor could be incorporated into the Japanese chestnut or the Chinese chestnut there would be a greater demand for uncooked chestnuts (Jaynes 1979). If the suckering could be eliminated, it may have promise as a dwarfing rootstock for choicer cultivars of chestnut (Bailey 1960) and should be broadly adapted since the Allegheny chinkapin occurs across a wide geographic range. The great drawback of the American chestnut was its small nut size and the added disadvantage that many nuts stuck fast in the bur at harvest and had to be removed by force (Smith 1950); the same can certainly be stated for the Allegheny chinkapin (Table 1). Because the nuts are small, difficult to harvest, and germinate at harvest time, chinkapins have limited potential as a commercial crop. However, their small tree size, precocity, and heavy production may be useful characteristics to breed into the commercial chestnut species. These chinkapin characteristics will facilitate the development of high-density chestnut production systems with earlier and higher yields than is possible with existing chestnut cultivars.

Since the chinkapin is adapted to a wide range of soils and site conditions, it should be considered for its wildlife value. The nuts are eaten by a number of small mammals such as squirrels, rabbits, deermice, and chipmunks, (Halls 1977). By cutting the stem at the ground surface, dense thickets can be established within a few years to provide food and cover for wildlife, especially grouse, bobwhite, and wild turkey.

A renowned horticulturist once remarked, "To hear about the attributes of the Allegheny chinkapin makes your mouth water but to see it makes your eyes water." According to Fuller (1896), "From present indications this tree will be well worthy of cultivation as an ornamental shade tree, even if we leave out of the account its rapid growth, productiveness, and delicious little nuts, which will be very acceptable for home use, if not, possessing any great commercial value." Ninety-six years later the economic potential of this crop still remains to be adequately demonstrated.

REFERENCES

Ashe, W.W. 1923. Further notes on trees and shrubs of the southeastern United States. Bul. Torrey Bot. Club. 50:359–363.

Ashe, W.W. 1924. Notes on woody plants. J. Elisha Mitchell Sci. Soc. 40:43–48.

Bailey, L.H. 1960. *Castanea*, p. 681–682 and Chestnut, p. 742–746. In: The standard cyclopedia of horticulture. Macmillan, New York.

Brooks, R.M. and H.P. Olmo. 1952. Chestnut, p. 50–52. In: Register of new fruit and nut varieties 1920–1950. Univ. California Press, Berkeley.

Brooks, R.M. and H. P. Olmo. 1972. Chestnut, p. 205–211. In: Register of new fruit and nut varieties. Univ. California Press, Berkeley.

Chandler, W.H. 1957. Edible nut tree, p. 418–457. In: Deciduous orchards. Lea and Febiger, Philadelphia.

Crandall, B.S., G.F. Gravatt, and M.M. Ryan. 1945. Root diseases of *Castanea* species and some coniferous and broadleaf nursery stocks, caused by *Phytophthora cinnamomi*. Phytopathology 35:162–180.

Crops Research Division–USDA. 1960. Index of plant diseases in the United States. Agr. Handb. 165. U.S. Government Printing Office, Washington, DC.

Forest Service–USDA. 1985. Insects of eastern forests. Misc. Publ. 1426. U.S. Government Printing Office, Washington, DC.

Fuller, A.S. 1896. The nut culturist, a treatise on the propagation, planting and cultivation of nut-bearing trees and shrubs adapted to the climate of the United States. Orange Judd Co., New York.

Gillespie, W.H. 1959. Beech family, p. 33–36. In: A compilation of edible wild plants of West Virginia. Scholar's Library, New York.

Graves, A.H. 1950. Relative blight resistance in species and hybrids of *Castanea*. Phytopathology 40:1125–1131.

Graves, A.H. 1961. Keys to chestnut species. Annu. Rpt. No. Nut Growers Assoc. 61:78–90.

Halls, L.K. 1977. Southern fruit-producing woody plants used by wildlife. U.S. Dept. Agr. Forest Serv. General Tech. Rpt. SO-16. New Orleans.

Hooker, W.V. 1967. Chinquapins in Oklahoma. Annu. Rpt. No. Nut Growers Assoc. 58:118–120.

Jaynes, R.A. 1975. Chestnuts, p. 490–503. In: J. Janick and J. Moore (eds.). Advances in fruit breeding. Purdue Univ. Press, West Lafayette, IN.

Jaynes, R.A. 1979. Chestnuts, p. 111–127. In: R.A. Jaynes (ed.). Nut tree culture in North America. Northern Nut Growers Assoc., Hamden, CT.

Johnson, G.P. 1987. Chinquapins: taxonomy, distribution, ecology, and importance. Annu. Rpt. No. Nut Growers Assoc. 78:58–62.

Johnson, G.P. 1988. Revision of *Castanea* sect. *Balanocastanon* (Fagaceae). J. Arnold Arbor. 69:25–49.

Krochmal, A. and C. Krochmal. 1982. Uncultivated nuts of the United States. U.S. Dept. Agr. Forest Service. Agr. Info. Bul. 450., Washington, DC.

McKay, J.W. 1942. Self-sterility in the Chinese chestnut (*C. mollissima*). Proc. Amer. Soc. Hort. Sci. 41:156–160.

Morris, R.T. 1914. Chestnut blight resistance. J. Hered. 5:26–29.

Paine, R.T. 1971. The measurement and application of the calorie to ecological problems. Annu. Rev. Ecol.

Systemics 2:145–164.

Pardo, R. 1978. National register of big trees. Amer. Forests 84(4):18–46.

Payne, J.A., J.D. Dutcher, and B.W. Wood. 1982. Chinkapins: A promising nut crop in the south? Annu. Rpt. No. Nut Growers Assoc. 73:23–26.

Payne, J.A., R.A. Jaynes, and S.J. Kays. 1983. Chinese chestnut production in the United States: practice, problems and possible solutions. Econ. Bot. 37:187–200.

Payne, J.A. and W.T. Johnson. 1979. Plant pests, p. 314–395. In: R.A. Jaynes (ed.). Nut tree culture in North America. Northern Nut Growers Assoc., Hamden, CT.

Porcher, F.P. 1970. Corylaceae (The nut tribe), p. 233–265. In: Resources of the southern fields and forests: medicinal, economical, and agricultural. Arno Press, New York.

Smith, J.R. 1950. Tree crops, a permanent agriculture. Devin–Adair, Old Greenwich, CT.

Stout, A.B. 1928. Dichogamy in flowering plants. Bul. Torrey Bot. Club 55:141–153.

Terrell, E.E. 1977. A checklist of names for 3,000 vascular plants of economic importance. USDA Handb. 505. U.S. Govt. Printing Office, Washington, DC.

Tucker, G.E. 1975. *Castanea pumila* var. *ozarkensis* (Ashe) Tucker, comb. nov. Proc. Ark. Acad. Sci. 29:67–69.

Vilkomerson, H. 1940. Flowering habits of the chestnut. Annu. Rpt. No. Nut Growers Assoc. 31:114–116.

Wallace, H.N. and P.H. Peacher. 1970. Chinkapin in Louisiana infected by *Endothia parasitica*. Plant Dis. Rptr. 54:713.

Woodroof, J.G. 1979. Tree nuts of less importance, p. 656–676. In: Tree nuts: production, processing, products. AVI, Westport, CT.

Pawpaw (*Asimina triloba*): a "Tropical" Fruit for Temperate Climates

M. Brett Callaway*

The pawpaw [*Asimina triloba* (L.) Dunal] is the largest fruit native to the United States (Darrow 1975). The genus *Asimina* is the only temperate climate representative of the tropical family Annonaceae. This family is famous for a number of fine fruit, including cherimoya (*Annona cherimola* Mill.), sugar apple (*Annona squamosa* L.), atemoya (*Annona squamosa* x *A. cherimola*), soursop (*Annona muricata* L.), custard apple (*Annona reticulata* L.), ilama (*Annona diversifolia* Safford), soncoya (*Annona purpurea* Moc. & Sesse), and biriba (*Rollinia mucosa* Baill.) (Morton, 1987). Of the nine species of Asimina found in the United States, *A. triloba* has the greatest potential for commercial fruit production. Other species are lacking in quality, size, hardiness, or other important characteristics. In addition to its promising potential for fruit production, certain parts of *A. triloba* plants contain asimicin, a compound with active pesticidal and neoplastic properties (Rupprecht et al. 1986, 1990; Ratnayake et al. 1993).

DISTRIBUTION

Fourteen species in the Annonaceae are native to the United States. These include nine species of *Asimina*, two species of *Deeringothamnus*, and three species of *Annona*. All *Asimina* species, excepting *A. parviflora* (Michx.) Dunal and *A. triloba*, are restricted to Florida and extreme southern portions of Georgia and Alabama (Callaway 1990). *Asimina parviflora* is distributed throughout the southeastern United States (Callaway 1990), while *A. triloba* is distributed over most of the eastern United States (Fig. 1) and even into extreme southern

---

*I acknowledge the helpful comments of Neal Peterson and Joe Hickman. Financial support during manuscript preparation was provided by USDA/CSRS Agreement No. KYX-10-91-17P to Kentucky State University.

Canada. *Deeringothamnus rugelii* (B.L. Robbins) Small and *D. pulchellus* Small are rare plants native only to Florida (Kral 1983). The *Annonas, A. glabra* L., *A. palustris* L., and *A. squamosa* L., are found only in extreme southern Florida (Small 1913; Wunderlin 1982). I am aware of fruiting plantings of pawpaws on four continents (North America, Asia, Australia, and Europe).

HORTICULTURE

Culture

Since no scientific work has been done on cultural requirements of pawpaws, the following discussion on culture is based largely on my personal observations. I prefer planting seed into Rootrainer book containers (see propagation section below) then transplanting 10 to 20 cm seedlings into tall pots. Plants are left in the tall pots until they reach 0.5 to 1.0 m in height before transplanting. Seedlings should be started in pots for several reasons. First, pawpaw seedlings are reported to be sensitive to ultraviolet light (Peterson 1991). However, following a season of growth in partial shade, they no longer seem to be affected by direct sunlight. Rather, they grow and produce better in full sun (Wilson and Schemske 1980). Pots may be conveniently grouped under shadecloth for a season before transplanting to permanent field locations. Second, pawpaws have a reputation of being difficult to transplant and this difficulty increases with plant size. Yet, small plants are more difficult to maintain under field conditions. There is a tradeoff between transplanting success and maintenance of plants in the field. Plants grown in containers to approximately 1 m in height before transplanting largely circumvent these problems. Finally, plants may reach bearing size sooner when grown in containers before transplanting to the field, since optimal growing conditions are often more easily provided to container-grown plants.

Plants appear to need a "rest" period. Seedlings germinated in the greenhouse in December ceased growth in February and did not resume growth until June, even though suitable growing conditions were maintained during the entire period.

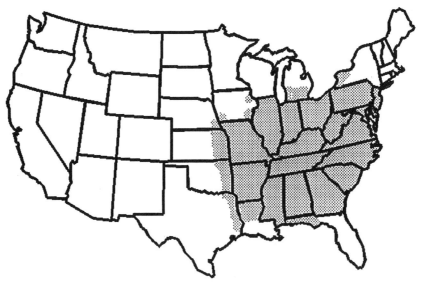

Fig. 1. Distribution of Asimina triloba in the United States. Source: Alabama (Clark 1971); Arkansas (Smith 1978); Florida (Kral 1960); Georgia (Jones and Coile 1988); Illinois (Mohlenbrock 1981); Indiana (Deam 1940); Iowa (Pammel and King 1930; The Great Plains Flora Association 1977; Stephens 1969); Kansas (The Great Plains Flora Association 1977; Stephens, 1969); Kentucky (Callaway unpublished; Johnson and Nicely, 1990; Kral, 1960); Louisana (Kral 1960); Maryland (Kral 1960); Michigan (Billington 1949); Mississippi (Kral 1960); Missouri (Steyermark 1963); Nebraska (Petersen 1912; The Great Plains Flora Association 1977); New Jersey (Hough 1983); New York (Bowden and Miller 1951); North Carolina (Radford et al. 1968); Ohio (Braun 1961); Oklahoma (Little 1981; The Great Plains Flora Association 1977); Pennsylvania (Bowden and Miller 1951; Kral, 1960); South Carolina (Radford et al. 1968); Tennessee (Kral 1960); Texas (Kral 1960; Simpson 1988); Virginia (Harvill et al. 1977); and West Virginia (Kral 1960).

Pawpaws appear to benefit from mulching with leaves, compost, or other material high in organic matter. Since their native habitat is river floodplains, they may be somewhat more sensitive to low soil moisture than other fruit trees. Pawpaws seem to be sensitive to low humidities and dry winds.

Seed Propagation

Seed should be removed from the fruit, cleaned, and placed in a polyethylene bag with damp sphagnum moss and should not be allowed to dry out. Seed should be stratified at 2° to 4°C for 60 to 100 days before planting (Thomson 1982; USDA 1948). Seed should be planted about 2.5 cm deep. The depth of Rootrainer books, commonly used in the propagation of forest trees, is especially desirable because of pawpaw's long taproot. Once seedlings reach a height of 10 to 20 cm they can be transplanted into tall pots (10 × 10 × 36 cm) with partially open bottoms and placed on greenhouse benches. Taproots growing out the bottom of these pots are "air-pruned."

The rate and percentage of seed germination is stimulated by bottom heat (27°C) (Fig. 2) with most seedlings emerging between 45 and 90 days after planting. Acid scarification reduced percent germination. Evert and Payne (1991) reported increased percent germination with increased shading.

Vegetative Propagation

The most reliable and commonly used method of vegetative propagation is chip-budding. Root cuttings have been used successfully (USDA 1948), but softwood propagation methods (those using cuttings from soft, succulent, new growth) have not been satisfactorily developed. I was able to generate shoots in vitro from leaf explants using a modified a medium developed for tissue culture of *Annona* spp. (Nair et al. 1984a,b).

Fruit Description, Composition, and Processing

Fruit are produced in clusters and are oblong to banana-shaped, providing insight into the origin of one of *A. triloba*'s early names, "Indiana banana." Fruit size ranges from quite small (20 g) to over 450 g. Skin is typically smooth and thin, ranging in color from green to bright yellow at maturity and turning brown or black after a frost. The fruit may be eaten when it becomes soft although some prefer to wait until after the skin has darkened. Flesh is custard-like in texture with flavor resembling cherimoya (*Annona cherimola*) or soursop (*Annona muricata*). Flesh color is typically orange but infrequently may be white (Callaway 1991). Large fruit usually have 10 to 15 large black seeds.

Peterson et al. (1982) evaluated the composition of pawpaw fruit (Table 1) and concluded that the fruit have a high nutritional quality compared to temperate fruits such as apple, peach, and grape. All commercially important fruit in the Annonaceae have relatively short shelf-lives. As Annonas are used in juices, ice cream, and other processed products similar processing may also be applicable to pawpaws.

Cultivars

A list of past and present cultivars has been compiled by Callaway (1990) and Peterson (1991). Many early cultivars have been lost over the years as the owners of nurseries and collections pass away. To date, there have been a total of 68 cultivars developed (Table 2). Only about 19 are commercially available (Table 3). Most are available in limited quantities from only one or two nurseries. The information available on these cultivars is based on the personal observations of very few persons; replicated yield tests have not been carried out. 'Overleese' and 'Sunflower' are probably the most widely grown cultivars and are generally considered to be among the highest quality. Relatively few nurseries sell pawpaw, although those who do, find it difficult to supply the demand.

Pests

Flyspeck (*Zygophiala jamaicensis* Mason) has been reported on fruit in Japan (Nasu and Kunoh 1987). A leaf spot caused by a complex of pathogens [*Mycocentrospora asiminae* (Ellis & Kellerm.) Deighton, *Rhopaloconidium asiminae* (Ellis & Morg.) Petr., and *Phyllosticta asiminae* Ellis & Kellerm.] has also been reported (Peterson 1991). None of these diseases caused significant damage to the fruit. Three lepidopterans have been reported to damage *Asimina* spp. *Eurytides marcellus* Cramer and *Omphalocera munroei* Martin feed on

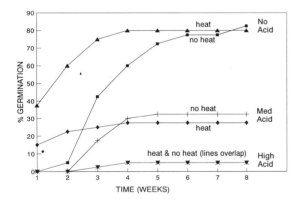

Fig. 2. Rate of germination over time as influenced by bottom heat (27°C) and acid scarification with 36N sulfuric acid.

Table 1. Composition of raw, unpeeled pawpaw fruit based on the edible portion (Peterson et al. 1982; Peterson 1991, and pers. commun.).

Constituent	Range
Proximates (g/100 g)	
Ash	0.6–0.7
Carbohydrate	16.8–22.4
Fat	0.6–1.4
Fiber	1.4–3.5
Food energy (Kcal/100 g)	77–89
Protein	0.8–1.4
Water	69.5–77.0
Vitamins (mg/100 g)	
A (IU/100 g)	66–1.5
C	7.6–20.9
Niacin	1.1–1.2
Riboflavin	0.09–0.09
Thiamin	0.01–0.01
Minerals (mg/100 g)	
Calcium	53–76
Copper	0.4–0.6
Iron	6.8–7.2
Magnesium	109–120
Manganese	2.5–2.6
Phosphorus	43–53
Potassium	314–368
Sulfur	62–78
Zinc	0.9–0.9
Fatty Acids (% of total)	
Linoleic	8.1–9.0
Linolenic	16.9–24.4
Oleic	23.3–38.0
Palmitic	18.6–24.4
Palmitoleic	5.8–10.2
Sugars (g/100 g)	
Fructose	1.3–2.8
Glucose	1.8–4.0
Sucrose	6.0–13.3
Essential Amino Acids (g/100 g of protein)	
Arginine	3.00–3.83
Histidine	1.55–2.19
Isoleucine	4.7–6.8
Leucine	5.8–8.2
Lysine	4.2–6.3
Methionine	0.9–1.4
Phenylalanine	3.7–4.9
Threonine	3.2–4.6
Tryptophan	0.4–0.9
Valine	4.2–6.0

Table 2. Descriptions of pawpaw cultivars.

Name	Description	Place of origin	Pedigree	Reference
Arkansas Beauty		AR	Selected from wild	Anon. 1917; Pape 1965
Betty Wirt	Fruit weighs up to 454 g, but averages 160 g	Wirt County, WV	Selected from wild	Bartholomew 1962; Pape 1965
Buckman	White flesh color, mild flavor; late to very late maturity		Selected by B. Buckman	Zimmerman 1938; Zimmerman 1941
Cheatwood		Gallia, OH	Selected from wild by J. Cheatwood	Anon. 1917
Cheely		Iuka, IL	Selected from wild by J. Cheely	Anon. 1917
Cox's Favorite			Selected from wild	Anon. 1917
Davis*	Fruit 115 g, up to 12 cm long; yellow-fleshed; ripens 1st week of October in MI; green skin; seed large; keeps well in cold storage	Bellevue, MI	Selected from wild by Corwin Davis around 1959	Brooks and Olmo 1972; Davis 1982; L. Davis pers. commun.
Dr. Potter	Small fruit size; mild flavor, ships fairly well; late maturity; rich yellow flesh	Julietta, IN	Selected from wild by B.S. Potter	Anon. 1917
Duck				Vines 1960
Early Best			Selected from wild by W.C. Stout	Anon. 1917
Early Cluster		IN	Selected from wild	Anon. 1917
Early Gold			Selected from wild	Zimmerman 1938
Endicott		Villa Ridge, IL	Selected from wild by G. Endicott	Anon. 1917
Fairchild	Early maturity		Selected by David Fairchild from 'Ketter' seed	Zimmerman 1938; Zimmerman 1941
Ford Amend*	Slightly smaller and earlier than 'Sunflower'; matures late Sept. in OR; flesh orange; skin greenish-yellow	Portland, OR	Selected by Ford Amend around 1950 from a seedling of unknown parentage Zimmerman seed	M. Dolan pers. commun.
G-2				Peterson 1991
Gable		PA	Selected from wild by J. Gable	Zimmerman 1938; Zimmerman 1941
Glaser		Evansville, IN	Selected by P. Glaser	Thomson 1982
Hann		AR	Selected from wild	Anon. 1917
Hengst			Selected from wild	Peterson 1991
Holtwood			Selected from wild by W. Hoopes	Vines 1960
Hope's August	Early maturity	Paint, OH	Selected from wild by A. Hope	Anon. 1917; Zimmerman 1941
Hope's September		Paint, OH	Selected from wild by A. Hope	Anon. 1917
Jumbo				Zimmerman 1941
Kercheval	Late to very late maturity			Pape 1965

Table 2. Continued.

Name	Description	Place of origin	Pedigree	Reference
Ketter	Matures evenly; skin comparatively thick & tough; does not discolor markedly; flesh medium yellow; mild but rich flavor, neither insipid nor cloying; large yellow fruit; early maturity	Ironton, OH	Selected by Mrs. F. Ketter	Anon. 1917; Zimmerman 1941
Kirsten*		Aliquippa, PA	Tom Mansell seedling 'Taytoo' x 'Overleese'	J.S. Akin pers. commun.
Kurle	Small-medium in size; yellow flesh and skin	MI	Seedling by R. Kurle from 'Davis'	Kurle 1982
Lawvere				Pape 1965
Little Rosie			Selected by R. Glaser	Glaser 1982
Long John		Evansville, IN	Selected by B. Buckman	Zimmerman 1938
M-1	Small fruit size		Selected by J. McKay from 'G-2' seedling	Peterson 1991
Mango*		Tifton, GA	Selected by Major Collins	J. Gordon pers. commun.; Peterson 1991
Martin	Large fruit size (Zimmerman says small size); flesh yellow & of superior quality (Zimmerman says skin tough); withstands cold well	Springfield, OH	Selected from wild by S.C. Martin	Anon. 1917; Zimmerman 1941
Mary Foos Johnson*	Similar to 'Sunflower'; original located at the North Wilamette Expt. Sta., Auroe, OR		Seedling given to North Wilamette Expt. Sta. by Ms. Mary Foos Johnson	Pape 1965
Mason/WLW*		Mason, OH	Selected from wild by E.J. Downing	Peterson 1991
Middletown		Middletown, OH	Selected from wild by E.J. Downing	Peterson 1991
Mitchell*	Fruit medium-size; skin slightly yellow; flesh golden; flavor "superb"	Jefferson Co., IL	Selected from wild by Joe Hickman	J. Hickman pers. commun.
Mudge			Selected from wild	Pape 1965
NC-1*	Fruit 340 g; few seed; yellow flesh and skin; thin skin; early, maturing Sept. 15 in Ontario	Ontario, Canada	Selected by R.D. Campbell around 1976 from 'Davis' x 'Overleese'	R.D. Campbell pers. commun.; L. Davis pers. commun.
Osborne	Late to very late maturity		Selected from wild	Zimmerman 1938; Zimmerman 1941

Table 2. Continued.

Name	Description	Place of origin	Pedigree	Reference
Oswald	Fruit 340 g; bears in clusters of 3 to 5; ripens 1st week of Oct. in MI	Hagerstown, MD	Selected from wild by E. Oswald	Anon. 1917
Overleese*		Rushville, IN	Selected from wild by W.B. Ward around 1950	Davis 1982; Davis 1986; Pape 1965; Peterson 1991
PA-Golden*	Flesh golden; skin yellow; matures mid-Sept. in Amherst, NY	Amherst, NY	Seedling selected by John Gordon around 1982 from seed originating from George Slate collection.	J. Gordon pers. commun.
Prolific*	Fruit 200–225 g; yellow flesh; ripens 1st week of Oct. in MI	Bellevue, MI	Seedling from Corwin Davis orchard	Davis 1986; L. Davis pers. commun.
Propst Early			Selected from wild	Anon. 1917
Rebecca's Gold*	Fruit kidney-shaped, 85–170 g; flesh yellow	CA	Selected by J.M. Riley in 1974 from Corwin Davis seed	J.S. Akin pers. commun.; California Rare Fruit Growers 1982; M. Dolan pers. commun.; Peterson 1991
Rees	Flesh pale yellow and of good flavor; not a large fruit size	Pleasanton, KS	Selected from wild by W. Rees	Anon. 1917
Roach		Dekalb, MO	Selected from wild by J.C. Roach	Anon. 1917
SAA-Overleese*	Fruit 285 g, rounded shape; flesh yellow, skin green; few seed; matures mid-Oct. in Amherst, NY	Amherst, NY	Seedling selected by John Gordon around 1982 from 'Overleese' seed.	J. Gordon pers. commun.
SAA-Zimmerman*	Fruit 170–225 g; few seed; yellow flesh and skin	Amherst, NY	Seedling selected by John Gordon around 1982 from seed originating from G.A. Zimmerman collection.	J. Gordon pers. commun.
Schriber		WV	Selected from wild	Zimmerman 1938
Scott			Selected from wild by C.S. Scott	Anon. 1917
Shannondale Silver Creek	Late to very late maturity Medium sized fruit	Millstedt, IL or Silver Creek, NY		Zimmerman 1938; Zimmerman 1941 J. Gordon pers. commun.; Thomson 1982
Sunflower*	Fruit up to 225 g; butter-color flesh; skin yellowish; few seed; ripens 1st week of Oct. in MI	Chanute, KS	Selected from wild by Milo Gibson around 1970	Davis 1979; Davis 1982; Davis 1983b; Davis 1986
Sweet Alice*		Mentor, OH	Selected by Homer Jacobs of the Holden Arboretum in 1934	Peterson 1991; Thomson 1982
Talbot	Fruit 285 g; flesh yellow, overall quality average	Linton, IN	Chance seedling selected about 1950 by John Talbot from Corwin Davis seed.	R.D. Campbell pers. commun.

Table 2. Continued.

Name	Description	Place of origin	Pedigree	Reference
Taylor	Not the same as 'Taylor' described below; flesh light color, mild flavor, late to very late maturity		Selected from wild	Zimmerman 1938; Zimmerman 1941
Taylor*	Small fruit; bears up to 7 fruit in a cluster; yellow flesh, green skin; ripens 1st week of Oct. in MI	Eaton Rapids, MI	Selected from wild by Corwin Davis in 1968	Davis 1969; Davis 1982; Davis 1983b; Davis 1986; L. Davis pers. commun.
Taytwo*	Fruit up to 285 g; begins ripening 10th of Oct. in MI; skin light green when ripe; flesh yellow; sometimes spelled 'Taytoo'	Eaton Rapids, MI	Selected from wild by Corwin Davis in 1968	Davis 1969; Davis 1982; Davis 1983b; Davis 1986; L. Davis pers. commun.; Mansell 1986
Tiedke	Late to very late maturity		Selected from wild	Zimmerman 1938; Zimmerman 1941
Uncle Tom	Probably the first named variety on record; ripens mid-Sept. in IN; fruit sets singly and in pairs	Cartersburg, IN	Selected from wild by J.A. Little around 1896	Little 1905
Van Der Bogart	Very similar to PA-Golden; matures mid-Sept. in Ithaca, NY	Ithaca, NY	Selected by Francis Van Der Bogart around 1970 from seed originating from the G.A. Zimmerman collection.	J. Gordon pers. commun.
Vena	Possibly the same as 'Talbot'	Linton, IN?		R.D. Campbell pers. commun.
Wells*	Fruit 340–400 g; skin green; flesh orange	Salem, IN	Selected from wild by David Wells in 1990	Callaway 1991
Wilson*	Fruit medium-size; skin yellow; flesh golden	On Black Mountain in Harlan County KY	Selected from wild by John Creech	J. Hickman pers. commun.
Zimmerman			G.A. Zimmerman seed	Peterson 1991

* These cultivars are commercially available.

Table 3. Suppliers of pawpaw cultivars.

J.S. Akin Sherwood's Greenhouses P.O. Box 6 Sibley, LA 71073	Phone: (318) 377-3653 Cultivars: Davis, Mango, Overleese, Rebecca's Gold, Sunflower, Sweet Alice, and Wilson Send Self-Addressed Stamped Envelope for price list
Hector Black Hidden Springs Nursery Rt. 14, Box 159 Cookville, TN 38501	Phone (615) 268-9889 Cultivars: Sunflower and Taylor. Catalog $0.40
Corwin and Letha Davis 20865 Junction Road Bellevue, MI 49021	Phone (616) 781-7402 Cultivars: Davis, Overleese, Prolific, Sunflower, Taylor, and Taytwo Include Self-Addressed Stamped Envelope.
Michael Dolan Burnt Ridge Nursery and Orchards 432 Burnt Ridge Rd. Onalaska, WA 98570	Phone: (206) 985-2873 Cultivars: Sunflower and Ford Amend. Send Self-Addressed Stamped Envelope for free catalog
J.H. Gordon, Jr. 1385 Campbell Blvd. Amherst, NY 14228-1404	Phone (716) 691-9371 Cultivars: PA-Golden, SAA-Overleese, and SAA-Zimmerman
Louisiana Nursery Rt. 7, Box 43 Opelousas, LA 70570	Phone: (318) 948-3696 Cultivars: Mitchell, Overleese, and Wilson. Catalog $5.00
Northwoods Nursery 28696 S. Cramer Rd. Molalla, OR 97038	Phone (503) 651-3737 Cultivars: Mary Foos Johnson, Prolific, Rebecca's Gold, Sunflower, and Wells
Oregon Exotics Rare Fruit Nursery Jerry Black 1065 Messinger Rd. Grants Pass, OR 97527	Phone: (503) 846-7578 Cultivar: W.L.W. Mason
Robert Seip Lennilea Farm Nursery R.D. 1, Box 683 Alburtis, PA 18011	Phone (215) 845-2077 Cultivars: Mango, Sunflower, and Sweet Alice

the leaves (Damman 1986). *Talponia plummeriana* Busck bores into the peduncle of flowers, causing serious loss of flowers in some years (Allard 1955). Fruit may also be eaten by wildlife including birds, foxes, opossums, squirrels, and raccoons.

Research Needs

Collection and testing of germplasm are needed. Since only 19 cultivars are available, wild germplasm remains an important source of genetic material for cultivar development and improvement. Superior selections from the wild should continue to be propagated and sold by nurserymen for home and commercial plantings. There is a great need for testing superior genotypes (wild selections, breeding lines, and cultivars) throughout the potential growing region to provide sound recommendations for growers.

Basic information is needed on the inheritance of commercially important traits, such as flowering behavior, fruit size, productivity, and maturity. This information is critical for the development of efficient, effective genetic improvement programs.

Basic horticultural information on such cultural practices as irrigation, fertilization, and pest control practices is also lacking. Information on pollination biology is needed. Wilson and Schemske (1980) demonstrated that fruit production on wild trees was limited by inadequate pollination. Only 0.41% of flowers set fruit on naturally pollinated plants in the wild, while as many as 17% of hand-pollinated flowers set fruit. A better understanding of the agents and mechanisms responsible for pawpaw pollination is needed to ensure reliable fruit set.

REFERENCES

Allard, H.A. 1955. The native pawpaw. Atlantic Naturalist 10:197–203.

Anonymous. 1917. The best papaws. J. Hered. 8:21–33.

Bartholemew, E.A. 1962. Possibilities of the papaw. Northern Nut Growers Assoc. Annu. Rpt. 53:71–74.

Billington, C. 1949. Shrubs of Michigan. 2nd ed. Cranbrook Institute of Science. Bul. No. 20.

Bowden, W.M. and B. Miller. 1951. Distribution of the pawpaw, *Asimina triloba* (L.) Dunal, in Southern Ontario. Can. Field-Naturalist 65:27–31.

Braun, E.L. 1961. The woody plants of Ohio. Ohio State Univ. Press, Columbus, OH. p. 148–149.

Brooks, R.M. and M.P. Olmo. 1972. Register of new fruit and nut varieties. 2nd ed. Univ. of California Press, Berkeley.

California Rare Fruit Growers. 1982. Fruit registration listing. California Rare Fruit Growers 1982 Yearb. California Rare Fruit Growers, The Fullerton Arboretum, California State Univ., Fullerton.

Callaway, M.B. 1990. The pawpaw (*Asimina triloba*). Kentucky State Univ. Pub. CRS-HORT1-901T.

Callaway, M.B. 1991. Germplasm collection using public contests—The *Asimina triloba* example. HortScience 26:722.

Clark, R.C. 1971. The woody plants of Alabama. Ann. Missouri Botanical Garden 58:99–242.

Damman, A.J. 1986. Facultative interactions between two lepidopteran herbivores of *Asimina*. Oecologia 78:214–219.

Darrow, G.M. 1975. Minor temperate fruits, p. 276–277. In: J. Janick and J.N. Moore (eds.). Advances in fruit breeding. Purdue Univ. Press, West Lafayette, IN.

Davis, C. 1969. Hunting for better paw paws. Northern Nut Growers Assoc. Annu. Rpt. 60:107–108.

Davis, C. 1979. Update on pawpaws. Northern Nut Growers Assoc. Annu. Rpt. 70:82–84.

Davis, C. 1982. The paw paw in southern Michigan. In: California Rare Fruit Growers 1982 Yearb. Fullerton. p. 38–41.

Davis, C. 1983. Pawpaw: The forgotten fruit. (revised 11-15-83). Mimeo. 20865 Junction Road, Bellevue, MI.

Deam, C.C. 1940. Flora of Indiana. Dept. of Conservation, Div. of Forestry, Indianapolis, IN. p. 478–479.

Evert, D.R. and J.A. Payne. 1991. Germination of *Asimina triloba* and *A. parviflora*. HortScience 26:777.

Glaser, R. 1982. The pawpaw in Indiana, p. 36. In: California rare fruit growers 1982 yearb. Fullerton.

Harvill, A.M., C.E. Stevens, and D.M.E. Ware. 1977. Atlas of the Virginia flora, Part 1. Virginia Botanical Associates, Farmville.

Hough, M.Y. 1983. New Jersey wild plants. Harmony Press, Harmony, NJ.

Johnson, G.P. and K.A. Nicely. 1990. The Magnoliales of Kentucky. Trans. Kentucky Acad. Sci. 51:14–17.

Jones, S.B. and N.C. Coile. 1988. The distribution of the vascular flora of Georgia. Dept. Botany, Univ. of Georgia, Athens.

Kral, R. 1983. A report on some rare, threatened, or endangered forest-related vascular plants of the south. USDA Forest Service Southern Region, Tech. Pub. R8-TP-2. p. 448–457.

Kral, R. 1960. A revision of *Asimina* and *Deeringothamnus* (Annonaceae). Brittonia 12:233–278.

Kurle, R. 1982. The paw paw in Illinois, p. 32–35. In: California rare fruit growers 1982 yearb. Fullerton.

Little, E.L. 1981. Forest trees of Oklahoma, p. 111. Oklahoma Forestry Div., State Dept. Agr. Pub. 1, (Revised ed. 12), Oklahoma City.

Little, J.A. 1905. A treatise on the Pawpaw. Orville G. Swindler, Clayton, IN.

Mansell, T. 1986. The advantages of self-rooted pawpaws. Pomona 19:62–63.

Mohlenbrock, R.H. 1981. The illustrated flora of Illinois: flowering plants, magnolias to pitcher plants. So. Illinois Univ. Press, Carbondale. p. 11–13.

Morton, J.F. 1987. Fruits of warm climates. Published by author.

Nair, S., P.K. Gupta, and A.F. Mascarenhas. 1984a. In vitro propagation of *Annona* hybrid (*Annona squamosa* L. x *Annona cherimola* L.). Indian J. Hort. 41:160–165.

Nair, S., P.K. Gupta, M.V. Shirgurkar, and A.F. Mascarenhas. 1984b. In vitro organogenesis from leaf explants of *Annona squamosa* Linn. Plant Cell Tissue Organ Culture 3:29–40.

Nasu, H. and H. Kunoh. 1987. Scanning electron microscopy of flyspeck of apple, pear, Japanese persimmon, plum, Chinese quince, and pawpaw. Plant Dis. 71:361–364.

Pammel, L.H. and C.M. King. 1930. Honey plants of Iowa. Iowa Geological Survey, Bul. 7, Iowa Geological Survey, Des Moines. p. 185–186.

Pape, E. 1965. The pawpaw. Northern Nut Growers Assoc. Annu. Rpt. 56:103–106.

Peterson, N.F. 1912. Flora of Nebraska. Published by author.

Peterson, R.N. 1991. Pawpaw (*Asimina*), p. 567–600. In: J.N. Moore and J.R. Ballington (eds.). Genetic resources of temperate fruit and nut crops. Intl. Soc. Hort. Sci., Wageningen.

Peterson, R.N., J.P. Cherry, and J.G. Simmons. 1982. Composition of pawpaw (*Asimina triloba*) fruit. Northern Nut Growers Assoc. Annu. Rpt. 73:97–107.

Radford, A.E., H.F. Ahles, and C.R. Bell. 1968. Manual of the vascular flora of the Carolinas, p. 475–477. Univ. North Carolina Press, Chapel Hill.

Ratnayake, S., J.K. Rupprecht, W.M. Potter, and J.L. McLaughlin. 1993. Evaluation of various parts of the paw paw tree, *Asimina triloba* (Annonaceae), as commercial sources of the pesticidal annonaceous acetogenins. In: J. Janick and J.E. Simon (eds.). Progress in new crops. Wiley, New York.

Rupprecht, J.K., C.-J. Chang, J.M. Cassady, and J.L. McLaughlin. 1986. Asimicin, a new cytotoxic and pesticidal acetogenin from the pawpaw, *Asimina triloba* (Annonaceae). Heterocycles 24:1197–1201.

Rupprecht, J.K., Y.-H. Hui, and J.L. McLaughlin. 1990. Annonaceous acetogenins: A review. J. Nat. Prod. 53:237–278.

Simpson, B.J. 1988. A field guide of Texas trees. Texas Monthly Press, Austin.

Small, J.K. 1913. Flora of the Florida keys. Published by author.

Smith, E.B. 1978. An annotated list of the vascular plants of Arkansas, p. 9–10. Published by author.

Steyermark, J.A. 1963. Flora of Missouri. The Iowa State University Press, Ames. p. 671–674.

The Great Plains Flora Association. 1977. Atlas of the flora of the great plains, p. 14. The Iowa State University Press, Ames, IA.

Thomson, P.H. 1982. The paw paw, p. 5–31. In: California rare fruit growers, 1982 yearb. California Rare Fruit Growers, Fullerton.

USDA. 1948. *Asimina triloba* (L.) Dunal, pawpaw, p. 92. In: woody-plant seed manual. USDA, Washington, DC. Misc. Publ. 654.

Vines, R.A. 1960. Custard-apple family (Annonaceae). p. 289–291. In: Trees, shrubs, and woody vines of the southwest. University of Texas Press.

Wilson, M.F. and D.W. Schemske. 1980. Pollinator limitation, fruit production, and floral display in pawpaw (*Asimina triloba*). Bul. Torrey Bot. Club 107:401–408.

Wunderlin, R.P. 1982. Guide to the vascular plants of Central Florida. Univ. Presses of Florida, Tampa. p. 188–189.

Zimmerman, G.A. 1938. The papaw. Northern Nut Growers Assoc. Annu. Rpt. 29:99–102.

Zimmerman, G.A. 1941. Hybrids of the American pawpaw. J. Hered. 32:83–91.

Saskatoon Berry: A Fruit Crop for the Prairies

G. Mazza and C.G. Davidson

The saskatoon (*Amelanchier alnifolia* Nutt., Rosaceae) is a fruit bearing shrub native to the southern Yukon and Northwest Territories, the Canadian prairies and the northern plains of the United States (Harris 1972). It is extremely adaptable and grows under a wide range of environmental conditions. Saskatoon plants begin to bear fruit when they are two to four years old and with proper management can yield 8 to 10 tonnes of fruit per hectare (Harris 1972; St. Pierre 1991). The fruit, usually called a berry, is actually a pome. Saskatoon berries were originally used as a major food source by the native people and early settlers of the North American prairies and, until recently, could be picked only in the wild (Harris 1972). In the past two decades, however, there has been increasing interest in utilizing this berry as a unique western Canadian fruit crop. Today, there are 100 to 200 ha of saskatoons on the Canadian prairies in production and 200 to 400 ha planted but still too young to produce significant quantities. Many of the most profitable orchards are near urban centers where a pick-your-own system is used to harvest and market the berries. Plants have access to irrigation and are grown under favorable environmental conditions to ensure high fruit yield and quality.

CULTIVARS

Many cultivars have been named by horticulturists over the years. These have been primarily chance seedlings that have been selected for superior plant and/or fruit characteristics. Currently, 'Smoky' is recommended for production of good quality, medium-sized fruit, and 'Honeywood' for large fruit of fair quality. Other cultivars include: 'Forestburg', 'Moonlake', 'Northline', 'Parkhill', 'Regent', 'Success', 'Porter', 'Thiessen', 'Altaglow', and 'Sturgeon'. 'Smoky', the most widely grown cultivar, has medium-sized, fleshy, round, sweet, mild-flavored fruit growing in clusters (Fig. 1). Selected physico-chemical characteristics of five cultivars are listed in Table 1.

PROPAGATION

Saskatoons can be propagated from seed, divisions, root cuttings, softwood cuttings, and cuttings from etiolated shoots (Nelson 1987). In vitro propagation of 'Northline', 'Pembina', 'Smoky', and 'Thiessen' saskatoon berries has been reported (Harris 1980; Pruski et al. 1990). However, rooting and post-rooting dormancy remains a problem for some cultivars. Growing saskatoons from seed is relatively simple, but plants grown from seed differ from parent in size and fruit characteristics (Davidson and Mazza 1991).

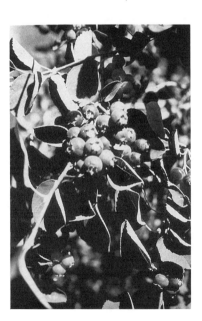

Fig. 1. 'Smoky' saskatoon berries at maturity.

CULTURE

Soils

A comparison of plantings in sandy loam vs clay loam indicates much better success in the former. A slight slope to provide for both air and water drainage is also important. This is in agreement with the natural habitat of the saskatoon which is often found in sandy and other well drained locales.

Spacing

Row planting in contrast to spaced single plants has led to the best plant establishment and growth. Rows planted 3.5 to 4 m apart with plants 1 m within rows led to a high plant population with abundant in-row suckering. Over the row mechanical harvesters require a minimum of 5 m, while pull-type harvesters require 6 m spacing.

Irrigation and Fertility

Irrigation under normally dry prairie conditions is essential for plant establishment, and to maximize growth and fruit yield. Both trickle and overhead irrigation systems are acceptable. While trickle irrigation is generally more economical and efficient, particularly with wide row spacing, overhead irrigation can provide frost protection and crop cooling. While fertility requirements have not been investigated, fall applications are not recommended since these may reduce winter-hardiness of plants.

Weed Control

Row cultivation can give relatively easy weed control if long rows are used at a spacing which enables use of various size cultivators as the planting grows. Currently, only the herbicide linuron is registered for use in saskatoon production in Canada. On an experimental basis, pre-plant incorporated trifluralin at 2.2 to 4.4 kg ai/ha provided excellent control of weeds at planting. Post-plant dormant application of linuron has provided nearly full season control of annual grasses and broad leafed weeds. Fall application is preferred. Spring application must be made prior to budbreak and must be followed by rain or irrigation.

Pruning

Saskatoon plants begin to bear fruit when they are 2 to 4 years old. The fruit is produced on the previous year's growth and on older wood. Usually young, vigorous branches yield the highest quality fruit. Pruning should be done in early spring after the danger of severe cold weather is past and before the plants start to grow. Removal of all weak, diseased, damaged and low branches as well as thinning of the center growth to keep it open is recommended. Generally, major pruning is not required until the plants are 6 to 8 years old.

Pests

A number of insects and diseases can damage the plants and fruit. Important insects that feed on flower buds, flowers, and fruit include lygus (*Lygus* sp.), saskatoon budmoth (*Epinota bicordana*), saskatoon sawfly (*Hoplocampa montanicola*), apple curculio (*Anthonomas quadrigibbus*), and a leaf rolling caterpillar (*Argyrotaenia*

Table 1. Physico-chemical characteristics of five saskatoon cultivars.

Cultivar	10 Berry weight (g)	pH	Titratable acidity (% malic acid)	Total solids (% dry wt)	Soluble solids (% sucrose)	SS/Ac	Anthocyanin content (mg/100 g berries)
Honeywood	12.7	3.8	0.54	25.6	18.7	34.7	114
Northline	8.0	3.9	0.45	25.1	16.1	35.5	111
Porter	7.8	3.8	0.56	22.7	16.3	29.5	108
Regent	6.8	4.4	0.29	20.8	14.8	52.8	72
Smoky	10.1	4.5	0.25	27.0	16.3	66.2	68

quadrifasciana) (St. Pierre 1989, 1991). In Canada, only deltamethrim (Decis) is registered for use, and it is effective in the control of such insects as the budmoth, cherry shoot borer, apple curculio, and saskatoon sawfly. Saskatoons are also attacked by various fungi and a few bacteria, but so far no viruses or mycoplasmas are known (Davidson 1987). Important diseases include saskatoon-juniper rust (*Symnosporangium* sp.), leaf and berry spots (*Entomosporium* sp.), dieback and cankers (*Cytospora* sp., *Nectria* sp.,), blackleaf and witches broom (*Apiosporina* sp.), brown rot (*Monilinia amelanchieris*), and fireblight [*Erwinia amylovora* (Burrill) Winslow et al.] (St. Pierre 1991). Control procedures include pruning to remove infected parts, site selection (especially for saskatoon-juniper rusts) and agronomic practices (irrigation and cultivation).

Harvesting

Saskatoon fruit grows in clusters. The fruit ripens almost evenly and the whole crop can usually be picked at one time. Yields of up to 10 tonnes/ha can be obtained with proper management.

The fruit can be picked by hand, or mechanically, using a hand-operated vibrator or a self-propelled blueberry harvester. For the fresh fruit market, the fruit should not be overripe or crushed, torn, or bruised.

FRUIT COMPOSITION

The nutritional value of saskatoon berries on a dry weight basis is listed in Table 2. Saskatoon berries contain higher levels of protein, fat, and fiber than most other fruit. Tuba et al. (1944) indicated that fresh saskatoon berries might be a useful source of vitamin C. Panther and Wolfe (1972), however, reported a negligible ascorbic acid content and that an ascorbic acid oxidizing enzyme system was present in the berries.

Total solids content ranges from 20 to 29.4% fresh weight with 15.9 to 23.4% sucrose and 8 to 12% reducing sugars (Mazza 1979, 1982). Wolfe and Wood (1971) found that the sugar content increases slowly as the fruit matures and then accelerates markedly before ripening. Their results also indicated that fructose content decreased rather markedly (25%) after the fruit ripened while the glucose content remained unchanged. Berry pH values range from 4.2 to 4.4 and titratable acidity values (% malic acid) from 0.36 to 0.49% (Mazza 1979; Green and Mazza 1986). The predominant acid in saskatoon berries is malic (Wolfe and Wood 1972) and the predominant aroma component is benzaldehyde (Mazza and Hodgins 1985). There are at least four anthocyanins

Table 2. Nutritional composition of 'Smoky' saskatoon berries.

Nutrient	Composition (% dry wt±SD)
Protein	9.7±1.3
Fat	4.2±0.5
Fiber	19.0±3.0
Calcium	0.44±0.06
Phosphorous	0.16±0.02
Potassium	1.22±0.16
Magnesium	0.20±0.03
Sulfur	0.06±0.02
Iron	67.0±11.7
Sodium	31.8±7.7
Manganese	67.0±11.8
Copper	7.2±0.7
Zinc	16.5±2.8
Barium	34.8±4.9
Molybdenum	0.4±0.0
Aluminum	74.5±13.2
Carotene	29.7±5.0

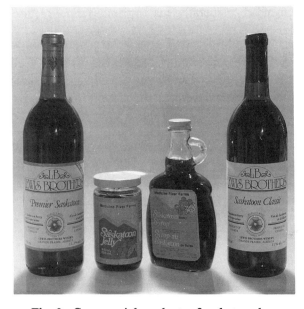

Fig. 2. Commercial products of saskatoon berry.

in ripe saskatoon berries; cyanidin 3-galactoside accounts for about 61% and 3-glucoside for 21% of total anthocyanins (Mazza 1986).

PROSPECTS

The saskatoon berry is a very new commercial fruit, yet several food processors are already using wild and cultivated berries in their food products (Fig. 2). There seems to be considerable potential for expansion of production and processing of saskatoon berry as many processors and distributors have reported they would use large quantities of this unique fruit if they had an assured supply at a reasonable price. For successful mass production of saskatoons, however, consistently higher yields and quality and improved pest control are required. This can only be achieved through increased research efforts.

REFERENCES

Davidson, C.G. and G. Mazza. 1991. Variability of fruit quality and plant height in populations of saskatoon berries (*Amelanchier alnifolia* Nutt.). Fruit Var. J. 45:162–165.

Davidson, J.G.N. 1987. The principal diseases of commercial saskatoons. Agr. Forestry Bul., Univ. of Alberta. Spring, 1987, 6–7.

Green, R.C. and G. Mazza. 1986. Relationships between anthocyanins, total phenolics, carbohydrates, acidity and colour of saskatoon berries. Can. Inst. Food Sci. Technol. J. 19:107–113.

Harris, R.E. 1972. The saskatoon. Agr. Can. Publication 1246.

Harris, R.E. 1980. Propagation of Amelanchier, *Amelanchier alnifolia* cv. Smoky in vitro. West. Can. Soc. Hort. Sci. 19:32–34.

Mazza, G. 1979. Development and consumer evaluation of a native fruit product. Can. Inst. Food Sci. Technol. J. 12(4):166–169.

Mazza, G. 1982. Chemical composition of Saskatoon berries (*Amelanchier alnifolia* Nutt.). J. Food Sci. 47:1730–1731.

Mazza, G. 1986. Anthocyanins and other phenolic compounds of saskatoon berries (*Amelanchier alnifolia* Nutt.). J. Food Sci. 51:1260–1264.

Mazza, G. and M.W. Hodgins. 1985. Benzaldehyde, a major aroma component of saskatoon berries. HortScience. 20:742–744.

Nelson, S.H. 1987. Effects of stock plant etiolation on the rooting of saskatoon berries (*Amelanchier alnifolia* Nutt.) cutting. Can. J. Plant Sci. 67:299–303.

Panther, M. and F.H. Wolfe. 1972. Studies on the degradation of ascorbic acid by saskatoon berry juice. Can. Inst. Food Sci. Technol. J. 5(2):93–96.

Pruski, K., J. Nowak, and G. Grainger. 1990. Micropropagation of four cultivars of saskatoon berry (*Amelanchier alnifolia* Nutt.). Plant Cell Tissue Organ Culture 21:103–109.

St. Pierre, R.G. 1989. Magnitude, timing and causes of immature fruit loss in *Amelanchier alnifolia* (Rosaceae). Can. J. Bot. 67:726–731.

St. Pierre, R.G. 1991. Growing saskatoons: A manual for orchardists. Univ. of Saskatchewan, Saskatoon, Saskatchewan.

Tuba, J., G. Hunter, and L.L. Kennedy. 1944. On sources of vitamin C. II. Alberta native fruits. Can. J. Res. 22(2):33–37.

Wolfe, F.H. and F.W. Wood. 1972. Non-volatile organic acid and sugar composition of saskatoon berries during ripening. Can. Inst. Food Sci. Technol. J. 4:29–30.

The Potential for Domestication and Utilization of Native Plums in Kansas

William Reid and Karen L.B. Gast

During the 19th century, Great Plains settlers demonstrated great interest in the domestication and utilization of North American plum species (*Prunus* spp.) (Bailey 1898; Goff 1897). In central and western Kansas, native plums represented the most reliable source of fresh fruit for many farm families (Kindscher 1987). By 1901, 305 native plum cultivars had been described, including 37 inter-specific hybrids (Waugh 1901). Interest in native plums waned during the 20th century, as mechanized farming and an increasingly efficient transportation system ushered in an age of agricultural specialization. By 1990, only five crops (wheat, maize, sorghum, soybeans, and hay) accounted for nearly 99% of the value of crops produced in Kansas (Byram 1990). Today, the decline in profits earned from producing traditional grain and forage crops has lead many farmers to search for new crops with greater profit potential. This search for agricultural diversification in the wheat belt has rekindled an interest in the domestication and utilization of native plums as a high value, speciality crop.

Eight species of native plum are found in Kansas, including *P. americana* Marsh., *P. angustifolia* Marsh., *P. besseyi* Bailey, *P. gracilis* Engelm. & Gray, *P. hortulana* Bailey, *P. mexicana* S. Wats., *P. munsoniana* Wight & Hedrick, and *P. rivularis* Scheele (Great Plains Flora Assn. 1986). Of these species, *P. americana*, *P. angustifolia*, *P. hortulana*, and *P. munsoniana*, are collected locally and processed into jams, jellies, and preserves in home kitchens. One species, *P. angustifolia*, has recently become the basis for a growing cottage industry in Kansas.

BOTANY

Prunus angustifolia can be found growing from Maryland to Florida in the east then westward to Kansas, Oklahoma, and Texas (Little 1977). The discontinuous distribution of *P. angustifolia* (Fig. 1) led Sargent (1965) to speculate that this species originated in the west and was moved eastward by native Americans and has since become naturalized in the southeastern United States.

Also known as the sandhill plum in Kansas (Stephens 1973), *P. angustifolia* forms large thickets in the sandy pastures of the central and western portions of the state. Large fruit size, small narrow leaves, and a dwarfed appearance led nineteenth century botanists to label the sandhill plum *P. angustifolia watsoni*, to distinguish it from the Chickasaw plum, *P. angustifolia*, common in southeastern states (Waugh 1903). Although modern botanists do not recognize the sandhill plum as a separate sub-species or botanical variety, the Kansas population

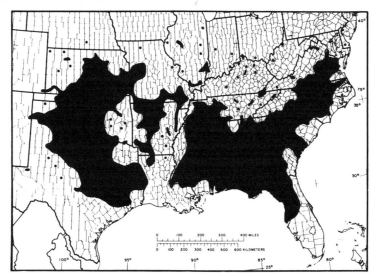

Fig. 1. The distribution of *Prunus angustifolia* in North America (Little 1977).

of *P. angustifolia* seems uniquely adapted for growth in a climate characterized by high heat (40°C) and drought in summer and bitter cold (–30°C) in mid-winter.

The sandhill plum is a much-branched shrub usually less than 2 m high. Thickets up to 20 m across are quickly formed by root suckers. Bright yellow-green leaves that are folded lengthwise help make sandhill plum colonies easily recognizable in the prairies of Kansas. Leaves are simple, alternate, and narrowly elliptical. Twigs are slender, red, glabrous, and often end in a spine. Many branches grow in a distinctive zig-zag pattern. Small white flowers emerge in early April before leaf burst. Flowers have 5 white rounded petals, 20 stamens, and a single egg-shaped ovary. Fruits ripen from early July to late August. Fruits are globose, average 2.1 cm across, and vary in skin color from orange-yellow to deep red (Fig. 2).

GENETIC DIVERSITY

In 1990, we initiated a study to measure the genetic diversity of *P. angustifolia* in Kansas by establishing a planting of 120 seedlings. Bushes used in this study were produced from seed collected from a native plum population located near Pratt, Kansas in 1988. Fifty-nine bushes produced their first fruit crop in 1991. Fruit weight varied from 2.6 to 13.8 g and fruit skin color from yellow to dark red. The orange-yellow flesh of sandhill plums contained from 9.0 to 19.4% soluble solids and were highly acid averaging pH 3.2.

One bush produced fruit that averaged 2.7 cm in diameter as compared to 'Methley', a Japanese plum, which averaged 3.0 cm in diameter (Norton et al. 1990). However, fruit size in sandhill plum is strongly influenced by crop load (Fig. 3). Differences in total bush yield accounted for 44% of the variation in fruit size with the remaining variation in fruit size due to genetic differences.

The selection of sandhill plum cultivars high in soluble solids is very important to the Kansas plum processing industry. Our seedling sandhill plum population averaged 14.3% soluble solids compared to an average of 17% for 9 Japanese plum cultivars (Norton et al. 1990). We did identify individual sandhill plum bushes that produced fruit containing 19.4% soluble solids.

Fruit was harvested from our seedling planting from July 3 to Sept. 11 with the majority of fruit harvested during late July and early August. The harvest season per bush varied from 1 to 7 weeks and averaged 3.6 weeks. The heaviest yielding bushes had the longest harvest season and produced over 4 kg of fruit.

Bush form varied widely. In the year prior to our first fruit crop, bushes could be easily rated as either prostrate, spreading, bushy, or upright. Precocity in sandhill plum seems closely associated with the prostrate growth form. The highest yielding bushes in the first year of fruiting were those that grew nearly horizontally (Fig.

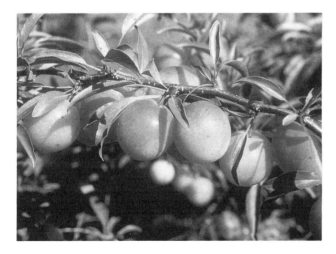

Fig. 2. Sandhill plum fruits are borne in clusters of 1 to 3. The fruits pictured here were light orange with a red blush and averaged 2.5 cm in diameter.

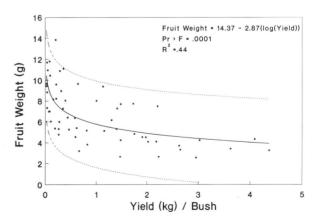

Fig. 3. The relationship between yield and fruit weight of 59 seedling sandhill plum bushes. The regression line (solid line) is bounded by 95% confidence limits (dashed lines).

4) but this growth form is the least desirable horticulturally. Fruit-laden limbs dropping on the ground were more prone to fruit rots and were difficult to harvest.

Evidence of bacterial spot infection caused by *Xanthomomas campestris* pv. *pruni* (Smith) Dye could be found on all bushes in the planting. Disease severity increased with fruit yield because of the negative influence of fruit production on vegetative growth. Those bushes with little or no fruit crop were able to outgrow the spread of the bacterial infection.

POTENTIAL FOR DOMESTICATION

Cultivar Development

Observations of the small sample of sandhill plum germplasm described above indicate that sufficient genetic diversity exists within the species for rapid crop improvement. Increased fruit size and higher soluble solids would lead the list of objectives for developing sandhill plum cultivars suited for the processing industry. Additional crop improvement objectives should include a condensed ripening season, an upright growth form, and resistance to bacterial spot.

A limited search of rural Pratt County, Kansas identified two thickets of that produced ample quantities of sandhill plums averaging 2.6 and 2.7 cm in diameter. A more detailed search should yield a sufficient number of superior individuals to begin screening for possible commercial cultivars.

Rootstocks

Prolific root suckering by *P. angustifolia* will make the commercial culture of this plum on its own roots impractical. Fortunately, *P. angustifolia* is graft-compatible with many of the non-suckering rootstocks that have been developed for other diploid plum species (Okie 1987). Growth and yield responses of sandhill plums propagated onto these Prunus rootstocks are not documented.

Pest Problems

The sandhill plum is susceptible to many of the same pests that attack commercial peach and plum orchards. Plum curculio, *Conotrachelus nenuphar* Herbst, is the primary insect pest of sandhill plum. Fruit drop and fruit damage caused by this insect must be controlled if commercial plantings of the sandhill plum are to be successful. Major disease problems include brown rot [*Monilinia fructicola* (Wint.) Honey] of the fruit and bacterial leaf spot (*Xanthomonas campestris* pv. *pruni* (Smith) Dye). There seems to be little natural resistance to either of these diseases within *P. angustifolia*. However, bacterial spot resistance has been identified in *P. cerarsifera* Ehrh. (Byrne 1989).

Chemical controls for the major pests of sandhill plum are widely available. Since sandhill plum is legally a plum, growers may apply any pesticide registered for use on European and Japanese plums for control of insect, disease, and weed pests.

Mechanical Harvest

Acceptance of sandhill plum as a crop in Kansas would depend in part on the availability of mechanical harvesting equipment. Fortunately, the dimensions and growth habit of the sandhill plum are close to those of the highbush blueberry. Harvesters developed for the blueberry industry should be easily adapted to sandhill plum harvest.

SANDHILL PLUM PRODUCT DEVELOPMENT

Sandhill plum jelly has been a regional favorite ever since the early settlers discovered abundant plum thickets on the Kansas prairie (Kindscher 1987). Until recently, sandhill plum jams and jellies were produced only in rural family kitchens for home consumption. With the rapid rise of consumer interest in regional and/or speciality foods, two Kansas food companies have begun manufacturing sandhill plum products for distribution nationally. Fruit is collected from uncultivated thickets and purchased for $1.10/kg. Products manufactured from the sandhill plum are marketed as uniquely Kansan and command as much as $17.50/kg.

Sandhill plums make distinctive fruit products that are often described as pleasingly tart with an apricot-like flavor. Besides the traditional jams and jellies, four additional Sandhill plum products have been developed

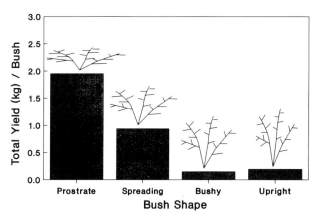

Fig. 4. The relationship between bush shape and fruit yield among 120 sandhill plum seedlings.

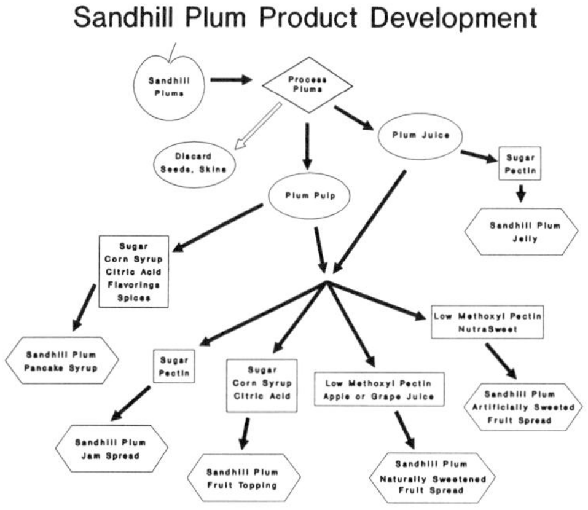

Fig. 5. A flow diagram for the manufacturing process of six sandhill plum products currently being produced in Kansas. Items enclosed in an oval represent ingredients derived from the sandhill plum. Additional ingredients are enclosed in rectangles, and final products are enclosed in hexagons.

by the Value-Added Center at Kansas State University. These include a pancake syrup, a fruit topping for ice-cream, a naturally sweetened fruit spread, and an artificially sweetened fruit spread. The manufacturing process for all six Sandhill plum products is outlined in Fig. 5.

CONCLUSIONS

Continued expansion of the sandhill plum industry will depend on the domestication of *P. angustifolia*. The rich genetic diversity found both within this species and among all native Kansas plums offer tremendous opportunities for crop development. Improvements in fruit size, soluble solids, and bush form can be made rapidly through careful examination of seedling populations. The domesticated Sandhill plum of the future is envisioned as a bush fruit adaptable to mechanical harvest with technology borrowed from the blueberry industry. Successful domestication and market development will provide Kansas farmers with an additional crop and allow them to reap the economic benefits of agricultural diversification.

REFERENCES

Bailey, L.H. 1898. Sketch of the evolution of our native fruits. Macmillan, New York.

Byram, T.J. 1990. Kansas farm facts 1990. Kansas State Board of Agr., Topeka.

Byrne, D.H. 1989. Inbreeding, coancestry, and founding clones of Japanese-type plums of California and the southeastern United States. J. Amer. Soc. Hort. Sci. 114:699–705.

Goff, E.S. 1897. The culture of native plums in the northwest. Wis. Agr. Expt. Sta. Bul. 63.

Great Plains Flora Association. 1986. Flora of the Great Plains. Univ. Press of Kansas, Lawrence.

Kindscher, K. 1987. Edible wild plants of the prairie, an ethnobotanical guide. Univ. Press of Kansas, Lawrence.

Little, E.L. 1977. Atlas of United States trees. Vol. 4. Minor eastern hardwoods. USDA For. Serv. Misc. Pub. 1342.

Norton, J.D., G.E. Boyhan, D.A. Smith, and B.R. Abrahams. 1990. 'AU-Rubrum' plum. HortScience 25:1311–1312.

Okie, W.R. 1987. Plum rootstocks, p. 321-360. In: R.C. Rom and R.F. Carlson (eds.). Rootstocks for fruit crops. Wiley, New York.

Sargent, C.S. 1965. Manual of trees of North America. Vol. 2. Dover Pub., New York.

Stephens, H.A. 1973. Woody plants of the north central plains. Univ. Press of Kansas, Lawrence.

Waugh, F.A. 1901. Plums and plum culture. Orange Judd, New York.

Waugh, F.A. 1903. Systematic pomology. Orange Judd, New York.

Commercialization of the Cloudberry (*Rubus chamaemorus* L.) in Norway

Kåre Rapp, S. Kristine Næss, and Harry Jan Swartz

The cloudberry, *Rubus chamaemorus* L., Rosaceae, is a small herbaceous bramble common to peat bogs in the northern hemisphere (Fig. 1). The berry has a strong musky flavor, quite distinct from that of any of the other bramble crops, and is highly prized as a dessert berry in Scandinavia. Recently, demand for the development of the cloudberry as a commercially viable crop has increased in northern Norway where many districts are struggling to maintain a viable economy.

PLANT DESCRIPTION

Distribution

The cloudberry is a circumpolar, subarctic species. It can be found as far north as 78°30' N in Svalbard, Norway and its distribution extends south to 44°N in New Hampshire, U.S.A. (Resvoll 1929). It is a common plant in northern Norway, and is also found in the highland areas and mountains farther south.

Morphology

The cloudberry is a dioecious perennial herb. The plant spreads mainly by means of an extensive rhizome system. Annual shoots consisting of from one to four lobed leaves may terminate in a single staminate or pistillate flower. Insect pollination is required for fruit set to occur in most places though wind pollination may also contribute to fruit set in coastal windswept areas.

In Norway, the cloudberry begins ripening in the end of July or early August. The berry, resembling a large amber raspberry, consists of from 5 to 25 drupelets. The cloudberry contains from 50 to over 150 mg ascorbic acid per 100 g fruit (Nordness and Werenskiold 1951; Heller 1981). It is also rich in benzoic acid (Honkanen and Pyysalo 1976) and can therefore be easily stored for several weeks or longer under normal refrigeration. For these reasons the cloudberry was favored in the prevention of scurvy by Norwegian sailors and North American Eskimos (Faegri 1970; Heller 1981).

COMMERCIALIZATION PROSPECTS

Although the cloudberry is a common plant throughout northern Norway, the Norwegians are unable to satisfy their domestic demand for the berry. In some years, 200 to 300 tons of cloudberries are imported from

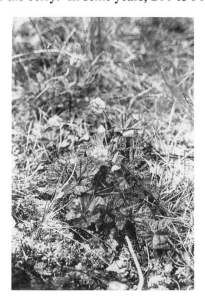

Fig. 1. The cloudberry.

Finland. The cloudberry harvest in the wild is highly unpredictable due to the unstable weather conditions prevailing in the beginning of June when the cloudberry flowers. Early frost in August may also destroy the crop in some years. In general, cloudberry yields from bog plants are very low, only averaging about 20 kg/ha. Domestication of the cloudberry would not only help fill the market demand for the berry but would also provide an attractive crop for use in boggy areas where little else of agricultural value can be grown. Several growers organizations have now been formed in Norway and a consultant has been employed at Holt Research Station, Tromsø, Norway (69°29'N) to study the commercialization potential of the crop and set forth research priorities.

Progress

Bog management. A number of bog management practices have been developed which can lead to greatly increased yields. Plowing furrows into a bog with a spacing of from 1 to 5 m leads to an increase in cloudberry proliferation and can reduce the incidence of spring freezes (Lid et al. 1961; Østgard 1964; Makinen and Oikarinen 1974; Rapp 1982). Fertilization of the bog with superphosphates or complete fertilizers (300 kg/ha) can increase yields per hectare by an average of 50 kg when the fertilizer is placed at a depth of 20 to 25 cm (Rapp 1989). Fertilizers applied to the surface of the bog or at greater depths tend to benefit other bog species at the expense of the cloudberry. In windswept areas, short fences may be useful in settling the snow in the winter to delay the blossoming period and therefore avoid spring frost injury. The use of windrows also leads to an increase in the activity of pollinating insects and has increased yields (Østgard 1964).

Genotype improvement. A prerequisite for the success of any of these bog management practices is the existence of a good stand of pistillate (fruit bearing) plants. In most cloudberry producing bogs, less than 25% of the flowering shoots are pistillate (Lid et al. 1967). Even among seedling populations there is an overabundance of male plants (Rapp 1987). Current research is aimed at the breeding of higher yielding pistillate or hermaphrodite cultivars and the development of efficient propagation methods.

The development of cloudberry cultivars is well underway at the Holt Research Station in northern Norway. Hundreds of seedlings from several different environments have been screened for high flower production and large berry size (Rapp 1988). Further performance evaluations have been made on promising selections in square meter plots where their ability to spread and become rapidly established can also be assessed. From these, two superior pistillate clones (An 267 and If 542), and two superior staminate clones (An 30 and An 257), have now been selected for cultivar release.

The development of hermaphrodite cultivars is an important goal in the domestication of the cloudberry. Occasionally, hermaphrodite flowers can be found in the wild. Several plants bearing such flowers have been collected for evaluation. Unfortunately, sex expression in these plants varies from year to year and also from flower to flower within a clone. Plants with hermaphroditic tendencies are currently being used as parents in the cloudberry breeding program in an attempt to develop stable hermaphrodite cloudberry cultivars.

Several crosses between cloudberry and other *Rubus* species including a hybrid blackberry, red raspberry clones, and several Asiatic ideobats have produced plants with overall general *chamaemorus* morphology (thornless, herbaceous, non-elongating) however, leaf pattern is definitely hybrid. The blackberry × cloudberry cross is much more vigorous than other hybrids and cloudberries.

Rapid and good seed germination is important to the success of a cloudberry breeding program. Normally cloudberry seed require 6 to 8 months cold stratification before germinating and germination rates are often well below 50% (Rantala 1976). By removing the endocarp and seed coat from fresh cloudberry seed, we have obtained in vitro germination rates of 75 to 85% four weeks after culture initiation.

Plant propagation. The cloudberry is difficult to propagate relative to other bramble species. Large turfs must be dug when collecting selections from the wild to ensure transplant survival. Further propagation of the selection can be made through the use of rhizome cuttings. The success rate with rhizome cuttings has been greatly improved by increasing the length of the cutting from about 7 cm to 15 to 20 cm. The best results have been obtained when the rhizome cuttings are taken in May or August (Rapp 1986). Although the cloudberry proliferates readily in tissue culture, explant rooting remains a major problem.

REFERENCES

Faegri, K. 1970. Norges planter (in Norwegian). J.V. Caappelens Press, Oslo, Norway.

Heller, C.A. 1981. Wild edible and poisonous plants of Alaska. 8th ed. Cooperative Extension Service, Univ. of Alaska, Fairbanks.

Honkanen, E. and T. Pyysalo. 1976. The aroma of cloudberries (*Rubus chamaemorus* L.). Z. Lebensm. Unters. Forsch. 160:393–400.

Lid, J., O. Lie, and A. Løddesøl. 1961. Orienterende forsøk med dyrking av molte. Medd. Det norske Myrselskap 59:1–26.

Makinen, Y. and H. Oikarinen. 1974. Cultivation of cloudberry in fennoscandia. Rpt. Kevo. Subarctic Res. 11:90–102.

Nordness, E. and B.Q. Werenskiold. 1951. The variation of the ascorbic acid content in raw and preserved cloudberries. *Rubus chamaemorus* L. Food Res. 17:117–122.

Østgard, O. 1964. Molteundersøkelser i Nord-Norge. Forsk. Fors. Landbr. 15:409–444.

Rantala, E. 1976. Sexual reproduction in the cloudberry. Ann. Agr. Fenn. 15:295–303.

Rapp, K. 1982. Kultivering av moltemyr. In: Landbrukets Årbok 1981. Tanum-Norli Press, Oslo, Norway.

Rapp, K. 1986. Vegetativ oppformering av molte (*Rubus chamaemorus* L.). Jord og Myr 10:1–11.

Rapp, K. 1987. Om kjønnsfordeling of kjønnsdifferensiering hos molte (*Rubus chamaemorus* L.). Jord og Myr 11:1–11.

Rapp, K. 1988. Foredling i molte. Inf. SFL Holt 16:67–70.

Rapp, K. 1989. Gjødsling til molte (*Rubus chamaemorus* L.) Jord og Myr 14:109–129.

Resvoll, T. 1929. *Rubus chamaemorus* L., a morphological-biological study. Nyt Mag. Naturvit. 67:55–129.

VEGETABLES

New Directions in Salad Crops: New Forms, New Tools, and Old Philosophy

Edward J. Ryder and William Waycott

Salad crops as such are not new. We are, however, finding new ways of using salad vegetables and they are turning up in new forms and colors. Familiar salad vegetables for one group of people may be quite new to another. There are even a few salad vegetables that would qualify as new in the narrowest sense, such as wild species and non-domestic plants that are now consumed as salad greens. The objective of this paper is to discuss new directions and trends in salad crops, as well as some new approaches in our research. We will also briefly discuss trends in plant breeding research that we consider to be unfortunate for the development on few and improved cultivars.

NEW DIRECTIONS IN USE AND FORM

Usage in the United States and Europe

Profound changes in the use of lettuce and other saladcrops have been taking place in the United States, western Europe, and several other parts of the world. The most surprising change has been the adoption of crisphead or iceberg lettuce in countries where it was hardly used before. In England, for example, people consumed mostly butterhead lettuce until the late 1970s. At that time, only about 3% of the lettuce was of the iceberg type. Then, the British discovered iceberg lettuce and it now comprises about 80% of the lettuce consumed in Britain. Similar changes have occurred in the Scandinavian countries and are beginning in other countries as well.

On the other hand, we in the United States have rediscovered that not all lettuce heads are round, crisp, and hard and once again are eating romaine, butterhead, and leaf lettuces, not to mention endive and escarole (*Cichorium endivia*), and spinach (*Spinacia oleracea*). In addition, we have discovered Little Gem, a Latin type lettuce, part cos and part butterhead, which is small, crisp, and sweet. We have discovered radicchio, a red Italian chicory (*C. intybus* L.); mizuna, a leafy vegetable from Japan (*Brassica japonica* L.); and rocket (*Eruca sativa* Mill.), formerly found in the wild, but now known in the cultivated form as arugula. Mizuna, arugula, and spinach are often found in a salad mixture called mezclun, which is made up of tiny lettuce leaves of various shapes and colors and other salad greens.

Variation in Form and Appearance

The proliferation of form and color existing in lettuce germplasm is quite astounding. Some relatively new variations in form and color can be seen now in commercial lettuce fields. In a recent planting of more than 400 lettuce Plant Introduction (PI) accessions, we found lines with leaves that ranged from dark green to light green, from deep crimson to light pink, as well as yellows and golds, and even blue teal. One line had plants with red rhubarb-like stems, another had plants that resembled balls of frilly green lace. (Table 1).

There are other crops we may see in the near future. Stem lettuce is a type found in both China and Egypt. The Chinese peel and cook the stems; the Egyptians eat them raw like a stalk of celery. This form probably originated in Egypt and was carried overland to eastern Asia many years ago. There are similar forms from Central Asia as well. Zuckerhut, also known as Pan di Zucchero or Sugarloaf, is an elongated, green chicory which heads nicely in late summer and has a milder flavor than radicchio.

Salad vegetables may be lightly processed. These are chopped or shredded prewashed leaves that are packaged for the consumer. About 12% of the harvested crop of iceberg lettuce is prepared in this way. MacDonalds alone purchases 2% of the entire United States iceberg lettuce crop in the chopped form.

Several kinds of miniaturized vegetables are appearing in market produce bins. These include carrots, watermelons, squashes, pumpkins, bok choi, and tomatoes. Soon mini-iceberg lettuce will join this group on the

Table 1. Partial list of lettuce USDA Plant Introductions (PI) with unusual color and form variants.

USDA PI number	Origin	Description
177418	Turkey	Dark green leaves
169511	Turkey	Pale green leaves
249536	Spain	Crimson leaves
206965	Turkey	Intense red leaves
271476	India	Light red leaves
289042C[z]	Hungary	Yellow leaves
220524	Afghanistan	Blue-green leaves, red stem
178923	Turkey	Tiny head, frilly green leaves
183234	Egypt	Large green leaves

[z]Subsample of 289042.

market. Mini-iceberg is an intriguing byproduct from one of our gibberellin biosynthetic studies. Germinating seeds of a genetic early flowering line were treated with ethyl methanesulfonate. Among the segregating progeny were several dwarf forms, which flowered early, but had smaller leaves and considerably shortened stems. One dwarf was crossed with a standard iceberg lettuce cultivar and among the progeny was an iceberg lettuce about one-fourth the size of a normal head, but otherwise normal in appearance. A press release about this material has generated considerable publicity in media as diverse as *Wall Street Journal* and *National Enquirer*. We will release this material early in 1992 and it should be available on the market by early 1993. We assume it will appeal mostly to single people or others, who, for some reason, cannot seem to get through a whole head of regular lettuce with dispatch.

Roots and Seeds

Most crops are produced for their above-ground parts and researchers often have neglected the contribution of roots to yield and quality. This has been true in lettuce research, at least until recent years. The modern butterhead and crisphead types of the United States and Western Europe generally have long narrow taproots and a relatively sparse secondary system. Recently, we examined roots of over 400 accessions of *L. sativa* and found substantial variation in root structure. Of specific interest were a number of cos (Romaine) types from Turkey and a stem lettuce from China. These root systems were characterized by more extensive branching off the tap root and may have longer tap roots. Two wild species were also studied, *L. serriola* and *L. saligna*. These species had similar root designs with several stout secondary roots and finer tertiary roots. However, they did not closely resemble the cos or stem lettuce root systems. We believe that selection on the basis of root structure may affect shoot development and reaction to injurious root colonizing organisms. Understanding the nature of root structures may also help in water and nutrient uptake studies.

Lettuce seed was probably used by the ancient Egyptians as a source of edible oil. One type of lettuce in our collection has a primitive, almost wild, shoot architecture. Although these plants resemble wild species, they have features which indicate they were selected for seed characteristics. The seeds of these plants are unusually large and germinate at high temperatures, compared to most cultivated lettuces. The plants also flower rapidly on multiple stems, producing large quantities of seeds. Research on the chemistry and quality of this oil is in progress today in modern Egypt (Shoeb et al. 1969; Ramadan 1976).

NEW DIRECTIONS IN TECHNIQUE AND TECHNOLOGY

Plant breeders frequently make the point that plant breeding is a long term proposition, requiring not only time, but perseverance and dedication. At the same time, we do look for ways to make the job easier and/or faster. In lettuce breeding, we have some tools that enable us to do that.

Genetic Engineering

Several new ways of altering plant genotypes have appeared over the past 15 years. Some of these are very promising and recent results indicate they will be useful additions to a breeder's set of tools. The potential of plant transformation is particularly exciting. In a sense, it is the ultimate backcross procedure. Ideally, one can transfer useful genes into a desired genotype, with little or no modification of the original phenotype. Results of studies with non-functional marker genes and genes for herbicide and pest resistance, hormone regulation, and nutritional enhancement, point towards phenomenal changes for plant genomic science. However, biotechnology is expensive and to do breeding work with an emphasis in this area may not be cost effective in the long term. Nevertheless, one can not afford to ignore the prospects.

We use transformation as a tool in lettuce breeding. Aside from the need to discover, clone, and incorporate needed genes for disease and insect resistance, we are particularly interested in genes which control lettuce growth and development. These include genes, such as those for early flowering and induction of stem elongation, which perceive day length and other environmental cues and thus, affect rate of growth. If these genes could be cloned and transferred to other species, they might be highly useful as backcross breeding aids.

Biotechnology is also making our job of detecting variation among lettuces much easier. We use RFLP and RAPD analysis to identify major differences between species as well as minor differences between and within lettuce cultivars. With this information, we are able to determine similarities, which should be useful for cultivar fingerprinting. It also may be useful in identifying duplicate accessions that we may wish to purge from our collection. These methods can also be used to map genes in preparation for cloning.

Backcross Procedures

One preferred breeding method in our lettuce program is the backcross procedure, for transferring single genes to a desirable recurrent parent. This procedure requires repeated crosses. Crossing can be difficult in lettuce, because of its flower structure. Each flower is a composite of several florets consisting of a single ligulate petal and a reproductive structure consisting of a tube formed by fused anthers, surrounding a single style with a bipartite stigma. The style elongates as the anthers shed pollen on their interior surfaces. The stigmas emerge from the top of the tube, covered with pollen. It is important to remove the pollen before it can germinate and replace it with pollen from the male parent. Some procedures have been developed by which one can maximize the proportion of hybrid to selfed seeds (Oliver 1910; Ryder and Johnson 1974).

Despite the difficulty of making crosses, backcrossing is an excellent means of conserving a valuable genotype. This is important in lettuce, as cultivar groups tend to last for many years. In this century, the Western iceberg lettuce industry has, in the main, been based upon four cultivar groups: New York types in the 1910s and 1920s, Imperial types in the 1930s and 1940s, Great Lakes types in the 1950s, 1960s, and early 1970s, and the Salinas types starting in the late 1970s and still in use. Historically, cultivar types last for many years. This longevity lends itself to a program of combining useful genes within manageable population sizes.

If more than one desirable gene is available for backcrossing, each can be backcrossed into the same desirable cultivar in parallel programs. At the completion of the backcross programs, the modified forms can then be crossed to each other and progeny selected with the contributed genes. The similarity of the respective populations insures that the number of other genes segregating is relatively less and the populations required will be smaller.

Lettuce breeders have a unique genetic tool that can reduce drastically the total time required to complete a backcross program. Several years ago, two partially dominant genes for flowering time, *Ef-1 ef-1* and *Ef-2 ef-2*, were identified. In the double-dominant condition, these genes reduce flowering time in head lettuce from, 140 days to 45 days (Ryder 1983, 1988). These time periods are specific to summer conditions in the greenhouse at our location and may vary in other locations. Because of the partial dominance, flowering times can be accurately predicted for all nine genotypes (Table 2).

The partial dominance of the early flowering trait means that the desired heterozygous segregants are identifiable. They are early, but not as early as the double-dominant. And, the preserved heterozygosity means that the early allele can be eliminated in favor of the late one at the end of the program. A modified backcross procedure was developed, with these genes as a vehicle to transfer useful genes to a recurrent parent in half the

Table 2. Days to first flower for all genotypes of two flowering time genes. Planted 13 July in greenhouse, Salinas, California.

Genotype	Range (days)
Ef-1 Ef-1 Ef-2 Ef-2	43–49
Ef-1 Ef-1 Ef-2 ef-2	52–57
Ef-1 Ef-1 ef-2 ef-2	59–76
Ef-1 ef-1 Ef-2 Ef-2	49–54
Ef-1 ef-1 Ef-2 ef-2	60–73
Ef-1 ef-1 ef-2 ef-2	74–88
ef-1 ef-1 Ef-2 Ef-2	93–118
ef-1 ef-1 Ef-2 ef-2	119–134
ef-1 ef-1 ef-2 ef-2	137–143

time required with backcrossing of normal late flowering cultivars (Ryder 1985). This method is being used to transfer a lettuce mosaic resistance gene to the cultivars 'Prizehead' and 'Salinas'. Also, an early flowering line was used during the breeding of the mini-lettuce. Similar genes exist in and may be similarly useful in other species.

Hybrids

F_1 hybrids have been important in many cross-pollinated species. In recent years, hybrids have also become increasingly important in some self-pollinated crops, such as tomatoes. We have observed apparent heterosis in lettuce, principally as increased seedling size, compared to the parents, but we have no data to support this observation. However, F_1 hybrids will probably not be important in our lettuce work. The reason for this is primarily functional. Lettuce pollen is sticky and cannot be carried by the wind. And, there are no known insect species that work lettuce flowers effectively to transfer pollen. Therefore, hand pollination is necessary to make a cross. The lettuce flower is a composite of 12 to 20 florets. Each pollination will yield a maximum of 12 to 20 seeds, some of which may result from selfing. Modern planting methods require 250,000 seeds to sow one hectare of lettuce, which would require at least 12,500 pollinations to produce enough seed. It is clear, that with present technology, the task is quite daunting. There is, of course, the possibility that one can create a single hybrid plant and then multiply it in cell culture. However, one runs the risk of somaclonal variation induced in tissue culture which could quickly alter a pure genotype.

Heterosis exists in many crops, but a major factor in the interest in F_1 hybrids among most seed companies is to conceal the identity of the hybrid parents, even though the biological and agricultural benefits of the hybrid may be limited.

Heterosis, as in the F_1 hybrid, is probably due to the accumulation of favorable alleles (Jinks 1983). The prevailing view is that a cross between two diverse genotypes gives the benefit of one set of dominant alleles from one parent and another set from the other parent. It is important also to consider that there may be recessive genes that are beneficial. In lettuce, for example, two important disease resistance alleles are recessive; *mo* against lettuce mosaic and *cor* against corky root rot. At each locus in which one parent has the dominant allele and the other has the recessive, it is necessary to fix the recessive alleles in the inbred populations in order to save the recessive effect in the hybrid. Population improvement is also necessary to save both alleles at each additive locus, to prevent loss of about half the effect at the locus, if it remained in the heterozygous condition. Population improvement is also useful to preserve epistatic effects.

In self-pollinated species, hybrid combinations are less likely to be superior to their parents for the vast majority of traits. The primary reason for the use of hybrids in self pollinated species is therefore, protection of the parents' identity. Some authors have expressed doubts over the usefulness of hybrids for self-pollinated crops, such as wheat and barley (Simmonds 1979; Wilson and Driscoll 1983).

Whither Plant Breeding?

We are advocates of cultivar development without economic gain as the primary motivation. As private sector breeding increases its market share and as public breeding institutions are scaled down or closed altogether, emphasis on basic and fundamental research as a foundation for cultivar development is sure to fade. Just as the F_1 hybrid has become a tool for profits, a similar phenomenon appears to be developing in the world of biotechnology. There are, as cited earlier, many important aspects of biotechnology that merit serious discussion. Yet, can we afford to limit our scope and purpose, continuing to sacrifice public plant breeding programs on the altar of financial gain. One of the tools of sacrifice is the dogma that the province of the public sector is basic research and that practical breeding, or the development of marketable products, is the province of private industry.

We believe that the current loss of public programs has lead to an ever narrowing set of breeding goals, whose principal criteria are to enable the development of profitable, protected products as fast as possible. Profit generation is a perfectly acceptable function of private industry. The problem is that it may not properly serve science, agriculture, humankind, or our society, particularly in the years to come.

Agriculture is biology in the environment; it is complex, ever shifting, and constantly interactive. Problems in agricultural research are often difficult, complex subjects, requiring intense study over an extended period, with limited concern for the financial gain. Private industry cannot and will not deal with many of these types of problems, e.g., the study of gibberellin biosynthesis and root branching in lettuce, which demand long-term commitments with uncertain conclusions. As public plant breeding programs disappear, or operate at the behest of the private sector, these difficult, lengthy, unpromising problems will simply continue to accumulate. Significant knowledge will remain buried and we will lose the commitment to probe important genetic potential in plants. Yet the probing of these concepts would permit us to answer important questions as well as to discover and develop new ideas essential for maintaining the high agricultural productivity we have known and come to rely on for the past several decades.

REFERENCES

Jinks, J.L. 1983. Biometrical genetics of heterosis, p. 1–46. In: R. Frankel (ed.). Heterosis, reappraisal of theory and practice. Springer–Verlag, Berlin.

Oliver, G.W. 1910. New methods of plant breeding. U.S. Bur. Plant Ind. Bul. 167.

Ramadan, A.A.S. 1976. Characteristics of prickly lettuce seed oil in relation to methods of extraction. Die Nahrung 20:579–583.

Ryder, E.J. 1983. Inheritance, linkage and gene interaction studies in lettuce. J. Amer. Soc. Hort. Sci. 108:985–991.

Ryder, E.J. 1985. Use of early flowering genes to reduce generation time in backcrossing, with specific application to lettuce breeding. J. Amer. Soc. Hort. Sci. 110:570–573

Ryder, E.J. 1988. Early flowering in lettuce as influenced by a second flowering time gene and seasonal variation. J. Amer. Soc. Hort. Sci. 113:456–460.

Ryder, E.J. and A.S. Johnson. 1974. Mist depollination of lettuce flowers. HortScience 9:584.

Shoeb, Z.E., F. Osman, Z.H.M. El-Kirdassy, and M.H. Eissa. 1969. Studies and evaluation of Egyptian lettuce seeds *Lactuca scariola* L. Grasas y Aceites 20:125–128.

Simmonds, N.W. 1979. Principles of crop improvement. Longman, London.

Wilson, P. and C.J. Driscoll. 1983. Hybrid wheat, p. 94–123. In: R. Frankel (ed.). Heterosis: Reappraisal of theory and practice. Springer–Verlag, Berlin.

Root Vegetables: New Uses for Old Crops

Wanda W. Collins

Vegetables grown for their edible roots or tubers encompass a wide range of starchy root crops, some of which are true botanical roots and others which are tubers or corms. The most economically significant root crops globally include potato (*Solanum tuberosum* L.), sweetpotato (also spelled sweet potato) [*Ipomoea batatas* (L) Lam.], cassava (*Manihot esculenta* Crantz), yams (*Dioscorea* spp.), and aroids [principally *Colocasia esculenta* (L.) Schott var. *esculenta* and *Xanthosoma* spp.]. Although traditionally, root vegetables have been considered low status and generally unimportant crops by consumers, governmental organizations, and researchers, on a global scale they account for three of the seven most important food crops in the world (FAO 1989).

Of these five majors root crops, only potato and sweetpotato are grown to any extent in the United States, and of these two, sweetpotato has the greatest potential for increased usage and consumption. However, there are other starchy root vegetables grown in various areas of the world where they are of local economic and cultural importance and which could conceivably be considered potential new crops for domestic consumption (O'Hair 1990a,b). Among the most promising may be some of the Andean root crops (Sperling and King 1990). In addition, apios (*Apios americana*), has received attention as a potential new crop. Apios is unique among the root and tuber crops mentioned in that it fixes nitrogen and also produces edible tubers, fleshy roots, and seeds (Putnam et al. 1991). Tubers are high in protein and carbohydrates (Walter et al. 1986) and are preferred by some to the domestic potato, *Solanum tuberosum*. The potential of apios as a new crop has been described by Reynolds et al. (1990).

DISTRIBUTION AND PRODUCTION OF MAJOR ROOT VEGETABLES

Most root vegetables are produced in developing countries. In developed countries, 99% of root production is in potato (Rhoades and Horton 1990). Fresh weight production of the five major root vegetables (potato, sweetpotato, cassava, yams, and aroids) is listed in Table 1 and compared with the other major crops which are produced at a level of 100 million tonnes globally. Potatoes, cassava, and sweetpotato rank among the seven major, global food crops which are produced at that level. Yams and aroids are produced at a much lower level, but are important staple food crops on a regional level.

Sweetpotatoes and potatoes are produced in the United States (Table 1). Cassava, yams, and aroids are long season crops requiring one to two years for maturity which precludes their being grown in any significant amount in the continental United States. Although some short-season types are available, they still require six months or more for maturity. There are some experimental results indicating that yams could be successfully produced domestically (Marsh 1991).

USE OF ROOT VEGETABLES IN THE UNITED STATES

Cassava, Yams, and Aroids

There is little consumption or consumer familiarity with cassava, yams, or aroids in the United States outside of ethnic populations. This status is not likely to change except for increased consumption by steadily increasing ethnic populations. They are, however, imported into the United States from the Caribbean and Latin America and are available for consumption. Quality of imported products is generally poor unless purchased immediately from a local market. Once the product reaches grocery shelves, it is generally well below fresh quality standards.

Studies in Missouri have shown that yams can be produced in that state by starting them in a greenhouse for six weeks followed by about 22 weeks in the field (Marsh 1988). Yield per plant was much lower than those obtained in tropical growing areas (3.5 kg/plant as opposed to 20 to 30 kg/plant) but yams were of good marketable quality.

Table 1. Production of major world food crops and root crops[z].

Crop	Global production (000 tons)	United States production (000 tons)
Wheat	538,056	55,407
Rice	506,291	7,007
Maize	470,318	191,197
Barley	168,964	8,784
Potato	276,740	16,659
Sweetpotato	133,234	542
Cassava	147,500	---
Yam	23,459	---
Aroids	5,814	3
Root crops total	590,176	17,204

[z]Source: FAO 1989 Production Yearbook (FAO 1990)

Potato

Potatoes have been the most widely used root vegetable grown in the United States; current per capita consumption is about 56.4 kg. Quality is excellent, consumption is high, and there are a multitude of products available to the consumer. Potatoes are used in many ways as a vegetable and as a snack food. Even so, new types of potatoes are being introduced to the fresh market for consumers to try. Among these are yellow potatoes and blue potatoes. The unique characteristics of these potatoes are novelty traits which may capture a very small portion of present markets. They do represent a potential for specialty markets at very high prices.

Sweetpotato

Sweetpotatoes are consumed in the United States on a much smaller scale than potatoes with the per capita consumption now about 5.8 kg. Quality is excellent but few products are available. Normally sweetpotatoes can be purchased fresh, canned (whole or cut), as a reconstituted patty, and in baby food. They are most often used in pies or as a candied vegetable. Use is seasonal revolving around Thanksgiving, Christmas, and Easter. This seasonality has been a major problem in marketing efforts to increase consumption. In the past, various products have been developed from sweetpotatoes, such as chips and fries, but none have been successful.

Sweetpotato does have the potential for increased production and consumption. Sweetpotato germplasm, like that of potato, is diverse with many types with different flesh colors, skin colors, textural properties, and nutritional components. There is excellent potential for the development of new products and new types of sweetpotatoes to fit various demands of different consumer groups. Breeding efforts in the United States have focused almost exclusively on a single phenotype: a sweet vegetable type (luxury type) which has copper skin, deep orange flesh (high carotene), sweetness, and moist texture (Collins 1987). The American public, through surveys, has expressed a flexibility of choice for some attributes, but the desired marketing type has remained the same. Although this type can still be greatly improved through breeding efforts, it is unlikely that the demand for the luxury type of sweetpotato will increase significantly unless new uses and products are developed.

POTENTIAL FOR INCREASED USE AND PRODUCTION OF SWEETPOTATOES

Ethnic Markets

Populations of ethnic cultural groups in the United States are substantial and continue to increase (Marsh 1991). Opportunities exist for American growers in the United States to produce different types of sweetpotatoes for those markets. Unlike cassava, aroids, and yams, importation of sweetpotatoes into the United States is prohibited by law. Hence, there is little or no supply for potential ethnic markets because the type of sweetpotato demanded by those markets is different from the normal phenotype which is now the major focus of domestic commercial sweetpotato production. Preferred types are red or white skinned, cream to white flesh, non-sweet or very slightly sweet, and dry in texture. Consumers in these groups are more accustomed to eating sweetpotato as a carbohydrate energy source (staple or supplemental staple type) than as a dessert or sweet vegetable (luxury type).

Staple, supplemental staple, and luxury types of sweetpotatoes were described by Villareal (1981) and further characterized by Collins (1987). Desired traits for each type are very different and breeding programs must have specific programs for developing acceptable cultivars of these types.

Some efforts do exist to meet the demands of ethnic markets. In Florida, "boniatoes," white-fleshed, dry, firm textured sweetpotatoes, have been produced for many years for the Hispanic market. Cultivars used in this production have been brought into Florida from nearby Caribbean islands, such as Cuba (O'Hair et al. 1983), and have not been improved for United States growing conditions. A new Japanese clone recently entered the domestic market and is being grown in California and North Carolina. This cultivar may not be ideally suited to domestic growing conditions. There is ample opportunity for breeders to respond to the need for new phenotypes to meet new market opportunities. No surveys have been conducted to assess potential demand, but it could equal as much as 25% of current production if the crop is properly marketed. Market feasibility studies would establish the extent of the potential market, and should they be positive, convince growers of the profitability of producing this type of sweetpotato.

The North Carolina State University sweetpotato breeding program has a small project underway to develop the type of sweetpotato described. The variability in sweetpotato is great enough so that almost any type desired can be constructed with proper breeding procedures. Several clones with different characteristics are in various stages of testing. There are also several research projects underway to study specific characteristics which are important in breeding clones with the necessary traits, such as studies on the heritability and factors affecting ß-amylase activity which lead to non-sweet types. Non-sweetness has proved to be one of the most difficult traits to incorporate in these clones even though non-sweet types exist in the breeding materials. Results of preliminary tests indicate that sweetness and the perception of sweetness is very complex and that lowering ß-amylase activity alone may not necessarily lead to non-sweet sweetpotatoes.

Development of New Value-added Products

The range of variability in sweetpotatoes is so great that many different phenotypes can be made available for special product development depending on the characteristics needed. Often it is difficult to determine, even through trial and error, what the best characteristics are for particular products. Value-added products such as french fries, chips, and flakes, have been developed from sweetpotato but none has been successfully marketed for any length of time. Much effort has been devoted to sweetpotato fries. However, consumer comments often refer to the sweetness, texture, and oil content as problems. The products developed, such as fries, have always been developed from the existing single phenotype grown in the United States today and this may be a major reason for the disappointing results with such products.

Sweetpotato in Breads and Flours

There have been efforts in the private sector to capitalize on the enormous potential for sweetpotato products. At least one patent has been granted for producing sweetpotato bread and flour composed of 100% sweetpotato. These products are marketed as hypoallergenic for people who cannot tolerate grain breads and flours. The price is quite high (approximately $12/lb. for flour and up to $17 for a loaf of bread) as is demand. The inventor in this case has surmounted the problems normally associated with increased amounts of sweetpotato flour in breads. A "boniato" type sweetpotato from Florida is used to make these products. As the process is patented, it is not available for general production at present. Several other patents are pending for other processes involving sweetpotato (K. Slimak pers. commun.).

Where wheat has to be imported or can be grown only with extensive inputs (such as in developing countries), sweetpotato is a viable alternative component for breads and flours. There are disadvantages such as reduced loaf volume and decreased storage life (Keya and Hadziye 1990), but the reduced costs and decreased dependability on imports may outweigh the disadvantages. The acceptability of component breads and flours is excellent with as much as 10 to 15% content of sweetpotato flour (Sammy 1984). Some researchers have reported using up to 25% sweetpotato flour with no adverse consumer reaction. In the United States, where wheat is plentiful and relatively inexpensive, this alternative use of sweetpotato does not appear to be economically justified except as a specialty product.

Use as Animal Feed or an Animal Feed Supplement

Sweetpotato is used as an animal feed and supplement in developing countries (Gohl 1981). Both vines and roots are used. Starch and protein digestibility of raw sweetpotatoes has been cited as an obstacle to increased use for animal feed. Trypsin inhibitor has been implicated in poor protein digestibility. Genetic variability does exist for level of trypsin inhibitor activity and genotypes with no measurable activity are available. In the United States, competition with maize (*Zea mays* L.) is a major impediment to increased usage of sweetpotato for animal feeds and supplements although interest is growing in the potential use as a component in chicken feed.

POTENTIAL FOR NEW MINOR ROOT CROPS

Recently, much attention has been focused on minor crops which are very important to the culture and subsistence of local farmers in many parts of the world. Concern has been raised about the future security of the genetic resources of these minor crops. In particular, recent attention has been focused on the Andean root and tuber crops. In addition to potatoes, several roots and tubers have played a significant role in the Andean culture and are cultivated in that area. Two of these which are more well known than others could be domestically grown. A third is lesser known but could also have some potential for production.

Oca (*Oxalis tuberosa* Molina, Oxalidaceae) is probably the most well known root vegetable other than potato in the Andean region. It is quite unusual in appearance with a brightly colored edible tuber and a pleasant mild flavor. Oxalic acid is a component of the tubers, but levels are generally not higher than those found in some other popular crops (S. O'Hair pers. commun.). Oca is commercially produced in Peru and has been commercialized in New Zealand (Yamaguchi 1983). A number of clones are grown and many accessions have been collected (S. O'Hair pers. commun.).

A second Andean root vegetable, ulluco or olluco or ullucu(s) (*Ullucus tuberosus* Caldas, Bassellaceae) is also grown commercially in the Andean regions of Peru. This is also a crop of wide genetic diversity with perhaps 50 to 70 clones being grown in the Andean region (S. O'Hair pers. commun.). External colors of tubers can be white, yellow, green, or magenta; the plants are frost resistant and require 140 to 150 days for tuber development (Yamaguchi 1983).

Mashua or anu (*Tropaeolum tuberosum* Ruiz & Pav. Family Tropaeolaceae) is a third Andean root vegetable and is related to the ornamental nasturtium. It is not commercially produced on the same scale as the other two crops. Consequently, it is not as well known as the other two. It is said to have medicinal properties and some cultivars may have pesticide properties (S. O'Hair pers. commun.).

Each of the three Andean root vegetables can be eaten fresh or dehydrated. All are used in the Andean region, along with potato, to make chuo, a dehydrated and frozen product which can last several years and serves as a secure food source when necessary. Each has the potential to be grown in certain areas of temperate climates.

FUTURE PROSPECTS

There are several opportunities for increased production and usage of root and tuber crops in the United States. Of the five major root crops, sweetpotato has the greatest potential for new uses and increased production. As sweetpotatoes cannot be imported in the United States, there is no significant current supply for specific types of sweetpotatoes suited to ethnic cultural preferences. Growers in North Carolina, who produce over 30% of the sweetpotatoes in the United States, have been reluctant to begin production of new types for ethnic markets. Market feasibility studies need to be undertaken to determine the potential markets.

With respect to new and unknown root crops, three Andean root crops, oca, ulluco, and mashua, offer potential for new production. However, a lack of funds to investigate the possibilities may preclude any development.

REFERENCES

Collins, W.W. 1987. Improvement of nutritional and edible qualities of sweetpotato for human consumption, p. 221–226. In: Exploration, maintenance and utilization of sweet potato genetic resources: Report of the first sweet potato planning conference, International Potato Center, Lima, Peru.

FAO. 1990. 1989 production yearbook. Rome, Italy.

Gohl, B. 1981. Tropical feeds. FAO, Rome, Italy.

Keya, E.L. and D. Hadziyev. 1990. p. 188–196. In: R.H. Howeler (ed.). Proc. 8th Symposium of the International Society for Tropical Root Crops. Oct. 30–Nov. 5, 1988. Bangkok, Thailand, 1990.

Marsh, D.B. 1988. Production of specialty crops for ethnic markets in the United States. HortScience 23:628.

Marsh, D.B. 1991. Ethnic crop production: An overview and implications for Missouri. HortScience 26:1133–1135.

O'Hair, S.K. 1990a. Tropical root and tuber crops. Hort. Rev. 12:157–196.

O'Hair, S.K. 1990b. Tropical root and tuber crops, p. 424–428. In: J. Janick and J.E. Simon (eds.). Advances in new crops. Timber Press, Portland, OR.

O'Hair, S.K., R. McSorley, J.L. Parrado, and R.F. Matthews. 1983. The production and qualities of Cuban sweetpotato cultivars in Florida. Proc. Amer. Soc. Hort. Sci. Tropical Region 27:35–41.

Reynolds, B.D., W.J. Blackmon, E. Wickremesinhe, M.H. Wells, and R.J. Constantin. 1990. Domestication of *Apios americana*, p. 436–442. In: J. Janick and J.E. Simon (eds.). Advances in new crops. Timber Press, Portland, OR.

Rhoades, R. and D. Horton. 1990. p. 8–19. In: R.H. Howeler (ed.). Proc. 8th Symposium of the International Society for Tropical Root Crops. Oct. 30–Nov. 5, 1988. Bangkok, Thailand.

Sammy, G.S. 1984. The processing potential or tropical root crops. Proc. Caribbean Regional Workshop on Tropical Root Crops, Jamaica, April 10–16, 1983. p. 199.

Sperling, C.R. and S.R. King. 1990. Andean tuber crops: worldwide potential, p. 428–435. In: J. Janick and J.E. Simon (eds.). Advances in new crops. Timber Press, Portland, OR.

Villareal, R.L. 1981. Sweet potato. Proc. First International Symposium. Asian Vegetable Research and Development Center, Tainan, Taiwan. p. 3–16.

Walter, W.M., E.M. Croom, G.L. Catignani, and W.C. Thresher. 1986. Compositional study of *Apios princena* tubers. J. Agr. Food Chem. 34:39–41.

Yamaguchi, M. 1983. World vegetables: Principles, production and nutritive values. AVI, Westport, CT.

New Opportunities in the Cucurbitaceae*

Timothy J. Ng

The Cucurbitaceae consists of nearly 100 genera and over 750 species (Yamaguchi 1983). Although most have Old World origins (Whitaker and Davis 1962), many species originated in the New World and at least seven genera have origins in both hemispheres (Esquinas-Alcazar and Gulick 1983). There is tremendous genetic diversity within the family, and the range of adaptation for cucurbit species includes tropical and subtropical regions, arid deserts, and temperate locations. A few species are adaptable to production at elevations as high as 2000 m.

The genetic diversity in cucurbits extends to both vegetative and reproductive characteristics. There is considerable range in the monoploid (x) chromosome number (Jeffrey 1990), including 7 (*Cucumis sativus*), 11 (*Citrullus* spp., *Momordica* spp., *Lagenaria* spp., *Sechium* spp., and *Trichosanthes* spp.), 12 (*Benincasa hispida*, *Coccinia cordifolia*, *Cucumis* spp. other than *C. sativus*, and *Praecitrullus fistulosus*), 13 (*Luffa* spp.), and 20 (*Cucurbita* spp.).

Archaeological evidence has indicated that cucurbits were present in ancient and prehistoric cultures. *Lagenaria* was associated with man as early as 12,000 BC in Peru (Esquinas-Alcazar and Gulick 1983). Archaeological expeditions in the Oaxaca region of Mexico have reported Cucurbita pepo to be associated with man as early as 8500 BC and cultivated by 4050 BC (Esquinas-Alcazar and Gulick 1983). Written Chinese records describing the use of cultivated cucurbits have been found from as early as 685 BC (Herklots 1972). American Indians cultivated squash in pre-Columbian times (Whitaker and Davis 1962), and chayote was a common vegetable among the Aztecs prior to the Spanish conquest (Herklots 1972). Depending upon the species, virtually all parts of the plant can be used for food, including leaves, shoots, roots, flowers, seeds, and immature and mature fruits. Starch can be extracted from roots, and the seeds are a rich source of oils and proteins (Jacks et al. 1972). In addition, some cucurbits have been used for ornamental purposes (e.g., gourds), for utensils (e.g., bowls, ladles, sponges, boxes, birdhouses, musical instruments), and for fuel and pharmacological uses in certain areas of the world.

NEW OPPORTUNITIES WITH COMMONLY GROWN CUCURBITS

Cucurbit crops commonly grown in the United States include cucumber (*Cucumis sativus*), melon (*Cucumis melo*), watermelon (*Citrullus lanatus*), and squash and pumpkin (*Cucurbita* spp.). Due to intensive breeding efforts, particularly with cucumber and melon, numerous new cultivars have been developed, some of them quite different from the traditional forms for these crops.

Cucumbers have been traditionally grown for either pickling or slicing purposes. Newer forms which are increasing in importance include hothouse cucumbers, which are elongated, seedless, and "burpless" (putatively reducing eructation). Nerson et al. (1990) reported on the development of melofon, a genotype of *Cucumis melo* which is suitable for pickle production.

Until recently, melon production has been limited in most parts of the United States to the reticulated (netted), orange-fleshed muskmelon. However, the smooth-skinned, green-fleshed honeydews have increased in popularity over the past decade, and varied displays of casaba and canary (smooth-skinned with yellow or mottled rinds, white-fleshed), Persian (lightly-netted, pink-fleshed), and crenshaw (smooth-skinned, pale orange-fleshed) melons are becoming an increasingly common sight in major markets. The genetic diversity within the species for fruit characteristics has resulted in recent cultivar developments such as orange-fleshed honeydews and green-fleshed netted melons. Additionally, producers are showing interest in forms cultivated in other countries, including the smooth-skinned, delicately-fleshed "Charentais" types in Europe and the dark green smooth-skinned "hami gua" melons of Asia.

---

*Scientific Article No. A6250, Contribution No. 8419 of the Maryland Agricultural Experiment Station.

Watermelon types have traditionally been red-fleshed and seeded. There is genetic variation for flesh color in the species, however, and colors can range from white or yellow to orange, depending upon the genetic constitution. Yellow-fleshed cultivars are now available, and there may be a market for white-fleshed cultivars if quality could be assured, since consumers tend to associate white flesh with immaturity. A relatively recent development in watermelon breeding has been the use of ploidy manipulations to produce seedless triploid genotypes (Kihara 1951). A number of seedless cultivars have been developed, but they tend to be more susceptible to physiological problems such as poor seed germination and hollow heart. In northwest China, edible seed watermelons are an important crop (Zhang and Jiang 1990); these melons are small in size (2.5 to 3.5 kg) with low soluble solids content, but have a high ratio of seed to flesh in the fruits. The seeds are roasted before eating.

Squash, derived from Algonquin Indian "askoot asquash" which means "eaten green," is a generic term to describe cultivars of four *Cucurbita* species: *C. argyrosperma* (= *C. mixta*), *C. maxima*, *C. moschata*, and *C. pepo*. These species are New World in origin, with all but *C. maxima* originating in central to southern Mexico (*C. maxima* originated in South America and was the only species not cultivated in the United States until post-Columbian times). Traditional forms of the *Cucurbita* spp. include summer squash, winter squash, pumpkins, and gourds. Production has recently increased with specialty forms such as spaghetti squash (*C. pepo*), whose internal flesh texture resembles strands of spaghetti following cooking. Another specialty crop is calabaza (*C. moschata*), a hard-shelled squash with bright orange, fine-grained flesh and excellent nutritive properties (Wessel-Beaver and Varela 1991). There has also been recent interest in edible pumpkin seed, particularly in genotypes with the hull-less trait (Loy 1990).

Although the new forms of these commonly grown cucurbits represent an increase of diversity within each commodity, they will probably not expand the market substantially (with the exception of niche markets) since consumers will probably elect to purchase them in place of the more traditional forms. Where the true opportunity for increased diversity and market growth exists is with cucurbit crops which are grown on an international scale, but are cultivated to only a limited extent in the United States.

CUCURBITS OF POTENTIAL ECONOMIC IMPORTANCE

Although by no means exhaustive, Table 1 lists cucurbit species which are cultivated to a significant extent in other parts of the world. Loosely grouped according to Old World and New World origins, Table 1 also lists the more frequently used common names for each of these species, along with growth habit and the parts of the plant which are used on an economic basis. Many of these species are described in detail by Chakravarty (1990), Herklots (1972), Tindall (1983), Whitaker (1990), Whitaker and Davis (1962), and Yamaguchi (1983).

Old World Cucurbits

Benincasa hispida. The winter melon has been reported to have been grown as a vegetable in China since 500 AD; even today, however, it is cultivated little outside of Asia. It was one of two cucurbit species identified by the National Academy of Sciences (1975) as being an underexploited tropical crop. Exhibiting relatively rapid growth, *B. hispida* grows best in temperate climates with adequate but not excessive rainfall. In Sri Lanka, the plant produces fruit from seed in two months during the rainy season. The distribution of staminate and pistillate flowers is influenced by temperature and daylength. Plants may be grown recumbent or trellised.

The mature fruit is the primary harvested plant part, although seeds are sometimes extracted, fried and eaten like pumpkin seeds. The fruit is covered by a white, chalky wax which deters microorganisms and helps impart an extraordinary longevity to the melon. Winter melon fruits can be stored for as long as a year without refrigeration. Fruits may weight up to 35 kg and consist of more than 96% water. They are usually sold whole in domestic markets, but are commonly displayed and sold by the slice in Asian markets. Somewhat bland in flavor when eaten fresh, the flesh is often used to make soup stock. Canned winter melon soup and dehydrated winter melon slices represent two of the processed products made from this species.

Citrullus colocynthis. A relative of watermelon, egusi is native to tropical Africa and highly drought tolerant. Productivity is enhanced during dry, sunny periods and reduced during periods of excessive rainfall and

Table 1. Old World and New World cucurbit species with potential for cultivation in the United States[z].

Species	Origin	Common names	Primary plant parts used	Other plant parts used	Growth habit
Old World					
Benincasa hispida (Thunb.) Cogn.	SE Asia & Indonesia	Winter melon, ash pumpkin, wax gourd, white gourd, dong gua, tallow gourd	Mature fruits	Young leaves, flower buds, seeds, immature fruits	Annual
Citrullus colocynthis (L.) Schrad.	Tropical Africa	Egusi	Seeds		Annual
Coccinia cordifolia Cogn.	Trop. Asia & Africa	Ivy gourd, scarlet-fruited gourd	Leaves, shoots, immature fruits (preserved)	Mature fruits	Semi-perennial
Cucumis anguria L.	Tropical Africa	West Indian gherkin, bur gherkin, maroon cucumber	Immature fruits		Annual
Lagenaria siceraria (Mol.) Standl.	Tropical Africa	Bottle gourd, calabash gourd, white-flowered gourd, trumpet gourd, Zucca melon	Young fruits, mature fruits[y]	Young shoots, young leaves, seeds	Annual
Luffa acutangula (L.) Roxb.	India	Angled loofah, towel gourd, dish-cloth gourd, ridged gourd, silk gourd, long okra, ribbed loofah, ribbed gourd	Immature fruits, leaves		Annual
Luffa aegyptiaca Muell.	India	Smooth loofah, dish-cloth gourd, vegetable sponge, sponge gourd, rag gourd, hechima	Immature fruits, mature fruits[y]		Annual
Momordica charantia L.	Tropical Africa	Bitter melon, balsam pear, carilla fruit, carilla gourd, bitter gourd, alligator pear	Immature fruits, young shoots	Young leaves,	Annual
Praecitrullus fistulosus (Stocks) Pang.	Tropical Africa	Round melon, squash melon	Mature fruit	Seeds	Annual
Telfairia occidentalis Hook. f.	Tropical Africa	Fluted gourd, fluted pumpkin	Female shoots, seeds		Perennial

Table 1. Continued.

Species	Origin	Common names	Primary plant parts used	Other plant parts used	Growth habit
Telfairia pedata (Sims) Hook.	Tropical Africa	Oyster nut, fluted pumpkin, Zanzibar oil vine	Seeds		Perennial
Trichosanthes cucumerina L.	India	Snake gourd, club gourd	Immature fruits, young shoots	Young leaves mature fruits	Annual
New World					
Cucurbita ficifolia Bouche	Central Mexico	Fig-leaved gourd, Malabar gourd	Mature fruits, seeds	Immature fruits	Annual
Cucurbita foetidissima HBK	Mexico & Southern US	Buffalo gourd, mock orange, stinking wild gourd, chilicote	Mature fruits[y]	Roots[y], seeds	Perennial
Cyclanthera pedata Schrad.	South America	Korila, wild cucumber, caihua, achoccha	Immature fruits	Shoots	Annual
Sechium edule (Jacq.) Sw.	So. Mexico & Central America	Chayote, choyote, cho-cho, christophine, choke, choko, sou-sou, chaka plant, chayotl vegetable pear, mirliton	Immature fruits, tubers, seeds	Young leaves, young tendrils	Perennial

[z]Modified from Chakravarty 1990; Herklots 1972; Tindall 1983; Whitaker 1990; Whitaker and Davis 1962; and Yamaguchi 1983.
[y]Non-food uses such as soaps, fuels, sponges, utensils, containers, musical instruments.

high humidity. It is suitable for production in "marginal growing areas." The fruits are extremely bitter, but the seeds are can be removed and roasted as an edible commodity (Soliman et al. 1985). The seeds are rich in oils, which can be extracted for cooking purposes, and the seeds can also be ground into a powder and used as a soup thickener or flavoring agent (Badifu and Ogunsua 1991).

Coccinia cordifolia. Ivy gourd is a semi-perennial which grows best under conditions of adequate rainfall and high humidity. One of the few dioecious cucurbits, with a hetermorphic (XY) chromosome pair determining sex, it produces best when a 1:10 ratio of male to females is used. Plants are commonly trellised. The leaves, shoots, and immature fruits are cooked and eaten; mature fruits are sometimes preserved.

Cucumis anguria. The West Indian gherkin grows and is used in a similar fashion as the cucumber. It was introduced into the United States in the early 1800s, but remains cultivated to only a limited extent. Oval in shape with a round cross-section, it has a highly warted skin, long spines and a large cavity with many seeds.

Lagenaria siceraria. The origin of the bottle gourd is acknowledged to be Africa, although archaeological evidence has placed it in Peru around 12000 BC, in Thailand about 8000 BC, and in Zambia around 2000 BC (Esquinas-Alcazar and Gulick 1983). It has traveled widely, perhaps because the hard, dry skin of the mature fruits is impervious to water; they are capable of floating on salt water for the better part of a year without any loss in seed viability (Herklots 1972; Tindall 1983). Tolerant to a wide range of rainfall, it may be grown either on the ground or trellised.

Young fruits are used as a cooked vegetable similar to zucchini. The flesh is white, firm, and has an excellent texture and a mild taste. Young shoots and leaves can be cooked, and seeds can be used in soups. Flesh of immature fruits can also be used in making icing for cakes, and the hard skin is sometimes sliced into thin, dry strips for cooking.

Some forms of *L. siceraria* are grown for non-food uses. Mature fruits, whose inside may be poisonous, contain an extremely hard and waterproof rind when dried. They can be used as multi-purpose containers (bowls, boxes, water jugs, cups, planters), utensils (ladles, pipes), musical instruments (e.g., sitars), floats for fishnets and rafts, or for ornamental purposes such as masks or native artifacts. Designs lightly scratched into the skin of developing fruit will develop into scars that remain intact in the mature fruits.

Luffa acutangula. The angled loofah is commonly grown in hot, humid tropical areas in Asia. Plants are generally grown on a trellis. Immature fruits, which are dark green with tender ridges, are used in soups and curries or as a cooked vegetable. They generally grow up to 0.6 m in length, and the flesh is spongy although the skin is coarse. The mature fruits are bitter and inedible, but the fibrous skeleton can be used as a sponge. However, the reticulated inner tissue is not as easily separated from the outer skin and inner flesh as *L. aegyptiaca* (= *L. cylindrica*).

Luffa aegyptiaca. Along with *Lagenaria siceraria*, *L. aegyptiaca* probably has the most diverse uses of any of the cultivated cucurbits. Immature fruits of the non-bitter genotypes are eaten fresh, cooked, or in soups, although they are inferior to immature *L. acutangula* fruits. The mature fruits are the source of the spongy reticulated material known as the domestic loofah. These loofahs are used for sponges and filters, and for stuffing pillows, saddles, and slippers. They can also be used for insulation and are attractive sources for packing materials because of their biodegradability. There is an increasing interest in domestic production (Davis 1991) since the United States is the major market and imports millions of loofahs from Asia each year.

Normally, mature fruits are left on vine to dry and the dry, thin outer skin is removed. The fruit is then soaked in running water for several days, after which the softer tissue is removed. After further soaking, then drying, the seeds are shaken out and the loofah is bleached either chemically or by the sun prior to marketing.

Momordica charantia. The bitter melon is adapted to a wide variation of climates, although production is best in hot, humid areas such as tropical Asia. The bitter immature fruits are usually soaked to remove some of the bitterness, then boiled or fried. Volatile components released during cooking enhance the flavor (Binder et al. 1989). Bitter melons can also be pickled or used in curries. Relative to other cucurbits, the fruit is highly nutritious due to the iron and ascorbic acid content. Plants are usually trellised, and fruits are protected from flies by tying a paper cylinder around the stalk. Some forms have bright red seeds due to a high lycopene content; Yen and Hwang (1985) have proposed using this pigment as an artificial food colorant.

Praecitrullus fistulosus. Primarily grown in India, the round melon was long considered to be *Citrullus lanatus* but was recently given its own taxonomic category due in part to its difference in monoploid chromosome number (Sujatha and Seshadri 1989). Growth conditions and requirements are similar to those of watermelon, but the entire immature fruit is used as a cooked vegetable. The seeds can also be removed and eaten.

Telfairia occidentalis. A dioecious perennial grown at elevations up to 2,000 m in West Africa, the fluted gourd is drought tolerant and is usually trellised. Shoots from the female plants can be cooked and eaten (Lucas 1988). The fruits are large (up to 13 kg) and inedible, but the seeds contain up to 30% protein and can be boiled and eaten, or ground into powder for soup. Seeds can also be fermented for several days and eaten as a slurry (Badifu and Ogunsua 1991).

Telfairia pedata. The oyster nut is a perennial grown in Central and East Africa. It is drought tolerant, can grow at elevations up to 2,000 m, requires 18 months to flowering, and is usually trellised. It produces very large, long, flat seeds which taste similar to almonds when roasted.

Trichosanthes cucumerina. The snake melon is an annual which requires high levels of soil moisture and trellising. A long growing season is necessary, and the flowers open late in the afternoon. Immature fruits are usually harvested when they are 0.3 to 0.4 m long; mature fruits can grow up to 1.5 m in length. Some of the fruits remain straight, while others may curl to resemble a snake. Immature fruits are boiled and eaten, while mature fruits are used in soups.

New World Cucurbits

Cucurbita ficifolia. The fig-leaved gourd grows in temperate highlands at elevations up to 2,000 m. One of the earliest cultivated plants in America, archaeological evidence indicates it was cultivated in Peru around 3000 BC (Herklots 1972). The immature fruits can be prepared and eaten similar to summer squash. Mature fruits can be preserved, and the black seeds are edible. In Latin America, the flesh is impregnated with sugar to make a candy or it can be fermented to make beer (Whitaker 1990).

Cucurbita foetidissima. Identified as an underexploited tropical crop by the National Academy of Sciences (1975), the buffalo gourd has multiple food and non-food uses (Bemis et al. 1975; Gathman and Bemis 1990). It is a perennial and is found growing wild in marginal lands in the southwestern United States. Some plants have been reported to be over 40 years old. It has a very large, fleshy storage root which can grow to depths up to 5 m and weigh as much as 30 kg after two growing seasons. Roots of older plants can weigh over 100 kg. Buffalo gourd primarily reproduces by asexual reproduction, but also produces small yellow, hard shelled fruits which are considered inedible.

American Indians have used the ripe fruit as a soap substitute and as ceremonial rattles. The seeds, which contain an abundant quantity of polyunsaturated fats and protein, are edible. The large storage roots contain large amounts of starch (up to 56% of the dry weight), and can also be used as fuel. Air-dried roots burn with the heat equivalent of wood and are being tested in Afghanistan as an alternative fuel to decrease deforestation (Winrock International 1991).

Cyclanthera pedata. Korila is relatively cold tolerant and adapted to elevations up to 2,000 m, but is also easy to cultivate in the tropics and subtropics. It is currently cultivated in the Carribean and in Central and South America. The foliage is glabrous and odoriferous. Fruits are pale green, flattened, and mostly hollow. The seed cavity is spongy, and the seeds are attached to a single placenta. Seeds are usually removed and the fruits are eaten raw or cooked. They are often used stuffed with meat, fish or cheese, then baked and eaten similar to stuffed peppers. The shoots are also edible.

Sechium edule. Chayote was a common vegetable among the Aztecs prior to Spanish conquest of Mexico. It is still one of the most widely cultivated of the cucurbits in Costa Rica. It requires high levels of soil moisture and can grow at elevations up to 1,500 m. Unlike most cucurbits, it has a daylength requirement of 12 to 12.5 h for flowering. The plants grow best on hillsides and are usually trellised. Parthenocarpic fruit set can be induced by gibberellin.

Unlike other cucurbits, the fruit contain only a single, large seed. The immature fruits can be eaten raw in salads and provide a good source of vitamin C (Herklots 1972). They can also be boiled, fried, steamed, or stuffed and baked. Young leaves and tendrils are also eaten, and seeds can be sauteed in butter as a delicacy. The large storage roots represent a rich source of starch (Chakravarty 1990).

POTENTIAL BIOCHEMICAL AND MEDICINAL USES

Cucurbits are a well-recognized source of secondary metabolites. The cucurbitacins, tetracyclic triterpenoids which impart a bitter flavor to many cucurbits, have been well-studied as attractants of beetles such as *Diabrotica* (Whitaker and Davis 1962). Alkaloids have been reported in *Momordica*, and saponins have been found in *Cucurbita*, *Citrullus*, *Lagenaria*, and *Momordica* (Schultes 1990).

As biochemical isolation techniques become more sophisticated and refined, new compounds of interest are being isolated. For instance, Mukherjee et al. (1986) isolated amarinin from *Luffa amara*; amarinin inhibits plant cell growth in culture, and its action cannot be overcome with gibberellin.

Perhaps of greatest current interest are the compounds of potential medicinal interest present within cucurbits. Table 2 lists reported pharmacological properties of many cultivated cucurbits; similar properties have been ascribed to other cucurbit species not currently under cultivation (Schultes 1990). Putative properties include purgative actions and treatment for physical ailments, diseases, and infectious organisms. "Infusions" (minced tissue suitable for steeping) of selected cucurbits are sold in some markets and reported to be able to alleviate or cure certain human ailments.

Recently, abortifacient proteins with ribosome-inhibiting properties have been isolated from several cucurbit species (Ng et al. 1991). Some of these species have been used to induce second trimester abortions in China since the 1920s. The abortifacient proteins include momorcharin (from *Momordica charantia*), luffaculin

Table 2. Putative medicinal and pharmacological properties of cultivated cucurbits[z].

Species	Purgative	Therapeutic medications		Infectious organisms	Other purported uses
		Physical ailments	Diseases		
Benincasa hispida	Diuretic, laxative	Dermatological, fever	Epilepsy, gonorrhea	Intestinal worms	Aphrodisiac
Citrulus colocynthis		Paralysis, muscle spasms			
Citrullus lanatus	Diuretic	Liver	Malaria		
Cucumis anguria		Stomach, edema, hemorrhoids		Ringworm	Freckle removal
Cucumis melo	Emetic			Intestinal worms	
Cucurbita maxima				Intestinal worms	
Cucurbita moschata & *Cucurbita pepo*	Diuretic	Ulcers, fever, jaundice	Measles, smallpox	Intestinal worms	
Lagenaria siceraria	Laxative	Kidney, flatulence, dermatological		Intestinal worms	
Luffa acutangula	Emetic	Stomach, fever		Intestinal worms	
Luffa cylindrica	Emetic, laxative	Asthma, sinusitis		Intestinal worms	Abortifacient
Momordica charantia	Laxative, emetic, emmenogogue	Colic, arthritis, hypertension, colds & fever, kidney & liver	Eczema, herpes, influenza, diabetes	Intestinal worms	Aphrodisiac
Sechium edule	Diuretic	Bladder, intestinal, hypertension, arteriosclerosis, dermatological,			

[z]Modified from Chakravarty 1990; Herklots 1972; Morton 1971; Nagao et al. 1991; Ng et al. 1991; Schultes 1990.

(from *Luffa operculata*), trichosanthin (from *Trichosanthes kirilowii*), and beta-trichosanthin (from *Trichosanthes cucumeroides*). Trichosanthin is of particular interest because its ribosome-inhibiting properties have been shown to be effective in inhibiting the replication of human immunodeficiency virus (HIV) in infected lymphocyte and phagocyte cells, indicating potential as a therapeutic agent for AIDS (McGrath et al. 1989). These proteins vary in their level of action and effectiveness, and further germplasm evaluation of cultivated and wild species may identify related compounds with greater efficacy for ribosome inactivation.

GERMPLASM RESOURCES

Few of these Old World and New World species have been subjected to major, intensive breeding efforts. However, extensive germplasm collections are maintained by the USDA Plant Germplasm System at the Plant Introduction Station in Iowa (Clark et al. 1991) and by the Vavilov Institute in Leningrad, USSR (Robinson 1989). Another major germplasm repository is maintained by the Peoples' Republic of China (Robinson 1989), and smaller gene banks are located in Mexico, India, Spain, Nigeria, Costa Rica, and the Philippines (Esquinas-Alcazar and Gulick 1983). These germplasm collections represent a valuable resource for breeding adapted cultivars of these exotic cucurbits for domestic production.

REFERENCES

Badifu, G.I.O. and A.O. Ogunsua. 1991. Chemical composition of kernels from some species of Cucurbitaceae grown in Nigeria. Plant Foods Human Nutr. 41:35–44.

Bemis, W.P., L.C. Curtis, C.W. Weber, J.W. Berry, and J.M. Nelson. 1975. The buffalo gourd (*Cucurbita foetidissima* HBK): a potential crop for the production of protein, oil, and starch on arid lands. Office Agr., Tech. Assistance Bureau, USAID Washington, DC.

Binder, R.G., R.A. Flath, and T.R. Mon. 1989. Volatile components of bittermelon. J. Agr. Food Chem. 37:418–420.

Chakravarty, H.L. 1990. Cucurbits of India and their role in the development of vegetable crops, p. 325–334. In: D.M. Bates, R.W. Robinson, and C. Jeffrey (eds.). Biology and utilization of the Cucurbitaceae. Cornell Univ. Press, Ithaca, NY.

Clark, R.L., M.P. Widrlechner, K.R. Reitsma, and C.C. Block. 1991. Cucurbit germplasm at the North Central Regional Plant Introduction Station, Ames, Iowa. HortScience 26:326,450–451.

Davis, J.M. 1991. Development of a production system for Luffa sponge gourds. HortScience 26:708 (Abstr.)

Esquinas-Alcazar, J.T. and P.J. Gulick. 1983. Genetic resources of Cucurbitaceae. Int. Board for Plant Genet. Resources, Rome.

Gathman, A.C. and W.P. Bemis. 1990. Domestication of buffalo gourd, *Cucurbita foetidissima*, p. 318–324. In: D.M. Bates, R.W. Robinson, and C. Jeffrey (eds.). Biology and utilization of the Cucurbitaceae. Cornell Univ. Press, Ithaca, NY.

Herklots, G.A.C. 1972. Vegetables in south-east Asia. George Allen & Unwin, London.

Jacks, T.H., T.P. Hensarling, and L.Y. Yatsu. 1972. Cucurbit seeds: I. Characterizations and uses of oils and proteins, a review. Econ. Bot. 26:135–141.

Jeffrey, C. 1990. Systematics of the Cucurbitaceae: An overview, p. 3–28. In: D.M. Bates, R.W. Robinson, and C. Jeffrey (eds.). Biology and utilization of the Cucurbitaceae. Cornell Univ. Press, Ithaca.

Kihara, H. 1951. Triploid watermelons. Proc. Amer. Soc. Hort. Sci. 58:217–230.

Loy, J.B. 1990. Hull-less seeded pumpkins: a new edible snackseed crop, p. 403–407. In: J. Janick and J.E. Simon (eds.). Advances in new crops. Timber Press, Portland, OR.

Lucas, E.O. 1988. The potential of leaf vegetables in Nigeria. Outlook Agr. 17:163–168.

McGrath, M.S., K.M. Hwang, S.E. Caldwell, I. Gaston, K.C. Luk, P. Wu, V.L. Ng, S. Crowe, J. Daniels, J. Marsh, T. Deinhart, P.V. Lekas, J. Vennari, H.W. Yeung, and J.D. Lifson. 1989. GLQ223: an inhibitor of human immunodeficiency virus replication in acutely and chronically infected cells of lymphocyte and mononuclear phagocyte lineage. Proc. Natl. Acad. Sci. (USA) 86:2844–2848.

Morton, J.F. 1971. The wax gourd, a year-round Florida vegetable with unusual keeping quality. Proc. Fla. State Hort. Soc. 81:104–109.

Mukherjee, S., A.K. Shaw, S.N. Ganguly, T. Ganguly, and P.K. Saha. 1986. Amarinin: a new growth inhibitor from *Luffa amara*. Plant Cell Physiol. 27:935–938.

Nagao, T., R. Tanaka, Y. Iwase, H. Hanazono, and H. Okabe. 1991. Studies on the constituents of *Luffa acutangula* Roxb. I. Structures of acutosides A-G, oleanane-type triterpene saponins isolated from the herb. Chem. Pharm. Bul. 39:599–606.

National Academy of Sciences. 1975. Underexploited tropical plants with promising economic value. Natl. Acad. Sci., Washington, DC.

Nerson, H., H.S. Paris, and M. Edelstein. 1990. Melofon: a new crop for concentrated yield of pickles, p. 399–402. In: J. Janick and J.E. Simon (eds.). Advances in new crops. Timber Press, Portland, OR.

Ng, T.B., Z. Feng, W.W. Li, and H.W. Yeung. 1991. Improved isolation and further characterization of beta-trichosanthin, a ribosome-inactivating and abortifacient protein from tubers of *Trichosanthes cucumeroides* (Cucurbitaceae). Int. J. Biochem. 23:561–567.

Robinson, R.W. 1989. Genetic resouces of the Cucurbitaceae, p. 85a–85j. In: C.E. Thomas (ed.). Proc. Cucurbitaceae '89: Evaluation and enhancement of cucurbit germplasm. USDA Vegetable Lab., Charleston, SC.

Schultes, R.E. 1990. Biodynamic cucurbits in the New World tropics, p. 307–317. In: D.M. Bates, R.W. Robinson, and C. Jeffrey (eds.). Biology and utilization of the Cucurbitaceae. Cornell Univ. Press, Ithaca, NY.

Soliman, M.A., A.A. El Sawy, H.M. Fadel, F. Osman, and A.M. Gad. 1985. Volatile components of roasted *Citrullus colocynthis* var. *colocynthoides*. Agr. Biol. Chem. Tokyo 49:269–275.

Sujatha, V.S. and V.S. Seshadri. 1989. Taxonomic position of round melon (*Praecitrullus fistulosus*). Cucurbit Genet. Coop. Rpt. 12:86–88.

Tindall, H.D. 1983. Vegetables in the tropics. AVI, Westport, CT.

Wessel-Beaver, L. and F. Varela. 1991. Performance of parents and progenies in Caribbean x temperate crosses of *Cucurbita moschata*. HortScience 26:740. (Abstr.)

Whitaker, T.W. 1990. Cucurbits of potential economic importance, p. 318–324. In: D.M. Bates, R.W. Robinson, and C. Jeffrey (eds.) Biology and utilization of the Cucurbitaceae. Cornell Univ. Press, Ithaca.

Whitaker, T.W. and G.N. Davis. 1962. Cucurbits. Interscience Publishers, Inc., New York.

Winrock International. 1991. Development: the changing landscape—Winrock International Annual Report 1990. Winrock International, Morrilton, AR.

Yamaguchi, M. 1983. World vegetables. AVI, Westport.

Yen, G.C. and L.S. Hwang. 1985. Lycopene from the seeds of ripe bitter melon (*Momordica charantia*) as a potential red food colorant. II. Storage stability, preparation of powdered lycopene and food applications. J. Chin. Agr. Chem. Soc. 23:151–161.

Zhang, X. and Y. Jiang. 1990. Edible seed watermelons (*Citrullus lanatus* (Thunb.) Matsum. & Nakai) in northwest China. Cucurbit Genet. Coop. Rpt. 13:40–42.

Specialty Melons for the Fresh Market*

James E. Simon, Mario R. Morales, and Denys J. Charles

Indiana is an important producer of muskmelons and watermelons, ranking third in muskmelons in the United States after California and Arizona. In 1987, more than 1,133 ha (2,800 acres) of muskmelons and more than 2,145 ha (5,300 acres) of watermelons were harvested in Indiana mainly in the southwest region with a combined farm value of more than $10 million (Census of Agriculture 1987; Sullivan 1989). Recent marketing studies indicate that significant growth in melon production and specialty cucurbits could occur in the Midwest due to increased market demand (Sullivan 1989). Our objective was to examine the adaptability of specialty melons to the Midwest. The study presented here is focused on seedless and yellow watermelons and green-fleshed muskmelons with the long range goal to utilize the existing agricultural and industrial infrastructure of southwestern Indiana to introduce and market new specialty melons.

Seedless watermelons were originally developed in 1939 by Kihara and Nishiyama (1947). These are triploids produced by crossing colchicine-induced tetraploids with diploids (Andrus et al. 1971). Intensive breeding and development by O.J. Eigsti, Goshen, Indiana, led to the Tri-X-313 series of seedless watermelons that became the domestic industry standard and later, the germplasm utilized by SunWorld Seedless, national marketers of seedless watermelons. In the past, problems of seedless melons included poor germination and emergence, high seed costs, poor yields, and irregular quality. Several of these problems have been overcome and the profusion of new seedless cultivars attests to the recent attention that this crop has received from private seed companies. Seedless watermelons may not only partially substitute for the purchase and consumption of regular seeded watermelons, but also have the potential to penetrate new consumer markets to which seeded watermelons were previously limited including nursing homes, hospitals, and other institutions.

Yellow-fleshed watermelons have received only minor market interest in the past partially due to the lack of cultivars with high quality fruit as well as consumer resistance to the yellow color. Many cultivars have had problems with cracking or hollow-heart, mealy texture, or nonuniform fruit. Greater consumer acceptance of nonred watermelons is evident by the recent inclusion of yellow-fleshed watermelons in the produce section of general large chain supermarkets.

Green-fleshed muskmelons for export to Europe were originally developed by plant breeders in Israel. These melons differ from the traditional orange-fleshed, netted 'Western' and 'Eastern' melons in both exterior and interior color. They have a nonridged yellow-gold to green exterior, a green-flesh interior with a creamy texture and very sweet flavor. The texture and flavor is different from the green-fleshed 'Honeydew' melon, which has a pale yellow/white exterior and is difficult to commercially grow in the Midwest and Eastern states.

METHODOLOGY

Since 1987, specialty melons trials have been conducted annually in southwestern Indiana at the Southwest Purdue Agricultural Center, Vincennes, to identify domestic and foreign cultivars that are adapted to Midwestern conditions and which could have strong consumer interest (Simon 1984, 1985, 1986, 1987; Simon et al. 1988, 1989, 1990, 1991). Results presented here are mainly confined to the 1991 field trials. Average yields of four seedless watermelon and four green-fleshed muskmelon cultivars evaluated in the 1989, 1990, and 1991 field trials is also presented. Seeds of seedless watermelon, yellow-fleshed watermelon, and green-fleshed muskmelon were sown in plastic trays inside a greenhouse on Apr. 29, May 6, and May 2 of 1991, respectively, and transplanted

---

*Journal Paper No. 13,226, Purdue Univ. Agr. Expt. Sta., West Lafayette, IN 47907-1165. This research was supported in parts by grants from the Indiana Business Modernization and Technology Corporation, Indianapolis, the Purdue University Cooperative Extension Service, and the seed companies of Abbott & Cobb), American SunWorld Seedless, Asgrow Seed Co., Baker Brothers Seeds, Harris Moran Seed Co., Hazera Seed Co., Hollar Seeds, Mikado Seeds, PetoSeed Co., Rogers Northrup King, Sakata Seeds. We thank Harry Paris and Zvi Karchi, ARO/Israel for their green-fleshed melon germplasm, Meb Lang and Tom Mouzin, Purdue, who assisted us in the field work and to Daniella Simon and Kevin Vonderwell, who participated in the quality evaluations of each fruit.

into the field on May 22. Seedless, yellow-fleshed, and green-fleshed melon cultivars were evaluated in 3 separate trials, using a completely randomized block design with three replications in each study. Watermelon plots consisted of single rows, 142 cm in length, with 7 plants per row (plants 20 cm apart within the row), and rows 25 cm apart. 'Crimson Sweet' was used as the pollinator in the seedless watermelon trial and planted in every sixth row plus the guard rows. Muskmelon plots consisted of single rows, 142 cm in length, with 14 plants per row (plants 10 cm apart within the row), and rows 25 cm apart. All rows were covered with black plastic mulch and trickle irrigated. Production practices for fertilization, weed, insect, and pest control have been described previously (Latin et al. 1991). The Purdue VARTEST computer program for variety testing was used for statistical analysis.

RESULTS AND CONCLUSIONS

Seedless and Yellow Watermelons

High yielding and high quality seedless and yellow watermelons (with excellent flavor, appearance with high total soluble solids) can be produced in the Midwest (Tables 1, 2, 4), with yield and quality influenced greatly by the selected cultivar. Several new seedless cultivars including 'King of Hearts', 'Queen of Hearts' (Petoseed Co., Inc.), 'Crimson Trio' and Scarlet Trio' (Rogers NK Seed Co.), and 'Tiffany' (Asgrow Seed Co.) compare favorably in yield and quality to the standard 'Tri-X-313', 'Sunrise', and 'Triplesweet' cultivars of SunWorld Seedless. With the inclusion of pollinating cultivars, seedless watermelons can be grown in a manner similar to regular watermelons. The continued proliferation in seedless watermelons will lead to an even greater number of red- and yellow-fleshed cultivars which will vary in size and shape from the rounded striped 'Crimson Sweet' type to the striped blocky 'Jubilee type', and to the dark nonstriped small rounded 'Sugar Baby' fruit type. Promising melons need to be screened for disease resistance prior to introduction. The seedless watermelon 'Quality' (Known-You-Seed) appeared quite promising with regard to yield and quality in our initial trials, but later was shown to be very susceptible to fusarium and thus, eliminated from our studies.

The yellow watermelon cultivars 'Sunshine' and 'Yellow Cutie' did not exhibit cracking and were relatively uniform in external appearance. Most yellow cultivars however, had a mealy texture and a light yellow flesh color. While yellow-fleshed watermelons can be now produced commercially, further improvement in fruit quality is needed. Fruits need to exhibit greater uniformity and a deeper, brighter, and more uniform yellow color.

Green-Fleshed Muskmelons

Green-fleshed muskmelons had an attractive golden to yellow exterior at maturity and continue to show great promise as a specialty melon (Table 3 and 4). These melons are very high yielding and many evaluated appear as tolerant as the orange-fleshed muskmelons to diseases such as fusarium wilt, endemic in Midwest production areas. These fruit have a creamy texture and very sweet flavor, with total soluble solids content as high as 15.4 % (Table 3). The aromatic volatiles, which are in part responsible for the fruits' aroma, appear similar for both orange and these green-flesh melons suggesting that differences in taste and flavor may be more related to individual sugars than differences in volatile compounds.

'Makdimmon' (Hazera Ltd., marketed in the United States as 'Mediterranean Delight' by Aristogenes), 'Rocky Sweet', (Hollar Seeds), and 'Galia' produced the highest quality fruit and are recommended for production in our area. However, while production techniques are similar to traditional muskmelons, harvesting and postharvest handling procedures differ. Greater care is needed in handling and packing, as the rinds of the green-fleshed fruit are thin and susceptible to bruising. The fruit of most green-flesh cultivars ripen over a very concentrated time period which requires greater care in the scheduling of field planting. Shelf life of these fruit also appear to be shorter. These cultivars may also differ in their tolerance to wet soil conditions and appear to respond best under drier growing conditions with irrigation. Further inprovements in their resistance to fusaruim wilt is required.

Specialty melons such as seedless and yellow watermelons, and green-fleshed muskmelons are very well adapted to Indiana growing conditions. High yields were obtained from seedless and green-fleshed melons over

Table 1. Comparison of yield and quality of seedless watermelon in southwestern Indiana, 1991.

Cultivar	Seed[z] source	Fresh wt (t/ha)	Total fruit (No./ha)	Avg. fruit weight (kg)	% of fruit harvested 7/29	% of fruit harvested 8/19	Soluble solids (%)	Flavor[y] rating (1–5)	Cracking[x] rating (0–5)	Uniformity[w] rating (1–5)
King of Hearts	PS	34.9	4549	7.7	40	60	11.2	3	0	3
Sunrise	AM	33.2	4164	8.0	41	59	9.8	3	0	4
Tripesweet	AM	31.6	4102	7.8	47	53	10.8	4	0	4
5032	AC	31.4	3845	8.2	35	65	11.0	3	0	3
NVH 4256	RG/NK	31.1	3588	8.6	44	56	10.2	4	0	4
Red Baron	MK	29.7	4932	6.0	27	73	11.0	3	0	4
Queen of Hearts	PS	27.4	3588	7.6	42	58	10.8	3	0	4
Scarlet Trio	RG/NK	27.1	3205	8.5	35	65	11.4	4	0	4
M-7	MK	26.9	4356	6.2	40	60	10.6	3	0	4
Nova	SK	26.5	3971	6.6	37	63	10.8	3	0	3
SWM 8702	SK	24.2	3138	8.0	40	60	10.0	3	1	4
Crimson Trio	RG/NK	23.0	2627	8.8	50	50	11.2	3	0	4
Tiffany	AS	22.5	2819	8.0	43	57	11.4	4	2	3
Tri-x-313	AM	21.7	2498	8.7	48	52	10.6	3	1	3
Laurel	GB	16.9	2115	8.0	38	62	11.8	2	3	3
SWM 8802	SK	16.4	2370	7.0	51	49	9.0	2	0	3
Grand mean		26.5	3492	7.7	41	59				
BLSD[v] (k = 100)		NSD	2478	0.6	NSD	NSD				
CV (%)		32.6	31	5.5	32	22				

[z]Abbott and Cobb Inc. (AC), American Sunmelon (AM), Asgrow Seed Co. (AS), Green Barn Seed Co. (GB), Mikado Seed Growers Co. (MK), Petoseed Co. (PS), Rogers Northrup King (RG/NK), Sakata Seed America Inc. (SK).
[y]Flavor: 1 = very poor and unacceptable, 3 = acceptable, 5 = excellent.
[x]Cracking: 0 = no cracking, 5 = severe cracking at stem end.
[w]Fruit uniformity: 1 = fruit very variable, 5 = fruit uniform in appearance.
[v]BLSD = Waller-Duncan Bayesian k-ratio t test.

Table 2. Comparison of yield and quality of yellow-fleshed watermelon in southwestern Indiana, 1991.

Cultivar	Seed[z] source	Fresh wt (MT/ha)	Total fruit (No./ha)	Avg. fruit weight (kg)	% of fruit harvested		Soluble solids (%)	Flavor[y] rating (1-5)	Cracking[x] rating (0-5)	Uniformity[w] rating (1-5)
					7/29	8/19				
NVH 4299	NK	61.1	4678	13.1	3	97	10.0	3	2	3
Sunshine	JS	29.4	5446	5.5	2	98	11.0	4	0	4
Yellow Doll	LI	27.5	8330	3.3	2	98	11.2	3	1	4
Yellow Baby	ST	27.3	7047	3.9	2	98	11.4	4	1	4
Yellow Baby	HM	22.8	5318	4.3	2	98	10.4	4	1	3
Yellow Cutie	SK	14.6	6279	2.3	2	98	10.8	3	0	4
Grand mean		30.4	6183	5.4						
BLSD[v] (k = 100)		11.2	1769	1.1	NSD	NSD				
CV (%)		21.2	15	12.8	47	1				

[z]Harris Moran Seed Co. (HM), Johnny's Selected Seeds (JS), Liberty Seed Co. (LI), Rogers Northrup King (RG/NK), Sakata Seed America Inc. (SK), Stokes Seeds Inc. (ST).
[y]Flavor: 1 = very poor and unacceptable, 3 = acceptable, 5 = excellent.
[x]Cracking: 0 = no cracking, 5 = severe cracking at stem end.
[w]Fruit uniformity: 1 = fruit very variable, 5 = fruit uniform in appearance.
[v]BLSD = Waller-Duncan Bayesian k-ratio t test.

Table 3. Comparison of yield and quality of green-fleshed muskmelon in southwestern Indiana, 1991.

Cultivar	Seed[z] source	Days to harvest	Fresh wt (MT/ha)	Total fruit (No./ha)	Avg. fruit weight (kg)	% of fruit harvested			Soluble solids (%)	Flavor[y] rating (1–5)
						7/08–7/14	7/15–7/24	7/25–8/05		
Makdimmon	HZ	67	41.1	18900	2.2	54	9	38	11.4	5
Delicate	IS	90	38.0	11317	3.4	33	50	17	15.4	3
Galia	IS	90	36.5	14307	2.6	49	41	10	12.2	3
Emerald Jewel	SK	76	35.4	15802	2.3	1	33	66	12.5	4
Galia 5	IS	90	34.4	14628	2.4	50	41	9	6.4	1
Passport	HL	67	34.0	16338	2.1	65	18	17	9.9	3
Caribe	RG/NK	75	33.9	15698	2.2	0	75	25	6.0	1
Amur	SK	74	31.2	13240	2.4	2	60	37	ND[x]	ND
PSX 24487	PS	70	31.0	16870	1.8	7	69	24	14.0	4
Galia 4	IS	90	30.9	15592	2.0	80	18	2	9.2	2
Concorde	AS	71	28.2	18898	1.5	5	77	18	13.4	3
Qalya	IS	68	27.1	13027	2.1	42	52	5	10.0	4
Rocky Sweet	HL	67	26.7	12175	2.2	45	39	15	13.8	5
Gallicum	PS	67	25.2	11423	2.2	36	56	8	13.2	4
Ogen	BB	75	23.2	12706	1.8	0	51	49	12.9	4
Grand mean		76	31.8	14728	2.2	31	46	23		
BLSD[w] (k = 100)		3	11.1	5528	0.2	16	19	15		
CV (%)		3	17.3	18	6.8	32	26	41		

[z]Asgrow Seed Co. (AS), Bakker Brothers Inc. (BB), Hollar & Co. (HL), Hazera Seed Ltd. (HZ), Dept. of Vegetable Crops, Haifa, Israel (IS), Petoseed Co. (PS), Rogers Northrup King, (RG/NK), Sakata Seed America Inc. (SK).
[y]Flavor: 1 = very poor and unacceptable, 3 = acceptable, 5 = excellent.
[x]ND = not determined.
[w]BLSD = Waller-Duncan Bayesian k-ratio t test.

Table 4. Yield comparisons of seedless watermelons and green-fleshed muskmelons grown in southwestern Indiana for three years (from 1989 to 1991).

	Fresh fruit yield							
	MT/ha[z]				No./ha			
Cultivar	1989	1990	1991	Mean	1989	1990	1991	Mean
Seedless watermelons								
King of Hearts	36.0	47.6	34.9	39.5	4357	5830	4549	4912
Sunrise	35.9	45.9	33.2	38.3	4229	5958	4165	4784
Tri-X-313	32.7	52.3	21.7	35.6	3716	6279	2499	4165
Queen of Hearts	37.1	40.8	27.4	35.1	4805	5382	3588	4592
Mean				37.1				4613
LSD (5%)				NSD				NSD
CV %				14.8				16.5
Green-fleshed muskmelons								
Makdimmon	40.7	50.4	41.1	44.1a	15483	20289	18900	18224
PSX-24487	34.5	41.0	30.9	35.5ab	23385	18473	16872	19577
Galia	21.3	39.3	36.5	32.4b	10465	20502	14309	15092
Rocky Sweet	19.5	46.1	26.7	30.8b	8970	17406	12173	12850
Mean				35.7				16436
LSD (5%)				11.4				NSD
CV %				14.5				19.2

[z]MT/ha spanned by the same letter are not significantly different NSD.

a three year period from 1989 to 1991 (Table 4). The high quality fruit of selected cultivars would more than meet market expectations and make these specialty melons an attractive new fresh product that can be handled and marketed within the existing agricultural and industrial infrastructure of southwestern Indiana.

REFERENCES

Andrus, C.F., V.S. Seshadri, and P.C. Grimball. 1971. Production of seedless watermelons. USDA/ARS Tech. Bul. No. 1425. Washington, DC.

Census of Agriculture. 1987. United States: Summary and state data. vol. 1. Geographic Area Series AC87-A-51. U.S. Dept. of Commerce, Bureau of the Census. Issued 1989:358–359.

Kihara, H. and I. Nishiyama. 1947. An application of sterility of autotriploid to the breeding of seedless watermelons. Seiken Ziho 3(III):5–15.

Latin, R.X., R.E. Foster, and J.E. Simon. 1991. Indiana vegetable production guide for commercial growers. Purdue Univ. Coop. Ext. Serv. ID-56.

Simon, J. (ed.). 1984. Indiana vegetable cultivar trials of 1984. Purdue Univ. Coop. Ext. Serv. Veg. Crops Memo 1984:1(1). West Lafayette, IN.

Simon, J. (ed.). 1985. Indiana vegetable cultivar trials of 1985. Purdue Univ. Coop. Ext. Serv. Veg. Crops Rpt. 1. West Lafayette, IN.

Simon, J. (ed.). 1986. Indiana vegetable cultivar trials of 1986. Purdue Univ. Agr. Expt. Sta. Bul. 517. West Lafayette, IN.

Simon, J. (ed.). 1987. Midwestern vegetable variety trial report for 1987. Purdue Univ. Agr. Expt. Sta. Bul. 528. West Lafayette, IN.

Simon, J.E., D.D. Daniels, and E. Cebert (eds.). 1988. Midwestern vegetable variety trial report for 1988. Purdue Univ. Agr. Expt. Sta. Bul. 551. West Lafayette, IN.

Simon, J.E., E. Cebert, and D.D. Daniels (eds.). 1989. Midwestern vegetable variety trial report for 1989. Purdue Univ. Agr. Expt. Sta. Bul. 577. West Lafayette, IN.

Simon, J.E., D.D. Daniels, and M.R. Morales (eds.). 1990. Midwestern vegetable variety trial report for 1990. Purdue Univ. Agr. Expt. Sta. Bul. 600. West Lafayette, IN.

Simon, J.E., M.R. Morales, and D.D. Daniels (eds.). 1991. Midwestern vegetable variety trial report for 1991. Purdue Univ. Agr. Expt. Sta. Bul. 627, West Lafayette, IN.

Sullivan, G. 1990. Economic and market feasibility for fruit and vegetable industry expansion in southwestern Indiana. Report for the Vincennes Area Community Development Corporation. Vincennes, IN.

Germination, Fruit Development, Yield, and Postharvest Characteristics of *Cucumis metuliferus**

A. Benzioni, S. Mendlinger, M. Ventura, and S. Huyskens

Cucumis metuliferus Mey. (the African horned cucumber, kiwano, melano) is endemic to the semi-arid regions of southern and central Africa, where it is eaten as a supplement by the local population (Bruecher 1977; Keith and Renew 1968). The plant is a monoecious, climbing annual with staminate flowers typically appearing several days before pistillate flowers. The ellipsoid fruit is bright yellow-orange in color when mature and shaped like a short stout cucumber with many blunt thorns on its surface. The mesocarp is green and consists of juicy bland-tasting tissue. *Cucumis metuliferus* is exported as a speciality fruit from New Zealand, Kenya, and Israel to Europe, and its market is expanding. Several problems associated with agrotechniques and fruit quality have emerged in the course of commercialization. Some of the problems encountered include poor germination, too small fruits at some locations, rapid fruit deterioration during cold storage under humid conditions, and failure of fruits to develop the desirable uniform orange color. In this paper, we report on efforts to improve conditions for successful germination, the effect of sowing dates on crop development, as well as fruit ripening in the field and in storage, and the effects of ethylene application to fruits in order to establish optimum harvest time, storage, and shipping conditions.

METHODOLOGY

Germination Experiment

Percentage and rate of germination were examined at 8°, 12°, 20°, 25°, 35°, 40°, and 45°C. Seeds were placed between two layers of wet cotton in petri dishes that were scored daily over a period of 24 days for germination. Germination under saline conditions of 0, 20, 50, and 80 mM NaCl was examined at 30°C.

Date of Planting Experiment

Seeds were sown on sandy loess at the Sha'ar Hanegev Experimental Station (northern Negev, Israel) on Mar. 15, Apr. 15, and June 3, 1988 at a density of 10,000 plants/ha. The field was dripirrigated twice a week at 2 liters/hr, with amounts calculated to replenish 40% of evapotranspiration till first flower stage, and 80% thereafter. Cultural measures (fertigation and disease and pest control schedules) were similar to the local practice for melons. A single harvest when almost all fruits were ripe (after color break, i.e. when skin shifts from dark green to pale yellow), was carried out on June 30 and on Sept. 16 for the first and second sowing dates, respectively. Plants sown in June failed to produce fruit prior to October and thus, were not harvested. At each harvest, a 10-m^2 plot was harvested from each bed and all fruits collected and divided according to fruit weight into large (>200 g) and small (<200 g).

---

*This work was supported by the GIARA program file No 864393. We gratefully acknowledge the excellent technical work of S. Avni and the styling of A. Sen and I. Mureinik.

Fruit Development
About 65 flowers were tagged and hand pollinated at anthesis. Fruits were picked 33, 37, 45, 51, and 61 days after pollination (DAP) for determination of fruit constituents.

Fruit Constituents
Total soluble solids (TSS), pH, electrical conductivity (EC), and reducing sugars (Sumner 1921) were determined in the fruit jelly. Pigments were extracted from the peel by a 4 acetone:5 hexane mixture.

Ethylene Treatments
Fruits were picked when whitish green, at about the turning point. Ethylene was applied by exposing fruits for 24 h to 160 µl ethylene. Treated and control fruits were then stored at 20°C for two months for further ripening and samples of fruits were removed periodically for analysis.

Storage
Yellow-orange fruits were stored at temperatures of 4°, 8°, 12°, 20° and 24°C. In addition, green fruits at about the turning point were picked and stored at 20°C. Every week, fruits were evaluated and overripe, soft, or damaged specimens were discarded.

RESULTS

Germination
Optimal temperatures for germination were 20° to 35°C where 95 to 100% of the seeds completed germination in three to eight days (Table 1). At 12°C, germination commenced at day 16, reaching a final count of 90% on day 24, and at 8°C was completely inhibited. At very high temperatures (40° and 45°C) percentage germination was greatly reduced, although enough seeds germinated to indicate possible genetic variation for heat tolerance (Table 1). Germination was unaffected by salinity of up to 50 mM NaCl.

Table 1. Germination percentage of *Cucumis metuliferus* seeds at eight temperatures and four NaCl concentrations[z].

Variable	Time till maximum germination (days)	Final germination (%)
Temp. (°C)		
8	---	0
12	24	90
20	8	100
25	3	100
30	3	100
35	5	100
40	20	35
45	2	15
NaCl (mM)		
0	3	100
20	3	100
50	12	100
80	24	100

[z]Germination tests used 10 seeds and two replications (15 seeds at 30°C for NaCl test)

Yields

March sown plants covered the beds in about six weeks and began to flower and set fruits in eight weeks. Vines of plants sown on the second date (Apr. 15) covered the beds only after ten weeks, although here too flowering began eight weeks from sowing. Fruit development was slower in the April sowing and although the number of fruits/ha was similar (271,000 versus 245,000 for the March planting), many fruits were smaller (Table 2). The plants sown on 3 June failed to grow well, and by the end of the experiment in October had neither covered the beds nor flowered. The plants of the March sowing yielded over 46 Mg/ha of fruits (Table 2). More than 60% of these fruits were large (>200 g) and would command premium prices in the market. The yield for the second sowing date was 28 Mg/ha, of which only 25% consisted of fruits classified as large; nearly half the fruits were very small and of non-commercial size (Table 2).

Fruit Development.

Maximal fruit weight of 205±57 g was reached by 33 DAP. The main period of fruit ripening on the plant in terms of changes in fruit constituents and color occurred between 37 and 51 DAP (Fig. 1, 2). During this time, both total soluble solids (TSS) and reducing sugar levels increased in fruits attached to the plant, peaking at about 50 DAP (Fig 1). The ripening period was also characterized by changes in the color of the fruit peel, with absorbance of light at wavelengths of 663 and 431 nm decreasing with time indicating loss of chlorophyll, and with absorbance at 442 and 470 nm increasing, indicating carotenoids production (Fig. 2).

Ethylene Application

Application of ethylene to fruits at the breaker stage resulted in fruits progressing from green to yellow within

Table 2. Fruit size fruit number and fruit yield of *Cucumis metuliferus* at different sowing dates[z].

Sowing date	Yield (Mg/ha)			Fruit number (1000/ha)		
	>200	<200	Total	>200	<200	Total
March 15	27.9a	18.5a	46.4a	107a	138b	245a
April 15	7.0b	21.2a	28.2b	31b	239a	271a

[z]Mean separation in columns by Duncan multiple range test, 5% level.

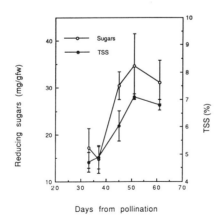

Fig. 1. Accumulation of reducing sugars and changes in soluble solids (TSS) in fruits maturing in the field. Fruits were picked at different stages of development. Values are means ±SE of five fruits.

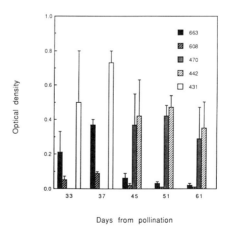

Fig. 2. Pigment profile changes in the fruit peel during fruit development in the field. Values are means ±SE of 5 fruits.

Fig. 3. Effect of 24 h of exposure to ethylene on pigment profiles of fruits during storage at 20°C. Each value is the mean of 5 to 6 fruits. Bar indicates the critical range according to the Tukey test.

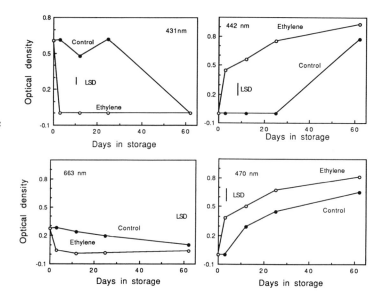

Table 3. Effect of ethylene (160 ppm), applied for 24 h, on fruit constituents during storage. Values are means±SE for 5 to 7 fruits.

Maturity at harvest	Storage (days)	Ethylene treatment	Fresh weight (g/fruit)	pH	EC (dS/m)	Acidity (μeq/gfw)	TSS (%)	Reducing sugars (mg/gfw)	Water loss (%)
Mature green	0		225±12	4.06±0.02	4.82±0.30	91±5	4.76±0.19	16.10±0.70	0.0
Mature green	3	+	198± 5	4.15±0.04	4.14±0.17	96±8	4.57±0.21	22.08±2.27	0.5
Mature green			199±12	4.22±0.05	4.11±0.10	88±6	4.33±0.19	19.96±1.02	0.8
Mature green	12	+	234±15	4.12±0.04	4.09±0.22	103±5	4.53±0.19	28.42±0.96	1.3
Mature green			202±17	4.21±0.06	3.72±0.12	85±9	4.02±0.38	21.12±2.60	1.4
Mature green	25	+	214±20	4.21±0.05	4.22±0.12	82±8	4.60±0.29	30.04±3.50	3.3
Mature green			219±10	4.18±0.05	4.14±0.16	81±8	4.93±0.30	30.18±4.04	2.8
Mature green	61	+	212±14	4.29±0.03	3.79±0.49	74±2	4.40±0.07	26.84±1.06	7.6
Mature green			211± 8	4.89±0.05	4.11±0.32	76±8	4.73±0.49	25.56±1.88	6.6
Yellow orange	0		236±10	4.24±0.02	3.41±0.14	96±3	6.19±0.14	41.62±3.20	0.0

Table 4. Effect of storage temperature and maturity at harvest on shelf life of *Cucumis metuliferus*. At each temperature 24 fruits were scored once a week; spoiled fruits were discarded.

Maturity at harvest	Storage temperature (°C)	Spoiled fruits (%) after storage					
		30d	37d	45d	55d	75d	90d
Ripe	4	17	89	100	100	100	100
Ripe	8	25	58	92	100	100	100
Ripe	12	60	60	100	100	100	100
Ripe	20	0	30	30	30	35	35
Ripe	24	0	0	0	0	0	0
Mature green	20	0	0	0	0	0	0
Mature green	24	0	0	0	0	0	0

three days of treatment (Fig. 3). Non-ethylene treated fruits took much longer to change color and at day 60 still appeared slightly green and less mature than ethylene-treated fruits. From the changes observed in the absorption peaks during ripening, it appears that in ethylene-treated fruits the absorbance at 431 nm disappeared three days after treatment while it took more than 30 days to fade in untreated fruits. The decline in the 431 nm peak was followed in all fruits by the development of a peak at 442 nm (Fig. 3). In some of the ethylene-treated fruits a new absorption band appeared at 420 nm, and fruits were more orange than yellow. No absorption at this wavelength was detected in fruits of the control group (data not presented). The TSS levels remained stable during storage and were unaffected by ethylene treatment. Reducing sugars of both treated and non treated fruits rose during storage from 16 to 25 to 30 mg/g fresh weight (Table 3). The rise in reducing sugars during storage was not enhanced by ethylene treatment and occurred within 12 days of commencement of storage. Electrical conductivity (EC) did not change during storage, and a decline in acidity and a rise in pH were observed (Table 3). Fruits from the same experiment allowed to ripen in the field had a higher final content of reducing sugars on a fresh weight basis, 42 mg/g vs 25 to 30 mg/g in storage (Table 3).

Storage

Fruits picked after the initiation of ripening (yellow color detectable) kept well at 20° and 24°C. All fruits kept at 24°C and 70% of those kept at 20°C were still firm and undamaged after three months of storage (Table 4). Cold storage at 4° or 8°C resulted in much shorter shelflife, and at 4°C chilling symptoms in the form of opaque spots on the fruit surface appeared (Table 4).

CONCLUSIONS

The best time for sowing *C. metuliferus* at our sites would be mid-March to early April. Fruits require about 35 days to mature green and another two weeks to full maturity. Ethylene enhances ripening similarly to its effect on 'Honey Dew' melons and its application may be of agronomic use, enabling growers to harvest at the breaker stage and store fruit for a longer period (McGlasson and Pratt 1964; Pratt et al. 1977). Fruits could be treated with ethylene just before marketing to induce a pleasing, uniform orange color on their arrival at the market.

The fruit has an exceptional long shelflife at temperatures of 20° to 24°C which makes it eminently suitable for development as a new exotic or ornamental crop. However, further research aimed at breeding or selecting for tastier genotypes is essential since the present unsatisfactory taste limits the potential market.

REFERENCES

Bruecher, H. 1977. Cucurbitaceae, p. 258–297. In: Tropische Nutzpflanzen. Springer Verlag, Berlin.

Keith, M.E. and A. Renew. 1975. Notes on some edible wild plants found in the Kalahari. Gemsbok Park. Koedoe 18:1–12.

McGlasson, W.B. and H.K. Pratt. 1964. Effect of ethylene on cantaloupe fruits harvested at various ages. Plant Physiol. 39:120–127.

Pratt, H.K., J.D. Goeschel, and F.W. Martin. 1977. Fruit growth and development, ripening and the role of ethylene in the 'honey dew' muskmelon. J. Amer. Hort. Sci. 102:203–210.

Sumner, J.B. 1921. Dinitrosalicylic acid: A reagent for estimation of sugar in normal and diabetic urine. J. Biol. Chem. 47:5–9.

Evaluation of *Cucumis metuliferus* as a Specialty Crop for Missouri

Dyremple B. Marsh

African Horned Cucumber (*Cucumis metuliferus* E. Mey. ex Naud. Cucurbitaceae), is a vining plant that produces an edible fruit for human consumption. The common name kiwano, was given to the fruits by promoters in New Zealand in order to market the crop in Japan and the United States (Morton 1987; Sweet 1987). Presently, kiwano is marketed as a specialty crop throughout the United States (Fig. 1). Part of its success is due to effective marketing techniques by specialty producers, packers, and the significant increase in the importation of exotic fruits and vegetables into the United States.

Seeds from 26 *Cucumis metuliferus* plant introductions obtained from the North Central Regional Plant Introduction Station, Ames, Iowa, were planted in the greenhouse Mar. 28, 1990, evaluated for number of leaves and vine length, and transplanted in the field on May 28 at Lincoln University's George Washington Carver Farm, Jefferson City, Missouri in three row plots with 1.4 m between 36 m long rows and 1 m between plants within rows. Before transplanting, the plots were fertilized with a 13N–5.6P–10.8K fertilizer to meet soil test recommendations. Plots were irrigated with a sprinkler system when necessary. At harvest, kiwano accessions were evaluated for fruit length, fruit width, fruit weight, and number of fruits per plant.

Cucumis metuliferus accessions seedlings varied significantly in the number of leaves and length of vines generated from the main stem (Table 1). Fruit numbers per plant varied from 101 for PI 414716 to 14 for PI 482441 (Table 1). Fruit production was concentrated within 50 cm of the main stem, thus, reducing the effect of vine length on total number of fruit produced. There were significant variations in fruit weight and fruit size between *Cucumis metuliferus* accessions (Table 1). The ripe fruit color was bright orange rind with a dark green interior. These colors varied only slightly between plant introductions. There were incidents of fusarium wilt in several of the accessions (PI numbers 292190, 482441, 482453, 482456, and 526241). Selections of accessions (482442, 482454, 482444, and 526240) showing resistance to *Fusarium oxysporum* will be evaluated in further studies.

Selection of 10 *Cucumis metuliferus* accessions were evaluated on the basis of superior yield, disease resistance, and plant vigor. The accessions showing most promise were PI's 482444, 414716, 482455, 526240, and 482454. Crop yields were encouraging in 1990, however, concerns remain regarding the resistance of accessions to fusarium wilt.

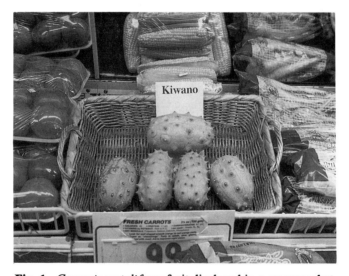

Fig. 1. *Cucumis metuliferus* fruit displayed in a supermarket in Jefferson City, Missouri.

Table 1. Growth and Yield of *Cucumis metuliferus* North Central Plant Introduction Accessions grown in Missouri, 1990.

Cucumis accessions (PI)	Greenhouse evaluation (pretransplant)		Field evaluation			
	Vine length (cm)	No. leaves/ seedling	Fruit size (cm)		Fruit wt (g)	No. fruit/ plant
			Length	Width		
292190	15.4	7	10	6	25	16
414716*	11.0	8	7	4	16	101
482435	18.2	8	11	6	30	28
482441	22.0	10	12	5	14	14
482442*	10.9	7	11	5	18	55
482443*	16.4	8	10	5	12	20
482444*	23.9	9	11	6	27	95
482446*	31.9	9	9	4	25	55
482448	25.4	8	8	4	26	18
482449	15.6	8	10	7	31	19
482450	18.5	8	11	6	15	23
482451*	17.2	8	12	6	18	23
482452*	20.6	9	10	5	23	95
482453	10.3	7	10	7	22	17
482454*	15.2	7	7	4	28	40
482455*	29.4	9	11	6	24	85
482456	19.9	7	12	5	28	19
482458	16.4	7	10	5	18	20
482459	13.3	7	9	6	24	19
482460	17.9	8	7	6	18	34
482462*	22.4	9	7	4	13	18
526240	35.1	10	10	5	25	37
526241	17.5	8	11	4	18	16
526242	14.0	8	12	5	21	18
LSD .05	6.4	NS	2	2	40	12

Cucumis accessions selected for further evaluation on the basis of growth and yield.

REFERENCES

Clark, R., M.P. Widrlechner, K.R. Reitsma, and C.C. Block. 1991. Cucurbit germplasm at the North Central Regional Plant Introduction Station, Ames, Iowa. HortScience 26:326, 451.

Marsh, D.B. 1988. Production of specialty crops for ethnic markets in the United States. HortScience 23:628.

Morton, J.F. 1987. The horn cucumber alias "Kiwano" (*Cucumis metuliferus*, Cucurbitaceae) Econ. Bot. 41:325–326.

Sweet, C. 1987. Kiwano: Can It make it here in the U.S.? California Grower 24:23–24.

Luffa Sponge Gourds: A Potential Crop for Small Farms

Jeanine M. Davis and Charles D. DeCourley

The fibrous interiors of fruits from the luffa sponge gourd (*Luffa aegyptiaca* Mill.) are used primarily as bath sponges but also as pot scrubbers, filters, packing material, and for making crafts. Currently, almost all luffa used in the United States is imported from Taiwan, China, Korea, El Salvador, Guatemala, Mexico, Venezuela, and Columbia. C.D. DeCourley conducted a survey of wholesale luffa buyers that revealed that luffa is imported as a raw dried product and as finished products such as bath mitts. Luffa sales are reported in inches. The survey showed that over 10 million inches (25×10^6 cm) of raw luffa, with a wholesale value of over \$0.5 million, are imported each year. Approximately 9 million inches (23×10^6 cm) are imported as luffa products. These value added products have a retail value of over \$4 million. Changing economic conditions and an increasing demand for luffa products, however, have also created the potential for viable domestic production.

Luffa is closely related to cucumber and has similar cultural requirements. It is a tropical plant, however, which requires a longer growing season than most cucurbits grown in North America. The objective of this study was to develop a production system for luffa grown in the temperate climates of North Carolina and Missouri.

PRODUCTION

Planting date, planting method, in-row spacing and pruning were studied in western North Carolina. In 1989, three planting dates (May 29, June 12, and June 26) and two planting methods (direct seeding vs. transplanting) were examined. Plants were trained to a single-curtain trellis and grown on raised beds with black plastic mulch and drip irrigation. Rows were spaced 1.5 m apart and plants were spaced 45.7 cm apart in the row. Highest yields, earliest maturity, and largest sponges were obtained when plants were transplanted and set early (Table 1). In 1990, three in-row spacings (31, 61, and 91 cm) and three pruning treatments (no pruning, removing the first four laterals, and topping the main stem at node 6) were examined. Plants were grown on trellises with rows spaced 1.5 m apart. The highest yields of marketable gourds were obtained when plants were spaced 31 cm apart in the row and the first four laterals were removed (Fig. 1). Although this treatment did not provide the largest gourds, there was no difference in yields of gourds in the size category most requested by buyers, i.e., gourds 31 to 61 cm long and 7.5 to 10 cm in diameter.

Table 1. Influence of planting date and planting method on yield and size of luffa gourds.

Planting date	Planting method	No. gourds/ha × 10³		Fruit size (cm)	
		1st harvest	Total harvest	Length	Diameter
May 29	Transplant	46.8	91.2	36.6	8.4
June 12	Transplant	32.8	81.8	36.0	8.3
June 26	Transplant	20.7	74.5	35.1	7.6
May 29	Direct seed	20.7	74.0	36.6	8.2
June 12	Direct seed	11.0	67.0	35.4	7.4
June 26	Direct seed	4.6	63.0	34.4	7.2

There is no significant difference in sponge length. Main effect differences (planting date and planting method) for yield and diameter are significant at P = 0.01. Interactions were not significant.

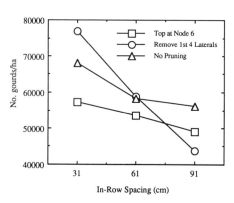

Fig. 1. Influence of spacing and pruning on luffa gourd yields.

Trellis systems and seed sources were also studied in Missouri. To produce straight, well-formed, disease-free gourds, luffa must be grown on a trellis. A sturdy trellis that permits good light penetration and air circulation is required. In 1990, three trellis systems were evaluated; a single curtain system, the Geneva double curtain (three wires formed a "V" at the top of the trellis) and the Lincoln system (four wires across the top of "T" posts). The Lincoln system was preferred because it provided the best support; the fruit hung free beneath the vines, resulting in a high percentage of straight fruit with few blemishes; and the fruit matured early.

Commercially available luffa seeds are rarely identified by cultivar, making it difficult to obtain seed that will produce gourds with desired characteristics. In 1990, seeds from 20 sources were grown. Days to maturity, yields, gourd size, and fiber quality varied considerably between seed lots. Number of gourds per plant ranged from 3.5 to 20. Average gourd length varied from 48 to 79 cm and the diameter from 7 to 11 cm. Days from fruit set to fruit maturity ranged from 53 to 88 days and was highly variable within each seed lot. Because luffa is open pollinated and crosses easily, further trials must be conducted on the seed collected from the most promising selections to determine if the quality can be maintained from year to year.

The skin, pulp, and seeds must be removed from the gourds before marketing. The skin and pulp are removed by soaking the gourds in water. The skins are easiest to remove from gourds that are mature when they begin to dry. An effective method for removing seeds is to shake them out manually. This method, however, is labor intensive and time-consuming. If a light colored sponge is desired, cleaned sponges may be soaked briefly in a 10% bleach solution.

MARKETING

Sponges with different fiber densities and textures are required for making different products. A subjective grading system with five grades based on fiber density, texture, and appearance was developed by C.D. DeCourley to assist buyers, growers, and researchers. J.M. Davis used an AgVision monochrome system (Decagon Devices, Inc., Pullman, WA) to provide a quantitative evaluation. AgVision is a computer controlled video system designed for digital image analysis. Using this system, the area occupied by fibers in a 50 cm^2 section of the outer wall of a luffa sponge was determined. Sponge samples from the seed source trials in Missouri were evaluated by three luffa buyers from the cosmetic industry and three researchers. In general, the buyers gave the samples lower quality ratings than did the researchers. All samples with a poor subjective rating also had a low rating with the AgVision system. A better grading system needs to be developed for both industry and research use.

The largest market for luffa is the cosmetic industry which uses luffa in various bath and cosmetic products. A small market for luffa sponges also exists at farmers' markets, gift shops, and to crafters. Wholesale buyers of luffa have indicated a willingness to purchase domestically grown luffa if the quality and prices are competitive with the imported product and the supply is consistent.

CONCLUSIONS AND RECOMMENDATIONS

Luffa gourds could be a new crop for a few American growers. Companies currently importing luffa are interested in domestic production. The known market will only support about 20 to 30 ha, but wholesale buyers indicate that demand is increasing. Presently, it is not known if high quality luffa can be produced at a price that is competitive with imported luffa. Before doing an economic feasibility study, a reliable production system needs to be developed. Based on the research and demonstrations conducted in North Carolina and Missouri, we currently recommend that growers start small and have a marketing plan before planting. Fertilizer recommendations for trellised cucumbers and pest control for gourds should be followed until specific studies on luffa are conducted. Seed should be obtained from sponges that are the quality desired by the buyer. Four to five week old transplants should be planted as soon after the last frost as possible. Plants should be spaced 31 cm apart in the row and the first four laterals removed. Irrigation is essential and mulch beneficial. A sturdy trellis is needed, preferably one that will allow the gourds to hang free. One or two bee hives should be placed near the field. Gourds should be removed from the field as soon as they are dry.

Population Density and Soil pH Effects on Vegetable Amaranth Production

Bharat P. Singh and Wayne F. Whitehead

The genus *Amaranthus* consists of nearly 60 species which can be broadly categorized into grain, green leaf vegetable, and weed types. Cultivation of amaranth (*Amaranthus* spp.) for their leaves dates back to more than 2,000 years. Presently, amaranth is extensively grown as a green leaf vegetable in many tropical countries (National Research Council 1984). The leaves are mostly consumed as pot-herb either alone or in combination with other vegetables and/or meat. Amaranth leaves are good source of dietary fiber and contains high amounts of proteins, vitamins, and minerals (Makus and Davis 1984; Teutonico and Knorr 1985; Willis et al. 1984).

Amaranth species utilized as a vegetable generally have short plants with wide leaves and small inflorescence (Huang 1980). Two species, *A tricolor* and *A. dubius* have the desired characteristics for the vegetable type and are commonly grown for this purpose in Asia, West Africa, and the Caribbean. A third species, *A. cruentus* is grown both for leaves and grain. The production of *A. cruentus* for leaves is most prevalent in humid tropical Africa (National Research Council 1984).

In the United States, amaranth is seldom used as a vegetable and production is limited to a few ethnic growers. Most greens grown in the United States prefer cool weather and perform poorly during hot summer months. There is a need to introduce leafy vegetables which can successfully be grown during the summer months. Amaranth may be such a candidate to fill this niche. Abbott and Campbell (1982) and Makus and Davis (1984) obtained high green yields from amaranth produced during summer months in Maryland and Arkansas, respectively. Sealy et al. (1990) reported that a West African cultivar 'Ibondwe' yielded 14 t/ha in central Texas and was comparable to spinach in taste. The object of this study was to establish optimum soil pH and intra-row plant spacing for amaranth production.

SOIL PH

The greenhouse experiment was conducted during November–December 1990, to compare the growth of amaranth at 6.4, 5.3, and 4.7 soil pH using Dothan sandy loam soil (fine loamy, siliceous, thermic, Plinthic Paleudult). Seeds of 'Hinchoy' were started in flats and 11-day-old seedlings were transplanted in thirty 3-liter pots, ten of each soil pH. The pots were arranged on the greenhouse benches in a randomized complete block design. The greenhouse was held at 32±3°C day/24±2°C night. Photoperiod was kept at 14 h and supplemental lighting was provided with fluorescent lamps. Five week old plants were harvested and the number of branches and leaves on the plants were counted. Plants were then separated into root, stem, and leaf portions and the fresh weight of plant components were determined. Leaf areas was measured with an area meter (LI-COR Model 3100, Lincoln, Nebraska). All plant parts were dried at 70°C in a forced air oven to a constant weight. The above experiment was repeated during January–February 1991.

Plants grown in pH 6.4 soil were significantly taller and had greater leaf area than plants grown in pH 5.3 or 4.7 soil (Table 1). There was a significant decrease in all above ground plant parts with each increase in soil acidity. The top fresh weight of plants grown in 5.3 and 4.7 pH soil were 27 and 73% lower, respectively, than plants grown in 6.4 pH soil. Campbell and Foy (1987) screened four grain amaranth populations of *A. cruentus*, *A. hypochondriacus*, and *A. hybridus* and also found that each performed poorly in Tatum soil (clayey, mixed, thermic, typic Hapludults) at 4.8 pH. Makus (1989) found that growth of vegetable amaranth was restricted in low pH Enders soil (clayey, mixed, thermic, typic Hapludults).

INTRA-ROW PLANT SPACING

A field experiment to compare the performance of amaranth at six intra-row plant spacings was conducted during summer of 1990. The genotype, RRC 241 was planted on a Dothan sandy loam soil (fine loamy, siliceous, thermic, Plinthic Paleudult) in 5 m long and 90 cm wide rows at six plant spacing of 4, 8, 16, 24, 32, and 40 cm in completely randomized blocks with three replications. Weeding was done mechanically and plots were irrigated as needed. The crop was harvested 40 days after planting. Data on plant height, branch number, and leaf number were obtained from five random plants from each plot. Plants were then separated into stem, petiole, and leaf parts. Plant component fresh weight was recorded and leaf area of two plants/plot was measured. Holes were made by a cork borer in the leaf blades of two random plants and 50 leaf discs were collected. The cumulative leaf area of the discs were measured and the leaf discs were dried to a constant weight at 70°C to calculate the specific leaf weight (unit dry weight/unit leaf area).

The tallest plants were produced in the closest spacing (Table 2). The relationship of plant height to intra-row spacing was quadratic in nature. The highest leaf number and maximum leaf area were obtained with the widest spacing. The regression of specific leaf weight on intra-row spacing was non-significant indicating that intra-row spacing did not affect leaf thickness. The maximum stem, petiole, and leaf fresh weights were produced in the widest spacing; minimum values were produced in closest spacing. As a result, the widest spacing had the

Table 1. Growth parameters of amaranth at three soil pH levels[z]

Soil pH	Plant height (cm)	Branch (no./plant)	Leaf (no./plant)	Leaf area (cm²/plant)	Plant weight (g/plant)			
					Top		Root	
					Fresh	Dry	Fresh	Dry
6.4	18.3a[y]	8.5a	47.1a	1343a	49.5a	3.8a	19.8a	2.3a
5.3	16.0b	7.2b	42.4a	1011b	36.3b	2.8b	16.6b	1.8a
4.7	10.2c	5.3c	28.5b	412c	13.3c	1.0c	4.2c	0.6b

[z]Experiments 1 and 2 combined.
[y]Mean separation within column by Duncan's multiple range test, $P = 0.05$.

Table 2. Growth parameters of amaranth at six intra-row plant spacings.

Intra-row spacing (cm)	Plant height (cm)	Branch (no./plant)	Leaf (no./plant)	Leaf area (cm²/plant)	Specific leaf weight (mg/cm²)	Plant fresh wt (g/plant)			Yield (kg/m²)
						Stem	Petiole	Leaf	
4	29.3	5.3	35.3	873	4.43	18.9	6.0	24.2	1.50
8	23.0	6.7	56.3	1420	5.54	21.2	8.9	51.9	1.15
16	21.7	8.0	69.7	1598	6.10	25.4	10.9	55.9	0.66
24	15.3	6.0	63.7	1370	3.05	18.4	8.2	52.4	0.41
32	16.0	7.0	65.7	1368	4.16	19.5	8.5	49.4	0.29
40	20.7	6.7	70.0	1882	4.16	27.7	14.5	65.7	0.35
Significance[z]	Q**[y]	NS[x]	C**[w]	C**[v]	NS[u]	NS[t]	C**[s]	C**[r]	Q**[q]

[z]C = cubic, Q = quadratic, L = linear
[y]$R^2 = 0.71$
[x]$R^2 = 0.03$
[w]$R^2 = 0.59$
[v]$R^2 = 0.80$
[u]$R^2 = 0.04$
[t]$R^2 = 0.06$
[s]$R^2 = 0.75$
[r]$R^2 = 0.66$
[q]$R^2 = 0.96$
NS, *, ** Nonsignificant or significant at $P = 0.05$ or 0.01, respectively.

highest and the closest spacing the lowest per plant fresh weight among the six intra-row spacings. On an unit area basis, however, green yield increased quadratically as intra-row spacing decreased. The coefficient of determination (R^2) of green yield with intra-row spacing was 0.96, indicating that 96% of the total variation in the mean yields could be explained by the quadratic regression equation.

CONCLUSIONS

Our results show that growth of vegetable amaranth was adversely affected by soil pHs of 5.3 and 4.7. A soil with pH of 6.4 could produce high yielding vegetable amaranth. Green yield increased quadratically as intra-row spacing decreased. Maximum yield at 4 cm spacing within row was 1.50 kg/m^2.

REFERENCES

Abbott, J.A. and T.A. Campbell. 1982. Sensory evaluation of vegetable amaranth (*Amaranthus* spp.). HortScience 17:409–410.

Campbell, T.A. and C.D. Foy. 1987. Selection of grain Amaranthus species for tolerance to excess aluminum in an acid soil. J. Plant Nutr. 10:249–260.

Huang, P.C. 1980. A study of the taxonomy of edible amaranth: an investigation of amaranth both of botanical and horticultural characteristics. Proc. 2nd Amaranth Conf. Rodale Press, Emmaus, PA. p. 142–150.

Makus, D.J. 1989. Aluminum accumulation in vegetable amaranth in soil with adjusted pH values. HortScience 24:460–463.

Makus, D.J. and D.R. Davis. 1984. A mid-summer crop for fresh greens or canning; vegetable amaranth. Ark. Farm Res. 33:10.

National Research Council. 1984. Amaranth: modern prospects for an ancient crop. National Academy Press, Washington, DC.

Sealy, R.L., E.L. McWilliams, J. Novak, F. Fong, and C.M. Kenerley. 1990. Vegetable amaranth: cultivar selection for summer production in the south, p. 396–398. In: J. Janick and J.E. Simon (eds.). Advances in new crops. Timber Press, Portland, OR.

Teutonico, R.A. and D. Knorr. 1985. Amaranth: composition, properties and applications of a rediscovered food crop. Food Tech. 39(4):49–60.

Willis, R.B.H., A.W.K. Wong, F.M. Scriven, and H. Greenfield. 1984. Nutrient composition of chinese vegetables. J. Agr. Food Chem. 32:413–416.

Comparison of Somatic and Sexual Interspecific Hybridization for the Development of New Brassica Vegetable Crops

Richard H. Ozminkowski, Jr. and Pablo S. Jourdan

The success of an allopolyploid, whether natural (*Brassica napus* L., *Nicotiana tabacum* L., *Triticum aestivum* L.) or synthetic (triticale, hakuran) is based in part on the variability within the original parent individuals (Dewey 1980). The genus *Brassica*, is a classic example of allopolyploid speciation (Fig. 1); it is extremely diverse in morphology encompassing many economically important crops. The natural allotetraploid *B. napus* has been produced from its diploid progenitor species (*B. oleracea* L. and *B. rapa* L.) by sexual interspecific hybridization for the development of the leafy vegetable crop 'Hakuran' (Nishi 1980), and by somatic hybridization (Jourdan et al. 1989) in attempts to transfer various nuclear and cytoplasmic traits between the species. This makes *B. napus* a model system for a comparison of sexual and somatic hybridization systems for the development of new crops.

Diploid cells used in somatic hybridization are not subject to the allelic segregation found in gamete formation nor the unilateral inheritance of cytoplasm as generally seen in sexual hybridization; therefore, somatic hybrids should retain any heterozygosity of the parents and allow for rearrangement of cytoplasm. The use of highly heterozygous parents in somatic hybridizations could incorporate high degrees of variation in the offspring (= F_2) of a single somatic hybrid not possible with sexual hybridization. Relatively homozygous lines have generally served as parents to resynthesized *B. napus*, thus impeding the exploitation of the high morphological variability within the parental species. Such variation is essential for new crop development and therefore requires that hybrids be produced from several different parent combinations in order to provide sufficient variation for cultivar development of a new crop.

The current study was designed to maximize the heterozygosity in a population of resynthesized allotetraploid *B. napus*, so as to maintain high variability in subsequent generations for the development and breeding of new crops. The primary objectives are to provide novel and supplemental variation for breeding vegetable-type *B. napus*, and to determine which method of resynthesis, sexual or somatic, would be more effective for doing so.

METHODOLOGY

Plant Material

Intraspecific F_1 hybrids between cultigens within the diploid progenitor species (*B. oleracea* and *B. rapa*) were produced by bud pollination in the greenhouse (Fig. 2). Each vegetable parent [cauliflower (*B. oleracea* ssp. *botrytis*), turnip (*B. rapa* ssp. *rapifera*), and chinese cabbage (*B. rapa* ssp. *pekinensis*)] was selected for its

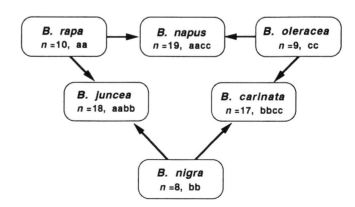

Fig. 1. Nuclear genomic relationships among selected *Brassica* species (adapted from U 1935). Species at intersections of the triangle are the diploid progenitor species of the respective allotetraploid species upon each side. Lower case letters represent the species nuclear genome composition.

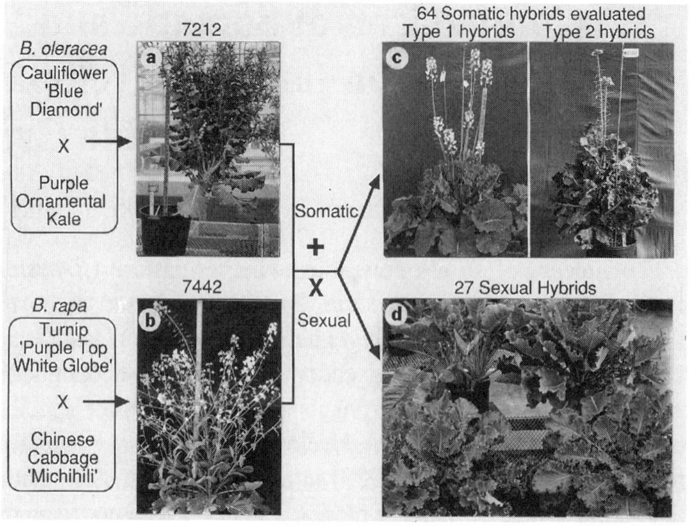

Fig. 2. Pedigree of (c) somatic and (d) sexual interspecific hybrids between (a) *B. oleracea* and (b) *B. rapa*.

distinctive morphological character whereas purple ornamental kale (*B. oleracea* ssp. *acephala*) was selected for its excellent regeneration from protoplasts. All cultigens had yellow flowers except cauliflower's which were white.

Production of Somatic Hybrids (R_0) and Their F_2 (= R_1) Populations

Production of the somatic hybrids followed standard protocols (Jourdan et al. 1989). Leaf tissue served as the protoplast source for somatic hybridization involving individual *B. rapa* and *B. oleracea* species-parent plants (Fig. 2). The latter's protoplasts were treated with iodoacetate prior to fusion by the polyethylene glycol method.

Somatic F_2 seed from bud self-pollinations were started in the greenhouse from three Type 1 (see Results) somatic hybrids. Seeds of the diploid parental lines 7212 (*B. oleracea*) and 7442 (*B. rapa*) were also started. Five-week-old seedlings were transplanted at ca. 0.6 m intervals in rows 1.6 m apart on raised beds. Plants were evaluated for various morphological characters on a 1 to 5 rating scale [plant habit, branching, leaf shape, undulation, vesture, leaf crinkle (internal bubbling of the leaf), leaf color, and rib color]. Leaf shape was classified as described by Gomez-Campo (1980) ranging from lyrate to heavily lobed (divided). Approximately, 350 F_2 plants from each of two somatic hybrids were used for frequency analysis.

Production of Sexual Hybrids

Reciprocal interspecific bud pollinations were made between the same species-parent individuals used in the fusion experiment (Fig. 2) during the months of November and December, under natural lighting in the greenhouse. Thirteen to 18 days after pollination, ovules were aseptically removed from the silique and placed in the liquid medium (MS_Q) of Quazi (1988) with the omission of tri-potassium phosphate. Cultures were incubated in dim light (60 µmol m^{-2}s^{-1}) on a gyratory shaker (33 rpm). Two to three weeks later, torpedo stage embryos were transferred to solid B5G1 medium [B5 media with 0.1 mg/liter gibberellic acid (GA_3), 0.8% washed agar] and grown at 4°C with 8/16 h light/dark periods for 10 days. Once developed, shoots were proliferated on a modified solid Murashige and Skoog (MS) medium (B5 vitamins) with 0.2 mg/liter 6-benzylamino purine (BA) and then maintained on hormone-free MS medium until placement into soil. Sexual hybrids were identified by intermediate morphology and glucose phosphate isomerase (GPI) and phosphoglucomutase (PGM) isoenzyme banding patterns using cellulose acetate electrophoresis (Hebert and Beaton 1989).

RESULTS AND DISCUSSION

Somatic Hybrids

Two types of somatic hybrids were produced (Fig. 2) and have been characterized previously (Ozminkowski and Jourdan 1991). Type 1 hybrids were uniform, vigorous, near-rosette in habit, with divided pubescent leaves, and white, fertile flowers. Flow cytometry analysis of nuclear DNA content indicated that these plants had a genome size similar to natural *B. napus*. Type 2 hybrids were variable in appearance, rugose, less vigorous, with distinct internodes, and near lyrate leaf shape; mature plants were nearly glabrous. These plants had low fertility and were chimeric (white and yellow) for flower color; flow cytometry data suggested that these plants had higher ploidy levels than natural *B. napus* making them less useful in a breeding program. No somatic hybrids were found to contain only the *B. oleracea* RFLP markers for either mitochondria or chloroplasts while many contained only the *B. rapa* markers. Several hybrids were found to contain the chloroplast and/or mitochondria RFLPs of both parents, suggesting either mixed or recombinant organellar genomes.

The somatic hybrids did not appear to be of any economic value per se. However, every somatic hybrid contained an allele at each locus from four diverse cultivated forms of *Brassica* allowing extensive segregation in the F_2 generation; the production of F_2 seed of the Type 1 hybrids was not a limiting factor.

Somatic F_2 (= R_1) Generation

Field-grown F_2 plants of the Type 1 hybrids were uniformly vigorous. Distinct morphologies became apparent about 4 weeks after planting. The morphological variability seen in the F_2 populations was sufficiently large to permit further intrapopulation crossing and selection for forms appealing to the consumer (e.g. glabrous, heading, good color). Several morphologies were found in the somatic F_2 population which show potential for new plant development (Fig. 3). Variation in leaf morphology is illustrated in Fig. 4.

When individual plant characters were evaluated, most of the plants were intermediate between the two species-parents though the frequencies were skewed in favor of *B. rapa*; this may be a contribution of the predominantly *B. rapa* cytoplasm or of more dominant *B. rapa* nuclear alleles. However, somatic hybrids containing only *B. oleracea* cytoplasm were not obtained for comparison. Most F_2 plants exhibited less extreme pubescence than the *B. rapa* parent, although several were seen with higher levels. Several glabrous plants were found, a character more favorable for marketing. Many plants displayed leaf undulation and crinkle more extreme than either species-parent. Plants with rib color that was much darker purple than either parent line were also found in this population. Leaf color was the only evaluated character to favor the blue-green *B. oleracea* parent. Only three F_2 plants flowered within five months after planting, thus preventing the analysis of fertility and segregation of flower color (all three had white flowers).

Sexual Hybrids

Twenty-seven embryos produced sexual hybrid plants (Table 1). Most (19 of 27) hybrid embryos produced greater than 20 shoots allowing clones of 11 to be placed in the field. Each sexual hybrid was unique in morphology (Figs. 2 and 5), as would be expected since allelic segregation occurred during gamete formation. Hybrids were very vigorous both in the greenhouse and field. All sexual hybrids were pubescent. Only four hybrids, all field-grown, have flowered five months after transplanting and are segregating for flower color though all flowers were small and sterile. Analysis of organelle-specific RFLPs suggested only maternal inheritance of cytoplasm.

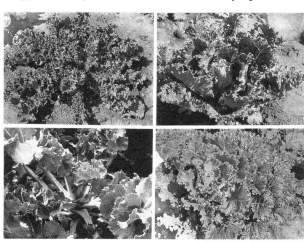

Fig. 3. Four somatic F_2 individuals exhibiting promising morphologies for development of new vegetables.

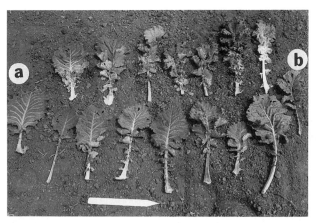
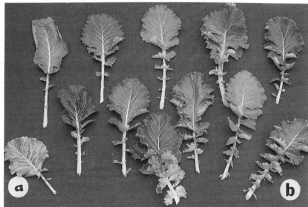

Fig. 4. Leaf variability of two parent lines a) 7212 and b) 7442 and the F_2 population (all others) of 2 somatic hybrids between these lines (stake = 30 cm).

Fig. 5. Leaf variability among sexual hybrids between heterozygous *B. oleracea* a) and *B. rapa* lines. b) Type 1 somatic hybrid leaf.

Table 1. Sexual F_1 hybrid plants produced by hybridizations between *B. oleracea* and *B. rapa* via ovule culture.

Cross	No. of pollinations made	No. of siliques cultured	No. of ovules cultured	No. of embryos developed	No. of hybrids produced	No. of maternal escapes
B. rapa x *B. oleracea*	603	176	~600	17	8	4
B. oleracea x *B. rapa*	188	12	114	40	19	3

DNA quantification through flow cytometry indicate these plants are allodiploids and therefore must have their genomes doubled to restore fertility. The result should be fully homozygous, inbred lines containing only one allele from each locus of each species. Thus, only those types produced in the hybrid generation are available for continued development without the production of additional interspecific hybrids. Few if any sexual hybrids displayed an economically favorable morphology per se; no glabrous or heading type plants were produced. This may be due to the limited number of sexual hybrids produced, an inherent difficulty to sexual hybridization between these two species.

CONCLUSION

The parents used in the synthesis of a novel or natural allopolyploid crop should contain maximum levels of variation to provide a germplasm resource sufficient for the development of new forms with a minimal number of resynthesis experiments. Using *Brassica*, we have compared two methods of producing allopolyploid species, sexual and somatic interspecific hybridization, for the development of new vegetables. Many independent sexual hybrids were necessary to represent only a fraction of the variability observed in the F_2 population of a single somatic hybrid produced from the same heterozygous parents. Since interspecific hybrids are often difficult to produce, maximal variability in fewer individual hybrids can be a tremendous savings in resources. Somatic hybridization can result in highly heterozygous hybrids and, in addition, offers the opportunity for novel organelle rearrangements which can lead to unique cytoplasmic male sterility systems (Jourdan et al. 1989); sexual hybridization generally produces hybrids containing maternal cytoplasm. Organelle analysis of the somatic and sexual hybrids produced in this study did support this hypothesis.

The availability of efficient techniques for protoplast regeneration and fusion in an increasing number of crops will allow plant breeders to choose between sexual and somatic hybridization for the production of interspecific hybrids based upon the individual breeding program objectives. We have shown in this study that, when a primary objective involves the production of new allopolyploid crops or to substantially increase the variability within existing allopolyploid species, somatic hybridization is the preferred method because high variability can be obtained among progeny from a single fertile somatic hybrid. The use of parent plants heterozygous for quantitative trait loci (QTL) involving yield or stress resistance permits combination of several alleles at each QTL in every somatic hybrid which would allow high genetic gain from subsequent selection. Conversely, if the objective is to introgress a simply-inherited trait into an existing crop, sexual hybridization may be preferred.

REFERENCES

Dewey, D.R. 1980. Some applications and misapplications of induced polyploidy to plant breeding, p. 445–470. In: W.H. Lewis (ed.). Polyploidy: biological relevance. vol 13. Basic life sciences. Plenum Press, NY.

Gomez-Campo, C. 1980. Morphology and morpho-taxonomy of the tribe *Brassiceae*, p. 3–31. In: S. Tsunoda, K. Hinata, and C. Gomez-Campo (eds.). Brassica crops and wild allies: biology and breeding. Japan Scientific Societies Press, Tokyo.

Hebert, P.D.N. and M.J. Beaton. 1989. Methodologies for allozyme analysis using cellulose acetate electrophoresis: a practical handbook. Helena Laboratories Inc. Beaumont, TX.

Jourdan, P.S., E.D. Earle, and M.A. Mutschler. 1989. Synthesis of male sterile, triazine-resistant *Brassica napus* by somatic hybridization between cytoplasmic male sterile *B. oleracea* and atrazine-resistant *B. campestris*. Theor. Appl. Genet. 78:445–455.

Nishi, S. 1980. Differentiation of Brassica crops in Asia and the breeding of 'hakuran', a newly synthesized leafy vegetable, p. 133–150. In: S. Tsunoda, K. Hinata, and C. Gomez-Campo (eds.). *Brassica* crops and wild allies: biology and breeding. Japan Scientific Societies Press, Tokyo.

Ozminkowski, R.H., Jr. and P.J. Jourdan. 1991. Characterization of *Brassica napus* resynthesized by interspecific somatic hybridization from highly heterozygous parents. HortScience 26:740 (Abstr. 425).

Quazi, M.H. 1988. Interspecific hybrids between *Brassica napus* L. and *B. oleracea* L. developed by embryo culture. Theor. Appl. Genet. 75:309–318.

U, N. 1935. Genomic analysis in *Brassica* with special reference to the experimental formation of *B. napus* and peculiar mode of fertilization. Japan. J. Bot. 7:309–452.

Evaluating Chinese Cabbage Cultivars for High Temperature Tolerance

I-Mo Fu, Carol Shennan, and Gregory E. Welbaum

Chinese cabbage [*Brassica campestris* L., *Pekinensis* group (Lour), Brassicaceae] has been an important vegetable in eastern Asia for many centuries (Li 1981). Chinese cabbage is an annual with only a few characteristics in common with cabbage (*B. oleracea* L., *Capitata* group). There are both heading and nonheading types of Chinese cabbage. Plants of nonheading types have several thick, white petioles with smooth, dark green leaf blades arranged in a tight cluster. Heading types generally produce an elongated, compact head comprised of wrinkled leaves with broad veins. Chinese cabbage is becoming increasingly popular in the United States due to a growing Asian population and a greater appreciation of the crop in general. The strong market demand has many vegetable growers interested in Chinese cabbage production. However, Chinese cabbage, unlike common cultivars of cabbage, is intolerant of warm temperatures. This may limit the development of Chinese cabbage as an alternative crop in much of the United States. Loose head formation, tip burn, and soft rot are major problems often encountered when Chinese cabbage is grown at high temperatures (Kuo and Tsay 1981; Fritz and Honma 1987). Experiments were conducted in Virginia and California to determine whether cultivars differ with respect to their susceptibility to premature bolting and high temperatures, whether mulching treatments affect heat tolerance, and which planting dates are optimal for Chinese cabbage production.

METHODOLOGY

In Davis, California, five heat-tolerant cultivars of Chinese cabbage (ASVEG #1, Blues, B14, B40, and China Express) were evaluated. In April, June, August, and September of 1988, transplants at the six leaf stage were set in double rows 51 cm apart on 102 cm raised beds with an in-row spacing of 31 cm. Three mulch treatments were employed: control (bare ground), straw, and clear plastic. The experimental design was a randomized complete block with split plots, with mulch treatments assigned to blocks and replicated 3 times and cultivars assigned to plots. The frequency of irrigation was based on tensiometer and neutron probe measurements. The following parameters were recorded at harvest: average head weight; the percentage of harvestable heads, bolting heads, diseased heads, and loose heads; and head solidity (Opeña and Lo 1981).

In Virginia, the cultivars China Flash, China Express, Tropical Quick, Mei Qing Choi, Joi Choi, Springtime, Kasumi, China Pride, and Summertime were evaluated. Two replications of each cultivar were organized in a completely randomized design. Transplants were set in double rows 46 cm apart with an in-row spacing of 31 cm in 1990 (mid-April and late July) and 1991 (mid-June). Fertilizer (10N–4.3P–8.3K) was row-banded at the rate of 85 kg/ha before planting, and a drench consisting of 9N–19.4P–12.5K fertilizer (4 g/liter) and the insecticide, Diazinon (0.7 g/liter), was applied at a rate of 250 ml/plant after transplanting. A Bravo/Ridomil drench was applied during development to combat head rot. Plots were harvested 61 and 68 days after transplanting.

RESULTS AND DISCUSSION

California Trials

The mean daily temperature for the April transplanting was 16.0°C, while the mean maximum daily temperature was 24.5°C. Only 28% of all April transplants produced harvestable heads largely due to a disease rate of 45% and the fact that 12% of the plants bolted prematurely. The mean daily temperature for the June transplanting was 24.8°C. Only 20% of all June transplants produced harvestable heads due to soft rot and tipburn. In August, the mean daily temperature dropped to 21.7°C, and 66% of all plants produced harvestable heads. The mean daily temperature for the September transplanting was 15.5°C, and the harvestable yield was 93%. Heat-tolerant cultivars from the April and June transplanting dates could not be identified because all cultivars produced a relatively low percentage of harvestable heads. Conversely, temperatures following the September transplanting were nearly ideal for Chinese cabbage production, so heat-tolerant cultivars could not be detected. Temperatures after the August transplanting were intermediate between those following the June and September transplantings, revealing significant differences among cultivars for all characteristics except the percentage of bolting and diseased heads (Table 1A).

The cultivar 'ASVEG #1' produced a high percentage of disease resistant, solid heads (Table 1B). The cultivar 'Bl4' was similar to 'ASVEG #1'. The head quality of 'China Express' was very good, but a high percentage of plants failed to form heads (Table 1B). There was also a significant cultivar by mulch interaction that was probably caused by the inconsistent response of cultivars to mulch treatments, making it impossible to draw simple conclusions about differences among the percentages of loose and harvestable heads (Table 1A). There were also significant differences among mulch treatments for the percentage of diseased heads, but a highly significant cultivar by mulch interaction makes it impossible to draw simple conclusions about these differences. There were no significant differences among the mulch treatments for head weight, the percentage of bolting plants, or head solidity (Table 1C).

Virginia Trials

There were significant differences among cultivars for the percentage of harvestable and bolting heads in June 1990 (Table 2). In some cases, the low percentage of harvestable heads was due to tipburn, soft rot, and bolting. The development of disease symptoms corresponded with an increase in the mean maximum daily temperature in April (21.2±0.7°C), May (21.4±0.8°C), and June (25.6±0.8°C). However, 'China Flash', 'China Express', and 'Kasumi' did not bolt and showed a lower frequency of head rot than other cultivars. Heads harvested in early October from the July transplanting did not bolt and had fewer incidences of head rot (not shown).

Table 1. Performance of mulched and unmulched Chinese cabbage cultivars, Davis, California, August, 1988[z].

Variable	Head weight (g)	Harvestable heads (%)	Bolting heads (%)	Diseased heads (%)	Loose heads (%)	Solidity[x] (g/cm^3)
A. Analysis of cultivar and mulch treatments						
Cultivar	*	**	NS	NS	**	**
Mulch	NS	*	NS	*	*	NS
Cult × mul	NS	*	ns	**	*	NS
B. Variation in cultivar performance[y]						
ASVEG	771ab	84	2	10	4	0.69a
Blues	961ab	27	0	19	54	0.49b
B14	782ab	75	0	23	3	0.55ab
B40	744b	51	0	16	22	0.41b
China Exp.	1002a	56	0	14	31	0.52b
C. Effect of mulch treatment[y]						
Control	894	66	1	10	16	0.49
Plastic	888	60	0	18	32	0.53
Straw	777	50	0	20	20	0.58

NS, *, ** Nonsignificant, significant at P = 0.05, and 0.01, respectively.
[z]N = 15, 9, 15, for Tables A, B, and C, respective.
[y]mean separation by Tukey's Studentized Range (HSD) Test.
[x]Solidity = mean head wt (g)/volume of head (cm^3); volume (cm^3) is estimated as (0.524)(head width)(head height).

Table 2. Performance of Chinese cabbage cultivars, June harvest, Blacksburg, Virginia, 1990.

Cultivar (Seed Co.)	Head weight (kg±SE)	Harvestable heads (%)	Bolting heads (%)	Plant height (cm±SE)	Plant diameter (cm±SE)	Comments
Mei Qing Choi (Sakata)	0.54±0.08	7	35	23.3±1.9	9.7±0.3	Light green petioles and foliage, a nonheading pak choi type. Soft rot af fected about 65% of the plants, resulting low in the harvestable yield.
Joi Choi (Sakata)	1.09±0.13	79	5	37.3±0.9	14.3±0.7	A nonheading pak choi type with dark green foliage and white petioles. Attractive large plants were less susceptible to soft rot compared to 'Mei Qing Choi'.
China Flash (Sakata)	1.85±0.17	80	0	28.9±0.6	17.0±0.5	Medium green napa type. Very compact plants produced medium sized heads. About 20% were affected by head rot. Recommended for further trial in Virginia.
Tropical Quick (Sakata)	0.44±0.97	0	100	39.2±2.2	10.4±0.6	Medium green tropical heading type. Plants bolted early in development. Does not appear to be adapted to Virginia.
China Express (Sakata)	1.56±0.10	85	0	30.2±0.6	16.5±0.8	Similar in appearance to 'China Flash'. Only a few plantswere affected by rot. Plants held well in the field without splitting. Recommended for further trial in Virginia.
Springtime (Stokes)	0.96±0.05	55	15	24.6±1.2	11.7±0.4	Light green napa type. Early maturing but susceptible to tipburn, soft rot, and splitting. May have some value as an early season cultivar.
Kasumi (Stokes)	2.14±0.13	90	0	26.9±0.6	19.2±0.7	Medium green napa type. Compact plants produced uniform extremely solid heads with little head rot. Recommended for further trial in Virginia.
China Pride (Stokes)	1.97±0.22	0	60	34.2±3.7	18.7±01.1	Large dark green napa type. Most plants bolted prematurely before head formation.
Summertime (Stokes)	1.39±0.08	50	0	32.6±0.8	15.1±0.3	Late maturing medium green napa type. Plants lacked uniformity and were susceptible to head rot.
LSD .05	0.45	24	29	3.1	2.8	

In 1991, Chinese cabbage was transplanted to the field in late June. Temperatures as high as 33°C were recorded on several occasions during head formation in July and August. The occurrence of head rot and tipburn were much greater than for the early June harvest from the previous year. The percentage of harvestable heads ranged from 25 to 72% in 1991 (not shown). In Virginia, soft rot may have been promoted by overhead irrigation and poor drainage, yet, in California where raised beds and furrow irrigation were used, soft rot was also a serious problem. Raised beds, in some instances, have been shown to be beneficial in reducing the incidence and spread of soft rot (Fritz and Honma 1987).

CONCLUSIONS

As reported by Palada et al. (1987), premature bolting is a problem with spring but not fall crops. In this study, several cultivars were found to be resistant to bolting (Table 1). There were also differences in heat tolerance among cultivars, although no cultivar was sufficiently resistant to be productive in mid-summer at either location. The highest incidence of diseased heads occurred in plantings that matured under high temperature conditions in mid-summer in both Virginia and California. In both locations, best results were obtained when Chinese cabbage was grown as a fall crop. This is in contrast to results showing that Chinese cabbage can be successfully grown as a spring crop (Palada et al. 1987). The cultivar 'ASVEG #1' performed well in California and has also performed well in other locations (Fritz and Honma 1987).

REFERENCES

Fritz, V.A. and S. Honma. 1987. The effect of raised beds, population densities, and planting date on the incidence of bacterial soft rot in Chinese cabbage. J. Amer. Soc. Hort. Sci. 112:41–44.

Kuo, C.G. and J.S. Tsay. 1981. Physiological responses of Chinese cabbage under high temperature, p. 217–224. In: N.S. Talekar and T.D. Griggs (eds.). Chinese cabbage. Proc. First Int. Symp. Asian Vegetable Research and Development Center, Shanhua, Tainan, Taiwan.

Li, C.W. 1981. The origin, evolution, taxonomy, and hybridization of Chinese cabbage, p. 3–10. In: N.S. Talekar and T.D. Griggs (eds.). Chinese cabbage. Proc. First Int. Symp. Asian Vegetable Research and Development Center, Shanhua, Tainan, Taiwan.

Opeña, R.T. and S.H. Lo. 1980. Procedures for Chinese cabbage evaluation trials. Asian Vegetable Research and Development Center, Int. Coop. Guide 80-144.

Palada, M.C., S. Ganser, and R.R. Harwood. 1987. Cultivar evaluation for early and extended production of Chinese cabbage in eastern Pennsylvania. HortScience 22:1260–1262.

Brussels Sprouts as an Alternative Crop for Southwest Virginia

Gregory E. Welbaum

Although over 750 ha of summer cabbage are produced annually in Southwest Virginia (Vavrina 1988), the cabbage industry in this region often suffers from low market prices due to excess production and inadequate marketing strategies. Replacing cabbage hectareage with another high value crop, such as Brussels sprouts, could raise cabbage prices by limiting production and provide additional income from a second crop. Brussels sprouts have much greater cold hardiness than cabbage and other alternative vegetable crops being considered for the region. The introduction of Brussels sprouts would allow growers to produce a vegetable crop in the fall and early winter when labor is more readily available and other vegetables are out of season. Since cabbage and Brussels sprouts require similar cultural practices, Brussels sprouts production would require only a modest investment in new harvesting equipment and minimal retraining of growers and farm laborers.

METHODOLOGY

Nine Brussels sprouts (*Brassica oleracea* L., Gemmifera group) cultivars were evaluated for growth and yield for the first time in Southwest Virginia: 'Rider', 'Golfer', and 'Boxer' (Seed Way Inc., P.O. 250, Hall, NY 14463); 'Pilar', 'Lunet', 'RS88032', and 'Dolmic' (Royal Sluis, 1293 Harkins Road, Salinas, CA 93901); 'Royal Marvel' and 'Prince Marvel' (Sakata Seeds America Inc., P.O. Box 880, 18095 Serene Drive, Morgan Hill, CA 95038).

Plants were grown in Speedling polystyrene trays in a greenhouse for six weeks and transplanted to a field at the Virginia Tech Horticulture Farm near Christiansburg on July, 25 1990. About 15 g of fertilizer

(10N–4.3P–8.3K) were placed beneath each plant during transplanting, and a soil drench consisting of 9N–19.4P–12.5K fertilizer (4 g/liter) plus the insecticide, Diazinon (0.7 g/liter), was applied at a rate of 250 ml per plant after transplanting. Plants were set in double rows 30 cm apart with an in-row spacing of 60 centimeters. Each cultivar was transplanted into double rows 15 m long in an unreplicated block. Overhead irrigation was applied as required and fungicide and insecticide treatments were applied in accordance with recommended procedures (Anon. 1990). On Nov. 30, 127 days after transplanting, 10 to 12 plants of each cultivar were randomly harvested. The unharvested plants were evaluated periodically throughout the winter to assess holding ability and freeze tolerance.

RESULTS AND DISCUSSION

Results of the trial are summarized in Table 1. All cultivars grew slowly during August and early September due to the high temperatures. Brussels sprouts that mature during warm weather in the summer and early fall often have a strong, disagreeable flavor, while plants that mature under cooler fall conditions, particularly after frost, have a milder flavor. In this study, even the early maturing cultivars such as 'Dolmic' and 'Prince Marvel' had experienced temperatures of –5°C before maturation in early November, and none of the sprouts sampled from any of the cultivars had a strong flavor.

'Dolmic', 'Golfer', and 'Rider' produced a significant percentage of large, loose sprouts. Large sprout size may be a characteristic of these cultivars or an indication of excessive nitrogen fertilization. 'Boxer', 'Lunet', 'Royal Marvel', and 'RS88032' exhibited excellent sprout quality. However, 'Royal Marvel' was the only high-yielding cultivar with excellent sprout quality. 'Royal Marvel' yielded 17.9 t/ha, about 14% greater than the average yield for Brussels sprouts in the United States (Lorenz and Maynard 1988).

Brussels sprouts are slow to mature and are known to be susceptible to a wide range of insect pests. An early season infestation of diamondback moth (*Plutella xylostella* L.) did considerable damage and required the application of insecticides. However, after the first killing frost in October, insects were no longer a problem and many of the later maturing cultivars, such as 'Lunet' and 'RS88032', matured in near perfect condition without further use of insecticides. The cultivar 'RS88032' matured in late December, after the harvest data in Table 1 had been collected. The optimal harvest date for 'RS88032' should have been on January 1.

Brussels sprouts characteristically have a long storage life if maintained under optimum conditions. In this study, Brussels sprouts were stored at 3°C and greater than 90% relative humidity for two weeks with no reduction in quality.

Plants remaining in the field throughout the winter were assessed for cold hardiness. As of Jan. 1, an estimated 90% of the sprouts for all cultivars were still marketable. During the month of January, the percentage of unmarketable sprouts for 'Prince Marvel', 'Dolmic', and 'Royal Marvel' increased as the outer leaves began to yellow. On two occasions in mid-January, temperatures dropped below –10°C. This resulted in freeze damage to exposed sprouts near the bottom of all plants that had dropped their lower leaves. Sprouts protected by foliage near the top of the plant were not damaged. In early February, plants were exposed to –12°C. The exposed sprouts received more damage, but surprisingly, many of the sprouts protected by foliage sustained only minor damage. In mid-February, most plants began to decline, and few marketable sprouts remained after this date. The winter of 1990–91 was uncharacteristically mild, and the Brussels sprout harvest period could be significantly reduced in other years with colder winters.

The sprouts of some cultivars are very difficult to remove from the plant by hand. Large scale production is extremely tedious and time consuming without mechanical harvesting equipment. Intact stalks can be cut at soil level and fed through a sprout stripper which removes the sprout from the stalk. Multitrade Inc. (P.O. Box 58, 1610 AB Bovenkarspel, the Netherlands) markets a sprout stripper that attaches to a tractor's three-point hitch and runs off power takeoff. The Multitrade Brussels sprout stripper sells for $4,352, including shipping charges from the Netherlands. More sophisticated and expensive harvesters are made by Mali-Ploeger B.V. of the Netherlands and are distributed in the United States by Agro Gold Inc. (Route 1, P.O. Box 299 B, Homer, IL 62849).

Table 1. Performance of Brussels sprouts cultivars, Blacksburg, Virginia, 1990–1991.

Cultivar (Seed Co.)	Plant height (cm)	No. marketable sprouts/plant	Marketable weight (g) Sprouts/plant	Marketable weight (g) Sprout	Sprout dimensions (mm ±SE)	Comments
Boxer (Seedway)	47.1	46.1	283	6.1	30.2±0.8 × 22.5±0.5	Light green, solid sprouts were produced on tall, late maturing plants. Sprout quality was high, but plants were not highly productive. Matured 125 days after transplanting. Very difficult to hand harvest.
Dolmic (Royal Sluis)	35.6	35.0	324	9.3	36.4±0.5 × 26.2±0.7	Small plants produced large sprouts that were not solid. Matured 115 days after transplanting. Very difficult to hand harvest.
Golfer (Seedway)	47.3	33.8	331	9.8	35.5±0.6 × 29.4±0.3	Sprouts were large, light green, and lacked uniformity. Some sprouts were large and not solid. Sprouts held well on the plant and were easily hand harvested.
Lunet (Royal Sluis)	37.6	40.6	232	5.7±0.2	27.9±0.2 × 22.4±0.3	Very attractive small, dark green, solid sprouts were produced on short plants. Sprout quality was very high but productivity was low. Late maturing sprouts held well in the field and tolerated cold weather.
Pilar (Royal Sluis)	39.4	46.7	348	7.4	32.9±0.7 × 24.7±0.6	Large, light green sprouts were produced on medium sized plants. Plants were very productive. Sprout quality was somewhat lacking, because the sprouts were not solid. Matured 125 days after transplanting. Easy to hand harvest.
Prince Marvel (Sakata)	36.6	45.9	324	7.1	32.4±0.7 × 25.9±0.3	Small sprouts were produced on compact plants. Both plants and sprouts have distinct red leaf veins. Sprouts near the top of the plant developed slowly. Suitable for hand harvest 180 days after transplanting.
Rider (Seedway)	38.6	39.7	308	7.7	32.7±0.5 × 26.5±0.6	Sprout size was variable. Many sprouts were large but not solid. Sprouts held well in the field. Suitable for hand harvest.
RS88032 (Royal Sluis)	49.9	38.4	258	6.7	30.3±1.0 × 29.4±0.3	Very large late maturing plants. Later harvests in mid-Dec. produced yields in excess of 300 g per plant. Performed well under cool conditions and held well in the field. High quality, uniform sprouts were light green in color. Difficult to hand harvest.
Royal Marvel (Sakata)	38.1	49.1	358	7.1	32.7±0.3 × 23.8±0.4	Similar to 'Prince Marvel'. Short compact plants produced uniform, high quality sprouts. Easily hand harvested 115 days after transplanting.
LSD .05	2.3	3.7	22	1.1		

CONCLUSIONS

Brussels sprouts are more cold hardy than the other alternative vegetable crops being considered for Virginia, thus permitting commercial vegetable production to continue into December. In this study, 'Royal Marvel' was particularly impressive, because it combined good sprout quality with high yields. More information is needed on the market potential of Brussels sprouts before this crop can be recommended to growers. A suitable mechanical harvester is necessary for efficient, large scale production of Brussels sprouts.

REFERENCES

Anon. 1990. Commercial vegetable production recommendations, Virginia, Virginia Cooperative Extension Service, Pub. 456–420.

Lorenz, O.A. and D.N. Maynard. 1988. Knott's handbook for vegetable growers. 3rd ed. Wiley-Interscience, New York.

Vavrina, C.S. 1988. Vegetables on increase in region. Southwest Farm Press. April 20.

Fennel: A New Specialty Vegetable for the Fresh Market*

Mario R. Morales, Denys J. Charles, and James E. Simon

Finocchio or Florence fennel (*Foeniculum vulgare* Mill. ssp. *vulgare* var. *azoricum* Mill. Thell, Apiaceae), is being marketed as "anise" in supermarkets throughout the United States. While many cultivars of fennel are grown for the aromatic seed and foliage, finocchio fennel is produced for the enlarged bulb (thickened leaf bases) (Simon et al. 1984). The bulbs are becoming increasingly popular as an specialty vegetable where the bulbs are either consumed raw or prepared by baking, blanching, or boiling. The bulbs are sold as "anise" because of the strong "licorice" or "anise" aroma. Increased consumption and demand for the fresh product offers expanded opportunities for American growers yet very little information is available for potential producers on production or varietal selection (Morales et al. 1991). Fennel, a perennial herb grown as an annual, has a tendency to bolt, a periodic problem with the splitting of the bulb and formation of excessive side shoots within the bulb. Yet, high quality bulbs should be firm, white, sweet, and whole with a minimum diameter of not less than 5 cm (Seelig 1974). The objective of this project was to evaluate fennel cultivars for yield and quality.

METHODOLOGY

Commercial seed of ten fennel cultivars was sown on Apr. 4 of 1990 and 1991. Seedlings were grown in a greenhouse for 38 days and then transplanted to the field onto raised beds on May 11 in 1990 and May 14 in 1991. The experiment was planted in a completely randomized block design with three replications consisting of single row plots. Rows were 1 m apart, 15 cm between plants and 27 plants/plot in 1990 and, 10 cm between plants and 15 plants/plot in 1991. Plants (Fig. 1) were harvested on July 17 in 1990 and Aug. 2 in 1991. In late May and June of 1991, black swallowtail caterpillars (*Pappio* sp.) were observed feeding on the leaves of the young transplants and manually removed from the plants. The middle 13 plants from each plot were harvested and the roots from each plant discarded. Five representative bulbs per plot were selected for qualitative evaluation of quality and visual appearance (Fig. 2).

---

*Journal Paper No. 13,211, Purdue Univ. Agr. Expt. Sta., West Lafayette, IN 47907-1165. This research was supported in part by grants from the Indiana Business Modernization and Technology Corporation, Indianapolis, and the Purdue University Agricultural Experiment Station (Specialty Crops Grant No. 014-1165-0000-65178). We thank Tom DeBaggio and Jules Janick for providing us with some of the Italian germplasm.

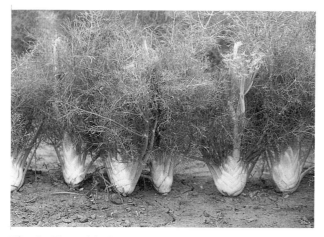

Fig. 1. Finocchio fennel plants growing in central Indiana.

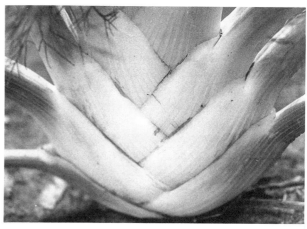

Fig. 2. Close-up of finocchio fennel 'bulb' cv. Zefa fino, comprised of thickened leaf bases formed at the base of the plant.

Table 1. Foliage and bulb means per plant of ten finocchio fennel cultivars grown in central Indiana for two growing seasons, 1990–1991.

Cultivar	Seed source	Foliage weight (g/plant)	Bulb Characteristics			
			Weight (g)	Length (cm)	Width (cm)	Circumference (cm)
Zefa fino	RS[z]	111	75a[y]	14.1a	9.8a	10.8a
Zefa fino	JS	106	74a	13.8a	10.0a	21.5a
Wandenromen	RS	144	58b	14.8a	8.9ab	18.9b
Romano precoce	FM&C	130	58b	14.4a	8.9ab	18.6b
Romanesco, Urbe	SAIS	132	57b	15.1a	8.9ab	18.9b
Grossissimo mammuth	FM&C	135	54bc	14.7a	8.8ab	18.5bc
Romagna	SAIS	134	48bc	14.2a	8.3bc	17.5bcd
Parma, Fucino	SAIS	113	45bc	14.3a	7.6c	16.7cd
Florence	CP	132	42c	13.8a	7.9bc	16.6d
Mantovano	SAIS	116	41c	12.2b	8.1bc	17.6bcd
Grand mean		125	55	14.1	8.7	18.5
CV		22	20	8.5	10.5	7.7

[z]Seed sources were RS = Royal Sluis, Holland; JS = Johnny's Selected Seeds, Albion, Maine; SAIS = Societa Agricola Italiana Sementi, Cesena (FO), Italy; FM&C = Faraone Mennella & Co., Pagani (SA), Italy; C = Companion Plants, Athens, Ohio.

[y]Values followed by same letter are not significantly different at P = 0.05.

RESULTS AND CONCLUSION

Significant variation among cultivars in bulb yield, bulb dimensions, days to 50% bolting, plant height, and number of side shoots was observed (Table 1, 2). The cultivar 'Zefa fino', from Royal Sluis and Johnny's Seed Company, was the highest in bulb weight, the lowest in foliage yield, and the second lowest in plant height, indicating an increased allocation of carbohydrates into the bulbs rather than to the foliage. 'Zefa fino' had significantly greater bulb circumference than the other cultivars (Table 1). Disease and insect damage to the bulbs was minimal and not different among cultivars (Table 2). Bulb width and circumference were correlated with bulb weight (Table 3).

Table 2. Characteristics of ten finocchio fennel cultivars grown in central Indiana, 1991.

Cultivar	Seed source	Days to 50% bolting	Plant height (cm)	Disease[x] damage	Insect[x] damage	No. side shoots
Zefa fino	RS[y]	114a[z]	41cd	1.3ab	0.0	5.1b
Zefa fino	JS	116a	42cd	1.1ab	0.3	5.1b
Wandenromen	RS	103bcd	52a	1.1ab	0.0	7.2a
Romano precoce	FM&C	107b	48ab	0.8ab	0.0	5.5ab
Romanesco, Urbe	SAIS	106bc	49a	1.1ab	0.2	6.0ab
Grossissimo mammuth	FM&C	106bc	50a	0.7b	0.0	5.6ab
Romagna	SAIS	102bcd	49a	1.1ab	0.2	6.7ab
Parma, Fucino	SAIS	101cd	45bc	1.2ab	0.2	5.1b
Florence	CP	100d	53a	0.8ab	0.2	6.3ab
Mantovano	SAIS	100d	40d	1.7a	0.0	5.6ab
Grand mean		105.5	47	1.1	0.1	5.8
cv		2.7	4			17.3

[x]Based on visual estimation of damage rating scale from 0 (no damage) to 5 (severe damage).
[y]Seed sources were RS = Royal Sluis, Holland; JS = Johnny's Selected Seeds, Albion, Maine; SAIS = Societa Agricola Italiana Sementi, Cesena (FO), Italy; FM&C = Faraone Mennella & Co., Pagani (SA), Italy; CP = Companion Plants, Athens, Ohio.
[z]Values followed by same letter are not significantly different at P = 0.05.

Table 3. Correlations of plant characteristics from ten finocchio fennel cultivars grown in 1990 and 1991.

Traits	Bulb wt.	Bulb length	Bulb width	circumference	Bulb 50% bolting[z]	Days to Plant height[z]
Foliage weight	0.48**	0.18	0.58**	0.60**	–0.29	0.36
Bulb weight		0.24	0.70**	0.84**	0.46**	0.04
Bulb length			0.23	0.22	–0.01	0.22
Bulb width				0.92**	0.47**	0.02
Bulb circumference					0.54**	–0.16
Days to 50% bolting						–0.36

*, ** Significance different from zero at P = 0.05 and 0.01, respectively.
[z]Data from only 1991.

'Zefa fino' also showed significant differences from the other cultivars in days to 50% bolting. The later maturity of this cultivar is highly desirable because a longer vegetative period permits the plant to produce larger and heavier bulbs. 'Zefa fino' had the lowest number of side shoots on the bulbs, an undesirable genetic trait among some cultivars.

The time from sowing in the greenhouse to harvest was 104 days in 1990 and 120 days in 1991; time from field transplanting to harvest was 67 days in 1990 and 80 days in 1991. Average growing season of direct seeded fennel in California ranges from 110 to 125 days (Seelig 1974). 'Zefa fino' had the greatest bulb weight and circumference. Because the width and thickness of finocchio fennel bulbs continues to increase over time (Suhonen and Kokkonen 1990), the determination of the optimum harvest period is difficult. While bulbs from all cultivars met the minimum requirement for bulb size (Seelig 1974), significant differences in visual appearance and shape suggests that genotype is very important in bulb quality. The most attractive appearance among the cultivars evaluated was 'Zefa fino', whose bulbs were white, firm, highly aromatic with no visual discolorations.

REFERENCES

Ahmed, A., A.A. Farooqi, and K.M. Bojappa. 1988. Effect of nutrients and spacings on growth, yield and essential oil content in fennel (*Foeniculum vulgare* Mill.). Indian Perfumer 32(4):301–305.

Morales, M., D. Charles, and J. Simon. 1991. Cultivation of finocchio fennel. Herb, spice, and medicinal plant digest. Coop. Ext. Serv. Univ. of Massachusetts, Amherst 9(1):1–4.

Seelig, R.A. 1974. Anise. Fruit and vegetable facts and pointers. United Fresh Fruit & Veg. Assoc., Alexandria, VA.

Simon, J.E., A.F. Chadwick, and L.E. Craker. 1984. Herbs: An indexed bibliography 1971–1980; the scientific literature on selected herbs, and aromatic and medicinal plants of the temperate zone. Archon Books, Hamden, CT.

Suhonen, I. and L. Kokkonen. 1990. The effect of planting date on growth, seed stalk development and yield of sweet fennel. J. Agr. Sci. Finland 62:237–244.

Essential Oil Content and Chemical Composition of Finocchio Fennel*

Denys J. Charles, Mario R. Morales, and James E. Simon

Finnochio or Florence fennel (*Foeniculum vulgare* Mill. subsp. *vulgare* var. *azoricum* Mill. Thell, Apiaceae), develops an edible bulb, a thickened base of leaves, which is becoming increasingly popular as a specialty vegetable in the United States (Simon 1990). Marketed for many years in Europe, the bulbs are either consumed fresh, or prepared by baking, blanching, or boiling. In the United States, the bulbs are marketed as "anise" because of the high concentration of anethole and methyl chavicol (estragole), components in the essential oil responsible for the anise aroma.

Finocchio fennel is closely related to sweet and bitter fennel commercially produced for either the seed, which is used as a spice, or the essential oil extracted from the seed. The essential oil of sweet fennel is used in cosmetics, pharmaceuticals, perfumery, and as a food additive. Extensive research has been conducted on the chemical composition of volatile oils of sweet fennel, var. *dulce* (Karlsen et al. 1969; Tsvetkov 1970; Ashraf and Bhatty 1975; Ravid et al. 1983; Akgul 1986; Katsiotis 1988); and bitter fennel, var. *vulgare* (Rothbacher and Kraus 1970; Trenkle 1972; Kraus and Hammerschmidt 1980; Arslan et al. 1989).

Karlsen et al. (1969) reported the major constituents of sweet fennel (var. *dulce*) and bitter fennel (var. *vulgare*) to include anethole, estragole, and fenchone plus an additional 18 compounds extracted in the monoterpene fraction of the fruit. The minor constituents accounted for 1 to 5% of the total oil of the volatile oil and included: α–pinene, camphene, ß–pinene, α–phellandrene, myrcene, limonene, ß–phellandrene, γ–terpinene, *cis*-ocimene, terpinolene, and p-cymene (listed in order of elution). Significant differences in oil composition between var. *dulce* and *vulgare* were noted (Karlsen et al. 1969). Katsiotis (1988) reported that the major oil constituent of sweet fennel fruit was *trans*-anethole (>83%), followed by relative minor amounts of estragole, fenchone, p-anisaldehyde and limonene (at relative concentrations from <1 to <5%) with only minor amounts of *cis*-anethole (<1.0%). The degree of comminution rather than the hydrodistillation period or distillation rate was found to influence the oil composition of sweet fennel fruit (Katsiotis 1988). Seed oil composition was reported to be influenced by growing region (Arslan et al. 1989).

Despite the extensive information on sweet and bitter fennel, little information is available on the chemical composition of finocchio fennel and the differences, if any, between the bulbs and the foliage which can be

---

*Journal Paper No. 13,178, Purdue Univ. Agr. Expt. Sta., West Lafayette, IN 47907-1165. This research was supported in part by grants from the Indiana Business Modernization and Technology Corporation, Indianapolis and the Purdue University Agricultural Experiment Station (Specialty Crops Grant No. 014-1165-0000-65178).

marketed separately in the fresh green form. Here, we report the chemical composition of the volatile oils from the bulbs of 16 commercially available cultivars of Finnochio fennel.

METHODOLOGY

Seeds from 16 cultivars of finocchio fennel were sown in the greenhouse at Purdue University on 4 Apr., and transplanted into the field at the O'Neall Vegetable Memorial Research Farm (Lafayette, Indiana) on 11 May. A preplant application of nitrogen (112 kg/ha) was applied prior to transplanting. The soil, an Oakley loam with a neutral soil pH, was prepared in raised beds (15 cm in height). Overhead irrigation was applied as needed.

Plants were placed into a randomized block design with three replications consisting of single row plots (3 m length, rows 1 m apart, plants 9 cm apart). A single harvest (July 17) was taken after all cultivars had begun to flower. Essential oils from the bulbs and foliage were extracted by hydrodistillation (1 h) with a modified clevenger trap (Charles and Simon 1990). The essential oil content was determined on a volume to fresh weight basis. Essential oil constituents were identified on the basis of retention time and coinjection with authentic compounds using a Varian 3700 gas chromatograph (GC) equipped with FID and an electronic 4270 integrator. A fused silica capillary column (12 m × 0.2 mm i.d) with an OV 101 (Varian, polydimethylsiloxane) bonded phase was used. Direct injection of 0.5 µl samples with He as a carrier gas and oven temperature held isothermal at 80°C for 2 min, and then programmed to increase at 3°C/min, to 160°C gave complete elution of all peaks (sensitivity 1010; attenuation 16). The injector and detector temperatures were 180° and 300°C, respectively. Identification of all compounds were verified by analyzing both standards (α-pinene, myrcene, limonene, γ-terpinene, fenchone, methyl chavicol, fenchyl acetate, and anethole) and essential oil samples by GC/mass spectroscopy as previously described (Simon and Quinn 1988; Charles et al. 1990). The mass spectroscopy conditions were as follows: ionization voltage, 70 eV; emission current, 40 uA; scan rate, 1 scan/s, mass range, 40 to 500 Da; ion source temperature, 160°C.

RESULTS AND DISCUSSION

No significant differences were observed in the essential oil content extracted from the bulbs and foliage of the different cultivars. The content of essential oil from the bulbs and foliage of different cultivars averaged 0.05% (volume/fresh weight). Essential oil yield from bulbs and foliage is very low compared to the oil yield reported (Embong et al. 1977) from sweet and bitter fennel fruit (2 to 6%).

The major essential oil constituents in the bulbs of finocchio fennel were anethole and limonene, comprising >80% of the oil (Table 1). In most cultivars, anethole was higher than limonene, except in 'Zefa fino' and 'Mantovano' where limonene was higher. Other chemical constituents in the bulb oil included α-pinene, myrcene, γ-terpinene, fenchone, methyl chavicol, and fenchyl acetate. The composition of essential oil from the foliage was similar to that found in the bulbs but, limonene was always higher than anethole in the foliage (Table 2).

The compounds present in the essential oils obtained from finocchio fennel bulbs and foliage are similar to those reported for sweet and bitter fennel but, the relative percentages of compounds such as anethole and limonene differ. Arslan et al. (1989) reported the percentage of anethole to be 86 to 88% in sweet fennel oil and 74% in bitter fennel oil while limonene was only 4 and 2% respectively in sweet and bitter fennel oil. Embong et al. (1977) working with *Foeniculum vulgare* var. *dulce* reported anethole as 69% in fruit oil and 39% in herb oil, the relative percentage of limonene being 8 and 20% in the fruit and herb oil. Finnochio fennel appears to contain lower anethole and higher limonene concentrations compared to sweet fennel and bitter fennel oil extracted from seeds and fruit. The bulbs and foliage of finocchio fennel also contain relatively higher concentrations of fenchyl acetate compared to the fruit of sweet fennel. This finocchio fennel oil could be designated as limonene-enriched, as suggested by Toth (1967) rather than a sweet or bitter oil.

While finocchio fennel bulbs contain higher concentrations of anethole, than that reported from sweet fennel foliage (Embong et al. 1977), the foliage of finocchio fennel is also highly aromatic. As foliage of sweet fennel is marketed as a fresh herb, called fennel weed or fennel herb, the possibility of marketing both the bulb and the fresh-cut foliage from the same plant of finocchio fennel remains an intriguing yet unexplored possibility.

Table 1. Major essential oil constituents in the bulbs of finocchio fennel 1990.

Cultivar	Essential oil constituents[z] (% total essential oil)							
	α-Pinene	Myrcene	Limonene	γ-Terpinene	Fenchone	Methyl chavicol[y]	Fenchyl acetate	Anethole
Cristallino Bianco	1.16	0.96	40.64	0.82	0.50	1.45	2.78	48.51
Firenze grosso dolce	1.41	1.05	39.03	1.30	0.78	1.35	4.59	42.90
Firenze tondo	1.27	1.00	37.90	0.83	0.23	1.42	5.60	48.31
Florence	1.19	0.91	40.69	1.09	0.29	1.43	4.80	45.60
Grossissimo Mammuth	0.92	0.83	33.92	1.18	0.51	1.48	3.55	50.38
Mantovano	0.51	0.74	53.95	3.36	0.00	0.82	4.61	28.92
Napoli gigante	1.16	0.95	34.62	1.32	0.67	1.74	4.91	51.16
Napoli tardivo	0.83	0.96	35.51	0.74	0.39	1.54	7.89	48.70
Parma sel. Fucino	1.50	1.08	37.96	1.62	0.15	1.45	5.08	47.80
Perfezione tondo	0.92	0.86	30.94	0.77	0.37	1.64	2.44	55.69
Romagna	2.26	1.13	34.22	1.56	0.34	1.43	6.08	47.34
Romanesco sel Urbe	1.12	0.89	41.18	0.98	0.12	1.44	4.37	46.99
Romano precoce	1.38	1.19	36.94	0.77	0.61	1.52	4.74	48.13
Sicilia grosso	1.18	1.15	42.96	0.97	0.72	1.42	3.71	45.37
Wadenromen	1.59	1.12	42.95	0.93	0.67	1.45	3.76	44.96
Wadenromen grosso	1.15	1.02	38.82	1.60	0.47	1.46	3.31	47.79
Zefa fino	0.56	0.79	41.81	1.92	0.16	1.28	4.36	43.08
Zefa fino	1.22	1.05	46.60	2.01	0.41	1.21	5.00	37.14

[z]Data based on three replications of 5 bulbs/replication.
[y]Also called estragole.

Table 2. Major essential oil constituents of the foliage of finocchio fennel, 1990.

Cultivar (source)	Essential oil constituents[z] (% total essential oil±SD)							
	α-Pinene	Myrcene	Limonene	γ-Terpinene	Fenchone	Methyl chavicol[y]	Fenchyl acetate	Anethole
Grossissimo Mammuth (FM&C)[x]	1.62±1.0	1.34±0.12	66.1±2.7	0.66±0.26	0.6±0.2	0.9±0.11	1.8±0.4	24.8±3.3
Mantovano (SAIS)	0.73±0.42	0.98±0.14	63.6±4.6	0.97±0.24	0.2±0.16	1.1±0.12	2.6±0.7	25.5±5.9
Zefa Fino (JS)	0.97±0.62	0.94±0.10	62.7±2.8	0.14±0.2	0.3±0.23	1.1±0.27	2.8±0.9	28.1±12.7

[z]Listed from left to right in order of elution.
[y]Also called estragole.
[x]FM&C = Faraone Mennella & Co.; SAIS = Societa Agricola Italiana Sementi; JS = Johnny's Selected Seeds.

REFERENCES

Akgul, A. 1986. Studies on the essential oils from Turkish fennel seeds (*Foeniculum vulgare* M. var. *dulce*). Prog. in Essential Oil Res. Walter de Gruyter & Co., Berlin. p. 487–489.

Arslan, N., A. Bayrak, and A. Akgul. 1989. The yield and components of essential oil in fennels of different origin (*Foeniculum vulgare* Mill.) grown in Ankara conditions. Herba Hungarica 28(3):27–31.

Ashraf, M. and M.K. Bhatty. 1975. Studies on the essential oils of the Pakistani species of the family Umbelliferae, Part II. *Foeniculum vulgare* M. (Fennel) seed oil. Pakistan J. Sci. Ind. Res. 18:236–240.

Charles, D.J. and J.E. Simon. 1990. Comparison of extraction methods for the rapid determination of essential oil content and composition of basil (*Ocimum* spp.). J. Amer. Soc. Hort. Sci. 115:458–462.

Charles, D.J., J.E. Simon, and K.V. Wood. 1990. Essential oil constituents of *Ocimum micranthum* Willd. J. Agr. Food Chem. 38:120–122.

Embong, M.B., D. Hadziyer, and S. Molnar. 1977. Essential oils from spices grown in Alberta. Fennel oil (*Foeniculum vulgare* var. *dulce*). Can. J. Plant Sci. 57:829–837.

Karlsen, J., A. Baerheim Svendsen, B. Chingova, and G. Zolotovitch. 1969. Studies on the fruits of *Foeniculum* species and their essential oil. Planta Med. 17:281–293.

Katsiotis, S.T. 1988. Study of different parameters influencing the composition of hydrodistilled sweet fennel oil. Flavour Fragrance J. 4:221–224.

Kraus, A. and F.-J. Hammerschmidt. 1980. An investigation of fennel oils. DRAGOCO-Report 27(2):31.

Ravid, U., E. Putievsky, and N. Snir. 1983. The volatile components of oleoresins and the essential oils of *Foeniculum vulgare* in Israel. J. Nat. Prod. 46:848–851.

Rothbacher, H. and A. Kraus. 1970. Terpenkohlenwasserstoffe in rumanischem Fenchelol. Pharmazie 25:566–567.

Simon, J.E. and J. Quinn. 1988. Characterization of essential oil of parsley. J. Agr. Food Chem. 36:467–472.

Simon, J.E. 1990. Essential oils and culinary herbs, p. 472–483. In: J. Janick and J.E. Simon (eds.). Advances in new crops. Timber Press, Portland, OR.

Toth, L. 1967. Untersuchungen uber das atherische Ol von Foeniculum vulgare II. Veranderungen der verschiedenen Fenchelole vor und nach der Ernte. Planta Med. 15:371–389.

Trenkle, K. 1972. Neuere Untersuchungen an Fenchel (*Foeniculum vulgare*, M.) II. Das atherische Ol von Frucht, Kraut und Wurzel fruktifizierenden Pflanzen. Pharmazie 27:319–324.

Tsvetkov, R. 1970. Study on the fruit quality of some umbelliferous essential oil plants. Planta Med. 18:350–353.

Effect of Nitrogen Nutrition on Roselle

E.G. Rhoden, P. David, and T. Small

Roselle (*Hibiscus sabdariffa* L. Malvaceae) is a short-day annual plant that closely resembles cranberry (*Vaccinium* spp.) in flavor (Morton 1987). Roselle, believed to originate from India where it is cultivated as an annual, is being introduced as a potential new crop for the southern United States; certain types are currently grown in Florida for their edible fruits. The growth pattern is that of an erect, bushy, herbaceous shrub which can grow to heights of 2.4 m. The leaves are borne alternately on the stem with red or green veins and long or short petioles.

In many parts of the world, the leaves are consumed as a green vegetable and the stem is a possible source of pulp for the paper industry. According to Adamson et al. (1975), roselle is the only new crop introduced in the southern United States as a pulp source that shows a high level of resistance to nematodes. Roselle is propagated from seeds and cuttings. Seeds planted for the production of fleshy calyxes are drilled in 1 m × 1 m rows. However, if grown for fiber and pulp, a spacing of 30 to 46 cm × 30 to 46 cm is used to reduce branching. Harvesting fruits may cause latent buds to develop thereby extending the growth period of the plant. This enhanced growth period coupled with higher applications of nitrogen could further increase the dry matter production of the plant, a desirable improvement. However, little information is available on the commercial production of roselle as a pulp crop.

Most crops grown in the southern United States require high rates of nitrogenous fertilizer for optimum yields, but the nutritional requirements of roselle are unknown (Adamson et al. 1979; Panchoo and Rhoden 1990). When roselle is grown for its calyxes, only half the recommended amounts of fertilizer for vegetables is applied. Excessive ammonia encourages vegetative growth and reduces fruit production. Therefore, increasing the rate of nitrogen application coupled with higher planting densities could be a method of utilizing the roselle plant as a pulp and fiber crop. Small and Rhoden (1991) obtained increased dry matter production with increased applications of ammonium nitrate. The objective of this study was to determine the response of roselle to early applications of nitrogenous fertilizer.

METHODOLOGY

A pot experiment was conducted to evaluate roselle plants in the greenhouse at the George Washington Carver Agricultural Experiment Station at Tuskegee University, Alabama. Five seeds were planted in 13 cm diameter polyethylene pot and thinned to one plant per pot two weeks after seedling emergence. The pots were arranged in a complete randomized design with split-plot arrangement of treatments and replicated four times. The growth medium for the experiment was a coarse fritted clay (Moltan Plus Company, Middleton, TN).

Starting at emergence, each pot was supplied with a base solution of 750 ml containing 3.4 g of 20N–8.6P–16.6K fertilizer/liter each week. At six weeks after emergence, all plants continued receiving the base amount of N–P–K fertilizer, while one-third received 250 ml of 20 g ammonium nitrate and another one-third received 250 ml of 40 g/liter solution. Plants showing any visible signs of water stress were supplied with added amounts of deionized distilled water.

Plant height and stem diameter were determined weekly. Each week, plants were harvested and then separated into roots and stems. Plants were oven-dried at 70°C for 72 h to determine dry matter production. The regular macro-Kjeldahl method was used form determining organic nitrogen (AOAC 1984).

RESULTS AND DISCUSSION

Increased nitrogen application did not cause an increase in plant height of roselle. There was no significant increase in dry matter production three weeks after additional nitrogen application. As plants matured, an additional 20 or 40 g of ammonium nitrate/liter gave significant increases in dry matter production and stem diameter (Fig. 1).

Nitrogen application affected root to shoot ratio. Initially, plants receiving only the base amount of nitrogen had root to shoot ratio of 6:1. However, as plants receiving the base amount of nutrients matured, there was a

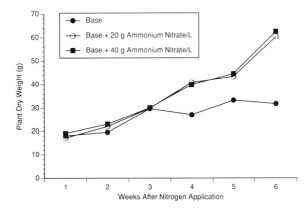
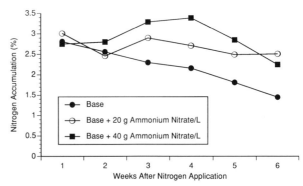

Fig. 1. Effect of nitrogen application on plant dry matter of roselle. Base solution was 3.4 g of 20N–8.6P–16.6K/ liter (750 ml weekly). Additional nitrogen applied to plants 6 weeks after germination at 250 ml of 20 or 40 g ammonium nitrate/liter.

Fig. 2. Effect of application rate on nitrogen accumulation in roselle. Base solution was 3.4 g of 20N–8.6P–16.6K/liter (750 ml weekly). Additional nitrogen applied to plants 6 weeks after germination at 250 ml of 20 or 40 g ammonium nitrate/liter.

decrease in the ratio to 2.5:1. The shoot to root ratio for plants receiving added levels of ammonium nitrate increased from a low of 4:1, one week after initial application, to a high of 6:1 four weeks after additional ammonium nitrate. Nitrogen accumulation increased with increasing amounts of applied nitrogen (Fig 2). Percent nitrogen accumulation decreased with maturity probably due to the dilution effects of increasing dry matter content. This study indicates that roselle responds to nitrogen at the early stages of development. Further studies are needed to quantify nutrient interactions.

REFERENCES

AOAC. 1984. Official methods of analysis. 14th ed. Assoc. of Official Anal. Chem., Washington, DC.

Adamson, W.C., J.A. Martin, and N.A. Minton. 1975. Rotation of kenaf and roselle on lands infected with root-knot nematodes. Plant Dis. Rptr. 59:130–132.

Adamson, W.C., F.L. Long, and M.O. Bagby. 1979. Effect of nitrogen fertilization on yield, composition and quality of kenaf. Agron. J. 71:11–14.

Morton, J.F. 1987. Roselle, p. 281–286. In: C.F. Dowling (ed.). Fruits of warm climates. Media, Inc., Greensboro, NC.

Panchoo, L. and E.G. Rhoden. 1990. Effect of transplant timing and terminal bud removal on sorrel. Caribbean Food Crop Soc. Proc. 26:245–254.

Small, T. and E.G. Rhoden. 1991. Production and nitrogen uptake of rozelle. HortScience 26:738 (Abstr).

Dry Edible Beans: A New Crop Opportunity for the East North Central Region

Glenn H. Sullivan and Lonni R. Davenport

Dry edible bean production in the United States increased from 0.8 million tonnes in 1970 to 1.5 million tonnes in 1990 (Table 1). Production expansion during this period was led by a 21% increase in domestic consumption and a 153% increase in export trade (USDA 1990). The most common commercial classes of dry beans grown in the United States include: small red, kidney, pinto, navy, and great northern (*Phaseolus vulgaris*); small lima (*P. lunatus*); and large lima (*P. limensis*). The largest share of domestic dry edible bean production in 1990 was comprised of pinto and navy beans, with 42 and 20% of total United States production, respectively (Table 2).

The dry bean industry is characterized by high regional concentration in production and processing (Fig. 1). However, production concentration is geographically dislocated from dry bean processing facilities. Dry bean processors are located predominantly in the eastern regions of the United States and Canada, while production expansion between 1970 and 1990 has accrued in the western regions (Table 1). This geographic dislocation between production and processing, combined with changing economic conditions within the industry, has forced dry bean processor to consider strategies for procuring supplies from areas with greater geo-economic relevance to their processing facilities and final demand.

PRODUCTION AND MARKET CONSIDERATIONS

With the exception of Michigan in the East North Central Region (ENCR), dry edible bean production has concentrated in the western regions of the United States (Table 1). Michigan led the nation in dry bean production in 1990, with about 17% of total production; followed by North Dakota and Nebraska with about 15% each. During the period 1970 to 1990, production in the West North Central Region (WNCR) increased 413%, followed by the Mountain Region (MR) at 96% (Table 1). Total dry bean production in the ENCR decreased 11.5% during this period.

Table 1. Dry edible bean production, by state and region.

Region State	1970 Production (tonnes)	1970 Value ($1000)	1980 Production (tonnes)	1980 Value ($1000)	1990 Production (tonnes)	1990 Value[z] ($1000)
East North Central						
Michigan	279,100	59,684	351,631	204,653	246,985	143,204
Mountain						
Colorado	90,630	14,985	105,326	66,641	193,914	120,128
Idaho	89,541	15,595	151,003	94,211	161,482	97,544
Wyoming	23,043	3,861	40,416	24,681	43,772	23,160
Pacific						
California	120,930	31,992	172,958	124,685	140,979	113,442
Washington	29,938	6,006	48,989	29,700	41,368	23,712
West North Central						
North Dakota	18,280	2,660	121,474	66,147	227,027	125,125
Nebraska	70,218	12,384	123,833	73,437	226,981	128,102
Other	67,541	13,165	96,798	53,292	188,471	116,257
United States	789,219	160,332	1,212,427	737,447	1,470,979	906,391

[z]Estimated. Source: NASS/USDA, CED/ERS, TVS-252, November 1990; TVS-253, April 1991; TVS-254, August 1991.

Table 2. Dry edible bean production, by commercial class of bean.

	Production (tonnes)		
Class	1970	1980	1990
Baby Lima	21,682	20,276	24,948
Large Lima	25,311	34,383	20,866
Great Northern	64,865	96,209	128,006
Pinto	244,218	468,705	613,382
Navy	234,965	259,323	299,059
Red Kidney[z]	59,059	79,698	106,777
Other	139,119	253,835	277,603
Total	789,219	1,212,427	1,470,979

[z]Not comparable to previous years, 1990 estimates include both light red and dark red kidneys. Source: NASS/USDA, CED/ERS, TVS-252, November 1990; TVS-253, April 1991; TVS-254, August 1991.

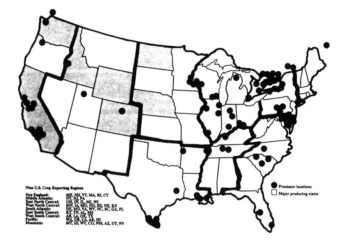

Fig. 1. Dry beans production and processor locations.

Pinto beans comprise the largest volume of any dry bean class produced for human consumption in the United States (Table 2). Total pinto bean production increased 151% between 1970 and 1990, with North Dakota and Colorado accounting for almost half of the crop. Exports and rising domestic demand for ethnic foods have contributed significantly to continued production expansion in pinto beans.

Navy beans accounted for the second largest volume of dry edible bean production in 1990, however, their domestic share of total production has declined (Table 2). This decline resulted primarily from lower export demand in Canada and the United Kingdom since 1980. Michigan's overall decline in dry bean production between 1980 and 1990 was directly attributed to weaker market demand for navy beans. Michigan accounts for over 50% of all navy bean production in the United States.

Food service industry demand in the United States has generated new production opportunities for dry bean classes not previously grown in large quantities, including small red, small white, and pink beans (*P. vulgaris*); blackeye pea (*Vigna unguiculata*); and garbanzo/chickpea (*Cicer arietinum*). Next to pinto beans, these specialty dry bean classes collectively generated the highest rate of domestic production expansion between 1970 and 1990 (Table 2). The small red dry bean class currently exhibits the greatest demand growth, and the greatest potential for production expansion in the ENCR.

ECONOMIC CONSIDERATIONS

Total farm value of dry edible bean production in the United States was estimated at $906 million in 1990; up from $737 million in 1980 (USDA 1991). While producers in the ENCR accounted for only 17% of the farmgate value for all domestic dry bean production in 1990, they are strategically positioned geographically and economically to significantly expand production (Sullivan 1990). Nearly two-thirds of all dry bean processors are located in the eastern regions of the United States, with the largest concentration in the ENCR and Ontario, Canada (Fig. 1). In addition, western dry bean production and transportation costs since 1987 have continued to increase at rates greater than consumer prices, thus encouraging eastern processors to lower costs by developing supply alternatives in closer proximity to their processing operations.

Potential net returns from dry edible beans as an alternative crop favor production expansion in the ENCR (Westcott and Zepp 1989). At current yields, gross receipts of $576/acre ($1,423/ha) are possible. Net returns at this level compete favorably with maize and soybean production under midwestern conditions in most years. Assuming designation by the Secretary of Agriculture under the triple-base statutes of the 1990 Farm Bill, producers in the ENCR could further increase their competitive position. Producers could substitute dry bean crops for a portion of their program area without accruing future crop base penalties. Under this program provision, the breakeven price for dry edible bean production would be consistently lower for ENCR producers than for producers in western regions (Westcott and Zepp 1989). While dry bean prices have been well above $16.50 per hundredweight ($363.66/t) over the last ten years (Table 3), prices at this level would still generate net returns that are competitive with maize in the ENCR. By comparison, dry bean prices would have to consistently exceed $24 per hundredweight ($529/t) to profitably compete with maize production in most western regions. This price level would also encourage the expansion of dry bean imports into the United States.

FUTURE PROSPECTS

Studies conducted by the Purdue Center for New Crops, in cooperation with the Brooks Foods Division of Curtice–Burns, Inc., confirmed that market and production opportunities existed for selected dry bean classes in the ENCR; particularly for the small red bean class. These studies further confirmed that dry edible bean production expansion in the ENCR has not been slowed by economic factors, but rather by lack of cultivars adapted to regional climatic and cultural conditions.

A statewide research and development initiative is geared to expand dry edible bean production in Indiana. The Indiana Business Modernization and Technology Corporation, and the Indiana Commissioner of Agriculture's Value–Added Grants Program provided development grants to help accomplish the objectives of this program initiative. Brooks Foods has provided the industry leadership for developing, testing, multiplying and

Table 3. Average annual grower price by dry edible bean commercial class ($/tonnes).

Class	1981/82	1985/86	1989/90
Great Northern	586.70	595.79	726.54
Pinto	392.93	487.08	893.24
Small Reds	463.93	512.44	737.57
Pinks	397.56	505.61	775.28
Baby Lima	590.49	449.38	742.42
Large Lima	814.09	515.97	949.47
Blackeye Pea	687.30	503.62	686.64
Small Whites	---	451.80	644.96
Lt. Red Kidney	692.15	590.94	947.04
Garbanzo (chickpea)	1,046.27	766.67	795.12
Navy	702.95	409.24	657.53

Source: NASS/USDA, CED/ERS, TVS-252, November 1990; TVS-253, April 1991; TVS-254, August 1991.

commercializing small red bean cultivars that can be adapted to farming conditions in Indiana and the ENCR. Promising cultivar selections were made and multiplied in cooperation with Asgrow Seed Company in 1990 for further field testing in 1991 and 1992. Seed multiplication for limited commercial plantings has been targeted for 1993, with full commercialization by Brooks Foods expected in 1994. Market and economic feasibility assessments indicate that these initiatives could increase dry edible bean production in the ENCR by 37 thousand tonnes annually (Sullivan 1990). This level of expansion translates into nearly 45 thousand acres (18,225 ha) of new production opportunities for growers.

REFERENCES

Bureau of the Census, U.S. Dept. of Commerce. 1987. Census of agriculture, Geographic Area Series, Volume 1, Part 14 and 51.

Michigan State Univ. 1984. Estimated crop and livestock budgets for Michigan. Staff Rpt. #446. Dept. of Agr. Econ., East Lansing.

Sullivan, G.H. 1990. Economic feasibility for producing dry edible beans in Indiana. Report for Indiana Business Modernization and Technology Corp., Indianapolis, IN.

United States Dept. of Agriculture, Economic Research Serv. 1990. Vegetable and specialties situation and outlook yearbook. TVS-252.

United States Dept. of Agriculture, Economic Research Serv. 1991. Vegetable and specialties situation and outlook report. TVS-253.

United States Dept. of Agriculture, Economic Research Serv. 1991. Vegetable and specialties situation and outlook report. TVS-254.

Westcott, P.C. and G. Zepp. 1989. Effects of the triple base proposal on planting decisions for potatoes and dry edible beans. Vegetable and specialties situation and outlook report. USDA/ERS, TVS-248.

Plant Configuration and Population Effects on Yield of Azuki Bean in Washington State

A.N. Hang, D.C. McClary, G.C. Gilliland, and T.A. Lumpkin

Azuki [*Vigna angularis* (Willd.) Ohwi & Ohashi] is an edible legume grown and used for centuries primarily in the East Asian countries of Japan, Korea, China, and Taiwan. Azuki seed is principally used in confectionery products. Seeds are cooked and mixed with varying portions of sugar and other ingredients to produce *an* which is used as pastry filling in traditional Oriental confections (Breene and Hardman 1989). Demand for high quality azuki seed has been well documented since 1960. Only 5% of the demand for azuki can be met by Japanese growers and seeds imported from other Asian countries do not appear to meet Japan's standards for quality. After several years of testing on the sandy soils of central Minnesota (Cox 1978) and our studies on the silt loam soils of central Washington state, we have concluded that azuki can be produced in the United States. Azuki may be an alternative crop that producers can rotate with small grains and alfalfa. There is limited production information in English available to growers or cultivars adapted to central Washington state growing conditions. Selection, testing and best management practices are needed before large hectarages can be committed to azuki production for the export market. The purpose of this study was to evaluate plant population and/or field configuration best suited for commercial production under irrigation for optimum use of land, solar radiation, and field equipment.

METHODOLOGY

The field experiment was conducted at Washington State University's Irrigated Agriculture Research center, Prosser in central Washington which is 46°15'N, 119°45'W and is 275 m in elevation. This site averages

160 frost-free days and 190 mm of precipitation annually, mostly during the winter months. The plot was on a silt loam soil (coarse-silty, mixed, mesic, Xerollic Camborthids) and no fertilizers were added during the growing season because of nutrient carryover N and P of 105 and 54 kg ha^{-1}. A randomized complete block split split plot design was used consisting of 3 blocks or main factors, i.e., plant density of 5, 7.5, and 10 cm apart within row; two subplot factors, i.e., 28 and 56 cm row spacings; and four subsubplot cultivars, i.e., 'Erimo', 'Adzuki Express', 'Hatsune', and 'Takara'. Each subsubplot was 2.3 by 6.1 m. The seed bed was deep plowed (25 to 30 cm) as needed, disked and harrowed before applying trifluralin (α,α,α-trifluoro-2,6-dinitro-N,N-dipropyl-p-toluidine; at a rate of 0.84 kg ha^{-1}) for weed control. Beans were planted 2.5 cm deep on May 17, 1990. Plots were sprinkler irrigated as needed for optimum growth. Aldicarb 10G [2-methyl-2(methylthio)propionaldehyde O-(methylcarbamoyl)oxime] was applied on July 13, 1990 at the rate of 16.8 kg ha^{-1} following dry bean specifications for two spotted-spider mite (*Tetranychus urticae* L.) control. Plots were hand harvested from randomly selected 1.1 by 2.0 m areas and threshed by a stationary combine for yield calculation.

RESULTS AND DISCUSSION

Monthly temperatures in 1990 were cooler than average in May and October and warmer during the rest of the growing season. Because of the cool weather, seedlings did not emerged until 12 days after planting. Like other dry edible beans, azuki requires warm temperatures to germinate and grow. Azuki was also reported to be sensitive to extreme weather conditions (D. Burke pers. commun.). 'Hatsune' was an early maturing cultivar and was harvested a week to 10 days earlier than 'Erimo' and 'Takara'. 'Adzuki Express' is a late maturing cultivar; a large percentage of pods of this cultivar was green when other cultivars were harvested.

'Erimo', a Japanese cultivar responded very well to row spacing between 18 and 56 cm. It yielded best on 56 cm versus 28 cm row spacing. The highest yield for this cultivar was 3,660 kg/ha at 352,360 plants/ha compared to 2,270 kg/ha from treatment 28 cm row spacing by 7.5 cm. Average yields from the 56 cm row plots and across within row spacing treatments were significantly higher than for 28 cm row plots, 3,530 vs 2,570 kg/ha (Table 1). Close spacing within the row changed the structure of 'Erimo'; plants were taller, and internodes were longer. After one year testing, we found that 'Erimo' performed best at 56 cm row spacing, and it outyielded the narrow row spacing by 950 kg/ha. At the 56 cm row spacing, 'Erimo' yielded best when planted 5 cm apart.

'Adzuki Express', an American cultivar, did equally well when grown in either 28 or 56 cm rows. However, highest yield of 3,230 kg/ha was achieved in treatment 28 by 5 cm or 704,720 plants/ha (plant row spacing interaction was significant at P = 0.06). 'Adzuki Express' is a late maturing cultivar; green pods and high bean

Table 1. Plant configuration and density effects on azuki yield at Washington State University, Irrigated Agriculture Research Center, Prosser, 1990.

Spacing (cm)		No. plants/ha (000)	Yield (t/ha)			
Row	Plant		'Erimo'	'Azuki Express'	'Hatsune'	'Takara'
28	5.1	705	2.91	3.23	4.07	3.22
	7.6	470	2.27	2.33	3.01	3.65
	10.2	352	2.54	2.45	3.03	2.82
	Mean		2.57	2.68	3.37	3.23
56	5.1	352	3.66	2.50	2.91	2.86
	7.6	235	3.54	2.98	2.97	3.08
	10.2	176	3.38	2.65	3.32	2.68
	Mean		3.53	2.71	3.07	2.87
Overall Mean			3.05	2.96	3.22	3.05
LSD (0.05)			0.74	0.81	NS	0.65
P: Row spacing			0.01	NS	NS	0.08
Plant spacing			NS	NS	NS	NS
Row × Plant inter.			NS	0.06	NS	NS

moisture were observed at harvest and it may require harvest 10 to 15 days later than 'Erimo'. 'Adzuki Express' had the lowest yield among the 4 cultivars tested.

'Hatsune', an early maturing Japanese cultivar performed best with 28 cm row and produced the highest yield of 4,065 kg/ha at 28 by 5 cm within row spacing (704,720 plants/ha). Average yields of 28 cm row plots were 300 kg/ha higher than those of the 56 cm spacing. 'Hatsune' was the highest yielding among all the tested cultivars.

'Takara', an old Japanese cultivar performed best in 28 cm row versus 56 cm row spacing and yielded 360 kg/ha more beans than those of the 56 cm row plots. Yield of this cultivar was optimum at 3,645 kg/ha with 28 by 7.5 cm (469,814 plants/ha).

We can suggest, on the basis of this first year data, that 'Hatsune' is well adapted to central Washington growing conditions followed by 'Erimo' and 'Takara'. 'Adzuki Express' was the lowest yielding and latest maturing cultivar tested in this location. 'Hatsune' and 'Takara' yield well with 28 cm row spacing while 'Erimo' yielded best at 56 cm row. 'Adzuki Express' did not respond to plant or row spacings tested in this study. Azuki yield in this study was comparable to the other dry edible beans grown in Washington State and was within the range of azuki yield grown in Minnesota (Cox 1978) and in Japan (McClary et al. 1989).

REFERENCES

Breene, B. and L. Hardman. 1989. Anatomy of the specialty crop: The azuki bean experience, p. 1–3. In: BioOptions 1(2). Newsletter of the Center for Alternative Plant and Animal products.

Cox, M. 1978. Minnesota farmers may have found lucrative new crop. Wall Street J. Oct. 5, 1978.

McClary, D.C., T.L. Raney, and T.A. Lumpkin. 1989. Japanese foodmarketing channels: A case study of azuki bean products. IMPACT Inform. Series 29. College of Agr. and Home Econ. Washington State Univ.

University of Minnesota. 1986. Varietal trials of farm crops: Pulse crops. Agr. Expt. Sta., St. Paul, MN.

Herbicides for Azuki Production*

D.C. McClary, A.N. Hang, G.C. Gilliland, J.M. Babcock, T.A. Lumpkin, A.G. Ogg, and L.K. Tanigoshi

Research and limited production of azuki, *Vigna angularis* (Willd.) Ohwi & Ohashi, has been conducted in Washington State since 1987. Farmers reported that several herbicides used commonly in *Phaseolus* spp. bean production were phytotoxic to azuki. Inadequate weed control were also observed in commercial azuki fields and is a limiting factor to commercialization. Greenhouse and field herbicide evaluation studies were initiated to identify herbicides that provide effective control of common eastern Washington weeds and which were not phytotoxic to azuki.

METHODOLOGY

Greenhouse Study

The trial was conducted from Dec. 7, 1988 to Jan. 19, 1989, and consisted of a total of 13 treatments, one pot per replication, four pots per treatment in a completely randomized design. Azuki seeds first were screened for uniformity of size and freedom from mechanical damage and then approximately 500 unblemished seeds of uniform size were imbibed with water for two days to identify those that were hard-seeded. Five imbibed seeds

---

*We acknowledge the IMPACT (International Marketing Program for Agricultural Commodities and Trade) Center, Washington State University, Pullman WA for providing major financial support to conduct this research project and ongoing herbicide evaluation studies.

without radicle protrusion were sown in each 20 cm diameter pot filled with herbicide-treated air-dried Warden silt loam (coarse-silty, mixed, mesic, Xerollic, Camborthid) for the seven preplant treatments; initial planting for five preemergence treatments, the nontreated check and one post emergence treatment were sown into air-dried soil only. The preemergence treatments were incorporated by hand to label specification for depth while the post emergence treatment was applied after the first trifoliates was fully expanded with a CO_2 backpack sprayer calibrated to deliver an equivalent of 252 liters/ha. Pots were maintained in a greenhouse that provided 12 hours of supplemental lighting using 400 watt high pressure sodium vapor bulbs and temperatures of 20°C (day) and 15°C (night). Subirrigation was used until seedling emergence to prevent soil crusting and then pots were irrigated overhead on demand. Fertilized water was applied once a week; pots were randomly rotated twice a week. Dates of individual hypocotyl (damaged and healthy) emergence, final healthy seedling number, plant height, leaf area index, shoot, and root total dry matter weight were recorded. Hypocotyl emergence data per pot was converted into speed of emergence rates using Maguire's (1962) formula Ni/Ti where Ni = ith number of seedlings present (i = 1) and Ti = ith days after planting (i = 1). Rates were then divided by the hypothetically perfect speed of emergence rate of five based on all five azuki seeds per pot germinating and emerging one day after sowing.

Field Studies

Two trials were conducted in 1990, using overhead or rill irrigation, at Prosser, WA (elevation: 300 m; location: 46° 15'N, 119° 50' W) on Warden silt loam. Four preplant incorporated herbicide treatments were tested along with checks in a completely randomized design replicated three times for the overhead irrigation trial; a total of 12 treatments were evaluated under rill irrigation using a randomized complete block design with four replications. Split plots for both trials within each treatment measured 2.3 m wide (four 56 cm rows) by 4.6 m long and were seeded with either 'Erimo' and 'Hatsune', two commercial Japanese azuki cultivars. Treatments were applied to both trials on 22 May, to preirrigated soil at a spray volume of 127 liters/ha and then incorporated to a depth of 7.6 cm. Planting on May 29 was at the rate of 237,000 seeds/ha. Glyphosate was applied preemergence on 8 June, in 127 liters/ha spray volume to four overhead irrigation herbicide treatments. Bentazon was applied on 22 June, to 2 rill trial treatments when first seedling trifoliates were emerging. Approximately 46 cm of total water was available to plants in the overhead trial during the growing season (40 h × 1.42 cm/h × 80% efficiency) while rill irrigation trial azuki had about 31 cm available water (102 cm for seven 36 h set × 30% efficiency). 'Hatsune' was harvested on Sept. 20 and 'Erimo' on 4 Oct.; both cultivars were thrashed on Oct. 10–12 with a Hedge 140 combine. Weekly emergence counts, days to anthesis, qualitative assessments of phytotoxicity and efficacy, the total dry matter weight ratio of azuki-to-weeds, seed yield, and ratio of treatment-to-handweeded check seed yield were recorded.

RESULTS AND DISCUSSION

Greenhouse Study

Azuki treated with chloramben, metolachlor, EPTC + ethalfluralin, and ethalfluralin (0.84 kg ai/ha) emerged faster compared to nontreated plants (Table 1). The checks also had significantly lower emergence percentages than the pendimethalin, ethalfluralin (1.45 kg ai/ha), and chloramben treatments. These results suggest that some herbicides might improve early azuki stand establishment by suppressing soil pathogens. Chloramben, however, caused distortions and enlargements of some seedling hypocotyls. Ethalfluralin (1.45 kg ai/ha), metolachlor + ethalfluralin, EPTC + ethalfluralin, EPTC, and EPTC + trifluralin treatments stunted azuki seedlings as compared to nontreated plants. Metolachlor + ethalfluralin treated azuki had significantly lower root weights as compared to nontreated seedlings. EPTC alone, in combination with ethalfluralin or trifluralin, and the four week post planting application of bentazon reduced azuki growth as compared to the checks. Pendimethalin (1.12 kg ai/ha), imazethepyr (0.053 kg ai/ha), ethalfluralin (0.84 kg ai/ha), and trifluralin (0.84 kg ai/ha) were not phytotoxic to azuki seedlings grown in the greenhouse.

Table 1. Results of greenhouse herbicide treatments on azuki[z].

Treatments	Speed of emergence[y]	No. final plants	Plant height (cm)	Leaf area index (cm^2)	Root weight (g)	Shoot weight (g)
Preplant						
Ethalfluralin (0.84)	0.40ab	4.5abc	21.7abcd	111bcd	0.055ab	0.40a
Ethalfluralin (1.45)	0.36abc	4.8ab	14.5d	98bcd	0.049abc	0.27b
Trifluralin (0.84)	0.37abc	4.0abcd	25.3abc	180a	0.051ab	0.39a
Chloramben (2.52)	0.46a	4.8ab	27.3ab	135abc	0.057a	0.38a
EPTC (3.36)	0.23d	3.0de	1.7e	3e	0.038abcd	0.03c
EPTC (3.36) + Ethalfluralin (0.84)	0.41ab	4.3abcd	2.6e	3e	0.031bcde	0.05c
EPTC (3.36) + Trifluralin (0.84)	0.28bcd	3.0de	0.9e	0e	0.020de	0.01c
Preemergence						
Metolachlor (1.96)	0.41ab	2.5e	18.5cd	85cd	0.025cde	0.22b
Pendimethalin (1.12)	0.34abcd	5.0a	22.9abcd	159ab	0.039abcd	0.42a
Imazethepyr (0.053)	0.37abc	4.5abc	29.6a	160ab	0.060a	0.46a
Metolachlor (1.96) + Ethalfluralin (0.84)	0.22d	2.3e	4.3e	22e	0.001e	0.04c
Pendimethalin (1.12) + Imazethepyr (0.053)	0.31bcd	4.0abcd	19.9bcd	151ab	0.031bcde	0.38a
Post emergence						
Bentazon (1.12)	0.30bcd	3.5bcde	18.5cd	53de	0.025cde	0.19b
Check	0.26cd	3.3cde	23.9abc	139abc	0.044abcd	0.41a

[z]Means within each column following by the same letter are not significantly different by LSD at 0.05.
[y]Speed of emergence per pot divided by the perfect emergence rate of five.

Field Studies

Overhead irrigation herbicide trial. Average azuki seed yields ranged from 211 kg/ha in the nonweeded checks to 3,165 kg/ha for handweeded treatments. Pendimethalin+imazethepyr was significantly less effective in controlling all weeds, especially barnyard grass, *Echinochloa crusgalli* (L.) Beauv., than ethalfluralin+imazethepyr (Table 2). There were no other significant differences among treatments for seedling emergence, days to anthesis, number of harvest plants, phytotoxic effects, the ratio of azuki-to-weed dry matter weights, azuki seed yield, and the ratio of treatment-to-handweeded check yield. The insignificant differences in phytotoxicity and yield between treatments with or without imazethepyr demonstrate that azuki has a high tolerance for this herbicide which was mistakenly applied at a rate ten times the recommended label specifications. 'Erimo' had a significantly higher ratio of treatment-to-handweeded check seed yield than 'Hatsune'; 'Hatsune' produced significantly higher yields than 'Erimo' in the handweeded checks but yield differences between varieties under the four different herbicide treatments were insignificant.

Rill irrigation herbicide trial. Azuki seed yields ranged from 665 kg/ha for the nonweeded checks to 2,203 kg/ha for the handweeded checks. There were significantly fewer plants 5.3 m^2 at harvest in ethalfluralin + imazethepyr and pendimethalin + bentazon treated plots as compared to the handweeded checks (Table 3). There were no significant differences in early season seedling counts among these three treatments suggesting that ethalfluralin + imazethepyr and pendimethalin + entazon caused some seedlings to die from either direct herbicide related phytotoxicity or diseases aided by herbicide damage/stress to seedlings. Both imazethepyr treatments, pendimethalin + imazethepyr, ethalfluralin + imazethepyr, and pendimethalin + bentazon treatments caused excessive azuki injury. Weed control in imazethepyr (0.53 kg ai/ha) and trifluralin plots were significantly less effective than that in handweeded check plots, especially for *E. crusgalli*.

Table 2. Results of herbicide treatments under overhead irrigation on azuki[z].

Treatments[y] (kg ai·ha⁻¹)	Plant number (5.3 m²)	Phytotoxicty rating (%)[x]	Efficacy rating (%)[x]	AzukiTDM/ Weed TDM	Yield (kg/ha)	Treatment/ handwd ck. (kg ai/ha)
Ethalfluralin (1.45) + Glyphosate (0.43)	24a	3.2b	95.3ab	1043ab	3404a	1.14a
Ethalfluralin (1.12) + Imazethepyr (0.35) + Glyphosate (0.43)	21a	38.6a	99.1a	2189a	2378b	0.77b
Pendimethalin (0.84) + Imazethepyr (0.35) + Glyphosate (0.43)	23a	21.5ab	89.9b	3b	2861ab	0.90ab
Trifluralin (0.84) + Imazethepyr (0.35) + Glyphosate (0.43)	18a	6.8ab	97.5ab	34b	3087ab	1.01ab
Handweeded check	26a	---	100a	179ab	3331a	1.00

[z]Means within each column followed by the same letter are not significantly different by LSD at 0.05. Only efficacy data is significantly different using protected LSD procedures requiring an initial analysis of varian (ANOVA) type 1 error probability of less than 0.1.
[y]Ethalfluralin, imazethepyr, pendimethalin, and trifluralin were preplant incorporated; Glyphosate (kg ai·ha⁻¹) with a 5% nonionic surfactant (X-77) was applied preemergent to azuki.
[x]Qualitative analysis of:
 Phytotoxicity: (0% = no crop injury; 100% = complete crop injury).
 Herbicide efficacy: (0% = no weed control; 100% = complete weed control).

Table 3. Results of herbicide treatments under rill irrigation on azuki[z].

Treatments[y] (kg ai·ha⁻¹)	Plant number (5.3 m²)	Phytotoxicty rating (%)[x]	Efficacy rating (%)[x]	AzukiTDM/ Weed TDM	Yield (kg/ha)	Treatment/ handwd ck. (kg ai/ha)
Ethalfluralin (1.45)	14abcde	7c	98.3ab	686b	2333a	1.16a
Ethalfluralin (1.12) +Imazethepyr (0.35)	10.4e	30ab	99.8a	1004ab	1706ab	0.79abc
Ethalfluralin (0.84) +Bentazon (0.84)	17.3ab	17bc	98.7ab	567b	2044a	1.05abc
Imazethepyr (0.53)	16abcd	49a	86.4b	9b	1252b	0.72abc
Imazethepyr (0.35)	12.8cde	33ab	98.4ab	1061ab	1994a	0.98abc
Pendimethalin (1.12)	15abcd	11bc	98.2ab	1196ab	1988a	1.06ab
Pendimethalin (0.84) +Imazethepyr (0.35)	13bcde	33ab	97.4ab	912b	1130b	0.65bc
Pendimethalin (0.84) +Bentazon (0.84)	11.8de	32ab	98.3ab	10b	1230b	0.61c
Trifluralin (0.84)	17.9a	7c	92.9b	753b	2029a	1.07ab
Handweeded check	17abc	---	100a	2801a	2203a	1.00+

[z]Means within each column followed by the same letter are not significantly different by LSD at 0.05.
[y]All herbicides were preplant incorporated except for Bentazon which was applied post emergent.
[x]Qualitative analysis of:
 Phytotoxicity: (0% = no crop injury; 100% = complete crop injury).
 Herbicide efficacy: (0% = no weed control; 100% = complete weed control).

A partitioning of yield with orthogonal contrasts demonstrated that azuki treated with either ethalfluralin or pendimethalin alone yielded significantly better than azuki in which these two herbicides were applied in combination with either imazethepyr or bentazon; azuki treated with either ethalfluralin alone or in combination with imazethepyr or bentazon yielded significantly more than azuki treated with pendimethalin in combination with both of these other herbicides as well as alone. Differences in emergence counts, days from sowing to anthesis, the ratio of azuki-to-weed total dry matter weight and yield ratio of treatments-to-handweeded checks among treatments were not significant at the 5% level. 'Hatsune' had a significantly higher ratio of treatment-to-handweeded check seed yield than 'Erimo' in this trial which is the opposite of the overhead irrigation results; significant varietal differences in water requirements during the growing season might account for this result and is being studied at this time.

Washington State azuki producers can use ethalfluralin (1.46 kg ai/ha), which is registered for use on dry edible beans such as azuki, to minimize phytotoxicity and maximize weed control in azuki production but not in combination with bentazon. The mistaken preplant incorporation of imazthapyra at rates ten times labeled rates without any phytotoxicity suggests that this herbicide has potential for azuki production, but must be field tested first at recommended rates.

REFERENCES

Maguire, J.D. 1962. Speed of germination: Aid in selection and evaluation for seedling emergence and vigor. Crop Sci. 2:176–177.

Range of Yield Components and Phenotypic Correlations in Tepary Beans (*Phaseolus acutifolius*) Under Dryland Conditions

Sathyanarayanaiah Kuruvadi and Isaac Sanchez Valdez

The genus Phaseolus mainly comprises four cultivated species: *P. vulgaris*, *P. coccineus*, *P. acutifolius*, and *P. lunatus* (Smartt 1979). Tepary bean (*P. acutifolius*) is highly resistant to drought (Nabhan and Felger 1978), useful as a source of disease, and drought resistance through interspecific hybridization with the common bean (Thomas et al. 1983). This species is distributed in the arid and semiarid regions namely: Arizona and New Mexico in the United States; and Baja California, Sonora, Chihuahua, Sinaloa, and Durango in Mexico. Seeds contain 23 to 25% proteins and produce higher yields when compared to several legume crops under extreme drought conditions. This legume possesses a broad spectrum of variability for yield and its components and has potential to become a new commercial crop. Tepary bean has not been extensively studied with respect to genetics, breeding, physiology, and agronomy. The objective of this investigation was to study the range of variability of yield and its components and to estimate phenotypic correlations between different pairs of characters.

METHODOLOGY

Sixteen accessions of tepary bean with a broad spectrum of variability were originally collected from five provinces in Mexico: 10 from Sonora (accession number 65, 74, 79, 84, 86, 99, 106, 112, 113, 121); two from Chihuahua (127, 129); and one each from Chiapas (39), Morelos (44), Campeche (49); and accession 46 from Guatemala. Four control cultivars ('Chapingo 24', 'Chapingo 25', PI 231638, and PI 319551) were included for comparison. All lines were seeded in a randomized block design with three replications at the Agricultural Experimental Station, Francisco I. Madero, Durango, Mexico. Each plot consisted of 4 rows, 6 m long, 76 cm between rows and 10 cm between plants within a row. Seeding was done in the first week of July during the monsoon season. Plant growth depended entirely upon natural precipitation and neither fertilizer nor irrigation were applied. The total precipitation received during the crop period was 48.9 cm. A five-plant random sample was taken in the middle two rows in each plot and observations were recorded on biometrical characters.

RESULTS AND DISCUSSION

Significant differences were found in yield, pods/plant, seed/pod, 100 seed weight, plant height, days to flower, and physiological maturity between genotypes revealing considerable genetic variability for these traits. Seed yield varied from 255 to 553 kg/ha with a mean of 387 kg/ha (Table 1). Line 86 produced the maximum grain yield (533 kg/ha) followed by the accession 106 (519 kg/ha). These two genotypes manifested 11.1 and 4.2% higher grain yield over the best check (PI 319551) and also demonstrated drought resistance based on grain yield.

Yield is a product of several yield components including the number of pods/plant, seeds/pod and seed weight. These components are generally the product of sequential development processes (Heinrich et al. 1983). The complex character yield has to be improved by improving the yield components. The number of pods/plant, a very important yield component, ranged from 8.1 to 37.1 among genotypes with a mean of 23.3. This trait showed very wide variation. Line 121 produced the maximum number of pods/plant (37.1) and lines 106, 113, 86, and 84 produced between 29 to 35 pods/plant. Normally pods/plant will have a tendency to increase with environmental improvements.

The number of seed/pod is a very prominent character, influencing yielding ability. This trait ranged from 3.1 to 5.8 with the check cultivar, 'Chapingo 24', recording the highest value. Other promising lines include accession 127, 49, and PI 319551. The variation for 100 seed weight was relatively narrow (10.6 to 12.8 g); accessions 49, 84, 6, 121, and PI 231638 had higher seed weights. Lines 49, 79, 86, 99, 113, and PI 231638 were

Table 1. Mean values for different agronomic characters in tepary beans under dryland conditions.

Accesion number and cultivar	Seed yield (kg/ha)	No. pods per plant	No. seeds per pod	100 seed weight (g)	Plant height (cm)	Days to flower	Days to maturity
39	327	8.1	3.1	11.1	12.9	68.7	110
44	476	9.8	4.4	12.2	14.3	59.3	110
46	337	4.5	3.3	11.0	13.3	68.0	107
49	255	27.7	5.4	14.3	13.1	58.7	94
65	353	21.3	5.2	11.3	13.6	62.3	100
74	369	24.3	5.2	11.3	17.5	63.0	105
79	370	19.1	5.3	10.6	14.0	51.0	95
84	364	28.7	4.7	12.8	18.4	52.3	89
86	553	30.2	4.6	12.7	16.0	49.7	94
99	379	23.5	5.1	11.8	14.8	57.3	96
106	519	35.2	5.1	11.7	18.0	53.7	97
112	350	22.8	5.2	11.9	15.8	58.0	103
113	362	32.9	4.3	12.1	13.7	52.7	93
121	484	37.1	4.5	12.3	14.5	51.0	96
127	334	20.4	5.6	11.6	17.4	62.7	103
129	453	23.0	5.1	11.6	14.9	60.7	103
Chapingo 24	331	22.6	5.8	11.3	13.9	53.3	94
Chapingo 25	296	19.3	5.2	11.2	17.9	60.0	108
PI 231638	338	23.1	5.1	12.5	13.4	51.7	94
PI 319551	498	31.2	5.4	11.9	13.3	53.7	100
Mean	387	23.3	4.8	11.9	15.0	57.6	99
DMS 5%	101	9.3	0.5	1.1	4.2	13.2	13

the earliest in maturity. A combination of desirable traits were not centered in a single genotype but were distributed over several genotypes. Hybridization between genotypes with higher grain yield and superior lines for yield components could result in desirable recombinations in the progeny.

The broad-sense heritability estimates were 0.998 for seed weight, 0.936 for pods/plant, and 0.886 for seeds/pod, indicating that these characters are amenable to selection. Grain yield was highly significant and positively associated with pods/plant and seed weight. Weber and Moorthy (1952) and Johnson et al. (1955) obtained positive and significant correlations between yield and seed weight in soybeans. Kuruvadi and Escobar (1987) observed association between yield and pods/plant in common bean. Selection for pods/plant, seed/pod, and seed weight individually or simultaneously should increase yielding ability of the genotypes provided they are not inversely correlated.

REFERENCES

Heinrich, G.M., C.A. Francis, and J.D. Eastin. 1983. Stability of sorghum yield components across diverse environments. Crop Sci. 23:209–212.

Johnson, H.W., H.F. Robinson, and R.E. Comstock. 1955. Genotypic and phenotypic correlations in soybeans and their implications in selection. Agron. J. 47:477–483.

Kuruvadi, S., and C.M.H. Escobar. 1987. Papel de componentes de rendimiento, correlaciones y sus implicaciones en el mejoramiento genetico de frijol (*P. vulgaris*). Agraria 3(1):1–15.

Nabhan, G.P. and R.S. Felger. 1978. Teparies in southwestern north America. A biogeographical and ethnohistorical study of *P. acutifolius*. Econ. Bot. 32:2–19.

Smartt, J. 1979. Interspecific hybridization in the grain legumes. A review. Econ. Bot. 33:329–337.

Thomas, C.V., R.M. Manshardt, and J.G. Waines. 1983. Teparies as a source of useful traits for improving common beans. Desert Plants 5:43–48.

Weber, C.R. and B.R. Moorthy. 1952. Heritable and nonheritable relationships and variability of oil content and agronomic characters in the F_2 generation of soybean crosses. Agron. J. 44:202–209.

Pigeonpeas: Potential New Crop for the Southeastern United States

Sharad C. Phatak, Ram G. Nadimpalli, Suresh C. Tiwari, and Harbans L. Bhardwaj

Pigeonpea [*Cajanus cajan* (L.) Millsp.] is one of the oldest food crops and ranks fifth in importance among edible legumes of the world (Morton 1976; Salunkhe et al. 1986). Pigeonpea grows well in tropical and subtropical environments extending between 30°N and 30°S latitude with a temperature range of 20° to 40°C (Sinha 1977). It is widely grown in about 14 countries in over 4 million ha. The major producers of pigeonpea in the world includes India, followed by Uganda, Tanzania, Kenya, Malawi, Ethiopia, and Mozambique in Africa; the Dominican Republic, Puerto Rica, and the West Indies in the Caribbean region and Latin America; Burma, Thailand, Indonesia, and the Philippines in Asia; and Australia (Sinha 1977). Several countries in Africa (in the central, western, and southern regions), North America, Central America, and South America have been identified as potential areas for pigeonpea production.

IMPORTANCE AND USES

Pigeonpea is used for food, feed, and fuel. Pigeonpea produces more nitrogen from plant biomass per unit area of land than many other legumes although it usually produces fewer nodules than legumes (Onim 1987). Pigeonpea can fix about 70 kg N/ha per season by symbiosis until the mid-pod-fill stage. This is around 88% of the total nitrogen content of the plant at that stage of growth. The residual effect on a following cereal crop can be as much as 40 kg N/ha (Nene 1987). Rarely does the plant need to be inoculated because it can nodulate on *Rhizobium* naturally present in most soils (Faris 1983). Pigeonpea has been used as a green manure crop. It grows well even in soils with a low phosphorus level. The plant is remarkably hardy to both low temperatures (as low as 5° to 10°C) and high temperatures (up to 40°C) and, thus, is an ideal crop to fit into cropping systems of in many parts of the world (Sinha 1977).

Pigeonpea is normally grown as an annual shrub, but is a perennial in which plants may grow for several years and develop into small trees. It gives additional yield after the first harvest if sufficient moisture is available, and it has great flexibility in a wide range of cropping systems. The crop has a wide range of maturity (80 to 250 days) and time to maturity is greatly affected by temperature and photoperiod. Thus, there exists maturity types of pigeonpea for many different cropping systems. Pigeonpea is a superb intercrop for planting with cereals and other crops. However, short-duration types have been developed in Australia and India that mature in less than 100 days with a yield potential of over 5,000 kg/ha and can be grown as sole crop in multiple cropping systems.

NUTRITIVE VALUE

Pigeonpea is a rich source of proteins, carbohydrates, and certain minerals. The protein content of commonly grown pigeonpea cultivars ranges between 17.9 and 24.3 g/100 g (Salunkhe et al. 1986) for whole grain samples, and between 21.1 and 28.1 g/100 g for split seed. Wild species of pigeonpea have been found to be a very promising source of high-protein and several high-protein genotypes have been developed with a protein content as high as 32.5% (Singh et al. 1990). These high-protein genotypes contain protein content on average by nearly 20% higher than the normal genotypes (Saxena et al. 1987; Reddy et al. 1979). The high-protein genotypes also contain significantly higher (about 25%) sulphur-containing amino acids, namely methionine and cystine (Singh et al. 1990). Pigeonpea seeds contain about 57.3 to 58.7% carbohydrate, 1.2 to 8.1% crude fiber, and 0.6 to 3.8% lipids (Sinha 1977). Pigeonpea is a good source of dietary minerals such as calcium, phosphorus, magnesium, iron, sulphur, and potassium (Table 1). It is also a good source of soluble vitamins, especially thiamin, riboflavin, niacin, and choline (Table 1).

Pigeonpea is most widely eaten in the form of split seeds and used in this way, it contains protein with an amino acid profile similar to that of soybean (Singh et al. 1990). Green pods and green seeds are also consumed as a vegetable. Vegetable pigeonpea types are important in Central America s well as in Western and Eastern Africa, where green peas are consumed as soups, etc. (Morton 1976). Vegetable types, generally large podded

Table 1. Mineral and vitamin contents of pigeonpea (Sinha 1977).

Mineral/vitamin	Range	Mean
Minerals	(mg/100g)	
Calcium	57–276	166.5
Total P	131.8–600	365.9
Phytin P	153–236	194.5
Magnesium	16–300	158
Iron	3.5–16.6	10.1
Sodium	---	28.5
Potassium	---	1104
Copper	---	1.25
Sulfur	---	177
Chlorine	---	5
Vitamins		
Thiamin	0.45–0.80	0.63
Riboflavin	0.13–0.19	0.16
Niacin	2.9–3.22	3.1
Folic acid	---	0.1
Choline	---	18.3
	($\mu g/100g$)	
Carotene	66–132	99

with large, sweet-tasting green seeds are preferred in Puerto Rico. Canned pigeonpeas are marketed in certain parts of the world (Morton 1976).

By-products of split and shrivelled seed are used as livestock feed. The present high cost of animal sources of protein feeds, such as fish and bonemeal, makes pigeonpea ideal to be used as a good plant protein substitute as it is less expensive. Pigeonpea provides an excellent forage for livestock and there is a great scope for selecting cultivars with not only higher grain yields but also higher forage yields and crude protein. It has a high percentage of crude protein (28.2 to 36.7). Pigeonpea stems are used as fuel wood in the energy-short villages of several African countries. Stems are also used for fencing crop fields, and in weaving cribs and baskets. Tall, perennial pigeonpeas are often also used as live fences in Africa and the Caribbean. Pigeonpea is also used in folk medicine in India, Argentina, and Cuba (Morton 1976).

POTENTIAL FOR PRODUCTION IN THE UNITED STATES

The United States National Technical Information Service prepared a report for the U.S. National Science Foundation in 1978, in which the need to introduce pigeonpea into the United States for large-scale production was stressed. Realizing the importance of its market potential and uses, we started evaluating a pigeonpea advanced breeding line that we received from the International Crops Research Institute for Semi-Arid Tropics (ICRISAT) in 1988. Pigeonpeas are a good alternative crop with low fertilizer requirements and with minimum pesticide need. Over sixty breeding lines have been evaluated during the last four years at Tifton, Georgia, and Lorman, Mississippi. Old cultivars with short-day requirements for flowering failed to mature before frost damage in October–November. However, new breeding lines less sensitive (e.g. ICPL 86005, ICPL 8501 etc.) to day length, flowered and produced a crop before frost. We have identified 6 breeding lines (ICPL 86005, ICPL 8501, ICPL 84023, ICPL 85046, ICPL 86015, and UPAS 120) producing over 4,000 kg/ha in 100 to 110 days, compared to the average world yield of pigeonpea of 700 kg/ha. Two or three breeding lines will be named and released in 1992.

REFERENCES

Faris, D.G. 1983. ICRISAT's research on pigeonpea, p. 17–20. In: Grain legumes in Asia. ICRISAT, Patancheru, India.

Morton, J.F. 1976. The pigeon pea (*Cajanus cajan* Millsp.), a high-protein, tropical legume. HortScience 11:11–19.

Nene, Y.L. 1987. Overview of pulses research at ICRISAT, p. 7–12. In: Adaptation of chickpea and pigeonpea to abiotic stresses. ICRISAT, Patancheru, India.

Onim, J.F.M. 1987. Multiple uses of pigeonpea, p. 115–120. In: Research on grain legumes in eastern and central Africa. International Livestock Centre for Africa (ILCA), Addis Ababa, Ethiopia.

Reddy, L.J., J.M. Green, S.S. Bisen, U. Singh, and R. Jambunathan. 1979. Seed protein studies on *Cajanus cajan* L., *Atylosia* spp, and some hybrid derivatives, p. 105–117. In: Seed protein improvement in cereals and grain legumes. vol. 2. IAEA/FAO, Neuherberg.

Salunkhe, D.K., J.K. Chavan, and S.S. Kadam. 1986. Pigeonpea as important food source. CRC Critical Review in Food Sci. and Nutrition 23(2):103–141.

Saxena, K.B., D.G. Faris, and S.C. Gupta. 1986. The potential of early maturing pigeonpea hybrids, p. 290. In: ACIAR Proc. on Legume Crop Improvement. Canberra, Australia.

Saxena, K.B., D.G. Faris, U. Singh, and R.V. Kumar. 1987. Relationship between seed size and protein content in newly developed high protein lines of pigeonpea. Plant Foods Hum. Nutr. 36:335–340.

Singh, U., R. Jambunathan, K.B. Saxena, and N. Subrahmanyam. 1990. Nutritional quality evaluation of newly developed high-protein genotypes of pigeonpea (*Cajanus cajan* L.). J. Sci. Food Agr. 50:201–209.

Sinha S.K. 1977. Food legumes: distribution, adaptability and biology of yield, p. 1–102. In: FAO plant production and protection paper 3. FAO, Rome.

FLORAL AND LANDSCAPE CROPS

New Hybrid Ornithogalums and Orchids

R.J. Griesbach, F. Meyer, and H. Koopowitz

NEW HYBRID ORNITHOGALUMS

A joint breeding program to improve *Ornithogalum* was started in the Spring of 1988 by the United States Department of Agriculture's Florist and Nursery Crops Laboratory of Beltsville, Maryland (USDA) and the University of California at Irvine Arboretum (UCI). The selection of the genus *Ornithogalum*, Liliacea, for a breeding program was based on several factors such as the need for improving the existing cut-flower crop, the need to develop new pot-plant types, and the existence of a large collection of species at UCI. We wanted to extend the color spectrum of the commercial cut flower types, presently only white, to include yellows, oranges, and pastels of these colors. We also wanted to expand the range of growth habits, flowering times, and the arrangement of the flowers on the stem in order to develop both pot-plant cultivars and novel cut-flower types.

Ornithogalum thyrsoides Jacq., the most commonly grown species, is characterized by a tall 20 to 100 cm raceme containing between 10 and 20, 3 to 5 cm flowers. The petals and sepals are nearly white [Royal Horticultural Society (RHS) Color Chart 4D] sometimes with a dark green or brown center which fades with age (Obermeyer 1978). *Ornithogalum thyrsoides* produces a very tight cluster of upright terminal flowers with short pedicels on a strong stem with short internodes between the flowers. Another species, *O. dubium* Houtt. is noted for its bright yellow (RHS 7A) to deep orange (RHS 28A) colored flowers. *Ornithogalum dubium* produces a short 10 to 20 cm raceme, containing between 10 and 20, 2 to 3 cm flowers (Obermeyer 1978). *Ornithogalum dubium* produces an inflorescence with long weak pedicels and long internodes between the flowers.

Our goal was to create interspecific hybrids between *O. dubium* and *O. thyrsoides*. Preliminary experiments suggested that mature seed could not be produced through classical sexual hybridization. In vitro, ovule-rescue was used to obtain seedlings (Meyer et al. 1991).

BREEDING METHODS

Ovaries were harvested 3 to 21 days after pollination (DAP). Between 10 and 14 DAP was optimal for ovule rescue. The seed capsules were surface sterilized in 1.5% NaOCl (30% laundry bleach) for 30 min and the ovules were aseptically removed. The excised ovules were then cultured in vitro. We were able to retrieve plants from ovaries harvested prior to the optimal 10 to 14 DAP, but the percentage of viable plants retrieved was extremely low. The medium consisted of 1/2 strength Murashige & Skoog salt and vitamins (MS) and 30 g/liter of sucrose and 6.5 g/liter of agar adjusted to 5.8 pH prior to autoclaving (Griesbach et al. 1992). After two to three months on this medium, the developing plants were large enough to be removed from culture and acclimated in the greenhouse. Flowering occurred after 6 to 9 months.

Specific clones were propagated via tissue culture (Griesbach et al. 1992). Mature but non-senescent leaves were harvested from plants before flowering and disinfected in 20% bleach for 20 min, rinsed twice in sterile water and cut into 2×1 cm sections. The leaf pieces were placed on a medium containing full strength MS salts, vitamins, and sugar supplemented with 1 mg/liter benzylaminopurine (BA). Within 3 weeks, 5 to 20 bulbous-plantlets developed at the cut surfaces. These plantlets continued to proliferate through off-shoots and were rooted on a hormone-free MS medium.

BREEDING RESULTS

Several hundred seedlings from 40 different crosses flowered (Meyer et al. 1991). Thirty-one of these crosses involved interspecific hybrids. Thirteen of these were F_1 hybrids; 11 were F_1-backcross hybrids; and 7 were F_2 hybrids. Nine intraspecific crosses were produced. Five of these were F_1 hybrids; 3 were F_1-backcross hybrids; and 1 was an F_2 hybrid.

Ornithogalum dubium produced flowers which ranged in color from dark yellow (RHS 7A) to dark orange (RHS 28B). Intraspecific F_1 hybrids were yellow-flowered and F_2 hybrids segregated for yellow and orange colors. No clear segregation patterns could be discerned.

Primary hybrids between *O. thyrsoides* and *O. dubium* produced flowers which were either light yellow (RHS 11C) or light orange (RHS 14D) depending upon the clones used. The gross morphology of the primary hybrids was intermediate between both parents, although the height of the flower stem and flower size tended to approach that of the larger parent. All of the primary hybrids had varying degrees of fertility, which provided the opportunity to generate successive generations.

The F_1 primary hybrids were either sibling crossed to produce an F_2 or back crossed with the highly colored species and hybrids. This effort was aimed at the continued introgression of deep, saturated colors into tall, cut-flower type species. We expected recombination and segregation to introgress both the saturated colors into the tall types and pastel colors into the dwarf types.

Of the over 200 F_2 segregates, no plants were found to have darkly colored or pure white flowers. In fact, the color range of the F_2 generation was very similar to that found in the F_1. However, in backcross hybrids of *O. dubium* to the F_1 primary hybrid, a wide range of colors from nearly white (RHS 4D) to dark orange (RHS 28A) or butter yellow (RHS 24B) were also found. A wide range of inflorescence types were obtained in the backcross hybrids. Tall, intermediate, and short inflorescences were found with either short, intermediate, or long internodes.

PROSPECTS

Several hybrids are now being multiplied in vitro in order to obtain a large quantity of plants for trials as cut flowers or pot plants. Some of these crosses produced 12 flower spikes from 4 to 5 bulbs in a single 10 cm pot. Such studies will also determine whether *Ornithogalum* can be commercially produced as a tissue-culture plug. We anticipate that pot plant *Ornithogalum* will be very successful as new crop and that the orange-colored cut flowered types will greatly expand the currently limited market for this crop.

CURRENT TRENDS IN POT PLANT ORCHIDS

Phalaenopsis hybrids are currently the most popular, pot-plant orchids. Sales at the Dutch Auctions has increased several hundred percent each year over the last few years. Plants are being produced in Europe, the United States, and Southeast Asia. The popularity of these hybrids is due to their short generation time of approximately two years, their ease of growth and flowering and the wide diversity of flowers colors. A new trend in *Phalaenopsis* breeding is in the development of dwarf, multiple flowering types.

Instead of producing a dozen or so 10 cm flowers on a 100 cm inflorescence, these new hybrids produce over 50, smaller 5 cm flowers on 50 cm long, laterally branched inflorescences.

REFERENCES

Griesbach, R.J., F. Meyer, and H. Koopowitz. 1992. Interspecific hybridization in *Ornithogalum*. J. Hered. (in press).

Meyer, F., R.J. Griesbach, and H. Koopowitz. 1991. Inter- and intra-specific hybridization in the genus *Ornithogalum*. Herbertia 46:129-139.

Obermeyer, A. 1978. Ornithogalum: a revision of the southern african species. Bothalea 12:323-376.

New Bedding Plants

Lowell C. Ewart

New floricultural crops have been defined by Roh and Lawson (1990) as "a newly discovered genera or species; newly introduced cultivars of plants grown in earlier years, but forgotten or without complete cultural information; plants that are cultivated in foreign countries but have not been introduced in the United States; or crops that can be produced with new production technologies that can enhance crop quality and shorten the total production time." If this classification is followed, new bedding plants fit the definition of new crops very well.

There has been a renewed interest to bring new bedding crops to market in the last five years. The trend is to introduce new perennial, bulb, and wildflower plants in addition to annuals for the bedding plant and landscape industries. This trend will likely continue well into the next century, especially with bedding plants and garden plants leading all other floriculture crops with a wholesale value of $971 million in 1990 (Agr. Stat. Board 1991). This represents an 8% gain over 1989, and reflects a yearly increase that has remained unbroken for over 10 years.

NEW CROPS FOR CONSIDERATION

The following taxa selections are either under evaluation or have recently been released for bedding plant sales. Additional new bedding plants are listed in Table 1.

Begonia

Begonia MSB-1 is a hybrid derived from inbreds developed from crossing *Begonia* x *semperflorens-cultorum* Hort. with *Begonia schmidtiana* Regel. The purpose was to develop material suitable for hanging basket production from seed rather than from cuttings. The plants grow fast, have a nice spreading, branched habit, and the flower color is a bright red. Evaluations have been excellent.

Canna

Canna x 'Tropical Rose' is an All-America Selections Flower Award Winner for 1992, the first canna ever to receive this award. 'Tropical Rose' is an improved dwarf canna that can be sold as young potted plants from seed sown 6 to 8 weeks prior to selling and which reaches heights of 76 cm (Sutherland 1991). Usually, cannas are grown from rhizomes rather than from seed. The soft rose-colored blooms appear the first of July and continue the rest of the summer in the Midwest.

Table 1. Examples of other new cultivars and species that show potential for bedding plant sales.

Taxa	Comments
Annuals	
Calandrinia x 'Bogota'	Very dwarf, heat tolerant, violet rose color
Centaurea x 'Blue Midget'	Dwarf, free flowering
Gaillardia x 'Red Plume'	Dwarf, heat tolerant, excellent flower production
Gaillardia x 'Yellow Sun'	Dwarf, heat tolerant
Impatiens x 'Spectra'	Dwarf New Guinea-type from seed
Lisianthus x 'Blue Lisa'	Dwarf, deep blue
Nasturtium x 'Tip Top'	Dwarf, in single colors or as a mix
Sanvitalia x 'Double Sprite Yellow'	Double flowers, heat tolerant
Perennials	
Claytonia verginica L.	Wildflower
Dicentra Cucullaria (L.) Bernh.	Wildflower
Lychnis x 'Molten Lava'	Dwarf, deep red
Platycodon x 'Sentimental Blue'	Dwarf, large flowered

Catharanthus

Catharanthus roseus (L.) G. Don still commonly known as vinca, has had several new additions due, in great part, to the work of R.D. Parker of the University of Connecticut. The cultivars 'Parasol' and 'Pretty In Rose' are both 1991 All-America Selections Bedding Plant Award Winners, and 'Pretty in White' is a 1992 All-American Selections Award Winner in this category.

'Parasol' improves on the cultivar 'Little Bright Eye' for flower size and flower quality. The large 4 to 5 cm blooms are pure white with a red center. The blooms have overlapping petals creating a full round flower. 'Parasol' exhibits heat and drought tolerance, and is an excellent landscape subject.

'Pretty in Rose' is a new deep rose, almost purple, color now available for the first time in vinca; whereas, 'Pretty in White' is a beautiful white with a small cream-colored eye. Both of these cultivars bloom all summer long and perform best in full sun. In combination with other annuals, they are perfectly suited to hanging baskets, planters, or patio urns.

These cultivars were derived from species and escaped 'wild' accessions (R.D. Parker pers. commun.). The collection, which began in 1978, contains material principally from Madagascar and Mauritius, but also contains material collected in Brazil, India, Mexico, Portugal, and South Africa.

Craspedia

Craspedia x 'Drumstick' is new to horticultural cultivation. This native from Australia is easily grown from seed. It is a green pack item and blooms approximately 170 days from seeding. The 3 cm globular flowering heads of golden yellow are held atop long, wiry stems about 60 cm tall. The excellent cutting stems rise from compact rosettes of ground level foliage. The flowers have very good durability either fresh or dried.

Gomphrena

Gomphrena x 'Strawberry Field' is the first true strawberry-red red gomphrena and is a beautiful, continuous blooming annual. The 3.5 cm blooms are borne in profusion on 60 cm stems, and they are delightful in bouquets either fresh or dried. It is a green pack item and starts to bloom approximately 90 days from seeding and will bloom all summer.

Hosta

Hosta selection MSH-1 (Fig. 1) was found growing among what appeared to be a variable group of seedlings in an old abandoned garden. The plants are very dwarf, early flowering with 26 cm flower stalks with light purple flowers. The plant silhouette is on the order of *Hosta lancifolia* Engl., but much smaller. The plants, in regular perennial fashion, bloom the second year from seed in early June in the Midwest and are excellent as a rock garden subject.

Iris

Dwarf bearded iris (*Iris pumila* L.) (Fig. 2) are beautiful in the spring and are usually purchased as rhizomes in late summer. They can now be produced as a spring sales, pot plant item (E.J. Holcomb pers. commun.) by storing potted rhizomes at 7°C for 8 weeks. There are many cultivars with various colors that bloom in about 25 days after storage and produce more flowering stalks per pot if the plants are grown under high pressure sodium lighting. These dwarf iris are excellent for rock garden or edging use, blooming in late April to early May. They are best grown in full sun in a well drained location.

Kalanchoe

Kalanchoe MSK-20, a selection developed for hanging basket production, was derived from crossing *Kalanchoe* x 'Jingle Bells' with *Kalanchoe manginii* Hamet. & Perr. B, and can be produced from cuttings or from seed. The plants need 5 weeks of short days to induce flowering. The critical photoperiod is 12 h, but the optimum is 9 h. The habit of the plant is more like *K. Manginii*, only larger. The 2.5 cm long, trumpet shaped, red flowers are borne in profusion on the ends of the branches. The natural flowering time is December through March in the United States.

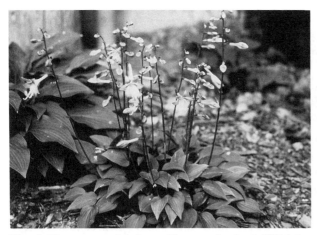

Fig. 1. Three-year-old plant of hosta selection MSH-1 in bloom.

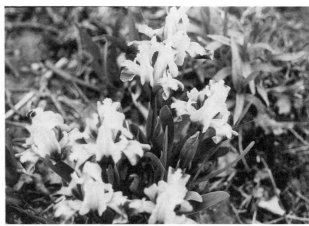

Fig. 2. May flowering selection of *Iris pumila*.

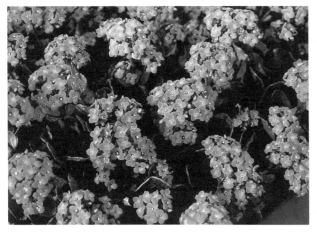

Fig. 3. Kalanchoe selection MSK-1 in bloom from seed.

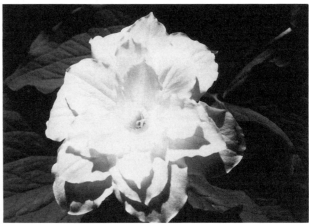

Fig. 4. Double flowering form of *Trillium grandiflorum*.

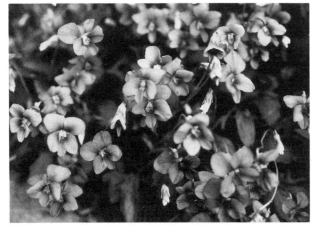

Fig. 5. Violet selection MSV-1 in bloom in early May.

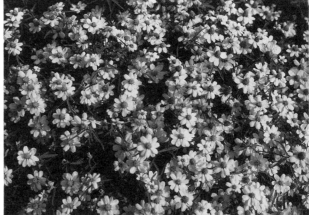

Fig. 6. *Zinnia angustifolia* cultivar 'White Star' in full bloom.

Kalanchoe MSK-1 (Fig. 3), 2, and 4, selections from crosses within *Kalanchoe blossfeldiana* Poelln., are produced from seed and are intended for mass market sales. The plants require short days for flower induction. The colors of MSK-1, 2, and 4 are orange scarlet, hot pink, and apricot-yellow, respectively. The individual flowers have a spread of 17 mm, and the natural flowering time is December through April in the United States.

Rhodohypoxis

Rhodohypoxis bourii (Bak.) Nel., known as the Starlet Flower, is native to South Africa and hardy only into zone 8. Grown from rhizomes, it has been used as a rock garden plant. It is suitable as an attractive spring pot plant, ready for sale 5 to 6 weeks from potting. The flower colors range from white, pale pink to red, and the flowers, each comprising 6 petals, meet at the center with no eye. The slender stems produce a succession of 2 cm flowers. The plants can be enjoyed as a patio subject or planted out in the garden, but should be removed before freezing temperatures are experienced. The rhizomes can reflower after 8 to 10 weeks of storage at 4°C (Bay City Flower Co. pers. commun.). Production of this crop is still somewhat hampered by the limited number of rhizomes available each year.

Salvia

'Lady in Red' salvia, an All-America Selections Flower Award Winner for 1992, is derived from *Salvia coccinea* Juss. ex J. Murr., sometimes called Texas sage. The bright red flowers, which attract humming birds and butterflies, are borne in loose whorls along a spike above the foliage. Mature plant height is 60 cm. 'Lady in Red' can be produced as a flowering bedding plant, using the same culture as for *Salvia splendens* F. Sellow ex Roem. & Schult (Sutherland 1991). Crop time from sowing to initial bloom is about 10 to 12 weeks, and the plants will flower all summer long.

Steirodiscus

Steirodiscus x 'Gold Rush' has a beautiful yellow, daisy-like flower about 2.5 cm in diameter. In full bloom, the flowers cover the entire plant which grows to 12 to 18 cm in height (Hamrick 1989). It is produced from seed and will grow well at 15° to 21°C. The plants, however, require a cool night temperature of 2° to 5°C and 15°C days to flower. Temperatures over 26°C will result in poor growth and shorten the bloom period. In general, the crop time is 12 weeks (American Takii Inc. pers. commun.).

Trillium

A double flowered form of *Trillium grandiflorum* (Michx.) Salisb. ('Flore Pleno') (Fig. 4) is quite rare as a commercial item. The single flowered type at one time was forced as a pot plant, but went out of style. Now, with the renewed interest in wildflowers in the landscape, such items have become popular again. The plants, however, are now protected in some states and cannot be dug from the wild. The double flowering form can be propagated vegetatively, but at a premium price. Potted up during the summer previous to spring sales and stored overwinter, this plant sells itself when in bloom at a garden center outlet. The double flowers have a good 2 to 3 weeks duration time which adds to their value for spring sales. The plants can be enjoyed best, however, if planted as soon as possible into the landscape.

Viola

Violet MSV-1 (Fig. 5) is of hybrid derivation from within the wild *Viola* stemless, blue, cut-leaved group. In the spring, the plants are covered with blue flowers that are held above the foliage forming a beautiful blue carpet. Propagation is by seed or division. Violets are photoperiodic (Mastalerz 1977), producing conspicuous clasmogamous flowers under short day, and inconspicuous clestogamous flowers under long day conditions. It should be possible to keep the plants flowering year-round by manipulating photoperiod and temperature. This should allow sales of flowering plants for landscape use from spring through most of the summer.

Zinnia

The most economic important garden zinnia (*Zinnia elegans* Jacq.) is very susceptible to several leaf diseases. *Zinnia angustifolia* HBK, however, is virtually disease free. Until now only the orange flowered cultivar 'Classic' was available. A new white flowered cultivar 'Star White' (Fig. 6) has been introduced. The single, daisy-like flowers measure about 2.5 cm and appear in mass on plants reaching 35 cm. The plants thrive in hot, dry conditions and carry the same disease resistance found in *Z. angustifolia* (Burpee pers. commun.). The plants bloom all summer and are propagated from seed.

CONCLUSION

The plants highlighted represent an interesting and colorful group of new plants that should find a home in the garden for years to come. They are an example of what new crops can do for increasing the interest of color and diversity in the landscape.

REFERENCES

Agricultural Statistical Board. 1991. Floriculture crops, 1990 Summary. Washington, DC., USDA, NASS. Arp. Sp Cr 6–1 (91).

Hamrick, D. 1989. 1989 International pack trials report. Grower Talks 53(3):32–67.

Mastalerz, J.W. 1977. The greenhouse environment. Wiley, New York.

Roh, M.S. and R.H. Lawson. 1990. New floriculture crops, p. 448–453. In: J. Janick and J.E. Simon (eds.). Advances in new crops. Timber Press, Portland, OR.

Sutherland, L. 1991. AAS winners span the spectrum in fresh, bright colors. Grower Talks 55(2):73–79.

A Program for the Selection and Introduction of New Plants for the Urban Landscape

Bruce Macdonald

The aim of this paper is to outline an innovative plant introduction program through which a university botanical garden in close cooperation with the British Columbia Nursery Trades Association (BCNTA) and the British Columbia Society of Landscape Architects (BCSLA) is able to evaluate, select, and introduce new and improved plant material into the nursery trade and the urban landscape.

DEVELOPING GOALS AND OBJECTIVES

Under the leadership of Roy L. Taylor, then Director of the University of British Columbia Botanical Garden, a 12-member committee was formed in 1980 and included representatives from growers, wholesalers, landscape contractors, and architects, as well as Botanical Garden staff. Initial meetings addressed the needs of a program for innovative plant introduction for urban landscape plants and set the overall objectives of what was subsequently named the Plant Introduction Scheme of the Botanical Garden of the University of British Columbia (PISBG). These needs, justification, and objectives were as follows:

- The BC nursery industry was undergoing considerable expansion. Growers saw the need for BC to develop superior plant material to increase sales into the North American and overseas markets.
- Rapidly increasing housing starts resulted in increased demand from the retail sector. There was a need to encourage greater local production or much of this demand would be met by American and European imports.
- A need for a greater diversity of plant material for residential, municipal, and highway landscapes.
- An opportunity for the Botanical Garden to utilize its collections for the financial benefit of local industry. In doing so, the Garden would cease to be a static "living museum" and become a higher profile, more dynamic member of the horticultural profession.
- To develop and enhance a close liaison between an academic institution, the nursery industry, and the landscape profession, where, traditionally, there had been little communication.

The development of a superior, successful introduction program demanded a close and critical evaluation of past and current programs of other institutions and companies. Assessments of successes and failures, costs and returns, and staff and time requirements led to the committee establishing:

- a model or framework of procedures from initial selection and evaluation to the release and marketing of an introduction (see Fig. 1);
- the criteria for selecting a plant for the program;
- recommended sources of funding to establish the program and ways to provide on-going revenue for its continuation and development;
- innovative ways for the promotion and marketing of new introductions.

FUNDING—GRANT AGENCIES, INDUSTRY, AND ROYALTIES

The committee quickly realized the necessity of "seed funding" to make improvements and additions to the Garden's nursery, to provide additional staff, and to establish an effective marketing and promotional program. Matching funds totalling CDN $300,000 were received from the Devonian Foundation of Calgary, which supported new horticultural projects in Western Canada, and Science Council of British Columbia—the major function for the latter is to fund research and development that directly benefits industry. At the request of the Science Council, a consultant was employed to assess the projected benefit to the nursery industry. Arcus Consulting Ltd. of Vancouver concluded that: "This analysis indicates a program of substantial benefit to the nursery trades industry of British Columbia. Further, the analysis indicates a program capable of generating positive cash flows one year after the first commercial sale of plants provided by the PISBG and within fours years of the commencement of the scheme."

There are two main sources of revenue. Firstly, the sale of stock/mother plants of new introductions to participating nurseries. Secondly, payment of royalties by nurseries propagating PISBG introductions. Each new introduction is registered with the Canadian Ornamental Plant Foundation (COPF) and royalties are paid on a quarterly basis. Royalties range from 4.0 cents to 34.0 cents per cutting or scion bud. COPF retains 10% and 90% is returned to the Botanical Garden for the continuation of the program.

PISBG plants registered with COPF include: *Anagallis monelli* 'Pacific Blue', *Arctostaphylos uva-ursi* 'Vancouver Jade', *Artemisia stelleriana* 'Silver Brocade', *Clematis* 'Blue Ravine', *Genista pilosa* 'Vancouver Gold', *Penstemon fruticosus* 'Purple Haze', *Potentilla fruticosa* 'Yellow Gem', *Ribes sanguineum* 'White Icicle', *Rubus calycinoides* 'Emerald Carpet', *Sorbus hupehensis* 'Pink Pagoda', and *Viburnum plicatum* 'Summer Snowflake'.

Recently, Canadian Plant Breeders' Rights legislation has been passed by the federal government. This will provide much greater protection for new cultivars in the future.

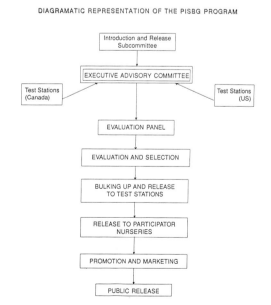

Fig. 1. Diagrammatic representation of the PISBG program.

STRUCTURE AND PROCEDURES OF THE PROGRAM

There are five parts to the program—evaluation and selection, propagation and distribution to participating nurseries, contract and royalty payments, test sites, and promotion and marketing.

Evaluation and Selection

The UBC Botanical Garden contains over 15,000 different accessions, thus providing a wide basis for selection. The three Garden areas that have provided the major sources of introductions are the Asian, Alpine and BC Native Garden components. The selection process begins with a 32-member evaluation panel which meets annually to review some 12 to 17 potential introductions. The panel is diverse, comprising representatives from retailers, wholesalers, landscape architects and contractors, parks boards, and retired members of the nursery industry. Recently, evaluations have been carried out with smaller specialist groups, e.g., landscape architects, to advise the committee on what they feel will be the trend in plant materials for the next five to ten years.

Each panel member completes an assessment form for each plant and its potential as an introduction. The form includes reasons for or against its selection, information on ease of production, possible uses in the landscape, and potential sales. Slides are used to illustrate plant characteristics during different seasons.

Subsequently, the forms are analyzed and reviewed by the evaluation committee which makes the final selections. The final choice of one to three plants per annum is made by the nursery industry and not the Botanical Garden. Experience has shown that it is far more effective to release a few good plants per year to the industry than numerous new plants—in the latter case there is a risk that they will be quickly relegated to collectors' items again, and momentum and energy lost could have been more efficiently used in developing other plants.

Propagation and Distribution to Participating Nurseries

The next phase is for the Botanical Garden's nursery to multiply the new selections to produce 600 to 1000 stock/mother plants. During this process, research and development work is carried out on propagation and growing and on developing recommendations for the extension service and growers. Once a sufficient number of plants has been produced, they are sold at a premium price to the participating nurseries. The PISBG program commenced with nine participating nurseries and today there are 42 nurseries, with associate nurseries in five different countries—England, France, the United States, Holland, and New Zealand.

Contracts and Royalties

A contract is sent to each participating nursery for consideration prior to the release of the stock/mother plants. Among the details included with the contract are colored photographs, production and cultural details, market potential, and the price of the plants. A major portion of this contract involves the date for public release and the royalty to be paid. For the program to work successfully, it is essential that no plants are sold prior to the release date and that sufficient quantities of plants are available for marketing.

Test Sites

A priority of the committee was the establishment of test sites to assess plants in areas of diverse climatic conditions. Winter hardiness was an obvious concern, but data on drought resistance and heat and humidity tolerance were also collected. Currently, there are seven test sites across Canada and six sites in the United States.

The plants are sent for testing prior to release. The length of testing is dependent on the species. For example, a little-known species from South America requires considerably more testing than a new cultivar of the widely grown shrub, *Potentilla fruticosa*. It is also important to trial plants under commercial conditions which are difficult to create at the Botanical Garden. Greater emphasis will be given evaluating new plants from propagation to marketing in selected nurseries in BC prior to general marketing.

The value of a test site to PISBG is dependent on goodwill, the ability of the staff to care for the plants correctly, and the return of accurate information.

Promotion, Publicity, and Marketing

Careful planning with the industry is essential to create an effective promotion, publicity, and marketing strategy.

Important features of this phase include:
- the production and distribution of colored information sheets and posters to landscape architects, retailers, and wholesalers, giving details of the plant's habit, culture, uses, and sales potential;
- the design and printing of colorful, custom-designed picture labels which will be attached to all plants for retail sale;
- participation in nursery trade shows across North America;
- pre-release of plants to high-profile landscaping projects;
- provision of press releases and articles to the media, trade journals, and garden magazines;
- investigation of licensing agreements in other countries where patents, trademarks, and plant breeders' rights exist;
- selection of an easily identifiable cultivar name for new plants is essential for mass marketing, customer recognition, and program profile.

FUTURE DEVELOPMENTS

The success of the PISBG program has led to a number of international awards, and this, in turn, has given the plants wider recognition. An example is the recent signing of a licensing agreement with a consortium of United Kingdom growers to market plants in Europe. The BC nursery industry has established the Henry M. Eddie Plant Development Foundation, named after one of the province's pioneer nurserymen and plant breeders. The aim is to provide an endowment of CDN $1 million, the interest from which will be used to fund programs in plant breeding, new plant development, and plant exploration.

The continuing success of a plant introduction program depends on new plants coming into production on an on-going basis. With this in mind, the Botanical Garden has recently received funding for the collection and evaluation of lesser known and improved forms of native plants. The collections made so far are considerable, thus, providing a valuable germplasm pool for future research.

CONCLUSIONS

The 13 introductions from the PISBG program have already resulted in over 5 million plants being produced world-wide for sale. More than 600,000 plants of the ground cover *Arctostaphylos uva-ursi* 'Vancouver Jade' were propagated in BC during 1991. New plants from PISBG have been exported to the United States, Holland, Denmark, France, New Zealand, Japan, and Korea. Not every introduction is expected to be a success, due to changes in consumer demand, unforeseeable pest and disease problems, and revisions of plant health regulations in provinces, states, and other countries.

Botanical gardens and arboreta are a unique source for potential plant introductions for the nursery industry and urban landscape. The University of British Columbia Plant Introduction Scheme has demonstrated that an institution can effectively cooperate with the nursery and landscape professions to commercially utilize their collections and research for mutual benefit. Detailed attention to planning, liaison with key personnel, promotion, marketing, and, not least, a clear consensus on the selection of the correct plant for introduction are vital for a program's success.

REFERENCES

Macdonald, A.B. 1985. A plant introduction scheme for new and recommended plants from British Columbia, Canada. Proc. Int. Plant Prop. Soc. 35:411–417.

Macdonald, A.B. 1988. Worthy introductions of western Canada. Amer. Nurseryman 167:122–124.

Taylor, R.L. 1983. University of British Columbia Botanical Garden Plant Introduction Scheme: an opportunity for a new relationship between nurseries and the public garden. Proc. Int. Plant Prop. Soc. 33:121–125.

Cliff Brake Fern: A Native Texas Fern with Landscaping Potential

Ramsey L. Sealy and Steve Bostic

Cliff Brake Fern [*Pellaea ovata* (Desv.) Weath.] is a native Texas fern that is found in nature on dry ledges and slopes of limestone outcroppings, calcareous rocks, or granite. It is frequently found on cliffs or at their bases; but also grows well in open rocky woodlands (Correll and Johnston 1979). Because of its tolerance to high temperatures, bright light, and alkaline conditions, cliff break fern might be well adapted to being incorporated into the xeriscape. Cliff break fern thrives in rich, well-drained soil (Hoshizaki 1975), and should be adaptable to many landscape situations.

Cliff Brake Fern has an attractive color, ranging from dark green to grayish-green (Jones 1987) and it has an interesting fine, open texture due to its peculiar rachis and costa structure (Lellinger 1985). Cliff break fern and other *Pellaea* spp. have been grown on trellises and in hanging baskets in greenhouses in the Northeast (Foster 1964), but its use in southern landscapes has been ignored. Because of the plant's apparent wide ecological adaptability and its ornamental qualities, *P. ovata* deserves consideration for use in the landscape and, in particular, in the xeriscape.

DESCRIPTION OF THE PLANT

P. ovata is a member of the Polypodiaceae, subfamily Gymnogrammeoidae, and tribe Cheilantheae (Tryon and Tryon 1973). Within the genus *Pellaea*, *P. ovata* is in the section Pellaea (Tryon and Tryon 1982).

P. ovata has slender rhizomes. Its leaves (fronds) may grow to 1 m or more in length and are divaricately bipinnate to tripinnate (Correll and Johnston 1979). There are 3 to 20 stalked pinnules on each pinna; the leaflets are 2 cm long and 1.5 cm wide and are ovate to oblong in shape with cordate to truncate bases (Correll and Johnston 1979) (Fig. 1). The petioles and rachises are pale tan-colored; the stalk is hard, dark, and polished (Hoshizaki 1975). The rachises and rachillae zigzag, often quite dramatically (Bailey and Bailey 1976). The zigzag pattern may all be in one plane or in several planes. Sori are borne in a marginal band along the blades and are covered by the reflexed margins of the pinnules (Bailey and Bailey 1976). The range of *P. ovata* is similar to that of several other American species of Pellaea, extending from the southwestern United States south to Argentina (Tryon and Tryon 1982).

The entire genus is adapted to relatively xeric conditions. The partially underground stems are covered with scales and have the capacity to survive light ground fires (Tryon and Tryon 1982). Further, the apogamous gametophytes do not require free water for fertilization (Tryon and Tryon 1982). New plants can be established during short moist periods because of rapid spore germination and sporophyte initiation (Tryon and Tryon 1982). *P. ovata* can tolerate and even thrive in moderate shade (as in open woodlands), but it may grow slowly under dense shade (Clute 1938). It is equally well adapted to full sun conditions (Hoshizaki 1975). *P. ovata* is native to areas with both very thin alkaline soils and areas with rich woodland soils (Clute 1938). *P. ovata* tolerates extremely hot summers (highs at 40°C or more) and can withstand at least brief periods of below freezing temperatures (periods of –17°C are reported with survival) (Hoshizaki 1975).

UTILITY IN THE LANDSCAPE

Several attributes recommend *P. ovata* as a xeriscape plant. These include its drought resistance and its tolerance of both alkaline soils and high temperatures. Cliff brake fern responds well to regular irrigation, but can thrive with neglect and occasional watering. We have observed that with even prolonged wilting, mature fronds of *P. ovata* revive with watering. Overwatering can kill cliff brake fern, and so it should not be placed with plants that have high water needs (Hoshizaki 1975). Since the fern is tolerant of both full sun and moderate shade, it can be used throughout the landscape in most light environments, except dense shade. Because it also grows well in rich woodland soils, *P. ovata* should be adaptable to many landscape schemes besides a xeriscape one. Some morphological characteristics make cliff break fern an interesting addition to the landscape (Fig. 2). The

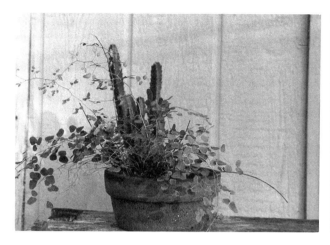
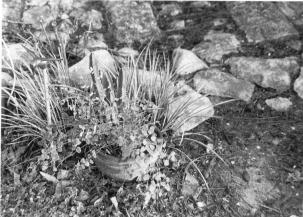

Fig. 1. A specimen of *Pellaea ovata*.　　Fig. 2. Use of *Pellaea ovata* in the landscape.

generic name *Pellaea* comes from a Greek word meaning "dusky" (Bailey and Bailey 1976), and the pinnules of *P. ovata* are somewhat to very glaucous. The small size of the leaflets (pinnules) and the open, zigzag character of the rachis allows *P. ovata* to lend an interesting open, light texture to the landscape. Cliff break fern can be effectively used in the landscape as a specimen plant, both potted or in the soil, and as part of a border, either by itself or in a mixed border.

Further popularization of *P. ovata* as a landscape plant will require determination of the limits of the fern's cold (freeze) tolerance, the extent of both drought and water-logging tolerance, information on the effect of different levels of shade on Cliff Break Fern's growth and survivability, and knowledge of the long-term adaptability of this new plant to the home landscape.

REFERENCES

Clute, W.N. 1938. Our ferns, their haunts, habits and folklore. 2nd ed. Lippincott, New York.

Correll, D.S., and M.C. Johnston. 1979. Manual of the vascular plants of Texas. The Univ. of Texas at Dallas, Richardson.

Foster, F.G. 1964. The gardener's fern book. Van Nostrand, Princeton, NJ.

Hoshizaki, B.J. 1975. Fern grower's manual. Knopf, New York.

Jones, D.L. 1987. Encyclopaedia of ferns. Timber Press, Portland, OR.

Lellinger, D.B. 1985. A field guide of the ferns and fern-allies of the United States and Canada. Smithsonian Institution Press, Washington, DC.

Staff of the Bailey Hortorium. 1976. Hortus III, Revised. Macmillan, New York.

Tryon, R.M., Jr. and A.F. Tryon. 1973. Geography, spores, and evolutionary relations in the cheilanthoid ferns, p. 145-153. In: A.C. Jermy, J.A. Crabbe, and B.A. Thomas (eds.). The phylogeny and classification of the ferns. Academic Press, London.

Tryon, R.M., Jr. and A.F. Tryon. 1982. Ferns and allied plants. Springer–Verlag, New York.

AROMATIC, SPICES, MEDICINAL, AND OTHERS

Herbs, Spices, and Condiments

Nicolas Verlet*

Herbs and spices cannot be really considered as "new crops," as they have been used and produced for many centuries. Nevertheless, herbs have been receiving a lot of positive media attention, and this has contributed to an expansion in the cultivation of herbs during the last decade. In order to get a better idea of the potential herb, spice, and condiment market in the United States, this paper will preview the increasing consumption, the competitiveness of the international supply, and the new markets for herbs.

THE DEMAND

All available date indicate a regular increase in the market for natural products. Between 1987 and 1990, the annual growth in the market for perfumery ingredients has been estimated to be 6%, for food aroma 8.5%, and for raw essential oils 7.5%. The consumption of herbs has risen in France from 10,000 t in 1970 to 32,000 t in 1990. American imports of spices and herbs which were 112,000 t in 1969, were 238,000 t in 1990. The demand for natural aromas remains very strong, and consequently herbs and spices, as well as other natural sources of aroma are preferred to synthetics in the food industry (more than 87% of the aromas used by Nestlé, one of the largest food companies in the world, are from natural origin). In the long term, the future of herbs and spices is closely related to a foodtasting war pitting the "MacDonalds" and other fast/convenience food companies against those seeking high quality food. Fortunately, while MacDonalds has opened an advanced post in Moscow and while fast foods have invaded the Champs Elysées, the spicy ethnic foods have counter-attacked through the east and west coasts of the United States. The industrial processes used in food manufacturing are currently unable to preserve the original tastes of the basic ingredients. Herbs and spices are therefore, more and more useful as flavor ingredients in food preparation.

THE SUPPLY

In the past, trade in herbs had the same degree of importance as trade in gold and precious stones. Twenty five hundred years ago, Heroditus described caravans of 500 elephants, 1,000 dromedaries, and 2,000 horses, escorted by 4,000 mounted soldiers, being used in the transport of rhubarb, cloves, cinnamon, and asa foetida from China, in a round trip, that took four full years (Delaveau 1989). While the relative importance of spices have declined, production and trade have become highly competitive.

The agricultural sector today faces tremendous difficulties. Long term cycles appear to determine commodity prices. The 1970s were characterized by the idea of shortage, related to overpopulation and the petroleum crisis. With the 1980s came oversupply and a fall in prices for the major commodities. In developing countries, the financial return for traditional exports, such as cocoa and coffee, has reached historically low levels. In Europe, an oversupply depresses prices for cereals and other alternative crops. The Eastern European countries, searching more than ever, for foreign currency to be used in the reconstruction of their economies, are attempting to export herbs. Development programs have been initiated throughout the world in the field of herbs and spices, as well as essential oils and medicinal plants. This increasing competition represents new sources of supply for traders. It is also a partial explanation for the decline in prices.

The situation, however, differs according to species, quality requirement, and level of mechanization. The "tropical" spices are produced in developing countries, often with a strong domestic market. Traditional producers of spices, such as India, have to face new competitors in Malaysia and Indonesia. Some herbs have been introduced in these countries, only for export purposes and the supply has increased where optimum production factors exists. Some countries have been able to maintain a monopolistic situation on the international market with specialty production, such as Egypt with basil and India with celery seeds. Bay leaves (*Laurus*

---

*I thank Lyle Craker for his assistance with the subtleties of the English language, and Jim Simon for his fruitful collaboration.

nobilis) are a good illustration of a market commodity having a monopolistic producer with Turkey supplying more than 90% of the world market. Since 1977, the average import of bay leaves into Germany has been 250 t, more than 93% is of Turkish origin. Similar figures for the United States are 450 t (93%), for France 200 t (87%), and for Great Britain 100 t (91%). Many countries have tried to penetrate the bay leaf market offering prices significantly below the Turkish prices. New producers, however, cannot maintain their positions more than one or two years at these price level. Due to the nuclear accident of Chernobyl and supply shortages, the prices of bay were exceptionally high in 1986 and 1987. The percentage of bay leaves coming from Turkey fell to 78% with the benefit going to Spain, Morocco, and Yugoslavia, but Turkey had recovered 99% of the American market by 1988 (Table 1).

The competition is more open for other species when technology and production practices may either increase the yield, reduce the production costs, or allow a better quality at a higher price. The oregano market is particularly interesting with the competition of three major producers (Mexico, Greece, and Turkey), where production is mainly from wild harvesting and the labor cost is the determinant. Israel has been very successful with oregano, introducing selected cultivars and mechanization and able to market at a price very similar to that of Turkey (Fig. 1). Thyme is another example of increasing competitiveness. The world leader in production of thyme leaves is Spain (2, 000 t/year). Most of the harvesting comes from wild plants of different species. In 1970, a few producers started to cultivate thyme in France, benefiting from research on breeding and selection. Clonal selections now combine regular quality with high yield. Since the beginning, the initiative has been supported by Ducros, the main trader in Europe, who has contracted with domestic producers at a relatively high price. This price has enabled production level to reach 100 t of dried leaves per year. The problem is now how to expand. Further expansion of thyme cultivation cannot be considered at current prices and the demand for quality thyme is now satisfied. Any expansion of production will induce a fall in price, progressively reaching the Spanish price (Fig. 2). This is the limit of a development based on better quality standards.

There are a number of herbs such as parsley, dill, and tarragon which are mainly produced and used in industrialized countries. A combination of good cultivars, dehydration processes, and intensive cultivation techniques have allowed these countries a dominant place in the dried market for these plants.

Table 1. Sources and prices of bay laurel (*Laurus nobilis* L.) imports into the United States[z].

Year	Turkey (%)	($/kg)	Other countries
1978	88	1.34	Yugoslavia (10%, $0.55)
1979	96	1.55	Greece (3%, $1.18)
1980	96	1.81	Greece (2%, $1.20)
1981	91	1.70	Albania (5%, $0.94)
1982	96	1.26	India (2%, $0.85)
1983	96	1.32	Greece (4%, $1.05)
1984	100	0.91	
1985	98	1.19	China (1%, $3.4)
1986	83	1.48	Portugal (4%, $1.42) Albania (2%, $2.50) Spain (1%, $3,11) Morocco (1%, $2.91)
1987	78	2.41	Germany (7%, $2,74) Spain (5%, $2.91) Portugal (3%, $1.75) Morocco (1%, $2.10) Yugoslavia (1%, $1.26)
1988	99	1.58	Mexico (1%, 1.26)

[z]Modified from USDA 1978–1988 U.S. Essential oil trade.

NEW MARKET FOR HERBS

The traditional dried form of herbs and spices is threatened in the future by new processing and preserving methods. Fresh herbs are now cultivated for use as ingredients in large scale food preparation (e.g. vinegars, mustards). New markets for fresh herbs primarily exist in restaurants, but small packages for the consumer are also commanding an increasing market share. Supermarket chains are seeking assurance of a steady, year-round supply of fresh herbs. Yet, storage and transportation of fresh material are costly especially over long distances. These markets represent new opportunities for producers in consuming countries. Nevertheless, the growers starting production face relatively expensive investments, especially during the winter period. Supply from warm countries, shipped by aircraft, is now on the market and relatively inexpensive (the shipping cost from Israel to New York is $1/kg). Frozen herbs are playing an increasing role in the food industry. The appearance of a whole range of consumer frozen products is something new, but it is difficult for new producers to take a place in the frozen market because of the technology and the high investments required.

OPPORTUNITIES FOR THE NORTH AMERICAN AGRICULTURE

It is useful to first present a brief view of production in Europe (Table 2). While herbs are not included in the Common Agricultural Policy of the European Common Market, the situation is very similar for producers in Europe and the United States. Aromatic plants are cultivated now in America for many purposes. Fresh herb production is well developed across the country. California, which benefits from good weather conditions can and does produce many herbs. Production on the East Coast has the advantage of being close to the consumer (e.g. parsley production in New Jersey). Phytofarm of America, located near Chicago, has established a controlled environment facility, where herbs are produced 365 days a year without influence from seasonal variations in temperature and light. At this facility a central computer monitors growing conditions such as temperature, carbon

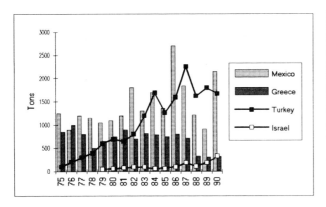   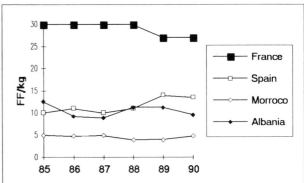

Fig. 1. Imports of oregano into the United States.   **Fig. 2.** Thyme price in the French market.

Table 2. Estimation of West European production of herbs[z].

Country	Area (ha)	Herb
Spain	28,000	Anise, saffron, mint, cumin, poppy, datura
France	20,000	Lavandin, poppy, clary sage, parsley, tarragon, thyme
Italy	2,800	Mint, tarragon, orris, sage
Netherlands	2,200	Poppy, parsley, caraway, digitalis, evening primrose
Denmark	2,000	Caraway
Germany	2,000	Mint, parsley, thyme, balm
U.K.	800	Parsley, evening primrose

[z]Modified from ONIPPAM 1990.

dioxide levels, lighting schedules, allowing for rapid growth without pesticides or herbicides (Wallick 1988). The USDA publishes a weekly National Wholesale Herb Market New Report containing price quotes which cover wholesale herb sales to retailers in 18 major cities (USDA 1989).

Large farms, dealing with vegetable dehydration, are producing dried herbs on a large scale. The domestic production of dried herbs is currently covering only a very small part of the demand. Some growers, like those in Arizona, have obtained good prices for sage, basil, and a few other herbs (approximately $6/kg, more than twice the international price). The domestic production of dried herbs is bought by traders concerned for a higher quality and a more secure supply. In the example of thyme, the demand for domestic production is rather small, and new producers may not expect a high price if the domestic cultivation of dried herbs increases substantially. Organic production allows a better margin of profit, especially for well managed farms like Trout Lake farm in Washington State where 200 ha of herbs are organically grown. Weed control in this type of production system is a crucial point for it is often difficult, after a mechanized harvest, to clean weeds from the final dried produce.

Unfortunately, there are few technical production guides available, and few breeding programs have been initiated. Successful development in production of herbs and spices requires good control of cultivation practices, of postharvest processing and storage, and of marketing technique. Consequently, success calls for active producers, open to innovation and in a permanent dialogue with researchers and consumers.

We have witnessed an increasing role for fresh and frozen herbs at the expense of the traditional dried form. In addition to the well-known oleoresins, more and more sophisticated forms of material and marketing are going to be used in the food industry. Today we have supercritical CO_2 extracts, isolates from essential oils, and aromas produced by cell cultures or other biotechnological processes. A "new" crop, unfortunately, quickly can become an "out of date" crop!

REFERENCES

Delaveau, P. 1987. Les épices. Paris.

Greenhalgh, P. 1979. The market for culinary herbs. Trop. Prod. Inst., London.

International Trade Center. 1982. Market for medicinal plants and their derivatives. UNCTAD GATT, Geneva.

ONIPPAM. 1990. Le commerce des plantes aromatiques et médicinales. Volx.

USDA. 1989. National wholesale herb market news report. USDA Agr. Mktg. Service. Fruit Veg. Mkt. News. Chicago. (issued weekly).

Verlet N. 1990. The world herbs and essential oils economy. 23rd Int. Hort. Congr. Florence, Italy.

Wallick, K. 1988. The phytofarm system of controlled environment herb production. Proc. Deuxiémes Rencontres Plantes Aromatiques et Médicinales. Dec. 5–7 1998, Nyons, France.

A Planning Scheme to Evaluate New Aromatic Plants for the Flavor and Fragrance Industries

Brian M. Lawrence

There are approximately 300 natural products used as raw materials in the flavor and fragrance industry. These raw materials can be found in the form of essential oils, extracts, oleoresins, concretes, absolutes, resinoids, and tinctures to name the major groups. Of these materials, about half are produced from cultivated plants while the remaining 50% are obtained either as by-products of a primary industry or are harvested from natural wild plants. Raw materials such as galbanum or opopanax are not distilled or extracted within close proximity where grown so these will not enter this discussion as they have little relevance as new crops.

The major portion of this discussion will be directed towards essential oil bearing plants. The 20 major oils in the world market are presented in Table 1. Accurate production figures are available for those oils produced in the United States (Simon 1990), but production statistics from third world countries and even some western countries are more obscure. Previous surveys of essential oils include those of Lawrence 1985 and the ITC (Anon 1986). The large volumes of oil produced suggest an economic potential for essential oil bearing plants as new crops.

The traditional view of essential oil production is that of simple farming or collection followed by oil distillation or extraction. Both intrinsic factors (genotype, state of maturity, part of plant harvested) and extrinsic factors (light, temperature, water, nutrients) will strongly influence the oil yield and composition (Bernath 1986; Lawrence 1986). Within a single clone, the intrinsic factors can be fixed whereas the extrinsic factors cannot.

In this paper, a crop development planning scheme is proposed which will be directed specifically towards the commercialization of essential oil species in the families Lamiaceae (Labiatae) (Table 2), Apiaceae (Umbelliferae) (Table 3), and Asteraceae (Compositae) (Table 4).

Table 1. The world's 20 top essential oils.

Essential oil	Species	Volume (t)	Value ($\times 10^6$)
Orange	*Citrus sinensis* (L.) Osbeck	26,000	58.5
Cornmint	*Mentha arvensis* L. f. *piperascens* Malinv. ex Holmes	4,300	34.4
Eucalyptus cineole-type	*Eucalyptus globulus* Labill., *E. polybractea* R.T. Baker and other Eucalyptus species	3,728	29.8
Citronella	*Cymbopogon winterianus* Jowitt and *C. nardus* (L.) Rendle	2,830	10.8
Peppermint	*Mentha* ×*piperita* L.	2,367	28.4
Lemon	*Citrus limon* (L.) N.L. Burm.	2,158	21.6
Eucalyptus citronellal-type	*Eucalyptus citriodora* Hook.	2,092	7.3
Clove leaf	*Syzygium aromaticum* (L.) Merr. and L.M. Perry	1,915	7.7
Cedarwood (US)	*Juniperus virginiana* L. and *J. ashei* Buchholz	1,640	9.8
Litsea cubeba	*Litsea cubeba* (Lour.) Pers.	1,005	17.1
Sassafras (Brazil)	*Ocotea pretiosa* (Nees) Benth.	1,000	4.0
Lime distilled (Brazil)	*Citrus aurantifolia* (Christm. & Panz.) Swingle	973	7.3
Native spearmint	*Mentha spicata* L.	851	17.0
Cedarwood (Chinese)	*Chamaecyparis funebris* (Endl.) Franco	800	3.2
Lavandin	*Lavandula intermedia* Emeric ex Loisel	768	6.1
Sassafras (Chinese)	*Cinnamomum micranthum* (Hayata) Hayata	750	3.0
Camphor	*Cinnamomum camphora* (L.) J. Presl.	725	3.6
Coriander	*Coriandrum sativum* L.	710	49.7
Grapefruit	*Citrus paradisi* Macfady	694	13.9
Patchouli	*Pogostemon cablin* (Blanco) Benth.	563	6.8

NEW CROP SELECTION

Prior to any market survey or crop selection, a knowledge is required of the micro-environment, the land, and water resources, natural flora and fauna, and local agricultural skills and problems. These include annual record of the maximum and minimum temperatures on a 24 hour basis, photoperiod, rainfall, soil type, pH, nutrient and humus content, and water holding capacity.

It is useful to know what irrigation methods are used locally, what are the local sources of water, and what is the normal frequency of irrigation and the quantity of water applied for specific crops for what periods of time. What is the normal field size? Is full mechanization feasible? What are the main local agricultural problems? What are the local pest disease and weed problems? What are the normal crops and cropping priorities. In the United States, much of this information along with some of the environmental data is readily available from the State Department of Agriculture or County Cooperative Extension Service.

An economic survey of oil production must be compiled. A crop development scheme for establishment and implementation of an essential oil crop development program using eastern North Carolina as an example of a site will be discussed. For essential oils a laboratory which possesses the capability of running labscale distillations, physico-chemical parameter measurements, and gas chromatographic analyses should be in place as well as a commercial scale steam distillation facility. It must be remembered that essential oils, which are natural mixtures of secondary plant products, are raw materials used in the flavor and fragrance industries. As a result, there are some economic questions that require accurate answers:

Table 2. Worldwide production of the major essential oils of the Lamiaceae.

Essential oil	Species	Volume	Value
Major essential oils		*(t)*	*($×10⁶)*
Cornmint	*Mentha arvensis* L. f. *piperascens* Malinv. ex Holmes	4,300	34.4
Peppermint	*Mentha ×piperita* L.	2,367	28.4
Native spearmint	*Mentha spicata* L.	851	17.0
Lavandin	*Lavandula intermedia* Emeric ex Loisel	768	6.1
Patchouli	*Pogostemon cablin* (Blanco) Benth.	563	6.8
Scotch spearmint	*Mentha gracilis* Sole	530	10.6
Lavender	*Lavandula angustifolia* Mill.	362	7.2
Rosemary	*Rosmarinus officinalis* L.	295	3.5
Clary sage	*Salvia sclarea* L.	70	5.6
Spike lavender	*Lavandula latifolia* Medik.	64	1.0
Ocimum	*Ocimum gratissimum* L. gratissimum	50	0.8
Basil	*Ocimum basilicum* L.	43	2.8
Marjoram	*Origanum majorana* L.	62	1.2
Sage	*Salvia officinalis* L.	35	1.8
Thyme	*Thymus zygis* L. and *T. vulgaris* L.	29	1.5
Minor essential oils		*(kg)*	*($×10³)*
Wild thyme	*Thymus pulegioides* L.	2,000	100
Monarda (geraniol type)	*Monarda fistulosa* var. *menthaefolia* (J. Graham) Fernald	2,000	40
Hyssop	*Hyssopus officinalis* L.	1,800	32
Perilla	*Perilla frutescens* (L.) Britton	1,500	1800
Savory	*Satureja montana* L.	1,500	90
Monarda (thymol type)	*Monarda citriodora*	100	5
Ocimum canum	*Ocimum canum* Sims	100	5
Catnip	*Nepeta cataria* L.	100	unknown
Melissa	*Melissa officinalis* L.	100	4
Ninde	*Aeollanthus gamwelliae* G. Taylor	<50	unknown
American pennyroyal	*Hedeoma pulegioides* (L.) Pers.	<50	unknown

1. Which oils are in short supply and which are in over supply?
2. Are there any current use trends for individual oils?
3. Which oils are subject to adulteration?
4. What oils are subject to climatic or political problems?

To answer these questions with today's information, the main essential oils which I have found to be in short supply are patchouli, hyssop, lemon balm, sage (Lamiaceae), blue chamomile, tagetes, yarrow, (Asteraceae) and galbanum, lovage herb, parsley herb (Apiaceae), whereas the oils in oversupply are spike lavender (Lamiaceae) and fennel (Apiaceae). The only current use trend in the oils of the three families other than those noted above is a decrease in lavender oil. All oils that possess components for which synthetic counterparts are readily available are subject to adulteration even if the chirality of the synthetic adulterant does not match that of the natural compound. Essential oils are produced in a variety of temperate and tropical parts of the world. Any oils that can be produced in the Peoples Republic of China can have a substantial impact of their supply and demand because they may be sold on the world market or they may be stockpiled below production costs or to elevate market price. I have seen this over the last decade with cornmint and citronella oils. In the former Soviet Union, eastern Europe, and other countries desperate for international currency, essential oils are often bartered into the Western world. I believe that much of the coriander oil produced in the former Soviet Union found its way into western countries via the barter route.

Assuming the decision is made that the essential oil production facility can be built and in this case study will be located in eastern North Carolina and the appropriate information is available that will help make a selection of which plants to grow, a set of action steps to become a commercial essential oil producer is needed. Let me propose a 5-stage development plan as follows:

Stage 1: Screening plants in small plots
Stage 2: Evaluation of trial rows

Table 3. Worldwide production of essential oils of the Asteraceae.

Essential oil	Species	Volume	Value
Major essential oils		*(t)*	*($×10⁶)*
Armoise	*Artemisia herba-alba* Asso	32	1.1
Tagetes	*Tagetes minuta* L.	11.9	1.2
Tarragon	*Artemisia dracunculus* L.	9.9	0.8
Roman chamomile	*Anthemis nobilis* L.	6.0	3.6
Wormwood	*Artemisia absinthum* L.	6.0	0.2
Blue chamomile	*Chamomilla recutita* (L.) Rauschert	4.3	2.2
Wild chamomile	*Ormenis mixta* Dumort. and *O. multicaulis* Braun-Blanq & Maire	2.0	<0.1
Muhuhu	*Brachylaena hutchinsii* Hutch.	2.0	<0.1
Artemisis martima	*Artemisia maritima* L.	1.0	<0.1
Davana	*Artemisia pallens* Wall. ex DC	1.0	0.3
Minor essential oils		*(kg)*	*($×10³)*
Yarrow	*Achillea millefolium* L.	800	88
Artemisia afra	*Artemisia afra* Jacq.	750	51
Artemisia annua	*Artemisia annua* L.	600	16
Helichrysum	*Helichrysum stoechas* (L.) Monech and *H. italicum* (Roth) G. Don	300	81
Santolina	*Santolina chamaecyparissus* L.	300	unknown
Balsamite	*Chrysanthemum balsamita* L.	100	3.5
Elecampane	*Inula helenium* L.	100	unknown
Ereocephalus	*Ereocephalus punctulatus* DC	50	unknown
Pteronia	*Pteronia incana* DC	50	unknown
Artemisia vestita	*Artemisia vestita* Wallich	50	unknown
Tansy	*Tanacetum vulgare* L.	<50	unknown

Stage 3:   Small scale experimental plantings
Stage 4:   Mini-commercialization
Stage 5:   Full-scale commercialization

STAGE 1: SCREENING OF PLANTS IN SMALL PLOTS

Questions that need to answered during this stage include:
- Will the plant grow well in this environment?
- Are there any climatic restrictions?
- Can the plant be reproduced successfully?
- Can the plant be rotated with other cash crops currently produced?
- What are potential problems?
- What are the projected economics?

The workload associated with this stage can be summarized as follows: prepare experimental garden, acquire seeds/plants, propagate seedlings/cuttings, plant garden, keep records, culture plants, study growth habits, maintain history on individual plants, harvest plants, steam distill plants, record yield, and conduct chemical analysis on promising oils. It is important to isolate plants for seed production that cross pollinate, eliminate any that show signs of disease, have insect pest problems, or that indicate mixed populations. Plants of little potential should be removed. A dossier must be maintained on all plants in the field.

At the same time as stage 1 screening is underway, economic dossiers on each promising species should be prepared. An example of a dossier for caraway can be seen in Table 5. Depending upon the species a plant may have to be grown in stage 1 for more than one year as all pertinent information may not be obtained. Assuming a species has potential, it is most likely that the best genotype has not been grown. A range of oil yields that were

Table 4. Worldwide production of essential oils of the Apiaceae.

Essential oil	Species	Volume	Value
Major essential oils		*(t)*	*($×10⁶)*
Coriander	*Coriandrum sativum* L.	710	49.5
Sweet fennel	*Foeniculum vulgare* Mill. var. dulce	255	7.7
Dill weed	*Anethum graveolens* L.	114	0.8
Celery seed	*Apium graveolens* L.	30	1.5
Caraway	*Carum carvi* L.	29	1.0
Bitter fennel	*Foeniculum vulgare* Mill. var. *vulgare*	28	0.7
Anise	*Pimpinella anisum* L.	26	0.7
Ajowan	*Trachyspermum copticum* (L.) Link	25	0.3
Indian dill seed	*Anethum sowa* Roxb. ex Flem.	25	0.1
European dill seed	*Anethum graveolens*	23	0.2
Cumin	*Cuminum cyminum* L.	15	0.9
Minor essential oils		*(kg)*	*($×10³)*
Carrot seed	*Daucus carota* L.	8,800	1230
Parsley seed	*Petroselinum crispum* (Mill.) Nym. ex A.W. Hill	8,300	1162
Angelica root	*Angelica archangelica*	4,400	3080
Parsley herb	*Petroselinum crispum*	4,000	560
Asafoetida	*Ferula assafoetida* L.	3,000	1035
Lovage root	*Levisticum officinale* L.	2,000	1600
Lovage herb	*Levisticum officinale* L.	1,500	712
Lovage seed	*Levisticum officinale* L.	900	unknown
Angelica seed	*Angelica archangelica*	800	880
Celery herb	*Apium graveolens*	800	60
Ammoniac gum	*Dorema ammoniacum* D. Don	200	unknown

obtained from various cultivars of some selected species grown over a 2-year period is presented in Table 6. These results clearly demonstrate that selection of a specific strain or chemotype with the highest oil yield (assuming an acceptable chemical composition) is imperative to maximize an economic return.

Before proceeding from stage 1 to stage 2, positive answers to the following questions are needed.
- Will the plant grow well in this environment?
- Does the oil yield appear promising?
- Does the oil composition indicate potential market acceptability?
- Is there a potential market for the oil?
- Is the oil a new geographic source for an existing oil?
- Is the oil a currently unknown commodity?
- Is the oil a source of a potentially marketable aroma chemical?
- Is there a uniqueness in the oil?
- Is the chemical composition of the oil normal?
- Is the oil subject to synthetic replacement?
- Is the oil vulnerable to speculation?
- Is there any American competition for the oil?
- What is the market size for the oil?
- What are the origin distributions of competitive oils versus markets?

STAGE 2: EVALUATION OF TRIAL ROWS

The following questions need to be answered in this trial row stage:
- What is optimum method of reproduction?
- Does planting date affect plant growth?
- What is optimum spacing in and between plants?
- What is the projected oil yield per unit acre?
- What is the best method for reproduction?
- At what maturity stage is the highest quantity of good quality oil produced?
- What is the diurnal fluctuation in oil yield?

The workload associated with this stage in the development plan can be summarized as follows: prepare the land, plan layout for trial rows, propagate plants, plant trial rows, determine alternate propagation methods, and keep records. For selected species, plant at various dates and spacings, determine good crop culture, monitor effect of stress on plants, and examine plants closely for problems. Finally, harvest plants at distinct stages of maturity and determine oil yield. Determine oil composition of oils obtained from plants harvested at various times. An example of the seasonal changes in chemical composition as the plant matures can be seen in Table 7. Finally, determine change in oil yield and composition of most promising species over a 24-hour period at optimum oil production time.

Table 5. A crop dossier for caraway (*Carum carvi* L.).

Where cultivated:	Netherlands, Poland, Hungary, Bulgaria, Australia
Grows wild in:	Europe and W. Asia
General plant information:	Biennial, Umbelliferae Temperate, seed and oil market
Market size:	3,600 to 4,500 kg oil (USA), 303 t seed (USA)
Price:	$33 to 35/kg oil (USA), $1.00 to 1.06/kg seed (USA)
Where used:	Mostly in flavors, also as a source of d-carvone
Sensitivities:	Seed yield, oil content in seed, shatterability, photoperiodic affect on oil composition, water requirements

Before proceeding from stage 2 to stage 3, positive answers on another set of questions are necessary:
- Can the plant be successfully reproduced?
- Is there a definite market potential for the oil?
- Does the crop exhibit an economic potential?
- What is the current market price of the oil?
- What is the current market supply situation?
- What are the market and usage trends for the oil?
- Would an extract of the plant material be a marketable commodity?
- Is there any value in the spent material?
- Is there any need for capital expenditure?
- Is the odor of the oil acceptable to the essential oil user?
- Does the trial quantity of oil meet physico-chemical specifications?

Table 6. Essential oil yield ranges for various commercially important species.

Species	Common name	Oil yield range (%)	No. samples
Foeniculum vulgare	Sweet and bitter fennel	1.3–9.8	50
Daucus carota	Carrot seed	0.05–7.15	84
Coriandrum sativum	Coriander	0.10–1.40	101
Ocimum basilicum	Basil	0.01–0.30	102
Salvia officinalis	Sage	0.04–0.17	19
Rosmarinus officinalis	Rosemary	0.20–1.19	31
Hyssopus officinalis	Hyssop	0.06–0.38	35
Tanacetum vulgare	Tansy	0.02–0.29	12
Mentha pulegium	Pennyroyal	0.10–0.38	12
Carum carvi	Caraway	3.2–7.4	10

Table 7. Comparative chemical composition of *Coriandrum sativum* L. at various stages of maturity.

Compound	Stages of plant maturity^z					
	1	2	3	4	5	6
Octanal	1.20	1.20	0.85	0.66	0.44	0.35
Nonanal	0.51	0.20	0.11	0.05	0.05	0.08
Decanal	30.0	18.09	11.91	6.30	6.24	1.61
Camphor	.08	trace	0.52	1.26	2.18	2.44
(E)-2-Decenal	20.6	46.5	46.5	40.6	30.2	3.9
Dodecanal	3.30	1.67	0.96	0.64	0.52	0.41
(E)-2-Undecenal	2.56	2.17	1.39	---	---	---
Tridecanal	3.07	1.87	2.02	0.92	1.08	0.46
(E)-2-Dodecanal	7.63	8.14	5.95	4.59	4.78	2.49
Tetradecanal	0.68	0.30	0.12	0.15	0.11	0.15
(E)-2-Tridecenal	0.49	0.21	0.14	0.09	0.09	0.13
(E)-2-Tetradecenal	4.45	2.57	1.73	1.53	1.59	1.73
Linalool	0.34	4.27	17.47	30.05	40.88	60.37
Geraniol	0.19	0.11	0.35	0.71	0.93	1.42
Geranyl acetate	4.17	0.78	0.76	0.69	0.69	0.66

^{z}Stages of maturity: 1 = floral initiation; 2 = nearly full flowering; 3 = full flowering, primary umbel young green fruit; 4 = past full flowering 50% flower, 50% fruit; 5 = full green fruit; 6 = brown fruit on lower umbels, green fruit on upper umbels; --- = not detected.

A considerable number of tasks require completion in order to adequately answer these questions. Assuming a positive answer, then the cultivar of the selected species can proceed to the next stage.

STAGE 3: SMALL SCALE EXPERIMENTAL ACREAGE

The following questions that need to be answered during this stage:
- What is the potential for mechanization?
- What are the best fertilizer, herbicide, pesticide, and irrigation practices?
- What is the best crop rotational scheme?
- What is the potential marketability of the oil?
- What is the economic potential?

The workload associated with this stage is to treat the cultivar of the selected species as a small farm crop by performing all farming practices using commercial mechanical equipment. At this stage in the life of the crop, replicated experiments should be performed so that fertilizer, irrigation, herbicide, and pesticide regimes can be established. At harvest time, the plants should be distilled using commercial or pilot scale equipment rather than laboratory equipment so that accurate yields per unit area can be obtained. Once the oil has been produced (presumably in kilogram quantities), then it should be circulated to user companies so that trade acceptability can be assessed. Also during this stage, a more detailed report on the market of the oil should be prepared. Finally, based on the costs associated with the trial acreage, a detailed economic analysis of oil production should be performed.

Assuming everything looks promising through this stage, before proceeding to stage 4, the following questions must now be answered.
- Is there a market demand for the oil?
- Is the production of this essential oil profitable?
- Can the crop be successfully mechanized?
- What are the optimum fertilizer, herbicide, pesticide, and irrigation practices?
- With what cash crops will the crops rotate?
- What is the optimum distillation time?
- What is the potential marketability of the oil?
- What is the return on the investment for establishing this new essential oil crop?

Once the cultivar of the selected species demonstrates potential as suggested by this planning scheme, the next step is mini-commercialization.

STAGE 4: MINI-COMMERCIALIZATION

By this stage two major questions need to be answered:
- Is this a commercially viable essential oil crop?
- What are the new problems that must be overcome?

The workload associated with this stage is often dependent upon the amount of seed, or propagates that are available to plant. It is recommended that a minimum of 2 ha (ca. 5 acres) be planted because an important factor to determine at this stage are the fixed costs associated with producing oil from the cultivar of the selected species at various hectarages (4, 20, 40, 400 ha). With this information in hand, an accurate picture of the economic viability of the crop can be obtained. With the yield information, it will be valuable to determine the area that it would take to plant and produce 1, 5, or 10.0% of the world market demands for this oil. This information will put the oil production statistics in perspective and may point out some potential vulnerability especially if the production facility becomes an essential oil monoculture.

Before proceeding from stage 4 to stage 5, a final set of questions need to be answered:
- Is there a market acceptance for this oil?
- Is the final profitability study favorable for the establishment of this essential oil crop?
- What are the costs associated with various crop sizes and is there an optimum crop size to maximize profit?

- How many hectares need to be devoted to the new crop to supply 1 to 10% of the world essential oil needs?

Assuming that all of the previously encountered questions can be answered favorably and the data collected was accurate, then the expansion to a large-scale production is the final stage in the development plan.

STAGE 5: FULL COMMERCIALIZATION

Once a crop is in full-scale commercial production, the area grown will be determined by the ease and ability to market the oil profitably. Although in this stage of the plan, the crop will move from the research phase into the maintenance and improvement stage, there are some tasks that should not be overlooked. This includes increase in oil yield, decrease in cost of oil production, increase processing efficiency to improve oil quality as the market demands, and maximize the market and profit position.

Based on the world market supply and demand and industry trends, the oils that could prove economically viable for production in North America include: sage, marjoram, hyssop and Melissa (Lamiaceae), blue chamomile, davana and tarragon (Asteraceae), lovage herb/root/seed, and parsley herb (Apiaceae).

REFERENCES

Anon. 1986. Essential oils and oleoresins: A study of selected producers and major markets. Int. Trade Centre, UNCTAD/GATT, Geneva.

Bernath, J. 1986. Production ecology of secondary plant products, p. 185–234. In: L.E. Craker and J.E. Simon (eds.). Herbs, spices, and medicinal plants: Recent advances in Botany, Horticulture and Pharmacology. Vol. 1. Oryx Press, Phoenix, AZ.

Lawrence, B.M. 1985. A review of the world production of essential oils (1984). Perfum. Flav. 10:1–16.

Lawrence, B.M. 1986. Essential oil production: A discussion of influencing factors, p. 363–369. In: T.H. Parliament and R. Croteau (eds.). Biogeneration of aromas. ACS Symposium Series 317 Amer. Chem. Soc., Washington, DC.

Simon, J.E. 1990. Essential oils and culinary herbs, p. 472–483. In: J. Janick and J.E. Simon (eds.). Advances in new crops. Timber Press, Portland, OR.

Monarda: A Source of Geraniol, Linalool, Thymol and Carvacrol-rich Essential Oils

G. Mazza, F.A. Kiehn, and H.H. Marshall

Monarda, commonly known as horsemint, bee balm, or wild bergamot, belongs to the mint family, Lamiaceae (Labiatae). It is an erect aromatic annual or perennial herb widely distributed throughout North America (Bailey 1977). Several of the 17 to 18 species of this genus have been utilized as ornamental plants, food and flavoring additives, and for medicinal purposes. The essential oil components of the leaves have been used to determine genetic relationships between species (Scora 1967). Plants of a given species from different geographical regions may, however, yield strikingly different oils.

Monarda fistulosa L., native to the Canadian prairies, is drought tolerant, winter hardy, and may yield an essential oil high in geraniol content (Marshall and Scora 1972; Mazza et al. 1987). When this native species is crossed with *M. didyma*, vigorous hybrids, yielding essential oils rich in geraniol, linalool, thymol, carvacrol, 1,8-cineole, and other terpenes can be produced. In the present study, the content and composition of the nitrogen extracted volatiles and hydrodistillated oils from eight winter-hardy, powdery mildew, and rust-resistant hybrids were determined, with the aim of developing new alternative crops for Canadian agriculture.

METHODOLOGY

A plantation of over 500 hybrids and clones of *M. fistulosa* var. *menthaefolia* and *M. didyma* 'Cambridge Scarlet', planted at approximately 10,000 plants/ha was established at Agriculture Canada Research Station, Morden, Manitoba, Canada in 1981. Plants were allowed to establish and grow under dryland culture, as described previously (Marshall and Chubey 1983). In 1987, all surviving plants (about 20% of the original number of plants) were analyzed for volatile constituents and eight of these clones were selected for possible commercial exploitation. These eight clones were propagated by softwood stem cuttings taken at the end of May, and field planted the end of June, 1988. In 1989 and 1990, 10 to 20 plants from each clone were harvested between July 5 and July 10, when the plants were in full bloom. After harvest, the whole plants (stems, leaves, and flowers) were cut into 2 cm lengths, weighed for yield determination and stored separately at $-20°C$ in sealed plastic bags until used.

The essential oil was extracted by hydrodistillation of the plant material using 600 g in a 5 liter round-bottomed flask with distilled, deionized water (2,400 ml), and a receiver for oils lighter than water. The distillation period was 2 h, and the essential oil content was determined on an oil weight to dry tissue weight basis. Headspace volatiles of the chopped plant material were extracted and concentrated by passing a stream of purified nitrogen (80 ml/min for 15 h; $21\pm1°C$) over the samples. The volatiles were adsorbed onto Tenax GC traps prepared by packing 100 ± 2 mg of 60–80 mesh Tenax GC into a 65 mm i.d. $\times$ 12 cm Pyrex tubing between pesticide grade silanized glass wool plugs. Monarda volatiles were subsequently eluted from the Tenax GC traps with 1 ml of freshly redistilled diethyl ether. Essential oil and headspace samples were analyzed using a Varian Model 3400 gas chromatograph equipped with a flame ionization detector (FID). A 30 m $\times$ 0.25 mm i.d. fused silica capillary column packed with 1 µm J&W DB-5 [polymethyl(5% phenyl) siloxane] was used for the separation of volatiles. The operating conditions were: injection port temperature, 230°C; detector temperature 250°C; column temperature programmed at 60°C for 0 min, 60° to 104°C at 4°C/min, 104° to 182°C at 6°C/min and at 182°C for 6 min; carrier gas flow rate, 1 ml He/min; linear velocity 24 cm/s.

Identification of the compounds was made by combined gas chromatography mass spectrometry (GC/MS) and by comparing retention times of monarda components with those of authentic compounds. A Finnigan MAT 90 mass spectrometer coupled with a Varian Model 3400 gas chromatograph was used for GC/MS analyses.

RESULTS AND DISCUSSION

The composition of the oils obtained by hydrodistillation of the plant material varied significantly among different hybrids (Fig. 1, Table 1). Six cyclic terpenes, including α-phellandrene, α-pinene, and camphene were present in oils of seven of the eight hybrids and ß-pinene ranged from 0.56 to 13.8% of the oil from these hybrids. The oil from the 'Morden #3' hybrid had practically no cyclic terpenes; however, analysis of the headspace of this hybrid revealed significant levels of these compounds (Table 2). Geraniol accounted for well over 90% of the composition of the oil from the hybrid, 'Morden #3'. Other components found in this oil at 0.5% level or higher included linalool, ß-myrcene, linalyl acetate, and a sesquiterpene, tentatively identified as germacrene-D. Presently, the chief natural source for geraniol is citronella oil, wherein it occurs with citronellal and citronellol and from which it is separated by fraction distillation (Kirk-Othmer 1983). The geraniol-rich 'Morden #3' originated from a cross between a geraniol race of *M. fistulosa* var. *menthaefolia* native to southern Manitoba, and the progeny of colchicine treated selection 65-5 (Fig. 2). 'Morden #3' was recommended for use as a commercial and competitive source of geraniol earlier (Marshall and Chubey 1983; Mazza et al. 1987), and over 70 ha are presently grown in southern Alberta for geraniol production. Geraniol is used in perfumery for its rosy scent, and in food products as a flavor ingredient. The essential oil of selection 75-1A contained over 73% carvacrol, while selection 75-1B oil contained 31% thymol (Table 1).

Table 1. Chemical composition of essential oils of *Monarda* selections[z].

		Relative composition (% of total oil)							
Peak[y]	Constituent	Morden #3	Marshalls Delight	75-1A	75-1B	84-2	80-1B	80-1A	L87-1
1	α-Thujene	tr	0.7	2.1	1.4	2.3	1.1	0.8	0.6
2	α-Pinene	---[x]	0.6	0.6	1.7	0.6	2.4	0.3	0.3
3	Camphene	---	0.3	0.1	1.2	0.1	1.5	0.2	0.2
4	ß-Pinene	0.3	7.6	0.6	8.7	1.4	13.8	1.7	0.8
5	1-Hepten-3-ol	tr	0.7	0.1	1.6	0.3	2.3	0.1	0.3
6	ß-Myrcene	1.4	1.6	2.4	2.5	2.5	2.7	1.2	0.9
7	α-Phellondrene	tr	0.1	0.4	0.2	0.4	0.2	0.1	0.1
8	α-Terpenene	tr	0.9	2.2	2.1	3.9	1.3	1.2	0.5
9	p-Cymene/Limonene	tr	1.3	6.0	3.0	4.2	1.7	2.5	0.6
10	1,8-Cineole	0.1	4.8	1.0	14.1	1.0	22.2	0.5	0.4
11	Unknown ($C_{12}H_{20}O_2$)	0.3	0.1	0.1	1.0	0.1	0.9	0.1	0.1
12	Ocimene	0.7	5.9	8.1	5.9	27.1	6.2	6.9	2.3
13	Bornyl acetate	tr	0.5	0.1	1.2	0.1	1.7	0.1	0.1
14	Linalool	1.1	49.8	0.1	1.5	0.3	0.4	45.7	67.0
15	Borneol	tr	0.3	tr	2.0	tr	2.0	0.2	0.3
16	Terpinen-4-ol	tr	0.7	0.8	1.0	0.5	1.1	0.5	0.3
17	α-Terpineol	tr	3.4	0.1	7.8	0.1	12.0	0.1	0.1
18	$C_{10}H_{12}O_2$	0.6	tr	---	5.4	0.1	tr	---	---
19	Nerol[y]	0.4	---	---	tr	3.3	0.1	---	tr
20	Geraniol	92.6	1.5	0.1	tr	---	---	0.1	tr
21	Neral	0.2	---	---	---	---	---	tr	---
22	Thymol	tr	0.5	0.3	31.1	0.1	3.1	1.4	0.4
23	Carvacrol	tr	17.8	73.5	3.8	49.6	22.3	33.3	22.4
24	Geranial	0.4	0.1	0.1	tr	0.1	0.1	0.1	tr
25	Jasmone	0.1	0.1	0.1	0.1	0.1	0.1	0.1	tr
26	ß-Caryophellene	0.2	0.4	0.1	0.4	0.4	0.5	0.3	0.2
27	Germacrene-D	0.8	1.0	0.5	0.5	0.7	0.7	1.3	0.8
Yield of oil (g/100 f.wt.)		1.2	0.6	1.1	0.6	1.1	0.7	0.8	1.0

[z]Identification for compounds 1, 4, 7, 13, 17, 18, 21, 25, 26, and 27 based on GC–MS data only.
[y]Refers to peak number in Fig. 1. Listed in order of elution.
[x]not detected.

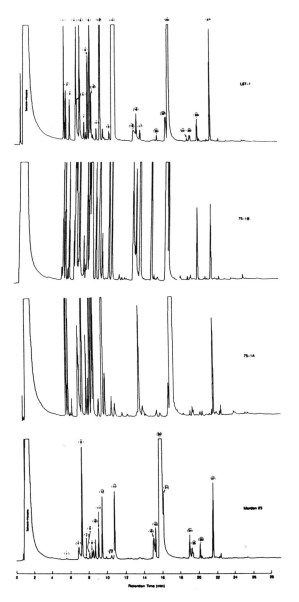

Fig. 1. Chromatograms of essential oils from four *Monarda* selections. For peak designation see Table 1.

Fig. 2. Pedigree of *Monarda* selections.

Table 2. Volatile composition of the essential oil of geraniol-rich 'Morden #3' monarda[z].

Peak[y]	Essential oil constituent	Relative composition (% of total essential oil)	
		Oil	Headspace
1	α-Thujene	tr	1.3
2	α-Pinene	---[x]	0.5
3	Camphene	---	0.1
4	ß-Pinene	0.3	6.0
5	1-Hepten-3-ol	tr	1.1
6	Myrcene	1.4	14.6
7	α-Phellandrene	tr	0.2
8	α-Terpenene	tr	7.2
9	p-Cymene/Limonene	tr	0.4
10	1,8-Cineole	0.1	0.2
11	Unknown ($C_{12}H_{20}O_2$)	0.2	1.1
12	Ocimene	0.7	8.6
13	Bornyl acetate	tr	tr
14	Linalool	1.1	3.0
15	Borneol	tr	0.1
16	Terpinen-4-ol	tr	0.3
17	α-Terpineol	tr	0.2
18	$C_{10}H_{12}O_2$	0.6	1.2
19	Nerol	0.4	3.5
20	Geraniol	92.6	39.5
21	Neral	0.2	3.6
22	Thymol	tr	tr
23	Carvacrol	tr	tr
24	Geranial	0.4	0.5
25	Jasmone	0.1	0.3
26	ß-Caryophellene	0.2	0.7
27	Germacrene-D	0.8	2.5

[z]Identification for compounds 1, 4, 7, 13, 17, 18, 21, 25, 26, and 27 based on GC-MS data only.
[y]Refers to peak number in Fig. 1. Listed in order of elution.
[x]Not detected.

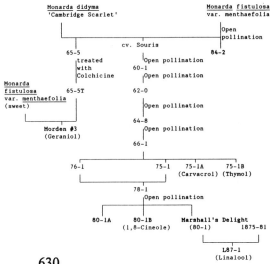

Linalool represented 45.7% of selection 80-1A, 49.8% of 'Marshall's Delight', and 67.0% of selection L87-1 essential oil (Table 1). This substantiates the close relationship existing between these three selections (Fig. 2); however, the other closely related selection, 80-1B, had only 0.4% of linalool, and a high amount of carvacrol (22.3%), 1,8-cineole (22.2%), ß-pinene (13.8%), and ocimene (6.2%). Therefore, a definite genetic segregation appears to have occured.

The oxygenated terpene, 1,8-cineole, occurred in all samples and represented 4.8, 14.1, and 22.2% of the oils from 'Marshall's Delight', '75-1B', and '80-1B' Monarda, respectively. 1,8-Cineole, also known as eucalyptol, cajuputoal, 1,8-oxido-p-menthane, or 1,8-epoxy-p-menthane, occurs in numerous essential oils (about 270) and is used widely in pharmaceutical preparations and food products such as beverages, ice cream, candies, baked goods, and chewing gum.

Propagation of these selections of monarda can easily be achieved through crown divisions, but this method is cumbersome and inefficient. A more effective and rapid method of propagation has been found to be through plant cuttings of actively growing stems. Stem cuttings, approximately 10 to 12 cm in length, are taken and all but two leaves removed, including the shoot tip. The bases of the cuttings are dipped in 1,000 ppm IBA rooting compound and placed in sand in a misting chamber. Cuttings taken in early June when the plants are actively growing produce root initials within one week and are ready for transplanting within 14 to 16 days. Propagation by tissue culture has also been successfully carried out in our laboratory using leaf cuttings.

Weeds do not pose a problem in the production of monarda. Herbicides such as trifluralin, terbacil, solan, and paraquat used together with good cultural practices can maintain a weed-free plantation. Trifluralin (1.12 kg/ha) should be used pre-plant incorporated when monarda is established. In the second year and every year thereafter, paraquat can be applied before the monarda shoots reach a height of 5 cm, to kill the early spring weeds. Application of herbicides in a commercial field, however, should only be used if the chemicals are legally registered for such use on this crop. This also kills off the monarda shoots. Application of terbacil (1.68 kg/ha) and 1 to 2 cm of irrigation should follow.

Rust, *Puccinia mentha*, is the major disease of *Monarda*. It has caused defoliation, girdling of stems, and degeneration of plants. The disease is spread by aerial rust spores under cool, cloudy, moist weather conditions. Relatively good control has been achieved by applying a contact herbicide, paraquat, in early spring when the monarda shoots are only about 5 cm tall to destroy all vegetation and thereby remove the required host for the spores.

Essential oil yield varies from about 0.65 to 1.2 g/100 g of fresh plant material (Table 1), or depending on the hybrid, 60 to 125 kg of oil/ha. As a result, it is our believe that four of these hybrids of monarda may have the potential of becoming commercial sources of geraniol, linalool, tymol, and carvacrol.

REFERENCES

Bailey, L.H. 1977. Manual of cultivated plants, p. 859. 16th ed. Macmillan, New York.

Furia, T.E. and N. Bellanca. 1975. Fenaroli's handbook of flavor ingredients. 2nd ed. vol 2. CRC Press, Boca Raton, FL. p. 83, 91, 460, 556.

Guenther, E. 1949. The essential oils. vols. II and III. Van Nostrand, New York. p. 708–713.

Kirk-Othmer. 1983. Encyclopedia of chemical technology. 3rd ed. Wiley, New York. p. 709–732.

Marshall, H.H. and B.B. Chubey. 1983. *Monarda* for geraniol production. Agr. Can., Canadex No. 268.10.

Marshall, H.H. and R.W. Scora. 1972. A new chemical race *of Monarda* fistulosa (Labiatae). Can. J. Bot. 50:1945–1849.

Mazza, G., B.B. Chubey, and F. Kiehn. 1987. Essential oil of *Monarda fistulosa* L. var. *menthaefolia*. Flavour Fragr. J. 2:129–132.

Scora, R.W. 1967. Study of the essential leaf oils of the genus *Monarda* (Labiatae). Amer. J. Bot. 54:446–452.

New Aromatic Lemon Basil Germplasm*

Mario R. Morales, Denys J. Charles, and James E. Simon

Basil (*Ocimum basilicum* L., Lamiaceae) has long been acclaimed for its diversity as a source of essential oils, its flavor and delicacy as a spice, and its beauty and fragrance as an ornamental (Simon et al. 1990). Basil is extensively used by the perfume, pharmacy, and food industries for its natural aroma and flavor (Darrah 1980; Simon et al. 1984). There are many variants of basil which exhibit a wide range of leaf color (green to dark purple), flower and bract color (red, white, lavender, or purple), and which vary in growth characteristics and aroma making it an increasingly popular culinary and ornamental herb. Basils are annual plants and, generally, flowering commences about 80 days after planting in late spring. The flowers as well as the leaves are highly aromatic.

Most basils are grown as culinary herbs primarily because of their unique aromas and fragrances, which can be strikingly similar to the aroma of cinnamon, licorice, lemon as well as the more traditional sweet basil aroma which is mainly due to a combination of linalool, methyl chavicol, and 1,8-cineole. Basils, which exhibit a lemon aroma (due to the presence of citral), are commercially available and are characterized by their small stature, early flowering, small and narrow leaves, and low essential oil and citral contents. In 1988, we compared three field-grown lemon basil cultivars, and found that the citral content in the essential oil was 12.6% (Companion Plants), 14.4% (Lake Valley), and 32.4% (Burpee Seeds). In 1989, we identified a single robust and tall plant with a very strong and distinct lemon fragrance within our germplasm collection. This individual plant was found within an extensive intermated germplasm collection of *Ocimum* spp. and served as the parent to derive a new type of lemon basil for the culinary and ornamental herb market. We were also interested in comparing the effect of steam versus hydrodistillation on oil yield and composition.

METHODOLOGY

In 1989, an individual plant with strong lemon aroma and a distinct upright growth habit with larger leaves than previously found on available lemon basil cultivars was identified in a genetically broadbase germplasm collection of basil (*Ocimum* spp.) growing at Lafayette, Indiana (Oakley silt loam soil). The selected plant was potted and placed in a greenhouse, isolated from all other basils. Selfed seed (S_1) was collected in March, 1990, and sown in the greenhouse on Apr. 20, 1990. One month later, the 80 plants obtained were transplanted into the field, eight rows of ten plants each. At full bloom (July 16), the foliage and flowers of each plant were harvested (from 20 to 25 cm above ground), and immediately dried at 37°C in a forced air dryer for 15 days. Essential oils were extracted by hydrodistillation via clevenger trap according to Charles and Simon (1990). Oil content was measured volumetrically (% v/dry wt), and oils stored in Teflon sealed silica vials at 2°C in the dark. Essential oil composition was determined using a Varian 3700 GC equipped with FID and a Varian electronic 4270 integrator as reported (Charles and Simon 1990). Identification of citral (= neral and geranial) was verified by the use of standards and with a Finnigan 4000 GC/MS as described (Charles et al. 1990; Simon and Quinn 1988).

From among the 80 field-grown plants in 1990, five plants were selected for further development based on plant type, visual appearance, essential oil content, aroma, and citral content. These plants were vegetatively propagated and greenhouse-grown in isolation during the Fall of 1990 and second generation selfed seed (S_2) collected in March 1991. These five lines and remnant seed of the original plant (check) were field evaluated in a completely randomized block design with three replications in 1991. Each line was transplanted into five-row plots, ten plants per row, 46 cm between plants and 91 cm between rows on May 22, 1991 (Fig. 1). Plant height was estimated by measuring two random plants from each of the five rows. A relative measure of the leaf size from each line was estimated by collecting two fully mature leaves from a randomly selected plant in each of the five rows per plot and measuring the total leaf area using a LI-COR Model 3100 area meter. From July 9 to 23,

---

*Journal paper no. 13,177, Purdue Univ. Agr. Expt. Sta., West Lafayette, IN 49707-1165. This research was supported in part by grants from the Indiana Business Modernization and Technology Corporation, Indianapolis, and the Purdue University Agricultural Experiment Station (Specialty Crops Grant No. 014-1165-0000-65178).

when plants where in full bloom (Fig. 2), the three central rows were harvested in bulk, cutting the plants at ground level, and all the biomass weighed fresh and then immediately distilled to collect the essential oils using a 500-liter portable steam distillation unit (Alkire and Simon 1990) at 0.56 kg/cm^2 for 2 h. On July 12, ten plants from the first row of each 5-row plot were individually harvested, cutting them 20 to 25 cm above ground, dried at 37°C in a forced air dryer from 15 to 20 days and the oil extracted using 40- to 75-g samples in 2-liter clevenger trap hydrodistillation units ran for 1.25 h. Oils were stored and analyzed as described earlier. The last row of each 5-row plot was left for seed collection.

RESULTS

In 1990, plants were first evaluated for visual appearance and aroma. Plants which had foliar discolorations, exhibited disease symptoms or any other irregularities were rogued. Variation was high in all growth and oil characteristics in the segregating lemon basil population in 1990. Mean growth characteristics were as follows: plant height 55 cm; fresh weight 256 g; dry weight 31.4 g; oil yield 0.69% (v/dw); and citral content 67.2% of total essential oil. Five plants (Plant No. 47, 48, 75, 77, and 78) with 76.4 to 78.7% citral and 0.44 to 0.75% (v/dw) essential oil content were selected.

In 1991, significant differences among the five lines (S_2) and plants derived from selfed seed from the original plant (check) were observed for foliage yield, plant height, days to 50% flowering, uniformity, and essential oil yield (hydrodistillation) (Table 1, 2). The lines did not vary from the original plant selection in relative leaf size and citral content as extracted by steam distillation.

While citral content in the hydrodistilled oil did not vary among the five lines, all were significantly higher (average 13%) than the original parent check (Table 2). On average, the five selected lines of the second generation plants yielded 53% more oil than the original plant check (via hydrodistillation) and the plants were significantly taller (Tables 1, 2).

While the steam and hydrodistillation methods yielded the same amount of essential oils (1.1 ml/m^2), the citral content in the hydrodistilled oil was 50% higher than from steam distillation. Citral could have been lost in the actual physical collection of the oil with the steam distillation unit, but whether the citral was lost or chemically altered is as yet unknown (Table 2). The correlation for essential oil yield between steam and hydrodistillation was highly significant (r = 0.74**) whereas, there was no correlation between the extraction methods for citral content (r = 0.20), due to the lack of complete citral recovery from steam distillation.

Citral content was about 14% lower in all lines and the check in 1991 compared to 1990, which we presume was due to the more stressful season with average high day and night temperatures. The effect of seasonal differences on citral content is unknown. The original plant (check) flowered about 4 to 7 days later than the selected lines. Lines 75, 77, and 47 were most uniform (Table 1). Essential oil yield correlated positively with plant height and foliage fresh weight and negatively with days to 50% flowering (Table 3).

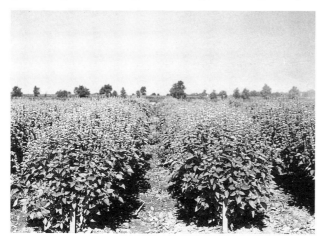

Fig. 1. Flowering plants of lemon basil germplasm grown in Central Indiana.

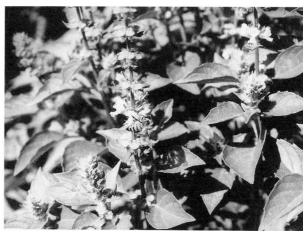

Fig. 2. Close-up of an individual plant of lemon basil.

Table 1. Growth and yield characteristics of second generation lemon basil lines evaluated in 1991.

Lines	Foliage yield		Plant height (cm)	No. days to 50% flowering	Leaf area[y] (cm^2)	Uniformity[x] estimate
	Area fresh wt[z] (kg/plot)	Plant dry wt (g/plant)				
75	25ab[w]	110a	62a	75a	19.7	1.7a
77	27a	112a	65a	77a	17.2	1.7a
47	28a	105ab	62a	74a	18.6	1.3a
78	24ab	94bc	58b	76a	18.5	3.3b
48	22b	100ab	62a	76a	17.8	2.7b
Check[v]	24ab	81c	53c	81b	19.3	5.0c
Mean	25	100	60	77	18.5	2.6
LSD (5%)	4	15	3	3	NSD	0.9
CV	8	9	2	2	9.4	19.4

[z]Based on harvesting 30 plants; plot size = 12.54 m^2.
[y]Based on 10 leaves/plot.
[x]Phenotype uniformity, based on visual estimating, 1 = very uniform; 5 = wide plant to plant variation.
[w]No significant differences between means with same letter.
[v]Seed from the original single plant identified in 1989.

Table 2. Effect of the extraction method on the essential oil yield and citral content of five second-generation sister lemon basil lines and the parent line evaluated in 1991.

	Extraction method				
	Steam distillation		Hydrodistillation		
	Essential oil yield (ml/m^2)	Citral content[z] (% of total oil)	Essential oil yield		Citral content[z] (% of total oil)
Lines			(ml/m^2)	(% v/dw)	
75	1.5a[y]	48	1.3a	0.81a	65a
77	1.4ab	49	1.2a	0.79ab	68a
47	1.2ab	42	1.2a	0.80a	68a
78	1.1ab	45	1.2a	0.87a	68a
48	1.0bc	38	1.2a	0.79ab	65a
Check	0.6c	43	0.8b	0.59b	59b
Mean	1.1	44	1.1	0.77	66
LSD (5%)	0.4	NSD	0.3	0.20	5
CV	19.5	14	14.1	14.80	4

[z]Citral contents of each line from first generation of selfed seed were 78.7% (P75), 77.0% (P77), 76.8% (P47), 76.5% (P48), and 76.4% (P78), and citral content of original plant was 67%, in 1990. Citral content from the hydrodistilled oil was about 14% lower in 1991 than in 1990.
[y]No significant differences between means with same letter.

Table 3. Correlation coefficients between five lemon basil traits of selected lines evaluated in 1991.

Trait	Essential oil yield[z]	Plant height	Days to 50% flowering	Leaf area
Foliage fresh weight	0.47*	0.26	−0.18	0.02
Essential oil yield[z]		0.72**	−0.56*	0.04
Plant height			−0.54*	−0.27
Days to 50% flowering				0.13

[z]Extracted by steam distillation.
*,**Levels of significance different from zero at probabilities of 0.05 and 0.01, respectively.

CONCLUSIONS

After two cycles of selfing and selection, we identified five uniform lines of lemon basil with desirable aromatic, horticultural, and ornamental characteristics. This is the first report of a tall highly aromatic lemon basil that has potential as an ornamental culinary herb. Plants exhibited a strong pleasant lemon aroma, and compared to commercially available lemon basil cultivars, had larger leaf size (similar to sweet basil genotypes), and taller stature. Both the available cultivars and the new lemon basils described here, have attractive white flowers (Fig. 2) which continue to bloom as the plants continue to grow until frost. Each line had a distinct lemon fragrance with a minimum citral content of 65% in 1991. All the lines were highly aromatic with essential oil contents of 0.79 to 0.87% (v/dw) in 1991. Each line was highly vigorous with plants reaching heights of 58 to 65 cm in 1991 (Fig. 1, 2). All five lines appear superior to the original plant (check), with lines 75, 77, and 47 the most aromatic, vigorous, and uniform.

REFERENCES

Alkire, B.H. and J.E. Simon. 1990. Construction and design of a portable steam distillation unit for peppermint and spearmint. In: Proc. 1990 Mint Industry Research Council (MIRC), Annual MIRC Meeting, Las Vegas, NV. January, 1991.

Charles, D.J. and J.E. Simon. 1990. Comparison of extraction methods for the rapid determination of essential oil content and composition of basil (*Ocimum* spp.). J. Amer. Soc. Hort. Sci. 115:458–462.

Charles, D.J., J.E. Simon, and K.V. Wood. 1990. Essential oil constituents of *Ocimum micranthum* Willd. J. Agr. Food Chem. 38:120–122.

Darrah, H.H. 1984. The cultivated basils. Buckeye Printing Company, Independence, MO.

Simon, J.E. and J. Quinn. 1988. Characterization of essential oil of parsley. J. Agr. Food Chem. 36:467–472.

Simon, J.E., A.F. Chadwick, and L.E. Craker. 1984. Herbs: An indexed bibliography 1971–1980; the scientific literature on selected herbs, and aromatic and medicinal plants of the temperate zone. Archon Books, Hamden, CT.

Simon, J.E., J. Quinn, and R.G. Murray. 1990. Basil: a source of essential oils, p. 484–489. In: J. Janick and J.E. Simon (eds.). Advances in new crops. Timber Press, Portland, OR.

Nitrogen Application Affects Yield and Content of the Active Substances in Camomile Genotypes

Wudeneh Letchamo

Camomile [*Chamomilla recutita*,(L.), Rausch.] is an important medicinal plant, whose multitherapeutic, cosmetic, and nutritional values have been established through years of traditional and scientific applications (Mann and Staba 1986; Schilcher 1987). Reports concerning the effect of nitrogen on growth, yield, and content of the active substances in camomile is contradictory and fragmentary. The objectives of this study was to compare the response of a diploid and two tetraploid camomile genotypes to low and high levels of nitrogen fertilization. A two year (1986–1987) pot experiment was conducted with three camomile genotypes under 5 different N levels.

METHODOLOGY

Seeds of three camomile genotypes, a diploid ($2n=18$), and two tetraploids (BK2-39, and R-43 $2n=36$) were obtained from the breeding program of the Institute of Agronomy and Plant Breeding I, Justus Liebig University, Giessen. The essential oil composition and morphology of these lines were previously described (Letchamo and Vömel 1989; Letchamo 1990).

Seedlings were raised in a greenhouse and transferred to 5 liter Mitscherlich pots filled with 2.0 kg of soil (RH loess serosiom) and 4.0 kg of sand. Four plants/pot with 8 replications of each variant were planted in spring 1986 and 1987. Five levels of N (NH_4NO_3) were used as follows. N0 = no nitrogen, N1 = 0.4 g N/pot, N2 = 0.8 g N/pot N3 = 1.2 g N/pot and N4 = 1.6 g N/pot. During planting, we applied 1.5 g/pot $CaCO_3$, 5.0 g/pot Fe, 5.0 g/pot Mn, 2.5 g/pot Cu, 2.5 g/pot Zn, 0.5 g/pot B, and 0.05 g/pot Mo. The flowers were hand harvested at the medium stage of their development (Letchamo 1990) and dried at 38°C for 72 h. Circulatory steam distillation (2.0 g of the dry sample) was carried out in a Neoclevenger type apparatus (in 500 ml volume round bottomed flask with 300 ml deionized water) for 2 h using n-Pentan as a distillation receiver (Hölzl and Demuth 1979). The essential oil content was determined gravimetrically. Essential oil samples were diluted in 1 ml toluol and analyzed using Carlo Erba Instruments, Model GC-6000 Vega Series-2; equipped with a flame ionization detector (FID) interfaced with a Spectrophysics Integrator Sp. San Jose California for chromatography data acquisition, processing, and quantitation. A 30 m × 0.25 mm id fused silica capillary column packed with a stationary phase of 0.25 µm thickness was used for the separation of volatiles. Carrier gas flow rate was 30 ml N/min; sample size was 1 µl direct injection with Hamilton Microliter syringe. Injector system was split-splitless with 1:20 ratio. Injection port temperature was 220°C, detector oven temperature was adjusted to 240°C. Column temperature was programmed at 120°C for 0 min., 120° to 150°C at 30°C/min for 2 min., 150° to 175°C, 10 min., 175°C to 220°C at 30°C/min. n-Hexadecane was used as an internal standard. The data were analyzed using analysis of variance following established statistical procedures (Dospechov 1979; Köhler et al. 1984) using SPSS/pc+.

RESULTS AND DISCUSSION

Morphological Changes and Flower Yield

Plant height, the straw yield, number of productive tillers, primary branches, and volume of the flower heads significantly increased due to the increased levels of N application (Fig. 1,2). Similar results were reported by Franz and Kirsch (1974) and Meawad et al. (1984) by applying N with K and some growth regulators at different levels respectively. Maximum response for straw was not reached by BK2-39 and R-43 even at N4 (Fig. 1,2). The straw yield of tetraploids, however, showed a significant growth with increased N application up to N4 (Fig. 2). A remarkably relaxed vegetative growth with thick leaves and branches was observed particularly by BK2-39 and R-43 at N4. At this N concentration the two tetraploid genotypes flowered ca. 8 days later than the control and lower levels of nitrogen (N1, N2, and N3) and remained dark green throughout the vegetation period.

The number of the flower heads and the drug yield (g/pot) significantly increased due to additional levels of nitrogen application in all the genotypes (Fig. 3). The drug and straw yield of the diploid did not show much difference between N3 and N4. A difference of 1.9 and 6.1 g/pot between N3 and N4 was obtained for drug and straw, respectively. The maximum drug yield response for this genotype was reached at N3, as further additions of N did not result in further increase (Fig. 3). Similarly, the drug yield difference between N3 and N4 was only 0.8 g/pot of the tetraploid BK2-39, with a maximum being at N3. The weight of individual flower heads increased only up to N2 in the diploid and BK2-39 and up to N3 in R-43. The difference was 11.2 g/pot for BK2-39 and 11.8 g/pot for R-43.

Essential Oil Content and Composition

Nitrogen fertilization increased the percentage (Table 1) and absolute yield of essential oil (Fig. 3). The contribution of N to the essential oil increment was 42% in the diploid, 25% in BK2-39, and 27% in R-43. There was no change in the composition of the essential oil due to the differences in N levels. A sample chromatogram of a tetraploid camomile essential oil is shown in Fig. 4.

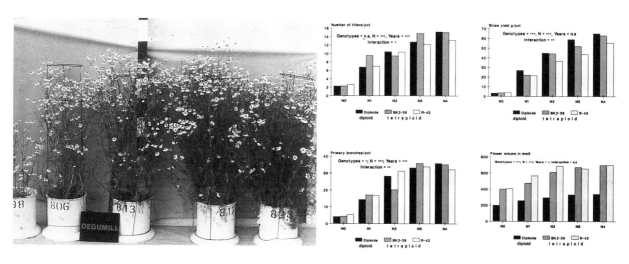

Fig. 1. Diploid camomile plants under pot experiment, R. Holzhausen summer 1987.

Fig. 2. Effect of N on morphological parameters and straw yield (dry matter) in camomile genotypes.

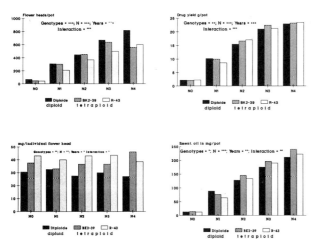

Fig. 3. Effect of N on yield parameters and drug (g/pot) and essential oil (mg/pot) yield of camomile genotypes.

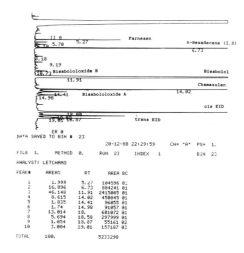

Fig. 4. Gas-chromatogram of tetraploid camomile essential oil.

Table 1. Effect of nitrogen on the content of essential oil (%) and active substances (mg/100 g drug) in camomile genotypes (a mean of 2 years), Rauischholzhausen, 1986–87.

Genotype	NH_4NO_3 (g/pot)	Essential oil (%)	Bisabolol (mg/100 g)	Chamazulen (mg/100 g)	cis-EID[z] (mg/100g)	trans-EID[z] (mg/100 g)
Diploid ($2n = 18$)						
N0	0.0	0.62	126	56.5	16.4	11.5
N1	0.4	0.85	185	71.0	25.4	21.1
N2	0.8	0.82	199	77.0	35.2	22.0
N3	1.2	0.83	203	78.0	24.8	16.8
N4	1.6	0.96	187	58.0	30.8	20.0
Significance: N		*	**	**	*	*
Regression: L		0.19*** (0.64)[y]	149*** (2.0)	2.4NS (0.06)	7.6* (0.40)	3.2NS (0.25)
Q		0.00NS (−0.01)	−71*** (−1.6)	−33.1** (−1.4)	−11.3* (−0.99)	−8.3* (−1.08)
a		0.62***	129***	66.2***	20.7***	15.7***
r		0.62***	0.64***	0.61NS	0.40*	0.25NS
Tetraploid BK2-39 ($2n = 36$)						
N0	0.0	0.69	178	59.5	44.3	23.5
N1	0.4	0.78	213	77.0	38.8	19.3
N2	0.8	0.89	205	101.0	39.5	19.1
N3	1.2	0.87	238	87.5	55.6	22.8
N4	1.6	0.92	229	76.0	56.8	24.8
Significance: N		*	**	**	*	*
Regression: L		0.15*** (0.50)	32.2** (0.41)	61.9** (1.27)	9.5* (0.34)	1.5NS (0.16)
Q		−0.13NS (−0.69)	−20.5NS (−0.44)	−31.9* (−1.09)	11.2NS (0.68)	7.3** (1.31)
a		0.69***	186.3***	59.0***	39.0***	23.0***
r		0.50***	0.41**	0.38*	0.34*	0.41*
Tetraploid R-43 ($2n = 36$)						
N0	0.0	0.61	177	52.5	46.0	20.6
N1	0.4	0.76	205	68.5	41.2	20.4
N2	0.8	0.80	224	88.0	41.0	24.7
N3	1.2	0.88	255	89.5	47.4	24.2
N4	1.6	0.85	229	83.0	56.9	29.2
Significance: N		*	**	**	*	*
Regression: L		0.14*** (0.52)	38.7* (0.36)	67.7** (1.47)	6.2NS (0.24)	4.9** (0.40)
Q		0.13NS (−0.79)	−42.0NS (0.65)	−31.9* (−1.09)	13.9NS (0.93)	1.9NS (0.25)
a		0.66***	186.5***	51.9***	41.2***	20.6***
r		0.52***	0.36*	0.52**	0.24NS	0.17*

[z]cis-trans-En-In-Dicycloether.
L = Linear; Q = Quadratic.
[y]( ) Values in brackets represent beta.
Significant at $P < 0.05$*; 0.01**; 0.001*** level respectively.
NS = Not significant.

(-)-α-Bisabolol, Chamazulen and *cis-trans*-En-In-Dicycloether (EID) Content

The lowest content of (-)-α-bisabolol in the diploid and tetraploids was achieved at N0 whereas the highest content was obtained at N3 from all the genotypes. With further increment of N levels (N4), a declining effect in (-)-α-bisabolol content was observed (Table 1). The overall application of N contributed to 41% increment in the diploid, 19% in BK2-39, and 17% in R-43.

Similarly, the lowest chamazulen content for all the genotypes was at N0 (Table 1) with a peak at intermediate N level depending on genotype. These results were in agreement with field experiments of Meawad et al. (1984). The overall contribution of N to Chamazulen increment was 17% in the diploid, 15% in BK2-39 and 28% in R-43.

The highest content of *cis-trans*-EID in the diploid was achieved at N2. The lowest value was recorded at N0. Further increment of N levels to N3 and N4 to the diploid brought about a decline in *cis-trans*-EID content (Table 1). However, the highest *cis-trans*-EID content in the tetraploids was obtained at N4, but a reasonably high concentration of *cis-trans*-EID was obtained at N0 in tetraploids (Table 1). The general contribution of N application for *cis*-EID was about 24% in the diploid, 12% in BK2-39 and 13% in R-43. This value for *trans*-EID was 16% for the diploid and 17% for BK2-39 and R-43.

We conclude that nitrogen application during growing conditions has a positive effect on the yield of camomile genotypes and favors the content of its active substances but, the response is affected by genotype. Establishment of the optimum level of N should be a compromise between drug yield, content of the essential oil, and the active substances in the flower heads.

REFERENCES

Dospechov, B.A. 1979. Statistical methods in field experiments (in Russian). Kolos press, Moscow.

Franz, Ch. and C. Kirsch. 1974. Growth and flower-bud-formation of *Matricaria chamomilla* L. in dependence on varied nitrogen and potassium nutrition (in German). Hort. Sci. 21:11–19.

Hölzl, J. and G. Demuth. 1979. Influence of ecological factors on the composition of the essential oil and flavonoids in *Matricaria chamomilla* of different origin (in German). Planta medica 27:37–45.

Köhler, W.G., Schachtel, and P. Volske. 1984. Biometry. Introduction to statistics for biologists and agricultural scientists (in German). Springer–Verlag, Berlin.

Letchamo, W. and A. Vömel. 1989. The relationship between ploidy levels and certain morphological characteristics of *Chamomilla recutita*. Planta Medica 55:527–528.

Letchamo, W. 1990. Genotypic and phenotypic variation in floral development of different genotypes of camomile. Herba Hungarica 29:34–40.

Mann, C. and E.J. Staba. 1986. The chemistry, pharmacology, and commercial formulations of chamomile, p. 235–280. In: L.E. Craker and J.E. Simon (eds.). Herbs, spices, and medicinal plants: Recent advances in botany, horticulture and pharmacology. vol. 1. Oryx Press, Phoenix, AZ.

Meawad, A.A., A.E. Awad, and A. Afify. 1984. The combined effect of N-fertilization and some growth regulators on camomile plants. Acta Hort. 144:123–133.

Schilcher, H. 1987. The camomile. A hand book for practitioners, pharmacists and other natural scientists (in German). Wissenschaftliche Verlagsgesselschaft mbH, Stuttgart.

Effect of Water Stress and Post-Harvest Handling on Artemisinin Content in the Leaves of *Artemisia Annua* L.*

Denys J. Charles, James E. Simon, Clinton C. Shock, Erik B.G. Feibert, and Robin M. Smith

Artemisia annua L., (Asteraceae) is a highly aromatic annual herb that has potential value as a source of artemisinin and essential oils (Simon et al. 1990). Artemisinin is a secondary plant product that has been found to have strong anti-malarial properties with little or no side effects (Klayman 1985). New anti-malarial drugs are important due to the increasing resistance of the malaria causing protozoans to current drugs (WHO 1981). Extensive research has been carried out over the last decade towards the characterization, isolation, synthesis, and pharmacology of artemisinin and its derivatives because of their effectiveness against both chloroquine and mafloquine resistant *Plasmodium falciparum* associated with cerebral malaria (Klayman 1985; Schmid and Hofheinz 1983; Xu et al. 1986). While artemisinin can be synthesized, the synthetic compound is unlikely to be economically competitive with the naturally produced compound (Schmid and Hofheinz 1983; Xu et al. 1986). Of the total artemisinin in the plant, 89% is found in the leaves (Charles et al. 1989).

For several years, we have been evaluating the plant's production potential, determining its horticultural characteristics, and developing a rapid assay to determine artemisinin content from crude plant materials for use in selection and breeding (Shock and Stieber 1987; Charles et al. 1990; Simon et al. 1990). Essential oil composition was also characterized in order to evaluate *Artemisia annua* as a source of aroma chemicals for the fragrance industry (Charles et al. 1991). Selection of lines for high artemisinin content began in 1989 at Purdue University and Oregon State University at the Malheur Experiment Station.

Artemisinin is unstable due to its endoperoxy group and the chemical analysis is difficult. Most secondary products can be altered by environmental factors as well as post-harvest handling practices, yet little is known about the stability of artemisinin when subjected to either pre- or post-harvest environmental changes. The objective of this study was to examine the influence of soil water stress and drying techniques on the retention of artemisinin.

METHODOLOGY

This report consists of three studies conducted in Ontario, Oregon. The first, a preliminary field trial, conducted in 1989, examined whether the time of harvest could influence artemisinin content. Seeds were sown in the greenhouse on March 30 and transplanted to the field Owyhee silt loam on May 3 into 1.12 m rows with 0.91 m between plants. Mechanical cultivation and manual hoeing kept the field weed free. The trial was fertilized with a total of 167 kg N/ha as broadcast urea and water-run UAN (urea ammonium nitrate). Leaf samples were collected from 20 plants in each of 27 lines on 3 harvest dates. All leaf samples were air dried in the shade and the stems removed by hand.

The next two studies were conducted in 1990 on a Greenleaf silt loam with a pH of 6.7, 1.6% organic matter, 28 meq/100 g CEC, 17 ppm potassium, 1996 ppm calcium, 362 ppm magnesium, 186 ppm sodium, 1.5 ppm zinc, 7.2 ppm iron, 26.7 ppm manganese, 1.1 ppm copper, and 0.5 ppm boron. The herbicides, Dual (2.2 kg ai/ha) and Treflan (0.56 kg ai/ha) were preplant incorporated on 2 May for weed control. Seeds were greenhouse sown on 29 Apr. and transplanted to the field on 29 May. Plants were 0.5 m apart, with 1.12 m between rows. For the water stress study, each plot consisted of three rows wide and 27 m long with 4 replications in a randomized complete block design. The crop was irrigated regularly with furrow irrigation. The crop was fertilized June 25 with 167 kg/ha of N in the form of urea. N-Serve at 0.84 kg ai/ha had been applied on the urea immediately before fertilization to conserve nitrogen.

---

*The authors gratefully acknowledge financial support for 1989 and 1990 research provided by the Malheur County Regional Economic Development Strategy Board. Oregon Agricultural Experiment Station, Technical Paper No. 9812; and from the Purdue Agricultural Experiment Station.

Treatments for the water stress trial were imposed in July. After July 1, the timing of irrigations (frequency and duration) was based on the soil water potential according to treatment criteria. The four treatments consisted of plots irrigated so as to maintain low, mild, moderate water stress, and low stress followed by mild then moderate stress (Table 1). Soil water potential was monitored in each plot with the use of four granular matrix sensors (Watermark Soil Moisture Sensors, Model 200X, Irrometer Inc., Riverside, CA) with two sensors placed 15 cm deep and two sensors placed 45 cm deep in the planted row within the harvest area of each plot. Criterion for irrigation of a plot was based on the average water potential of the four sensors in each plot. Granular matrix sensor resistance was calibrated against tensiometer measurements of soil water potential in the field. Sensors were read several times a week and before all irrigations.

Leaf samples for artemisinin content were collected from 12 plants in the center of each plot on 20 Aug., 5 Sept. (first bud), and Sept. 5 (onset of flowering) from the soil water stress study. A total of 12 contiguous plants from the center rows of each plot were harvested on Sept. 17 from the soil water stress study to determine fresh weight yield. Plants were harvested at the soil surface. Plant height, fresh weight, plant dry weight, dry leaf weight, leaf to stem ratio, and artemisinin content were determined.

Six drying treatments were examined: sun dried, sun dried shaded in paper bag, air dried indoors, and artificial drying using forced air heat at 30°, 50°, and 80°C (Table 2). For each drying treatment, plant samples were dried for 0, 12, 24, 36, and 48 h. To reduce error from interplant variation, composite samples consisting of branches from thirty adjacent plants were used for every treatment in each of five replicates. Air temperature, relative humidity, and sample temperatures were determined, except at 80°C where relative humidity was not determined. Leaves from each treatment were evaluated for water and artemisinin content. All artemisinin concentrations reported are based on the harvest of all leaves from whole plants.

Table 1. Water stress treatments for *Artemisia annua* at Ontario, Oregon, 1990.

Treatment	Irrigation criteria (kPa)	Timing
Low stress	−50	from July 1
Mild stress	−100	from July 1
Moderate stress	−150	from July 1
Stress before harvest	−50	from July to 8 Aug.
then	−150	from Aug. 8 to Sept. 5

Plants harvested on Aug. 20, Sept. 5, and Sept 17.

Table 2. Effects of six drying treatments and four durations on the artemisinin content in *Artemisia annua* leaves, 1990.

Drying method	Avg. air RH (%)	Air temp. (°C) avg.	Air temp. (°C) max.	Sample temp. (°C) avg.	Sample temp. (°C) max.	Artemisinin content (% dry weight) 12h	24h	36h	48h
Sun	30.9	23.5	30.0	25.0	42.2	0.08±0.06	0.09±0.03	0.10±0.03	0.12±0.06
Air dried outside	30.9	23.5	30.0	24.4	35.6	0.15±0.12	0.17±0.10	0.04±0.02	0.08±0.02
Air dried inside	35.6	23.2	28.9	19.5	22.8	0.15±0.07	0.19±0.08	0.12±0.09	0.09±0.06
30°C	52.8	32.1	35.0	31.9	34.4	0.07±0.05	0.06±0.01	0.06±0.01	0.05±0.03
50°C	36.3	49.6	53.9	49.5	52.8	0.05±0.02	0.05±0.02	0.06±0.02	0.12±0.08
80°C	ND	79.9	80.0	70.9	80.0	0.13±0.11	0.08±0.04	0.06±0.02	0.06±0.03

Plants harvested on Aug. 20, Sept. 5, and Sept 17.

RESULTS AND DISCUSSION

Harvest date had a significant effect on artemisinin content, with July 26 harvest giving the highest artemisinin content (Table 3). Higher artemisinin content well before flower bud formation was not expected and a further examination of seasonal changes in artemisinin accumulation is needed. However, this data and our current studies do show that artemisinin content does change within the plant over the growing season. We expected that the increase in artemisinin content would have been related to the contribution of flowers.

Stress has been shown to induce the synthesis of a number of secondary or natural plant products (Fluck 1955; Gershenzon 1984). To investigate the possible effect of water stress on the accumulation of artemisinin, four different water stress treatments were investigated. Artemisinin content was determined for plants harvested on Aug. 20, Sept. 5, and Sept. 17. Season long (July 1 to Sept. 17) water stress was not related to artemisinin content, plant or leaf yields. Water stress during the two weeks before harvest was associated with reduced plant height ($p = 0.014$). Regression analysis revealed that greater soil water stress (lower soil water potential) during the two weeks before harvest lead to reduced leaf artemisinin content (Fig. 1).

Since postharvest handling of artemisia plants could affect artemisinin content, six drying techniques over different time periods were examined to identify the best drying method. Drying method and duration had highly significant effects on leaf moisture (Fig. 2, 3). Artemisinin contents were retained to a greater extent when plants were dried under ambient conditions compared to forced air at 30° to 80°C, except when dried at 80°C for the shortest time period (12 h) (Table 2). Prolonged drying generally resulted in further losses in artemisinin. In conclusion, these results strongly suggest that both plant water status and post-harvest handling can influence the retention of artemisinin.

Table 3. Artemisinin content in air dried leaves at different harvest dates[z], 1989.

Harvest date	Days after planting	Growth stage	Artemisinin content[y] (% dry wt)
June 30	90	Active growth	0.06
July 26	117	Active growth	0.15
September 5	158	Visible flower bud	0.06
LSD (0.05)			0.04

[z]Means are from 20 plants in each of 27 lines sampled on three dates.
[y]Only leaves were analyzed, flowers were not present.

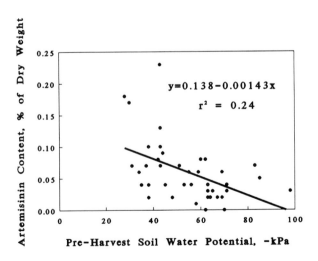

Fig. 1. Decline in artemisinin content from *Artemisia annua* with average soil water potential (x) two weeks before plant sampling ($P < 0.01$). Data are from all plant samples from the water stress trial at Ontario, Oregon, taken Aug. 20 and Sept. 5, 1990.

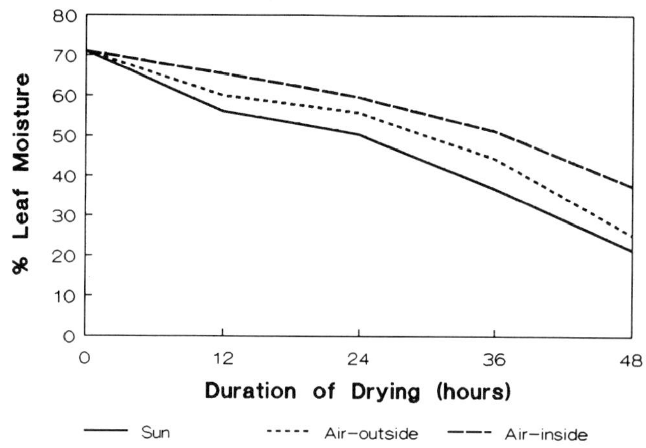

Fig. 2. Effects of different ambient air drying treatments on leaf moisture of *Artemisia annua*, LSD (0.05) = 4.1 for treatment × duration. For the air outside and air inside treatments, leaf material was placed in paper bags, Ontario, Oregon, 1990.

Fig. 3. Effect of different forced air drying treatments on leaf moisture of *Artemisia annua*, LSD (0.05) = 4.1 for treatment × duration, Ontario, Oregon, 1990.

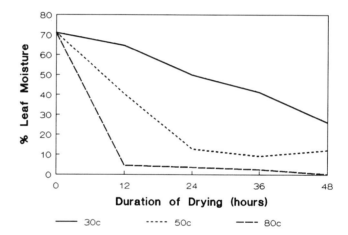

REFERENCES

Charles, D.J., J.E. Simon, K.V. Wood, and P. Heinstein. 1990. Germplasm variation in artemisinin content of *Artemisia annua* using an alternative method of artemisinin analysis from crude plant extracts. J. Nat. Prod. 53(1):157–160.

Charles, D.J., E. Cebert, and J.E. Simon. 1991. Characterization of the Essential oil of *Artemisia annua* L. J. Ess. Oil Res. 3:33–39.

Fluck, H. 1955. The influence of climate on the active principles in medicinal plants. J. Pharm. Pharmacol. 7:361–383.

Gershenzon, J. 1984. In: B.N. Timmerman, C. Steelnik, and F.A. Loewus (eds.). Phytochemical adaptations to stress. Recent advances in phytochemistry. vol. 18. Plenum Press, New York.

Klayman, D.L. 1985. Quinghaosu (artemisinin): an antimalarial drug from China. Science 228:1049–1055.

Schmid, G. and W. Hofheinz. 1983. Total synthesis of Qinghaosu. J. Amer. Chem. Soc. 105:624–625.

Shock, C.C. and T.S. Stieber. 1987. Productivity of *Artemisia annua* in the Treasure Valley. Oregon State Univ. Special Rpt. 814:115–123.

Simon, J.E., D. Charles, E. Cebert, L. Grant, J. Janick, and A. Whipkey. 1990. *Artemisia annua* L.: A promising aromatic and medicinal, p. 522–526. In: Janick, J. and J.E. Simon (eds.). Advances in new crops. Timber Press, Portland, OR.

World Health Organization. 1981. Report of the fourth meeting of the scientific working group on the chemotherapy of malaria. Beijing, People's Republic of China, October 6–10, 1981.

Xu, X., J. Zhu, D. Huang, and W. Zhou. 1986. Total synthesis of arteannuin and deoxyarteannuin. Tetrahedron 42:819–828.

Evaluation of the Pawpaw Tree, *Asimina triloba* (Annonaceae), as a Commercial Source of the Pesticidal Annonaceous Acetogenins*

Sunil Ratnayake, J. Kent Rupprecht, William M. Potter, and Jerry L. McLaughlin

The potent antitumor, pesticidal and/or insect antifeedant properties of the Annonaceous acetogenins have been previously reported (Rupprecht et al. 1986; Hui et al. 1989; Alkofahi et al. 1989) and patented (Mikolajczak et al. 1988, 1989). A recent compilation reviews the chemistry and biological actions, known to date, of this new class of diversely bioactive botanical compounds (Rupprecht et al. 1990). The Annonaceae is almost exclusively a tropical plant family and encompasses over 2000 species (Heywood 1978). However, the pawpaw (*Asimina triloba* Dunal) is a temperate representative and is an abundant native of eastern North America. Work on the seeds and stem bark of the pawpaw initially revealed pesticidal actions of the acetogenins and focused on asimicin (1), a major bioactive component of a complex mixture of these compounds (Rupprecht et al. 1986; Alkofahi et al. 1989).

Asimicin (1) (Fig. 1) was originally isolated from a 90% aqueous methanol partition fraction (Fig. 2) (F005) from the 95% ethanol extract of the stem bark of pawpaw (Mikolajczak et al. 1988). F005 is identical to the F020 as described in the initial patent of Mikolajczak et al. (1988). It was isolated via bioactivity-directed fractionation using a simple test involving lethality to brine shrimp larvae (*Artemia salina* Leach) (BST). Promising pesticidal activities paralleled the BST throughout the fractionation (Alkofahi et al. 1989) and included significant activity against blowfly larvae (*Colliphora vicina* Meig), two-spotted spider mite (*Tetranychus urticae* Koch), melon aphid (*Aphis gossyphii* Glover), mosquito larvae (*Aedes aegypti* Linnaeus), Mexican bean beetle (*Epilachna varivestis* Mulsant), striped cucumber beetle (*Acalymma vittatum* F.), and a free-living nematode [*Caenorhabditis elegans* (Maupas) Dougherty]. Subsequent testing of F005 has shown promising activities against a host of additional pests, especially those of horticultural concern.

Asimicin (1) contains eight chiral centers (256 possible stereoisomers) and, thus, is not a good candidate for commercial chemical synthesis. However, plant extracts, such as F005, containing a mixture of the bioactive acetogenins can be quickly and inexpensively prepared. As is true with the pyrethrins, such botanical mixtures often increase the pesticidal spectrum and are less likely to induce pest resistance after repeated application. Therefore, a plant extract, such as F005, would be a logical means for incorporation of the acetogenins into a pesticidal product. F005, obtained from the stem bark of pawpaw and suspended with 2% aqueous Tween 80

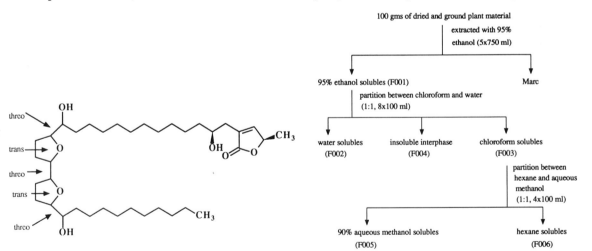

Fig. 1. Structure of asimicin.

Fig. 2. Scheme for extraction and partitioning of *Asimina triloba*.

---

*This work was supported by NIH/NCI RO1 grant no. CA 30909.

in the concentration range of 0.05 to 0.5% (500 to 5000 ppm), provides effective pesticidal action and plant protection in laboratory and field tests. Fig. 2 illustrates the protective effect of F005 against foliar damage on bush beans infested with bean leaf beetles (*Cerotoma trifurcata* Forster).

Asimina triloba is quite common as an understory shrub and small tree throughout the eastern United States, and the edible fruits, called "pawpaw" (Fig. 3), have generated considerable interest for commercial production (Callaway 1990). Over 18 million trees (3 to 13 cm diam) are growing in Indiana (Spencer et al. 1990), and other eastern states have similarly high populations. Thus, an evaluation of the relative biological potencies and percentage yields of standardized extracts from the various plant parts is needed. The development of such new, environmentally compatible, biologically degradable, botanically-derived, pesticides has become more desirable (Arnason et al. 1989).

METHODOLOGY

The plant material was collected in Indiana during July 1988 and October 1990 with the exception of the seeds which were collected in November 1989 from plantings at the University of Maryland, established in 1982 by R. Neal Peterson. The Indiana collections came from a single clone at the Horticultural Research Farm, Purdue University, and were identified by George R. Parker, Professor of Forestry. The unripe fruits were frozen and freeze-dried, while the seeds were air dried at room temperature. The other plant materials were dried in an oven at 40°C, and all of the materials were ground in a Wiley mill (unless otherwise stated, 4 mm mesh size was used in all cases). The woody collections were chipped and shredded (Mantis, Chipmate) prior to drying.

The dried plant materials (100 g) were then repeatedly extracted (Fig. 4) with 95% ethanol (5 × 750 ml). The combined extract was evaporated under reduced pressure (below 40°C) to provide a syrupy residue (F001). F001 was transferred to a 250 ml separatory funnel with a mixture of 100 ml of water and 100 ml of chloroform. After removal of the chloroform layer, the water layer was then extracted seven additional times with 100 ml portions of chloroform, and the combined layers were reduced under rotary vacuum (<40°C) to obtain the chloroform residue (F003). F003 was further partitioned between hexane and 10% water in methanol (1:1, 4 × 100 ml), and the solvents were evaporated under reduced pressure to afford the hexane solubles (F006) and the 90% aqueous methanol solubles (F005). The yield of F005 in grams from 100 g of plant material then directly corresponded to the percentage yields from the various plant parts.

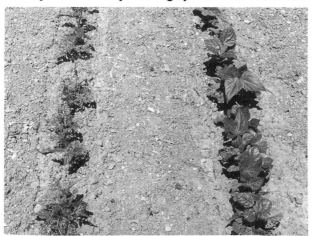

Fig. 3. Bush beans (cv. Blue Lake). The row on the left has a natural infestation with bean leaf beetles (*Cerotoma trifurcata* Forster). The row on the right was sprayed three times during a ten day period with 0.5% of F005 (F020), suspended with 2% Tween 80, in water. F005 (F020) is prepared from the bark of the pawpaw tree (*Asimina triloba*). Note the protective effect of the Annonaceous acetogenins in a field test against garden insects.

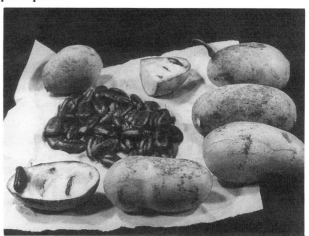

Fig. 4. Fruits and seeds of pawpaw (*Asimina triloba*).

The brine shrimp lethality bioassay (BST) (Meyer et al. 1982) was performed with the aqueous methanol soluble fractions (F005) as follows: 20 mg of each fraction was dissolved in 2 ml of methanol and 5, 50, and 500 µl amounts were transferred to 2 dram vials to correspond to 10, 100 and 1000 ppm concentrations; three vials were prepared for each concentration. These vials were dried overnight to permit evaporation of the methanol, and control vials were prepared using 500 µl of methanol alone. Ten brine shrimp larvae, taken 48 h after initiation of hatching in 3.8% aqueous sea salt brine (Instant Ocean, Metaframe) were added to each vial, and the final volume of each vial was adjusted to 5 ml using the artificial sea water. After 24 h, survivors were counted, and LC_{50} values with 95% confidence intervals were computed using a Finney's probit analysis program adapted to an IBM personal computer (discs of the program are available from J.L. McLaughlin).

RESULTS AND DISCUSSION

To access the pesticidal potential of the available biomass of *A. triloba*, various plant parts were collected and extracted in a standardized way (Fig. 4), and the resulting 90% aqueous methanol fractions (F005) were bioassayed in the BST. The percentage of F005 obtained from each plant part was also calculated, and this yield was correlated with the BST data to determine which plant part would yield the greatest quantity of an extract that could be suitably active for incorporation into a commercial product.

Table 1 shows the brine shrimp lethality of F005 for the various plant parts extracted and tested. The twigs, unripe fruit, seeds, root wood, and all the stem bark samples were the most active plant parts with LC_{50} values ranging from 0.042 to 0.104 ppm. These differences in activity, however, were not significant since the BST 95% confidence intervals all overlap. The BST activity of the root bark is very close to the above plant parts and is probably equivalent in activity even though there is a slight difference in the 95% confidence interval overlap between the root bark and the unripe fruit and root wood (D 0.01 ppm). The whole above-ground plant (leaves, stem, wood, and stem bark) and stems consisting of wood and bark were approximately 1/8 to 1/2 as active as the above plant parts. The BST of the wood and of the leaves were between 40 to 100 times and 500 to 1,200 times, respectively, less active than the most active plant parts. Furthermore, there were no significant differences in the bioactivities of the stem bark collected in July 1988 and October 1990, indicating that collections of bark made during the summer and fall are biologically equivalent and that the pesticidal constituents are stable over some period of time when the dried bark is stored.

The percentages of 90% aqueous methanol extractables (F005) of each plant part tested were also determined (Table 1). The unripe fruit, leaves, and seeds gave the highest percentages of F005. They would appear to be suitable sources of F005; however, the F005 from the leaves is the least active of the plant parts tested, and therefore, the leaves are a poor candidate for use. The extracts of the unripe fruit and seeds are extremely bioactive and also give a very high yield of F005; unfortunately, these plant parts represent the least available forms of biomass and are therefore unsuitable for commercial development. The root bark and stem bark afforded 1.96 to 2.72% yields into the 90% aqueous methanol extractables, and both plant parts possess potent brine shrimp activity. However, uprooting of the trees would destroy the stands and would require replanting on a commercial scale. When the stem bark was ground more finely (2 mm versus 4 mm sieves) the percentage of F005 increased by approximately 20%. The amount of 90% aqueous methanol extractables (F005) of the stem wood and bark, whole (above-ground) plant, root wood, and stem wood were 1.61, 1.60, 1.27, and 0.90%, respectively. The plant part which represents the best balance of yield and biological activity to its availability as a source of biomass is either the stem bark or the stem wood and stem bark in combination. Stripping of the bark is quite labor intensive; thus, mechanically chipping and shredding of the stem would be most practical.

To assess further the pesticidal potential of the combined stem wood and stem bark biomass, stems of various diameters were collected, chipped and shredded, dried, and pulverized, and standardized extracts were prepared; the BST was made on the F005 extract from stems of the different diameters. The percentage of F005 obtained and the brine shrimp activity were both inversely proportional to the stem diameter (Table 2). The activity of the smallest stems, 64 mm or less in diameter, was significantly greater than the other diameters tested.

Asimicin (1) and several other acetogenin compounds play the major role in the pesticidal activity. Asimicin alone gives BST LC_{50} values at 0.03 ppm (Rupprecht et al. 1986), whereas its stereoisomer, bullatacin gives LC_{50}

values at 0.00159 ppm (Hui et al. 1989). In addition to asimicin, bullatacin, bullatacinone, and trilobacin are all potent acetogenins recently isolated from F005 of pawpaw (Zhao et al. 1992). The variations of observed toxicity are probably due to quantitative variations of these and additional toxic acetogenins as distributed in different parts of the plant. The amounts of these compounds may also vary seasonally, but this variable has not been studied.

It is probable that the toxicities are higher in the twigs, unripe fruit, seeds, and bark because these are the plant parts which can be most easily damaged by herbivores, environmental pests and pathogens, and, therefore, for the purpose of defense, higher concentrations of the protective acetogenins may accumulate in these parts. The root (both bark and wood) may accumulate these compounds to avoid attack by nematodes and other soil pathogens.

In conclusion, the bioactivity of the *A. triloba* tree is concentrated mainly in the twigs, unripe fruits, seeds, root, and bark, but stems, especially those with the smallest diameters, are also significantly toxic. Therefore, the smaller aerial parts, minus the leaves, could be used as a biomass for the pesticidal extract. Finer milling would give more solubles while maintaining the level of the bioactivity. The stem bark collected in July showed more activity which, however, was not significantly different from the values of F005 obtained from the batch collected

Table 1. Brine shrimp lethality and percentage yields of F005 (90% aqueous methanol fraction) from various plant parts of *Asimina triloba*.

Plant part extracted	LC_{50} (ppm)[z]	Yield of F005 (%)
Twigs[y]	0.042 (0.02–0.09)	1.78
Unripe fruit[x]	0.060 (0.03–0.08)	5.11
Root wood[w]	0.060 (0.03–0.08)	1.27
Seed[v]	0.065 (0.03–0.10)	4.03
Stem bark[x,u]	0.077 (0.04–0.12)	2.71
Stem bark[y,u]	0.102 (0.06–0.15)	1.96
Stem bark[y]	0.104 (0.03–0.20)	2.52
Root bark[w]	0.135 (0.09–0.21)	2.72
Whole stem: wood, bark and leaves[y]	0.202 (0.14–0.31)	1.60
Stem wood[y]	4.86 (0.37–11.93)	0.90
Leaves[y]	53.6 (33–82)	4.36

[z]With 95% confidence intervals in parenthesis.
[y]Collected in October 1990.
[x]Collected in July 1988.
[w]Collected in November 1990.
[v]Collected in November 1989.
[u]Ground to a mesh size of 2 mm, all other samples were ground to a 4 mm mesh size.

Table 2. Variation of the percentage F005 (90% aqueous methanol solubles and brine shrimp lethality with differing stem diameters.

Stem diameter of extracted material (mm)	Percentage of F005	LC_{50} (ppm)[z]
251–500	1.36	0.36 (0.23–0.55)
189–250	1.45	0.22 (0.13–0.34)
65–188	1.76	0.22 (0.13–0.34)
0–64 (twigs)	1.78	0.04 (0.01–0.09)

[z]With 95% confidence intervals in parentheses.

in October from the same clone. It is possible that further screenings of wild populations of pawpaw could identify some clones with acceptably high levels of bioactivity in the leaves. The brine shrimp toxicity bioassay can be conveniently used as a rapid quality control measure of the total bioactivity of mixtures of the acetogenin compounds. Thus, the commercially used extract could be easily standardized as to bioactivity in furnishing a consistently bioactive product. A recent study with asimicin and F005 in the guinea pig maximization test showed only weak skin sensitization and suggested that few or no dermatologic problems are expected as a result of the pesticide use and human dermal contact (Avalos et al. 1992). Furthermore, in the Ames test, F005 was negative in nine of ten determinations with five histidine mutants of *Salmonella typhimurium* (Loeffler), with and without hepatic enzyme activation; such results are superior to many common substances, such as caffeine, and suggest that F005 is not a serious mutagen (P.E. Kirby pers. commun.). Mode of action studies in three separate laboratories have recently determined that F005, asimicin, and bullatacin are superb inhibitors (at subnanomolar concentrations) of Complex I in mitochondrial electron transport systems from several organisms; this is very similar to the site of action of rotenone, an established and approved botanical pesticide (J.T. Arnason; R. Hollingworth, C.E. Snipes pers. commun.).

REFERENCES

Alkofahi, A., J.K. Rupprecht, J.E. Anderson, J.L. McLaughlin, K. L. Mikolajczak, and B.A. Scott. 1989. Search for new pesticides from higher plants, p. 25–43. In: J.T. Arnason, B. J.R. Philogene, P. Morand (eds.). Insecticides of plant origin. Amer. Chem. Soc., Washington, DC.

Alvalos, J., J.K. Rupprecht, J.L. McLaughlin, and E. Rodriguez. 1992. Guinea pig maximization test of pawpaw, *Asimina triloba* (Annonaceae). Contact Dermatitis.

Arnason, J.T., B.J.R. Philogene, and P. Morand (eds.). 1989. Insecticides of plant origin. Amer. Chem. Soc., Washington, DC.

Callaway, M.B. 1990. The Pawpaw *Asimina triloba*). Kentucky State Univ., Frankfort, KY, Pub. CRS-Hort 1-901 T.

Heywood, V.H. 1978. Flowering plants of the world. University Press, Oxford.

Hui, Y.-H., J.K. Rupprecht, Y.-M. Liu, J.E. Anderson, D.L. Smith, C.-J. Chang, and J.L. McLaughlin. 1989. Bullatacin and bullatacinone: Two highly potent bioactive acetogenins from *Annona bullata*. J. Nat. Prod. 52: 463–477.

Meyer, B.N., N.R. Ferrigni, J.E. Putnam, L.B. Jacobsen, D.E. Nichols, and J.L. McLaughlin. 1982. Brine shrimp: A convenient general bioassay for active plant constituents. Planta Medica 45:31–34.

Mikolajczak, K.L., J.K. Rupprecht, and J.L. McLaughlin. 1988. Control of pests with acetogenins. U.S. Patent No. 4,721,727, issued January 1988.

Mikolajczak, K.L., J.K. Rupprecht, and J.L. McLaughlin. 1988. Control of pests with Annonaceous acetogenins. U.S. Patent No. 4,855,319, issued August 1989.

Ratnayake, S., J.K. Rupprecht, W.M. Potter, and J.L. McLaughlin. 1992. Evaluation of various parts of the pawpaw tree, *Asimina triloba* (Annonaceae), as commercial sources of the pesticidal Annonaceous acetogenins. J. Econ. Entomol.

Rupprecht, J.K., Y.-H. Hui, and J.L. McLaughlin. 1990. Annonaceous acetogenins: A review. J. Nat. Prod. 53: 237–278.

Rupprecht, J.K., C.-J. Chang, J.M. Cassady, J.L. McLaughlin, K.L. Mikolajczak, and D. Weisleder. 1986. Asimicin, a new cytotoxic and pesticidal acetogenin from the pawpaw, *Asimina triloba* (Annonaceae). Heterocycles 24:1197–1201.

Spencer, J.S. Jr., N.P. Kingsley, and R.W. Mayer. 1990. Indiana timber resources, 1986: An analysis. Resour. Bul. NC-113. St. Paul, MN. U.S. Department of Agriculture, Forest Service, North Central Forest Experimental Station, St. Paul, Minnesota.

Zhao, G.-X., Y.-H. Hui, J.K. Rupprecht, J.L. McLaughlin, and K.V. Wood. 1992. Additional bioactive compounds and trilobacin, a novel highly cytotoxic acetogenin, from the bark of *Asimina triloba* (Annonaceae). J. Nat. Prod. 55:347–356.

Tagetes minuta: A Potential New Herb from South America

Jacqueline A. Soule

The New World genus Tagetes (Asteraceae) includes the popular garden marigold, *Tagetes erecta* L. Other members of the genus are equally easy to cultivate, and have a long history of human use as beverages, condiments, ornamentals, as medicinal decoctions, and in ritual (Diaz 1976; Morton 1981; Nuttall 1920; Neher 1968). *Tagetes erecta* is used as a beverage in South Carolina (Crellin 1984) and in parts of the southern United States (Linares and Bye 1987). *Tagetes lucida* Cav. is a popular beverage in Mexico and Guatemala, where it is also used as a medicinal tea and in ritual (Linares and Bye 1987; O'Gorman 1961). *Tagetes minuta* L., a species native to southern South America, is used as a condiment, as a refreshing beverage, and for medicinal purposes (Manfred 1947; Freise 1934; Parodi 1959; Thays 1910). In each case, leaves, stems, and flowers are utilized. In recent years, there has been an increasing interest in using the herbal products of indigenous peoples (Anjaria 1989). Tagetes minuta could be another new herb brought to the world market.

BOTANY

Origin

Tagetes minuta is native to the temperate grasslands and montane regions of southern South America, including the countries of Argentina, Chile, Bolivia, Peru, and in the Chaco region of Paraguay (McVaugh 1943; Reiche 1903; Perkins 1912; Herrera 1941; Espinar 1967). *T. minuta* is often found growing in disturbed areas during early successional stages. This affinity for disturbed sites has allowed the species to colonize many areas around the world. Since the time of the Spanish Conquest, it has been introduced into Europe (Jordano and Ocana 1955), Asia (Cherpanov 1981), Africa (Hillard 1977), Madagascar (Humbert 1923), India (Rao et al. 1988), Australia (Webb 1948), and Hawaii (Hosaka 1954).

Morphology

Tagetes minuta is an erect annual herb reaching 1 to 2 m (Fig. 1). Leaves are slightly glossy green, and are pinnately dissected into 4 to 6 pairs of pinnae. Leaf margins are finely serrate. The undersurface of the leaves bear a number of small, punctate, multicellular glands, orangish in color, which exude a licorice-like aroma when ruptured. Glands may also be found on the stems and involucre bracts. Four or five fused involucre bracts surround each head. There are typically 3 to 5 yellow-orange ray florets, and 10 to 15 yellow-orange disk florets per capitula. The heads are small, 10 to 15 mm long, and including ray florets, 10 to 20 mm in diameter. The heads are borne in a clustered panicle of 20 to 80 capitula. The dark brown achenes are 10 to 12 mm long, with a pappus of 1 to 4 tiny scales and 0 to 2 retrosely serrulate awns which are 1 to 3 mm long.

ETHNOBOTANY

The New World peoples have been using *Tagetes minuta* as a flavorful beverage, a medicinal tea, and a condiment since pre-contact times (Rees 1817). The local names vary by region, most commonly found in the literature as; *chinchilla, chiquilla, chilca, zuico, suico,* or the Spanish term *anisillo*.

A beverage is prepared from *Tagetes minuta* by steeping a "half-handful" of the dried plant in hot water for 3 to 5 min. The beverage may be consumed warm or cooled, and may be sweetened to individual taste (Neher 1968).

For medicinal use, a decoction made by steeping a "double handful" of the dried plant in boiling water for 3 to 5 minutes is used as a remedy for the common cold; including upper and lower respiratory tract inflammations, and for digestive system complaints; stomach upset, diarrhea, and "liver" ailments. The decoction is consumed warm, and may be sweetened to individual taste (Neher 1968; Parodi 1959; Cavanilles 1802).

Tagetes minuta is used as a condiment in Chile and Argentina. It is popular in rice dishes and as a flavoring in stews. In northern Chile *suico* is so highly prized that many people actively collect wild populations to dry a sufficient supply to last the winter (Kennedy pers. commun.).

Tagetes minuta is often referred to as a weed. Cabrera (1971) states that ".... Spegazzini mentions that this plant is a common weed of cultivation in the lower Rio Negro Valley...." Spegazzini and Cabrera appear to not understand the native outlook on "weeds." The farmers view the "weeds" as a second crop. Many of the Latin American farmers who do not practice industrialized agriculture will leave volunteer plants of *Tagetes minuta* in their fields. This second crop is beneficial in several ways: first, rapid growth of *T. minuta* quickly shades out other plant species that may be of less use to the farmer, second, it can be harvested for personal use, or for sale in city markets, and third, has been reported to aid in the retention of humidity in the field (Jimenez-Osornio 1991).

Tagetes minuta is commercially grown and harvested for its essential oils which are used in the flavor and perfume industry as "Tagetes Oil." The oil is used in perfumes, and as a flavor component in most major food products, including cola beverages, alcoholic beverages, frozen dairy desserts, candy, baked goods, gelatins, puddings, condiments, and relishes (Leung 1980). Brazil is one major producer of *T. minuta* for Tagetes Oil (Craveiro et al. 1988). Worldwide production of the oil was around 1.5 tonnes in 1984 (Lawrence 1985).

CULTURE

General

Tagetes minuta grows readily from seed sown directly into the soil once the danger of frost has past (B.M. Lawrence unpub. report). Plant height varies with conditions. Based on studies of herbarium material from the

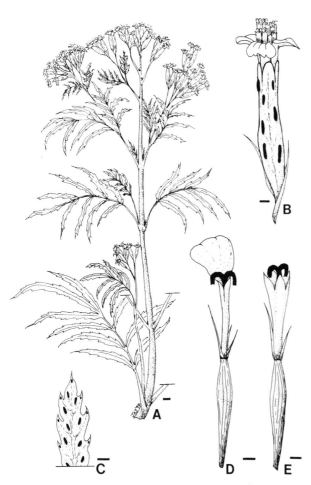

Fig. 1. *Tagetes minuta*, based on herbarium specimens at TEX/LL. (A) habit (B) head (C) leaf under surface (D) ray floret (E) disk floret. Bars: (A) 1 cm (B–E) 1 mm

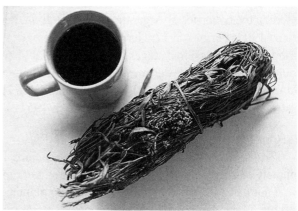

Fig. 2. *Tagetes minuta* purchased in a marketplace in Chile. The material was folded and wrapped with plastic twine while fresh.

Fig 3. Chemical formula of 7 thiophenes found in *Tagetes minuta* with antiviral activity. Alpha-T indicates alpha-thiophene, numbers indicate numbers in Hudson (1990).

University of Texas and Lundell Collection; Field Museum, Chicago; New York Botanic Garden; University of Arizona; Michigan State University; and California Academy of Sciences; single, open grown plants range from 0.5 to 1 m tall, yet when grown in dense stands, a height of 2 m can be reached.

Tagetes minuta thrives in full sun. Competition for sunlight can lead to tall spindly plants with a low biomass. Higher biomass is attained from spacing the plants 1 m apart, and removal of the apical meristem at 30 days to stimulate branching. Meristem removal may be done mechanically.

Pests

Pests do not appear to be a significant problem with *Tagetes minuta* in field culture. Red spider mite and root knot nematode are often serious pests on cultivated forms of *Tagetes erecta* (Steiner 1941). In field studies in Austin, Texas, these pests have not been found on *T. minuta* despite the presence of large populations of these pests on *T. erecta* at the same site.

Harvest

Harvest for use as a beverage or condiment is done manually by cutting the main stem at ground level, since the entire above-ground portion of the plant is considered useful. Plants over 1 m have individual branches cut off and dried. The plant material is folded and tied into bundles using twine, grasses, or a pliable branch of *T. minuta* (Fig. 2). The bundles are hung in a dry place, out of direct sunlight, to dry. Commercial hand harvesting is feasible due to low labor rates in South American countries. Since the whole plant is utilized, mechanical harvesting could be a viable option, and is used in essential oil production.

SECONDARY COMPOUNDS

Tagetes minuta is rich in many secondary compounds, including acyclic, monocyclic and bicyclic monoterpenes, sesquiterpenes, flavonoids, thiophenes, and aromatics (Rodriguez and Mabry 1977). There is evidence that the secondary compounds in *Tagetes* are effective deterrents of numerous organisms, including: fungi (Chan et al. 1975), fungi pathenogenic on humans (Camm et al. 1975), bacteria (Grover and Rao 1978), round worms in general (Loewe 1974), trematodes (Graham et al. 1980), nematodes (Grainge and Ahmed 1988), and numerous insect pests through several different mechanisms (Jacobsen 1990; Saxena and Koul 1982; Maradufu et al. 1978; Saxena and Srivastava 1973). Many closely related plant secondary compounds have demonstrated medicinal value in humans (Kennewell 1990; Korolkovas and Burckhalter 1976) In vivo human studies of the secondary compounds of *T. minuta* have not been reported, although other *Tagetes* species have proven medically safe and efficacious (Caceres et al. 1987).

Hethelyi et al. (1986), determined anti-microbial activity of five secondary compounds in *Tagetes minuta*; beta-ocimene, dihydrotagetone, tagetone, (Z)-ocimenone, and (E)-ocimenone. When tested on 40 strains of bacteria and fungi, the essential oil of *T. minuta* had a 100% inhibitory effect on Gram-positive bacteria, a 95% inhibitory effect on Gram-negative bacteria, and a 100% inhibitory effect on fungi.

Hudson (1990) tested the many different secondary compounds for anti-viral activity, and determined that thiophenes demonstrated the greatest anti-viral action at the lowest doses, and with the least toxicity overall. Of the thiophenes, molecules with two or more thiophene units showed the highest activity. In all cases, the best success was against viruses with envelopes. Hudson tested 32 thiophenes, evaluated their efficacy and determined the 10 most effective ones (Fig. 3). Atkinson et al. (1964) first reported the thiophenes found in *Tagetes minuta*. A comparison of Atkinson's results to those of Hudson, shows that 7 of the 10 most effective anti-viral thiophenes are found in *Tagetes minuta*.

The work of Hethelyi et al. (1986) and that of Hudson (1990) indicate that the use of *Tagetes minuta* as a medicinal beverage by indigenous people may have a valid biological basis, although in vivo work has not been published. Further work is warranted, and could be used to aid in the marketing of herbal products of *Tagetes minuta*.

Toxicology

There are some unsubstantiated reports of poisoning by *Tagetes minuta*. Watt and Breyer-Brandwijk (1932) mention that death of children in South Africa is reportedly due to allowing them to sleep next to *T. minuta* state: "Unfortunately no proper investigation of these occurrences have been made and one doubts very much whether the plant has been the cause of death." Given the high suspected rate of infanticide of female children in Africa a half-century ago, *T. minuta* as the cause of death is highly unlikely. Hurst (1942) mentions that in Australia, in 1935, the plant is suspected in the death of several cows, "but the evidence was rather weak." and states that "A large dose of the plant in the flowering stage had no effect on sheep."

Chandhoke and Ghatak (1969), working with experimental animals, determined that the oil of *Tagetes minuta* has hypotensive, bronchodilatory, spazmolytic, anti-inflammatory, and tranquilizing properties. These actions are in accordance with the reported folk use of the beverage as a medical decoction. Given that generations of South Americans have used *T. minuta* as a beverage and condiment, it seems that use in moderation causes no ill effects; however additional toxicology studies would be necessary prior to marketing the plant as a beverage.

FUTURE PROSPECTS

Tagetes minuta can be used for a hot or cold refreshing beverage. In taste tests at the University of Texas, subjects reported that the flavor is slightly sweet and anise-like, mild and not overpowering to the palate. Overall, the flavor was well received, although subject preference was significantly positively correlated to their preference for "black jelly beans or licorice."

Currently, many nations are actively seeking alternative cash crops to replace cultivation of illegal drug plants. Several species of Tagetes have been investigated, including *Tagetes minuta* (Bernal and Correa 1991; Arora 1989). *Tagetes minuta* as a herbal beverage has the potential to become a new crop for many of the hitherto drug growing areas, providing further research into the toxicology and marketing is conducted and remains promising.

REFERENCES

Anjaria, J.V. 1989. Herbal drugs: potential for industry and cash, p. 84–92. In: G.E. Wickens, N. Haq, and P. Day (eds.). New crops for food and industry. Chapman and Hall, London.

Arora, J.S. 1989. Marigolds, p. 713–731. In: T.K. Bose and L.P. Yadav (eds.). Commercial flowers. Naya Prokash, Calcutta.

Atkinson, R.E., R.F. Curtis, and G.T. Phillips. 1964. Bi-thienyl derivitives from *Tagetes minuta* L. Tetrahedron Lett. 43:3159–3162

Bernal, H.Y. and J.E. Correa. 1991. Especies vegetales promisorias: Compositae, *Tagetes*. Programa de recursos vegetales del convenio "Andres Bello" Bolivia, Colombia, Chile, Ecuador, Espana, Panama, Peru, y Venezuala. Santafe de Bogota, Colombia. p. 115–139.

Cabrera, A.L. 1971. Compositae. In: M.N. Correa (ed.). Flora Patagonica Coleccion Cientifica del Inta. Buenos Aires.

Caceres, A., L.M. Giron, S.R. Alvarado, and M.F. Torres. 1987. Screening of antimicrobial activity of plants popularly used in Guatemala for the treatment of dermatomucosal diseases. J. Ethnopharmacol. 20:223–237.

Camm, E.L., G.H.N. Towers, and J.C. Mitchell. 1975. UV-mediated antibiotic activity of some Compositeae species. Phytochemistry 14:2007–2011.

Chan, G.F.Q., G.H.N. Towers, and J.C. Mitchell. 1975. Ultraviolet-mediated antibiotic activity of thiophene compounds of *Tagetes*. Phytochemistry 14:2295–2296.

Chandhoke, N. and B.J.R. Ghatak. 1969. In vivo studies of the effects of *Tagetes* oil. Indian J. Med. Res. 57:864.

Cherpanov, S.K. 1981. Plantae Vasculares U.R.S.S. Navaka, Lenningrad.

Craveiro, C.C., F.J.A. Matos, M.I.L. Machado, and J.W. Alencar. 1988. Essential oils of *Tagetes minuta* from Brazil. Perfum. Flavor. 13(5):35–36.

Crellin, J.K. 1984. Traditional medicine in Southern Appalachia and some thoughts for the history of medicinal plants, p. 65–78. In: W.H. Hein (ed.). Botanical drugs of the Americas in the Old & New World. Wissenschaftliche Verlagsgesellschaft, Stuttgart.

Diaz, J.L. 1976. Usos de las plantas medicinales de Mexico. Instituto Mexicano para el Estudio de las Plantas Medicinals. Mexico.

Espinar, L.A. 1967. Las especias de *Tagetes* (Compositae) de la region central Argentina. Kurtziana 4:51–71.

Freise, F.W. 1934. Plantas Medicinales Brasileiras. Instituto Agronomico do Estado, Sao Paulo.

Gillet, J. and E. Paque. 1910. Plantes Principales de la region de Kisantu. Musee du Congo Belge, Botanique, Ser. 5. University of Natal Press, Pietermaritzburg. 1:1–57.

Graham, K., A. Graham, and G.H.N. Towers. 1980. Cercaricidal activity of phenylheptatriyne and alpha-tertienyl, naturally occuring compounds in species of the Asteraceae. Can. J. Zool. 58:1955–1958.

Grainge, M. and S. Ahmed. 1988. Handbook of plants with pest-control properties. Wiley, New York.

Grover, G.S., and J.T. Rao. 1978. In vitro antimicrobial studies of the essential oil of *Tagetes erecta*. Perfum. Flavor. 3(5):28.

Herrera, F.L. 1941. Sinopsis de la flora del Cuzco. Government of Peru, Lima.

Hethelyi, E., B. Danos, and P. Tetenyi. 1986. GC–MS analysis of the esssential oils of four *Tagetes* species and the anti-microbial activity of *Tagetes minuta*. Flav. Fragr. J. 1:169–173.

Hillard, O.M. 1977. Compositae in Natal. University of Natal Press, Pietermaritzburg.

Hosaka, E.Y. and A. Thistle. 1954. Noxious plants of the Hawaiian ranges. Ext. Bul. Univ. of Hawaii & U.S. Dept. Agr. 62.

Hudson, J.B. 1990. Antiviral compounds from plants. CRC Press, Inc., Boca Raton, FL.

Humbert, H. 1923. Les Composees de Madagascar. E. Lanier, Imprimerie, Caen.

Hurst, E. 1942. The poison plants of New South Wales. N.S.W. Poison Plants Comm. Univ. of Sydney.

Jacobson, M. 1990. Glossary of plants derived insect deterrents. CRC Press, Inc., Boca Raton, FL.

Jimenez-Osornio, J.J. 1991. Ethnoecology of *Chenopodium ambrosoides*. Amer. J. Bot. 76(6):139. (Abst.)

Jordano, D. and M. Ocana. 1955. Catalogo del herbario de los botanicos cordobeses Rafael de Leon y Galvez, Fr. Jose de Jesus Munoz Capilla, Rafael Entrenas, y Antonio Cabrera. Anales Inst. Bot. Cavanilles 14:597–720.

Kennewell, P.D. 1990. Comprehensive medicinal chemistry. Pergamon Press, Oxford, U.K.

Korolkovas, A. and J.H. Burckhalter. 1976. Essentials of medicinal plant chemistry. Wiley, New York.

Lawrence, B.M. 1985. A review of the world production of essential oils (1984). Perfum. Flavor. 10(5):1–16.

Leung, A.Y. 1980. Encyclopedia of common natural ingredients. Wiley, New York.

Linares, E. and R.A. Bye. 1987. A study of four medicinal plant complexes of Mexico and adjacent United States. J. Ethnopharmacol. 19:153–183.

Loewe, H. 1974. Recent advances in the medicinal chemistry of anthelminthics, p. 271–301. In: J. Maas (ed.). Medicinal chemistry IV. Elsevier., Amsterdam.

Manfred, L. 1947. 7000 Recetas Botanicas. Editorial Kier, Buenos Aires.

Maradufu, A., R. Lubega, and F. Dorn. 1978. Isolation of (5E)-ocimenone, a mosquito larvicide from *Tagetes minuta*. Llyodia 41(2):181–182.

McVaugh, R. 1943. Botanical collections of the La Plata expedition of 1853–1855. Brittonia 5(1):64–79.

Morton, J.F. 1981. Atlas of medicinal plants of Middle America. Chas. C. Thomas, Springfield, IL.

Neher, R.T. 1968. The ethnobotany of *Tagetes*. Econ. Bot. 22:317–325.

Nuttall, Z. 1920. Los Jardines del Antiguo Mexico. Sociedad Cientifica "Antonio Alzate", Mexico.

O'Gorman, H. 1961. Mexican flowering trees and plants. Ammex Associados, Mexico City.

Parodi, L.R. 1959. Enciclopedia Argentina de Agricultura y Jardineria. Editorial Acme S.A.C.I., Buenos Aires 1:845.

Perkins, J. 1912. Beitrage zur flora von Boliva. Bot. Jahrb. Syst. 49(1).

Rao, R.R., H.J. Chowdhery, P.K. Hajra, S. Kumar, P.C. Pant, B.D. Naithani, B.P. Uniyal, R. Mathur, and S.K. Mamgain. 1988. Flora Indicae Enumeratio—Asteraceae. Botanical Survey of India. Ser. 4. Government of India, New Delhi.

Rees, A. 1817. Tagetes. In: A. Rees (ed.). The Cyclopedia. London. 35 (1).

Reiche, C. 1903. Estudios criticos sobre la flora de Chile. Anales Univ. Chile 112:97–179.

Rodriguez, E. and T.J. Mabry. 1977. Tageteae—chemical review. In: V.H. Heywood, J.B. Harborne, and B.L. Turner (eds.). The biology and chemistry of the Compositeae. Academic Press, London.

Saxena, B.P. and J.B. Srivastava. 1973. *Tagetes minuta* L. oil: A new source of juvenile hormone mimicking substance. Indian J. Expt. Biol. 11(1):56–58.

Saxena, B.P. and O. Koul. 1982. Essential oils and insect control, p. 766–776. In: C.K. Atal and B.M. Kapur (eds.). Cultivation and utilization of aromatic plants. Council of Sci. Res., Jammu-Tawi, India.

Steiner, G. 1941. Nematodes parasitic on and associated with roots of marigolds (*Tagetes* hybrids). Proc. Biol. Soc. Wash. 54:31–34.

Thays, C. 1910. El jardin botanico de Buenos Aires. Buenos Aires.

Watt, J.M. and M.G. Breyer-Brandwijk. 1932. Medicinal and poisonous plants of Southern and Eastern Africa. E. & S. Livingstone Ltd., Edinburgh.

Webb, L.J. 1948. Guide to medicinal and poisonous plants of Queensland. Council for Sci. & Indust. Res., Melbourne.

Soft-Shell Crayfish: A New Crop for the Midwest*

Paul B. Brown

Crayfish production consistently ranks as one of the largest aquacultural industries in the United States, typically the second largest industry behind culture of channel catfish (USDA 1991). The primary production areas include Louisiana, Texas, Arkansas, and other southern states, and annual production ranges from 35 to 55 million kg (Huner and Barr 1984; Roberts and Harper 1988). However, supplies of fresh crayfish from those areas are seasonal, typically available from December through June (Huner 1990; Huner and Romaire 1990). Reproductive characteristics of native midwestern crayfish species are offset seasonally from crayfish in the South (Page 1985; Hobbs and Jass 1988); thus, production may be seasonally offset. Preliminary studies to date indicated that the production season in the Midwest will be June through November (Brown et al. 1990). Thus, midwestern farmers have an opportunity to fill a market niche with a native species at a time of year when there is no competition for fresh product.

Crayfish production can be divided into two distinct segments: hard- and soft-shell production (Huner 1990; Huner and Romaire 1990). Hard-shell producers market tail meat, similar to shrimp production, while soft-shell producers market the entire body, similar to soft-shell crab production. Soft-shell production requires a dependable source of relatively large, hard-shell crayfish.

Studies conducted in our laboratory have indicated significant potential for pond production of native species for the tail-meat market (Table 1). In our first attempt at producing the northern or fantail crayfish (*Orconectes viriles*), production levels were dependent on initial stocking strategy, but ranged from 323 to 807 kg/ha when fed agricultural forages (Brown et al. 1990), which compares favorably with average production levels in the South of 545 to 691 kg/ha (Roberts and Harper 1988). That initial study and two regional symposia on crayfish culture stimulated a great deal of interest in crayfish and construction of ponds was initiated. The next step in providing opportunities to midwestern farmers is evaluation of soft-shell production.

AQUACULTURE

Culture

A typical scenario in producing soft-shell crayfish involves collecting or harvesting hard-shell crayfish from wild populations or aquaculture ponds and transporting them to an indoor, controlled molting facility. Groups of crayfish are then stocked into relatively shallow tanks (<0.3 m), fed any of a variety of feeds including potatoes, whole fish, carrots, or one of the new formulated diets for crustaceans, and premolt individuals are identified and moved to separate molting tanks (Culley et al. 1985). All crustaceans are cannibalistic, particularly when one of their cohorts molts in a communal tank; thus, identifying and moving premolt animals is an important economic

---

*This study was funded by the Indiana Corporation for Science and Technology (now the Business Modernization and Technology Corporation).

consideration.

Economics and Marketing

Soft-shell producers in the South purchase crayfish for $0.07 to 0.50 per kg, transport those animals to controlled, indoor tanks, and wait for the animal to molt, which typically takes 1 to 4 weeks. Soft-shell crayfish retail for $1.80 to $3.60 per kg. Thus, the profit margin and relatively quick turnover of product entices many farmers into soft-shell production.

Markets for crayfish have been expanding in recent years. The market in northern Europe is especially promising, as several festivals in the fall of each year are centered on consumption of crayfish, yet their native species have been decimated by an introduced fungal epidemic (Huner 1990). Southern producers can supply only frozen product during that portion of the year, whereas midwestern producers can supply fresh product.

Our objective in this research was to evaluate the potential of soft-shell production of crayfish using one of the more promising midwestern species, *O. viriles*. Specifically, we examined the effects of selected rearing temperatures on molting frequency.

METHODOLOGY

Northern crayfish were obtained in September from a producer in Indiana and transported to the Purdue University Aquacultural Research Laboratory. Those individuals weighed 20 to 55 g and pond water temperature was 19° to 24°C at the time of collection. Crayfish were divided into similar groups (equal numbers of male and female) and immediately stocked into crayfish molting trays (2.0 × 0.8 × 0.1 m). Water temperatures were set at either 20°, 25°, or 30°C using submersible chillers or heaters and triplicate tanks were used at each temperature.

Table 1. Mean production of northern crayfish (*Orconectes viriles*) in deep or shallow ponds[z].

Treatment	Production[y] ±SE (kg/ha)
Deep ponds	
Wheat straw	457±107
Corn silage	323±163
Negative control (no inputs)	422±216
Shallow ponds	
Wheat straw	807±41
Corn silage	784±101
Negative control (no inputs)	779±73

[z]Data from Brown et al. (1990).
[y]Means of three replications.

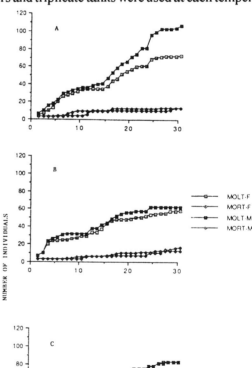

Fig. 1. Mean cumulative number of male (M) or female (F) crayfish that molted (molt) or died (mort) when reared at 20° (A), 25° (B), or 30°C (C).

All crayfish were fed a commercially-available crustacean diet (Zeigler Brothers, Gardners, PA) to satiation twice daily and individual premolt crayfish (those individuals within 1 to 2 days of molting) were removed to separate tanks. Cumulative molt and survival data were collected from each temperature treatment.

RESULTS AND DISCUSSION

Both male and female crayfish molted at the three temperatures; there were no significant differences among sex. Those reared at 20°C exhibited the largest number of successful molts and the fewest numbers of deaths (Fig. 1), while number of successful molts declined and numbers of deaths increased with increased temperatures. Differences observed at 20° vs. 30°C were significantly different ($P<0.05$). Unpublished data from our laboratory indicated that 25°C was optimal for juvenile *O. viriles* and weight gain of crayfish at 25°C was significantly higher than those reared at 20°C. Thus, optimal temperature for growth may decrease in older animals.

While the absolute numbers of crayfish that molted over the 30-day experimental period was higher at 20°C compared to higher temperatures, a higher percentage molted in a shorter period of time at 30°C than at lower temperatures. That molting activity was completed prior to significant increases in mortality. Thus, more rapid turnover of crayfish from molting facilities may be possible using controlled temperature manipulations.

Regardless of temperature, there was a biphasic response of molting activity. That response became more dramatic as temperature increased from 20° to 30°C. In general, a large number of crayfish molted within the first 5 to 10 days (as many as 64% of the population reared at 30°C), followed by a quiescent period, then another period of molting. This observation has important management implications. For example, if an economically-large segment of any population molts within a shorter period of time than expected (up to 4 weeks), then more rapid turnover of that commodity may be possible, thereby increasing the amount of marketable product through a production season. Several other factors such as length of photoperiod and water levels may influence molting frequency and synchronization within a given population.

SUMMARY

Native midwestern crayfish will molt in controlled situations and that molting is influenced by water temperature. Molting activity is relatively rapid, with a large percentage occurring within the first 10 days. The response, regardless of temperature, was biphasic and probably reflects individuals in different stages of the molt cycle when acquired. Those that were near stage E (ecdysis) in the molt cycle molted within the first 5 to 10 days, while those is earlier stages required approximately 15 days to molt. Management options are now available to aquaculturists that will allow more carefully manipulated molting activity patterns in populations of native midwestern crayfish. The results of this study should be considered promising and, coupled with ongoing studies in our laboratory, will facilitate growth of the crayfish industry in the Midwest.

REFERENCES

Brown, P.B., M.L. Hooe, and W.G. Blythe. 1990. Preliminary evaluation of production systems and forages for culture of *Orconectes viriles*, the northern or fantail crayfish. J. World Aquaculture Soc. 21:53–58.

Culley, D.D., M.Z. Said, and E. Rejmankova. 1985. Producing soft crawfish: a status report. Louisiana Sea Grant Program, Center for Wetland Resources, Baton Rouge.

Hobbs, H.H., III and J.P. Jass. 1988. The crayfishes and shrimp of Wisconsin. Milwaukee Public Museum, Milwaukee.

Huner, J.V. 1990. Biology, fisheries, and cultivation of freshwater crawfishes in the US. Rev. Aquatic Sci. 2:229–254.

Huner, J.V. and J.E. Barr. 1984. Red swamp crawfish: biology and exploitation. Louisiana Sea Grant Program, Louisiana State Univ., Baton Rouge.

Huner, J.V. and R.P. Romaire. 1990. Crawfish culture in the southeastern USA. World Aquaculture 21:58–65.

Page, L.M. 1985. The crayfishes and shrimps (Decapoda) of Illinois. Illinois Natural History Survey Bul. 33:335–448.

Roberts, K.J. and C.D. Harper. 1988. Seafood market trends. Louisiana Coop. Ext. Serv., Baton Rouge.

USDA. 1991. Aquaculture situation and outlook report. USDA, Commodity Economics Division, Economic Research Service. Washington, DC.

PART III
PATHS TOWARD COMMERCIALIZATION

INDUSTRY OUTLOOK

New Crops from a Seed Company Perspective

Carrol D. Bolen

Seed companies are often encouraged to become more involved in the development and commercialization of new crops. Seed industry response to requests for support have generally been viewed as lukewarm, at best. Although this response may seem unusual considering the fact that the seed industry is accustomed to making long-term investments in research and development, a thorough examination of the criteria used for investment decisions by seed companies sheds light on the difficulty of getting support for investment in new crops.

CRITERIA FOR INVESTMENT DECISIONS

Seed companies differ in the approach they use to make investment decisions. This will depend upon such factors as company size, interest in diversification, capital resources available, or willingness to take risks. However, most seed companies will look at a similar group of factors in making an investment decision. Comments here are those things generally considered by Pioneer Hi-Bred International, Inc.

Intellectual Property Protection

As we look at new opportunities, a key consideration is intellectual property protection. We must be convinced that we can adequately protect the investment made in research and development. Hybrid crops have generally given that protection, while self-pollinated crops have not. The Plant Variety Protection Act provides some protection, but the farmer exemption permitted by the Act is clearly a major limitation to investment in self-pollinated crops. For example, Pioneer started research and development of hard red winter wheat in 1970. After several years of marketing products during the 1980s, the program was dropped in December of 1989. Farmers had accepted our products which commanded a nice market share, but most of the seed was coming from farmers' bins rather than a Pioneer seed bag. We simply could not make enough money to get a reasonable return on our research investment. A similar scenario developed for our hard red spring wheat program. Cotton ginners saving and selling seed was a major reason we decided to terminate our cotton seed business in the United States.

Pioneer will likely not be interested in any new crop that doesn't have one of the following protection mechanisms: (1) capable of being hybridized; (2) an effective plant patent; (3) vertical integration through contract production.

Kenaf is a good example of a new crop that offers intellectual property protection through vertical integration. I've been impressed with the Kenaf International program and believe that system merits consideration in other new crops as well. Clearly, we plan to use a similar plan for some of the specialty products being developed at Pioneer. We intend to control a major portion of the value added chain.

Synergy with Existing Business

Businesses often expand into other areas because of synergistic effects. The seed industry is no exception. Pioneer started as a hybrid seed corn company and over a period of years successfully expanded into several other crops. The logic was that we could use our plant breeding technology and seed distribution channels as a competitive advantage. Generally speaking, this strategy has been effective. However, as we look at new crops, we must assess how important our strengths are in relation to what is needed to make the new crop successful.

I can recall evaluating triticale as a potential new crop for Pioneer in the mid-1980s. We started a full scale triticale breeding program in 1986 after determining there would be good synergy between triticale and our winter wheat program. Also, working with triticale should improve our chances of being successful in hybrid wheat development. However, we decided to get out of hard red winter and hard red spring wheat development in December of 1989 and as a consequence decided to drop triticale at the same time. So, synergy helped get Pioneer into triticale and synergy helped to get us out.

Canola is our most recent example of a new crop for Pioneer. The decision was made in 1988 to enter the canola seed market. We acquired the canola program of Biotechnica Canada, in 1989, and started our own research and development program in Europe. In 1990, we acquired Allelix Crop Technologies of Toronto,

Canada, a major developer of canola seed. The major reasons for our interest in canola are: (1) hybridization seems likely; (2) seed margins are good, especially in Europe; (3) canola oil is growing in popularity with consumers; (4) canola hectarage is significant worldwide and beginning to show growth in the United States; (5) we are already involved with other oilseed crops (soybeans, sunflowers) and needed canola to complete our involvement in the three major annual oilseeds; (6) seed can be marketed through existing distribution systems; (7) canola is a good crop for developing specialty oils which is a target of Pioneer.

Stage of Commercialization

Most "new crops" have been around for a long time. Some have been in commercial channels for years, but because of limited production are still considered new crops. Naturally, we are most interested in crops that are developed to the point where they have proven their commercial worth. This may be viewed by many as wanting the reward without the risk. However, we see the risk of too early an entry as being greater than the potential reward. Pioneer's position is that once a crop has proven its' potential, we can then become a player and obtain most of the benefits without much risk. That places the major responsibility for new crop development in the hands of public institutions. It is a role they have performed well over the years and should continue to perform. There does become a point when a new crop looks promising enough that a company like Pioneer will decide to become actively involved.

Market Potential

We must have some idea of the market potential for the new crop in order to determine our interest. Ideally, we like to see large volume potential with very good profit margin. Realistically, this seldom happens. Given a choice, we're more inclined to opt for low volume and high margin rather than high volume and low margin.

Financial Considerations

In dollar terms, we're seldom interested in looking at anything new unless it has the potential of contributing at least one million dollars in profit per year. We're not going to get very excited unless the long term potential is five million dollars or more per year.

Pioneer has a stated goal of 20% return on stockholders equity. Although this may sound like a high target, it is an accepted norm for many of the food industry companies. New crops are evaluated against the 20% return on equity (ROE) target. If the crop is still several years away from commercial scale-up, it is very difficult to invest much at this stage and show a long term 20% ROE unless there is a very good margin once the product comes to market.

Because of the large public ownership of seed companies that has resulted from consolidation within the industry, there is considerably more pressure on companies for good short to intermediate financial returns. This is not the best environment for considering investing in something that likely will not return a good profit for several years.

Alternative Opportunities

Seed companies generally have many investment options with limited resources available. Priorities must be established. Heading the list of priorities will generally be those items that protect or enhance the existing business. New opportunities will normally be secondary.

There are two growing investment areas which I believe will make it difficult to obtain funding for new crops. One is biotechnology in general, and the other modification of traditional crops. Most, if not all, seed companies that invest in research and development have maintained or increased their traditional plant breeding budgets while adding on a layer of biotechnology costs. In addition, Pioneer has begun a significant effort to modify the protein, oil, and starch profiles of several traditional crops.

I firmly believe that modification of major crops will prove to be tough competition for some of the product targets of new crops. Through a combination of traditional plant breeding, mutations, and biotechnology, we are seeing many opportunities for new products. For example, vegetable oils with a modified fatty acid profile or protein meal with a modified amino acid profile. These are much more exciting to us today than anything we've looked at in the new crops area. Perhaps one of the main reasons for this view is that we see a need to protect and an opportunity to enhance market share in our existing seed product lines.

SUMMARY

Although there are several new crops that show promise for commercialization, the seed industry has shown very little interest in supporting the development process. That trend is likely to continue for the following reasons: (1) there are few new crops success stories; (2) there are many investment alternatives; (3) new crops often take a long time to get a return on investment while the seed industry is looking to more short to intermediate needs; and (4) intellectual property protection is limited with many new crops.

Processing Tomatoes: Old Crop in a New Area

William Reinert*

Tomato production in the United States did not grow from 1986 to 1988 (Table 1). In September 1988, an early rain in California devastated the late crop and processing tomato growers lost well over 1 million tonnes of tomatoes to mold. This event coupled with severe world production problems and an increased demand for tomato based products in Campbell's created a severe shortage. Although the Campbell Soup Co. could potentially exhaust inventories prior to the next season, the decision was made to grow tomatoes in California's Imperial Valley for the first time, to supply paste 30 days earlier than normal. The following account will detail the steps necessary to produce this crop.

Table 1. United States processing tomato production.

Location	1986	1987	1988	1989	1990	1991
Production (tonnes)						
United States	6,085	6,897	6,722	8,604	9,388	9,864
California	5,879	6,080	5,940	7,788	8,442	8,975
New Jersey	47	51	38	29	52	43
Ohio	349	335	326	355	395	356
Other States	432	431	418	432	499	491
Area harvested (ha)						
United States	102,009	104,048	111,260	129,848	143,466	144,065
California	85,149	86,606	91,503	111,900	125,457	126,266
New Jersey	1,214	1,174	1,336	1,214	1,336	1,052
Ohio	5,590	6,475	7,163	7,082	6,920	7,163
Other States	9,656	9,794	11,295	10,462	9,753	9,583
Average yield (t/ha)						
United States	65.7	66.4	60.5	66.3	65.4	68.4
California	69.1	70.2	65.0	69.7	67.2	71.0
New Jersey	39.0	43.5	28.5	23.5	38.8	40.8
Ohio	58.3	51.6	45.5	50.2	56.9	49.8
Other States	43.0	43.9	37.2	44.8	51.1	43.9

---

*I thank Rick Orzalli from the Sacramento Agriculture Department for his tireless efforts in putting the entire Imperial Valley plan together.

RESULTS

The Campbell Agriculture Department went through a six step process to be prepared to produce tomatoes in the Spring of 1989 in the Imperial Valley. The six critical inputs for new area development included: (1) extension service; (2) grower association; (3) grower base; (4) inspection system; (5) transportation; (6) communication.

The extension system inputs in California are excellent. A Farm Advisor system exists throughout most counties and a station at the Imperial Valley was established over 20 years ago. A significant amount of weather history was available from the extension service which would prove important to identify when to plant so that a harvesting schedule could be developed. The Extension Service also had significant data on the location of various soil types in the Imperial County which aided in locating the sites for field production. We were also able to obtain additional information on the Valley's current crops, their relative value, and the crop rotation schedule. Tomatoes cannot follow certain crops because of potential herbicide carryover problems.

The California Process Tomato Growers Association (CTGA) had been established back in 1948. In 1988, there were approximately 570 California tomato growers, almost half of them CTGA members. There were eight CTGA members located in Imperial Valley. These eight growers established a set of contacts to begin working with which then allowed the Agriculture Department to begin developing a grower base. As the growers were being identified, a contract needed to be created which specifically detailed (1) total tonnage; (2) price per ton; (3) incentives; (4) timing (delivery schedule); (5) deductions and payment schedule. Most contracts are developed on a tonnage basis and the grower is responsible to calculate area requirements. In the Imperial Valley, the Campbell contract was on an area basis because of our lack of sufficient historical yield information. Incentives would include tomatoes with higher soluble solids and early production. A tomato cultivar program was developed based on the weather data and the type of tomato paste in shortest supply. The cultivars selected had to be extremely firm because of the long distance the tomatoes would have to be trucked. The delivery schedule also needed to be created. Normal production from Fresno usually started the first of July; therefore, production had to commence prior to July. The goal was to start harvesting in the Imperial Valley the first of June. The last consideration was to make sure that the farmers had all the specific farm equipment necessary for growing the processing tomatoes. Bed shapers, seeders, cultivators were some specific implements, but probably the most important piece was the custom tomato harvester. Very few harvesters were available in the Imperial Valley, but the California processing tomato industry was large enough to have developed a custom harvest industry. This custom harvesting industry trucked the machines to the Imperial Valley and was able to provide this critical service to the Imperial growers.

The state of California had created a marketing order to develop the Tomato Processing Advisory Board which set up an inspection system based on color, soluble solids, mold damage, and insect damage. After the tomatoes are harvested and loaded directly into open gondolas, the trucks are directed to the nearest state certified station. Each tomato load is sampled a minimum of four times with a plunger that is capable of taking 45 kg each cycle. The tomatoes are dumped into a bucket and brought to the station to have all the specific measurements performed. If the tomatoes did not meet state grade, loads were either sorted or dumped.

An elaborate transportation system was created to have the tomatoes hauled from the Imperial Valley to Campbell's nearest paste production plant in Stockton, 1,086 km (675 miles) away. To eliminate the need for two drivers per load, a double hub system was created. In this manner, one driver could complete one complete cycle and not exceed his allowable driving time. The double hub system created an extra station between Imperial and Stockton to act as a transfer point. This extra station had responsibility to weigh trucks and add tomatoes to maximize loads. The harvesting of tomatoes and transportation to the paste plants was done completely at night in order to avoid the deleterious effect of the Imperial Valley's high day temperatures on fruit quality.

The last input for the successful introduction of tomatoes into this new region is a real time computer-based information system. It was critical for maximum plant efficiency to process a specific number of loads per day; thus, it was necessary to know how many loads were to be harvested, when the loads were on the road and past the inspection station, and finally at the middle exchange station. An elaborate tagging system was installed to follow loads from Imperial to Stockton so a dispatcher could call up any terminal in the system and determine the number of loads at any particular step in the system.

Table 2. Tomato operations Imperial Valley—1989.

Variable	Planned	Actual
Start-up	June 5	June 6
Hectarage	745	745
Yield (t/ha)	75.3	80.5
Tonnes processed	56,087	59,991
Soluble solids (%)	4.5	4.97
Total tonnes 46% equiv. tomato paste	5,554	6,511
kg paste/tonne	99	109
No. of growers	10	10
Freight costs/tonne	$62.82	$65.82

DISCUSSION

Table 2 illustrates the plan versus the actual results accomplished by the Agriculture Department in Imperial Valley. In all measurable terms, the results equaled, if not exceeded the plan, except for freight costs. The increased yields and soluble solids were the two key items that allowed an extra 900 tonnes of paste to be manufactured at the Stockton plant. The overall savings for Campbell was estimated to be in excess of five million dollars. The most important point was that the June produced paste was shipped immediately to the various Campbell manufacturing plants in the United States to prevent a gap in the supply of red-based soups and tomato juice to the supermarket distribution system.

California growers responded quickly to the tomato paste shortage after 1988 (Table 1). By the end of the 1990 season, a 42% increase in harvested tonnage was accomplished by means of an additional 34,000 ha of tomatoes.

Pesticide Chemicals: An Industry Perspective on Minor Crop Uses

Robert F. Bischoff

Presently, there are almost no incentives for pesticide chemical manufacturers to develop their products for minor crop use applications. As a result of the regulatory process including the Federal Insecticide Fungicide and Rodenticide Act (FIFRA) of 1988, many minor crop uses are not being supported on product labeling because of excessive costs to develop supportive data packages and other factors that impact a product's regulatory status. Accordingly, minor crop growers will find fewer and fewer products available to control their various pest problems.

The purpose of this paper is to describe the commercialization process for new pesticide agrichemicals as followed by the basic manufacturers of these products, concerns that this industry has with minor crop uses, and finally some thoughts on how to provide incentives to the agrichemical producers to develop new and maintain existing minor crop uses on their pesticide product labeling.

COMMERCIALIZATION PROCESS FOR NEW AGRICULTURAL PESTICIDES

The development of new pesticide products is a very costly, time consuming and risky process that involves an extensive research and development component. From a research and development perspective, the process begins in the Discovery Laboratories, where teams of biologists and synthesis chemists prepare new chemicals and evaluate them for effectiveness in a greenhouse or small plot environment. Having determined that a new compound merits further testing, field research scientists evaluate the material under expected environmental use conditions by using larger test plots out-of-doors. Shortly before and concurrently to field testing, other testing is implemented by toxicologists to determine the impact on various mammalian and other non-target organisms and by residue, environmental, and metabolism chemists who study the effects of the potential chemicals on the environment. Formulation chemists and process engineers define the composition and process for preparing the end use formulations, i.e. liquid, granulars, etc., that are applied to the target crop(s). Technical Service and Development take field testing beyond the internal field testing facilities that a company has and serve as a technical interface between the company, the scientific community, and the customer. Finally, the regulatory function relying on data inputs from all of the various R&D laboratories secures approval for the first registration from the various federal and state regulatory agencies.

The process described above is driven by the need to satisfy data requirements as prescribed by federal and state regulatory agencies to support a new registration. These data requirements are listed by the Environmental Protection Agency (EPA) under Title 40 Code of Federal Regulations Part 158, and include product chemistry, environmental chemistry, residue chemistry, hazards to humans and domestic animals, reentry protection, hazards to wildlife and aquatic organisms, hazards to nontarget insects, spray drift evaluation, phytotoxicity to target and non-target plants, and more.

Because of the extensive testing required, the agrichemical industry has estimated that $40 to $60 million in development costs are incurred before the first registration of a new pesticide chemical is received, and that the process takes over seven years from discovery to registration. A recent analysis for five compounds in predevelopment at DowElanco shows an average anticipated expenditure of $46 million before first registration and sales occur. It is further estimated that only one in twenty thousand new chemicals tested in the discovery screening process survive as a new registered compound. The development process is clearly a high risk venture in that at any time during the development phase, an adverse finding in the tests being conducted (such as a toxicological or environmental one) can limit the number of potential end uses or result in the termination of the project.

For all these reasons, it is imperative that a discovery program focus its screening tests to identify various herbicides, insecticides, fungicides, etc., on the crops with the greatest market potential, namely corn, soybeans, wheat, cotton, and rice. There is little or no incentive for agrichemical companies to develop pesticides for lower valued markets including fruits, vegetables, and other minor crops.

PESTICIDES ON MINOR CROPS/CONCERNS AND ISSUES

Other than the innate costs associated with the development and maintenance of a data base to support pesticide registrations, there are a number of other factors that impact considerations of support for minor crop uses by pesticide chemical producers. In general, minor crops are higher in value (in terms of dollar return per unit area) than a rowcrop such as maize or soybeans. This represents a greater potential product liability to the seller of pesticide products, should a yield loss be linked to those products.

Another consideration involves the limited manpower, laboratory space, and funding that an agrichemical producer has available for research and development purposes and the balance to maintain between spending monies for new product development versus maintaining existing products. FIFRA '88 and other regulatory mandates have had a tremendous effect on this balance as reflected by the numerous voluntary cancellations regarding existing products and various minor crop uses.

Finally, there are concerns associated with dietary and non-dietary risk assessments. Sometimes, the impact on the reference dose (acceptable daily intake) is excessive and can prevent the pesticide chemical producer from registering on crops of higher market potential. In other cases, there may be a worker exposure issue particularly with many of the fruit and vegetable crops which may involve a high level of hand labor.

PESTICIDES ON MINOR CROPS/FUTURE OPPORTUNITIES

There is indeed a crisis situation concerning the availability of pesticide products for application on minor crops. However, there are a number of possible solutions or opportunities to consider as a means of mitigating or resolving this issue. Firstly, pesticide chemical manufacturers need incentives to seek minor crop uses for their products. This can be accomplished through the EPA registration process by reducing data requirements through the use of surrogate data, waiving tolerance and registration maintenance fees, and expediting the EPA review of a major crop submission if a minor crop use is included in the submission package.

Second, product liability concerns affecting the basic pesticide chemical suppliers have to be addressed. The use of indemnification/liability waiver agreements appear to be a step in the right direction.

Third, more aware and involved minor crop growers and grower groups are needed. When appropriate, this sector can pool its resources to fund data development in support of minor crop use registrations. Implied in this process is better communication and cooperation between pesticide chemical suppliers and the minor crop grower community.

Finally, additional funding is needed to support the IR-4 minor crop use program. Over time, the IR-4 program has been the most effective and prolific organization in terms of supporting new minor crop uses. With the advent of FIFRA '88, a considerable strain on the IR-4 budget developed causing additional funding needs.

SUMMARY

Many factors affect the pesticide registration process, resulting in fewer and fewer products available to the grower for the control of pests on minor crops. Presently, there are no incentives for pesticide chemical producers to develop or maintain minor crop uses on their product labeling. High costs and risks associated with developing and maintaining supportive data packages necessitate a focus on major crops such as corn, soybeans, cotton, rice, and wheat. Other concerns associated with minor crops include product liability claims, limited research and development resources, and possible unfavorable impacts on dietary and non-dietary risk assessments. Possible solutions to this crisis situation include incentives for pesticide chemical producers to pursue minor crop use registrations, product liability relief, a more involved minor crop grower community, and additional funding for the IR-4 program.

Medicinal Plants and the Pharmaceutical Industry

James A. Duke

There is a trend for synthetics to replace natural compounds in Prescription and Over the Counter (OTC) Pharmaceuticals. Today, ephedrine, salicylates, vitamins, and xanthines are mostly synthetic and steroids are often semisynthetic. While agreeing with Farnsworth and Bingel (1977) that 25% of modern prescription drugs contain at least one phytochemical, I suspect that only about 10% or our leading drugs (excluding the illicit drugs, cocaine, crack, hashish, heroin, marijuana, and opium) now contain phytochemicals still extracted directly from the higher plants.

I draw on four major sources to support this contention: (1) Products of America's largest pharmaceutical firms listed in the Physicians Desk Reference (PDR 1991), (2) Reanalysis of Farnsworth and Bingel (1977), (3) Canadian OTC Drugs (CPA 1988), and (4) Sittig's Encyclopedia (1988).

CLASSIFYING MAJOR DRUGS

If only about 10% of the 100 most important major drugs (Sittig 1988) and the PDR-listed drugs (PDR 1991) of major drug companies contain major compounds *still* derived from plants, we must clarify the 25% figure (Farnsworth and Bingel 1977) that conservationists have quoted and misquoted for twenty years. Emphasizing the constancy of this 25%, Farnsworth et al. (1985) reported: "In the USA, for example, 25% of all prescriptions dispensed from community pharmacies from 1959 to 1980 contained plant extracts or active principles prepared from higher plants. This figure (25%) did not vary by more than ±1.0% in any of the 22 years surveyed ... and in 1980 consumers in the USA paid more than $8,000 million for prescriptions containing active principles obtained from plants." However, about 15% of those 25% are now produced synthetically or semisynthetically and thus, no longer derived directly from natural sources. Farnsworth and Bingel's (1977) estimate remains correct if phrased as: 25% of modern prescription drugs contain at least one compound now *or once* derived *or patterned after compounds derived* from higher plants.

American consumers want natural drugs, believing natural drugs are safer than synthetics. The pharmaceutical firms seem to prefer synthetics or semisynthetics, in part due to proprietary economic reasons. The health of the drug company by necessity must concern the drug company before the health of the consumer. As noted in a recent International Trade Commission Study, "Between 1976 and 1990, the cost of developing a pharmaceutical product in the US increased from $54 million to $231 million. Only one out of every 4,000-10,000 compounds discovered can be marketed commercially—after which a company has less than ten years to partially recoup its R&D investment before its patent expires and generic manufacturers enter the market or a me-too drug is created by a competitor" (Chemical Marketing Reporter 1991). Such investments may lead pharmaceutical firms to prefer a proprietary synthetic or semisynthetic to a relatively less proprietary herbal or natural product. American pharmaceutical firms often seek the semisynthetic and avoid the natural compound, when, at least in some cases, the natural compound might be best. The pharmaceutical firm must consider several attributes including, safety, efficacy, reproducibility of results, patentability, and profitability. With at least $7,000 in public relations directed to each physician in this country by the pharmaceutical firms, the physicians may reflect the same priorities as the pharmaceutical firms. Consumers, National Institute of Health, Food and Drug Administration, and the government as a whole should seek the safest, cheapest, most efficacious drugs. Often, these could prove to be standardized herbs or relatively unpatentable natural products, placing the drug companies and the consumers and government's interests in conflict. More than 10% of Americans can't even afford modern medicine and/or insurance. Farnsworth (1990) estimates that about 64% of the world's population or 3.2 billion people use plants as drugs (largely unable to afford modern medicine). If their drugs are worth as much to them economically as modern medicine is to Americans, these plants are worth trillions of dollars.

What can be done to determine which natural alternatives are relatively safe, efficacious, and affordable to the majority of the world's citizenry? There must be some economic incentive for drug firms to investigate natural alternatives. Clearly, it would not make sense for a drug firm to invest $231 million proving that a widely grown ornamental could prevent migraine, when the drug firms are already reaping millions of dollars in the sale of proprietary migraine medications. If, on the other hand, drug companies by mandate, compared new synthetic drugs not only with placebo, but with one of the best herbal alternatives, e.g. feverfew for migraine, those drug companies could be given some marketing exclusivity on natural alternatives that the companies prove efficacious. As a society, we would feel safer in the knowledge that home-grown herbs had been proven efficacious, at least under the experimental conditions.

American consumers are calling for greater use of natural products (certainly they prefer natural antioxidants, cosmetics, dyes, food colors, and pesticides, if not medicines) while the pharmaceutical firms have moved towards the synthetic. It is hard to document the disdain for the natural compound among the druggists. Farnsworth notes, however (1990):

"Of all the pharmaceutical companies I know in the US that are interested in research on plant materials—and that's probably only four—none is interested in discovering active chemical structures which will be patented and marketed as drugs per se. They are looking for lead structures from which they would prepare analogues."

The only pharmaceutical firms that I know in the United States that are interested in natural products are Merck Sharp & Dohme (West Point, Pennsylvania), Eastman Pharmaceuticals (Rochester, New York), SmithKline Beecham (Pittsburg, Pennsylvania), and Glaxo (Research Triangle Park, North Carolina). There are several small start-up companies, getting into this area either from a mass screening viewpoint or from looking to ethnobotany e.g. Shaman Pharmaceuticals (see King 1991), to provide leads. This is a new trend: five years ago, there wasn't a single pharmaceutical company in the United States that had any interest in developing drugs from higher plants." (Farnsworth 1990).

PRODUCTS OF AMERICA'S LARGEST PHARMACEUTICAL FIRMS

Green consumerism has not yet reached the pharmaceutical industry. One might define a "green" pharmaceutical as one containing as its major ingredient a compound still commercially extracted from a higher plant. Estimated percentages of "green" products produced by some major pharmaceutical firms are tabulated in Table 1. Their drugs, as listed in PDR (1991), were evaluated to see what percentage still contained natural

Table 1. Some higher plants used in the drugs of major firms and estimated percentage of "green" drugs (after Valueline and Chemical Marketing Reporter).

Company	Projected earnings ($billion/1991)	Higher plants used	Natural (%)
Bristol-Myers	11.2	Mayapple, ephedra, yew	<10
Merck	8.6	Rauwolfia	<5
Pfizer	7.2	Rauwolfia	<5
Smith Kline Beecham		Pyrethrins	<1
American Home Products	7.1	Opium, quinine	30
Eli Lilly	5.9	Periwinkle, curare	17
Warner Lambert	5.0	Belladonna, ephedra	<5
Rhone Poulenc	3.7	Opium, rauwolfia	15
Schering-Plough	3.6	Ephedra	<5
Upjohn	3.4	Belladonna	<2
Marion Merrell Dow	2.8	Opium, quinine, nicotine	17
Syntex	1.8	(Barbasco formerly)	<1
Johnson & Johnson		Psyllium	10
G.B.Searle	1.4		

products as *one of the* major ingredients. The average for these firms is less than 10% "green." If all the once-natural compounds, or compounds patterned after once-natural, and excipients, such as acacia, candellila, carnauba, guar, tragacanth, are included, then more than 50% of their drugs contain some naturally occurring phytochemical. Thus, a sensu stricto interpretation (only still-natural phytochemicals as major ingredients), finds fewer that 10% natural or "green" pharmaceuticals. A sensu lato interpretation (containing a now-natural or once-natural phytochemical as a major *or minor* ingredient), finds more than half of modern pharmaceuticals are at least partially "green."

Reanalysis of Farnsworth and Bingel (1977)

Table 2, modified from Farnsworth and Bingel (1977) lists the major plant-derived phytochemicals in United States prescriptions two decades ago. Steroids are clearly the largest items in Table 2. From mare's urine as a source of steroids, we moved to temperate *Dioscorea villosa*, and then to tropical "barbasco" (*Dioscorea* spp.). After too many price hikes in the barbasco, the steroid industry largely went to semisynthetic modification of the phytosterols from temperate soybeans. In general, most modern steroids are now semisynthetic. Codeine, atropine, hyoscyamine, digoxin, digitoxin, pilocarpine, and quinidine are still derived from plants. Reserpine, pseudoephedrine, and ephedrine, count for 3% of those prescriptions cited by Farnsworth and Bingel (1977), and are sometimes produced synthetically, sometimes natural. Two-thirds of American ephedrine is synthetic, one-third from German, one-third from American factories, the other third being natural ephedrine from China. The relative share of the synthetic will probably increase in the future. Assume that half of our ephedrine, pseudoephedrine, and reserpine are synthetic and that all the steroids are now semisynthetic, subtract and find that, accepting these assumptions and no change in percentages, only 6.4% of our drugs have these natural ingredients, synthetic or semisynthetic compounds having replaced the natural compounds.

Analysis of Sittig's Encyclopedia

In his first Table, Sittig (1988) lists the top 100 generic pharmaceuticals in the United States in 1976. The top four items had sales over $100 million; the cutoff after 100 was at the 10 million sales level. Total United States sales of the top 100 was about $3 billion. Among the top 25 of Sittig, only one (4%), is clearly derived largely from higher plants, digoxin from temperate *Digitalis* as number 4. Theophylline once derived from subtropical *Camellia* (and possibly tropical *Theobroma*), at number 21, is still used but is almost if not exclusively synthesized. Methyldopa is synthesized, but could possibly be based on the legumes like *Mucuna* and *Vicia* which contain levodopa. Likewise, the hormones norethindrone, ethinyl estradiol, and conjugated estrogens appear to be wholly synthesized or semisynthetic but they could probably be derived from starting estrogenic compounds in palm and pine pollens or pomegranates. Tartaric acid and potassium chloride, e.g., also occur in higher plants but can be viewed as phytochemicals.

Farther down Sittig's top 100, there are even fewer clearly "green" drugs. There are several estrogenic or androgenic hormones, presumably largely semisynthetic. There are several antibiotics derived from lower plants. Some have salicylic or tartaric acids or maleic-acids, coumarin, ethanol, furfurylamines, triethylamines, guanidine, benzaldehyde, proline, piperidine, heptaldehydes, and some contain semisynthetic opiates. Natural products, if they are used, are often only minor elements in a bigger formula. Stretching to accept guaifenesin (largely guaiacol which could come from a tropical tree), warfarin sodium (based largely on 4-hydroxy-coumarin, which could come from a tropical tree), and "nicotine polacrillex" (presumably based on natural nicotine which could be obtained from tropical trees (*Duboisia*) or weeds (*Nicotiana*), only about 5% of the top hundred are based primarily on higher plant phytochemicals. Ten percent are antibiotics derived from lower plants, mostly bacteria by biotechnology. Only by counting all the "iffy" odds and ends can one stretch the percentage to 25% containing at least one compound that could conceivably be derived from a higher plant.

Analysis of Canadian OTC Evidence

A fourth line of evidence (CPA 1988) confirms Farnsworth's 25% figure sensu lato. As in the United States, Canadians share a desire to take more responsibility for their own health care. An aging population and the resulting strain on health care services will force consumers to take an even greater role in years to come (CPA 1988).

The product monographs appendix of the CPA Book lists hundreds of apparently approved medicines from A&C with Codeine to Zinkosalb, both of which contain salicylic compounds which the American Indians once derived from poplars, willows, and even wintergreens. Such compounds count in the Farnsworth 25%, even though they are now synthetic.

A&C with Codeine illustrates the problems one encounters in trying to make a survey of this type. It contains three major ingredients, the now-synthetic acetylsalicylic acid, the sometimes synthesized caffeine, and the still natural codeine. Thus, it clearly contains one natural ingredient, probably the most expensive ingredient, codeine, still derived from the opium poppy. The caffeine may be synthesized or may be a by-product of decaffeinated coffee. The acetylsalicylic-acid could fall into the category called semisynthetic, if derived by acetylation of natural salicylic acid, but today it is mostly a pure synthetic, involving the utilization of no higher plant phytochemicals.

A and D Ointment is equally problematic. Vitamins A & D, as all vitamins, could come from natural products. But most are not derived from higher plants and all are synthesized (Harold Newmark pers. commun.). A and D Ointment would be scored "non-green," the lanolin of course derived from animals. Vitamins should be scored non-phytochemical ("non-green") unless the monograph specifies that the vitamin is plant derived. Absorbine contains methyl-salicylate and menthol, both natural products, now largely synthesized. Excipients like the glycine and lactose in Acetest are, of course, not scored as major ingredients. Similarly homatropine, while related to atropine, is treated here as a synthetic. How should one score ACI-JEL vaginal buffer which contains some herbal excipients like tragacanth and acacia, and compounds that do occur in plants like acetic and ricinoleic acids which are cheaper as synthetics? Resorcinol is scored synthetic though it too can be derived from umbelliferone. Pseudoephedrine and ephedrine are sometimes synthesized. Although lidocaine is said to have been patterned after gramine, it is not a phytochemical. Aloe in After Burn certainly makes it score "green." Similarly the witch hazel, not the salicylic acid in Aknoderm, makes it score "green." Listerine Antiseptic contains 21.9% alcohol, 0.09% eucalyptol (cineole), 0.06% thymol, and 0.04% menthol (all derivable from plants but probably synthetic).

SCORING PHYTOMEDICINALS

This discussion illustrates the subjective nature of assigning economic values to a very complicated and

Table 2. Reanalysis of common phytochemicals in the United States containing plant derived higher drugs (Modified from Farnsworth and Bingel 1977).

Phytochemical	Percent of total Rxs
Steroids (95% from diosgenin)	14.7
Codeine	2.0
Atropine	1.5
Reserpine	1.5
Pseudoephedrine	0.9
Ephedrine	0.8
Hyoscyamine	0.8
Digoxin	0.7
Scopolamine	0.7
Digitoxin	0.3
Pilocarpine	0.3
Quinidine	0.2
Total	24.4

Table 3. Natural product patents.

Country	Number of patents	Percentage
Belgium	2	0.8
Brazil	1	0.4
China	14	5.6
Czechoslovakia	2	0.8
European	26	10.5
France	5	2.0
Germany	12	4.8
Hungary	1	0.4
International	13	5.2
Japan	148	59.6
Poland	2	0.8
United Kingdom	2	0.8
United States	13	5.2
Soviet Union	7	2.8

widely divergent phytomedicinal industry. A generous scoring, allowing all vitamins and amino-acids, acetic acid, lactose, as major or minor ingredients or excipients would give at least 50% "green." Thus, the final percentage of plants or plant-derived extracts in modern pharmaceuticals will ultimately depend upon your definition of phytomedicinal. Should such natural compounds as alcohol, vinegar, citric acid, resorcinol, be included, then well over 50%, perhaps 75% of medicines contain plant-derived phytochemicals. Only by counting all of the following major naturals could one score the Canadian OTC's as 25% "green" (CPA 1988): allantoin, benzoin, bran, caffeine, camphor, caprylic-acid, charcoal, cineole, citric-acid, codeine, cresol, ephedrine, guaiacol, lecithin, menthol, methylcellulose, methylmorphine, pectin, phenol, pseudephedrine, salicylates, sorbitol, tartaric-acid, turpentine, and undecylinic-acid.

The score could top 50% "green" if one counts minor ingredients, all vitamins and minerals which occur in higher plants, plus these other even more marginal compounds: acetic-acid, agar and alginates, alcohols, amino acids, all vitamins (even ascorbic acid), benzocaine, benzyl alcohol, benzyl benzoate, citrates, crotamiton, danthron and casanthranol (close to anthraquinoones), dextromorphinan and complex opiates, dextrose and other refined sugars, epinephrine, guaifenesin, homatropine, homosalate, hydrocortisone, hydroquinone, lactulose, lidocaine, paba, phenylephrine, resorcinol, selenium, and other minerals like sulfur, urease, and vanillylamide.

Some argue that we would be better with more natural product medicines and fewer synthetics. If reverting to natural medicines, which also prove safe and efficacious, could also help save the rain forest, there's one more reason to consider natural drugs. The government should consider requiring pharmaceutical firms not only to prove their new drugs safe and efficacious, but compare them not only to placebo, but also to one or more of the better herbal alternatives. If energy costs remain as they are or become less expensive, we should expect even more synthetics to replace naturals, in both Prescription and OTC drugs. If energy costs get more expensive, or if "green" consumers get louder, we may reverse the trend from natural to synthetic in this country.

Natural Product Patents

With American drug firms trending away from the natural product, the Japanese are increasing their share of the world's natural product patents. Surveys (Duke 1990) over the last four years have shown the Japanese percentage of the world's natural product patents surge from 40 to 60%. In 1990, at least among those natural-product patents reported in Phytotherapy Research, Japan obtained more than five times more than did the United States (Table 3.). As American consumer demand for the *natural* increases, the pharmaceutical dissatisfaction for the *natural* ironically also increases.

REFERENCES

Canadian Pharmaceutical Association (CPA). 1988. Self medication. 1785 Alta Vista Drive, Ottawa, Canada.
Farnsworth, N.R., O. Akerele, A.S. Bingel, D.D. Soejarto, and Z.G. Guo. 1985. Medicinal plants in therapy. Bul. World Health Org. 63(6):965–981.
Farnsworth, N.R. and A.S. Bingel. 1977. Problems and prospects of discovering new drugs from higher plants by pharmacological screening, p. 1–22. In: H. Wagner and P. Wolff (eds.). New natural products with pharmacological, biological or therapeutic activity. Springer-Verlag, New York.
Farnsworth, N.R. 1990. The role of ethnopharmacology in drug development, p. 2–11. In: D.J. Chadwick and J. Marsh (eds.). Bioactive compounds from plants. Ciba Foundation Symposium 154. Wiley, Chichester, UK.
International Trade Commission. 1991. Chemical Marketing Reporter Oct. 21 p. 31.
King, S.R. 1991. The source of our cures. Cultural Survival Quart. (Summer):19–22.
PDR. 1991. Physicians desk reference. 45th ed. Medical Economics Company, Oradell, NJ.
Sittig, M. 1988. Pharmaceutical manufacturing encyclopedia. 2nd ed. 2 vols. Noyes Publ., Park Ridge, NJ.

Phytomedicines as a New Crop Opportunity

Loren D. Israelsen

Phytomedicines, simply defined, are a special category of plant drugs. They are standardized, which means that certain compounds in the plant material are quantified and elucidated so as to have a replicable final product, batch after batch. One of the criticisms traditionally leveled against natural medicines is the lack of standard levels of biological materials from the natural plants.

In many parts of the world, the United States is considered a third world country when it comes to phytomedicines. Unfortunately, our European colleagues are far ahead of us; they have a multi-billion dollar industry in phytomedicines, whereas ours is only a two hundred million dollar industry. Even so, there are a lot of exciting developments in the United States. Over the last five years, I estimate that the American medicinal herb industry has grown at a rate exceeding 20% per year and this trend continues today.

Phytomedicines represent new crop opportunities for several reasons. First, the companies who use these products are very keen to get high quality, sanitary material. This is becoming quite a serious problem. One example we have seen quite recently relates to problems in Eastern Europe, the source of many of these plants. Would you buy plant material which has been growing next to a steel plant in Eastern Europe? Most people would not. The United States is a good growers market because it has a stable political environment, has many different growing climates and conditions, excellent choice of growers, and the ability to grow according to industrial specifications. The Appalachian region, in particular, is very rich in medicinal flora.

Of growing concern is the extinction of medicinal plant species in this country. Given the growing demand for these botanicals and current problems in over-collecting, it is quite likely that some of the last populations of these plants will be collected over the next five to ten years if we don't begin to cultivate them commercially. Finally, these specialty crops could provide profitable growing opportunities for small farmers. Some of these crops appear to be ideally suited to the small farmer.

IMPORTANT MEDICINAL PLANTS

Ginkgo biloba. The nuts of this tree are quite tasty when properly roasted. An extract (Fünfgeld 1988) derived from the leaf of this tree is the single largest selling drug in Germany and France today (Foster 1991). The extract is used for peripheral circulation and has the unique property of making red blood cells more elastic and selectively dilating capillaries. Consequently, this extract is used in Europe for treating conditions of tinnitus, vertigo, cold hands, cold feet, macular degeneration, and dementia. In order to meet the demand for the leaf, there is a 400 hectare farm in South Carolina which produces over a million kilograms of dried leaves a year. There are other plantations now being developed to meet the international demand for this product.

American ginseng (*Panax quinquifolium*). In Marathon County, Wisconsin, alone, this crop represents a one hundred million dollar a year crop (raw and finished product) which is primarily exported to China where it is widely used and appreciated. Oddly enough, we buy *Panax ginseng* from China because Americans prefer their material and they ours.

Saw palmetto (*Serenoa repens*). The berries of the Saw Palmetto are quite useful for benign prostatic hypertrophy. This is a very big pharmaceutical in Germany and France. There is a well developed industry in Florida which produces berries for export to Europe.

Goldenseal (*Hydrastis canadensis*). This is one of the fastest growing products in the United States in the natural products industry and used to be in the United States Pharmacopoeia until about 40 years ago. It is native to Appalachia and is one of the crops that is most threatened by extirpation because of growing demand. Ginseng growers in Wisconsin have been contacted to see if they could grow Goldenseal. To date, the project is showing signs of success, and it seems likely that a large percentage of this product will come from cultivated plots rather than naturally occurring populations.

Bloodroot (*Sanguanaria canadensis*). This is very popular and is the active ingredient in a toothpaste product called Viadent. It is used to control plaque and gingivitis (Bennet et al. 1990).

Siberian ginseng (*Eleutherococcus senticosus*). This is a very popular and interesting product. It is called an adaptogen. It was developed in Russia by Dr. Breckman. Adaptogens are body regulators which promote proper balance. Many medical doctors question this hypothesis, but there is a significant amount of empirical and clinical data from Russia to support this (Farnsworth et al. 1985).

Echinacea (*Echinacea purpurea*). This is a popular nonspecific immunostimulant in Germany and much of Europe. There are hundreds of hectares of cultivated Echinacea in Europe. There is also a large organic farm, Trout Lake Farm in Washington State, which grows significant amounts of this product. Echinacea is used as a preventative for colds and flues and is quite effective when used in this way. It is one of Europe's most popular natural products.

Milk thistle (*Silybum marianum*). This is used in Europe for liver conditions, treatment of acute mushroom poisoning, and other hepatoxic compounds.

Black cohosh (*Cimicifuga racemosa*). This is an interesting native American plant. It has a rich tradition among Native Americans and by people who live in the Appalachian region. It is used by women for regulation of hormonal cycles (Foster and Duke 1990).

Valerian (*Valeriana officinalus*). This is one of the more popular sleep aids in Europe and has been widely used for hundreds of years. There is no reason why this cannot be grown in the United States.

Feverfew (*Tanacetum parthenium*). Research in England has shown promising results in the treatment of migraine. A small amount of feverfew when taken orally can reduce the frequency and severity of migraine. It has great medical potential and could most definitely be grown in this country (Awang 1989).

St. John's wort (*Hypericum perforatum*). This is a popular European product. It has antiviral properties and also antidepressant properties (Hobbs 1988/1989).

Catnip (*Nepeta cataria*). Not only is it my cat's favorite play thing, but it is also used as a mild sedative (Tyler 1987). This is currently being grown in the United States as a sedative, although not commercially.

Pacific yew (*Taxus brevifolia*). At the moment, this is a most controversial and interesting phytomedicine. The pacific yew tree is the source of taxol which shows great promise for the treatment of ovarian and other cancers. However, there are not enough trees. These trees grow very slowly, and if harvested for taxol, the natural stands of the yew tree would be exhausted. The ability to obtain taxol from ornamental sources of *Taxus* as well as planting nurseries of the western yew for taxol extraction are underway.

Ginger (*Zingiber officinale*). It is not only a well known spice, but it has been proven to be as effective as dramamine in reducing nausea and motion sickness (Holtman et al. 1989). It has also been quite useful for pregnant women who are suffering nausea in early pregnancy and is quite safe (Bone et al. 1990).

CONCLUSIONS

In the United States, the policies of the Food and Drug Administration (FDA), historically, have been unhelpful to natural products. These plant products are polypharmaceutics, meaning they have multiple compounds, and FDA is not presently prepared to review products containing more than one compound. Demanding evidence that each individual component in an extract is safe and effective is a matter of scientific curiosity, but has little to do with the inherent questions of safety and effectiveness of the extract. Unfortunately, FDA still struggles with this concept.

The natural healthcare market is a very fast growing one. It is projected that at current inflation rates for health care, by the year 2030, health care costs could consume 100% of the gross national product. Something must be done. People are turning more and more to prevention and wellness programs, including natural medicines. As this trend develops, phytomedicines could become an important new alternative crop in the United States.

REFERENCES

Awang, D. 1989. Feverfew. Can. Pharm. J. 122(5):266–70.

Bennett, B.C., C.R. Bell, and R.T. Boulware. 1990. Geographic and variation in alkaloid content of *Sanguinaria canadensisi* (Papaveraceae). Rhodora 92(870):57–69.

Bone, M.E., D.J. Wilkinson, J.R. Young, J. McNeil, and S. Sharlton. 1990. Ginger-root—a new antiemetic. The effect of ginger root on postoperative nausea and vomiting after major gynaecological surgery. Anesthesia 45(8):669–671.

Farnsworth, N.R., A.D. Kinghom, D.D. Soejarto, and D.P. Waller. 1985. Siberian ginseng (*Eleutherococcus senticosus*): Current status as an adaptogen, p. 155–215. In: H. Wagner, H. Hikino, and N.R. Farnsworth (eds.). Economic and medicinal plant research. Vol. 1. Academic Press, Orlando, FL.

Foster, S. 1991. Ginkgo (*Ginkgo biloba*). American Botanical Council. Botanical Series #304. Austin, TX.

Foster, S. and J. Duke. 1990. A field guide to medicinal plants: Eastern and Central North America. Houghton Mifflin Co, Boston.

Fünfgeld, E.W. (ed). 1988. Rökan (*Ginkgo biloba*), recent results in pharmacology, and clinic. Springer-Verlag, Berlin.

Hobbs, C. 1988/1989. St. John's Wort *Hypericum perforatum*. L.A. Review. HerbalGram 18/19:24–33.

Holtman, S., A.H. Clarke, H. Schereer, and M. Hohn. 1989. The anti-motion sickness mechanism of ginger. Acta Otolaryngol (Stockh). 108:168–174.

Tyler, V.E. 1987. The new honest herbal. George F. Stickley Company, Philadelphia.

COMMERCIALIZATION

Commercializing Industrial Crops: The Industrial Component

AMERICAN ASSOCIATION OF INDUSTRIAL CROPS (AAIC) PANEL DISCUSSION

Introduction

Anson E. Thompson

U.S. Department of Agriculture, Agricultural Research Service

The primary focus of the Second National New Crops Symposium is on Exploration, Research, and Commercialization. The Association for the Advancement of Industrial Crops (AAIC), the organizer of this Panel Discussion Session, is structured to facilitate and address all aspects of developing and commercializing industrial crops. We know quite a lot, and are reasonably proficient and successful in our exploration and research efforts. However, the requirements for successful commercialization of the results of our research are the least understood and most difficult component to manage in the total system.

A diverse group of industrial leaders in new crops research and development have been brought together as panelists, and invited to present their own ideas on the role that industry must play in the total commercialization process of developing new and alternative industrial crops.

We know there is no one pathway or solution to the successful commercialization of new industrial crops. Hopefully, the ideas from these panelists and from the Symposium will better enable us to tailor a unique, successful solution to our individual sets of conditions and variables. Thus, our major objective is to exchange ideas on the possibilities and opportunities as well as constraints. By this process, we should be able to identify new courses of action that could move this essential developmental process forward to the mutual benefit of all participants, as well as the ultimate consumer.

Cooperative Research and Development Agreements Under the Technology Transfer Act of 1986

James T. Hall

USDA/ARS Office of Cooperative Interactions

We have all heard of the difficulties involved in getting new crops and industrial products made from them into commercial production and use. Research at a number of locations and organizations around the country has identified possible products that can be produced from new crops; e.g., high value oils, rubber, newsprint. While it is often possible to produce industrial products from new or even existing crops, the path to commercialization is not an easy nor straight forward one. Sometimes, we in the research community, talk blithely about technology transfer of our research findings, forgetting that the cost of commercialization for a new product or process is at least nine times the cost of doing the original research. In the case of a new crop and its intended products, the cost for commercialization may be even higher as a percentage of the total cost of introduction.

The expenses involved in developing new products often stymies commercial development by producers and processing firms. Industrial firms do not feel they can risk the tremendous investment that is necessary to accomplish the transfer of one of our ideas into a commercially viable, profit-making enterprise. One way to help overcome this problem is through cooperative research and development beyond the basic discoveries. Thus, I would like to discuss technology transfer, specifically Cooperative Research and Development Agreements, commonly referred to as CRADAs.

CRADAs were authorized under and are an implementation of the Federal Technology Transfer Act of 1986 (Public Law 99-502). The objectives of CRADAs is to help bridge the technology transfer gap between discoveries (technology in the rough in many cases) made in Federal laboratories like USDA/ARS, and the marketplace. The Federal government, by utilizing CRADAs, has put the "D" in R&D to get new products/processes on the market in order to improve American industry's competitive position in world markets.

USDA/ARS is one of the leaders, along with the National Institutes of Health (NIH), in their use of CRADAs. Despite the fact that ARS accounts for less than 1% of the total Federal R&D budget of over $70 billion, ARS has entered into more than 200 CRADAs since the first one was signed in July, 1987. All but a few are with individual industrial firms. Some early ones have already resulted in new products reaching the market including:

- A plant virus test kit sold in the United States and abroad.
- A system for in-ovo vaccination of chick embryos prior to hatch. This will eliminate the need to vaccinate each chick.
- The first biocontrol fungus to reduce/eliminate "damping-off" disease of bedding plants.
- An ultrasonic mixing device for use with atomic absorption equipment.

Interestingly, two of the above were CRADAs with very small firms (Agdia and Embrex), and two with large firms (W.R. Grace and Perkin–Elmer). Many more ARS developed products and processes are in the pipeline on their way to the market via CRADAs. Of course, not all or probably even a majority of CRADAs will result in commercial success, but a significant number will, and those that do, may have only reached the marketplace precisely due to the cooperative development strategy.

A Technology Transfer Agreement between a commercial firm and USDA/ARS will include provisions on:

1. Research, development, and commercialization to be done by each party. This is the "heart" of a CRADA because it is essentially a plan of work for the project agreed upon by ARS scientists and company scientists, or other company representatives. In a small company, this might be the owner/CEO.
2. What USDA-ARS will contribute. ARS can contribute anything it has in-kind such as personnel, equipment, supplies, land, laboratory space, etc., but the Technology Transfer Act precludes ARS from putting cash into the project; e.g., dollars to the cooperator or a third party.
3. What the commercial firm will contribute. The cooperator, most often a commercial firm, can put dollars into ARS to help pay costs that may not have been incurred if the CRADA project had not been undertaken. The firm can also provide in-kind services, materials, etc. of all kinds including personnel to work in ARS facilities on the project; e.g., provide a post-doc for a period of time. It must be noted that a firm cannot "hire" ARS to do contract research on technology it owns.
4. Confidentiality of findings or information that may be exchanged.
5. Publication of results. We insist that we be able to publish any results that derive from a CRADA.
6. Inventions. This is a most important provision. The ownership of these inventions and the right to license are spelled out in the CRADA. There are three categories of ownership of inventions as follows:
   a. They are owned by ARS if an invention is made strictly by an ARS employee or employees.
   b. They are jointly owned by ARS and the cooperating firm if the employees are both involved in making an invention.
   c. They are owned entirely by the cooperating firm if only their employees are involved in making an invention.
7. Copyrights are also covered, but at the present time computer software developed by ARS and other Federal laboratories cannot be copyrighted.
8. The liability of each party is spelled out. The remainder of a CRADA is mainly "boiler-plate" covering the points listed above. Most of these have been standard for years in other ARS cooperative research agreements; e.g., specific cooperative agreements, trust fund agreements, reimbursable agreements, etc.

There are several major benefits of Technology Transfer Agreements to commercial firms. A very important benefit is the first right to exclusive licenses on patented inventions made under the agreement. A major new feature of CRADAs compared with previous ARS cooperative research agreements is the "first right of refusal." This means that cooperators have first chance at a license to any potentially patentable technology developed that is owned or jointly owned by ARS. However, this does not apply to inventions related to the technology being addressed under a CRADA where the invention was made before the CRADA was signed.

Other benefits to the commercial firm are improved access to ARS scientists and facilities. As a firm's employees work more closely with ARS scientists, better access is almost guaranteed. They also have better access to expertise related to research results and inventions. The knowledge of an ARS scientist in regard to the fine points of problems and potential uses and benefits of a particular technology may be worth more than what is on paper or published in scientific journals. Of course, the most important benefit is the enhancement of profitability related to the development and marketing of new products and processes, which is the ultimate goal of the collaboration made possible by CRADAs.

There are also major benefits of the Technology Transfer Agreements to USDA/ARS. These arrangements significantly improve the opportunities for ARS to develop and transfer technology. It again puts the "D" in R&D. ARS also receives better feedback from industry on what research is needed. CRADAs require regular or at least frequent contact with industry representatives for operation of the CRADA, which provides more opportunity for feedback. ARS scientists and administrators also receive increased familiarity with problems related to commercialization of a product or process.

Another important benefit in these times of budgetary restraint is that scientists and ARS share licensing fees and royalties. There is a chance for funds returning to ARS to help finance more technology transfer. This provides a real incentive to scientists as the inventors receive 25% of any licensing fees and royalties paid to ARS by the licensee.

There are several steps that firms can take to initiate a Technology Transfer Agreement with USDA/ARS. First, the firm must learn of ARS research capabilities, programs, and results. These can be through contacts made at professional and scientific society meetings, published journals, and other ARS publications. One-on-one visits to laboratories to meet and discuss mutual interests with the scientists are useful. The USDA/ARS computer database TEKTRAN, which contains brief reports of the latest ARS research results, is another good source. TEKTRAN and most ARS publications also give information to facilitate contact with the ARS scientist who is responsible for the program of interest.

The next step is to work with the ARS scientist to develop the necessary plan of work for the cooperative research and development program. This would usually take the form of a brief, jointly written proposal. It is important that the draft proposal receives appropriate preliminary review and clearance within the private firm and within the ARS. Delays at this step can be avoided by both parties if proper attention to getting preliminary approval. The final step involves the joint approval of the cooperative research and development agreement that incorporates the proposed research plan. Final approval in many firms require processing through several levels just as in ARS, and this combination may take several weeks, or even months to complete. Careful preliminary discussion, planning, and agreement can significantly reduce the length of time involved in the final approval process.

A CRADA is a technique that has promise, but it is only one phase or a beginning of technology transfer. In the subsequent phases, there are other important activities such as assembling financial resources for further research and development, conducting marketing studies, pilot plant evaluations, scale up of production, and distribution activities.

CRADAs may not be applicable to all technologies. Involvement of other mechanisms such as the Agricultural Extension Service and other technology transfer entities is essential to the successful commercialization of viable new crop-related products and processes developed by ARS, the State Agricultural Experiment Stations, and industry.

Role of the New Uses Council

Raymond L. Burns
New Uses Council

The New Uses Council (NUC) was formulated within the past 15 months as an outgrowth of an effort by several State Departments of Agriculture from the 12 states that make up the Midwestern State Departments of Agriculture group. They were joined by the Southern State Departments of Agriculture, the Western State Departments of Agriculture, and several Federal governmental officials and private firms. Basically, it was formed to see if we could put in place an attitude among ourselves, in Washington, DC, and with other groups that would foster work toward the development of new uses and new products. After having organized and conducted two conferences and developed language for the 1990 Farm Bill, a Working Committee formally organized and incorporated into the New Uses Council. The NUC is a national, nonprofit association made up of both public and private sector individuals and agencies. The NUC was primarily formed to promote commercialization and use of nonfood industrial products made from agricultural commodities including crops, livestock, and forestry. Our methodology involves the organization of specific project consortia of business, government, and academia. We seek to encourage public policies and programs that assist in expanded activities in this area.

GOALS

How do we seek to go about accomplishing our objectives? We were not formed to be in competition with any other society or group that is in place. We are organized in an attempt to be an umbrella organization that brings together common interests, and to help all concerned in getting industrial products developed from agricultural materials. Although our focus is on industrial products, nonfood and nonfeed, this does not mean that we are anti-food or feed. It is just that we want to focus on the utilization of commodities that exist, and to bring on line new crops and new products of any nature.

We envision our role as one that helps foster the various interdisciplinary linkages that exist in the research and academic areas. We seek also those linkages that bridge over into and involve the business community. One of our roles is to encourage a focus on the eventual end users, and to bring research efforts into the marketplace. We want to build constituencies and a knowledge base among administrators within USDA/ARS, Land Grant, and other universities. They need to be sympathetic to the funding and utilization of programs. Often the administrator is the spigot as well as the funnel in regard to what can be done.

PROGRAMS

In several states, we have brought together state agencies, such as the Departments of Agriculture or Departments of Commerce, with University Deans and other administrators into one day retreats. We look together at all the industrial materials, scientists, and other resources available, how they are funded, and how they should be evaluated. We have found that the agricultural deans and state administrators did not really realize all that was ongoing. We believe that just sharing the focus of the importance of our work and the impediments of getting into the marketplace is a worthy goal and effort. There are other state administrators such as governors, heads of departments of commerce, and certainly state legislators that also need to be made aware of these new potentials and opportunities. We have worked with the U.S. Small Business Administration and Department of Commerce, who see this as a new opportunity for economic development in rural areas.

The New Uses Council has worked to a considerable extent with the USDA, the Congress, and other national entities to educate them about opportunities and needs. We believed it is necessary to get rid of some of the governmental impediments that were in our Farm Bills. These have prevented a producer of normal farm commodities, such as grains and soybeans, from growing a new crop or from developing research and opportunities for new uses of our traditional crops. In recognition of these constraints, an effort was undertaken to see if we could get new language in the 1990 Farm Bill. The New Uses Council contributed to and supported incorporation of Title XVI, Subtitle G—Alternative Agricultural Research Centers (AARC). This new legislation should significantly contribute to the development of new industrial uses and products from agricultural materials. We have just learned during this conference that Congress has agreed and the President has signed the Bill to appropriate $4.5 million for FY 1992. The guidelines in Subtitle G call for an appropriation of $485 million for AARC over the next decade. However, if we added up all the work that is now ongoing, we would be hard pressed to identify $2 to $3 million per year. This extrapolates to a 20 fold increase in effort in this direction, and we will continue to try to see that it happens.

Activities also are taking place in the private sector, including the various commodity groups. We need a good foundation or basis of support among such groups as the maize, soybean, and wheat growers and users. We need to educate them about the opportunities in this area, and gain their support. Some commodity groups are concerned that a new effort may diminish emphasis on their crop. We must build a constituency with them, and an awareness and a desire on their part to see that we are successful, and that our efforts are complimentary. It is extremely important that we develop good relations with them.

We need to work with our processors, both established and potential. We need to promote the processing of agricultural materials into either an intermediate feedstock or a consumer ready product, or our work on commercialization does not get into the marketplace.

Almost always, we need to seek and try to get adequate financing. If it is only a concept and only works on paper, but doesn't work enough to draw capital to it, it will not happen. Either established or newly formed companies will have to be successful in getting capitalized to do the job. Industry representatives talk in the terms of getting a 20% return on investment. I believe these new things are going to have to bring in 40% returns, or venture capitalists will not "buy in."

The New Uses Council sees our focus and efforts on getting new uses commercialized as not being a competitive effort, or an attempt to displace any existing activity. Our motives are to help "grease the slide" to bring in the eventual processors and marketers of the end use, to work closely with them to commercialize the process or product, and to get the needed financing. We do this by newsletters, and by holding conferences and meetings.

The 1992 Annual Meeting of the New Uses Council in St. Louis—Biobased Product Expo '92 "Expanding Markets for Agricultural & Forestry Materials" will be a major event. The Department of Energy has committed $50,000 to coparticipate in it. Substantial funds from the Office of the Secretary of Agriculture are committed, and funds from the U.S. Small Business Administration are anticipated. The Association for the Advancement of Industrial Crops (AAIC) will hold their annual meeting in conjunction, and will jointly participate in activities designed to further our mutual goals. The New Uses Council's primary role is to try to be an umbrella, to provide linkages, and bring together all individuals and groups that share our vision of developing new industrial uses and products from agricultural materials.

Commercializing New Crops: Measuring the Opportunity

Keith A. Walker

Agrigenetics Company

Efforts to develop new crop opportunities for American farmers and new uses for current crops have been going on for a number of years. Often great technical progress is made, but efforts stumble at the point where industry must become involved in the commercialization process. The failure to successfully pass the technology to industry has, in numerous cases, led to failure and frustration. Two questions often asked at this point are: Why isn't industry more interested in this opportunity? What can be done to attract industry's attention to this idea/product/process?

While there may not be a generally applicable answer to these questions, there is a guide-post that most companies use to measure a technological opportunity. The process called "Opportunity Analysis," whether completed formally or informally, is a part of every company's commercial development function, and contains within it the elements that form the motivators necessary to gain the interest of private enterprise. The perspective presented here is that scientists would benefit by understanding the framework of such an analysis, and could use it to improve the probability of commercial success of their ideas.

OPPORTUNITY ANALYSIS

Opportunity Analysis is a structured examination of an innovation in terms of what the business in that innovation would look like. Along the way, various marketing, manufacturing, technological and, ultimately, financial questions get answered. The business in the technology will ultimately be modeled. While the model may be right or wrong, its purpose is to serve as a guide for future questions. The uncertainties and risks can, however, be weighed against the potential financial rewards for final judgment.

Market Analysis

Market analysis is the key to the success or failure of an innovation. This, I am convinced, is true regardless of whether the innovation is driven by the strength of its technology or pulled through into the market. In recent years, we have all been told how important it is to stay close to the customer and their needs. A great deal has been written on the subject of marketing and market strategy. It is all very helpful, but for the innovator there are only a few questions of fundamental importance:

- Who is the customer for this innovation?
- Will the innovation compete on price or performance (is the product unique and differentiated)?
- How will the value the innovation brings be recognized and captured?
- How much is that value?

In answering these questions, the innovator will learn whether there is an immediate need for the product, or whether a market must be created. Also learned will be whether the product will compete on price, value, or service. Most importantly, the innovator should identify important quality attributes which, if incorporated into the product during development, can improve it marketability.

There is one other important element. In market assessment, if we never think beyond the current needs of the customer, then we may never find the truly unique and differentiated products that novel technology can provide. This approach to commercial development has recently been described by D.N. Peters as pioneer, fill-in, or lily-pad marketing. These strategies involve short step-outs from currently identified businesses or markets anticipating future needs and directions. Pioneer marketing requires a more intimate association between the technologist on the one hand and the marketer on the other. In my opinion, bridging the knowledge gap between these two disciplines is of greatest importance to much of the innovation necessary to the successful development of new crops.

Technology Component

The technology component is the element in the analysis with which we are most familiar. As scientists, we all have good instincts about what areas of scientific endeavor may create the kind of unique knowledge that builds toward successful innovations. There are two elements to consider in the technological component, however, which are often not dealt with on an ongoing basis as research proceeds. The first of these is the length of the research path for the innovation. Projects with more than one major technical hurdle diminish dramatically in their overall probability of success. The second element to consider is the cost of the research relative to the probability of a payback. This element becomes clearer as the research and market analysis proceed together.

Manufacturing Component

Evaluation of the ease of manufacturing of an innovation is not given the attention it might deserve, especially in early stage project analysis. Clearly, the more unique and differentiated the innovation is from anything in the market, the higher its value-in-use. The larger the potential gross margin in the product, the better the innovation will tolerate mistakes along the way to commercialization. In early stage projects, perhaps the best that can be accomplished is to define the tolerance limits for a product cost and measure the probability of success against those limits.

Financial Analysis

The last element in the opportunity analysis is to merge the information learned over the course of the analysis into a full set of pro-forma financials depicting the way the business in the innovation can work. This analysis would include revenues from product sales, cost of sales estimates, estimates of other business expenses, and R&D. Finally, net present and terminal values for the innovation can be calculated, even though these figures may only represent best estimates.

SUMMARY

It is often the case that the Opportunity Analysis cannot or need not have been completed in its entirety to make an informed decision regarding the potential of an innovation. In practice, it is often used in "bits and pieces" to focus on a critical step in a project. One of the major challenges in fitting new crops into the context of the Opportunity Analysis is the lack of critical information about one or more components of the proposed product. The analysis may, therefore, best be used in those circumstances to focus research and development on getting the answers to critical questions in a timely fashion.

Perspective From a Small Industrial Company

James H. Brown
Jojoba Growers and Processors, Inc.

As we go forward in the pursuit of commercializing products derived from new agricultural crops, we draw heavily on our previous experiences and those of others who have achieved some measures of success, or those who have reported failures. From the perspective of a small business, there is only a small margin of error allowable as we conduct our analysis and decide whether or not we should invest time and other resources into a venture based upon a new agricultural crop. My comments are specific to our own set of circumstances, although the thought process would be similar for another group facing the same issues. As a point of reference, I will draw heavily on our experiences with other agricultural crops we have looked to as a source of raw materials for industrialization such as jojoba, and now lesquerella.

THE PROCESS

Decisions of whether or not to pursue commercialization of products from new crops are reached as a result of both formal and informal evaluations of all aspects of the chain of resources required to deliver a profitable commodity to a buyer. For ourselves, a small company, we see a greater likelihood of success if we concentrate on products from new, as opposed to established crops. In fact, we believe that if a product or crop is already far down the road toward commercialization, we probably do not have a good chance to be a significant factor in the eventual supply chain. As a small business, we must create early equity and build upon that equity with the resources that we have available.

Our process of evaluation must lead us to the conclusion that we can deliver a value-added product or service to a buyer. Our focal point is not the creation of technical solutions, but the application of new or existing technologies in the development of a profitable business center. The literature is filled with examples of technically elegant solutions without economic commercial application. Small businesses such as ours cannot make many payrolls with reprints of papers we might publish.

RESOURCES

Our first step in the review process is generally a careful and objective evaluation of the resources we possess that can be applied toward achieving a first level of commercialization of the new product. We ask ourselves if the equities we have created with jojoba and other products can be effectively applied to achieve commercialization of the new product. At this stage, we are mindful that supply issues are usually far from being solved, and we admittedly focus on whether or not we think we can sell the new product at a profit.

In our view, the most significant resource a successful new product venture can have is a buyer. While a purchase order does not make an industry, it's a very good place to start.

In the case of jojoba, the distribution system we have created over the past 15 years, is oriented to the cosmetic and personal care industry. This industry also uses significant quantities of castor oil, which contains hydroxy fatty acids similar to lesquerella oil. Our evaluation concluded that lesquerella oil has an opportunity to achieve a first level of commercial use within the cosmetic industry. While lesquerella will initially command higher prices than castor, there are niche applications within the cosmetic industry where high price is accepted in exchange for uniqueness or perceived benefits such as mildness. The marketing and distribution system in place for jojoba can be effectively utilized to gain trial and acceptance of lesquerella and other botanical ingredients within the cosmetic industry.

Next, we must evaluate our resources in terms of our ability to participate in the eventual chain of supply for the new crop product. While an early pioneering effort in the development of a new industry is important, it can as often mean that you simply make a better target for your competitors.

With jojoba, those early efforts most closely tied to the marketplace have proven to be the most successful. Other factors contributing to effective longevity in the jojoba chain of supply have been related to the early development of various technologies associated with the agronomics or processing of jojoba. In the case of lesquerella, there are number of factors in place that we believe will enhance its likelihood of becoming a long lived new industrial crop.

First, and most important, is the fact that for the past seven or eight years, lesquerella has had an ongoing, albeit small, program of USDA/ARS sponsored genetic and agronomic research. This research has resulted in significant advances in the domestication of this wild species. Jojoba, despite the fact that it has been the most successful new industrial crop to be commercialized since castor, has suffered from the lack of public research funding.

Second, small business organizations such as ours now have USDA supported Small Business Innovative Research (SBIR) grant funding available specifically to develop new and/or improved technologies related to increased production of industrial products from agricultural materials. In addition, there is a small research effort underway within the USDA/ARS to conduct lesquerella product development and utilization research. Through grants, liberalized technology transfer policies, efforts of the USDA Office of Agricultural Materials, the New Uses Council, etc., small businesses such as ours have an enhanced opportunity to initiate new ventures with new crops, and achieve the first levels of commercialization. We also create new jobs and hopefully generate income and taxes to repay the national investment made through the USDA.

In a more intuitive process, we examine other factors that might influence the critical mass of effort that might be applied to new crops such as jojoba or lesquerella. Can the new crop be a substitute for an imported crop? Can the new crop be exported? Can it be grown in an area where it is likely to be a substitute for a crop requiring a lot of water, and/or other cultural inputs that might be detrimental to the environment? Can it replace a crop that is highly subsidized? Are there co-products and/or by-product opportunities with the new crop? While all of these factors are important considerations, none is more important than whether or not we believe we can develop an initial market for the new crop product.

Perspective from a Large Industrial Company

Joseph S. Boggs
The Procter & Gamble Company

Procter & Gamble's (P&G) chemical division is responsible for the making of oleochemicals from natural fats and oils for applications in our own non-food products (soaps, detergents, shampoos, deodorants), and for sale to the merchant market. My specific responsibility is for the R&D efforts supporting our current business brands—alchohols, glycerine, fatty acids, amines, and future surfactant developments.

My link to the "new crop" world comes from P&G's participation and support in the commercialization of *Cuphea*. Our company's involvement with *Cuphea* began in the early 1980s when P&G, along with Henkel KGaA and the USDA/ARS, co-sponsored a germplasm collection trip to Brazil for Shirley Graham of Kent State University, Ohio. Since 1984, we have supported *Cuphea* through an industry association called the Soap & Detergent Association (SDA). My role began in the summer of 1985, as Chairman of the Technical Subcommittee for the SDA; in effect, to be the technical liaison to this program for the Association.

The basic premise of the *Cuphea* project stem from the fact that seed oils of *Cuphea* species are uniquely high in the production of shorter chain triglycerides—specifically, and most interestingly to us, the lauric or C-12 oils. Presently, the only major source of lauric oils (coconut and palm kernel oil) come from Southeast Asia—the Philippines, Malaysia, and Indonesia. Lauric oils have unique properties that are desirable and/or essential to several American industrial and food applications.

Periodically, there have been major swings in the availability of these oils, generally due to weather conditions such as drought and typhoons. This, in turn, has resulted in significant price spikes occurring about one year in five. A major objective to domesticate *Cuphea* was to secure a domestic source of lauric oils and to be guaranteed an adequate supply at an affordable price. It would be prudent today, however, to acknowledge that since the *Cuphea* development began, there has been major palm kernel oil development work going on in Malaysia and Indonesia. This development may possibly shift the issue of availability and price from the periodic crisis level to that of a more manageable concern area; only time will tell.

A second major objective in developing *Cuphea* was not only to reduce dependency on a source that had a history of volatility of supply availability, but also to provide a domestic source of this oil that could benefit our country in several ways. First, it could provide another crop for the farmer that is not just a food replacement crop, but rather: (a) adds to their arsenal of options; and (b) might be growable on more marginal land, thereby helping the plight of the American farmer. Second, this is annually a half-billion dollar business that could help the United States balance of trade, and third, the expectations for any new development are that good spin-off developments and applications can occur. Certainly, with the wide range of chainlength properties available from the many *Cuphea* species this possibility clearly exists.

In short, there has been and continues to be a real industry need for domestically produced lauric oils. *Cuphea* represents a reasonable technical lead to meet that need, and together this can be a helpful business opportunity for the American farmer and the American economy.

Needs—leads—and business opportunities are three elements that are like the three legs of a stool. If one is missing or even a little short, the stool will not stand up. Another visual picture is a triangle with these three elements at the points. If you draw circles around the points, you have a real chance for a success only where the three overlap.

If there is anything that all R&D projects can suffer from, it is having an interesting technology that either doesn't fill a clear need or doesn't represent a good business opportunity. I call it the idea of a technology looking for a home! Thus, we need to be certain that we are not just working on an interesting new crop that may not speak to a clear need in the marketplace, or a clear opportunity for the farmer, or by the same token may not work for industry. If industry represents the need, the scientific community represents the technology or lead, and the opportunity benefits the American farmer and our economy, together the three parts of the triangle must stay linked. For a new crop idea to succeed, all three legs of the stool must be connected, that is we must be working together. Even with all three points overlapping, any new crop venture is a long shot proposition. Without visible good linkage of all three elements, there is little chance of successful commercialization. Many failed projects upon close examination can be demonstrated to have been short on one of these legs.

Working together means more than just good communication and verbal expression of interest. I would encourage, as we did in *Cuphea*, that all three parties (in this case academia, the USDA/ARS and industry), put hard dollars into the effort, until the program has a life of its own. Where there is an established crop you have an industry association supporting ideas, but for a new crop, sponsoring money may be hard to come by. However, money talks and shows the real strength of the interest. Without it, industry particularly can support a lot of avenues and ideas for study, but may pay only lip service to the outcome.

Cuphea has been and is still just a technology lead toward achieving a domestic source of lauric or short chain oils. The program has passed the embryonic stage. It has a viable life, and there has been much good progress on the technology, but clearly success has not yet been achieved. *Cuphea* development would not have reached this stage without a good balance of support from the needs, leads, and business opportunity components. In new crop work, industry, academia, and the USDA need each other and need to work hand-in-hand on program priorities to be certain the elements for success are really there and in proper balance.

Perspective from an Independent Industrial Consulting Company

R. Martin O'Shea

Smithers Scientific Services, Inc.

Smithers Scientific Services, Inc. has special expertise in the rubber industry, and provides consultation to clients both in this country and abroad. We are involved in preparing feasibility studies, forecasts and programs requiring expertise in marketing, marketing research, business development, inventory management, financial management, strategic planning and purchasing. In the capacity as Director of Marketing Research, I recently completed extensive research into the rubber industry in Western and Eastern Europe and the USSR, and on the demand for natural rubber in the United States in the event of a national emergency. The current and future status of commercialization of guayule as a new domestic rubber crop was thoroughly evaluated.

Developing potential end use markets for industrial crops such as guayule is more complex than it is for ornamental or food crops. After initial processing, ornamentals and food crops are usually sold directly to the consumer. Therefore, the success or failure of these crops usually rest with the ultimate consumer who can be influenced by costs, promotional or advertising campaigns, food "fads," nutritional values, and a variety of other factors over which the agricultural industry has some control. As examples, consider the changes in demand that have occurred over the past few years with items such as: Columbian ("mountain grown") coffee, tofu, whole bran, broccoli, kiwifruit, well-marbled beef, and "no cholesterol" foods.

Unlike foodstuffs and ornamentals, however, most industrial crops are not sold to end users. The ultimate consumers may not even know what raw materials are in the goods they buy, and certainly are influenced more by factors that are not directly attributable to the agricultural commodities.

This is the case with natural rubber extracted from guayule, or from the rubber tree, *Hevea brasiliensis*. Smithers has researched consumer behavior in the tire industry, and recognized that most consumers are very unsophisticated when it comes to making value judgments and other purchasing decisions on the tires they buy. Consumers buy because of brand or trade name recognition, price and then "perceived values" such as "performance," "safety," or other intangibles or factors the consumer cannot measure. Thus, the problem facing the agricultural industry with a product such as guayule rubber is how to market or sell the manufacturers on the benefits or advantages of the material that cannot be translated into greater sales, or sales at a higher unit price, to the end consumer.

To be marketable to the tire producers, guayule rubber must meet one of the following two criteria:
1. It must perform the same function as hevea rubber at a lower cost.
2. It must enhance performance at the same cost, or at least at no cost disadvantage.

And, of course, the cost/benefit factors must be sufficient to be an incentive to the producers to spend what could easily be millions of dollars in development, and in compounding and converting from hevea to guayule rubber.

Even if guayule proves to be a "drop-in" substitute for hevea, the tire producers may offer significant resistance to change. Until someone takes the first step to prove the worthiness of guayule rubber, there is too much potential risk to warrant using guayule without some significant economic advantage.

Therefore, guayule is stuck on the horns of a dilemma with regards to the commercialization efforts. To prove itself to the tire producers, there must be sufficient rubber available of consistent properties to satisfy all research needs up through long range, full factory trials and use in actual field conditions. Additionally, this rubber must be reasonably competitively priced, or at least have good prospects of being available in quantity at an attractive price in the future. However, to be available in the quantities needed for full trials requires extensive capital expenditures to develop the agricultural aspects of the business and the industrial infrastructure. Commercial entities are unwilling to risk the capital needed to produce the rubber unless it has already been proven to be commercially and technically feasible.

Obviously, to move guayule rubber and its co-products off dead center requires some innovative thinking. Guayule will not sell itself. If it is to become a commercial reality, something or somebody must champion the product in an industry that still suffers from the "NIH Syndrome"—Not Invented Here.

The trials done to date indicate that guayule rubber is a viable alternative to hevea rubber from a technical standpoint. Therefore, what is needed is the incentive for the initial capitalization required for it to be a commercial success. We feel this can best be accomplished by the support of the Department of Defense as a critical need in times of national emergency. A relatively modest expenditure now, properly applied, could be returned many times over once guayule rubber becomes a commercial reality.

Perspective from Europe

Louis J.M. van Soest
Centre for Plant Breeding and Reproductive Research

Major industrial crop commercialization activities involving public and private sectors are being pursued within the European Communities (EC). The range and scope of these activities in Europe can be illustrated by describing those related to the development of new oilseed crops. Vegetable Oils for Innovation in Chemical Industries (VOICI) is a multidisciplinary R&D program within the framework of the European Collaborative Linkage of Agriculture and Industry through Research (ECLAIR) program of the Commission of the European Communities. The objective of the program is to develop and evaluate some potential economically feasible vegetable oil crops for the chemical industries. VOICI includes 12 participants from four countries of the EC. The research conducted within VOICI includes the total production chain divided into three R&D clusters.

In addition to VOICI, a National Vegetable Oil Program (NOP) was started in The Netherlands in 1990. Some nine institutes of the Ministry of Agriculture, Nature Management, and Fisheries participate in this program. The research is conducted on eight potential vegetable oilseed crops. Several Dutch oil processing industries are involved in the advisory commission of the National Vegetable Oil Program.

VEGETABLE OILSEED CROPS INCLUDED IN VOICI

The vegetable oilseed crops concerned and their principal components are: Crambe (*Crambe abyssinica*, Brassicaceae)—erucic acid; Dimorphotheca (*Dimorphotheca pluvialis*, Asteraceae)—dimorphecolic acid; and Meadowfoam (*Limnanthes alba*, Limnanthaceae)—long chain fatty acids.

Information on yield and seed characteristics summarized in Table 1 were obtained from selected accessions grown in The Netherlands from 1988 to 1990 in trials and small scale cultivations. Compared to existing oilseed crops like rape seed and sunflower, the oil yield per hectare is rather low. Further crop development of these crops should be directed toward oil yield increases.

R&D CONDUCTED WITHIN THE THREE CLUSTERS

The VOICI program is funded 50% by the EC, and 50% by 12 partners. The participants included in the three clusters are both governmental organizations and private enterprises. The research conducted within VOICI includes the total production chain divided into the following three clusters.

Table 1. Yields and seed characteristics of three novel oilseed crops.

Crop	Yield (t/ha)	Oil (%)	Principal fatty acid	Principal fatty acid (%)
Crambe	2.0–3.0	28–36[z]	Erucic	56–62
Dimorphotheca	1.2–1.7	15–22	Dimorphecolic	55–64
Limnanthes	0.2–1.0	19–27	C20:1d5	60–62
			C22:1d13	13–26
			C22:2 d5,13	12–23

[z]Seeds plus hull.

Primary Production
- Exploitation of germplasm; introduction and collecting, preliminary evaluation, and conservation of germplasm (Government funding).
- Optimization of the growing and harvest techniques of selected industrial oilseed crops (Mix of government and private funding).
- Determination of production characteristics and potentials (Government funding).
- Breeding research for genetic adaptation and improvement of yield, quality, and yield security of the selected industrial oilseed crops (Government funding).
- Practical breeding to develop varieties of crambe and dimorphotheca (Private funding).
- Small and large scale seed production for practical crop investigation and production of seed for oil milling (Private funding).

Agro-technology
- Assessment of the relationship between storage and processing of oilseeds and oil quality, including analyses (Government funding).
- Development and evaluation of process equipment for supercritical CO_2 extraction (SCE) for selected oilseed crops (Private funding).
- Small scale oil production on basis batch processes (Mix of private and government funding).
- Industrial scale processing and refining of larger quantities of oils of selected crops (Private funding).

Industrial Processing and Application
- Evaluation of oils for oleochemicals (Private funding).
    - Splitting, distillation, and analysis of long chain and hydroxy fatty acids.
    - Derivation of amides and dimers of long chain fatty acids.
    - Devivalisation (hardening, waxy ester production) of hydroxy fatty acids.
    - Evaluation of oleochemicals for a range of intermediate products.
- Analysis and evaluation of selected oilseed crops for resin and lacquer formulations and testing of coatings based thereon (Private funding).
- Developing, testing, and performance rating of lubricants and additives based on vegetable oils (Private funding).
- Refining and development of chemical derivatives from meadowfoam (*Limnanthes*) oil, and cosmetic evaluation of the refined oil and derivatives (Private funding).

OVERCOMING CONSTRAINTS IN RELATION TO COMMERCIALIZATION

Programs to overcome major constraints for the ultimate commercialization of these crops can be summarized as follows:

- Broadening gene pools of the crops for further genetic improvement. Some limiting traits are asynchronous ripening and poor seed retention resulting in low yield in dimorphotheca and meadowfoam.
- Increase of disease resistance against fungal diseases and beet cyst nematodes in crambe.
- Increasing low oil content in dimorphotheca and meadowfoam.
- Optimal methods for refining oils, especially in dimorphotheca.
- Optimization of growing and harvesting methods for all crops.
- Utilization of meal, e.g. high levels of glucosinolates in crambe and meadowfoam, and low protein levels.
- Research of the industrial partners should reveal the potential utilization of the oils and their specific fatty acids. Particularly, the potential use of the hydroxy fatty acids of dimorphotheca, and the unique long chain fatty acids of meadowfoam need further application research by the industrial partners.

CONCLUSION

Research conducted in two large multidisciplinary vegetable oil programs have been the first steps to develop potential oil crops. Within the framework of VOICI industries, agricultural cooperatives, and research institutions of four EC countries are conducting research to evaluate the possibilities of three novel oil plants. The national program in The Netherlands includes nine governmental institutes, and conducts research on eight potential oilseed crops. Both programs are complementary and coordinated by the Centre for Plant Breeding and Reproduction Research (CPRO-DLO). There are intensive contacts with industries, a prerequisite for the final commercialization of the oils. The expected outcome of the programs is manifold and spreads over the entire production chain.

Open Discussion

Moderator: Duane L. Johnson
Colorado State University

Daniel Kugler, *USDA/CSRS Office of Agricultural Materials*

Dr. van Soest, you have projects in The Netherlands that alone are funded at levels that are higher than the total appropriation made to the new AARC—Alternative Agriculture Research and Commercialization Subtitle of our new Farm Bill. Would you comment on the general level of support for the commercialization in the European Community?

Louis van Soest, *Panelist*

It is very difficult to say exactly how much it is. The EC has several programs. One program, ECLAIR, concentrates on the linkage between agriculture and industry. Furthermore, there is the Bridge Program, and there are two or three programs on biotechnology where some industrial crop development is involved. Currently, the EC is about to start an Agro–Industry Program, which is mainly meant for diversification—not only crops, but also for animals. This program will be funded over the next four years (1992–1996) at a rate equivalent to about U.S. $300 million. Thus, about $400 million in total is directed to development of crop diversification for the next four years.

W.M.J. van Gelder, *Wageningen, The Netherlands*

Additional EC funds related to R&D on industrial utilization of agricultural crops would total to about $400 million, which is quite a large total. Many research programs are ongoing within the EC. In The Netherlands, we have programs on industrial utilization of carbohydrates, application of and utilization of fiber materials, protein crops preferably in the non-food, non-feed area, and oilseeds. Some of these programs are cooperative, involving the research institutes and universities to develop entirely new technologies and products. The research institutes and universities have been requested to be sure that industry expresses support for these projects. It is important that the developments being created will be used directly by industry.

The present situation in Europe in regard to agricultural raw materials from an industrial perspective is rather negative. Many agricultural raw materials are not properly characterized. We hardly know the structure, composition, and industry specifications for many materials. Our first step is to adequately characterize our raw materials, and working closely with industry, determine how these materials can be used. We believe this is primarily the task of the government, because most industries are not directly interested in the use of raw materials from agriculture as their current raw material supplies are satisfactory. We have to convince industry that there is a real opportunity from a price-performance point of view. When you reach that stage, you will then have close cooperation with industry. However, I see some differences in our situation compared to that in the United States in regard to the sharing of financial rewards from such cooperation. Our programs are primarily directed to finding an outlet for the excess agricultural raw materials. We therefore think that it is not strictly necessary that the government receives profits from the patents, even when they have been jointly developed. The surplus situation with respect to agricultural products is not a problem for industry. It is the problem of the agricultural sector.

Daniel Kugler, *USDA/CSRS Office of Agricultural Materials*

There are representatives on the Panel that have international operations. Does the level of support in Europe surprises you? Is the United States behind what is happening in Europe, and what do we do if that is the case?

Keith Walker, *Panelist*

I am not surprised at the level of support. From a very parochial perspective, I do not believe that Agrigenetics/Lubrizol corporation would see it as a race where somebody is ahead or behind. We look at our business on a world-wide basis. Some of the products we may develop from new crops we may only market in Europe. Lubrizol receives more than 50% of its current revenue dollars from offshore. So, we look at the whole world as a market. We believe that the United States Federal government has a unique responsibility relative to the interests of the American public, and it ought to represent those interests. We have a unique responsibility relative to our shareholders, and our global business interests.

James Brown, *Panelist*

My reaction would be to look at this situation in terms of the jojoba industry. I believe that jojoba is the most successful industrial crop commercialized since castor. Since the mid 1970s, there has only been less than $2 to 3 million total in public funds directed toward jojoba research. To me this only says that there is considerable potential in the further development of the industry given appropriate levels of R&D.

Robert Kleiman, *USDA/ARS*

One aspect we have not addressed is discovery. Everyone is using germplasm that was discovered in the 1960s. Of the some 300,000 species of plants we have only looked at 10 to 15,000. There are many new kinds of materials that may be useful for industry, American agriculture or for world agriculture. We are not taking full opportunity of this area. As for our role at the National Center for Agricultural Utilization Research (NCAUR) in Peoria, we have made some of these initial discoveries. We are now trying to utilize some of these materials that we have discovered, and are serving as a catalyst, pushing and cajoling others to recognize that there are some new materials out there that should be used. We try to give concrete examples of how these plant-based compounds may be used. I do agree with Dr. van Gelder that these materials must be characterized before industry will become interested.

Martin O'Shea, *Panelist*

One of the factors that has impeded R&D in some of the industrial crops has been the lack of germplasm. This directly affects the development and propagation of the crop itself, and the production of enough material to do the needed research for full commercialization. That is one of the roles in which the USDA is very effective.

Duane Johnson, *Moderator*

We need to remember that just because we look at one sample, and do not find what we want within a species, this does not imply a lack of variation. In general, large variation in specific chemical constituents within a species is to be expected.

Joseph Boggs, *Panelist*

I wish to follow up on some of the comments made by Robert Kleiman. In regard to the "needs, leads, and business opportunity factors" of which I previously spoke, I should emphasize that before you get ready to converge these concepts, there is a stage of work in the "leads area," that I call the "diverging stage." Exploring and looking for germplasm is the idea generation stage, and does not require combining the three components. We need that type of research first. However, the researcher needs to have an eye on what makes sense for a future, potential industry. Focus should not just be on what is solely of academic interest to the researcher.

Anson Thompson, *Panelist*

I would like to follow up on Joseph Boggs comments. The cuphea story is instructive. If the interest of industry had not been forthcoming, as expressed by the administrators of Procter & Gamble who came to the USDA and sold us on the need for more research leading to commercialization, we would not likely have started the research on our own. They clearly indicated their interest by offering to equally match USDA funds with those of their own. Actually it ended up with a unique, three-way funding involving USDA/ARS, the Soap & Detergent Association, and Oregon State University. There is always much competition for the limited amount of funds we do have. It is very difficult for us to work on certain things unless we have a real push or the expressed interest of industry. In this case, industry got our attention. We all thought cuphea had high potential, but the seed shattering aspect would be a terrible problem to overcome. It seems to have been a rather long haul since the cooperative program was started in 1983. Now it looks like there has been a major breakthrough in the development of nonshattering germplasm. Things are coming around, and it should not be difficult to sustain the necessary funding for continued research and successful commercialization. From my experience in this type of work, having someone from industry showing a strong, specific interest in ones research certainly facilitates gaining administrative and financial support.

Kenneth Carlson, *USDA/ARS*

I would like to ask the four industry oriented panelists, who have all worked a number of years in this area, whether you feel more or less encouraged in regard to the utilization of new or alternative crops after having participated in this Symposium.

Keith Walker, *Panelist*

From my own perspective, I am neither more or less encouraged. Our company has a strategy, it has an approach, and this meeting has been consistent and supports our own internal plan, direction, and views as to where we want to go and what we want to accomplish. So in that context, I am not any less encouraged than I was three days ago. In addition, I have come in contact with others here and have picked up some other new ideas. This has been a valuable conference for me. I have met several people that I want to talk to about some new opportunities. That is most important for me. My job is to put together different ideas and come up with a new approach or angle.

James Brown, *Panelist*

Overall, it has been very encouraging. We have had a good number of very positive discussions with both private individuals and companies, and persons from academic institutions from around the country and the world about the new interest we have in lesquerella and vernonia. We have discussed possible ways to cooperate and move commercialization forward. It has been discouraging from the standpoint of the jojoba industry. We have been trying for years to get public funding for additional research, but it has fallen on deaf ears. We do not intend to stop in our efforts, and hope that jojoba will remain an industry for this country. Unfortunately, we think it is probably headed South, the same way as castor, citrus, and other crops have done. I can see us holding a meeting 30 years from now trying to bring jojoba back to this country. So I guess I have had both encouragement and discouragement from this meeting.

Joseph Boggs, *Panelist*

In general, I am encouraged by the large attendance of people interested in and working on new crops. I think we sometimes get a little discouraged when we think of our national budget, and the percentage that goes to agriculture and of that which then goes to new crops research. You get to a very, very small number. If you compare that with the funding of other countries, and see the different proportions allocated, you wonder why new crops research continues to be underfunded. It is almost impossible to compete with all the other programs that get sponsored in the United States. However, I am almost an eternal optimist when I look at a group like this, and see for example just the progress that has been made on lesquerella, where pilot plant hectarage have been planted and things are beginning to happen. There is nothing like success to stimulate more funding for other new opportunities.

Martin O'Shea, *Panelist*

I am encouraged by this Symposium for several reasons. One is the breadth and depth of knowledge that has been brought to this conference. I think that the academic and scientific research that has been conducted and presented here is most impressive. Unfortunately, the industry that I represent had combined losses worldwide of about $2 billion in 1990, so they are starting to rival the United States national budget. That makes it difficult to take this kind of development and carry it forward on an industrial scale. However, eventually, the supply and demand situation on natural rubber will get to a point where it will no longer be a buyers market, even as oligopolistic as it is. Eventually, guayule will have a place as an industrial crop that will be very badly needed by all the world's industrialized economies. One of the things that is discouraging with new crops development is the tendency of governments to fund R&D on an annual cycle. A perennial crop like guayule takes a minimum of 18–24 months to mature. When you start funding annually, you just get going with the program when the funding gets cut off. If this happens, you can sit with the program dormant for a couple of years, before you can start all over again. This is not a very good way to fund a development program. I would certainly encourage legislative bodies responsible for these programs to be more far reaching in their thinking, and fund these on 4, 5, or 6 year cycles. This would help bring a program to fruition with the life cycle of the plant.

Keith Walker, *Panelist*

Many of you may be familiar with W. Edwards Deming, the management guru that helped make Japan what it is today. Many United States corporations are being "Demingized." One of Deming's major points is that of "constancy of purpose." Those in the government sector need to see to it that your administrators develop that kind of constancy and consistency in purpose. In my opinion, there is a more consistent, purposeful movement in Europe as compared to the United States. Perhaps they move later than we do in some cases, and perhaps the environment is not as entrepreneurial or as innovative. However, when you see both European companies and governments moving with a kind of constancy of purpose, which allows them to carry through on projects without deleterious interruptions, you have to be impressed.

This may be the time for all of us to examine whether a commercial development kind of function deserves to be developed and funded. This might be especially relevant with the USDA. The USDA puts out a voluminous amount of information. They make things available in terms of opportunities. That is wonderful, but it requires industry to locate the information and approach the USDA with a deal. If for some reason you happen to miss the newspaper that morning, you won't see it. There is a need for scientists and technologists who do these enormously innovative things, to have a group who can run their own opportunity analyses. They could then latch on to the most promising ones and sell them to industry. What happens now is that researchers, who should be in the laboratory, are forced to be in commercial development. I met an Agricultural Economist at a meeting this summer who was trying to sell a new development project and complained he did not know what he was. I replied he was a commercial developer, not an Agricultural Economist! It would be interesting if we could get university and public sector administrators to think about the possibilities of being a little more proactive.

James Brown, *Panelist*

I do not think that USDA does a very good job in communicating the real capabilities they do have, at least down to our levels. As we have become more and more involved in discussions on these new crops, we find a great number of opportunities to do mutual, cooperative work. We also have the opportunity to offer suggestions and comments to programs, especially at the initial stages of development. We could often save some time and energy if we have an early opportunity to comment. On the other hand, we can possibly move things along a lot faster if we know more about some of the resources available to us. Much of our previous lack of knowledge may have been our own fault. We are finding more and more opportunities that are out there, such as the CRADAs and the new Small Business Innovative Research (SBIR) grants in the area of industrial applications involving agricultural materials. It is especially helpful that these opportunities are specifically directed to organizations such as ours. As we become more involved, we feel that there are probably others who are equally uninformed. More could be done to communicate those types of opportunities to companies such as ourselves.

Louis van Soest, *Panelist*

In The Netherlands, we have a number of these national programs that are specifically focused on potential or new crops. Our Ministry of Agriculture, Nature Management, and Fisheries is now considering whether some of these programs, which will go up to 1994 or 1995, should be continued or terminated. The possibilities of future commercialization within 4 to 10 years is one of the major criteria.

James Hall, *Panelist*

I believe that in respect to development we are "preaching to the choir." If you want something to happen, you have to talk to the Congress and the upper administrative levels of the Department, because that is where decisions are made on the levels of funding. You cannot formulate and maintain a commercial development group like you are talking about within USDA on $50,000 a year. Keith Walker related that Lubrizol had about 230 staff in commercial development. What are their sales?

Keith Walker, *Panelist*

This is the number of staff in just one division, with sales of about $500 million.

James Hall, *Panelist*

In contrast, that is roughly about the same or actually a little less than the USDA/ARS total annual budget; about $600 million.

Keith Walker, *Panelist*

Our research budget at Lubrizol is about $100 million, so to be comparable, USDA/ARS should have over 1,000 commercial development people!!

Francis Nakayama, *USDA/ARS*

I think that one of the things that industry is missing is the failure to ask the right questions. We have a tremendous computer data base that covers both Federal and State agencies. For example, Robert Perdue requested information on vernonia harvesting. The key word he searched was vacuum. Lo and behold, the computer spewed out all the methods of harvesting different crops using a vacuum system. He is now using this to harvest his vernonia seed. There is a database available, and one simply needs to search the system. If you do not get the answer you need, you keep asking. Then you need to contact the right people. If you searched for the word cuphea, I am sure most of the names of those that have worked with cuphea would be listed along with their research and location. As an ARS scientist, we are obligated to spread our information, and we are requested to participate in technological transfer to private industry and to the consumer.

Robert Kleiman, *USDA/ARS*

We haven't had our heads in the sand completely over the years. Whenever we have found anything and when our research is completed, we have published in appropriate journals, attended and reported on our findings at appropriate meetings. If we have something in the oleochemical area we go to the oil chemist's meetings; if we have something in rubber, we go to the rubber technology people and give a talk. We are not hiding this technology. The only other thing I can think of is to take out an ad in the *Wall Street Journal*! Maybe that is what we should be doing. We have tried to promote or at least tell the industry and public that we are working in a variety of areas.

Martin O'Shea, *Panelist*

You will probably meet more resistance from industry, particularly highly competitive industries like the one I am involved in, when you start asking them questions, than you will when they start asking you questions. The tire industry can be surprisingly uncooperative when it comes to trying to find out what their current thoughts are concerning research and development projects. That is not information passed about very freely among the industry. So it is not entirely the fault or shortcoming of the USDA and various other governmental agencies when they try to promote these new things. In very many cases, industry is going to be less than cooperative talking about their thrust and specific nature of their research to you.

Anson Thompson, *Panelist*

I would like to elaborate on the comments of Francis Nakayama and Robert Kleiman. USDA researchers must prepare interpretive summaries every time we publish a paper in layman's language on what we have done, its purpose, what the outcome might be, and what the potential is for our findings. These things are available through James Hall's office in Beltsville through the TEKTRAN system.

James Hall, *Panelist*

This is available electronically to anyone that has a personal computer, a modem, and a telephone line.

Lewrene Glaser, *USDA/ERS*

We have been talking mainly about Federal programs. I would like to hear comments about different approaches in regard to State programs, whether offered by universities or various State agencies and organizations that have been developed to look at this problem.

Raymond Burns, *Panelist*

The New Uses Council has met with and brought together State agencies and Land Grant Universities in six states to date. I believe that if this had been done five years ago, only about a dozen ongoing industrial material projects would have been involved. In our recent meetings during the last few months, we have discovered scientists and projects numbering about 150. I believe that this type of developmental research is more popular and acceptable today, and scientists are not shunned for saying they are working on something other than food and fiber. There has always been scientists that have worked in areas that have led to industrial applications. However, to fully capitalize on this new opportunity, we need a lot of reapplication of talents, efforts, materials, and financial resources. Based on our small sample, I would surmise that essentially all of the States have ongoing programs of some magnitude. I believe it is coming into focus with greater clarity that industrial products from agricultural materials represent a real opportunity and challenge. One of our goals is to help gain support in State legislatures for companion programs to the Federal programs.

James Simon, *Purdue University*

Indiana has about 13 of 26 million total acres in crops, with about 10 million acres in maize or soybeans. The agricultural industry in the state represents a major economic force, but the risks involved in the economic dependency on a few major crops has lead the state as well as Purdue University to consider exploring the potential opportunity for new or additional crops and plant-based products.

In Indiana, we are fortunate to have a State Agency, the Indiana Business Modernization and Technology Corporation (BMT) that provided the initial funding and remains the major supporter of our New Crops Center at Purdue University. The BMT, formerly known as the Indiana Corporation for Science and Technology (CST), also co-sponsored and provided financial support to this Symposium as well as our first Symposium on New Crops held in 1988. We are pleased that this State Agency has the vision to recognize the economic potential for Indiana businesses in new crops and plant products. State funding is very closely linked with the commercialization of new crops and products. BMT is not interested in supporting research per se, but only in supporting research on specific projects that have already shown preliminary promise, and which can receive matching funds from private industry.

We also have a second State Agency, the Center for Value-Added Products, that funds and supports work on plant and animal based products and is focused to a larger extent on the commercialization of new products and processes for the food industry. Both of these funding opportunities are focused on the commercialization and the demonstration of potential economic gain to the state and could be classified more as economic development projects than merely "agricultural projects."

Both State Agencies have been very supportive to Agriculture. However, we have to convince them that determine whether support for specific projects should be committed for longer than a single year or single growing season, making R&D plans more efficient and realistic. We need, in particular, to take our case to them and educate them and others at the State House on the many new crop activities and the economic benefits of diversifying our agricultural base. We have found that most legislators and State personnel, who had previously been very much unaware of these activities and their potential for economic development, have become quite interested and supportive of such programs.

Lastly, support from the State has enabled us to generate additional funds from private industry, which allows us to leverage modest funds to accomplish larger objectives. State support should not be overlooked, but as we have found in Indiana, may take several years to develop.

Raymond Burns, *Panelist*

I would add that when we deal with State legislators and annual budgets, they demand instant success. They have a very short term and want something immediately to take home to their constituents. There are many competing interests within the districts they represent, and they are limited in what they can do. This is only amplified in the national Congress, and this problem will not disappear. We need a bigger, broader, more knowledgeable constituency. When working with a national commodity group, we frequently get pressures if we are working to bring on an industrial material that may bring competing byproducts into the marketplace. The staff of the commodity group is hired to make their commodity go, and represents parochial interests. Almost all farmers grow more than one commodity, and they could care less which commodity group is successful if on the whole they are successful. We have to continue to bridge these gaps.

Lyndon Drewlow, *Mikkelsens, Inc., Ashtabula, Ohio*

One of the plant explorations, a USDA/ARS–Longwood Gardens sponsored expedition in the late 1960s, collected 21 accessions of New Guinea Impatiens as a secondary product. These were turned over to private breeders in 1971. USDA/ARS, Longwood, and some university scientists worked on it initially to develop new germplasm and cultivars. In 1991 there was over 100 million cuttings sold worldwide. There are breeding programs in Israel, Germany, the United States, and probably The Netherlands. They have also been introduced into Australia, New Zealand, and Japan, all based on these 21 new accessions. I would estimate the current value of this new crop to be from $50 to 100 million, and this has all happened within the past 20 years with a crop that was not even in our marketplace. So, in the ornamental area, results can be very rapid and economically significant.

W.M.J. van Gelder, *Wageningen, The Netherlands*

There is a different attitude toward new crops in America and in Europe. In Europe, we need development very rapidly. We have big problems in regard to excess production. We all know there are international trade negotiations, and things have not gone too well so far. With respect to the price policy, the EC does not choose to let its farmers suffer from a too drastically decreasing income; especially not where it concerns small family farms. Therefore, the EC is urgently working to create new market outlets for agricultural products especially in the area of non-food/non-feed products, and providing a good funding base.

Summary and Conclusions

Joseph C. Roetheli
USDA/CSRS Office of Agricultural Materials

The panelists did an exceptional job of providing insights into the process of commercializing research advances that use agricultural materials in industrial products. Much could be gained from more sessions such as this, plus small informal sessions where a few private sector representatives meet with a group of researchers on a specific topic. Representatives of the private sector have a lot to offer to researchers in terms of how the private sector thinks and operates as well as knowing the needs in the marketplace.

The session's overriding theme was the need for an improved mechanism to bridge the gap between research advances developed by the public sector and those elements of the private sector that are willing to risk investment in a new product, process, or crop.

Opportunities exist to produce industrial products from agricultural materials. Commercial success would employ excess agricultural resources and spur rural economic development. New crops are one component in the equation. The panelists discussed techniques to capitalize on a crops potential and hence increase the return on investment to taxpayers for publicly funded research.

Research, development, and commercialization are required to transform potential for industrial products from agricultural materials into marketplace reality. The need for new crops for industrial feedstocks will be derived from demand in the marketplace for the final product. Several panelists spoke of need to focus on a market demand driven approach as opposed to a technology driven approach. This requires a change in attitude of how research priorities are developed. James Brown stressed the need for private firms, especially small ones, to identify a market first before working to perfect a technology or product. After specifically identifying and evaluating the market need, research then can be accurately and effectively targeted.

A necessary condition or prerequisite for a commercial success is for the product to be technically sound. However, sound research or technology is far from being sufficient for a product to be successful in the marketplace. James Hall thoroughly discussed the use of Cooperative Research and Development Agreements (CRADAs) for facilitating transfer of new technology developed in Federal laboratories to an appropriate private entity. He also discussed how CRADAs can be used to facilitate fruitful cooperative R&D efforts between Federal scientists and those in industry, which should improve the probability of successful commercialization of a product or process. Successful progress in moving a new product or crop toward the marketplace requires matching of an interested private firm to work with the appropriate cadre of multidisciplinary researchers. Identifying and obtaining the interest of the "right" private firm is a key element that is often overlooked in the process.

Keith Walker related the need to perform structured analysis to clearly identify potential and hindrances. This analysis is necessary to screen for opportunities with sufficient potential to recover the research and development costs as well as to generate an acceptable return. This assessment should cover the entire system of production through marketing needs for converting an industrial material into a viable industrial product.

Martin O'Shea noted that the private sector should identify the most promising market opportunities. He also shared views on how interactions occur when an oligopolistic situation exists. He noted the need for cooperation between the private and public sectors to reduce risk over the period of time required to commercialize a new product or process.

Commercializing a new product from a research idea typically requires a bare minimum of five years. James Hall accurately pointed out that the cost of development and demonstration are typically nearly 120 times the cost of the research itself.

Researchers need to be continually asking themselves and representatives of the private sector questions such as: What will the world of industrial products look like in one or two decades? Who will be interested in buying and who will be interested in manufacturing the product? What are the chances of commercial success? Is there a "demand pull" or is a product the result of "technology push?"

Joseph Boggs delineated elements needed to successfully commercialize a product from a new crop such as cuphea by analogy to a three legged stool. The three legs of this "stool" are: Need—identification of the market need; Lead—time needed to commercialize a product; and Opportunity—profitable business potential.

One way to think about finding the "right" combination of firm and researchers is to have a knowledgeable generalist to cultivate relationships with researchers and firms to seek workable matches. I serve in such a role at CSRS's Office of Agricultural Materials in the USDA. I perceive myself as a mutual fund manager for a portfolio of industrial products to be made from agricultural materials for which interest can be generated in private firms. Resources include research conducted in the public sector. The goal is to maximize return to the investors.

One of the most important components of matching the researchers with firms is face-to-face discussions especially with high level representatives of private firms. Building private-public partnerships is a "contact sport," requiring body contact, and is key to moving new products into the marketplace. Such contacts by several individuals have resulted in two private firms working with USDA on lesquerella development and a number with the crambe/industrial rapeseed effort.

Raymond Burns of the New Uses Council noted that use of agricultural materials for industrial feedstocks can fill market niches and use excess capacity that exists in agriculture. Diversifying into use of agricultural materials for industrial products opens new markets for farmers. New food products generally substitute for existing foods, and while perhaps improving diets, they do little to expand market opportunities for excess agricultural resources. The New Uses Council promotes use of industrial products from agricultural materials, and sees a weak link between public research and commercial production that needs to be strengthened. The Alternative Agricultural Research & Commercialization (AARC) Center may soon become an effective bridge in this regard.

In the past, a major gap has existed in funding and effort to move research advances to a point that commercial firms are willing to risk investment in production of new products. Our system, in effect, has been similar to a researcher taking a technical publication to one side of a gorge and throwing it into the air in hopes that the wind will carry it intact across the raging river to a private firm, and that someone in the private sector will then read it and act. AARC provides the framework for a bridge between the two sides of the gorge thereby allowing much more rapid and effective linkage between public research and commercial production by the private sector. The latter represents the foundation of our economic system. AARC authorizes private-public partnerships and encourages an integrated systems approach that is best accomplished by use of multidisciplinary teams.

In the United States, more private-public partnerships are needed on applied or adaptive work, including industrial uses of agricultural materials from new crops. The AARC targets this area. This assumes that the very basic research has already been conducted, a historical strength of the United States.

Congress appropriated $4.5 million for AARC in fiscal year 1992 for adaptive and applied work. Meanwhile, as noted by Louis van Soest, The Netherlands, a very small country relative to the United States, is investing significant funds in an effort to commercialize industrial crops. In addition to the funds Louis van Soest cited for industrial oilseed development, over $2 million per year of its own funds plus a similar amount from the European Community (EC) are being invested in work to commercialize one fiber crop, hemp. With increased emphasis on global markets and with the major gap that exists in funding between research advances and commercial production in the United States, the $4.5 million represents but a small start in what is required.

Research findings take on their real value when products are rapidly and successfully commercialized. Commercialization is required for the American taxpayer to receive a respectable return from the "mutual fund" composed of industrial products from agricultural materials.

Index to Species, Crops, and Crop Products

Abaca, 435
Abelia chinensis, 141
Abelmoschus
    esculentus, 18, 19, 416
    manihot, 19
Abyssinian mustard, 302
Acacia, 17
Acanthaceae, 170
Acanthoscelides, 17
Accha hausca, 171
Acer
    griseum, 145
    japonicum, 143
    maximowiczianum, 144
    palmatum, 143
Acha, 64
Achillea millefolium, 88, 101, 622
Actinidia
    chinensis, 58, 83, 146
    deliciosa, 51, 57–58, 83
Adzuki bean, 19
Aeollanthus gamwelliae, 621
Aeschynanthus, 70
African grasses, 294–298
African horned cucumber, 61, 553–559
African horned melon, 61
African oil palm, 64, 314, 466
African rice, 14
Agaricus, 86
Agavaceae, 441
Agave, 435, 436
    fourcroydes, 435, 441
    mapisaga, 441
    salmiana, 441
    sisalana, 435, 441
    tequilana, 441
Agropyron, 285
    cristatum, 149, 150
    desertorum, 149, 150
    fragile, 149
Aibika, 19
Ailanthus altissima, 140
Ajowan oil, 623
Albizia julibrissin, 146
Alfalfa, 97, 418
Algae, 19
Allegheny chinkapin, 500
Allium, 86, 169
    ampeloprasum, 86

    cepa, 86
Aloysia triphylla, 54
Amaranth, 7, 13, 14, 18, 19, 35, 72, 78, 93, 97, 102–105, 117, 211–218, 219–221, 562–564
Amaranthus, 19, 34, 71, 74, 211–218, 219–221, 562–564
    albus, 414
    caudatus, 211
    cruentus, 93, 211, 219, 221, 562
    dubius, 562
    hybridus, 211, 219, 562
    hyprochondriacus, 93, 211, 215, 219, 562
    palmeri, 211
    tricolor, 562
Amarun uchu, 170
Amaryllis, 87, 88
Amaryllis, 88
Amelanchier alnifolia, 516–519
American chinkapin, 500
American ginseng, 54, 86, 670
American pear, 83
American pennyroyal oil, 621
Amiruca panga, 171
Ammoniac gum oil, 623
Anacardiaceae, 496
Anagallis monelli, 609
    'Pacific Blue' 609
Ananas comosus, 465
Ancistrocladus abbreviatus, 164
Andia paju (caspi), 171
Andropogon
    gayanus, 16, 295
    gerardii, 152, 285
Anethum
    graveolens, 623
    sowa, 623
Angelica archangelica, 623
Angelica root oil, 623
Angled luffa, 84, 86
Anigozanthos, 70
Anise-leaved magnolia, 144
Anise oil, 623. See also Fennel
Annona
    cherimola, 56, 60, 83, 169, 451, 456, 505, 507
    diversifolia, 505
    glabra, 453, 506
    muricata, 505, 507

    palustris, 506
    purpurea, 505
    reticulata, 453, 505
    squamosa, 83, 451, 453, 456, 505, 506
Annonaceae, 452, 505
Anthemis nobilis, 622
Anthurium, 88
Anthurium, 88
Anu, 536
Apiaceae, 576, 620, 622, 623
Apios, 85, 86, 533
Apios americana, 86, 533
Apium graveolens, 623
Apocynaceae, 170
Apple, 51, 58–59, 109, 144, 156
Apple cactus, 486–491
Apricot, 83, 84, 156–158
Aquifoliaceae, 170
Aquilegia, 101
Arabidopsis thaliana, 188, 189
Araceae, 170
Arachis, 13, 14, 20
    hypogaea, 86, 257
    pintoi, 16, 470
Arctium lappa, 54
Arctostaphylos uva-ursi, 609
    'Vancover Jade', 609
Arecacea, 170
Aristida pungens, 64
Armangui, 171
Armoise oil, 622
Arnica montana, 54
Aroids, 13, 19, 533, 534
Aromatic plants, 620–627. See also entries under specific aromatic plants.
Arracacha, 20
Arracacia xanthorrhiza, 20
Artemisia
    absinthium, 101, 622
    afra, 622
    annua, 70, 622, 640–643
    dracunculus, 55, 622
    herba-alba, 622
    martima, 622
    pallens, 622
    stelleriana, 609
        'Silver Brocade', 609
    vestita, 622

Artichoke, 68
Artocarpus, 472
 altilis, 465
 heterophyllus, 456
Arugula, 528
Asafoetida, 616, 623
Asclepias
 speciosa, 428, 429, 430
 syriaca, 428, 430
Asian pear, 83, 84
Asimina
 parviflora, 505
 triloba, 83, 505–515, 644–648
Asparagus, 53, 84, 86
Asparagus bean, 84, 86
Asparagus officinalis, 86
Asplenium, 170
Assam Aur Aur, 472–474
Asteraceae, 170, 355, 389, 620, 622, 640, 649, 684
Astragalus, 48–49, 50
Astragalus adsurgens, 48–49, 50
Atemoya, 82, 83, 451–454, 455, 456, 457, 505
Auricularia polytricha, 55
Avena sativa, 310
Averrhoa carambola, 74, 75, 83, 448, 456
 'Arkin', 83, 448, 450
 'B-2', 448
 'B-10', 448
 'B-16', 448
 'B-17', 448
 'Dah Pon', 448, 450
 'Demak', 448
 'Fwang Tung', 448
 'Gold Star', 448, 450
 'Hew-1', 448
 'Kary', 448
 'Maha', 448
 'Mih Tao', 448
 'Newcomb', 448
 'Sri Kembangan', 448
 'Star King', 448
 'Tean Ma', 448
 'Thayer', 448
Avocado, 455, 456, 457
Ayacara, 171
Azalea, 141, 144
Azolla, 19
Azuki bean, 45–47, 49–50, 124, 588–594

Babaco, 60

Baby lima bean, 585, 586, 587
Bactris gasipaes, 169, 172, 465–472
Bahiagrass, 152
Balsamite, 622
Bambarra groundnut, 13, 19, 20, 65
Bamboo, 7
Banana, 14, 22, 455, 456, 457, 465
Banisteriopsis caapi, 170
Barbados cherry, 455, 456, 457
Barbasco, 666
Barley, 92, 97, 294, 534
Barnyard grass, 592
Barnyard millet, 18
Basella alba, 19
Basil, 324, 632–635
Basil oil, 621, 625, 632–635
Bay leaf, 616–617
Bean, 7, 8, 13, 14, 17, 19, 30, 41, 84, 87, 257, 279, 585–588
Beauty bush, 145
Bee balm, 628
Beet, 84
Begonia, 56, 604
Belgian endive, 85, 86, 109, 115, 117, 528
Belladonna, 666
Bell pepper, 86
Benincasa hispida, 19, 538, 539, 540, 544
Bergamot, 628
Bermudagrass, 152, 285, 294, 295, 296
Betula schmidtii, 145
Big bluestem, 152, 285
Bignoniaceae, 170
Biomass fuel crops, 287–288
Biriba, 505
Bison bison, 284
Bitter fennel, 623, 625
Bitter gourd, 19
Bixa orellana, 169
Black bean, 19
Black cohosh, 670
Blackea rosea, 170
Blackeye pea, 586, 587
Black locust, 72, 73, 432–435
Black mustard, 384, 385, 386
Black rush, 444
Black sapote, 455, 456, 457
Black truffle, 55
Bladderpod, 76–77, 100
Bloodroot, 670

Blueberry, 83, 84
Bluebunch wheatgrass, 151
Blue chamomile oil, 622
Blue corn, 228–230. *See also* Maize
Blue daze, 88
Blue-green algae, 19
Bok choy, 84, 85
Boletus edulis, 55
Bombara groundnut, 14
Boniato, 535
Bonsai, 143
Borage, 7, 36, 101, 106
Boraginaceae, 170
Borago officinalis, 101, 106
Bothriochloa, 285
Bottle gourd, 84, 86, 542
Bouteloua, 285
Brachiaria, 64
 decumbens, 295
 mutica, 295
Brachyaria
 brizantha, 16
 dictyoneura, 16
 humidicola, 16
Brachylaena hutchinsii, 622
Brambles, 83, 84
Brassica, 13, 71, 77, 565-569
 campestris, 92, 300, 308, 309, 311, 570–573
  'ASVEG #1', 571
  'ASVEG #2', 571
  'China Express', 570, 571, 572
  'China Flash', 570, 571, 572
  'China Pride', 570, 572
  'Joi Choi', 570, 572
  'Kasumi', 570, 571, 572
  'Mei Qing Choi', 570, 572
  'Spingtime', 570, 572
  'Summertime', 570, 572
  'Tropical Quick', 570, 572
 carinata, 302, 308, 309, 310
 chinensis, 68
 hirta, 77, 308, 309, 310, 311, 312, 313, 316
 japonica, 528
 juncea, 77, 302, 308, 309, 310, 311, 312
 kaber, 384
 napus, 32, 73, 92, 181–189, 300, 302, 303, 308, 314, 316, 565, 567

nigra, 302, 308, 309, 384
oleracea, 86, 88, 302, 565, 566, 567, 568, 570, 573-576
   'Boxer', 573, 574, 575
   'Dolmic', 573, 574, 575
   'Golfer', 573, 574, 575
   'Lunet', 573, 574, 575
   'Pilar', 573, 575
   'Prince Marvel', 573, 574, 575
   'Rider', 573, 574, 575
   'Royal Marvel', 573, 574, 575
   'RS88032', 574, 575
   subsp. *acephala*, 566
   subsp. *botrytis*, 565
pekinensis, 68, 570–573
rapa, 86, 302, 303, 565, 566, 567, 568
   subsp. *pekinensis*, 565
   subsp. *rapifera*, 565
tournefortii, 308, 309
Brassicaceae, 20, 170, 570, 684
Brazilian rubber tree, 192–195
Breadfruit, 465
Breadwheats, 15
Brier rose, 54
Broccoli, 85, 86, 109, 110, 683
Bromus inermis, 148, 284–285
Brosimum
   uleti, 169
   utile, 170
Browse, 14
Brugmansia arborea, 170
Brunfelsia
   chiricaspi, 170
   grandiflora, 170
Brussels sprouts, 85, 86, 109, 573–576
Bryophyllum ginnatum, 170
Buchloe dactyloides, 288
Buckwheat, 7, 244–254
Buffalo gourd, 101
Buffalograss, 288
Buffelgrass, 152, 295, 296
Bujiu panga, 171
Bulb flowers, 88, 89, 109
Bulb onion, 84, 85, 86
Bunch grape, 83
Bunchosia, 169
Burdock, 54
Burseraceae, 463
Bush chestnut, 500–505
Butio, 169

Butterfly pea, 19
Button mushroom, 55
Butum, 169

Cabbage, 14, 85, 86, 88, 109
   flowering, 88
Cacao, 475–478
Cactaceae, 486, 491
Cactus, 68, 69
Caesalpiniaceae, 170
Cajanus cajan, 14, 16, 19, 257, 597–599
Calabaza, 84, 86, 539
Caladium, 87, 88
Caladium, 88
Calathea, 88
Calathea, 87, 88
Calendula, 33, 106
   officinalis, 32, 33, 34, 42, 43, 44, 106
California bay, 176, 178, 179
Calla, 61
Calocarpum sapota, 456
Calvija harlingii, 169
Camelina, 314–322
Camelina
   sativa, 106–107, 314–315, 316, 317, 319
Camellia, 141
Camellia, 666
   japonica, 141
   reticulata, 141
Camomile, 636–639. *See also* Chamomile
Camphor oil, 620
Cana agria, 170
Canarium ovatum, 463
Canistel, 455, 456, 457
Canna, 604
Cannabis sativa, 35, 40
Canola. *See* Rapeseed/canola
Cape gooseberry, 60, 479
Capparidaceae, 170
Capsicum, 86, 132–139
   annuum, 86, 132, 133, 134, 135, 136, 137
      var. *aviculare*, 137
   baccatum, 133, 135
      var. *pendulum*, 134, 136, 137
   baccatum sensu lato, 132
   buforum, 133
   campylopodium, 133
   cardenasii, 133, 135, 136

chacoense, 133, 137
chinense, 133, 134–135, 136, 137
coccineum, 133
cornutum, 133
dimorphum, 133
dusenii, 133
eximium, 133, 135, 136, 137
frutescens, 134, 136, 137
geminifolium, 133
glapagoensis, 133
hookerianum, 133
lanceolatum, 133
leptopodum, 133
minutiflorum, 133
mirabile, 133
parvifolium, 133
praetermissum, 133, 137
pubescens, 132, 133, 134, 135, 136, 137
schottianum, 133
scolnikianum, 133
tovarii, 133
villosum, 133
Capulin cherry, 61
Carambola, 72, 74, 75, 78, 82, 83, 448–451, 455, 456, 457
   'Arkin', 83
   'Gefner', 83
Caraway, 31, 36, 55
Caraway oil, 623, 624, 625
Carbohydrate crops, 33–34, 40-41
Carica
   heilbornii, 60
   papaya, 456, 465
Carludovica palmata, 170
Carnation, 62
Carob (*Ceratonia siliqua*), 8
Carrot seed oil, 623, 625
Carthamus tinctorius, 100
Carum carvi, 36, 55, 623, 624, 625
Caryodendron orinocense, 169
Casimiroa, 483
   edulis, 456, 483–485
   emarginata, 483
   pringlei, 483
   pubescens, 483
   sapota, 483
   tetrameria, 483
   watsonii, 483
Cassava, 11, 13, 14, 19, 22, 533, 534
Cassia, 17
   rotundifolia, 470

Castanea
   alabamensis, 500
   alnifolia, 500
   arkansana, 500
   ashei, 500
   crenata, 56
   floridana, 500
   mollissima, 83
   ozarkensis, 500
   paucispina, 500
   pumila, 500-504
   sativa, 56
Castor bean, 30, 32, 380–383
Castor oil, 33
Catharanthus roseus, 165, 605
   'Parasol', 605
   'Pretty In Rose', 605
Catnip oil, 621, 670
Cauliflower, 85, 109, 566
Cecropia, 170
Cecropiaceae, 170
Cedarwood oil, 620
Celastraceae, 170
Celery herb oil, 623
Cenchrus
   biflorus, 64
   ciliaris, 152, 295, 296
Centipedegrass, 153
Centrosema
   acutifolium, 16
   brasilianum, 16
   macrocarpum, 16
   pubescens, 16
Cep, 55
Cepparis sola, 170
Ceratonia siliqua, 8
Cereals, 12, 14, 64, 93, 96, 97, 98, 198–210, 294
Cereus peruvianus, 486–491
Chamaecyparis
   unebris, 620
   obtusa, 143
   isifera, 143
Chamomile, 54. *See also* Camomile
Chamomilla recutita, 54, 622, 636–639
Charlock, 387
Chayote, 543–544
Chekkurmanis, 19
Chenopodium, 71
   berlandieri, 222
   hircinum, 222
   quinoa, 30, 34, 41, 107, 222–227, 328

'Amachuma', 224
'Apelawa', 224
Chenopods, 7
Cherimoya, 56, 60, 505
Cherry, 159
Cherry tomato, 85
Chestnut, 56
Chickpea, 14, 101, 256, 257–258, 259, 260, 262, 279, 586, 587
Chicorium intybus, 86, 87
Chicory, 68, 69, 528
Chili pepper, 132–139
Chinese cabbage, 18, 68, 85, 86, 109, 570–573
Chinese chestnut, 82, 83
Chinese ginseng, 54, 670
Chinese gooseberry, 146
Chinese okra, 84, 86
Chinese pear, 83
Chinkapin, 500–505
Chionanthus
   pygmaeus, 141
   retusus, 141
   virginicus, 141
Chiri panga, 171
Chloris gayana, 295
Chrysanthemum
   balsamita, 622
   cinerariaefolium, 70
   parthenium, 54
Chrysothamnus, 355
   nauseosus, 355–356
      subsp. *salicifolius*, 356, 357
      subsp. *viridulus*, 357
   viscidiflorus, 356
Chrytophyllum venezuelanense, 169
Chunchu, 171
Cicer, 14, 259
   arietinum, 14, 101, 256, 257–258, 259, 279, 586
   reticulatum, 259
Cichorium
   endivia, 528
   intybus, 34, 40, 68, 69
Cimicifuga racemosa, 670
Cinnamomum
   camphora, 620
   micranthum, 620
Cinnamon, 616
Citronella oil, 620
Citrullus, 538, 544
   colocynthis, 539, 540, 542, 544

   lanatus, 64, 87, 538, 544
Citrus
   aurantifolia, 620
   grandis, 456
   limon, 620
   paradisi, 620
   sinensis, 620
   'Tahiti', 456
Clarkia amoena
   subsp. *Whitneyi*, 88
Clary sage, 55, 621
Clausena lansium, 456
Clavija harlingii, 170
Clematis, 609
   'Blue Ravine', 609
Clibaduim asperum, 170
Cliff break fern, 612–613
Clitoria ternatea, 19
Cloudberry, 524–526
Clove, 22, 616
Clove leaf oil, 620
Clover, 51
Cluster bean, 84, 86
Coccinia
   cordifolia, 538, 540, 542
   grandis, 86, 87
Coccomyces hiemalis, 159
Cocoa, 475–477. *See also* Cacao
Coconut, 372, 465, 466
Coconut oil, 176
Cocos nucifera, 372, 465, 466
Cocoyam, 19
Coffea arabica, 64, 465
Coffee, 22, 64, 65, 465, 683
Cola, 65
Collards, 84, 86
Colocasia, 19, 170
   esculenta, 169, 465, 533
Columbine, 101
Columnea archidonae, 170
Commelinaceae, 170
Commelina erecta, 170
Common bean, 14, 17, 22, 257, 279
Common chinkapin, 500
Common gooseberry, 479
Compositae, 620. *See* Asteraceae
Condiments, 98
Coneflower, 54
Conringia orientalis, 384
Cordyline, 62
Coriander, 30, 33, 36, 55, 106
Coriander oil, 620, 623, 625
Coriandrum sativum, 32, 34, 55, 106, 620, 623, 625

Corida nodosa, 170
Cormels, 75
Corn, 228–230. *See also* Maize
Cornmint oil, 620, 621
Cotton, 65, 110, 277, 416
Cowpea, 14, 64, 65, 257
Crabgrass, 414
Craetaegus aestivalis, 83
Crambe, 30, 33, 71, 74, 76, 78, 94, 97, 384, 386, 684, 685
Crambe, 71, 72
    abyssinica, 33, 34, 42, 43, 44, 94, 316, 384, 684
Cranberry, 583
Crape myrtle, 88, 89
Craspedia, 605
Crassulaceae, 170
Crataegus monogyna, 54
Crayfish, 654–656
Creeping vervain, 87
Crested wheatgrass, 149
Crimson clover, 278
Crotalaria juncea, 70
Croton lechleri, 170
Crown vetch, 114
Cruciferae. *See* Brassicaceae
Cryptomeria japonica, 141
Cucumber, 85, 86, 110
Cucumis, 538
    anguria, 540, 542, 544
    melo, 86, 538, 544
    metuliferus, 61, 553–559
    sativus, 86, 538
Cucurbita, 87, 538, 544
    argyrosperma, 539
    ficifolia, 541, 543
    foetidissima, 101, 541, 543
    maxima, 539, 544
    moschata, 86, 539, 544
    pepo, 68, 69–70, 539, 544
Cucurbitaceae, 538–546
Cucurbits, 13
Cucu tsicta, 171
Cuilichi lulu, 171
Cumin oil, 623
Cuminum cyminum, 623
Cuphea, 30, 32, 33, 71, 72, 73, 74, 76, 77, 78, 176, 372–379, 682, 683, 688
    calophylla, 375
    glutinosa, 74
    ignea, 74
    laminuligera, 73, 77
    lanceolata, 77, 372, 373, 374, 375, 376
    eptopoda, 375
    lutea, 77
    tolucana, 77, 375
    viscosissima, 77, 372, 373, 374, 375, 376
    wrightii, 73, 77, 375
Curare, 666
Custard apple, 453, 505
Cyamopsis tetragonolobus, 86
Cyclanthaceae, 170
Cyclanthera pedata, 541, 543
Cymbopogon
    citratis, 86
    winterianus, 620
Cynara scolymus, 68
Cynodon
    dactylon, 152, 285, 294, 295, 296
    nlemfuensis, 295, 296
Cyphomandra betacea, 59

Dactylis glomerata, 148
Dactyloctenium, 64
Daffodil, 89
Dahlia, 62
Daikon, 84, 86
Dallisgrass, 152
Dandelion, 54
Dasylirion, 435, 436
Daucus carota, 623, 625
Davana oil, 622
Davidia involucrata, 143, 144
Dawn redwood, 146
Dawson's magnolia, 146
Deeringothamnus, 505
    pulchellus, 506
    rugelii, 506
Desmodium
    heterophyllum, 470
    ovalifolium, 16, 470
Dicentra spectabilis, 141
Digitalis, 666
Digitaria
    decumbens, 295, 296
    exilis, 64
    sanguinalis, 414
Dill, 617, 623
Dimorphotheca, 33, 44, 685, 686
    pluvialis, 30, 32, 33, 34, 43, 684
Dioscorea, 14, 19, 533, 666
    trifida, 169
    villosa, 666
Diospyros
    ebenaster, 456
    kaki, 83
    lotus, 83
Disparus, 86
Dolichos lablab, 8, 19, 86
Dorema ammoniacum, 623
Dove tree, 143, 144
Dry bean, 585–588
Duboisia, 667
Duckweed, 68
Dumduma, 171
Durian, 462
Durio, 472
    zibethinus, 462
Duroia hirsuta, 170
Dwarf chestnut, 500–505

Easter cactus, 68, 69
Eastern gamagrass, 285
Echinacea
    crusgalli, 592
    purpurea, 54, 670
Echinochloa, 18
Edamame soybean, 47–48, 49–50, 124
Eggplant, 13, 18, 84, 87
    'Little Fingers', 85
Elaeis guineensis, 64, 314, 372, 466
Elecampane, 622
Elephant garlic, 85, 86, 109
Elephant grass, 40
Eleusine coracana, 18, 64
Eleutherococcus senticosus, 670
Elytrigia repens, 151, 152
Emerald Carpet, 609
Empoasca, 17
Endive, 85, 86, 109, 115, 117, 528
English pea, 84, 86
Ennealophus, 56
Ephedra, 666
Eragrostis, 64, 285
    curvula, 153, 295, 296
    pilosa, 64
    tef, 64, 100, 231–234
Ereocephalus punctulatus, 622
Eromochloa ophiuroides, 153
Eruca, 77
    sativa, 308, 309, 528
Eryngium foetidum, 169
Erythroxylaceae, 170
Erythroxylum gracilipes, 170
Essential oil, 620–635
Ethanol, 394–399

Eucalyptus, 17, 620
  citriodora, 620
  globus, 620
Eucalyptus oil
  cineole-type, 620
  citronella-type, 620
Eucrosia, 70, 71
Euphorbia, 30, 32, 36, 107
  lagascae, 30, 32, 33, 34, 42, 43, 44, 107, 384, 386, 387–388
  lathyris, 32, 33
Euphorbiaceae, 170, 380
Euphoria longana, 456
Eurasian apple, 51
European dill seed oil, 623
Eustoma, 70
Euterpe, 466, 468
  edulis, 466, 467
  oleracea, 466, 467, 468
Evening primrose, 7, 36
Evolvus glomeratus grandiflorus, 88
Exochorda racemosa, 141

Faba bean, 41, 256, 257, 258, 259, 260, 262
Fabaceae, 170
Fagaceae, 432
Fagopyrum
  cymosum, 251
  esculentum, 7, 244–254
    'Mancan', 251–254
    'Manor', 251–254
    'Tokyo', 251–254
  sagittatum, 251
  tataricum, 251
Fanweed, 384–388
Feedstocks, 30
Feijoa, 59–60, 82, 83
Feijoa sellowiana, 59–60, 83
Fennel, 36, 107, 576–582, 623, 625
Fennel oil, 622
Fenugreek, 101, 106
Ferula assafoetida, 623
Festuca, 147
  arundinacea, 147–148, 284
    Alta', 147
Feverfew, 54, 670
Fiber crops, 35–36, 40, 41–42
Fiber sorghum, 35, 36
Ficus, 73
  carica, 83
Fieldbean, 114
Field pea, 256–257, 257, 258

Field pennycress, 385
Fig, 83, 84
Fig-leaved gourd, 543
Finger millet, 18, 64
Finocchio, 36, 107, 576-582
Firebush, 88
Flacourtiaceae, 170
Flax, 30, 35, 40, 41, 42, 43, 44, 94, 319, 320
Flor del sielo, 170
Flower bulbs. *See* Bulb flowers
Flower crops, 61–62
Flowering cabbage, 88
Flowering kale, 88
Flur huasca, 171
Foeniculum vulgare, 576, 579–582, 625
  'Cristallino Bianco', 581
  'CV', 577, 578
  'Firenze grosso dolce', 581
  'Firenze tondo', 581
  'Florence', 577, 578, 581
  'Grand mean', 577, 578
  'Grossissimo mammuth', 577, 578, 581
  'Montovano', 577, 578, 581
  'Napoli gigante', 581
  'Napoli tardivo', 581
  'Parma sel Fucino', 577, 578, 581
  'Perfezione tondo', 581
  'Romagna', 577, 578, 581
  'Romanesco sel Urbe', 577, 578, 581
  'Romano precoce', 577, 578, 581
  'Sicilia grosso', 581
  var. *dulce*, 107, 579, 580, 623
  var. *vulgare*, 576, 623
  'Wadenromen', 577, 578, 581
  'Wadenromen grosso', 581
  Zefa fino', 577, 578, 581
Fonio, 64
Forage crops, 14, 16, 72, 98, 147–154, 284–286
Forsythia
  ovata, 146
  viridissima, 141
Fortunella, 456
Foxglove, 36
Foxtail millet, 18
French tarragon, 55
Fruit crops, 82–84, 155–160. *See also* entries under specific fruit crops

Fuchsia, 56
Fungi, 55
Fusarium, 85

Galbanum oil, 622
Gallu caspi, 171
Gambagrass, 295
Garabatu yuyu, 169
Garbanzo bean, 101, 586, 587
Garcinia
  hombrioniana, 472–474
  mangostana, 472
Garlic, 109
  elephant, 85, 86
Genista pilosa, 609
  'Vancouver Gold', 609
Gerbera, 70
Gesneriaceae, 170
Gherkin, 542
Ginger root, 53, 54, 465, 670
Ginkgo biloba, 140, 669–670
Ginkgo tree, 140, 669–670
Ginseng, 54, 85, 86, 109, 670
Globe artichoke, 68
Glycine max, 14, 92, 257, 267, 277, 314, 418
Godetia, 87, 88
Goldenberry, 479–480
Golden-fleshed potato, 86
Golden larch, 141
Golden rain-tree, 140
Goldenseal, 54, 85, 86, 109, 670
Gomphrena, 605
Gooseberry, 146, 479
Gossypium hirsutum, 277, 416
Gourd, 19, 539
  bitter gourd, 19
  bottle gourd, 84, 86, 542
  buffalo gourd, 101
  fig-leaved gourd, 543
  ivy gourd, 84, 86, 542
  luffa sponge gourd, 84, 86, 560–561
  pointed gourd, 84, 86
  snake gourd, 19
  sponge gourd, 19
  wax gourd, 19
Grain, 93, 109
Grain legumes, 12
Grama grass, 285
Gramineae. *See* Poaceae
Grape, 83
Grapefruit, 455
Grapefuit oil, 620

Grasses, 14, 16, 36, 64, 127, 147–154, 284–298
Grasspea, 256, 257, 258, 259–260
Great northern bean, 585, 586, 587
Green-fleshed muskmelon, 547, 548, 551, 552
Green gram, 257
Green onion, 84, 86
Green shell bean, 84
Grevillea, 17
Grias neuberthii, 169, 170
Grindelia camporum, 107
Groundnut, 14, 65
Guar, 84, 86
Guarea cinnamomea, 170
Guava, 455, 456, 457, 465
Guayule, 7, 30, 70, 72, 73, 76, 78, 97, 100, 192, 194–195, 338–346, 349–355, 683–684
Guineagrass, 295
Guizotia abyssinica, 65, 107–108
Gumweed, 107
Gypsophila, 62

Hakuran, 565
Halocarpus biformis, 55
Hare's ear mustard, 384, 386, 387
Hawthorn, 54
Head lettuce, 85. *See also* Lettuce
Hebe, 62
Hedeoma pulegioides, 621
Helianthus
  annuus, 32, 114, 284, 314
  tuberosus, 34, 41
Helichrysum oil, 622
Helichrysum stoechas, 622
Helminthesporium maydis, xxi
Hemp, 31, 35, 36, 40, 41, 43, 44, 70
Hemp bast, 42
Henequen, 435
Heptacodium miconioides, 146
Herbs, 86, 616-619. *See also* entries under specific herb plants
Herrania, 169
  nitida, 169
Hesperaloe, 435–442
  funifera, 436, 437, 438, 439, 440, 441
  nocturna, 436, 437, 440
  parviflora, 436, 437
Hevea, 73, 338, 341
  brasiliensis, 192–195, 338,

349, 683
Hevea rubber tree, 22
Hibiscus
  cannabinus, 35, 68–69, 402, 409, 411, 413, 416
    'Cuba 2032', 417, 418, 419, 420
    'Everglades 41', 417, 418, 419, 420
    'Everglades 71', 417
    'Guatamala 4', 418, 419, 420
    'Guatamala 45', 417, 418, 419, 420
    'Guatamala 48', 417, 419, 420
    'Guatamala 51', 417, 418, 419
  sabdariffa, 583–584
Himatanthus lancifolius, 170
Hinoki cypress, 143
Holly, 88, 89
Homalanthus acuminatus, 163
Honesty, 30
Honeysuckle, 146
Hordeum, 14
  vulgare, 92
Horehound, 54
Horse gram, 257
Horsemint, 628
Hosta lancifolia, 605, 606
Huagra huanduj, 171
Huarangayura, 171
Huiqui huasca, 171
Hungarian broomgrass, 148
Husk tomato, 84, 86
Hyacinth, 84
Hyacinth bean, 19, 86, 257
Hydrastis canadensis, 54, 86, 670
Hylocereus, 491–495
  Alon, 492, 493
  costaricensis, 492, 493
  Equador, 492, 493, 494
  Katom, 492, 493
  paolyrhi, 492, 493
  polyrhizus, 492, 494, 495
Hyparrhenia rufa, 295
Hypericum perforatum, 54, 670
Hyptis pectinata, 170
Hyssop, 55
Hyssop oil, 621, 622, 625
Hyssopus officinalis, 55, 621, 625

Icsa nanai yura, 171

Ilama, 505
Ilex, 88
  guayuosa, 170
  pedunculosa, 144
Ilia huanga lumu, 171
Indian dill seed oil, 623
Indiangrass, 152, 285
Inga, 169
  edulis, 169
Inula helenium, 622
Ipomea
  aquatica, 19
  batatas, 169, 533
  batatus, 14
Iris, 605
  pumila, 605, 606
Ironweed, 384
Isla vapa yura, 171
Ivy gourd, 84, 86, 542

Jaboticaba, 455, 456, 457
Jack bean, 19
Jackfruit, 455, 456, 457
Jalapeño pepper, 84
Japanese crab apple, 143
Japanese maple, 143
Japanese muskmelon, 84, 86
Japanese wisteria, 143
Japanese yew, 143
Japanese zelkova, 143
Jaraguagrass, 295
Jelly fungus, 55
Jerusalem artichoke, 30, 34, 35, 41
Jessenia bataua, 169
Jojoba, 7, 30, 32, 33, 71, 72, 76, 78, 97, 100, 101, 358–362, 687, 688–689
Jujube, 83
Juncus roemerianus, 444
Juniperus virginiana, 620
Jute, 42

Kaber mustard, 387
Kalanchoe
  blossfeldiana, 606
  manginii, 605, 606
Kale (flowering), 88
Kangkong, 19
Kenaf, 8, 13, 30, 35, 68–69, 72, 75, 76, 78, 97, 402–421
Kentucky bluegrass, 148, 284
Kerstingiella geocarpa, 19, 65
Kersting's groundnut, 19
Kidney bean, 585, 586, 587

Kikuyugrass, 295
Kiwano, 61, 553–559
Kiwifruit, 51, 57-58, 82, 83, 84, 683
Kleingrass, 295, 296
Kobus magnolia, 143
Kodo millet, 13, 18
Koelreuteria paniculata, 140
Kolkwitzia amabilis, 145
Korean forsythia, 146
Korean stewartia, 145
Kowhai, 62
Krebs, 64
Kumquat, 455, 456, 457

Labiatae, 620
Lablab, 8, 84, 86
Lablab purpureus, 257
Lacebark pine, 141
Lachenallia, 70
Lactuca
   saligna, 529
   sativa, 86, 100, 529
   serriola, 529
Lagenaria, 538, 544
   siceraria, 19, 86, 540, 542, 544
Lagerstroemia, 88
Lamiaceae, 170, 620, 621, 622, 628, 632
Landscape plants, 140–147, 288, 608–613
Large lima bean, 585, 586, 587
Lathyrus, 16
   sativus, 256, 257, 258, 259–260
Lauki, 84, 86
Lauraceae, 170
Laurus nobilis, 616–617
Lavandin, 55
Lavandula
   angustifolia, 621
   intermedia, 620, 621
   latifolia, 621
Lavender, 36, 55
Lavender oil, 621
Lavandula
   angustifolia, 55
   intermedia, 55
   latifolia, 55
Lavandin oil, 620, 621
Lecythidaceae, 170
Leek, 84, 86
Legumes, 14, 16, 19, 65, 72, 96, 97, 98, 256–265. *See* Fabaceae

Leguminosae. *See* Fabaceae, Legumes
Lemon balm, 54, 622
Lemon basil, 632-635
Lemon grass, 84, 86
Lemon oil, 620
Lemon verbena, 54
Lens, 14, 20, 259
   culinaris, 101, 256, 257, 258, 259, 279–282
      'Eston', 279, 281
      'Laird', 279, 281
      subsp. *culinaris*, 259
      subsp. *odemensis*, 259
      subsp. *orientalis*, 259
   nigricans, 259
Lentil, 101, 257, 258, 259, 260, 261–262, 279–282
Lentin, 256
Lentinus edodes, 55
Lepidium meyenii, 20
Leptospermum, 62
Lesquerella, 71, 72, 73, 76, 78, 100, 362–371
   fendleri, 76–77, 362, 365–366, 367–371
Lettuce, 85, 86, 100, 109, 528–532
Leucaena, 17
Leucodendrons, 62
Levisticum officinale, 623
Leymus cinereus, 152
Liliacea, 602
Lilium regale, 146
Lima bean, 19, 257, 585, 587
Lime, 455, 457
Lime distilled oil, 620
Limnanthaceae, 684
Limnanthes, 33, 71, 72, 76, 78, 101, 685
   alba, 32, 33, 34, 42, 43, 44, 77, 684
   douglasii, 185, 186
Limonium, 62
Linseed, 32, 33
Linseed oil, 320
Linum usitatissimum, 35, 40, 319
Lisianthus, 70
Litichi chinensis, 456
Litsea cubeba, 620
Litsea cubeba oil, 620
Little bluestem, 285
Little millet, 18
Locust bean, 257
Loganiaceae, 170

Lolium perenne, 51
Lomariopsis, 170
Lonchocarpus nicou, 170
Longan, 68, 455, 456, 457
Longleaf pine, 444
Long-stalk holly, 144
Lonicera fragrantissima, 141
Lovage herb oil, 622, 623
Lovage root oil, 623
Lovage seed oil, 623
Lovegrass, 285
Luffa, 13, 19, 538
   acutangula, 86, 540, 542, 544
   aegyptiaca, 86, 540, 542, 560–561
   amara, 544
   cylindrica, 544
   operculata, 545
Luffa sponge gourd, 84, 86, 560–561
Lupin, 13, 93, 114, 115, 117, 257, 266-278
Lupine, 30, 41, 68, 69, 93, 97, 100
Lupinus, 257, 266, 277
   albus, 41, 68, 69, 93, 100, 266, 267, 268, 277–278
   augustifolius, 266, 267, 268, 277
   cosentenii, 266
   hispanicus, 278
   luteus, 266, 268, 277
   mutabilis, 100, 266, 267
Lustunda, 171
Luta luta, 171
Lychee, 68, 455, 456, 457
Lycopersicon esculentum, 87
Lycopersicon lycopersicum, 87
Lythraceae, 372

Maca, 20
Macadamia, 56, 464, 465
Macadamia
   integrifolia, 56, 465
   tetraphylla, 56
Machacui caparina, 171
Machacui mandi, 171
Machacui mishu, 171
Machi manga, 171
Macrotyloma uniflorum, 257
Magnolia, 144
Magnolia
   dawsoniana, 146
   kobus, 143
   salicifolia, 144
   sargentiana, 146
   stellata, 143

zennii, 146
Maidenhair tree, 140
Maize, 13, 14, 19, 22, 92, 94, 127, 203, 204, 205, 228–230, 277, 286, 294, 329, 333, 409, 534, 536, 663
Malabar spinach, 19
Malpighiaceae, 170
Malpighia glabra, 456
Malus
  domestica, 51, 58–59
    'Braeburn', 58
    'Gala', 58
    'Golden Delicious', 59
    'Granny Smith', 58
    'Royal Gala', 58
    'Splendour', 58
  floribunda, 143
  halliana, 143
  hupehensis, 146
  kirghisorum, 156
  niedzwetzkyana, 156
  sargentii, 144
  sierversii, 156
Malvaceae, 409, 416, 583
Mamey sapote, 455, 456, 457
Mangifera, 472
  indica, 456
Mango, 455, 456, 457
Mangow, 457
Manihot esculenta, 14, 533
Manilkara zapota, 456
Manool, 55
Mansoa standlevi, 169, 170, 173, 174
Marigold, 30, 389–393, 649–654
Marjoram oil, 621
Marrubium vulgare, 54
Marula, 496-499
Mashua, 20, 536
Mati muyu caspi, 171
Matisia cordata, 169, 172
Matsutake, 55
Mauritia flexusa, 169
Mayapple, 666
Mayhaw, 82, 83, 84
Maytenus krukowii, 170, 173, 174
Meadowfoam, 30, 71, 73, 76, 97, 101, 185, 186, 187, 684, 686
Medicago, 16
  sativa, 418
Medicinal plants. *See also* Pharmaceutical crops and entries under specific plants

Melano, 61, 553–559
Melastomaceae, 170
Meliaceae, 170
Melinis minutiflora, 295
Melissa officinalis, 54, 621
Melissa oil, 621
Melon, 128, 129, 538–539, 47–553
Mentha
  arvensis, 620, 621
  gracilis, 621
  piperita, 55, 620, 621
  pulegium, 625
  spicata, 55, 620, 621
Metasequoia glyptostroboides, 146
Meterosideros, 62
Milfoil, 101
Milk thistle, 670
Milkweed, 94, 422–431
Millet, 11, 14, 18, 65, 294
Mimosaceae, 170
Minor millets, 14, 18
Mint, 36, 55, 97, 620, 621
Miscanthus, 30, 35, 36
  sinensis, 36, 40
Mizuna, 528
Molassesgrass, 295
Momordica, 13, 538, 544
  charantia, 19, 540, 542, 544
Monarda, 628-631
  citriodora, 621
  didyma, 628
  fistulosa, 628
    var. *menthaefolia*, 621, 628, 629
  geraniol type, 621
  thymol type, 621
Monterey pine, 51
Moraceae, 170
Moss verbena, 87, 88
Moutan, 141
Mucuna pruriens, 19
Muhlenbergia
  capillaris, 444
  filipes, 444
Muhuhu oil, 622
Mungbean, 14, 18, 19, 257
Munu chupa, 171
Musa, 14, 456, 465, 472
  textilis, 435
Mushrooms, 85, 86, 109, 117
Muskmelon, 84, 86, 547, 548, 551, 552
Mustard, 115, 302, 384, 385, 386, 387

Myoga ginger, 53, 54
Myrciaria cauliflora, 456
Myroxylon balsamum, 170

Napa, 84, 85
Napiergrass, 295, 296
Naranjilla, 61
Nasturtium, 185, 186
Native spearmint oil, 620
Navy bean, 585, 586, 587
Neosprucea, 170
Nepeta cataria, 621, 670
Nephelium, 472
  aculeatum, 462
  compressum, 462
  lappaceum, 461
  laurinum, 462
  maingayi, 462
  muduseum, 462
  reticulatum, 462
  uncinatum, 462
Nerine, 61
Nerine, 61
New Zealand Christmas tree, 62
Nicotiana, 667
  tabacum, 565
Nicotine, 666
Niger, 107–108
Nikko maple, 144
Ninde oil, 621
Nolina, 435, 436
Nut crops, 155–160. *See also* entries under specific nut crops
Nutmeg, 22

Oats, 294, 310
Oca, 20, 61, 536
Ochnaceae, 170
Ocimum, 632
  basilicum, 169, 324, 621, 625, 632
  gratissimum, 621
Ocimum oil, 621
Ocium canum, 621
Ocotea
  pretiosa, 620
  quixos, 169
Oenothera, 36
Oil palm, 64, 314, 372
Oilseed, 30, 31, 32-33, 40, 41, 42–44, 65, 71, 96, 98, 100, 176, 181–191, 308–313, 684. *See also* entries under specific oilseeds

Okra, 18, 19, 84, 86, 416
Old world bluestem, 285
Onion, 18, 53, 84, 85, 86
Opium, 666
Opium poppy, 101
Orange browallia, 88
Orange oil, 620
Orchardgrass, 148
Orchidaceae, 170
Orconectes viriles, 654–656
Oregano, 55, 617, 618
Organic vegetables, 86
Oriental persimmon, 82, 83
Oriental vegetables, 86
Origanum
    majorana, 621
    vulgare, 55
Ormenis mixta, 622
Ornamental plants, 140–147, 288, 608–613
Ornithogalum, 70, 602–603
    dubium, 602–603
    thyrsoides, 602–603
Oryza, 14
    glaberrima, 14
Ourateae, 170, 173
Oxalidaceae, 448
Oxalis tuberosa, 20, 61, 536
Oyster mushroom, 85

Pachyrhizus erosus, 19
Pacific yew, 670
Paeonia suffruticosa, 141
Pagoda tree, 140
Pak choi, 68
Pala panga, 171
Palm, 466. *See also* Oil palm
Palmetto, 670
Palm heart, 465–472
Palm leaf, 444
Panax
    ginseng, 54, 670
    quinquefolius, 54, 86, 670
Pangolagrass, 295, 296
Panicum, 64
    coloratum, 295, 296
    laetum, 64
    maximum, 16, 295
    miliaceium, 18
    sumatrense, 18
    turgidum, 64
    virgatum, 152, 285
Papaver somniferum, 101
Papaya, 455, 456, 457, 465

Paperbark maple, 145
Paragrass, 295
Parkia, 257
Parsley, 617
Parsley oil, 623
    herb, 622
    seed, 623
Parthenium
    argentatum, 99-100, 192, 194–195, 343, 345, 347–348, 349, 352
    incanum, 343
    lozanianum, 347-348
Parvar, 84, 86
Pascopyrum smithii, 285
Paspalum
    dilatatum, 152
    notatum, 152
    scrobiculatum, 18
Passiflora, 83, 169, 172
    ampullacea, 481
    antioquiensis, 481
    cumbalensis, 482
    edulis, 456, 480
        f. *flavicarpa*, 480
    goudatiana, 482
    granadilla, 481
    ligularis, 481
    manicata, 482
    mixta, 482
    mollissima, 481, 482
    trifoliata, 482
    tripartita, 482
    trisecta, 482
Passifloraceae, 480
Passion fruit, 68, 82, 455, 456, 457, 480–483
Paste tomato, 85. *See also* Tomato
Patchouli oil, 620, 621, 622
Paullinia, 170, 173, 174
Pawpaw, 83, 84, 505-515, 644–648
Pea, 41, 86, 259, 260–261, 270, 279
Peach palm, 465
Pea eggplant, 84, 86
Peanut, 22, 84, 86, 257
Pear, 82, 83, 84
Pearl lupin, 100
Pearl millet, 14, 15–16, 64, 72, 74, 75, 78, 127, 128, 129, 152, 198–210, 294
Pejibaye, 465-472
Pellaea, 612

    ovata, 612–613
Pennisetum, 14
    clandestinum, 295
    glaucum, 14, 64, 75, 152, 198–210, 294
    monodii, 198
    purpureum, 198, 295, 296
    stenostachyum, 198
    violaceum, 198
Pennycress, 385
Pennyroyal oil, 625
Penstemon fruticosus, 609
    'Purple Haze', 609
Peony, 62
Pepino, 60
Pepper, 14, 18, 84, 85, 86, 132–139
Peppermint, 55
Peppermint oil, 620, 621
Perennial ryegrass, 51
Perilla, 322–328
Perilla, 322–323
    frutescens, 322, 621
Perilla oil, 621
Periwinkle, 666
Persea americana, 170, 456
Persimmon, 82, 83, 84
Pesticide chemicals, 662-664
Petroselinum crispum, 623
Pharmaceutical crops, 161–167, 170–171, 544–545, 636–639, 640–643, 644–648, 649–654, 664–671
Phaseolus, 7, 8, 13, 14, 17, 590
    acutifolius, 14, 594-596
        'Chapingo 24', 594, 595
        'Chapingo 25', 594, 595
        'PI 231638', 594, 595
        'PI 319551', 594, 595
    coccineus, 594
    limensis, 585
    lunatus, 257, 585, 594
    vulgaris, 14, 17, 114, 169, 257, 279, 585, 586, 594
Pheonix dactylifera, 64
Phleum pratense, 148–149
Phormium, 62
Physalis
    ixocarpa, 86, 87, 479
    peruviana, 60, 479
    pruinosa, 479
Phytolacca rivinoides, 169
Pigeonpea, 11, 14, 16, 19, 257, 597–599
Pigweed, 414

Pili nut, 463–464
Pimpinella anisum, 623
Pine, 51, 55
Pineapple, 465
Pineapple guava, 59-60, 82, 83
Pink bean, 587
Pink pine, 55
Pink trumpet vine, 88
Pinsha caliu, 171
Pinto bean, 585, 586, 587
Pinus
   bungeanus, 141
   palustris, 444
   radiata, 51
Piper, 170
   veneralense, 170
Piperaceae, 170
Piptademia pteroclada, 170
Piquin pepper, 84
Piri piri panga, 171
Pisum, 16
   fulvum, 259
   sativum, 41, 86, 256–257, 259, 270, 279
Pitaya, 491-495
Plantago ovata, 101, 108
Plantain, 14, 19, 456, 457, 465
Platycodon grandiflorus, 141
Plukenetia volubilis, 169
Plum, 83, 520-523
Poaceae, 294, 444
Poa pratensis, 148, 284
Podranea ricasoliana, 88
Pogostemon cablin, 620, 621
Pohutakawa, 62
Pointed gourd, 84, 86
Polymnia sonchifolia, 20, 61
Polypodiaceae, 170
Pomegranate, 82, 83
Pond apple, 453
Poppy, 36, 101
Potalia amara, 170, 173, 174
Potato, 13, 14, 19, 20, 22, 41, 86, 109, 533, 534
Potentilla fruticosa, 609, 610
   'Yellow Gem', 609
Pouruma cecropiaefolia, 169, 172, 173
Pouteria, 169
   caimito, 169
   campechiana, 456
Praecitrullus fistulosus, 538, 540, 543
Proso millet, 18

Protein crops, 41
Prunica granatum, 83
Prunus, 83, 520–523
   americana, 520
   angustifolia, 520, 521, 522
   avium, 159
   besseyi, 520
   capuli, 61
   cerasus, 159
   fruticosa, 159
   gracilis, 520
   hortulana, 520
   mexicana, 520
   munsoniana, 520
   rivularis, 520
   sargentii, 144
Psathyrostachys juncea, 150–151
Pseudolarix amabilis, 141
Pseudoroegneria
   spicata, 151
   stipifolia, 151
Psidium guajava, 456, 465
Psophocarpus tetragonolobus, 19, 87, 257
Psyllium, 101, 108, 666
Pteronia incana, 622
Puma yuyu, 171
Pummelo, 455, 456, 457
Pumpkin, 68, 69–70, 84, 87, 538, 539
Pupa huasca, 171
Puru panga, 171
Pyrethrin, 666
Pyrethrum, 70
Pyrus
   armeniaca, 83
   communis, 83
   pyrifolia, 83, 146
   serotina, 83
Pytomedicines, 669-671

Quackgrass, 151–152
Quihuin ambi, 171
Quihui yuyu, 170
Quinine, 666
Quinoa, 13, 31, 34, 35, 41, 78, 107, 222–227, 328–336

Rabbiteye blueberry, 83, 84
Radicchio, 84, 87, 528
Radicchio chicory, 68
Rambutan, 461–463
Rape, 30
Rapeseed/canola, 32, 33, 68, 71, 72, 73, 77, 78, 93, 94, 97, 102–105, 103, 109, 110, 111, 114, 117, 118, 127, 128, 300–301, 302–307, 314
Raphanus, 13
   sativum, 86
Rauwolfia, 666
Rayu paju, 171
Rayu palanda, 170
Red kidney bean, 585, 586, 587
Regal lily, 146
Rheum rhababarum, 87
Rhipsalidopsis gaertneri, 69
Rhizobium, 16
Rhizopus javanicus, 44
Rhodesgrass, 295
Rhododendron
   fortunei, 141
   kaempferi, 144
Rhodohypoxis bourii, 607
Rhubarb, 84, 87, 616
Ribes, 479
   sanguineum, 609
      'White Icicle', 609
Rice, 11, 12, 13, 14, 65, 294, 333, 534
Rice bean, 7, 19
Ricinus communis, 380
Rinus cumminis, 32
Robinia pseudoacacia, 73, 432
Rocket, 528
Rollinia mucosa, 505
Roman chamomile oil, 622
Root chicory, 30, 34, 35
Roots/tubers, 12, 13, 14, 19, 20, 76, 533–537. *See also entries under specific roots and tubers*
Rosa
   damascena, 55
   rugosa, 54
Rosaceae, 524
Rose, 36, 55
Rosehips, 54
Rosella, 13
Roselle, 78, 583–584
Rosemary oil, 621, 625
Rose verbena, 87, 88
Rosmarinus officinalis, 621, 625
Rosy periwinkle, 8
Rubber, 192–196, 338–357
Rubber tree, 22, 192–195, 349, 683
Rubiaceae, 170
Rubus, 83
   calycinoides, 609

Rubus, continued
    'Emerald Carpet', 609
  chamaemorus, 524–526
Russian thistle, 226
Russian wildrye, 150–151
Rutaceae, 483
Rye, 278
Ryegrass, 51

Sabal palmetto, 444
Saccharum officinarum, 465
Sacha huanduj, 171
Sacha limon, 171
Safflower, 65, 100, 187
Sage, 55, 101
Sage oil, 621, 622, 625
St. John's wort, 54, 670
Salad burnet, 101
Salsola pestifer, 226
Salvia
  coccinea, 607
  leucantha, 88
  officinalis, 55, 101, 621, 625
  sclarea, 55, 621
  splendens, 607
Sand bluestem, 152
Sandersonia, 61
Sandersonia auriantiaca, 61
Sandhill plum, 520-523
Sand pear, 83, 146
Sanguanaria canadensis, 670
Sanguisorba, 101
Sani papa, 169
Santa maria panga, 171
Santolina chamaecyparissus, 622
Sapindaceae, 170, 461
Sapodilla, 455, 456, 457
Sapote, 455, 456, 457, 483–485
Sargent cherry, 144
Sargent crab apple, 144
Sargent magnolia, 146
Sarsiliu, 171
Saskatoon berry, 516-519
Sassafras oil
  Brazil, 620
  China, 620
Satin flower, 87
Satureja
  hortensis, 101
  montana, 621
Sauropus androgynus, 19
Savory oil, 621
Sawara cypress, 143
Saw palmetto, 670

Schizachyrium scoparium, 285
Schmidt's birch, 145
Scholar's tree, 140
Sciadopitys verticillata, 143
Sclerocarya birrea
  subsp. *Caffra*, 496–499
Scotch spearmint, 621
Secale cereale, 278
Sechium, 538
  edule, 541, 543–544
Seedless watermelon, 84, 547, 548, 549, 552
Senna ruiziana, 170
Serenoa repens, 670
Sesame, 107
Sesamum indicum, 107
Sesbania, 17
Setaria
  anceps, 295
  italica, 18
Setariagrass, 295
Seven-son-flower, 146
Shia huasca, 171
Shia panga, 171
Shiitake mushroom, 85, 117
Shimbi, 169
Siberian ginseng, 670
Silk tree, 146
Silybum marianum, 54, 670
Simira, 170
Simmondsia chinensis, 32, 100, 101, 358, 360
Sinapis alba, 302, 308, 313
Sirlu panga, 171
Sisal, 42, 435
Sitimu panga, 171
Smilaceae, 170
Smilax, 170
Smooth broomgrass, 148, 284–285
Snake gourd, 19
Soft-shell crayfish, 654–656
Solanaceae, 170, 479
Solanum, 14, 54, 65
  aviculare, 54
  laciniatum, 54
  macrocarpon, 87
  mamosum, 170
  muricatum, 60
  quitoense, 61, 169
  torvum, 86
  tuberosum, 14, 86, 533
Soncoya, 505
Sophora, 62
  japonica, 140

Sorbus hupehensis, 609
  'Pink Pagoda', 609
Sorghastrum mutans, 152, 285
Sorghum, 14, 30, 34, 35, 36, 64, 65, 94, 109, 203, 204, 205, 277, 286, 294, 394–399
Sorghum, 64
  bicolor, 14, 34, 277, 294
  vulgare, 36
Sour cherry, 159
Soursop, 505, 507
Southern highbush blueberry, 83, 84
Soybean, 14, 47–48, 49–50, 92, 94, 117, 127, 128, 129, 204, 257, 267, 277, 314, 418, 663
Spaghetti squash, 539
Spearmint, 55, 621
Spearmint oil, 620, 621
Spelt, 93
Spike lavender, 55, 621, 622
Spilanthes, 170
Spinach, 226, 528. *See also* Malabar spinach
Spinacia oleracea, 226, 528
Sponge gourd, 19
Squash, 22, 53, 538, 539
Starch, 34
Stargrass, 295, 296
Starlet flower, 607
Star magnolia, 143
Steirodiscus, 607
Sterculia, 476
  urens, 476
Sterculiaceae, 475, 476
Stewartia koreana, 145
Stinkweed, 385
Stokes aster, 71, 78
Stokesia laevis, 70, 71
Streptosolen jamesonii, 88
Stylosanthes
  capitata, 16
  guianensis, 16
Sucuva, 171
Sugar apple, 82, 83, 451, 455, 456, 457, 505
Sugar beet, 41
Sugarcane, 7, 465
Sugars, 22, 34
Summer savory, 101
Summer squash, 539
Sunflower, 30, 32, 33, 94, 114, 115, 124, 284, 314
Sunn hemp, 70, 78

Supai caspi, 171
Supai chunda, 170
Surinamgrass, 295
Suru panga, 171
Swarzia simplex, 170
Sweet corn, 85, 87
Sweet fennel, 623, 625
Sweetgrass, 442–445
Sweet pea, 62
Sweet potato, 7, 13, 14, 20, 533, 534–536
Sweetsop, 83
Sweet sorghum, 30, 34, 35, 109, 394–399
Switchgrass, 152, 285, 286, 288
Syzygium
   aromaticum, 620
   samarangense, 456

Tabernaemontana sananho, 169, 170
Tagetes
   erecta, 389, 649
   lucida, 649
   minuta, 622, 649–654
Tagetes oil, 622
Tahiti lime, 456, 457
Tall fescue, 147-148, 284
Tamarillo, 59
Tanacetum
   parthenium, 670
   vulgare, 622, 625
Tanier, 72, 78
Tansy oil, 622, 625
Taraxacum officinale, 54
Taro, 465
Tarragon, 55, 617
Tarragon oil, 622
Tarwi, 100
Taxol, 161, 164–166
Taxus
   brevifolia, 164–165, 670
   chinensis, 165
   cuspidata, 143
   globosa, 165
   wallichiana, 165
   yunnanensis, 165
Tea crab, 146
Tef, 100, 231–234
Teffy amaranth, 97
Telfairia
   occidentalis, 65, 540, 543
   pedata, 541, 543
Teosinte, 14

Tepary bean, 17, 594–596
Thai eggplant, 84, 87
Theobroma, 666
   bicolor, 169, 172
   cacao, 475-478
Theophrastaceae, 170
Theophylline, 666
Thinopyrum, 285
Thistle, 54
Thlaspi arvense, 384
Thyme, 36, 55, 617
Thyme oil, 621
Thymus
   pulegioides, 621
   vulgaris, 55, 621
   zygis, 621
Tibouchina, 56
Timothy, 148–149
Tindora, 84, 87
Tobacco, 110
Tofu, 683
Tomatillo, 85, 87, 479
Tomato, 14, 18, 85, 86, 87, 128, 660–662
Trachyspermum copticum, 623
Tree chinkapin, 500
Tree of heaven, 140
Tree peony, 141
Trees, 17, 89, 140
Tree tomato, 59
Tricholoma matsutake, 55
Trichosanthes, 13, 538
   cucumerina, 19, 541, 543
   cucumeroides, 545
   dioica, 86
   kirilowii, 545
Trifolium, 16
   incarnatum, 278
   repens, 51
Trigonella, 16
   foenum-graecum, 101, 106
Trillium grandiflorum, 606, 607
Tripsacum dactyloides, 285
Tripscum, 14
Triticale, 93, 114, 565
Triticale, 11, 14, 15
   hexaploide, 93
Triticum, 14
   aestivum, 14, 277, 286, 565
      var. *spelta*, 93
   durum, 14
Tropaeolum
   majus, 185, 186
   tuberosum, 20, 536

Truffle, 55
Trumpet vine, 88
Tuber
   magnatum, 55
   melanosporum, 55
Tulips, 89
Tumble pigweed, 414
Turfgrass, 288

Ucsha, 169
Ulluco, 20, 536
Ullucus tuberosus, 20, 536
Umbelliferae, 620
Umbellularia californica, 176, 178, 179
Umbrella pine, 143
Urera caracasana, 171
Urticaceae, 171

Vaccinium, 583
   ashei, 83
   corymbosum, 83
Valerian, 36, 54, 670
Valeriana officianlis, 54, 670
Variegated thistle, 54
Vegetable crops, 18, 84–87. *See also entries under specific vegetable crops*
Vegetable oils, 7
Vegetable soybean, 18
Velvet bean, 19
Velvet sage, 88
Verbena, 87, 88
Verbena
   brasiliansis, 171
   canadiensis, 88
   rigida, 88
Verbenaceae, 171
Vernonia, 71, 72, 73, 76, 78, 362–367
   galamensis, 362, 363, 364, 384
Vervain, 87, 88
   'Polaris', 87
Vettiver grass, 8
Viburnum
   plicatum, 141, 609
      'Summer Snowflake', 609
   rytidophyllum, 146
Vicia, 14, 16, 259
   faba, 41, 256, 257, 258, 259
      subsp. *faba*, 259
      subsp. *paucijuga*, 259
Vigna, 14
   angularis, 19, 588–594

Vigna, continued
    'Adzuki Express', 589, 590
    'Erimo', 589, 590
    'Hatsune', 589, 590
    'Takara', 589, 590
   aureus, 257
   mungo, 19
   radiata, 19, 257
   sinensis, 64
   umbellata, 19
   unguiculata, 14, 18, 19, 257, 586
      subsp. *sesquipedalis*, 86, 87
Vinca, 87, 605
Viola, 607
Violet, 606, 607
Vitus aestivalis, 83
Voandezia, 14
   subterranea, 19, 65

Walnut, 157, 158–159
Wampee, 455, 456, 457
Wasabi, 53
Wasabia japonica, 53
Watermelon, 64, 65, 84, 538–539, 547–552
   seedless, 84, 87, 547, 548, 549, 552
   yellow-fleshed, 547, 548, 550
Wax gourd, 19
Wax jambu, 455, 456, 457
Waxy hulless barley, 92
Weeping lovegrass, 153, 295, 296
Weigela florida, 141
Western wheatgrass, 285
West Indian gherkin, 542

Wheat, 11, 12, 13, 15, 64, 94, 96, 97, 277, 286, 294, 333, 534
Wheatgrass, 285, 286
White clover, 51
White bean, 587
White lupine, 69, 93, 100
White sapote, 455, 456, 457, 483–485
White truffle, 55
Wild bergamot, 628
Wild cassava, 14
Wild chamomile oil, 622
Wild coffee, 65
Wild cola, 65
Wild cotton, 65
Wild cowpea, 65
Wildflowers, 117
Wild millet, 65
Wild mustard, 384, 386, 387
Wild potato, 14
Wild rice, 14, 65, 94, 114, 235–243, 284
Wildrye, 152
Wild sorghum, 65
Wild thyme oil, 621
Wild watermelon, 65
Willow-leaved magnolia, 144
Winged bean, 7, 8, 13, 19, 84, 257
   seedless, 87
Winter rapeseed, 73
Winter squash, 539
Wisteria
   loribunda, 143
   sinensis, 141
Witloof chicory, 68, 69, 86
Wormwood, 101
Wormwood oil, 622

Xanthosoma, 19, 72
   sagittifolium, 75, 76

Yacami panga, 171
Yacon, 20, 61
Yam, 14, 19, 533, 534
Yambean, 19
Yardlong bean, 18, 19, 84, 87
Yarrow, 88, 101
Yarrow oil, 622
Yellow-fleshed watermelon, 547, 548, 550
Yellow mustard, 302
Yucca, 435, 436, 441

Zabrotes, 17
Zantedeschia, 61
   aethiopica, 61
Zea mays, 14, 87, 92, 228–230, 277, 286, 329, 333, 409, 536
Zelkova serrata, 143
Zen magnolia, 146
Zingiber
   mioga, 53, 54
   officinale, 171, 465, 670
Zingiberaceae, 171
Zinnia
   angustifolia
      'Classic', 607
      'White Star', 606, 607
   elegans, 607
Zizania
   aquatica, 114, 235, 284
   latifolia, 235
   palustris, 94, 235–243
   texana, 235
Zizyphus, 83
Zoysia, 285
Zoysiagrass, 285

Index to Authors

Aksland, G.E. 277–278
Anderson, L. 176–181
Andrews, David J. 198–208, 208–210
Arquette, James G. 367–371
Asay, Kay H. 147–154
Auld, Dick L. 95–102, 308–314
Babcock, J.M. 590–594
Backhaus, Ralph A. 192–196
Balick, M.J. 167–174
BeMiller, James N. 389–393, 475–478
Benzioni, A. 553–557
Berti, Marisol T. 106–109
Bertram, Robert B. 11–22
Bhardwaj, Harbans L. 597–599
Bhat, R.B. 355–357
Bischoff, Robert F. 662–664
Bledsoe, Robert E. 416–421
Bleibaum, J. 176181
Boggs, Joseph S. 681–683
Bolen, Carrol D. 658–660
Bolotin, D. 167–174
Borrego, F. 343–345, 347–348
Bostic, Steve 612–613
Boyd, Michael R. 161–167
Bradley, V.L. 99–102
Breene, W.M. 314–322
Brenner, David M. 322–328
Brigham, Raymond D. 380–383
Brown, James H. 367–371, 680–681
Brown, Paul B. 654–656
Budin, J.T. 314–322
Burns, Raymond L. 677–678
Burton, Glenn W. 294–298
Callaway, M. Brett 505–515
Cardellina, John H., II 161–167
Carr, Patrick M. 384–388
Charles, Denys J. 547–553, 576–579, 579–582, 632–635, 640–643
Clark, R.L. 99–102
Clement, Charles R. 465–472
Cohen, Y. 167–174
Collins, Wanda W. 533–537
Conrad, John W. 24
Cook, Charles G. 411–412
Cornish, Katrina 192–196

Cragg, Gordon M. 161–167
Crane, Jonathan H. 448–460
Cundiff, John S. 394–399
Cuperus, F.P. 38–45
Davenport, Lonni R. 585–588
David, P. 583–584
Davidson, C.G. 516–519
Davies, H. Maelor 176–181
Davis, Jeanine M. 560–561
Dean, Bill B. 122–126
DeCourley, Charles D. 560–561
DeFrank, Joseph 465–472
Derksen, J.T.P. 38–45
Dierig, David A. 362–367
Douglas, James A. 51–57
Dufault, Robert J. 442–445
Duke, James A. 664–669
Eckhoff, J.L. 231–234
Eshbaugh, W. Hardy 132–139
Estilai, Ali 349–351
Evans, David W. 409–410
Ewart, Lowell C. 604–608
Fan, C. 176–181
Feibert, Erik B.G. 640–643
Field, L.A. 314–322
Figueira, Antonio 475–478
Foster, Michael 354–355
Fowler, Cary 22–27
Fowler, James L. 352–353
Friedman, J. 167–174
Fu, IMo 570–573
Gareau, R,M. 308–314
Gast, Karen L.B. 520–523
Gilbertson, Kenneth M. 231–234
Gilliland, G.C. 588–590, 590–594
Grever, Michael R. 161–167
Griesbach, Robert J. 602–603
Hall, James T. 674–676
Hang, An N. 409–410, 588–590, 590–594
Hannan, R.M. 99–102
Hanover, James W. 432–435
Haq, N. 511
Harlan, Jack R. 64–65
Hawkins, D.J. 176–181
Heikkinen, M.K. 308–314
Henderson, T.L. 219–221

Hess, W.M. 355–357
Hewett, Errol W. 57–64
Horbowicz, Marcin 244–250
Huang, J. 355–357
Huyskens, S. 553–557
Israelsen, Loren D. 669–671
Ito, Philip 465–472
Jackson, Mary 442–445
Janick, Jules xx, xxi, 127–129, 475–478
Jasso de Rodriguez, Diana 345–346
Jaworski, Casimir A. 300–301
Johnson, Duane L. 222–227, 228–230
Johnson, George P. 500–505
Johnson, R.C. 99–102
Jourdan, Pablo S. 565–569
Kiehn, F.A. 628–631
Kiula, Barnabas 208–210
Kleine, Greg 354–355
Knapp, Steven J. 372–379
Knudsen, Herbert D. 422–428, 428–431
Konovsky, J.C. 45–51
Koopowitz, H. 602–603
Koziol, Michael J. 328–336
Kumar, K. Anand 198–208
Kunst, Ljerka 181–191
Kuruvadi, Sathyanaravanaiah 343–345, 345–346, 347–348, 594–596
Lopez Benitez, Alfonso 343–345, 347–348
Lamberts, Mary 82–92
Larson, K.J. 45–51
Lawrence, Brian M. 620–627
Letchamo, Wudeneh 636–639
Lumpkin, Thomas A. 45–51, 122–126, 588–590, 590–594
Macdonald, Bruce 608–611
MacKenzie, Samuel L. 181–191
Manshardt, Richard M. 465–472
Marsh, Dyremple B. 558–559
Marshall, H.H. 628–631
Mask, Paul L. 277–278
Matus, A. 279–282
Mazza, G. 251–254, 516–519, 628–631,

McCain, Richard 479–486
McCann, Laura 114–119
McClary, Dean C. 45–51, 588–590, 590–594
McLaughlin, Jerry L. 644–648
McLaughlin, Steven P. 435–442
Medina, Ana L. 389–393
Mendlinger, S. 553–557
Mendosa, P. 167–174
Meyer, F. 602–603
Miller, Gregory 500–505
Mitra, N. Jha 228–230
Mizrahi, Yosef 486–491, 491–495, 496–499
Moore, Jaroy 354–355
Moore, K.J. 284–293
Morales, Mario R. 547–553, 576–579, 579–582, 632–635,
Muehlbauer, Fredrick J. 256–265
Mullins, G.L. 277–278
Muuse, B.G. 38–45
Myers, Robert L. 102–105, 120–121
Nadimpalli, Ram G. 597–599
Næss, S. Kristine 524–526
Nelson, J.M. 360–362
Nerd, Avinoam 486–491, 491–495, 496–499,
Ng, Timothy J. 538–546
O'Rourke, Desmond A. 122–126
O'Shea, R. Martin 683–684
Obendorf, Ralph L. 244–250
Oelke, Ervin A. 114–119, 235–243
Ogg, A.G. 590–594
Oplinger, Edward S. 92–95
Ozminkowski, Richard H., Jr. 565–569
Palzkill, David A. 358–359, 360–362
Pan, Zhiqang 192–196
Payne, Jerry. A. 500–505
Phatak, Sharad C. 300–301, 597–599
Potter, William M. 644–648

Putnam, Daniel H. 114–119, 266–277, 314–322
Rains, Glen C. 394–399
Rajewski, John F. 198–208, 208–210
Ramirez, F. 347–348
Rapp, Kåre 524–526
Ratnayake, Sunil 644–648
Raveh, Eran 491–495
Ravetta, Damian A. 358–359
Ray, Dennis T. 338–342
Reeves, D.W. 277–278
Reid, William 520–523
Reinert, William 660–662
Rhoden, E.G. 583–584
Rios, M. 167–174
Riveland, N. 219–221
Robinson, Frank E. 407–408
Roetheli, Joseph C. 693–694
Rupprecht, J. Kent 644–648
Ryder, Edward J. 528–532
Salvo, Stephen K. 442–445
Sanchez Valdez, Isaac 594–596
Schepartz, Saul 161–167
Schneiter, A.A. 106–109, 219–221
Schulz-Schaeffer, J.R. 211–218
Scott, Andrew W., Jr. 411–412
Sealy, Ramsey L. 612–613
Shands, Henry L. xx
Shannon, Michael C. 349–351
Sherman, Carol 570–573
Shock, Clinton C. 640–643
Simon, James E. xx, 547–553, 576–579, 579–582, 632–635, 640–643
Singh, Bharat P. 562–564
Slinkard, A.E. 279–282
Small, T. 583–584
Smith, Robin M. 640–643
Snader, Kenneth M. 161–167
Soule, Jacqueline A. 649–654
Sovero, Matti 302–307
Spongberg, Stephen A. 140–147

Stallknecht, Gilbert F. 211–218, 231–234
Stout, D.M. 99–102
Suffness, Matthew 161–167
Sullivan, Glenn H. 585–588
Swartz, Harry Jan 524–526
Tanigoshi, L.K. 590–594
Taylor, Charles S. 402–407
Taylor, David C. 181–191
Taylor, Douglas P. 244–250
Thompson, Anson E. xx, 362–367, 674
Thompson, Maxine M. 155–160
Tinggal, Hj. Serudin D. S. Hj. 472–474
Tinguely, Robert 352–353
Tiwari, Suresh C. 597–599
van Dam, J.E.G. 38–45
van Gelder, Willem M.J. 38–45
van Santen, E. 277–278
van Soest, Louis J.M. 30–38, 684–686
Vandenberg, A. 279–282
Ventura, M. 553–557
Verlet, Nicolas 616–619
Voelker, Toni A. 176–181
Vogel, Kenneth P. 284–293
Walker, Keith A. 678–680
Ward, Sarah M. 222–227
Waycott, William 528–532
Webber, Charles L., III 413–416, 416–421
Weber, D.J. 355–357
Weiss, Julia 486–491, 491–495
Welbaum, Gregory E. 109–111, 394–399, 570–573, 573–576
White, George A. 68–81
Whitehead, Wayne F. 562–564
Williams, Trevor 5–11
Witt, Merle D. 428–431
Worrell, A.C. 176–181
Zee, Francis T. 461–465, 465–472
Zeller, Richard D. 422–428